DRUG RESIDUES
IN FOODS

FOOD SCIENCE AND TECHNOLOGY

A Series of Monographs, Textbooks, and Reference Books

1. Flavor Research: Principles and Techniques, *R. Teranishi, I. Hornstein, P. Issenberg, and E. L. Wick*
2. Principles of Enzymology for the Food Sciences, *John R. Whitaker*
3. Low-Temperature Preservation of Foods and Living Matter, *Owen R. Fennema, William D. Powrie, and Elmer H. Marth*
4. Principles of Food Science
   Part I: Food Chemistry, *edited by Owen R. Fennema*
   Part II: Physical Methods of Food Preservation, *Marcus Karel, Owen R. Fennema, and Daryl B. Lund*
5. Food Emulsions, *edited by Stig E. Friberg*
6. Nutritional and Safety Aspects of Food Processing, *edited by Steven R. Tannenbaum*
7. Flavor Research: Recent Advances, *edited by R. Teranishi, Robert A. Flath, and Hiroshi Sugisawa*
8. Computer-Aided Techniques in Food Technology, *edited by Israel Saguy*
9. Handbook of Tropical Foods, *edited by Harvey T. Chan*
10. Antimicrobials in Foods, *edited by Alfred Larry Branen and P. Michael Davidson*
11. Food Constituents and Food Residues: Their Chromatographic Determination, *edited by James F. Lawrence*

Additional Volumes in Preparation

DRUG RESIDUES IN FOODS

Pharmacology, Food Safety, and Analysis

Nikolaos A. Botsoglou
Dimitrios J. Fletouris

Aristotle University
Thessaloniki, Greece

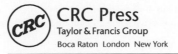

CRC Press
Taylor & Francis Group
Boca Raton London New York

CRC Press is an imprint of the
Taylor & Francis Group, an **informa** business

CRC Press
Taylor & Francis Group
6000 Broken Sound Parkway NW, Suite 300
Boca Raton, FL 33487-2742

First issued in paperback 2019

© 2001 by Taylor & Francis Group, LLC
CRC Press is an imprint of Taylor & Francis Group, an Informa business

No claim to original U.S. Government works

ISBN-13: 978-0-8247-8959-6 (hbk)
ISBN-13: 978-0-367-39792-0 (pbk)

Visit the Taylor & Francis Web site at
http://www.taylorandfrancis.com

and the CRC Press Web site at
http://www.crcpress.com

Σχόσας την φροντΙδα λεπτήν
κατά μΙκρόν περκρρόνεΙ τα πράγματα,
ορθώς δΙαΙρών καΙ σκοπών.
Κάν απορής τΙ των νοημάτων,
αφεΙς άπελθε, καΙ κατά την γνώμην πάλΙν,
κΙνησον αύθΙς αυτό καΙ ζυγώθρΙσον.

ΑΡΙΣΤΟΦΑΝΗΣ, ΝεφέλαΙ

Divide your thoughts to small places
and search the things around you one by one,
by dividing in the right way and examining them.
And if you reach a point and you stumble in one of your thoughts,
leave it and go elsewhere, and then back to the same bring your mind,
and re-evaluate it.

Aristophanes, Nephele

Preface

As protein needs for the growing world population expand, maximization of animal productivity has become a matter of major concern. Through improved technology, new animal hybrids are being developed, highly productive strains of livestock are being bred, and imported breeds are being introduced into new localities with the sole intention of increasing productivity and quality of animal products. Modern farming systems involving intensive rearing of animals in restricted areas are being optimized so that adequate supplies of food of animal origin for the increasing world population can be produced at reasonable prices.

The rearing conditions of a large number of animals in close confinement and the high stocking densities in intensive aquaculture could hardly be more favorable for the frequent incidence and rapid spread of diseases. Many practices in modern animal husbandry, such as livestock marketing, movement of very young animals, and certain forms of intensification, can further act as trigger factors for the initiation and development of clinical diseases. This has led to an increasing use of a great variety of drugs for therapeutic, preventive, or growth in promoting applications in animal and fish farming.

Drugs, however valuable for increasing food animal productivity they may be, present a concern for public health, considering the potential presence of their residues in the edible products of treated animals. Extra-label or illegal use of sometimes dangerous drugs in food animals are examples of applications that may cause a real health hazard.

Surveillance of animal-derived food for drug residues through toxicological and analytical investigations has stimulated public awareness during the last two decades, and in turn has forced all partners in the food chain and health authorities to apply control techniques in the various steps of production on the farm and in the slaughterhouse, in food-processing factories, and at sale points.

Currently, extensive research is carried out for an increasingly stringent and better defined interdisciplinary control. Regulatory authorities around the world demand progressively more information, not only on new drugs but also on older and established compounds where re-registration may be required to ensure that up-to-date standards of safety, quality, and efficacy are attained. New analytical methods are being developed for screening, quantification, and confirmation of residues in food as, in parallel with human medicine, innovative drugs are being introduced into animal farming, whereas the detection requirements for the parent drugs and/or their metabolites are frequently changed downward.

The relevant scientific information grows daily. With so extensive a literature, valuable pieces of information on the issue of drug residues in foods are scattered widely throughout the world. This book tries to bring together such information into one compact volume so as to give all the necessary knowledge to anyone who is involved in food production and the control of food safety.

Data are summarized in tables throughout the volume in the same way. An abundance of such material, along with figures and examples, makes this publication a solid reference book. Particular food safety issues—such as the fate of residues during food cooking—that, although important, are rarely considered in literature, are included also in this book. Apart from theses unique features, this book seeks to discuss analytical problems in current methodology, giving special emphasis to the more promising screening and confirmatory procedures for routine monitoring of drug residues in foods. Preference is given to recently developed automated multiresidue methods, and attempts are made, where feasible, to provide ideas for better approaches to existing analytical methodology.

The book contains 30 chapters covering topics related to drug residues in foods. It is divided into three parts. The first part, consisting of nine chapters, deals with the drugs potentially used in food-producing animals. Chapter 1 discusses drug usage, and Chapter 2 provides some important pharmacokinetic considerations on the fate of drugs in terrestrial and aquatic species. The next six chapters are dedicated to the most significant groups and sub-groups of drugs potentially used in food-producing animals. All the necessary information on the chemical structures of the parent drugs and their metabolites, dosages and routes of drug administration in the targeted species, and absorption, distribution, biotransformation, and excretion data are fully detailed for a rather high number of individual members within each sub-group. Special emphasis is given to the residue depletion profile of the potentially used drugs and their metabolites in all edible animal products. Chapter 9 discusses benefits versus risks of drug usage in food-producing animals, providing answers to frequently asked questions such as how to address the development of antimicrobial resistance.

The second part deals with the significance and control of drug residues in foods. Chapter 10 discusses the toxicological, pharmacological, technological, and other risks associated with the drug residues present in the edible animal products. Chapters 11 to 13, the reader can find information on the regulatory outlines all over the world, make an approach to the global harmonization issue of the regulatory requirements, and get an idea on the incidence of violative residues in the United States, Canada, Europe, and other countries. Factors of management and/or biological origin involved in food contamination are discussed in Chapter 14. Chapter 15 summarizes the cost of residues in the livestock industry, whereas Chapter 16 deals with the residue avoidance management. Chapter 17 reviews on the stability of residues during food storage, cooking, and processing. Consumer perception and concerns are discussed in Chapter 18.

Starting with a description of the analytical challenge in Chapter 19, the third part, which is devoted to analytical attitudes, proceeds with a detailed description in Chapter 20 of modern sample preparation procedures including solid-phase extraction, matrix solid-phase dispersion, use of restricted-access media, supercritical fluid extraction, and immunoaffinity cleanup. Flexible derivatization techniques including fluorescence, ultraviolet-visible, enzymatic, and photochemical derivatization procedures are presented in Chapter 21.

The next two chapters are dedicated to separation and detection techniques. Principles of liquid chromatography, gas chromatography, thin-layer chromatography, supercritical fluid chromatography, and capillary electrophoresis are reviewed in Chapter 22. Properties of microbiological, immunochemical, and all known physicochemical detection systems are discussed in Chapter 23. Modern confirmation techniques based on coupling chromatographic methods with diode array, mass spectrometric, and infrared spectroscopic detectors are surveyed in Chapter 24, while method validation parameters are examined in Chapter 25. Chapter 26 deals with major quality criteria for selecting an analytical method, interpretation of the analytical results, and strategies for monitoring the food supply for drug residues.

Chapters 27, 28, and 29 of Part III give an overview of all microbiological, immunochemical, and physicochemical methods presently available in the field of drug residue analysis. In addition, the relative advantages and disadvantages of the different methods are assessed. Particular emphasis is given to the most promising methods in terms of simplicity, rapidity, reliability, and applicability, and their analytical features are fully detailed. In the final chapter, future trends in the analysis of drug residues in foods are summarized.

The book is indented neither as a pharmacology text nor as a residues analysis text; tries to bridge that gap. Because so much specialist knowledge is now available, the real challenge is to try to encapsulate this, creating a stimulus and direction for greater in-depth study. Our objective is that the content of this book will serve as an invaluable tool to those with a professional interest in food safety such as food scientists and technologists, toxicologists, veterinarians, clinicians, food and analytical chemists, biologists and biochemists in state service, private laboratories, academic service, industry, and the regulatory sphere. This book is also intended for use as a primary textbook by those who wish to learn about the feed–animal–food chain contamination as part of their formal education, such as undergraduate, graduate, and postgraduate students. It will also be useful to scientists whose training is not primarily in analytical work but who are faced with the difficult task of analyzing food for drug residues.

We are indebted to all of our colleagues for their assistance with this work. Special appreciation is due to the efficient library service at Aristotle University of Thessaloniki. Finally, a word of thanks to our families for their understanding and constant encouragement to proceed in the face of a large task.

Nikolaos A. Botsoglou
Dimitries J. Fletuvris

Contents

PART II: RESIDUES IN FOOD

1

A General View of Drug Usage

1.1 INTRODUCTION

In modern farming practices, drugs are being used on a large scale. This is connected with the enormous increase and intensification of animal husbandry. In contrast to the traditional system of free-range husbandry, in which the animals were allowed to wander around wide areas of the farm in the open air to forage for food, the current intensive rearing of animals in restricted accommodation has inevitably increased the incidence and spread of diseases. Hence, there has been an increased need for using therapeutic agents.

Drugs are applied in animal husbandry for different reasons. They are used to cure or prevent diseases in animals, to increase feed efficiency and/or growth rate, and to sedate animals in order to minimize the effect of stress. Since not all applications are of therapeutic character, it is customary to term *veterinary drug* any pharmacologically active substance in animal husbandry, regardless of its purpose of use and mode of application (1). In this context, substances used for increasing feed efficiency and/or growth rate are also considered veterinary drugs.

As both human and veterinary medicine expand their armamentarium into more powerful classes of therapeutic agents, the range of drugs with a potential of use in food-producing animals is continuously widening. The Food Safety and Inspection Service (FSIS) of the US Department of Agriculture (USDA) has estimated that as many as 400 substances, not all of which are veterinary drugs, have the potential for use in food animal production (2).

1

1.2   CLASSIFICATION OF POTENTIALLY USED DRUGS

Drugs most commonly used for the treatment and prevention of diseases in food-producing animals can be classified into the major classes of antibacterials, anthelminthics, anticoccidials, and other antiprotozoals. A high number of subclasses, each containing a great variety of individual drugs, exists within each of these classes. Aminoglycosides and aminocyclitols, amphenicols, β-lactams, macrolides and lincosamides, nitrofurans, quinolones, sulfonamides and diaminopyrimidine potentiators, tetracyclines, and other compounds are all subclasses of the antibacterial class of drugs. Benzimidazoles, imidazothiazoles, organophosphates, tetrahydropyrimides, salicylanilides, substituted phenols, macrocyclic lactones, piperazine derivatives, and other compounds constitute the subclasses of the anthelminthic class of drugs. Benzamides, carbanilides, nitroimidazoles, polyether ionophores, quinolone derivatives, triazines, and other compounds make up the subclasses of the anticoccidial and other antiprotozoal class of drugs.

Other drugs of lesser therapeutic importance can be classified into a series of minor classes including the antifungals, β-adrenergic agonists, corticosteroids, diuretics, dyes, nonsteroidal anti-inflammatories, sedatives and β-blockers, and thyreostatics. It is important to note that some drugs within the classes mentioned have dual function and can properly be classified in more than one of the above classes. As a result, overlap between drug classes is not unusual.

Drugs within the classes of the antibacterials, anthelminthics, anticoccidials, and other antiprotozoals can be administered orally, parenterally, or topically. Some orally administered drugs can be incorporated in the feed for treatment of diseases. Although they are added in the feed, their use differs from what has become known as *feed additives*. One should differentiate between the high-level curative infeed medication of diseased animals and the low-level drug feeding of healthy animals to improve feed efficiency, promote growth, or prevent coccidiosis. For the latter application, a number of approved drugs can be incorporated in feeds and administered to animals without a veterinary prescription. However, the production of feeds containing such additives may only take place under strictly regulated conditions.

As important as the therapeutic drugs are for animal health, of far greater economic importance are the feed additives. They dominate the animal drug market, accounting for about 50% of the total. The group of feed additives includes specific antibiotics and synthetic antibacterials, collectively called antimicrobial growth promoters, as well as anticoccidial drugs. The class of the antimicrobial growth promoters can be classified into the subclasses of the organic arsenicals, peptide antibiotics, quinoxaline-1,4-dioxides, and other compounds, some of which have dual action and can properly be classified in one of the classes mentioned above.

Apart from the antimicrobial growth promoters, there have been some other hormonal-type compounds with anabolic activity that are administered usually in the form of implants. These compounds constitute the class of the anabolic hormonal-type growth promoters, which can be classified into the subclasses of the endogenous sex steroids, steroidal compounds not occurring naturally, nonsteroidal compounds not occurring naturally, and polypeptide hormones.

1.3 EXTENT OF DRUG USE

Specific market data on the extent of drug use are scarcely available because this information is usually considered proprietary. However, the use of veterinary drugs has become a daily event in intensive farming. It is estimated that about 80% of all food-producing animals in the United States normally receive some form of drug medication during their lifetime (3). It can, therefore, be taken for granted that drugs intended for food-producing animals are currently used throughout the world on a large scale.

There is no doubt that in terms of drug type, feed additive use is presently by far the most significant. In 1978, the nonmedical use of drugs in food-producing animals was estimated by the US International Trade Commission at about 5000–6000 tons (4). This figure, although valuable, cannot give a clear picture of the extent of use of feed additives, since it tends to blur the distinction between drugs such as growth promoters that are added in feeds at levels of a few parts per million and anticoccidials that are added at much higher levels. In addition, the differences in feed consumption by different animal species further shade the picture.

According to the Animal Health Institute of the United States, drug sales at the manufacturers' level for food-producing animals exceeded $2000 million in 1983, the feed additive market being about half of that total (5). A total of approximately 31.9 million pounds of antibiotics were produced, 58% being tetracyclines and penicillin G. Over half of this quantity was used in animal feeding stuffs. It was estimated that, in the United States, 75% of dairy calves, 60% of beef cattle, 75% of swine, and 80% of poultry received one or more drugs in their feed during their lifetime (6). Tetracyclines and penicillin G dominated the product lists in terms of total use, but tylosin, sulfonamides, nitrofurans, antimicrobial growth promoters, and the ionophore antibacterials were also highly significant.

In 1986, the animal drug market was estimated to be worth over $9000 million, with feed additives and therapeutics each contributing 45% of the total (6). The United States shared 28% of the market, and Western Europe 24.5%. A breakdown by animal usage showed that cattle formed 32%, with poultry making up 24%, swine 21%, sheep 10% and horses 4%.

After the United States, Japan is the second largest consumer of animal health products. In 1990, 110 feed additives were approved for use in Japan and production reached 78,000 tons estimated to be worth 60,000 million yen.

In 1991, North America and Western Europe represented more than half of the world market for veterinary drugs (at 56.8%) with estimated sales at manufacturers' level of 5606 million ecu (7). Other regions of the world including Asia/Pacific, Eastern Europe, Latin America, and Oceania registered sales of 1707, 1133, 0.938, 0.299, and 0.175 million ecu, respectively. A breakdown of the global market by animal usage showed that 27.1% was used for cattle, 29.6% for swine, 26.4% for poultry, 5.1% for sheep/goats, and 11.8% for companion animals including horses. A breakdown of the world veterinary drug market by product type showed that 18.6% were antibacterial and antifungal agents, 13.2% parasiticides, 42.2% feed additives, 14.8% other pharmaceuticals, and 11.1% biological agents (7).

1.4 METHODS OF MEDICATION

Unlike with humans and companions animals, for which the treatment of bacterial diseases is invariably directed at individual patients, antimicrobial therapy in food-producing animals can be applied on either an individual or herd/flock basis.

1.4.1 Individual Medication

Large food-producing animals that are generally held on less intensive farming, such as lactating cows suffering from mastitis, are usually treated individually. Topical, parenteral, intramammary, or oral via bolus or paste treatments are major routes of individual medication for cattle. Diseased animals from a large population, such as hogs and veal calves that frequently suffer from respiratory or gastrointestinal diseases during the later stages of the fattening process, are also treated individually. Another form of individual treatment is the injection of tranquillizers to hogs and steers to prevent losses from stress during transportation to the slaughterhouse.

1.4.2 Mass Medication

The concept of mass medication can hardly be accepted outside the agricultural field, but the experience of veterinary practitioners who treat large herds or flocks of animals fully supports this concept, especially in those areas of animal management where it is essential to keep all the animals at a level of optimal productivity (8).

Farm animals being managed under intensive systems are very susceptible to disease outbreaks since they are usually of the same age, often very immature, and are in constant contact with their feces. Epidemiological studies have shown that the introduction of a highly infectious disease into a large population of animals kept in the same pen will ultimately result in a large proportion of these animals becoming infected (9). The reasonable therapeutic approach to this problem is to treat the whole group as an individual. By this method, there will be no need to continually withdraw and treat individual animals, which would be very costly in time and also stressful to the animals due to frequent interference by the human attendants when catching animals for medication.

A further extension of mass medication is being referred to as prophylactic or preventive medication. Again, one should differentiate between the low-level medication of healthy animals to improve feed efficiency and promote growth, and the high-level curative medication of diseased animals.

Preventive medication does not apply to the individually housed animal but only to the group or herd of animals in which clinical disease has broken out in one or more individuals. Previous veterinary experience has indicated that if medication is not applied to that group or herd, there will be a continuing sequence of infected individuals accompanied by a prolonged period of suboptimal performance in the affected group of animals (10). Rapid cure of a herd infection will bring about a cessation of bacterial excretion, which will be advantageous to the remainder of the herd, and also prevent undue contamination of the farm environment. An example of preventive medication is dry-cow therapy: a slow-release antibiotic preparation is infused into the cow's udder at the end of a lactation cycle to overcome any residual infection and to protect against the establishment of new infection during the dry period and prior to the commencement of a new lactation cycle.

In general, the frequency of mass medication is higher in young animals because they are most sensitive to infections. Owing to this sensitivity, food animal production companies are always faced with disease problems when young growing animals, usually calves and piglets, are transferred from breeding to finisher units. This transfer, which often involves prolonged traveling, mixing of animals from different suppliers, and a diet change, may bring about a disturbance of the gastrointestinal flora, reorganization of social dominance, and redistribution of microorganisms of many species and types within the newly grouped animals. Such disturbances may result in serious health problems. A similar situation may also occur at weaning. Since these events are usually totally predictable, it is common practice to apply preventive medication as a starting therapy when such animals are brought in the grower/finisher units. Nevertheless, the decision to employ mass medication must never be taken lightly by food animal producers because of the cost of the drugs to treat a large population of animals and the problems that may arise with the need to adhere to the labeled withdrawal periods.

1.5 DOSAGE FORMS AND ROUTES OF ADMINISTRATION

Because of clinical need, the species involved, or the needs of herd- or flock-scale treatment, drug preparations for food-producing animals are presented in dosage forms that vary greatly. A plethora of different main dosage forms are available in the veterinary medicine market including ampoules, boluses, capsules, creams, foams, gels, granules, medicated premixes, oily solutions, ointments, pastes, powders, solutions, suspensions, tablets, and vaginal spirals and sponges.

The type of formulation influences the systemic availability of the drug from its dosage form (11), whereas the amount of the drug limits its use to only specific animal species because of the wide body-weight range in animals. There is no single optimal dose for any given drug; there are too many variables, including host resistance, bacterial virulence, and site of injection, to allow a single dosage recommendation to cover all situations. While many diseases can be treated using routine dosage levels, special situations may require an increase in dosage or even allow for a reduced dosage schedule. The cost of the preparation and the ease of administration are often major factors governing the compliance with instructions to administer the drug at the recommended dosage and intervals. There has generally been a tendency to use too-low dosage, which may be quite sufficient in some cases but often lead to erroneous conclusion that the drug is ineffective. Sometimes, the dosage may actually be appropriate but the dosage interval too long to sustain activity, or the interval appropriate but the dosage too low.

The dosage form of a drug preparation determines its route of administration. Veterinary drugs can be administered to food-producing animals by a variety of greatly differing ways including aural, dressing, infeed, intradermal, intramammary, intramuscular, intranasal, intraruminal, intraocular, intravaginal, intravenous, implants, inhalations, oral, per rectum, and subcutaneous routes of administration. When extravascular routes of administration are employed, absorption is the critical factor that determines the entry of a drug into the bloodstream. Since such a factor does not exist when the dose is introduced directly into the blood stream, intravenous routes of administration provide therapeutic serum concentrations sooner than extravascular routes with even an adequate rate of absorption. As a result, intravenous injection is often the most satisfactory route of administration for initiating therapy for animals with acute infections. Use of the intravenous route of administration is limited, however, by the lack of availability of parenteral preparations formulated appropriately for injection by this route.

For maintenance of therapeutic serum concentrations, intramuscular and subcutaneous or oral routes of administration are usually preferable. The intramuscular and subcutaneous routes are by far the most frequently used extravascular parenteral routes of drug administration in farm animals. Factors that influence drug absorption from intramuscular and subcutaneous injection sites include the physicochemical properties of the drug that govern its passage across the membrane separating the absorption site from the blood, the pH of the solution at the absorption site, and the local blood circulation. The less ionized and more lipophilic the drug, the greater the rate of absorption. An interesting application of this principle is treatment with prolonged-release drug preparations. The duration of the pharmacological effect is controlled by the rate of drug release from the dosage from rather than by the disposition kinetics of the drug. Another requirement is that the formulation of the parenteral preparation be such that its intramuscular injection does not cause tissue damage with persistence of residual concentrations at the injection site. Limited data appear to indicate that the extent of systemic availability of intramuscularly administered drugs can vary as widely between different sites as between intramuscular and subcutaneous sites.

Other less frequently used parenteral routes such as intra-articular or subconjuctival injections and intramammary or intrauterine infusions have limited application: they aim at directly placing high drug concentrations close to the site of infection. These routes of administration differ from the major parenteral routes in that absorption into the systemic circulation is not a prerequisite for delivery of drug to the site of action. When the infection site is relatively inaccessible, such as in the case of mastitis, the combined use of systemic and local delivery of drug to the site of infection may represent the optimum approach to treatment.

Most oral preparations are solid dosage forms that need to be dissolved before they can be absorbed. The inert ingredients of such dosage forms can have a profound effect on the dissolution of the active ingredient and thereby control its rate of absorption. In addition, the drug may be unstable in the gastrointestinal fluids, as in the case of penicillin G, or metabolized.

Metabolism may be mediated by intestinal microflora, epithelial enzymes, or liver enzymes preceding entry into the systemic circulation. Chloramphenicol is well absorbed when administered orally to calves less than 1 week old, but it is inactivated by microflora when administered to ruminants. Similar observations have been made after oral administration of amoxicillin, ampicillin, and cephalexin therapy in young calves (11). On the other hand, trimethoprim, which is extensively metabolized in the liver and may undergo some metabolism in the rumen, shows higher systemic availability in the newborn calf and kid, due probably to the lower metabolic activity in the neonatal animal.

In mass medication of nearly all food-producing animals, the most important route of drug administration is, by far, oral treatment through milk replacer, drinking water, or the feed; herds of cattle or sheep are mass-medicated with antiparasitics by topical or licking-block formulations. Oral treatment is effective if the drug is readily absorbed from the gastrointestinal tract or if the infection is located in the gut. Treatment through drinking water is a convenient route for diseased animals that do not eat well, although the large interanimal variability in water intake, the spilling of water, and consequently the high dosages that are necessary, are negative factors. For fish, oral treatment using a medicated bath is a very elegant route, while mass medication through drinking water or the feed prevails for poultry, swine, and fish.

Medicated premixes sometimes, present special problems due to incompatibility of the components in a formulation (12). For example, tetracyclines may be inactivated either by the drug carrier as in the case of premixes containing divalent ions such as calcium, or by the diluent as in the case of milk replacers that also contain calcium (13). Other drugs can be inactivated by complexation to particular components in the feed, as in the case of the thiophanate complexation to copper. Drug inactivation may also occur during feed preparations, as in the case of the conditioning/pelleting processes where high temperature and moisture conditions are applied.

When drug combinations are used, treatment failures may appear in cases in which the individual drugs contained in the preparation antagonize each other (such as in the case of combination of chloramphenicol and aminoglycosides) or induce cross-resistance (such as in the case of combination of chloramphenicol and tetracyclines) (14, 15). The effects of antibiotic combinations are specific for individual bacterial species and may have quite diverse effects ranging between synergism and antagonism of one another when utilized against different bacteria (16, 17). Nevertheless, there have been many disease situations in which the use of more than one antibacterial agents may be justified, particularly when a mixed bacterial population is involved.

REFERENCES

1. A. Somogyi, Food Addit. Contam., 1:81 (1984).
2. W.A. Moats, and M.B. Medina, in Veterinary Drug Residues, Food Safety (W.A. Moats, and M.B. Medina, Eds.), American Chemical Society, Washington, D.C., p. vii (1996).
3. R.C. Livingston, J. Assoc. Off. Anal. Chem., 68:966 (1985).
4. National Academy of Science, in The Effects on Human Health of Subtherapeutic Use of Antimicrobials in Animal Feeds, National Research Council, Report No 88, March (1981).
5. Animal Health Institute, Alexandria, VA, USA
6. N.T. Crosby, in Determination of Veterinary Residues in Food (N.T. Crosby, Ed.), Ellis Horwood, London, England (1991).
7. D.J.S. Miller, in Residues of Veterinary Drugs in Food, Proc. Euroresidue II Conf., Veldhoven, May 3–5, 1993 (N. Haagsma, A. Ruiter, and P.B. Czedik-Eysenberg, Eds.), Fac. Vet. Med., Univ. Utrecht, The Netherlands, p. 65 (1993).
8. J.R. Walton, Zbl. Vet. Med. A., 30:81 (1983).
9. G.C. Brander, and P.R. Ellis, in Animal and Human Health: The Control of Disease (G.C. Brander and P.R. Ellis, Eds.), Baillier Tindall, London, UK (1976).
10. G. Ziv, in Agricultural Uses of Antibiotics (W.A. Moats, Ed.), American Chemical Society, Washington, DC, p. 8 (1986).
11. J.D. Baggot, J. Am. Vet. Med. Assoc., 185:1076 (1984).
12. M.M.L. Aerts, in Residues of Veterinary Drugs in Edible Products. An Analytucal Approach, Thesis, University of Amsterdam (1990).

13. T.F. Sellers, and W.M. Marine, in Drill's Pharmacology in Medicine (J.R. DiPalma, Ed.), 3rd Edition, McGraw-Hill Book Co., New York, p. 1352 (1965).
14. E. Goren, Tijdschr. Diergeneesk., 108:350 (1983).
15. M. Pilloud, Schweiz. Arch. Tierheilk., 126:571 (1984).
16. G.E. Burrows, Bovine Pract., 15:99 (1980).
17. C.M. Stowe, J. Am. Vet. Med. Assoc., 185:1137 (1985).

2

Some Pharmacokinetic Considerations

The residues in edible products of treated animals do not necessarily constitute the pharmaceutical compounds initially administered to the animals. They may consist of various components including the parent compound and/or free metabolites, and metabolites covalently bound to macromolecules.

The ability of the treated animal to detoxify and eliminate the drug has a significant bearing on both the relative and absolute amount of any of these components likely to remain in tissues. The degree to which the drug is absorbed, the extent of drug distribution, the rate and extent of drug metabolism, and the rate of excretion of the parent compound and its various metabolites, all govern decidedly the total residue burden. Properties of drugs and biological membranes that together determine the qualitative and quantitative issues of the fate of drugs in terrestrial and aquatic species are briefly described below.

2.1 FATE OF DRUGS IN TERRESTRIAL SPECIES

2.1.1 Absorption

Absorption is described by determining the rate constant of drug passing into the bloodstream at successive time intervals after administration. Residues may be found in tissues after some or all of the drug has been systemically absorbed. Absorption is influenced by the properties of cell membranes, the physicochemical characteristics of the drug, and the route of drug administration (1).

11

It has long been established that all cell membranes in the body are composed of a fundamental structure called plasma membrane. This boundary surrounds single cells such as epithelial cells. More complex membranes such as intestinal epithelium and skin, are composed of multiples of this fundamental structure, which has been visualized as a bimolecular layer of lipid molecules with a monolayer of protein adsorbed into each surface. Cell membranes are further interspersed with small pores that can be protein line channels through the lipid layer or, simply, spaces between the lipid molecules. In membranes composed of many cells, the spaces between the cells constitute another kind of membrane pores (2).

As a result of this structure, many drugs can move across cell membranes by a process of simple diffusion. In this simple or passive diffusion process, the rate of transport of the drug is directly proportional to the membrane thickness, the cross-sectional area of the membrane exposed to the drug solution, and its concentration gradient across the membrane that results in a net movement of particles from the higher to the lower concentration. Lipid-soluble drugs move across the predominantly lipid cell membrane by passive diffusion, its relative speed being determined by the lipid solubility or, more precisely, the lipid to water partition coefficient of the drug. The greater this drug partition coefficient, the higher the concentration of the drug in the membrane, and the faster the diffusion. Many lipid-insoluble compounds of small molecular size can also diffuse rapidly across the cell membrane through the pores. Passage through the pores is a passive process called filtration because it involves flow of water that drags with it any soluble molecules whose dimensions are less than the pores, due to hydrostatic or osmotic differences across the membrane.

Filtration and diffusion passive processes cannot, however, explain the passage of all drugs through the cell membranes. This is due to the fact that cell membranes also possess specialized active transport mechanisms that facilitate entry of large lipid-insoluble molecules into the cell. With these mechanisms, not only is the transport process rapid but the drugs can move across the membranes against a concentration gradient (i.e., from low to high concentration). It is assumed that this transport is mediated by some carrier molecules in the membrane that complex with the solute at one surface of the membrane. Following complexation, the carrier–solute complex moves across the membrane, the solute is then released, and the carrier returns to the original surface where it can combine with another molecule of solute. Carriers show a specificity toward certain drugs, so not all drugs may be transported by this process. Since carrier molecules are available only in limited amounts in the cell membrane, saturation may end the process. Two main types of carrier-mediated transport mechanisms are known. The active transport is the process that can transport a substance against an concentration gradient but is blocked by metabolic inhibitors, whereas facilitated diffusion is the term applied to carrier-mediated transport that operates along a concentration gradient (i.e., from a higher to a lower concentration) and does not require energy (3).

Two other types of specialized transport mechanisms, pinocytosis and phagocytosis, may also account for the transmembrane movement of some macromolecules (2). In these complex processes, the cell engulfs a droplet of extracellular fluid or a particle of solid material such as a bacterium. The droplet or particle is completely surrounded by a portion of the cell membrane and the resulting vesicle becomes detached and moves into the cell cytoplasm.

Apart from the properties of the cell membranes, certain physicochemical characteristics of the drugs can significantly influence the rate of their absorption. Most drugs are either weak acids or bases that exist in solution as a mixture of ionized and nonionized forms. Nonionized forms are more lipophilic whereas ionized forms more hydrophilic. Consequently, the nonionized forma are lipid soluble and able to permeate rapidly across cell membranes. This process is known as passive nonionic diffusion.

On the other hand, the ionized forms, which tend to be less lipid soluble, cannot diffuse across the lipid phase of the cell membrane. Ionized molecules may also repelled from the cell surface by groups with similar charge, or may be attracted to it and held there by groups with opposite charge. Ionized drug forms are, sometimes, unable to be filtered even through the aqueous pores of the membranes due to their own size or to the size they attain after the attraction of water molecules.

Therefore, the ratio of the ionized to the nonionized form, which depends on the pKa of the drug and the pH of the medium, in any given tissue of the body is of major importance. When the pKa of the drug equals the pH of the medium, 50% of the drug is in the ionized form whereas 50% in the nonionized. As the nonionized portion crosses the membrane into the bloodstream, there may be a continuous redistribution of the remaining ionized form to the nonionized form, so that eventually all of the drug is absorbed by flux across the membrane. For drugs that ionize, it is also possible, under certain conditions, to find at equilibrium unequal concentrations of total ionized and nonionized drug on either side of the membrane. Only the nonionized molecules readily cross the lipid barrier and achieve the same equilibrium concentration on both sides of the membrane, the ionized molecules being virtually excluded from transmembrane diffusion.

Drugs are administered to animals by parenteral or enteral administration, and topical application. Parenteral administration bypasses the alimentary tract and can be effected by a variety of routes including intravenous, intramuscular, subcutaneous, intraperitoneal, or intrapleural injections; inhalation; and percutaneously. In intravenous injections, entry of drugs into the system depends only upon the rate of injection and not on absorption into the bloodstream. As a result, water-soluble poorly absorbed drugs may be readily administered.

Unlike with intravenous administration, absorption of drugs after intramuscular, subcutaneous, and intraperitoneal injection is influenced by several factors (4). The rate-limiting step for absorption is the rate of the blood flow in the tissue. Adequate circulation is needed to maintain the concentration gradient that is so critical to passive absorption or facilitated diffusion into the bloodstream. The higher the vascularity of the tissue, the better the absorption, because diffusion distances are decreased. The nature of the vehicle and the lipid solubility of the drug, where favorable, will also potentiate absorption. In general, the larger the molecule the longer the dissolution time, and consequently the higher the absorption time. The volume injected and the concentration of the drug in solution can also have varying effects upon absorption, depending upon the potential for the drug molecule to come into contact with the absorptive surface.

The advantages of administration by intramuscular injection are that the muscle can act as a depot, and the rate of disappearance of drug from the site of injection can be calculated. Inhalational, intranasal, and intratracheal administration are normally reserved for vapors and aerosols including anesthetics. Absorption is facilitated by small-sized particles, high lipid solubility, sufficient pulmonary blood flow, and a large absorptive surface area, as it is present in healthy lungs. Administration by these routes can be very rapid when several of the factors favoring increased absorption are combined.

With percutaneous administration, the drugs must pass through the stratum corneum, epidermal cells, sweat glands, sebaceous glands, or hair follicles before being absorbed. Only very lipid-soluble drugs will pass through intact skin. However, it is often difficult to obtain sufficient concentrations of the drug in the plasma or at the site of action to obtain the desired effect. Even when significant absorption has been demonstrated, it is often not reproducible because of intraspecies variability in transdermal absorption.

Enteral administration is utilized for drugs that may be absorbed via the intestinal tract. Oral and rectal administration are the usual routes. Absorption by these routes is highly species-specific and is affected by many factors. The presence of food in the stomach may reduce, increase, delay, or have no affect upon absorption, depending upon the drug formulation. The pH of the gastrointestinal fluid is most important in determining the percentage of the drug in the unionized form, thus favoring its absorption. The rate of splanchnic blood flow may enhance drug absorption and is influenced by the meal. Adequate motility is necessary to transport the drug to the area of optimal absorption. Physiological factors affecting absorption include posture of the animal, osmotic pressure, gastrointestinal content, and distention. Pathological factors affecting absorption include ulcers, obstructions, liver disease, trauma, and gastroenterostomies. Drugs administered rectally do not have to pass through the liver prior to entry into the systemic circulation, but absorption via the rectum is often incomplete and irregular.

When local effects are desired in the integument, synovium, central nervous system, mammary glands, or uterus, intradermal or topical, intra-articular, intrathecal, intramammary, or intrauterine administration may be most appropriate. The advantage of local administration is the ability to achieve a high concentration of drug at the immediate site of action. All of these routes, depending upon the drug preparation, however, have the potential for facilitating inadvertent systemic exposure.

2.1.2 Distribution

Whatever the route of administration, almost all therapeutic agents, once absorbed, reach their sites of action through the systemic circulation. From the bloodstream, the drug must traverse the various biological membranes and be dispatched to the body fluid compartments before its molecules can reach intracellular sites of action. Some drugs cannot pass all types of membranes and therefore are restricted in their distribution, whereas others pass through all membranes and become distributed throughout the various fluid compartments. The distribution is initially governed by the lipid solubility of the drug, the cardiac output, and the regional blood flow at the sites of administration and action. In addition, some drugs may accumulate in various areas as a result of binding, dissolving in fat, or an active transport mechanism. The accumulation can be at the site of action or, more often, in some other location. In the latter case, the site of accumulation may serve as a storage depot for the drug.

The fate of many drugs in the body is influenced by their binding tendency to plasma proteins (5). Only the fraction of the drug in the bloodstream that does not bind to albumin can leave the circulation to become distributed throughout the body, and reach the sites of action. On the other hand, the protein–drug complexes serve as a circulating drug reservoir that releases more drug to restore the equilibrium as the free drug diffuses out from the capillaries. In this way the plasma concentration of even highly bound drugs falls to low levels and eventually disappears. Once drug distribution is complete, the free-drug concentration throughout extracellular water equals that in serum water. It is not the total but rather the free-drug concentration in serum that correlates with the concentration at the sites of action. For highly bound drugs, the free-drug concentration in serum is only a small percentage of the total amount present.

For the majority of drugs, binding to albumin is quantitatively the most important and often accounts for almost all of the drug binding in plasma; only a few drugs show high affinity for other proteins; for example, the corticosteroids that exhibit a high binding tendency to globulins. The molecule of albumin presents multiple binding sites with differing affinities. Most of these sites show more extensive binding to weak acids than to weak bases by weak chemical bonds of the Van der Waals, hydrogen, or ionic type (6).

The extent of binding to albumin is influenced by the drug concentration and thus, in cases of overdose, a much higher percentage of drug than normal is available to leave the bloodstream. A decrease in the total albumin levels will generally increase the absolute total amount of drug present that is unbound and therefore available to leave the bloodstream, although the percentage fraction of the protein-bound remaining drug will often be constant. The concentration or the properties of serum albumin are altered in many diseases. Such changes can decrease the drug–albumin interaction. In other words, when the serum concentration of albumin or the drug-binding capacity of albumin molecules is abnormally low, a smaller proportion of a potential albumin-binding drug interacts with albumin than under normal conditions. Thus, the free drug concentration is greater than normal. A practical consequence of this is that the toxicity of drugs that are normally highly bound is greatly increased by hypoproteinemia.

One of the most important practical aspects of protein binding is the fact that drugs of similar or markedly dissimilar structure may compete for the same binding sites on the protein (7). Hence, multidrug therapy may lead to alteration in the plasma concentration and the rate of elimination of drugs, because of multiple competition for the plasma protein-binding sites.

Many drugs can partially displace one another from albumin, and this may lead to an intensification of the pharmacological action. Only when substances are extensively bound in plasma would displacement from binding sites release amounts of drug that, on distribution into other parts of the body, would significantly increase the concentration in the tissue. For drugs that are bound less than 80%, an alteration in protein binding of 5% will not significantly affect tissue concentrations of the free drug. However, when drugs are bound at a percentage greater than 95%, a 5% decrease in binding will result in doubling of the unbound fraction; in this case, the alteration in tissue concentration of the free drug is significant because this free drug will then be available for distribution to the tissues.

Drugs with high affinities for plasma albumin can also displace drugs with lower affinities. For example, sulfonamides bind to plasma proteins, but if phenylbutazone, which has a greater affinity for the binding sites, is administered, the concentration of the free sulfonamides in the plasma will increase due to drug displacement.

The greater the extent of binding to albumin, the less drug is available at any one time at the site of hepatic biotransformation and renal excretion. Consequently, extensive binding to plasma proteins can reduce the rate of elimination of drugs and also their metabolism or biotransformation, thus increasing the duration of action of a single dose of such drugs. The duration of action of some diuretics, sulfonamides, and tetracyclines tends to correlate well with their degree of protein binding.

Marked differences in the drug-binding capacity of plasma proteins exist among mammalian species. Variations in the plasma protein binding of drugs may contribute to the species differences in the tissue levels of the drugs, their toxicity, and overall kinetics, particularly if the binding is extensive.

Distribution of drugs to the tissues and the equilibration of drugs between blood and tissue are both affected by the regional blood flow. Liver, kidney, heart, and the brain are the most highly perfused tissues in the body and, therefore, are readily exposed to drugs. The pH of the receiving tissue affects absorption much the same as the pH of the absorptive surface affects transport, since entry of drugs into the cells is generally restricted to their lipid-soluble, nonionized forms. Thus, metabolites and ionized forms that are water-soluble will stay in the bloodstream to be transported to the kidneys for excretion, instead of being distributed to the tissues.

Since most drugs have pKa values between 3 and 11, they are, accordingly, partly ionized over the range of the physiological pH values. Their distribution and concentration in the various tissues are consequently markedly influenced by the pH of the tissues and the pKa of the particular drug. The implications of this type of distribution have significant practical effects on the passage of drugs across any of the membranes of the body where a pH gradient may exist, (e.g., across the mammary gland epithelium, the renal tubular epithelium, the salivary gland epithelium, and the ruminal, gastric, or intestinal epithelium). More striking effects are seen when a large pH difference exists (e.g., between plasma and gastric juice or between plasma and urine).

Many acidic drugs, such as sulfonamides, phenylbutazone, salicylates, and penicillins, are highly protein bound or too hydrophilic to diffuse across cell membranes and enter cellular water and adipose tissue in significant amounts. These drugs have low distribution in monogastric animals. Basic drugs tend to be widely distributed and to have particularly large distribution in ruminant animals because these drugs diffuse into the rumen and become trapped by ionization of ruminal liquor.

Drugs binding to tissues may produce areas of high drug concentration. Binding of drugs to proteins and other macromolecules is known to occur in almost every tissue of the body including bone and fat. This has been demonstrated with globulins, hemoglobin, mucopolysaccharides, nucleoproteins, phospholipids, and other compounds. This type of binding is usually reversible, and depot binding results simply in a drug reservoir. If the plasma concentration of a drug decreases, the drug may enter the plasma from these storage sites via a concentration gradient. Thus, aminoglycosides bound to proximal tubular cellular components can remain in the kidney for months after plasma concentrations have become undetectable. Without these storage pools, many drugs would be metabolized and excreted so rapidly that they would hardly have time to exert their pharmacological action.

The effect of binding and degree of ionization on the distribution of drugs in the animal body can be illustrated in the following example. When a weakly acidic drug (pKa 2) that is 50% protein-bound is administered orally to a sow, 91% will be unionized at the stomach pH 1, and thus readily absorbed. In the bloodstream, however, where the pH is 7, the drug will be 99.999% ionized, and thus will not readily pass through the blood vessels into the tissues. If the pKa of the drug is 6, the drug will virtually be 100% un-ionized in the stomach and 9% unionized in the blood, allowing for higher amounts to distribute to the tissues. If the sow is lactating and the pH of the milk is elevated because of an infection, only 1% in the milk will be nonionized, and as the drug crosses into the milk it may become ion trapped, favoring accumulation in the milk.

2.1.3 Biotransformation

Some drugs are eliminated from the body unchanged, but most drugs undergo biotransformation. Biotransformation enables a drug to be converted to forms readily excreted by the liver and kidney, whereas sometimes it enables a drug to be converted to an active form. These conversions almost always result in metabolites that are more polar than the parent drug.

The major site of drug biotransformation is the liver, where the smooth endoplasmic reticulum is probably the most important site of metabolism; biotransformation is mostly effected by cytochrome P-450, an NADPH-dependent microsomal enzyme system. Although the liver possesses the greatest capacity for biotransformation, kidney, lung, brain, adrenals, skin, blood, neurons, and gastrointestinal tract are also involved. Intestinal bacterial enzymes, rumen hydrolytic, and reduction microfloral enzymes also play a major role in the metabolism of enterically administered or excreted drugs. Biotransformed drugs delivered to the intestinal tract may, additionally, be converted to the parent drug form via enzymes from intestinal bacteria such as β-glucuronidase (4).

Two types of enzymatic pathways, the so-called phase I and phase II pathways, are generally implicated in drug biotransformation. Phase I pathways correspond to functionalization processes, whereas phase II correspond to biosynthetic or conjugative processes. Phase I functionalization processes include oxidation, reduction, hydrolysis, hydration, and isomerization reactions.

Oxidation reactions can produce hydroxylation on the aromatic rings, such as in the case of the steroids and thiabendazole, or on the aliphatic carbon chain such as in the case of pentobarbitone. They can also cause epoxidation, which leads to normally unstable intermediates that can be hydrolyzed by epoxide hydrolase to dihydrodiols. In addition, they can produce oxidative dealkylation at the alpha carbons of the alkyl groups attached to a nitrogen, sulfur, or oxygen atom of the drug molecule, as in the case of the macrolide antibiotics and trimethoprim. Moreover, they can induce oxidation of sulfur atoms to the corresponding sulfoxides, as in the case of bithionol, chlorpromazine, and oxfendazole, and/or oxidation of nitrogen atoms to the corresponding hydroxylamines or N-oxides, as in the case of trimethoprim.

Reduction reactions are responsible for the transformation of aldehyde and ketonic groups of drugs such as steroids, mebendazole, and zearalenone to the corresponding alcohols, and for the reduction of azo- and nitro-drugs. On the other hand, hydrolysis reactions lead to cleavage of ester and amide linkages and can proceed through a large number of nonspecific esterases and amidases.

Phase II biosynthetic or conjugative processes require energy to drive the reaction and to activate endogenous substrates as conjugating factors. Glucuronidation represents one of the major reactions leading to water-soluble compounds that are eliminated from the body into the urine and bile. Glucuronides are synthesized when endogenous glucuronic acid is used for drug conjugation. Numerous functional groups of the drugs such as aromatic alcohol groups for steroids, amine groups for sulfonamides, and sulfydryl groups for thiophenols are involved in this conjugation. For some drugs such as phenylbutazone, glucuronides can be formed from nucleophilic carbon atoms. Inactivation of the parent drug almost always occurs when the conjugations occur at hydroxyl, sulfydryl, carboxyl, or amino groups.

Sulfation is another main conjugation reaction in mammals for hydroxyl or amine groups of drugs. Sulfate conjugation is facilitated by sulfurases using endogenous thiosulfate and sulfate groups. Methylation at oxygen, sulfur, and nitrogen atoms is facilitated by methyltransferases using endogenous methionine as a methyl donor. Another main route of biotransformation for arylamines, aliphatic amines, and sulfonamides is N-acetylation. Glycine and glutamine are the amino acids involved in acetylation reactions in most mammalian species, but in ducks, geese, hens, and turkeys, ornithine is the amino acid mainly used for this conjugation (3). Polymorphism of acetylation for selected substrates has been reported in both humans and animals.

The rate of biotransformation is usually determined by the activity of the liver microsomal enzymes system. However, several drugs have the ability to stimulate not only their own metabolism but also the metabolism of other compounds. This increase in the rate of metabolism can be attributed primarily to a morphological proliferation of the endoplasmic reticulum, with concurrent increases in the quantity and turnover of the drug-metabolizing enzymes. The phenomenon of induction of drug metabolism has been demonstrated for several species including rabbits, trout, cattle, sheep, and swine (8), and for several drugs including chlorpromazine, estradiol, griseofulvin, phenobarbital, phenylbutazone, amprolium, and zoalene (9, 10).

Thus, tissue levels of amprolium and zoalene that can induce their own metabolism were higher in chickens at 3 weeks of dosing than at 8 weeks. This may explain, in part, why drugs such as these do not accumulate in body tissues and disappear so quickly following cessation of treatment. On the other hand, phenobarbital can induce the metabolism of other compounds; experimental animals given daily doses of this drug showed increased capacity to metabolize steroids (11).

It is also of importance to recognize that just as small quantities of drugs can induce increased drug-metabolizing capacity, small amounts of some other drugs inhibit the rate of biotransformation. This delayed biotransformation can be seen within minutes after administration of drugs such as chloramphenicol (9).

Apart from the site and route of administration, formulation, dosage, and duration of treatment, biotransformation is often also affected by several other factors including age, species differences, sex differences, diet, diseases, hormones, and environment. The activity of the liver microsomal enzymes is low in newborns and aging animals resulting in a slower rate of biotransformation. Species differences in dosage and response are often due to biotransformation differences. Inadequate protein intake approaching starvation may also decrease the rate of biotransformation (12). Diseases of the liver sometimes also interfere with the normal biotransformation capacity. In addition, increase in biotransformation may occur at high body temperatures because of an increase in the metabolic rate.

2.1.4   Excretion

Excretion is the process by which the parent drug and its metabolites are removed from the body fluids before elimination occurs. The most important site of drug excretion is the kidney. Extrarenal sites of excretion include the liver, lung, mammary gland, sweat gland, salivary glands, and intestinal mucosa.

Excretion of drugs through the kidney takes place primarily by glomerular filtration, although proximal tubular secretion and distal tubular absorption also occur. Glomerular filtration relies on the pore size and does not make any distinction between ionized and nonionized forms of the drugs. The rate of glomerular filtration varies among species, the driving force being the blood pressure. In glomerular filtration, the extent of protein binding is of great importance since drugs bound to tissue or serum proteins cannot be filtered by the renal glomerulus.

Proximal tubular secretion is an energy-dependent active-transport mechanism. Specific high-affinity proteins in the proximal tubule transport drugs into the tubule for elimination via the urine. These proteins can also remove acidic and basic drugs from plasma protein-binding sites and transport them into the tubule. Since it is carrier-mediated, this mechanism is a saturable system. Therefore, other drugs may also compete for transport where similar carriers are employed.

Distal tubular resorption occurs with many lipid-soluble or nonionized drugs. Reabsorption in the distal tubule can occur by active transport with saturation and competition, or by passive diffusion. Water is reabsorbed, thus producing a high concentration in the urine and a concentration gradient that favors drug resorption.

The pKa of the drug, the pH of the urine, and the rate of blood flow are all parameters affecting drug reabsorption. Where it is desirable to increase excretion of a drug, manipulation of the pH of urine to favor the ionized form of the drug may decrease reabsorption. When the tubular urine becomes alkaline, basic drugs tend to exist largely in the nonionized form. As the drugs become less polar, they are able to back-diffuse through the lipid cell membrane of the renal tubular epithelium into the blood and so increase their retention in the body.

On the other hand, acidic drugs tend to ionize under conditions of alkaline pH and so are unable to permeate the renal tubular epithelium and are preferentially excreted. The converse applies to conditions of acidic urinary pH. This has been demonstrated experimentally for many drugs; weak bases are excreted more rapidly in acidic urine, whereas weak acids are excreted more rapidly in alkaline urine. In the horse, phenylbutazone, which is a weak organic acid with a pKa of 4.6, has a more delayed clearance time under conditions of aciduria than under conditions of alkaline urine.

Renal insufficiency significantly affects drug excretion. Thus, a reduced dosage or an increased dosage interval may be necessary for drugs such as polymyxin, gentamicin, penicillins, lincomycin, tetracycline, kanamycin, vancomycin, clindamycin, nitrofurantoin, colistin, streptomycin, neomycin, erythromycin, and sulfonamides, in order to avoid high plasma levels. This is because the rate of excretion of these drugs is considerably inhibited in case of renal insufficiency. Switching to drugs such as docycycline, novobiocin, or chloramphenicol that are not primarily dependent upon renal excretion may aid in avoiding buildup of residues or dosage and interval adjustments (9).

Although most compounds are excreted primarily by renal mechanisms, some drugs are partially or completely excreted through the bile. Substances excreted through the bile are usually drug products biotransformed in the liver, they possess a high degree of polarity, and are often conjugated. There is an extensive species variation among animals in their general ability to secrete drugs in the bile. Chickens are characterized as good biliary excreters, whereas sheep and rabbits are characterized as moderate and poor excreters. As with all systems involved in drug disposition, consideration must be also given to the increased tissue accumulation that may occur with hepatic disease and parasites.

Part of the drug that enters the gut through the bile is eliminated via the feces or may be reabsorbed and then be excreted in the urine or returned to the gut through the bile. The latter cycle is called enterohepatic circulation because in this cycle the compounds may travel the route in progressively reducing amounts several times before elimination is completed. Reabsorption occurs when bacterial enzymes liberate the active drug from those conjugates in which the glucuronide moiety is attached via an oxygen group. Since some of the drug remains in the gut and part of the reabsorbed drug may be eliminated by another route, the concentration of the free drug in the body progressively declines.

Mammary transfer of drugs is also considerably affected by protein binding. Since only the unbound form of drugs can equilibrate between plasma and other body fluids, passage, for example, of penicillin across the mammary barrier would be expected to occur very slowly due to the high tendency of this compound to bind to plasma proteins. Passage of sulfonamides into bovine milk is also independent on the plasma concentration of the drug but it is greatly affected by the pH of the milk and the pKa of the drug (13). Acidity of milk favors mammary excretion of basic drugs but does not exclude acidic drugs. In cases of mastitis where the pH of the milk is less acidic, both the ionized fraction in the milk and the excretion via the milk are altered. After dosing normal and mastitic ewes with sulfamethazine, drug residues were significantly higher in the mastitic animals since the mastitic milk was considerably more alkaline than the milk of normal ewes (14).

In species where reabsorption of drugs from the gastrointestinal tract increases the half-life of elimination, salivary secretion represents another important excretion route. The large volume of alkaline saliva produced by ruminants offers the possibility of trapping the acidic drugs. Exhalation of products of drug metabolism, such as carbon dioxide and water, can also account for drug excretion.

2.2 FATE OF DRUGS IN AQUATIC SPECIES

Although drug biotransformation has been systematically studied in mammalian species for many years, similar investigations in aquatic species have lagged behind mammalian research. Only in the last decade has the importance of biotransformation in fish and crustaceans been recognized (15).

Fish possess a large number of unique features that differentiate them both structurally and functionally from other vertebrates. Many of these biological features, including the gills, blood circulation and blood characteristics, and hepatic, renal, and digestive functions, are critical to drug pharmacokinetics.

The gill, one of the most versatile organs in fish, is an important avenue for drug absorption and elimination. Elimination of drugs across the gill is highly dependent upon the lipophilicity and charge of the compound. Compounds that are moderately lipophilic and neutrally charged, are readily eliminated across the gill.

Blood pH in a variety of fish species has been shown to be higher than that typically reported in mammals. This is of importance since the ionization status of drugs is dependent on the pH of the transport blood and water, and the pKa of the particular compound. In the trout, for example, blood pH values average about 8.0 but if the fish is stressed by handling for a duration as short as 30 s, blood pH values average around 7.5 (16). Such factors may influence drug ionization in fish. Several other mechanisms, including the counter flow of blood and water, diffusion barriers, and lamellar recruitment, which serve to maximize extraction of oxygen from the water environment, also serve to promote drug transfer. Water-quality alterations in pH and hypoxia-induced respiratory adjustments can also alter the absorption and disposition of drugs in fish (17, 18).

The circulatory system of fish is also unique structurally and functionally. Structurally, the membranous nature of the vasculature makes for a friable high-capacitance system under low pressure. Low blood flows result in somewhat longer distributional phases for many drugs. Processes such as heart rate and stroke volume that influence drug distribution are themselves influenced by external factors such as temperature and stress. In addition, total plasma protein content differs in fish as compared to mammals. Total plasma protein in the trout and flounder is approximately one-half that of mammals such as dogs and cats. For many compounds protein binding is considerably lower in fish than their mammalian counterparts (19, 20).

Hepatic function is also important because fish liver can change dramatically in regard to its weight and chemical composition; changes in chemical composition concern mainly alterations in glycogen and lipid content. Seasonal gonadal maturation, time from last feeding, and response to stress may influence these parameters (21, 22). In addition, hepatic perfusion is poor in fish with rates accounting for 25–50% of those found in mammals. These features are important in regard to drug metabolism.

Fish are extremely good biliary concentrators of drugs. Molecular weight and polarity concerns for biliary elimination are basically similar to mammals, but bile formation in fish is nearly 50 times slower than mammals. As a result, fish have the capacity to biotransform a variety of substrates, although the rates generally observed are lower than in many mammalian species. Sufficient evidence exists to indicate that glucuronyl transferase, sulfotransferase, glutathione-S-transferase, and epoxide hydrolase activities in fish are, at least qualitatively, similar to those found in mammals (23, 24).

The kidney of most fish is primarily involved in hematopoiesis and osmoregulation. Fresh-water fish are hypertonic relative to the water. The continual osmotic uptake of water is balanced by production of as large amounts as 2–4 ml/kg/h of dilute urine. Salt-water fish, on the other hand, are hypotonic relative to their environment, resulting in body water loss. In response, marine species produce much smaller volumes of urine. Large differences exist among different fish species in regard to nephron structure to facilitate these functional responses. These features may influence the renal contribution to drug disposition: appreciable amounts of the administered drugs are excreted in the urine of fish in the form of the parent compound and/or its metabolites. A number of studies have demonstrated that glucuronide, sulfate, and taurine conjugates are excreted by the fish kidney as a result of anion/cation carrier-mediated mechanisms (25, 26).

Unlike fresh-water species, marine species drink appreciable quantities of water to maintain their hydration status and, therefore, can provide drug access to uptake by the gastrointestinal tract. However, regional pH of the gastrointestinal tract may vary considerably between fish species. For example, the pH of the stomach is much more alkaline in herbaceous than carnivorous fish.

On the other hand, crustacean species differ considerably from fish in their biological make-up. The hepatopancreas, antennal gland, intestine, and gill are the most important organs of drug metabolism in crustaceans. The high fat content of hepatopancreas, which is the major organ of metabolism and storage of nutrients, makes this organ a storage site for lipophilic drugs. The antennal glands are paired organs that function in urine formation, salt balance, and steroid biosynthesis (27). Crustacean gill and intestine are, on the other hand, organs with a not well defined role in drug metabolism and excretion (28).

Another major difference between crustacea and fish is the presence of shell, which appears to absorb certain xenobiotics (29). As a result, metabolism and excretion of lipophilic drugs and their metabolites are usually slower in crustaceans than in other species. Glucuronidation, a major pathway of drug conjugation in terrestrial and aquatic species, has not been definitely determined in crustacean tissues or excreta. Instead, conjugation of the hydroxyl groups of drugs with glucose has been detected in crustaceans (30). Like fish, crustaceans also conjugate carboxylic acids with taurine, but not with glycine (31). Other major pathways of drug conjugation processes including acetylation, sulfation, and glutathione conjugation are also found in crustaceans (32).

Following their formation in the hepatopancreas, metabolites are usually excreted in feces and urine, antennal gland, or other sites. Available data indicate that drugs that are readily soluble or can be biotransformed into water-soluble conjugates are more rapidly excreted from crustaceans than lipid-soluble drugs. Hence, very lipophilic drugs can be expected to attain much higher concentrations in the hepatopancreas than in other tissues, and to be slowly excreted in feces after metabolism to more polar metabolites.

REFERENCES

1. S.H. Curry, in Drug Disposition and Pharmacokinetics (S.H. Curry, Ed.), Blackwell Scientific Publications, Oxford (1977).
2. T.B. Barragry, in Veterinary Drug Therapy (T.B. Barragry, Ed.), Lea & Febiger, PA (1994).

3. J. Weissinger, and L.M. Crawford, in Animal Drugs and Human Health (L.M. Crawford and Don A. Franco, Eds.), Technomic Publishing Co., PA, USA (1994).
4. N.H. Booth, and L.E. McDonald, in Veterinary Pharmacology and Therapeutics (N.H. Booth and L.E. McDonald, Eds.), Iowa State University Press, Ames, IA (1982).
5. B.K. Martin, Nature, 207:274 (1965).
6. M.C. Meyer, and D.E. Guttman, J. Pharm. Sci., 57:895 (1968).
7. L.S. Goodman, and A. Gilman, in The Pharmacological Basis of Therapeutics (L.S. Goodman and A. Gilman, Eds.), MacMillan Publishing Co, New York (1985).
8. J.C. Street, R.W. Chadwick, M. Wang, and R.L. Phillips, J. Agric. Food Chem., 14: 545 (1966).
9. J. Weissinger, in Agents of Disease III—Veterinary Pharmacology and Toxicology, Course Syllabus, Colorado State University (1983).
10. J. Bruggeman, J. Schole, and J. Tiews, J. Agric. Food Chem., 11:367 (1963).
11. A.H. Conney, and A. Klutch, J. Biol. Chem., 238:1611 (1963).
12. R. Kato, T. Oshima, and S. Tonizawa, Jpn. J. Pharmacol., 18:356 (1968).
13. F. Rasmussen, Acta Pharmacol. Toxicol., 15:139 (1958).
14. E.A. Tunnicliff, and K.F. Swingle, Am. J. Vet. Res., 26:920 (1965).
15. K.M. Kleinow, M.O. James, and J.J. Lech, in Xenobiotics and Food-Producing Animals (D.H. Hutson, D.R. Hawkins, G.P. Paulson, and C.B. Struble, Eds.), American Chemical Society, Washington, DC, p. 98 (1992).
16. T.A. Heming, Am. J. Vet. Res., 50:93 (1989).
17. T. Endo, and M. Onozawa, Nippon Suisan Gak., 53:551 (1987).
18. J.M. McKim, and H.M. Goeden, Comp. Biochem. Physiol., 72C:65 (1982).
19. B.F. Droy, M.S. Goodrich, J.J. Lech, and K.M. Kleinow, Xenobiotica, 20:147 (1990).
20. K.S. Squibb, C.M.F. Michel, J.T. Zelikoff, and J.M. O'Connor, Vet. Human Toxicol., 30:31 (1988).
21. K.M. Kleinow, B.F. Droy, D.R. Buhler, and D.E. Williams, Toxicol. Appl. Pharm., 104:367 (1990).
22. M.R. Miller, D.E. Hinton, J.J. Blair, and J.J. Stegeman, Mar. Environ. Res., 24:37 (1988).
23. C.D. Klaasen, and G.L. Plaa, J. Appl. Physiol., 22:151 (1967).
24. W.H. Gingerich, L.J. Weber, and R.E. Larson, Comp. Biochem. Physiol., 58C:113 (1977).
25. M.O. James, and J.B. Pritchard, Drug Metabol. Disp., 15:665 (1987).
26. S.M. Plakas, and M.O. James, Drug Metabol. Disp., 18:552 (1990).
27. M.O. James, and K.T. Shiverick, Arch. Biochem. Biophys., 233:1 (1984).
28. M.O. James, J.D. Schell, M.G. Baron, and C-L. J. Li, Drug Metabol. Disp., 19:536 (1991).
29. M.G. Barron, C. Gedutis, and M.O. James, Xenobiotica, 18:269 (1988).
30. J.D. Schell, and M.O. James, J. Biochem. Toxicol., 4:133 (1989).
31. M.G. Barron, S.C. Hansen, and T. Ball, Drug Metabol. Disp., 19:163 (1991).
32. M.O. James, and M.G. Barron, Vet. Human Toxicol., 30:36 (1988).

3

Antibacterial Drugs

In principle, all drug preparations administered to food-producing animals may lead to residues in the edible tissues, milk, or eggs. In addition to the drug dosage, the levels of those residues depend on the period between administration and slaughter or collection of the animal products, the so-called withdrawal period, which, on its turn, depends on the pharmacokinetic profile of the drug.

Residues of antibacterial drugs in foodstuffs from animal origin could represent a hazard for the consumer of these products. Toxic effects are unlikely since residues will be present only at very low concentrations. Nevertheless, some substances must receive particular attention owing to their harmfulness. Allergic reactions may be also produced in sensitive or sensitized individuals. However, the principal hazardous effect is likely to be development of resistance strains of bacteria following the ingestion of subtherapeutic doses of antimicrobials. The resistance could be transferred to other bacteria. This could include transfer of resistance from nonpathogenic organisms to pathogenic organisms, which would then no longer respond to normal drug treatment. The illicit use of antibiotics could thus increase the risk of foodborne infection with antibiotic-resistant pathogenic bacteria contaminating food taken by humans.

A brief description of the antibacterial drugs potentially used in food-producing animals, along with their pharmacokinetic profiles, is provided here.

3.1. AMINOGLYCOSIDES AND AMINOCYCLITOLS

Aminoglycosides and aminocyclitols are antibiotics elaborated by bacteria of the genus *Streptomyces* and *Micromonospora* (1). Streptomycin, kanamycin, amikacin, neomycin, and apramycin are examples of antibiotics derived from the former species, in which case the compound name ends in the suffix -mycin, while gentamicin and sisomicin are antibiotics derived from the latter, in which case the compound name ends in the suffix -micin.

The structure of aminoglycosides consists of one or more amino sugar units in the form of a glycosamine and/or a disaccharide containing D-ribose, which are attached to a central aglycon moiety with glycosidic linkage (2). The central moiety, a saturated ring substituted with amine and hydroxyl groups, is 2-deoxys-treptamine in most aminoglycosides but streptidine in the streptomycin and dihy-drostreptomycin.

Aminocyclitols are closely related to aminoglycosides. They differ in that aminoglycosides contain amino sugars joined by a glycosidic link, while amino-cyclitols have the amino group on the cyclitol ring (3). The two major aminocycli-tols are spectinomycin and apramycin.

Most aminoglycosides are complexes of several almost identical compo-nents differing either in the degree of methylation of one amino sugar unit, as in the case of gentamicin, or in the stereochemistry of the disaccharide unit, as in the case of neomycin. Differences in the substitutions on the basic ring structures between the various aminoglycosides account for the relatively minor differences in antimicrobial spectra, patterns of resistance, and toxicity.

The aminoglycosides interfere with bacterial protein synthesis by binding irreversibly to ribosome and could cause cell membrane damage. They may be inactivated by bacterial resistant enzymes but bacteria could also display resis-tance through ribosomal modifications or by decreased uptake of antibiotic into the bacterial cell.

Aminoglycosides are widely distributed in the body after injection and little is absorbed from the gastrointestinal tract. However, inflammation or other lesions may increase absorption considerably (4). Aminoglycosides are not metabolized in the body but are bound and eliminated by renal glomerular filtration and excre-tion in the urine (5). Residues in the body tend to be concentrated in the kidney (6). When used at therapeutic dosages, ototoxicosis principally, but also nephro-toxicosis, allergy, and neuromuscular effects are the adverse effects of the amino-glycosides.

In food-producing animals, the most commonly used aminoglycosides and aminocyclitols are streptomycin, dihydrostreptomycin, gentamicin, neomycin, and spectinomycin, although other members of this family are used to a lesser degree. Several new aminoglycosides are available for human use or are being developed for human and veterinary use, such as paromomycin, dibecacin, and habecacin. The development of semisynthetic derivatives has resulted in drugs with lower toxicity and greater effectiveness. Kanamycin was synthetically modi-fied to produce tobramycin and amikacin, and sisomicin has been synthetically modified to produce netilmicin (7). The need to turn to other members of the aminoglycoside family is determined by the growing resistance of bacteria to the established drugs (8). Structures of selected aminoglycosides are shown in Figure 3.1.

Apramycin is a broad-spectrum aminocyclitol antibiotic and component of the nebramycin complex, produced by a strain of *Streptomyces tenebrarius*. Use of this antibiotic is specifically aimed at mass therapy of colibacillosis and salmonellosis in veal calves and swine. It is administered to calves by intramuscular or oral route at a dose of 20–40 mg/kg body weight/day for 5 days, and to swine via the drinking water at a dosage of 7.5–12.5 mg/kg bw/day for 7 days, or via the feed at a rate of 100 mg/kg feed for 28 days. It is further used for treatment of colibacillosis in lambs given orally at a dosage of 10 mg/kg bw/day for 3–5 days, and for treatment of *E. coli* septicemia in poultry administered in the drinking water at a concentration of 250–500 mg/L for 7 days. In contrast to other aminoglycosides, apramycin is not used in human medicine.

If apramycin is used, incorrectly, residues may be found in large concentrations in foodstuffs of animal origin and represent both a hazard for the consumer and a disruptive element for the manufacturing processes adopted by the food industry. Apramycin is poorly absorbed after oral administration, but is rapidly and effectively absorbed after parenteral administration and distributed through the extracellular fluid. Excretion is through the kidney, and the compound is found unchanged in the urine. More than 75% of the total residues found in liver and kidneys of animals slaughtered 5–6 days after treatment appear to be unmetabolized apramycin.

After oral administration to pigs of 20 mg apramycin/kg bw /day for 7 days, detectable residues were present only in kidney. One day after the treatment, residues in kidney were in the range 5800–15,300 parts per billion (ppb), declining to 2500–3100 ppb 7 days after treatment, and to below 210 ppb 14 days after treatment. Unlike with pigs, residues are much higher in calf tissues. Apramycin residues in calves given orally 20 mg/kg bw/day for 5 days declined from 2800 to 21,700 ppb in kidney, 100 ppb in fat, and 1200 ppb in the liver at 7 days after treatment to 200–9400 ppb in kidney, to less than 50 ppb in fat, and 400–700 ppb in the liver at 21 days after treatment.

Residues in tissues are, generally, much higher with parenteral than oral administration. Residues in calves given intramuscularly 20 mg apramycin /kg bw /day for 5 days declined from 296,600–435,300 ppb in kidney, 8700–14,700 ppb in liver, 6200 ppb in fat, 1900–3400 in muscle, and 23,600–65,100 at the injection site at 4 h after the last treatment to 1200–14,500 ppb in kidney, 3500–4200 ppb in liver, 400 ppb in fat, below 268 ppb in muscle, and less than 268–4600 ppb at the injection site at 28 days after treatment.

In broilers given drinking water containing 500 mg radiolabeled apramycin/ L for 5 days, mean total residues in kidney declined from 3230 ppb at 1 day after treatment to 1475 ppb 7 days later, and to 470 ppb 14 days after treatment. Over

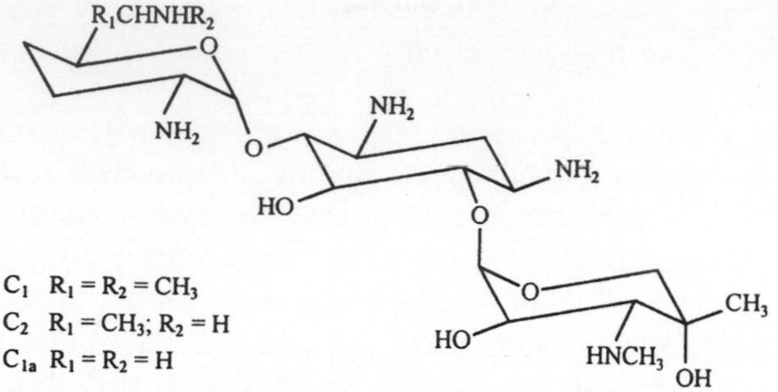

R$_1$CHNHR$_2$

Gentamicin C$_1$ R$_1$ = R$_2$ = CH$_3$
            C$_2$ R$_1$ = CH$_3$; R$_2$ = H
            C$_{1a}$ R$_1$ = R$_2$ = H

Gentamicin

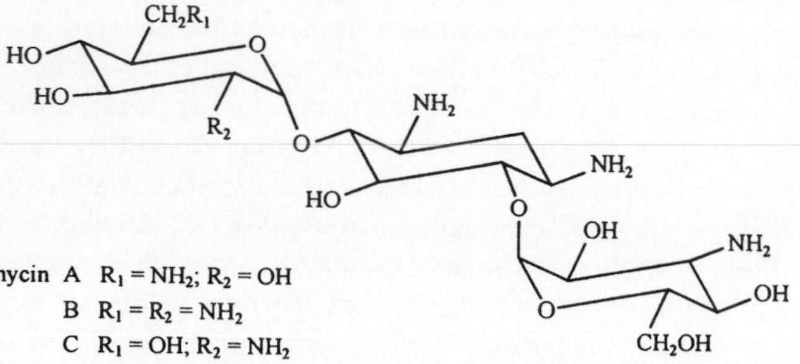

CH$_2$R$_1$

Kanamycin A R$_1$ = NH$_2$; R$_2$ = OH
           B R$_1$ = R$_2$ = NH$_2$
           C R$_1$ = OH; R$_2$ = NH$_2$

Kanamycin

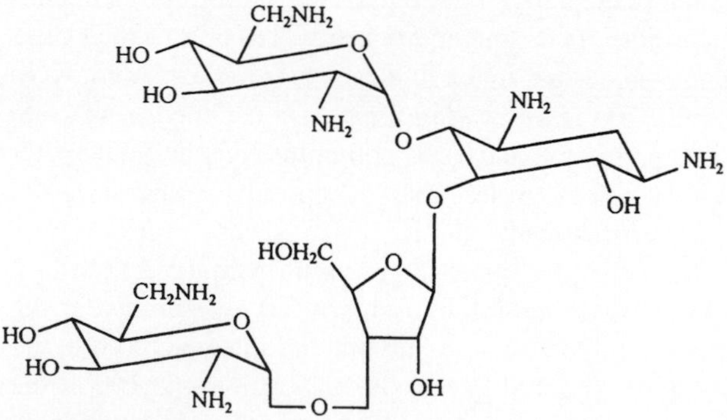

CH$_2$NH$_2$

CH$_2$NH$_2$

Neomycin B

FIG. 3.1 Chemical structures of commonly used aminoglycosides and amino-cyclitols.

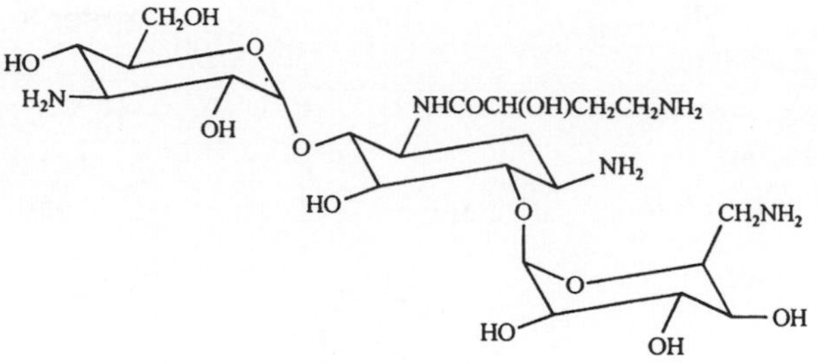

Amikacin

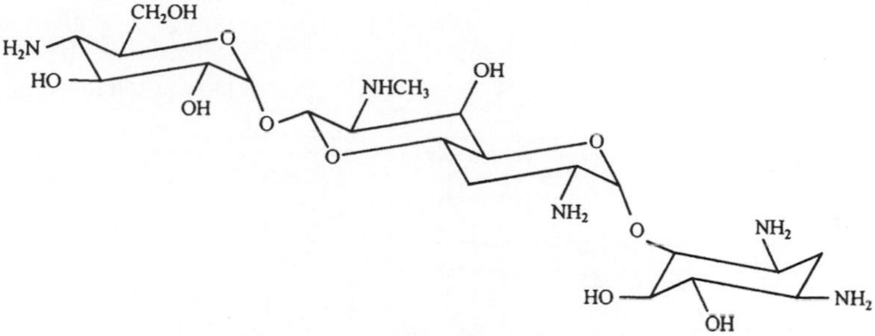

Apramycin

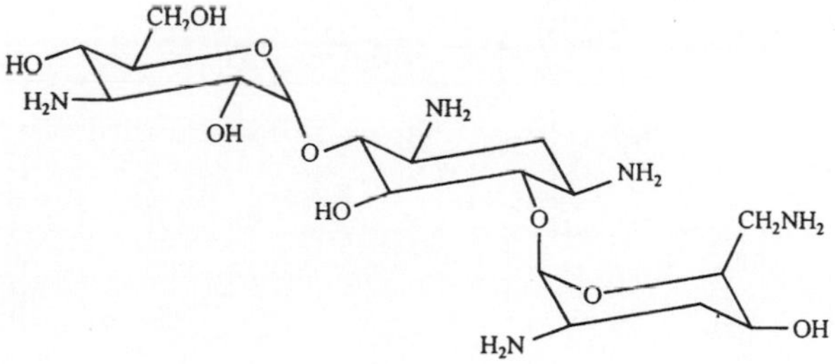

Tobramycin

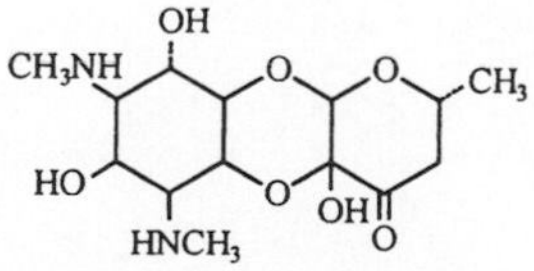

Spectinomycin

Fig. 3.1 *Continued*

31

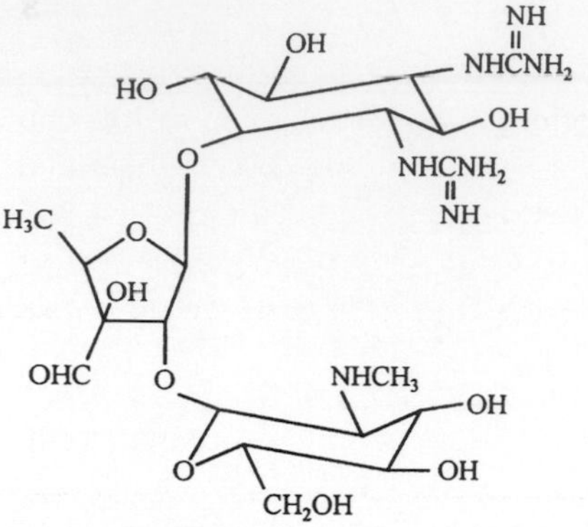

Streptomycin

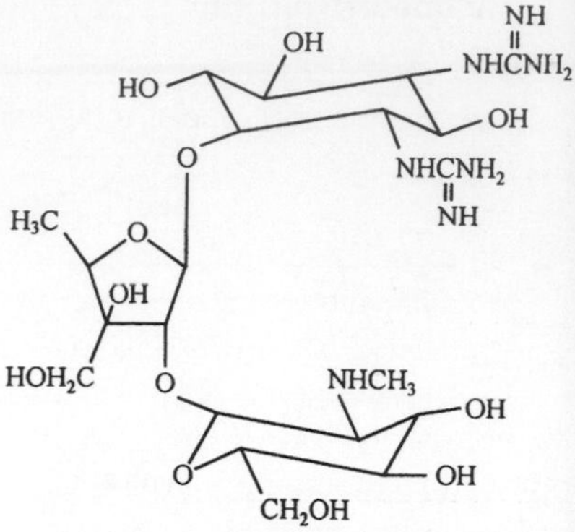

Dihydrostreptomycin

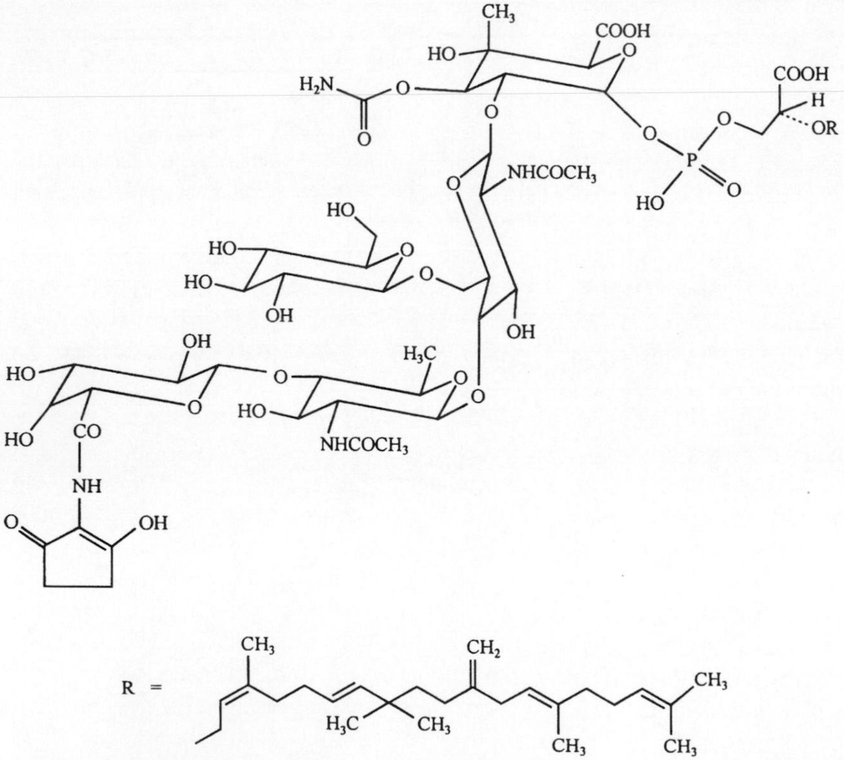

Bambermycin (moenomycin A)

Fig. 3.1 *Continued*

the same period, mean total residues in liver declined from 420 ppb to 150 ppb and finally to 80 ppb, whereas those in skin were from 70 ppb to 60 ppb and finally to 30 ppb. Mean total residues in muscle declined from 70 ppb at 1 day after treatment to 20 ppb at 7 days after treatment. Compositional analysis of total residues showed that more than 80% of the residues in liver and kidney consisted of unmetabolized apramycin.

Apramycin is authorized for use neither in laying hens nor in cattle or sheep producing milk for human consumption. When apramycin was administered intravenously and intramuscularly to lactating cows with clinically normal and acutely inflamed udders, and to lactating ewes with normal or subclinically infected udders, drug penetration into the milk from the acutely inflamed quarters of cows was extensive. Maximum concentrations in mastitic milk were more than 10-fold greater than those in normal milk (9). On the other hand, the drug had limited access to the milk produced by subclinically infected half-udders of ewes.

Bambermycin is an aminoglycoside complex produced by *Streptomyces bambergiensis* and related strains. This complex is also known as flavomycin, flavophospholipol, or moenomycin. It consists of at least four active components known as moenomycins A, B_1, B_2, and C; moenomycin A is the major component. Bambermycin, although possessing antibacterial activity, is used only as a growth-promoting agent in veterinary medicine. It is added to cattle, swine, poultry, and rabbit feeds at dosages ranging from 1 to 20 ppm.

Bambermycin is an antibiotic that, because of its heteropolar behavior, tends to form complexes. It is, therefore, a compound that is extremely difficult for animals to absorb. Balance studies proved that bambermycin is not absorbed but is excreted in the feces as the intact, biologically active drug. As a result, no withdrawal period is required.

Gentamicin is an aminoglycoside complex composed of three major components designated C_1, C_2, and C_{1a}. It is a generally utilized bactericidal agent with the broadest spectrum of activity among the aminoglycosides. Gentamicin is indicated for treatment of pigs with colibacillosis or swine dysentery at a dosage of 5 mg/kg bw intramuscularly or orally. It has been also used in cattle by intramammary infusion for treatment of mastitis, by intrauterine infusion for treatment of metritis, and parenterally for treatment of respiratory diseases. A popular treatment regimen combines gentamicin and penicillin. Apart from its ototoxic and nephrotoxic potential, gentamicin may also cause liver disturbances and both peripheral and central neuropathies including encephalopathy, lethargy, and convulsions.

The compound is poorly absorbed from the gastrointestinal tract. Gentamicin serum and tissues concentrations during and following intramuscular or oral administration of gentamicin (5 mg/kg bw twice daily) to calves showed that the drug was absorbed poorly after oral administration but rapidly after intramuscular injection (10).

After parenteral doses, gentamicin distributed into extracellular space but significant amounts penetrated the kidney and inner ear. There was negligible biotransformation of the drug following parenteral administration and unchanged gentamicin was excreted rapidly in the urine. After intramuscular injection, significant amounts penetrated into the kidney and liver, with only low levels being found in muscle and fat; residues in kidney depleted to below 0.08 ppm by day 14. Only low levels of residues, as determined by total radioactivity, were found in pigs given oral doses of radiolabeled gentamicin. The disposition of gentamicin after repeated oral administration to neonatal piglets with enterotoxemia was fully comparable to the disposition in healthy piglets, as indicated by the plasma and fecal levels observed during treatment (11). Also, the residue depletion in body tissues was fully comparable; at 14 and 28 days withdrawal, residue levels were <0.05 ppm in muscle, and <0.10 ppm in liver. At 14 days, kidney contained 0.17–0.27 ppm, whereas at 28 days than 0.15 ppm.

In dairy cattle given gentamicin by a intramuscular injection, intramammary infusion, or intrauterine infusion, milk was free of detectable residues at 60–84 h posttreatment. However, following repeated treatment over a period of 5 days, depletion of gentamicin residues to a concentration less than or equal to 30 ppb appeared at 228 h posttreatment (12). Therefore, illegal and extralabel use of the compound is likely to cause residues in milk.

In general gentamicin is excreted by the urinary route, and so has the drawback of binding to the kidney tissue, which in food-producing animals may give residues lasting over months (13). Thus, even the minor fraction absorbed after oral administration accumulates in the kidney and brings about concentrations far above the accepted residue concentrations. Following oral application, a long withdrawal period of more than 105 days before slaughter applies to the kidney, independent of application form. However, this precaution is not necessary for meat, and a much shorter withdrawal period of 5 days is observed in calves following oral application. Following intramuscular application to calves, the withdrawal period for meat should be prolonged to about 60 days.

Kanamycin is an aminoglycoside complex produced by *Streptomyces kanamyceticus*. It is comprised of three components, kanamycin A being the major component and kanamycins B and C minor congeners. Kanamycin is active against many pathogenic bacteria and has been used parenterally for treatment of bovine respiratory disease, mastitis, and other infectious conditions. A popular combination used in horses and cattle with respiratory disease is kanamycin and penicillin G. It is also used orally for treatment of bacterial enteritis because limited absorption occurs after oral administration.

Apart from its ototoxic and nephrotoxic potential, kanamycin may also cause liver disturbances and both peripheral and central neuropathies including encephalopathy, lethargy, and convulsions. Cochlear toxicity is more frequent than vestibular toxicity with kanamycin. Gastrointestinal disturbances have been reported following administration of kanamycin by mouth.

Kanamycin crosses placenta and is found in breast milk. When kanamycin was administered intramuscularly to cattle, sheep, and swine at dosages in the range 5–10 mg/kg bw at 12 h intervals, milk was free of the antibiotic 36 h after the last injection (14). However, kanamycin residues persisted longer in the kidney tissue.

Neomycin is an aminoglycoside complex produced by *Streptomyces fradiae*. It consists of three components: A, B, and C. Component B is the major component of commercial preparations of neomycin (over 90%). Framycetin, which is also known as soframycin, is merely the more pure B component of neomycin. Component C is present only in traces (< 1%) in the neomycin complex. Both B and C components of neomycin are chemically similar and biologically active.

Neomycin is administered orally for treatment of bacterial infections of cattle, sheep, pigs, goats, and poultry at a dosage of 10 mg/kg bw. It is also used as a feed additive for growth-promoting purposes. Neomycin is further available alone or in combination with other drugs such as oxytetracycline, oleandomycin, lincomycin, and prednisolone, in intramammary formulations for treatment of mastitis. There has been relatively little clinical use of neomycin parenterally in animals because of the compound's reported nephrotoxicity and ototoxicity.

Neomycin is particularly ototoxic and nephrotoxic when given parenterally. As with gentamicin and kanamycin, the nephrotoxicity may be reversible but the ototoxicity is usually irreversible and deafness may occur following oral administration, instillation into cavities, or topical use. It may block neuromuscular action and respiratory depression has been reported. Local treatments may cause hypersensitivity, rashes, pruritus, and anaphylaxis. Neomycin is not genotoxic.

Neomycin is poorly absorbed from the gastrointestinal tract, and has low absorption from the udder. In contrast, it is rapidly absorbed following parenteral administration. In all cases, it undergoes negligible biotransformation in the body. Orally administered neomycin is mainly excreted unchanged in the feces, whereas after parenteral administration it is excreted fairly rapidly in the urine. Neomycin must not be used parenterally in food-producing animals because of the prolonged persistence of its residues in edible tissues, eggs, and milk.

Spectinomycin is an aminocyclitol antibiotic produced by *Streptomyces spectabilis*. It is indicated for use via the oral and intramuscular or subcutaneous routes in the treatment of a variety of enteric, respiratory, and other infections of cattle, sheep, swine and poultry. Recommended dosages are 7.5–12.5 mg/kg bw for intramuscular injections and 1–5 mg/bird for subcutaneous injections in poultry. Spectinomycin is frequently combined with lincomycin and administered either intramuscularly at 15 mg/kg bw to calves, sheep, and swine (15), and at

30 mg/kg bw to poultry or orally at a dosage of 5–10 mg/kg bw in swine and 50–150 mg/kg feed in poultry.

Spectinomycin is a particularly valuable antibiotic because of its low toxicity. It may cause hepatic, renal, and hematological disturbances. Anaphylaxis has rarely been reported.

The absorption of spectinomycin is poor via the oral route, but rapid and extensive after intramuscular injection. It is not extensively metabolized in animals and rapidly excreted in the urine (16). Following subcutaneous injections of spectinomycin sulfate to cattle, 70–83% of the dose was excreted in the urine and 62–64% of this was parent spectinomycin (17). Several minor metabolites were found in the urine that consisted mostly of dihydroxyspectinomycin and two acetylated isomers, and an unusual ammoniated spectinomycin metabolite and its acetylated derivative. There was also some evidence, but it was not compelling, for a spectinomycin sulfate conjugate. Dihydrospectinomycin and parent spectinomycin were the only identifiable major components found in the liver and the kidney, respectively. Liver and kidney retained the highest concentrations of total residues throughout the 15-day withdrawal period.

Residue depletion studies with calves given intramuscular spectinomycin 30 mg/kg bw/day for 5 consecutive days showed that the average concentrations of the parent drug in liver, kidney, muscle, and fat were 4654, 43,053, 646, and less than 200 ppb, respectively, at 3 days, and 903, 2750, 200, and less than 27.1 ppb at 14 days after the last dose.

Residue depletion studies with piglets orally dosed with 30 mg spectinomycin/kg bw/day for 5 consecutive days showed that the average concentrations of the parent drug in liver, kidney, muscle, and skin/fat were 1030, 7700, less than 300, and less than 394 ppb, respectively, at 3 days, and less than 198, 500, 300, and 26 ppb, respectively, at 14 days postdosing. Broilers given water dosed at 50 mg spectinomycin/kg bw/day for 5 consecutive days were not found to contain detectable spectinomycin concentrations (limit of detection: 500 ppb for liver and kidney and 250 ppb for muscle and skin/fat) in any edible tissue even only 1 day after the last dose.

Passage of spectinomycin into milk is possibly limited by its high degree of ionization in serum and its low lipid solubility. Pertinent studies with similarly treated lactating cows showed spectinomycin levels in milk to average 1431, 439, and less than 100 ppb at the 12, 24, and 36 h milking.

Streptomycin and **dihydrostreptomycin** are aminoglycoside antibiotics closely related in structure, which are active against mainly gram-negative bacteria. Streptomycin is produced by certain strains of *Streptomyces griseus;* dihydrostreptomycin can be prepared by reduction of streptomycin.

They are active against many gram-negative bacteria but resistance develops rapidly and limits their use. Streptomycin and dihydrostreptomycin are less nephrotoxic than other aminoglycosides. They may cause neurological disturbances including optic neuritis and peripheral neuropathies. Hypersensitivity, severe dermatitis, and anaphylaxis have been reported.

Administration of streptomycin intramuscularly is the method of choice for treating systemic infections. Oral forms of streptomycin or dihydrostreptomycin, frequently combined with sulfonamide drugs and other compounds, are also used in animals for treatment of enteric infections. In addition, streptomycin is used as a feed additive for growth promotion purposes. In some countries, the combination of streptomycin with procaine penicillin is used as an initial nonspecific therapy in farm animals, and in intramammary applications for treatment of mastitis. Intramuscular dosages are in the range 5–10 mg/kg bw, while oral dosages are 20 mg/kg bw. Dihydrostreptomycin is also used in veterinary medicine in intramammary and topical treatments.

Results of pharmacokinetic studies of streptomycin are in most cases also applicable to dihydrostreptomycin and vice versa. In animals, the absorption of both streptomycin and dihydrostreptomycin is poor via the oral route but rapid after intramuscular administration. In cattle, peak serum levels were obtained 1 h after intramuscular injection of either streptomycin or dihydrostreptomycin (18), whereas serum concentrations produced in sheep and horses paralleled those obtained in cattle (19). As a result, most of an oral dose is recovered in the feces whereas most of a parenteral dose is recovered in the urine. However, if kidney function is severely impaired, little of an intramuscularly administered dose is excreted in the urine.

Unfortunately, streptomycin residues persist for long time at the site of injection and are also found in the kidney. Residue levels in other edible products of drug-treated sheep, pigs, and poultry were generally low and did not necessitate long withdrawal periods.

Analysis of bovine and swine kidney and muscle pairs from suspect Canadian slaughter animals has indicated an average difference in residue levels of 150/L and 164/L, respectively, for dihydrostreptomycin (20). Although dihydrostreptomycin is eliminated with the milk soon after its intramuscular administration to lactating cows, reaching residue levels in the range 0.05–0.13 ppb, it is not absorbed when given by the intramammary route and, thus, care must be taken to obey recommended withdrawal periods to avoid residues in milk.

3.2 AMPHENICOLS

Chloramphenicol, thiamphenicol, and florfenicol are broad-spectrum antibacterials with closely related chemical structures (Fig. 3.2). In thiamphenicol, the p-nitro group on the benzene ring of chloramphenicol is replaced with a methyl sulfonyl group. In florfenicol, the hydroxyl group on the side chain of thiamphenicol is replaced with a fluorine. They are all potent antibacterial agents acting

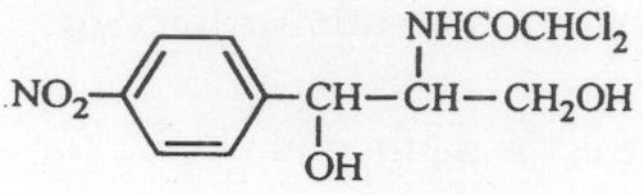

NO₂—⟨benzene ring⟩—CH—CH—CH₂OH with NHCOCHCl₂ above CH and OH below

Chloramphenicol

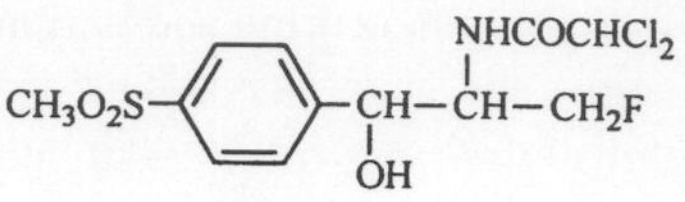

CH₃O₂S—⟨benzene ring⟩—CH—CH—CH₂F with NHCOCHCl₂ above CH and OH below

Florfenicol

CH₃O₂S—⟨benzene ring⟩—CH—CH—CH₂OH with NHCOCHCl₂ above CH and OH below

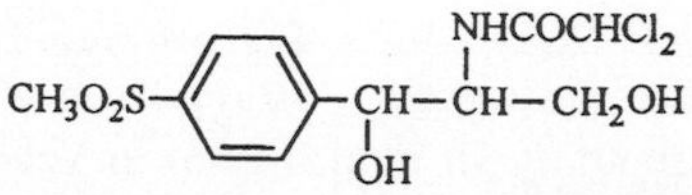

Thiamphenicol

FIG. 3.2 Chemical structures of commonly used amphenicols.

through interaction with ribosomes to inhibit organisms from synthesizing proteins (21).

Chloramphenicol is a highly active antibiotic that was first isolated from cultures of *Streptomyces venezuelae* but is now produced synthetically. It is unique among natural compounds in that it contains a nitrobenzene moiety. Chloramphenicol has been used both in treatment and prophylactically in food-producing animals for over 40 years, administered orally with the feed or drinking water to poultry, veal calves, swine, sheep, and lambs, and intramuscularly or intravenously to sheep, goats, pigs, and calves at a dosage of 2–4 mg/kg bw. In several countries, chloramphenicol has been also used in fish for the treatment of furunculoses on salmonids (22).

The most serious toxic effect of chloramphenicol is depression of the bone marrow, which is generally dose-related and reversible but is sometimes dose-unrelated, irreversible, and fatal in patients who are probably genetically predisposed (23). In newborn infants receiving large doses of chloramphenicol, a toxic syndrome has been reported, characterized by vomiting, hypothermia, cyanosis, and circulatory collapse followed by death. This syndrome may also rarely occur in adults and in infants born to mothers given chloramphenicol in pregnancy. Chloramphenicol may also cause neuritis, encephalopathy with dementia, and ototoxicity. Since chloramphenicol and its metabolites would be genotoxic, its use is restricted in many countries, while it is totally banned for use in food-producing animals within the European Union and United States (24, 25). Considerable concern has been voiced over the extralabel use of chloramphenicol in animals, and surveillance programs within many countries constantly monitor for residues of the drug.

In most species, chloramphenicol is rapidly and almost completely absorbed from the gastrointestinal tract. This route of administration provides antibiotic levels in blood comparable with or higher than the intramuscular or the subcutaneous routes. The only known exception is in ruminants in which the drug is destroyed by the rumen microflora.

Chloramphenicol is rapidly metabolized to its glucuronide conjugate in the liver of most species. In swine liver, kidney, and serum, more than one-half of the chloramphenicol present is in the conjugated form (26), but in muscles of swine, chicken, and calf, conjugated chloramphenicol is not observed (27). Six metabolites have been observed (28) in plasma and tissues of calves after oral administration of a single dose of 50 mg radiolabeled chloramphenicol/kg bw, the glucuronated metabolite being the major one in the plasma with a maximum concentration of 2.6 ppm at 3 h. Another metabolite identified as nitroaminopropanediol did not exceed 0.13 ppm; at 5 h post administration, the parent drug represented 88.7% of the total radioactivity in plasma, 74.2% in muscle, 61.5% in fat, 26.4% in liver, and 18.4% in kidney.

After infeed medication to swine, chloramphenicol was rapidly absorbed and declined rapidly thereafter due both to its rapid elimination and intensive metabolism (29). Chloramphenicol glucuronide was the main metabolite formed (30); deacetylchloramphenicol was also present although in minor quantities. No other metabolites such as nitrosochloramphenicol or dehydrochloramphenicol could be detected in the kidney that was the target tissue (31).

When chloramphenicol is administered parenterally, it rapidly enters the enterohepatic cycle, which is of significance because it prolongs the residence of the drug in the body. Deposition of chloramphenicol residues in animal tissues results from this prolongation of excretion. In diseased animals, residues of chloramphenicol can be detected for weeks after the initial administration.

Following intramuscular injection of chloramphenicol in sheep, the withdrawal period down to the level of 0.05 ppm was estimated at 14.4 days for the injection site, 6 days for noninjected muscle, 9 days for fat, 11 days for kidney, and 11 days for the liver (32). When chloramphenicol was administered to rabbits, muscle and kidney were the tissues containing the highest levels of the parent drug at 6 h postdosing, whereas at 24 h only muscle contained detectable amounts of residues (33).

The ability of liver to biotransform chloramphenicol has been also demonstrated in several fish species. In pertinent studies, various metabolic pathways were determined and chloramphenicol–glucuronide, chloramphenicol–base, chloramphenicol–alcohol, and chloramphenicol–oxamate were the main metabolites observed (34, 35). Following hepatic biotransformation, a large proportion of the administered dose was excreted in the urine.

Thiamphenicol is a synthetic chloramphenicol analogue with a molecular structure that appears to preserve the antibacterial properties, decrease markedly the metabolism by the liver, enhance kidney excretion, and eliminate the occurrence of aplastic anemia, although it is probably more liable to cause dose-dependent reversible depression of the bone marrow (15). These properties make it preferable in certain cases to chloramphenicol (36, 37).

Interest in the use of thiamphenicol in veterinary medicine, has grown recently. Thiamphenicol is intended for the treatment and control of respiratory and intestinal diseases in cattle and poultry where it is administered orally at dosages of 5000 mg/kg feed for 5 days (calves), 1000 mg/kg feed for 5 days (poultry), and 800 mg/2 drinking water for 5 days (poultry), or intramuscularly at dosages of 50 mg/kg bw for 7 days (cattle) and 70 mg/kg bw for 3 days (turkeys). In addition, it is intended for intramammary administration in both lactating and dry cows at a dosage of 10 mg/kg bw, and for intrauterine administration in cows at a dosage of 15 mg/kg bw. Thiamphenicol may also serve as a suitable replacement for other antibiotics that present long depletion times in aquaculture.

Following oral or parenteral administration, thiamphenicol is well absorbed and rapidly and extensively distributed in the tissues of most animal species. Thiamphenicol is primarily excreted in the urine but small amounts are found in feces as well. It is excreted almost entirely in the unchanged form. Unlike chloramphenicol, thiamphenicol may not be an optimal substrate for the hepatic microsomal enzyme glucuronyl transferase. In rabbits and rats, more than 90% of the administered dose was excreted unchanged. However, a higher level of glucuronidation occurred in swine.

Residue depletion studies in orally treated beef cattle showed that liver, kidney, and muscle contained 65–77 ppb, 50–115 ppb, and less than 20 ppb thiamphenicol, respectively, at 4 days after dosing, but less than 20 ppb at 10 days after dosing. Milk from dairy cows intramuscularly dosed with thiamphenicol contained residues $\geq$ 800 ppb 1 day after the cessation of treatment, but less than 20 ppb 48 h later.

Following treatment with thiamphenicol in drinking water, concentrations of the parent drug in liver, kidney, muscle, and skin/fat tissues of broiler chickens were 310.2 ppb, 386.2 ppb, 852.4 ppb, and 20100 ppb, respectively, 1 day after the cessation of treatment, dropping to 7–21 ppb, less than 3 ppb, 4.6–57.8 ppb, and 5100 ppb at 17 days after cessation of treatment. Eggs from laying hens exposed to thiamphenicol through their diet were found to contain 72–190 ppb and 20–43 ppb at 4 and 7 days after cessation of treatment, respectively. At day 9, none of the laid eggs contained more than 20 ppb thiamphenicol.

Residue depletion studies in sea bream administered once daily for 5 consecutive days feed medicated with 4 ppm thiamphenicol showed that residue levels in muscle, liver, and skin were 240 ppb, 380 ppb, and 180 ppb, respectively, at 1 day after treatment (38).

Florfenicol is a fluorinated derivative of thiamphenicol developed in the United States for use exclusively in veterinary medicine. It has been approved for treatment of bovine respiratory disease in the United States (39). Florfenicol has been also recently approved in Japan for use by the aquaculture industry to prevent yellowtail disease.

Florfenicol targets the bacterial ribosome and inhibits bacterial protein biosynthesis. Acquired resistance has been reported, the forms being ribosomal mutations and reduction of the cell permeability. The molecular structure of florfenicol precludes the possibility that its toxicity is associated with idiosyncratic anemia.

The pharmacokinetic characteristics of florfenicol have been described in goats (40), calves (41), and chickens (42). The efficacy of florfenicol in aquaculture has been also demonstrated against bacteria involved in some major fish pathologies, especially in salmon and trout (43, 44). Pharmacokinetic studies in Atlantic salmon indicated that the compound was well absorbed and distributed following oral administration (45). Tissue residue depletion studies after an oral daily administration of 10 mg/kg bw florfenicol in rainbow trout at 10°C for 10 days showed that muscle/skin tissue contained 150 ppb drug at 15 days after the last dose (46).

3.3 β-LACTAMS

The β-lactam antibiotics are the most widely used antimicrobial drugs in veterinary practice. They represent an enormous class of compounds, the discovery, chemistry, and biology of which have been well reviewed (47–49). Penicillin G and penicillin V are two of the naturally occurring penicillins belonging to the group of antibiotics collectively referred to as β-lactams. This group is further comprised of a great variety of semisynthetic penicillins including the cephalosporin antibiotics. All β-lactams have at their basic structure a β-lactam ring responsible for the antibacterial activity and variable side chains that account for the major differences in their chemical and pharmacological properties. The primary distinguishing structural difference between penicillins and cephalosporins is the ring system fused to the β-lactam ring. This is a five-membered thiazolidine ring for penicillins and a six-membered dihydrothiazine ring for cephalosporins.

All β-lactam antibiotics are bactericidal. They interfere with the synthesis of the bacterial wall by inhibiting the bacterial transpeptidase enzymes essential for the construction of peptidoglycan of the wall. Some β-lactams may be inactivated by the β-lactamases (penicillinases) produced by bacteria and, thus, the activity of both penicillins and cephalosporins can be determined by their ability to withstand the destructive action of β-lactamases also produced by the organism for its optimal protection. Bacterial resistance caused by β-lactamase production can be overcome by either modifying the β-lactam nucleus to produce a resistant antibiotic such as cloxacillin or by using combinations of β-lactams with naturally occurring compounds such as clavulanic acid or sulbactam that resemble penicillin structurally and are inhibitors of the β-lactamase enzymes (50).

3.3.1 Penicillins

Penicillins have been used in veterinary medicine for more than 30 years and still constitute the most important group of antibiotics. They can be classified in three distinct groups. The group of the natural penicillins includes penicillin G and penicillin V; the group of the penicillinase-resistant penicillins includes methicillin, nafcillin, oxacillin, cloxacillin, dicloxacillin, and mecillinam; the group of the broad-spectrum penicillins includes ampicillin, amoxicillin, and hetacillin (Fig. 3.3.1)

All penicillins have low toxicity in the normal sense of the word. The most common adverse effects of penicillins by far are hypersensitivity reactions and especially skin rashes. Gastrointestinal disturbances including diarrhea, nausea, and vomiting may sometimes also appear. No teratogenic effects have been reported.

Distribution of penicillin antibiotics is limited to extracellular fluids, but inflammation may enhance their distribution into tissues. Penicillins are actively transported in kidney, brain, and liver. Most penicillins undergo minimal hepatic metabolism and are cleared from the plasma primarily by renal excretion. Secretion of penicillins by the renal tubules results in high urine concentrations and rapid elimination from the body (50).

Penicillin G or benzylpenicillin is a natural penicillin produced by *Penicillium chrysogenum*. It is active against gram-positive bacteria and is administered by intravenous, intramuscular, intramammary, or subcutaneous injection. The oral route is not satisfactory because penicillin G is largely destroyed by gastric acid and bacterial action. It is used for therapy in all farm animal species with a dose range of 3–25 mg/kg bw. Major uses are for the control of mastitis in dairy cows and for treating infections of the gastrointestinal system and the urinary and respiratory tract.

The rates of absorption, clearance, and elimination of penicillin G are influenced by its formulation. Penicillin G is available in a number of different salts either with inorganic ions including sodium, potassium, or calcium or with organic cations including procaine and benzathine. These salts have differing solubilities and hence differing durations of action.

The sodium and potassium salts are rapidly absorbed but give effective plasma concentrations for no more than 4 h. The procaine salt has a lower solubility and forms, on injection, a depot that slowly releases penicillin G, maintaining effective concentrations for up to 24 h. After intramuscular treatment of swine

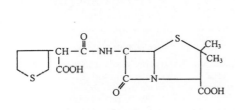

Benzylpenicillin

Phenoxymethylpenicillin

Methicillin

Amoxicillin

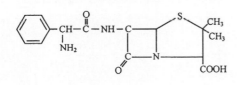

Ticarcillin

Piperacillin

Ampicillin

Carbenicillin

Hetacillin

Oxacillin

FIG. 3.3.1 Chemical structures of commonly used penicillins.

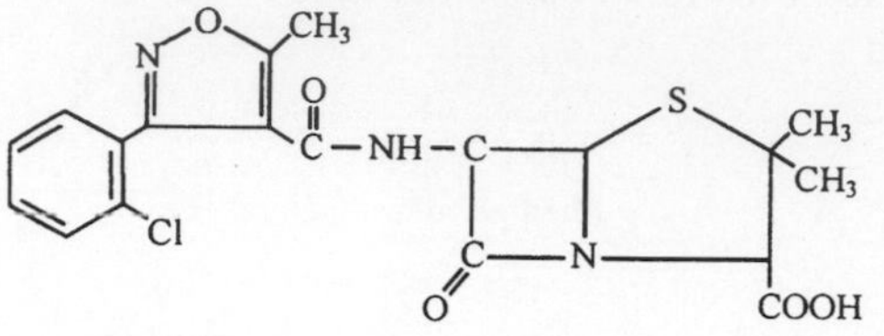

Cloxacillin

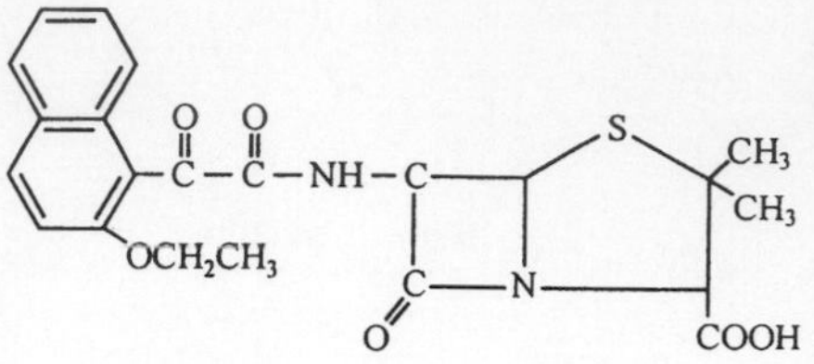

Nafcillin

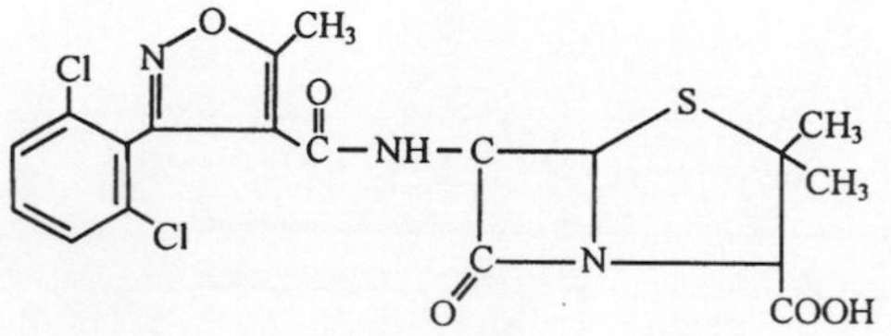

Dicloxacillin

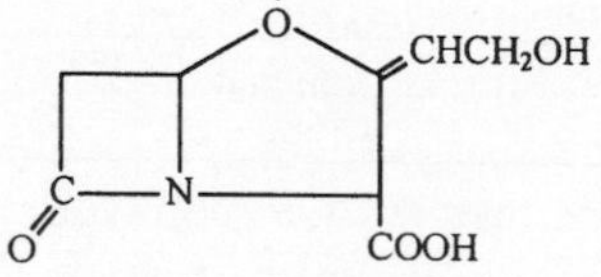

Clavulanic acid

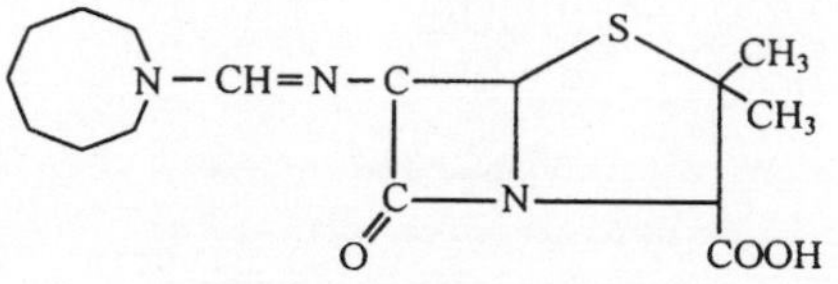

Mecillinam

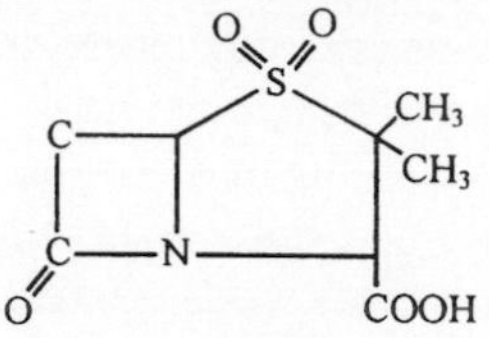

Sulbactam

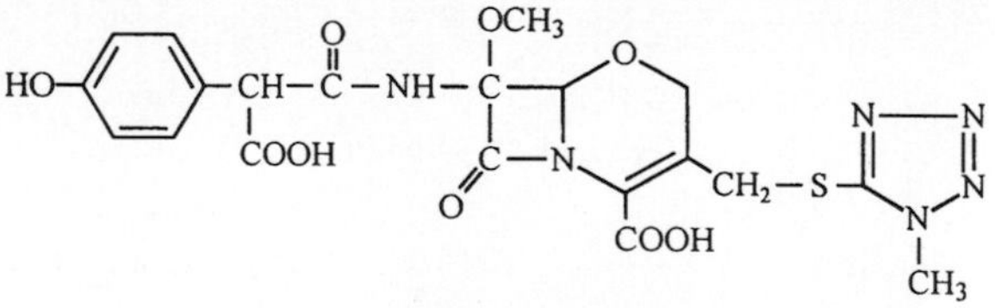

Moxalactam

FIG. 3.3.1 *Continued*

with procaine penicillin G, blood levels peaked 1 h after injection but were barely detectable 24 h after treatment (51). In another pertinent study in swine, blood serum and tissues except the injected muscle were free of detectable penicillin G at 24 h after treatment, whereas, by 48 h, the injected muscle was also essentially free of drug residues (52).

The benzathine salt is only slightly soluble and therefore has a prolonged action, but plasma concentrations are generally lower (53, 54). Hence, benzathine salt is usually used in conjunction with procaine salt, to give an initial high plasma level with prolonged activity. Numerous long-acting formulations in which penicillin G is combined with other antibiotics are also available for treatment of bovine mastitis. The need to use formulations containing benzathine penicillin G in food-producing animals has been questioned by Nouws (55), who reported that high penicillin G concentrations may remain at the injection sites for 3–10 weeks or even longer when benzathine or benethamine penicillin G is administered to pigs. On the other hand, detectable penicillin levels were found up to 120 h in tissues of chickens fed diets containing up to 500 ppm of benzathine penicillin (56).

The rates of absorption, clearance, and elimination of penicillin G are further influenced by the route of administration. Intramuscular and subcutaneous injections provide drug to the bloodstream more slowly, but maintain concentrations longer than the intravenous administration. Absorption of penicillin G from intramuscular or subcutaneous sites can be further slowed down by the use of the relatively insoluble procaine salt. When equivalent dosages of penicillin G and procaine penicillin G were injected parenterally, peak residues concentration in blood occurred after 2 h and the drug had cleared the blood by 8 following penicillin G administration. With the procaine penicillin G, peak residues concentration appeared 5 h after injection and the drug cleared the plasma 24 h after administration (57).

Penicillin G is readily absorbed into the bloodstream where it is partially bound to blood proteins. During the first few hours after injection of penicillin G, residue concentration was higher in the blood than in other tissues and milk, except liver and kidney. Thereafter, there was a more rapid drug clearance from the blood and the concentrations in tissues and milk became higher. Penicillin G was rapidly cleared from the blood through the kidneys and excreted unchanged, almost entirely into the urine.

Although it is not a major elimination route following intravenous or intramuscular injection of penicillin G to dairy cattle, milk constitutes a very important route of elimination following intramammary injection since most of the dose enters milk (58, 59). The persistence of residues in milk does depend on the formulation and route of administration, but, in a wide variety of trials, residues were not found to persist beyond 5 days after the end of treatment (59, 60). Transfer of penicillin G from treated to untreated quarters has also been observed in dairy cattle (59), and residues could be detected in most tissues sampled within 24 h following treatment.

Some workers have suggested (61) that subcutaneous injection of penicillin G in food-producing animals might have advantages over intramuscular injection to overcome the problem of drug residues in muscle tissues at the injection sites. A few practitioners prefer the subcutaneous route over the intramuscular route when giving large doses because the injections are easier to give and cause less muscle stiffness. However, subcutaneous injection of procaine penicillin G in cattle is an extralabel use in Canada for which withdrawal times are not available. The tissue depletion profiles of procaine penicillin G following intramuscular and subcutaneous injection have been investigated in beef steers (62). These studies demonstrated that the appropriate withdrawal period after extralabel intramuscular dosages of 24,000 and 66,000 IU/kg bw was 10 and 21 days, respectively.

When procaine penicillin G was intramuscularly injected in pigs at the approved (15,000 IU/kg bw) label dose once daily for 3 days, residues were not found in liver after 1 day of withdrawal, in muscle and fat after 2 days of withdrawal, in plasma after 4 days of withdrawal, in skin after 5 days of withdrawal, or in kidney and the injection sites after 8 days of withdrawal (63). When these pigs were given an extralabel dose at the 66,000 IU/kg bw level, residues were not found in liver after 2 days of withdrawal, in fat after 3 days of withdrawal, or in muscle, skin, plasma, or injection sites after 7 days of withdrawal.

Penicillin V or phenoxymethylpenicillin is a β-lactam antibiotic produced by *Penicillium notatum.* It is a biosynthetic penicillin that should be differentiated from the semisynthetic penicillins since it is produced by altering the composition of the medium where the mold is growing.

Like penicillin G, penicillin V is also available in a number of different salts either with inorganic ions including sodium, potassium, or calcium, or with organic cations including benzathine and hydrabramine. These salts have differing solubilities and hence differing duration of action.

This antibiotic is used as an economical oral treatment for gram-positive infections in farm animals at a dosage of 8 mg/kg bw because it has the property of being stable in the gastric acid, allowing it to be bioavailable by the oral route. It is well absorbed from the gastrointestinal tract and metabolized in the liver. Unchanged compound and metabolites are excreted in urine. Small amounts are also found in bile.

Ampicillin is a broad-spectrum semisynthetic antibiotic also inactivated by β-lactamases. The action and uses of ampicillin are like those of penicillin G but it has a broader spectrum of activity. It is active against a large number of gram-positive and gram-negative organisms and, thus, it is of high value in the treatment of several diseases in cattle, swine, sheep, horses, and poultry. Many prodrugs that are hydrolyzed to ampicillin in vivo also exist and are better absorbed from the gastrointestinal tract than ampicillin. Ampicillin is available in powder, tablet, cream, intramammary, and parenteral injection formulations.

Ampicillin is relatively stable in gastric acid secretion and well absorbed from the gastrointestinal tract. In most animal species, about 35% of an oral dose is absorbed, reaching peak serum levels within 1–2 h after dosing. It is widely distributed in body tissues and concentrated in liver and kidney. Ampicillin is excreted primarily in the unchanged form in the urine, and some may be excreted in the feces as well. Little ampicillin is excreted in milk, whereas high concentrations have been found in bile. Following oral administration to cattle, ampicillin may be returned to the intestinal lumen through enterohepatic circulation. This is of importance in residue depletion studies.

The disposition profile of ampicillin has been thoroughly investigated in honeybees, larvae, and honey and royal jelly from hives treated with 30 mg of ampicillin/hive in syrup or in paste (64). In hives given the antibiotic in syrup, high drug residue levels were found in honey, which lasted over 14 days beyond the detection limit of the analytical method. In hives given the same dosage of ampicillin in paste, relatively low residues were found in the honey. The distribution of the drug residues in young larvae and jelly, which was the food of the larvae, was very low as well.

Amoxicillin is a close analogue to ampicillin that is also inactivated by β-lactamases. The action and uses of amoxicillin are like those of ampicillin. Hence it is used against a wide variety of bacterial infections in farm animals including those of the gastrointestinal, respiratory, urinary, and mammary system. It is administered in the form of tablets, suspensions, powders, parenteral, and intra-mammary formulations at dosage rates of 10 mg/kg bw by the oral route and 7–15 mg/kg bw by the parenteral route.

After oral administration to preruminant calves and pigs, amoxicillin is absorbed better and has more rapid action and greater resistance to the gastric acid than ampicillin. Following amoxicillin administration, plasma levels are approximately twice those achieved by the same dosage of ampicillin. Unlike with ampicillin, food cannot impair absorption of amoxicillin. When given intravenously to calves, the elimination half-life is approximately 90 min, slightly longer than that of ampicillin.

Amoxicillin is widely distributed in body tissues and its metabolism is limited. Excretion of amoxicillin is through the kidney, resulting in high concentrations in both the kidney tissue and urine, where the levels may be 100-fold higher than that in serum. Concentrations in milk are 10 times lower than those in serum. Following intramuscular or subcutaneous injection to goats, levels of amoxicillin in milk were very close to the detection limit of 10 ppb within 24 h after the last dose (65).

When amoxicillin in addition to colistin was given subcutaneously to turkeys for 4 consecutive days, average drug concentrations in muscle and at the injection sites were about 389 and 440 ppb, respectively, 1 day after treatment withdrawal, with a subsequent rapid decline (66). The drug was undetectable in liver and kidney by 10 days posttreatment. When amoxicillin was administered orally to broilers for 5 consecutive days, no significant differences were observed between the elimination profiles in healthy and diseased birds (67). In all cases, kidney was the target tissue containing 2–7 ppm or less than 0.05 ppm at 1 h or 24 h, respectively, after the last treatment. Levels in muscle and fat were below the 0.05 ppm detection limit at 4 h after the last dosage, and in liver and skin at 8 h after the last dosage. The daily administration of amoxicillin to laying hens at a dosage of 16 mg/kg bw for 5 consecutive days was not found in another experiment capable of resulting in residues in eggs at concentrations above 0.007 ppm (68).

Hetacillin is a semisynthetic prodrug of ampicillin also inactivated by β-lactamases. It is more stable in the gastric acid than ampicillin and amoxicillin and, therefore, is absorbed best. Hetacillin is inactive per se, but after it enters the bloodstream it is metabolized to ampicillin and becomes active.

Oxacillin, cloxacillin, and dicloxacillin are all semisynthetic isoxazolyl penicillins suitably modified to be relatively resistant to hydrolysis by staphylococcal β-lactamase. They have the additional advantage of being stable in the presence of gastric acid, so they can be administered orally as well as parenterally.

Dicloxacillin is absorbed well from the gastrointestinal tract but the presence of food in the stomach reduces resorption. Although cloxacillin differs chemically from oxacillin only in the presence of a chlorine atom, their absorption profile after oral administration is not similar. Cloxacillin is more rapidly and effectively absorbed than oxacillin. However, absorption of all isoxazolyl penicillins is better when given by intramuscular injection. These agents can be also administered by intravenous, intrauterine, intra-articular, intrapleural, and intramammary injections.

Following absorption, all isoxazolyl penicillins are bound to plasma proteins in the circulation and are partly metabolized in the body. They cross the placenta and are found in breast milk. Parent drugs and their metabolites are principally excreted in the urine, whereas small amounts are also found in bile.

Oxacillin and cloxacillin are the most widely used isoxazolyl penicillins, the latter being particularly appropriate for treatment or prevention of bovine staphylococcal mastitis. Following intramammary treatment of a lactating cow with three successive infusions of 200 mg/48 h each of sodium cloxacillin, residues were present in milk (detection limit equal to 3 ppb) from the treated quarter for 60 h after the last infusion; crossover from treated to untreated quarter was also observed (59). When cloxacillin benzathine was administered by the intramammary route to dairy cows in the dry period at a dosage of 500 mg/quarter, cloxacillin residues were present neither in serum (<25 ppb) sampled after 5 days of drug administration nor in milk (<5 ppb), including the milk collected just after parturition (69). Therefore, this milk could be ingested by newborn calves or used for human consumption without any health risk even after cloxacillin treatment.

Methicillin is a semisynthetic penicillin that also resists the action of β-lactamases and, thus, is frequently used for penicillin G-resistant staphylococci. It is the first semisynthetic penicillin developed but it is poorly absorbed when given orally due to its instability in gastric acid. Absorption is better when it is administered intravenously or intramuscularly. Methicillin is principally eliminated in the urine but small amounts are also found in bile and other body fluids.

Nafcillin is a semisynthetic penicillin that is resistant to β-lactamases but can be largely inactivated by hepatic enzymes. It is the active ingredient in intramammary preparations intended for treatment of mastitis in dairy cows and prevention of mastitis during the dry period in cattle, sheep, and goats.

Nafcillin shows properties similar to those of oxacillin and cloxacillin. Thus, it is incompletely resorbed from the gastrointestinal tract especially when given after a meal. It crosses the placenta and is found in breast milk.

In dogs, absorption following oral administration tends to be poor. At similar oral doses, peak serum levels are lower and plasma levels are less persistent than those observed for methicillin. Following intramuscular administration, however, maximum concentrations in serum are reached within 30 min. In contrast to methicillin, liver is the main excretory pathway for nafcillin. Like most other penicillins, nafcillin undergoes biotransformation to a small extent. Parent compound and its metabolites are excreted in bile and urine. Concentrations of nafcillin in tissues tend to be higher and more persistent following parenteral administration than was the case for methicillin, obviously due to enterohepatic recirculation.

The presence of detectable levels in plasma and urine of treated cows indicates that nafcillin is absorbed systematically following intramammary administration. The major part of nafcillin is excreted in the milk, but a higher proportion of nafcillin is absorbed from the udder when nafcillin is administered at drying off. Residue depletion studies (70) with lactating cows showed that residues in all edible tissues were below 300 ppb at 72 h after cessation of treatment, while residues in milk were below 30 ppb from the fourth milking onwards, after cessation of the treatment.

Pregnant ewes and dairy goats given intramammary infusions with 100 mg nafcillin per teat immediately after the last milking prior to drying off, were not found to contain detectable (<15–20 ppb) residue concentrations in milk, irrespective of the length of the dry period and the interval between lambing and sampling. Detectable residue concentrations could not be observed in any edible tissues of these animals species.

Mecillinam is a semisynthetic penicillin with the unusual property of being a specific gram-negative antibiotic. It is used in form of a uterine bolus for prophylactic and therapeutic treatment of endometritis in cattle. Pharmacokinetic studies show that mecillinam is poorly absorbed following oral administration in laboratory animals and cattle.

Following parenteral administration to laboratory animals, the elimination half-life in plasma was 0.8–1.5 h, with the highest tissue concentrations appearing in kidney and liver. Mecillinam was excreted mainly through the urine within the first few hours after administration. Seven metabolites were found in dog urine, but only the formyl-6-aminopenicillanic acid could be identified.

In nonruminant calves given an oral dose of 15 mg/kg bw, only 1–3% of the dose was excreted in the first 24 h through urine. In contrast, when the same dose was administered intravenously, as much as 40–60% of the dose could be excreted in the first 24 h through urine.

Following intrauterine administration to postpartum cows, the maximum plasma concentrations of mecillinam within 1–4 h were generally low compared to the administered dose, indicating limited absorption of the drug from the uterine cavity; mecillinam residues could be only occasionally detected in milk from the first milking following treatment. Residue depletion studies in cattle after a single intrauterine administration of mecillinam showed that 12 h after treatment the concentrations of the parent drug in liver, kidney, muscle, and fat were all below the quantification limit of 50 ppb.

3.3.2 Cephalosporins

The cephalosporins are semisynthetic β-lactams derived from cephalosporin C, a natural antibiotic. Their active basic nucleus consists of a six-membered dihydrothiazine ring fused to a β-lactam ring (Fig. 3.3.2). Cephalosporins have some desirable quality characteristics that are generally deficient in penicillins. The popularity and usefulness of cephalosporins results from their resistance to many β-lactamases, their stability in acidic media, their wide spectrum of activity compared with penicillin G, and their wide safety margin. Similarly to penicillins, cephalosporins inhibit the synthesis of bacterial cell wall. They generally exhibit good activity against both gram-positive and gram-negative bacteria, and may be administered both orally and parenterally. The adverse effects associated with cephalosporins are similar to those described for penicillins.

The term ''generation'' has been primarily used as a means of classifying these antibiotics on the basis of their in vitro antibacterial potency and spectrum of activity. With the introduction of each cephalosporin generation, there was a loss of gram-positive but an increase in gram-negative activity, a widening of the spectrum, an enhancement of the resistance to β-lactamases, and a marked increase in cost (71, 72).

First-generation cephalosporins are the cephalosporins most often used in food-producing animals. Included in this group are cephapirin, cephacetrile, ceph-

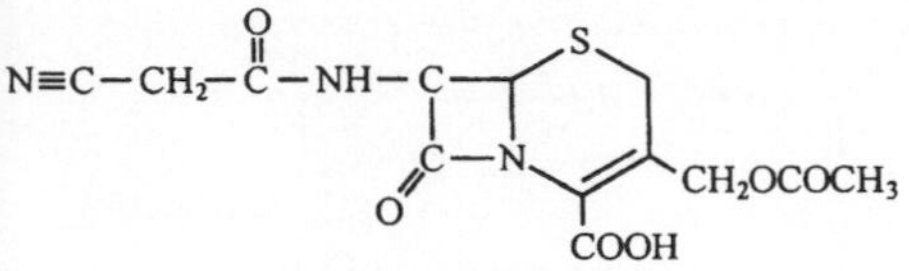

Cephacetrile

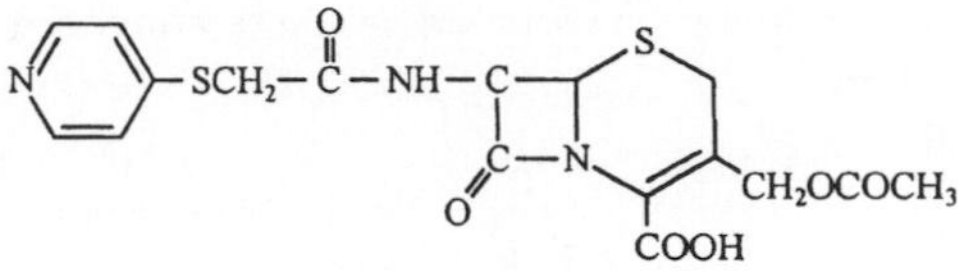

Cephapirin

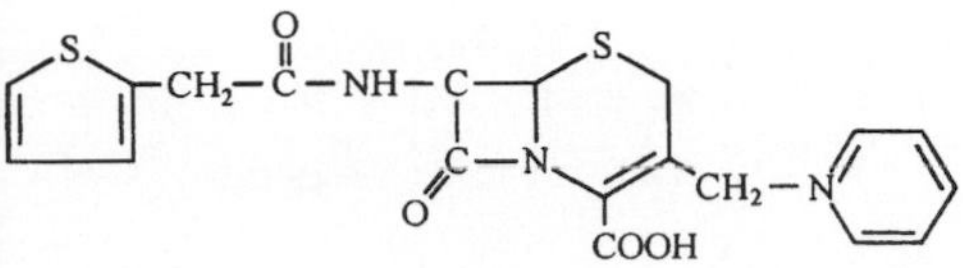

Cephaloridine

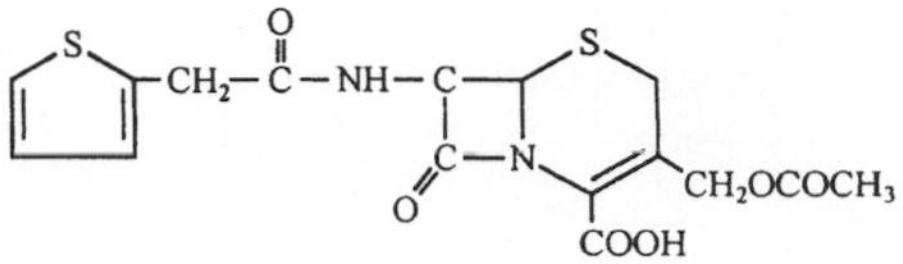

Cephalothin

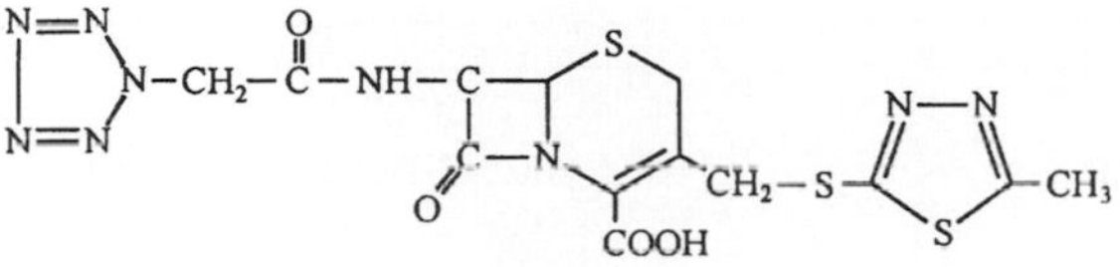

Cefazolin

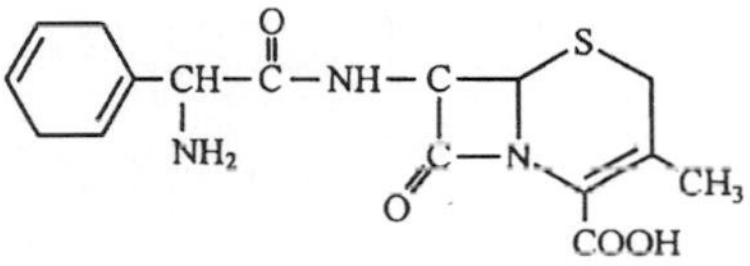

Cephradine

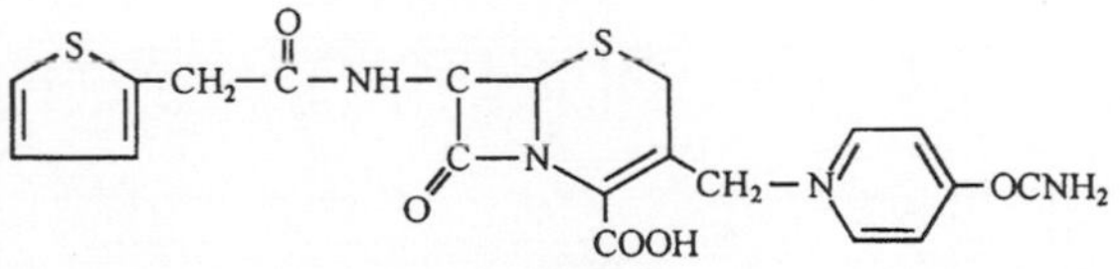

Cephalonium

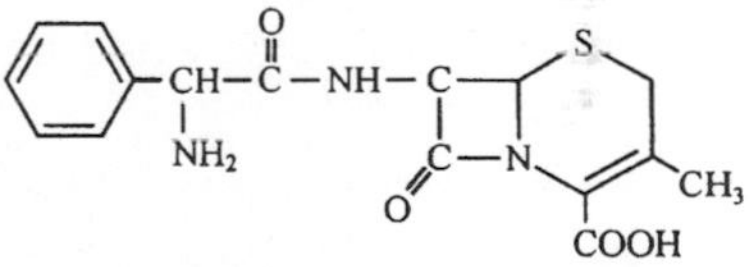

Cephalexin

FIG. 3.3.2 Chemical structures of commonly used cephalosporins.

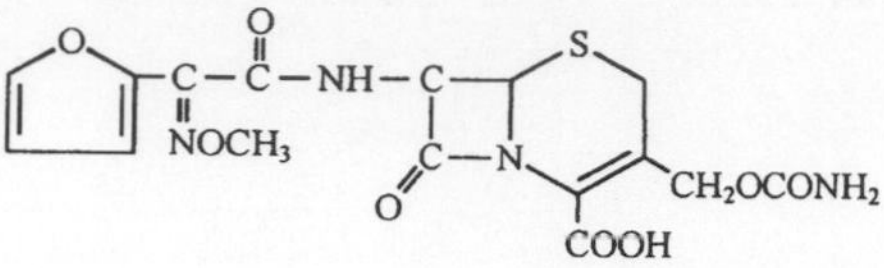

Cefuroxime

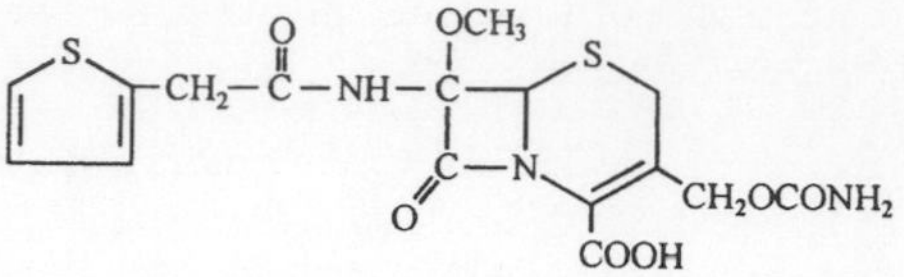

Cefoxitin

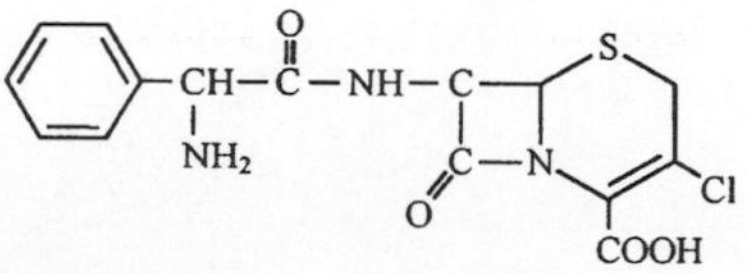

Cefaclor

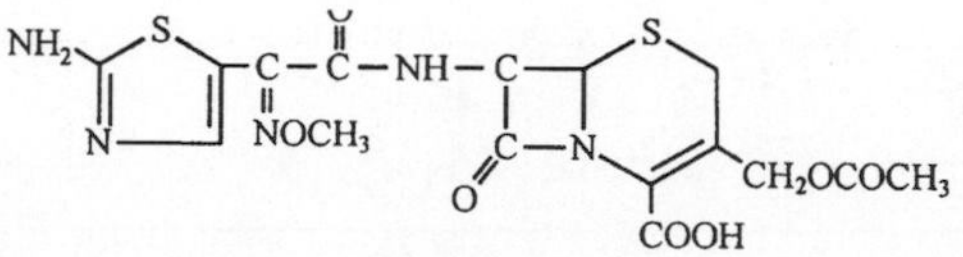

Cefotaxime

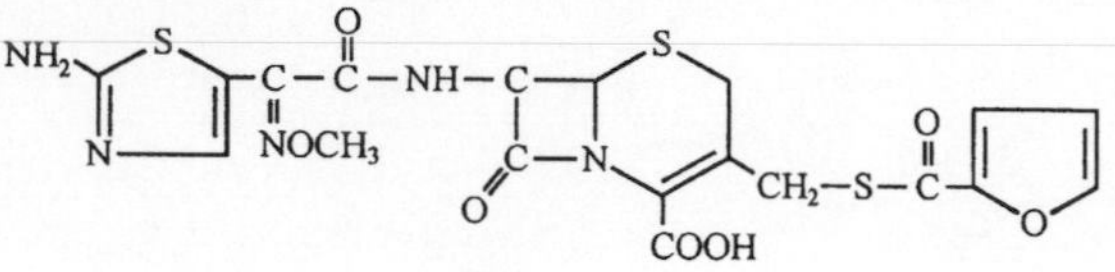

Ceftiofur

FIG. 3.3.2 *Continued*

alexin, cephalonium, cefazolin, cephalothin, cefadroxil, and cephradine. Second-generation cephalosporins include the parenteral agents cefoxitin and cefuroxime which, however, are used infrequently in veterinary medicine because of their high cost. Third-generation cephalosporins, such as cefoperazone, ceftiofur, and cefquinome, are reserved for specialized conditions such as antibiotic-resistant infections that are difficult to treat safety. However, their cost, which is often five to six times higher than that of first-generation cephalosporins, makes their use prohibitive for farm animals.

Cephapirin, a first-generation cephalosporin, is used in form of benzathine or sodium salts for intramammary treatment of mastitis in dry and lactating cows. In the United States, the benzathine intramammary formulations are sold for use by dairy farmers without a prescription. The benzathine salts are further used for intrauterine treatment of endometritis, whereas the sodium salts for parenteral treatment of infections in cattle, sheep, goats, and pigs at a dosage of 10 mg/kg bw.

Pharmacokinetic studies in mice, rats, and dogs showed that cephapirin was readily metabolized into desacetylcephapirin. The rate and the extent of this metabolism showed a decreasing tendency from rodents to dogs. In these species, the plasma elimination half-lives of cephapirin and desacetylcephapirin were 0.4–0.9 h. In dairy cows, cephapirin was mainly eliminated by the urinary route and, to a smaller extent, by the biliary route.

Residue depletion studies in dairy cows following intramuscular administration of 8.5 mg benzathine cephapirin/kg bw showed that residue levels in kidney, muscle, and liver were 1–5 ppm, less than 0.008–0.024 ppm, and less than 0.045 ppm, respectively, at 4.5 h postdosing (73). After intramuscular administration of 10 mg/kg bw sodium cephapirin to lactating cows, residue levels of 0.03–0.11 ppm were present in milk at 1–4 h, whereas 0.01 ppm were found from 4–8 h postdosing. In piglets, after intramuscular treatment with 20 mg/kg bw sodium cephapirin, residues could not be detected in liver, kidney, spleen, lung, and muscle at 24–120 h after treatment.

Following intramammary infusion of cephapirin to a lactating cow, the parent compound metabolized rapidly so that nearly similar levels of cephapirin and desacetylcephapirin appeared in milk 16 h after the medication (74–76). At 24 h, desacetylcephapirin was the major residue in milk. The concentration of the parent drug declined to below 0.005 ppm at the 64 h milking.

After intramammary administration of 381 mg benzathine cephapirin to dairy cows, residue levels in fat, muscle, udder, kidney, and liver were below the limit of detection (0.04 ppb) at day 21–42. Following intramammary administration of 261 mg sodium cephapirin in lactating cows, residue levels in milk were 5–20 ppm at first milking, up to 2.5 ppm at fourth milking, and below the limit of detection from the fifth milking onwards. After intramammary infusions of 500 mg benzathine cephapirin to dairy cows during the dry period, residue levels in milk were less than 0.02–0.13 ppm at fourth and fifth milking, and less than 0.02 ppm from sixth milking onward.

Cephacetrile is a first-generation cephalosporin used for the intramammary treatment of mastitis in lactating cows. Its antibacterial activity is similar to that of penicillin G but it is β-lactamase-resistant.

Oral bioavailability of cephacetrile appears to be rather low. In calves dosed orally with 20 mg cephacetrile/kg bw, only 3–15% of the dose was absorbed from the gastrointestinal tract. Following parenteral administration of cephacetrile to cattle, sheep, and goats, plasma elimination half-lives were shorter than 1 h. The drug was poorly metabolized, with desacetylcephacetrile and its lactone being the only metabolites detected. Cephacetrile was rapidly and almost exclusively excreted through the urine. In goats intramuscularly injected with 10 mg cephacetrile/kg bw, 80% of the dose was recovered in urine within 12 h and more than 90% within the first day after treatment.

Absorption through the udder is moderate; after intramammary administration of radiolabeled cephacetrile to cows, 54.6% of the dose was recovered in milk, 21% in urine and feces, and only 2.55 in tissues within 5 days. At 5 days posttreatment, kidney, udder, and liver contained total drug-related residues equivalent to 232, 227, and 33 ppb of cephacetrile, respectively. When lactating cows were treated with 250 mg intramammary cephacetrile/quarter twice at an interval of 24 h, mean residue concentrations in milk were 14257, 1860, 208, 20, and less than 5 ppb at the first, second, fifth, seventh, and ninth milking postdosing, respectively.

Cephalexin is a first-generation cephalosporin that can be given orally without its gastrointestinal absorption being altered by the presence of food in the stomach. Sodium cephalexin is indicated for treating infections of the gastrointestinal and respiratory tract in cattle, sheep, and swine at dosages in the range 7–10 mg/kg bw. With its monohydrate and benzathine formulations, cephalexin is also administered in intramammary form for treatment of mastitis in lactating (200 mg/quarter) and dry cows (375 mg/quarter).

Cephalexin is quickly absorbed and metabolized to unidentified compounds in cattle, sheep, and swine. It is principally excreted in urine but small amounts are also excreted by liver in bile. No detectable residues (limit of detection 60 ppb) were found in cows, in sheep and swine slaughtered at 4 and 10 days, respectively, after receiving intramuscularly 7 mg cephalexin sodium/kg bw/day for 5 consecutive days. No detectable residues were found in sheep and swine slaughtered 3 and 2 days, respectively, after receiving 10 mg cephalexin sodium/kg bw/day intramuscularly for 5 consecutive days.

Intramammary treatment of lactating cows with 200 mg cephalexin/quarter for four consecutive milkings resulted in cephalexin concentrations in the mammary tissue, kidney, liver, fat, and muscle of 513–1267, 553–1378, 47–94, 37–299, and less than 20–199 ppb, respectively, at 12 h after last treatment. At 4 days postdosing, cephalexin concentrations were 21–174, less than 20–24, and less than 20 ppb in the mammary tissue, kidney, and other tissues, respectively, whereas at 9 days these levels were 53–89 ppb in mammary tissue and less than 20 ppb in all other tissues. Cephalexin concentrations in milk were found to be up to 37,320 ppb during administration, but decreased from 1181–37,061 ppb at first milking to less than 10 ppb at the 13–15th milking after the last dosing.

Cephalonium, a first-generation cephalosporin, is exclusively used in veterinary medicine. It has a low solubility in water and so it is indicated for intramammary administration to cows for treating existing infections and preventing new infections during the dry period. However, this may lead to postcalving residues, which can persist beyond 4 days after calving (15).

Cefazolin is a first-generation cephalosporin with antibacterial activity similar to that of penicillin G but it is β-lactamase-resistant. It is poorly absorbed from the gastrointestinal tract and, thus, it is primarily administered parenterally. It is widely used for treatment of mastitis in lactating cows, sheep, and goats and for treatment at drying off by the intramammary route.

The adverse effects associated with cefazolin are generally similar to those described for penicillins. Cefazolin contains a methylthiodiazolethiol side chain and may further cause hypoprothrombinemia and a disulfiram-like reaction with alcohol similar to that seen with cephalosporins containing the related *N*-methylthiotetrazole side chain.

Absorption of cefazolin is poor: low concentrations were found in plasma and tissues after intramammary administration. It is bound to plasma proteins in the circulation and crosses the placenta. Metabolism of cefazolin is very limited and no major metabolites seem to occur. After parenteral administration to horse, nearly 100% of the dose was excreted unchanged in the urine within 24 h.

Depletion studies carried out in lactating cows showed that residues in milk were below 50 ppb at the seventh milking and below 25 ppb at the eighth milking after the last treatment (74). In tissues, cefazolin could be found only in kidney and liver at 3 h after last treatment, and also in kidney at very low concentrations at 24 h after treatment. Depletion studies carried out in cows at drying off showed that residues in udder declined from 3500–16,500 ppb at day 7 after treatment to 40 1400 ppb at day 14 after treatment. On day 21, residue levels varied from below the detection limit (25 ppb) to 600 ppb. Residues were not detected in the milk collected at the first and second milking after calving from cows treated at drying off 28–40 days before calving. No residues were detected in edible tissues sampled 21 days after the drying off treatment.

When ewes and goats were treated according to recommendations (78), cefazolin residues were below the limit of detection (25 ppb) in all milk samples collected at the three first milkings following parturition. For the ewes included in the study, the length of the dry period averaged 137 days; the corresponding figure for goats was 76 days. Residue levels in all edible tissues were below the detection limit at day 21 after treatment.

Cephalothin, a first-generation cephalosporin, is suitable for administration only by injection. It is more resistant to staphylococcal β-lactamase than other first-generation cephalosporins.

The most common adverse effects, as for penicillin G, are hypersensitivity reactions and especially skin rashes, urticaria, fever, and anaphylaxis. Cephalothin may cause renal failure, hepatitis, and jaundice. Gastrointestinal disturbances may also occur, particularly diarrhea, nausea, and vomiting.

Following injection, cephalothin is well and rapidly absorbed from intramuscular sites. It is widely distributed in body tissues and fluids and binds to plasma proteins. Cephalothin crosses the placenta and is found in breast milk. It is metabolized in the liver to the less active desacetylcephalosporin product, which is subsequently excreted, along with the parent compound, in the urine.

Cefoxitin is a second-generation cephalosporin that is both well absorbed by the intramuscular route and not metabolized in the body. It is stable not only to staphylococcal β-lactamase but also to gram-negative bacterial enzymes. This is due to the fact that cefoxitin is strictly a cephamycin rather than a cephalosporin, since it is derived by a chemical modification of the naturally occurring cephamycin (79). This difference in molecular structure gives cefoxitin its high degree of resistance to inactivation by bacterial cephalosporinases. Because of its effectiveness against many aerobic and anaerobic bacterial infections, cefoxitin is widely used in human and veterinary medicine to aid in the prevention of postoperative infections (80).

Cefuroxime is also a second-generation cephalosporin resistant to some β-lactamases. It is used in veterinary medicine in intramammary treatments. Cefuroxime axetil is also a prodrug active by the oral route. It is absorbed from the gastrointestinal tract and its absorption is enhanced if the compound is given after food. It is rapidly hydrolyzed in blood to cefuroxime.

Cefuroxime is widely distributed in the body, crosses the placenta, and is found in breast milk. It is bound to plasma proteins in the circulation. Cefuroxime is principally excreted unchanged in urine and small amounts are excreted by liver in bile.

Cefoperazone is a third-generation cephalosporin with activity against both gram-positive and gram-negative pathogens. It is suitable for use as an intramammary product in the treatment of bovine mastitis due to its broad-spectrum activity, nonirritant properties, and persistence at a significant level in the treated quarter of a cow for three to four milkings after a single intramammary infusion of 250 mg. It is also used in horses where, after intramuscular or intravenous administration, it attains serum, spongy bone, and urine concentrations above 1 ppm for at least 5 h (81).

The great biliary excretion of cefoperazone causes changes in bowel flora and diarrhea may often occur. Containing a N-methylthiotetrazole side chain, cefoperazone may also cause hypoprothrombinemia and a disulfiram-like reaction with alcohol (alcohol intolerance). This antibiotic should be avoided by patients receiving anticoagulants.

Cefoperazone is widely distributed in body tissues and fluids. It is bound to plasma proteins in the circulation. It is excreted primarily in the bile, and is also excreted in urine and poorly in breast milk. Cefoperazone is susceptible to the action of some β-lactamases, and thus may be given with a β-lactamase inhibitor.

Ceftiofur is a third-generation cephalosporin active against both gram-positive and gram-negative bacteria and is resistant to β-lactamases. It is administered intramuscularly to cattle, including lactating cows, at dosages of up to 2 mg/kg bw for up to 5 days, and to swine at dosages of up to 5 mg/kg bw for up to 3 days for control of respiratory tract bacterial infections.

Ceftiofur is absorbed poorly after oral administration but rapidly after intramuscular injection. In all species, ceftiofur was rapidly metabolized to desfuroylceftiofur and furoic acid. Desfuroylceftiofur occurred in the free form in the plasma of treated cattle but was covalently bound to plasma proteins in rats (82). Maximum blood concentrations of ceftiofur-related residues were achieved within 0.5 and 2 h of dosing. Unmetabolized ceftiofur was generally undetectable in blood within 2–4 h of dosing (83). More than 90% of the administered dose was excreted within 24 h of administration, mostly in urine. Residues in urine and feces were composed primarily of desfuroylceftiofur and desfuroylceftiofur cysteine disulfide, with small amounts of unmetabolized ceftiofur.

After intramuscular injections of radiolabeled ceftiofur to cattle and swine, the compound was absorbed rapidly into the blood and eliminated mostly in urine (84). The tissue in which highest residue concentrations were observed at 12 h after the last dose was the kidney. Most of the radioactivity was found in the form of the microbiologically active primary metabolite, desfuroylceftiofur, conjugated to macromolecules in plasma and tissues. Desfuroylceftiofur cysteine was also found in tissues, plasma, and urine, whereas the desfuroylceftiofur dimer was found in urine. It was suggested that since the binding of desfuroylceftiofur to biological molecules is reversible, all of the ceftiofur-related residues that contain the desfuroylceftiofur moiety have the potential to be microbiologically active.

Residue depletion studies in pigs after intramuscular administration of ceftiofur showed total residue concentrations of 590, 1190, 250, 400, and 1320 ppb in liver, kidney, muscle, skin/fat, and injection site, respectively, at 12 h after dosing. In cattle, intramuscular administration of radiolabeled ceftiofur resulted in total residue concentrations of 1294, 250, 60, and 60 ppb equivalents in liver; 3508, 853, 159, and 159 ppb equivalents in kidney; 208, 20, <10, and <10 ppb equivalents in muscle; 324, 37, <10, and <10 ppb equivalents in fat; and 3924, 766, 399, and 399 ppb equivalents at the injection site at 8 h, 3, 21, and 39 days withdrawal, respectively.

Milk from lactating cows intramuscularly injected with radiolabeled ceftiofur was found to contain 103 and 50 ppb of total residues at 12 and 24 h, respectively, postdosing. No parent ceftiofur could be detected in milk (85). Therefore, use of ceftiofur at the approved dosage and route is not expected to result in ceftiofur-related residues exceeding maximum residue limit (MRL) at any time postdosing, and no milk withdrawal periods need to be assigned for ceftiofur. In addition, ceftiofur residues are not hazardous to industrial cheese and yogurt starter cultures.

Cefquinome, a third-generation cephalosporin, has been developed solely for veterinary use. It is used for the treatment of respiratory tract diseases in cattle and swine by the intramuscular route at a dosage of 1 and 2 mg/kg bw/day, respectively, for 3–5 days. It is also administered in intramammary form for treatment of bacterial infections of the udder in lactating cows.

Absorption of orally administered cefquinome is poor, but absorption following intramuscular or subcutaneous administration proceeds relatively quickly. A small fraction of the intramammarily administered cefquinome is absorbed systemically. Distribution of cefquinome is not extensive; following parenteral administration of radiolabeled cefquinome the highest activities were found in injection-site tissues, kidney, and liver. Excretion of parenterally administered cefquinome is predominantly renal, while intramammarily administered cefquinome is excreted mainly in milk. Cefquinome is metabolically quite stable.

The residue profile of cefquinome in beef calves intramuscularly treated with the drug has been studied (86). The data were reminiscent of those form other cephalosporins and indicated that cefquinome was rapidly cleared, with detectable levels of significance seen at injection site, kidney, and liver tissues. However, the residues remaining after 12 h at the injection site, kidney, and liver were not antimicrobially active and/or bioavailable and no parent drug could be detected; 80–100% of these residues were bound residues.

Residue depletion studies (87) after intramammary administration of cefquinome to lactating cows showed that residues in edible tissues could be detected only in kidney at 24 h posttreatment and at concentrations below 200 ppb. High concentrations of cefquinome were found in milk at the first milking posttreatment, while at the 10th milking the residue concentrations in all milk samples were below 20 ppb.

Residue depletion studies in pigs given intramuscularly the recommended treatment regimen showed that injection sites contained up to 208 ppb cefquinome 24 h after the last injection, declining to no measurable amounts at 144 h. Kidney contained 88–293 ppb at 24 h, but no measurable residues at 48, 72, and 120 h after the treatment. Liver, fat, skin, and muscle excluding the injection site were not found to contain detectable cefquinome up to 72 h after treatment.

Clavulanic acid is produced by *Streptomyces clavuligerus* and is structurally related to penicillins. This naturally occurring compound is a specific and irreversible inhibitor of a wide range of bacterial β-lactamases and, therefore, can enhance the activity of penicillins and cephalosporins against many resistant organisms. Potassium clavulanate can be administered both orally and perenterally in combination with antibiotics sensitive to the action of β-lactamases.

Following oral treatment to calves, 34% of the dose is absorbed and peak concentration occurs within 3–4 h after dosing. Complete absorption occurs after intramuscular administration. Body clearance of clavulanic acid is significantly higher for chickens than for turkeys and pigeons (88). Biotransformation studies in dogs and humans show that the main identifiable compounds in urine of both species are the parent drug and its metabolite 1-amino-4-hydroxybutan-2-one.

The main excretion pathway is through the urine in both calves and swine. Residue depletion studies did not showed detectable (<0.01 ppm) residues in calves treated orally with 8 mg clavulanic acid–ampicillin formulation/kg bw *for* 3 *days* and slaughtered after 3 days; or in calves, pigs, and sheep treated *intramuscularly with* 1.75 *mg/kg bw for* 5 *days and slaughtered after* 10, 7, *and* 14 days, respectively.

Excretion in milk occurs to a limited extent, and the concentrations attained are lower that those detected in plasma. No detectable residues were found in cow milk at 24, 48, or 72 h after a 5 day intramuscular treatment of 1.75 mg/kg bw, or intramammary infusions of 50 mg of the drug in one or the four quarters of the udder.

Sulbactam is a penicillanic acid sulfone. It exhibits a weak antibacterial activity, and is an inhibitor of β-lactamases produced by some bacteria. Hence, it can enhance the activity of penicillins and cephalosporins against many resistant organisms when used in combination with these antibiotics. Sulbactam, although it has a spectrum similar to that of clavulanic acid, is, however, a less potent inhibitor.

Sodium sulbactam is poorly absorbed from the gastrointestinal tract and is administered parenterally in combination with ampicillin or cefoperazone. Its pharmacokinetics are similar to those of ampicillin.

3.4 MACROLIDES AND LINCOSAMIDES

The macrolide antibiotics are basic macrocyclic compounds that have a common 14-, 16-, or 17- membered macrocyclic lactone ring linked to one or more deoxy sugars, often amino sugars, by glycoside bonding (Fig. 3.4). Most macrolide antibiotics are compounds isolated from culture broth of *Streptomyces* strains. An exception is mirosamicin, which is produced by *Micromonospora*. They are highly effective against a wide range of gram-positive bacteria with limited or no activity against most gram-negative bacteria. They represent the most effective medicines against diseases produced by *Mycoplasma*.

Erythromycin and oleandomycin are examples with a 14-membered ring. The former is a mixture of three closely related compounds: erythromycin A, B, and C; erythromycin A is the major and most important component. The latter consists of a single component.

Spiramycin, kitasamycin, josamycin, desmycosin, mirosamicin, tilmicosin, and tylosin are examples with a 16-membered ring. Spiramycin consists of three components: spiramycin I, II, and III; spiramycin I is the major component. Kitasamycin consists of several components: leucomycin A_1, A_{3-9}, and A_{13}, the leucomycin A_5 being the major component (89). Josamycin is identical to the leucomycin A_3 (90), while tylosin consists of four components, tylosin A, B, C, and D, the major component being tylosin A. Tylosin B is identical to desmycosin,

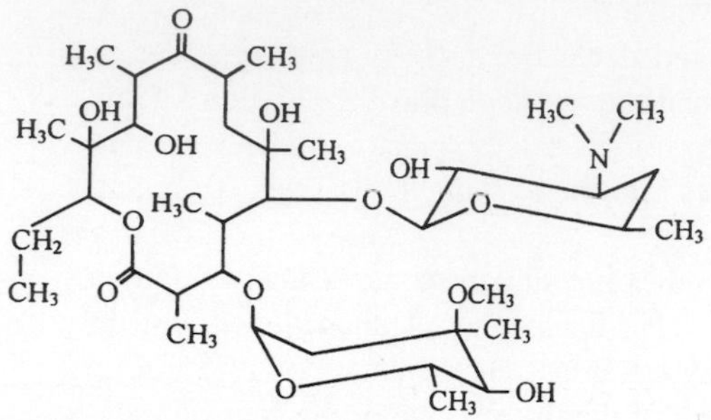

Erythromycin A

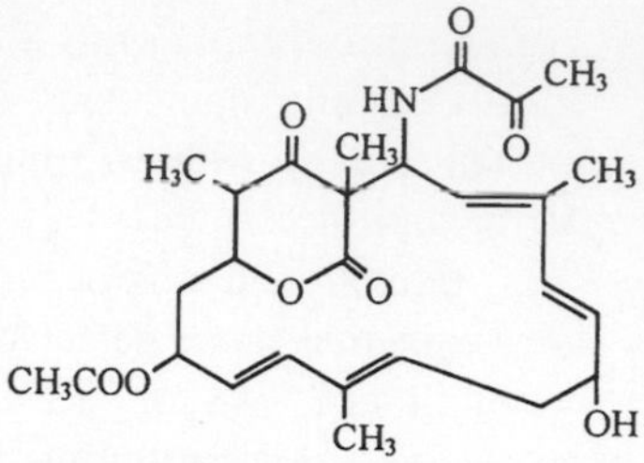

Sedecamycin

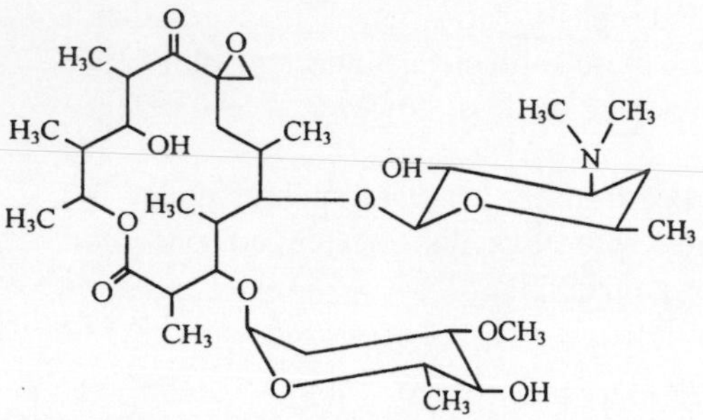

Oleandomycin

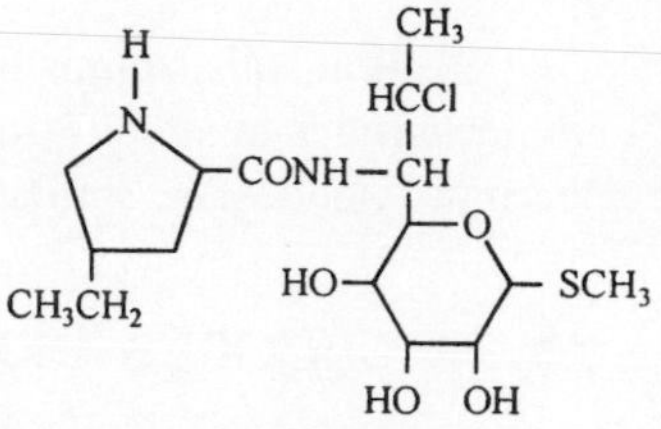

Pirlimycin

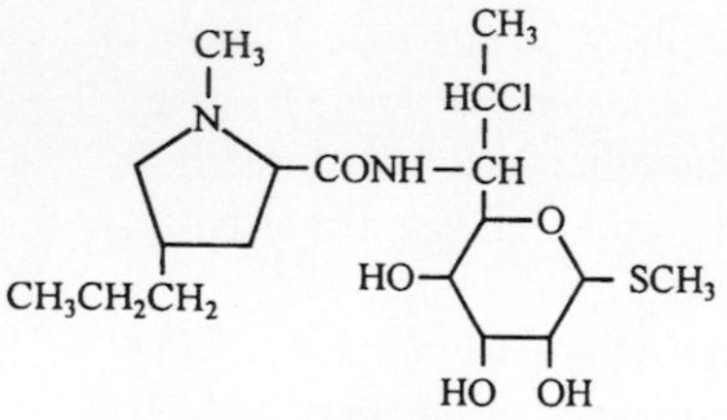

Clindamycin

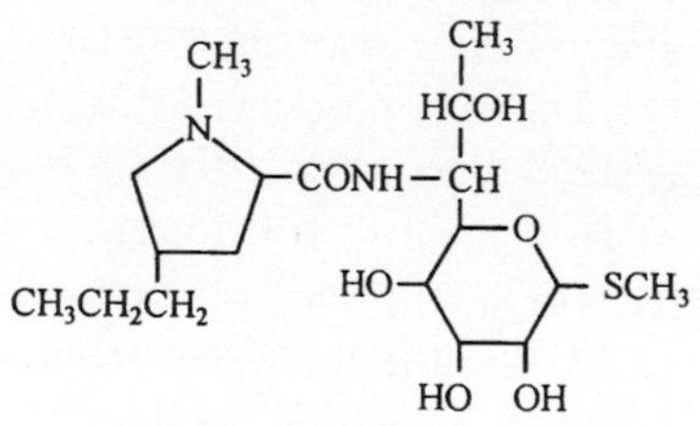

Lincomycin

FIG. 3.4   Chemical structures of commonly used macrolides and lincosamides.

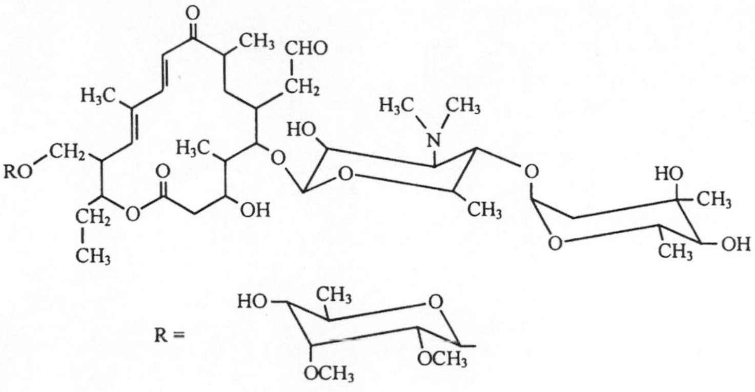

Tylosin

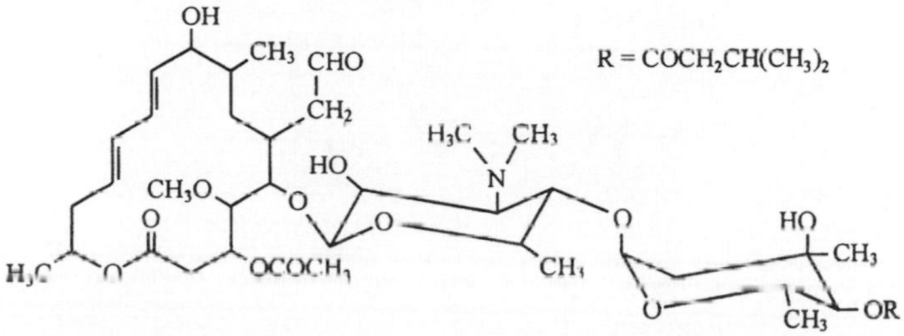

R = COCH₂CH(CH₃)₂

Josamycin

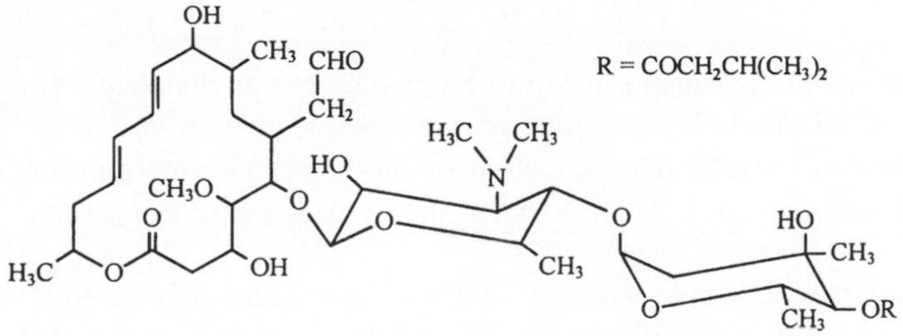

R = COCH₂CH(CH₃)₂

Kitasamycin

FIG. 3.4 *Continued*

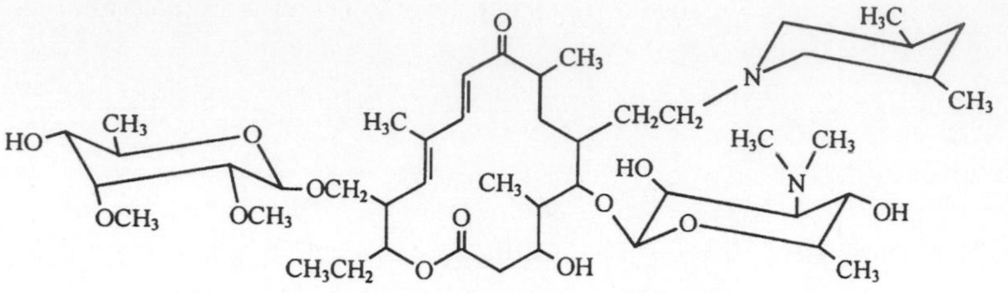

Tilmicosin

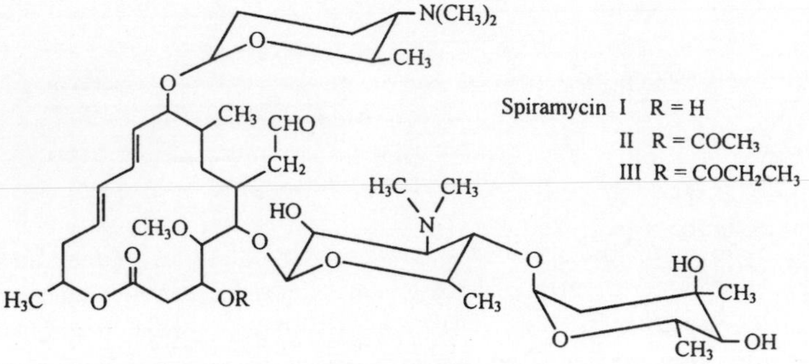

Spiramycin I   R = H
           II R = COCH₃
           III R = COCH₂CH₃

Spiramycin

FIG. 3.4 *Continued*

another macrolide antibiotic, which is the mild acid hydrolysis product of tylosin; further acid hydrolysis results in sugar mycarose and an inactive residue. Tilmicosin can be prepared by reductive amination of the C-20 aldehyde group of desmycosin (91). Mirosamicin is the principal of the five components of mycinamycins (92).

Sedecamycin is an example with a 17-membered ring that belongs to the lankacidin group of antibiotics. It is a neutral compound since, unlike other macrolides containing amino sugars, sedecamycin does not contain amino sugar moieties (93).

Macrolide antibiotics target the bacterial ribosome and inhibit the bacterial protein biosynthesis. Many gram-negative bacteria are inherently resistant to macrolides because their outer membrane is impermeable to macrolides. Several mechanisms of acquired resistance have been reported. In some cases, resistance is conferred by methylation of ribosomes by methylase enzymes, the genes of which are carried on plasmids or chromosomes. Some bacteria are also able to produce enzymes that inactivate macrolides either by destroying the macrocyclic nucleus or by attaching a conjugate onto the antibiotic. Resistance can also occur via a protein that increases drug efflux from bacteria. The macrolide antibiotics generally exhibit low toxicity (15).

In general, the macrolides are administered orally but sometimes also parenterally. All the members of this group are well absorbed and are distributed extensively in tissues, especially in the lungs, liver, and kidneys, with high tissue to plasma ratios. They are retained in the tissues for long periods after the levels in the blood have ceased to be detectable. Elimination of all macrolides occurs primarily through hepatic metabolism, which accounts for approximately 60% of an administered intravenous dose; the remainder is excreted in active form in the urine and bile. With oral and intramuscular administration, urinary excretion decreases, but biliary excretion and hepatic metabolism increase proportionally. Milk has often macrolide concentrations severalfold greater than in plasma (7).

Lincosamides constitute a small group of antibiotics that includes lincomycin, clindamycin, and pirlimycin. They are all monoglycosides with an amino acidlike side chain. Lincomycin, the parent compound of this group, contains a thiolated-D-erythro-α-D-galacto-octopyranoside that is joined to a proline via an amide linkage. Clindamycin is a semisynthetic derivative of lincomycin with a chlorine replacing a hydroxyl group at the seven position of the lincomycin molecule. Lincomycin and clindamycin are the best known members of this group of drugs. Pirlimycin is another semisynthetic derivative containing the chloro-sugar moiety of clindamycin and the modified amino acid residue, 4-ethyl-pipecolic acid.

Lincosamide antibiotics are highly effective against a wide range of gram-positive and anaerobic bacteria. They are generally inactive against gram-negative bacteria but are synergistic with aminoglycosides against these bacteria. Lincosamides are inhibitors of bacterial protein biosynthesis and block the bacterial ribosomes similarly to macrolides. Bacteria have developed resistance to the lincosamides. A common form of resistance arises from mutation of bacterial ribosome. The lincosamides may also inactivated by plasmid-mediated enzymes. Lincosamides appear to be safe compounds exhibiting generally low toxicity (15).

3.4.1 Macrolide Antibiotics

Tylosin (tylosin A) is a macrolide antibiotic produced by *Streptomyces fradiae*. Desmycosin (tylosin B), macrocin (tylosin C), and relomycin (tylosin D) are minor compounds also produced by this bacterial strain.

Tylosin is widely and exclusively used in veterinary medicine and is primarily directed against the chronic respiratory disease complex in chickens and infectious sinusitus in turkeys, although it is also effective for bovine respiratory and swine dysentery diseases. It is also used as a growth promoter for pigs. Tylosin can be administered orally either through the drinking water to chickens, turkeys, and pigs at a dosage of 0.2–0.5 mg/L; or through the feed to pigs at 20–40 mg/kg; subcutaneously in chickens; and intramuscularly to cattle, calves, and pigs at 2–10 mg/kg bw.

It is well absorbed by oral or parenteral routes and is excreted relatively slowly. Although tylosin is extensively metabolized, the parent compound always occurs in tissues at higher concentration than its metabolites (94). After oral administration of radiolabeled tylosin to swine, almost all of the radioactivity was excreted through the feces in the form of tylosin A, tylosin D, and dihydrodesmycosin; very low concentrations of these residues were also present in liver and kidney (95).

Residue depletion studies in pigs and cattle showed that the tissue in which the highest residue levels occur depends highly on the route of administration. Using injectable preparations of tylosin, higher and more persistent residue concentrations are found in kidney, excluding the injection site. However, using oral preparations, the highest residue concentrations are found in liver (95).

The route of administration also determines the level of the residues in the tissues; in general, oral dosing of animals results in lower residue concentrations than injections (96, 97). For that reason, detectable residues of parent tylosin cannot be found in swine liver unless the medicated feed contains at least 1000 ppm of the drug (98); residues of the parent compound are also undetectable in poultry tissues following oral administration of tylosin.

Tylosin in its unchanged form can pass into milk and eggs. When lactating cows were intramuscularly injected with 17.6 mg tylosin/kg bw for 5 days, residues of the parent drug persisted in milk for longer than 3 days after the final treatment, at a mean concentration of 0.03 ppm (99). Thus, milk taken from cows during treatment and for 96 h after the last treatment, must not be used as food. Tylosin must not be used in laying hens, whereas broilers must not be slaughtered for food within 3 days of injection or 1 day of oral treatment. In addition, turkeys and pigs must not be slaughtered for food within 5 and 21 days after treatment, respectively.

Tilmicosin is a macrolide antibiotic exclusively used in veterinary medicine and resembling tylosin. It is approved for treatment of respiratory diseases in beef cattle and sheep by the subcutaneous route (100, 101). It is also indicated for treatment and control of respiratory diseases associated with mycoplasma in broiler chickens, but not in laying hens. Of major significance is that in contrast to other macrolides, tilmicosin is not safe for use in swine since fatalities may occur at dosage as low as 20 mg/kg bw (7).

In cattle, treatment consists of 10 mg tilmicosin/kg bw as a single injection administered subcutaneously in the neck. This results in long-lived serum and tissue tilmicosin levels. Cattle dosed with radiolabeled tilmicosin excreted most of the dose in feces (102). Among edible tissues, liver and kidney contained the highest levels of radioactivity. Total residues that accumulated in liver were mostly composed of the parent compound and the N-desmethyl metabolite. Liver was the tissue with the highest and most slowly depleting residues; parent tilmicosin declined to less than 1 ppm by 28 days after treatment.

Because of this slow kinetic excretory pattern, tilmicosin is contraindicated for use in lactating animals. Rapid and extensive penetration of tilmicosin from blood into milk and slow elimination from the milk are among the characteristic kinetic features of the drug after intravenous and subcutaneous administration (103).

When tilmicosin was administered to six lactating cows as a single subcutaneous dosage of 10 mg/kg (104), residues in milk were higher than 25 ppb from 19 to 31 days postdosing. Following subcutaneous administration to sheep, a maximum concentration of 10247 ppb of tilmicosin was observed in milk at 8 h after dosing; by day 12, however, the concentration of tilmicosin was below the MRL of 50 ppb. The half-life of tilmicosin in milk was calculated to be approximately 24 h (105).

After oral administration of radiolabeled tilmicosin to broilers at dosage in the range 25–450 mg/L in water for 3–5 days, radioactivity was mainly distributed to liver and kidney and, to a lesser extent, to muscle and fat. The parent drug was the main residue in tissues, excreta, and bile, but partly desmethylated, hydroxylated, reduced, and sulfated metabolites could be also identified. Similar pharmacokinetic characteristics were also observed in cattle, swine, and sheep. In broilers treated with tilmicosin at the recommended dosage, residues of the parent drug in liver were 2.6 ppm at day 3 declining to 0.13 ppm at day 17; residue levels in kidney averaged 0.65 ppm at day 3 and declined via 0.08 ppm on day 10 to below 0.06 ppm thereafter. Residues in muscle, fat, and skin were approximately 0.10 ppm at day 3 and less than 0.014 ppm after day 14.

Sedecamycin is a macrolide primarily used for treating swine dysentery. As with most macrolides, sedecamycin is extensively metabolized in swine; 20 metabolites have been detected, the major ones being lankacidin C, lankacidinol, and lankacidinol A (106).

Both the parent drug and its metabolites disappear from all tissues at 1 day after treatment withdrawal. When pigs were fed diets containing 50–500 mg sedecamycin/kg for 14 or 28 days, liver contained the highest residue concentration 2 h after withdrawal of the diets. Muscle and fat, however, were free of drug residues even with the heavy-dosage 500 mg/kg medication.

Erythromycin is a macrolide antibiotic produced by *Streptomyces erythreus*. It is considered the most active macrolide for treatment of staphylococcal infections in cases of penicillin resistance. It is used parenterally at a dosage of 3–5 mg/kg bw, in intramammary form at 300 mg/quarter, and orally at 20–50 mg/kg bw. For treatment of mycoplasmal infections in poultry, an oral medication at 0.25 g/L of drinking water is also used. Erythromycin is the most acid-labile of the macrolides; the erythromycin base is unstable in gastric acid but some salts and esters are acid-resistant and are given orally.

Erythromycin is absorbed rapidly when administered orally. Peak serum concentration occurred 1–2 h after oral administration and 1–3 h after intramuscular use. In the latter case, peak serum concentrations were maintained for several hours and then decline slowly. Two hours after intramuscular administration, the highest concentrations were detected in liver, lungs and kidney.

Erythromycin distributes widely in the body with residue levels in tissues generally exceeding those in serum. Both hepatic and renal routes of elimination of erythromycin are significant and it undergoes enterohepatic circulation. Elimination of erythromycin in relatively high levels in the feces may follow its oral administration. As with almost all macrolides, the principal metabolic pathway of erythromycin is by N-desmethylation of the desosamine sugar (107).

Oleandomycin is a macrolide antibiotic produced by *Streptomyces antibioticus*. Oleandomycin and its triacetylated form, troleandomycin, are less effective than erythromycin against staphylococcal infections. They are usually administered orally or intravenously; intramuscular administration is avoided because of the pain and tissue irritation it induces. Oleandomycin is also used in intramammary treatments and as a feed additive for growth promotion purposes.

The toxicity of oleandomycin is quite low. Troleandomycin may cause hepatic disturbances and jaundice, liver function should be monitored in patients.

Oleandomycin is absorbed fairly slowly after oral administration, but troleandomycin is more rapidly and completely absorbed. Following absorption, troleandomycin is converted to several metabolites but oleandomycin is not metabolized (108). After both oral or parenteral administration, oleandomycin can be detected in many tissues including liver, kidney, spleen, heart, lungs, and bile.

Spiramycin is a macrolide–antibiotic complex produced by *Streptomyces ambofaciens*. It is used for the treatment and control of a number of bacterial and mycoplasmal infections in a variety of food-producing animals. Like tylosin, spiramycin has been used in many countries as a feed additive at low inclusion rates. It is available as spiramycin embonate for use in animal feed, and as the adipate for administration by parenteral routes.

Spiramycin is incompletely absorbed from the gastrointestinal tract, but widely distributed in tissues. After absorption, some portion of the drug is desmycarosylated into neospiramycin by gastric acid; neospiramycin does not differ from the parent drug in the antibacterial activity (109). Spiramycin is metabolized in the liver to active metabolites and excreted in bile but also in urine. It is found in breast milk. In raw milk, the neospiramycin level was 6–7% of the spiramycin content (110).

Data from the literature suggest that spiramycin produces more persistent residues than the other macrolides (95). However, due to the microbiological methods most often applied, uncertainties remain as to whether the activity measured comes from the parent drug or its metabolites. Young cattle injected with spiramycin at 30 mg/kg bw showed higher residue concentrations in the liver and kidney than in muscle and fat. Unlike with other tissues, residues in liver persisted for 28 days after treatment. Calves fed spiramycin at 25 mg/kg bw for 7 days also showed high residue concentrations in the liver and kidney, which declined below 0.1 ppm at 24 days after withdrawal. In contrast, residue levels in muscle and fat could not be detected at 3 days after treatment.

Residue studies following oral administration of spiramycin were also carried out in swine and poultry. The high residue levels found in swine liver and kidney declined to below 0.3 ppm at 10 days after treatment. The residue levels found in the liver of broilers given medicated feed (300 mg/kg of feed) for 10 days declined below 0.02 ppm at 8 days after the dietary administration.

Kitasamycin is a macrolide antibiotic intended for use in poultry and pigs. It is administered through the feed for the protection and treatment of chicken respiratory mycoplasmosis at a dosage of 500 mg/kg feed, and for protection and treatment of pig diarrhea at a dosage of 330 mg/kg feed.

Pharmacokinetic studies in pigs following a single oral administration of 20 mg kitasamycin/kg bw showed that the drug was rapidly absorbed and distributed in the body. A maximum plasma concentration of 4.5 ppm was attained within 0.5 h, the half-life in plasma being 0.7 h. Highest tissue residue concentrations (21 ppm) were detected in kidney within 1–2 h. The ratio of the maximum concentrations determined in kidney to that in liver was around 3:2.

In chickens given a single oral administration of 200 mg kitasamycin/kg bw, a maximum plasma concentration of 4 ppm was attained within 2 h, the half-life in plasma being 1.2 h. Highest tissue residue concentrations (40 ppm) were detected in liver within 2 h The ratio of the maximum concentrations determined in liver to that in kidney and in muscle was 12:8:1.

Residue depletion studies in pigs fed 330 mg kitasamycin/kg feed for 14 days showed that at zero withdrawal only liver (100 ppb) and kidney (60 ppb) contained detectable residues. One day after withdrawal of the treatment, residual antibiotic activity was detectable only in the liver. Residue depletion studies in chickens fed 500 mg kitasamycin/kg feed for 14 days showed that at zero withdrawal only liver (70 ppb) contained detectable residues. One day after withdrawal, residual antibiotic activity could not be detected in any tissue.

Josamycin is a macrolide antibiotic produced by *Streptomyces narbonensis* var. *josamyceticus*. It is used for the prevention and treatment of chronic respiratory diseases caused by mycoplasma and gram-positive germs in chickens and pigs by the oral route via drinking water or feed at a dosage of 9–18 mg/kg bw/day for 3–5 and up to 14 days, respectively.

Josamycin is absorbed from the gastrointestinal tract and concentrated in lungs. It is principally excreted in bile. In rats, 99% of the total radioactivity was excreted in urine and feces within 4 days after oral administration at a dosage of 400 mg radiolabeled josamycin/kg bw. A major metabolite, deisovalery-josa-mycin, representing 96% of the total urinary metabolites, was identified.

Residue depletion studies in chickens showed that 1 day after the end of treatment the concentrations of the microbiologically active residues in liver, kidney, and fat/skin were 490, 240, and 330–41,810 ppb, respectively. Eggs from laying hens similarly treated contained residues ranged from less than 100 ppb to 450 ppb during treatment and at 3 days after treatment.

Residue depletion studies in pigs showed that 2 days after the end of treat-ment the concentrations of microbiologically active residues in muscle, fat, skin, and kidney were from less than 100 ppb to 190 ppb, 4100 ppb, 780 ppb, and from less than 100 ppb to 1660 ppb, respectively.

3.4.2   Lincosamide Antibiotics

Lincomycin is an antibiotic produced by *Streptomyces lincolnensis*. It is used in monopreparations or in combination with other antibiotics such as spectinomycin, sulfamethazine, and gentamicin, for the initial treatment of mild to moderate staphylococcal infections in a variety of animal species. It can be administered orally to poultry at dosages equivalent to up to 50 mg/kg bw/day for up to 7 days, and to swine at dosages equivalent to up to 10 mg/kg bw/day for up to 21 days. In calves, sheep, goats, and swine, it can be administered intramuscularly at dosages of up to 15 mg/kg bw/day for up to 4–7 days. It is also added in feeds for growth-promoting purposes.

Lincomycin is reported to cause gastrointestinal disturbances including diarrhea, vomiting, nausea, and colitis that may prove fatal. Other adverse effects include skin rashes, urticaria, polyarthritis, hepatic damage, and hematological disturbances.

Lincomycin is readily absorbed when given orally but its resorption may be affected by the presence of food. It is also completely absorbed from intramus-cular sites. It is widely distributed in the body and does not appear to concentrate in any particular tissue. Pharmacokinetic studies indicate that bile is an important route of excretion. Lincomycin has been also shown to be excreted in the milk of lactating cows and goats (111). Metabolism of lincomycin in food-producing animals proceeds primarily through oxidation of the sulfur atom to the sulfoxide metabolite, demethylation to the N-desmethyl metabolite, and conversion of both metabolites to N-desmethyl lincomycin sulfoxide.

Residue depletion studies in laying hens given oral boluses of 0.55 mg radiolabeled lincomycin/12 h for 12 days showed that residual radioactivity in whole eggs was in the range 1.2–12.0 ppb lincomycin equivalents during the treatment period, and in the range 1–4 ppb equivalents 3 days after treatment; liver contained 141, 24, and 6 ppb equivalents; kidney 152, 21, and 6 ppb equivalents; muscle 20, 13, and 10 ppb equivalents; and skin/fat 19, 14, and 3 ppb equivalents at 4, 28, and 76 h after treatment, respectively.

When pigs were intramuscularly injected with lincomycin, liver contained 4710, 4860, 2480, 552, 65, and <17 ppb; kidney contained 20,900, 18,400, 7470, 1360, 239, and <60 ppb; and muscle contained 2460, 1840, 638, 85, <17, and <17 ppb lincomycin at 3, 6, 12, 24, 48, and 144 days after treatment, respectively. When pigs were given water containing 66 mg lincomycin/L for 7 days, liver contained 204, 105, 53, 17, and <17 ppb; kidney contained 647, 296, 161, <60, and <60 ppb; and muscle contained 42, 28, <17, <17, and <17 ppb lincomycin at 3, 6, 12, 24, and 48 days after treatment, respectively.

In sheep intramuscularly injected with 5 mg lincomycin/kg bw/day for 3 days, liver contained 4340, 27, <17, and <17 ppb lincomycin at 8 h, 7, 14, and 21 days after treatment, respectively. In lactating cows given intramammary lincomycin 200 mg/quarter, milk contained 64,000–150,000 ppb at 12 h, 4900–62,000 ppb at 24 h, < 200–3950 ppb at 36 h, and below 200 ppb at 48 h postdosing. In goats given 15 mg lincomycin/kg bw/day intramuscularly for 3 days, milk contained 2110 ppb at 24 h, 443 ppb at 36 h, 115 ppb at 48 h, and less than 100 ppb at 60 h and at all time points thereafter.

Clindamycin is a more potent drug than the parent lincomycin. It possesses neuromuscular blocking activity and should not be used with other compounds having similar activity. The indications for clindamycin treatment are the same as those for lincomycin. It is absorbed more rapidly orally, and its absorption is not affected by the presence of food in the gastrointestinal tract as happens with lincomycin.

Clindamycin is widely distributed in body fluids and tissues. It is bound to plasma proteins in the circulation. It crosses the placenta and appears in breast milk. Clindamycin is mostly metabolized in the liver and excreted in the bile and urine as parent drug and active metabolites (89). Similarly to lincomycin, metabolism of clindamycin proceeds primarily by oxidation of the sulfur atom to the sulfoxide metabolite and demethylation to the N-desmethyl metabolite (112).

Pirlimycin is a lincosamide recently approved by the US Food and Drug Administration for treatment of mastitis in dairy cattle (113, 114). It has excellent activity against *Staphylococcus aureus,* the principal organism responsible for mastitis in the dairy cow, and is administered as an aqueous gel by intramammary infusion (115).

Metabolism studies (116) in dairy cows treated twice at a 24 h interval with radiolabeled pirlimycin into all quarters at 200 mg/quarter by the intramammary route showed that the drug was readily absorbed from the udder; about 68% of the dose was excreted in the milk, urine, and feces as parent pirlimycin. About 4% appeared as pirlimycin sulfoxide generated by hepatic oxidation, and

was excreted in both urine and feces. Demethylation to the N-desmethyl metabolite was not observed (112).

Both pirlimycin and its sulfoxide metabolite were partially converted to
ribonucleotide adducts by gastrointestinal tract microflora and excreted in feces.
Such adducts have been well documented as products of antibiotic inactivation
by bacteria for a variety of substances including lincomycin and clindamycin
(117–119).

These polar adducts were apparently not reabsorbed since there was no
evidence of their presence in either milk or tissue. Total pirlimycin residues in
milk were 43.95 ppm 12 h after its last administration, but declined rapidly
thereafter to reach 0.09 ppm at 120 h after drug withdrawal. Muscle and fat
contained 0.10 and 0.22 ppm, respectively, on day 4, but no detectable residues
beyond day 6. Liver and kidney contained 9.18 and 1.96 ppm, respectively, on
day 4, and 0.50 and 0.01 ppm, respectively, on day 28.

In liver, a minor component of total residues was attributed to pirlimycin
itself while the bulk, 77%, was attributed to the sulfoxide metabolite (116). The
liver contained relatively higher concentrations of total pirlimycin residues than
other tissues, the sulfoxide metabolite accounting for approximately 62% of the
total residues.

3.5 NITROFURANS

The nitrofurans are synthetic antibacterial compounds, all containing in their
molecule a characteristic 5-nitrofuran ring (Fig. 3.5). Furazolidone, nitrofurazone,
furaltadone, and nitrofurantoin are all nitrofurans that have been widely used in
the prophylactic and therapeutic treatment of infections caused by bacteria and
protozoa in swine, cattle, poultry, rabbits, and fish. They have been also used as
feed additives in animal husbandry. They are very effective drugs and do not
appreciably contribute to the development of resistance (120).

Nitrofurans are metabolized in vivo to reduced forms responsible for the
effects exerted upon bacteria. These metabolites inhibit bacterial respiration, glucose metabolism, and ribosomal function, and may damage bacterial DNA.

Controversy regarding the use of nitrofurans in food-producing animals has
arisen during the last two decades because indications have appeared that residues
of these drugs may be mutagenic and tumorigenic (121, 122). Extensive toxicological studies showed that nitrofurazone was a carcinogenic but not genotoxic
agent, whereas furazolidone exhibited both carcinogenic and genotoxic properties
(123). As a result, systemic use of nitrofurans, as a chemical class, in food-
producing animals was prohibited in the United States and Europe, except for
topical applications (124). Because of the carcinogenic potential of these otherwise important antimicrobial drugs, interest in all nitrofurans has been further
lost in several other countries in the world.

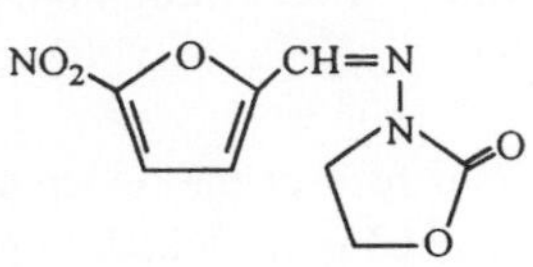

Furazolidone 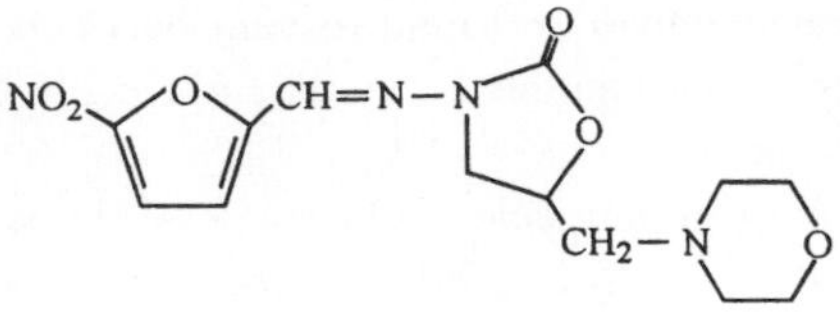   Furaltadone

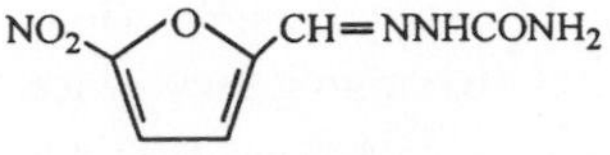

Nitrofurazone 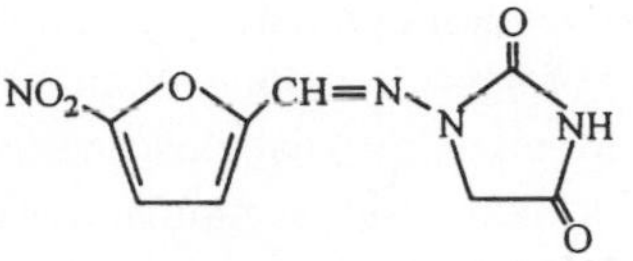   Nitrofurantoin

FIG. 3.5 Chemical structures of commonly used nitrofurans.

Furazolidone has been used for treatment of *Salmonella* infections in most farm animals. It has been also used as a feed additive for growth-promoting purposes. For poultry it was given in the feed at a level of 0.04% for 10 days, and in large animals at an oral dosage of 10–12 mg/kg bw for 5–7 days.

Furazolidone is extensively metabolized in animals after its absorption from the gastrointestinal tract (125). Immediately after its last administration to chickens and pigs, residual concentrations of the parent drug in muscle, kidney, and liver tissues were less than 0.5 ppb (126). In chicken and swine urine, the unchanged furazolidone occurred only in trace amounts, but a large number of metabolites, most of which could not be identified, appeared. Among those metabolites, the open-chain cyano metabolite, 3-(4-cyano-2-oxobutylideneamino)-2-oxazolidone, was most common in animal species.

Other residue depletion studies in pigs and calves given medicated feed at 300 mg/kg feed also showed that the parent drug is either absent or present at very low levels in muscle tissues, even at zero withdrawal (127, 128). In poultry treated with 440 mg furazolidone/kg feed, residues of the parent drug could be detected in muscle at very low ppb concentrations for up to 4 days after the cessation of treatment (129). When laying hens were given medicated feed for 28, 14, and 14 days, residues of the parent drug in the whole egg declined to 1 ppb at 9, 10, and 11 days for the 100 ppm, 200 ppm, and 400 ppm feeding level, respectively (130). In the same study, the deposition and clearance of residual furazolidone were found to vary between yolk and albumen; levels in albumen were lower than those in yolk and cleared rapidly while those in yolk took longer to clear.

In trout species held at 8–14°C and given medicated feed at the 35 ppm level for 20 days, residues of the parent compound accumulated in muscle during the medication period, reaching a maximum of 0.482 ppm at day 10 of medication (131). After withdrawal of the medication, residues fell rapidly to less than 0.075 ppm at day 10 posttreatment.

Residue depletion studies with radiolabeled furazolidone have shown that the almost complete degradation of the drug in the body resulted in formation of a variety of protein-bound metabolites that were not solvent-extractable. Thus, when pigs were given radiolabeled furazolidone orally at 16.5 mg/kg bw/day for 14 days (123), total residual radioactivity in liver, kidney, muscle, and fat accounted for 41.1 ppm, 34.4 ppm, 13.2 ppm, and 6.2 ppm furazolidone equivalents, respectively, at zero withdrawal (132). Total residues were substantially lower by 21 days withdrawal, but were still in the ppm range at 45 days withdrawal. Extraction of the incurred muscle tissue at 0 and 45 days withdrawal with organic solvents led to removal of 21.8 and 13.7% of the total radioactivity, respectively. In contrast, 44 and 8.3% of the total radioactivity was extracted from liver on days 0 and 45, respectively.

This nonextractable radioactivity was probably the result of covalent binding of the furazolidone intermediates to endogenous macromolecules. The bioavailability of these bound tissue residues from the above pig residue depletion study was determined by feeding rats lyophilized samples of liver and muscle tissues from animals sacrificed at 0 and 45 days after the last treatment (132). Results showed that the fraction of the bound residues bioavailable to rats was in the range 16–41%. The toxicological impact of these bioavailable bound residues has not been yet determined.

Nitrofurazone has been used as a wide-spectrum antimicrobial drug for prophylactic and therapeutic purposes in swine, cattle, sheep, goats, chickens, turkeys, and fish for many years. The drug is also available as a premix for inclusion in the feed for growth-promoting purposes, and as a piglet dosing pump at a dosage of 100 mg/day. It is also used at a concentration of 0.2% in a cream for treatment of topical bacterial infections.

In common with other nitrofurans, nitrofurazone is well absorbed from the gut following oral administration. Limited information is available on the extent of its biotransformation and on the identities of the metabolites produced. However, a comparison with other nitrofurans suggests that nitrofurazone also undergoes extensive biotransformation.

Following infeed administration of a commercial dose of the drug to chickens, residues of parent nitrofurazone were highest in the liver (113 ppb) and lowest in muscle (0.7–9 ppb) at zero withdrawal, whereas no residues of the parent drug could be detected at 2-day withdrawal. Following administration to laying hens of a medicated feed containing 100 mg/kg each nitrofurazone, furazolidone, nitrofurantoin, and furaltadone for 7 days, residues of nitrofurazone in egg yolk showed a maximum concentration of 0.5 ppm (129). In pig muscle, no residues could be detected at zero withdrawal after feeding of a commercial dose of nitrofurazone (123).

Furaltadone has been used primarily for treatment of poultry infected with salmonellosis, colibacillosis, coccidiosis, blackhead, and infectious synovitis at a dosage of 0.02–0.04% in the drinking water or feed for a maximum of 10 days. The drug has been also used in intramammary form to treat bovine mastitis at a dosage of 500 mg/quarter.

Following oral administration, furaltadone is well absorbed from the gastrointestinal tract. After administration to laying hens of a medicated feed containing 100 mg/kg each nitrofurazone, furazolidone, nitrofurantoin, and furaltadone for 7 days, residues of furaltadone in egg yolk showed a maximum concentration of 0.2 ppm (129).

Nitrofurantoin has been used as an urinary antiseptic in calves and horses at an oral dosage of 10 mg/kg bw/day. It is absorbed rapidly and completely from the gastrointestinal tract. About 40% of the drug is eliminated in the urine, while the remainder is catabolized.

When laying hens were fed a diet containing nitrofurantoin in addition to furazolidone, furaltadone and nitrofurazone at levels of 100, 100, 50, and 100 ppm in the feed, respectively, residues in the eggs laid between days 6 and 15 contained 84, 164, 171, and 20 ppb of the drugs, respectively (133).

3.6 QUINOLONES

Quinolones constitute an expanding group of synthetic antibiotics that are very effective in combating various diseases in animal husbandry and aquaculture. Although oxolinic acid and nalidixic acid, the earliest members of this group, showed activity against only gram-negative bacteria, the former has been by far the most widely used drug in fish farming for prophylaxis and treatment of bacterial fish disease during the last decade (134, 135).

Recent research on 4-quinolone-3-carboxylates has led to discovery of the fluoroquinolones, which are second-generation quinolones and include ciprofloxacin, danofloxacin, difloxacin, enrofloxacin, flumequine, marbofloxacin, norfloxacin, ofloxacin, and sarafloxacin. The main difference between classic quinolones and the fluoroquinolones is that the latter contain a fluorine atom at the C-3 position and a piperazinyl group at the C-7 position (Fig. 3.6).

The addition of either the fluorine or the piperazino moiety, or both, to the basic quinolone backbone enhances the overall antibacterial activity of the new compounds. Fluorine increases the activity against gram-positive pathogens,

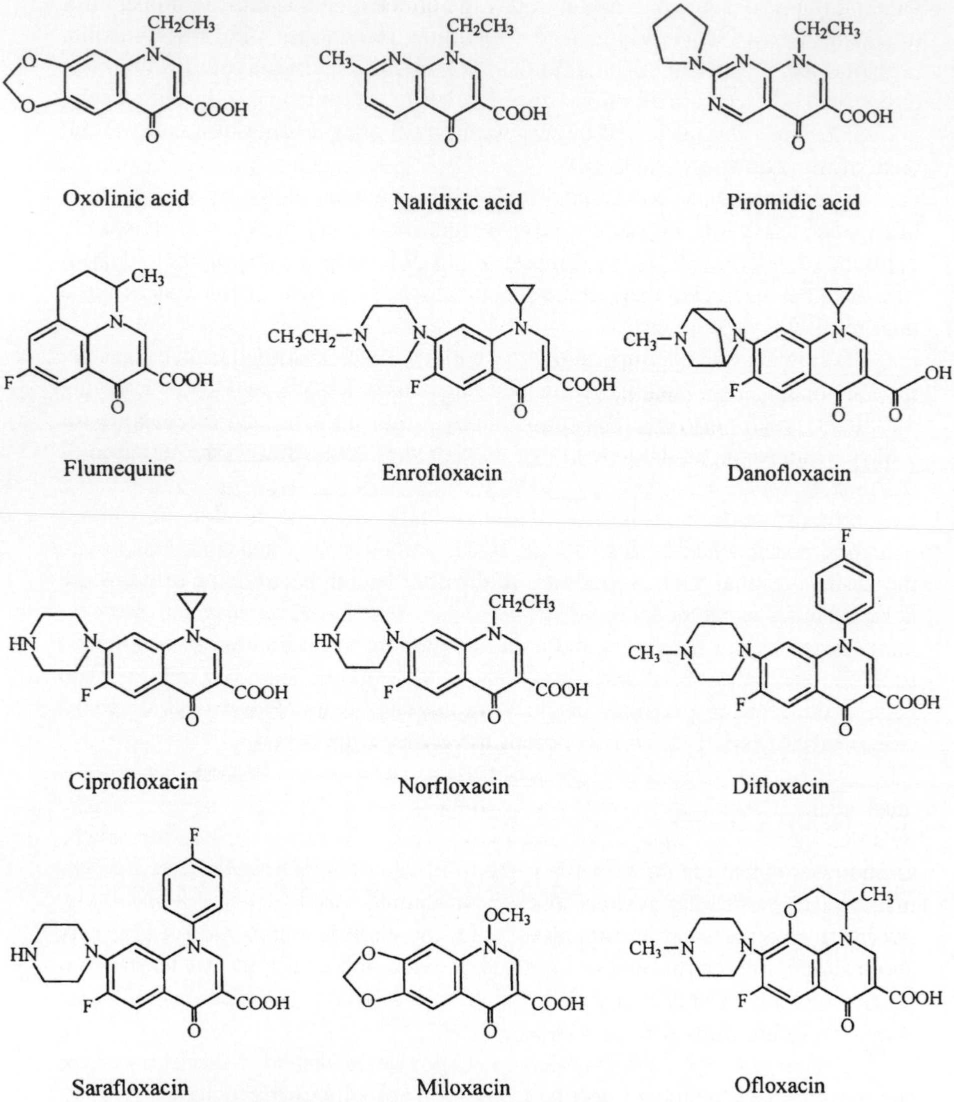

FIG. 3.6 Chemical structures of commonly used quinolones.

whereas the piperazino moiety improves the effectiveness against gram-negative organisms (136). The mode of action of quinolones is not entirely understood, but it has been demonstrated that they inhibit the action of bacterial DNA gyrase enzymes.

The main application of fluoroquinolones has been for gastrointestinal and respiratory infections. The US Food and Drug Administration has approved the therapeutic use of sarafloxacin in poultry, making this the first approved fluroquinolone in food animals (137). Other members of this class of drugs have been petitioned for similar use. Although not approved for use in treatment of infections in cows, enrofloxacin is the most commonly used fluroquinolone in the European Union (138).

Gastrointestinal disturbances including nausea, vomiting, and diarrhea are the most frequent adverse affects of quinolone antibiotics. Headache, visual disturbances, and insomnia have been reported. Rashes, pruritus and epidermal necrolysis have sometimes also occurred. Quinolones are not recommended for children, adolescents, and pregnant and breastfeeding women because they cause joint erosions in immature animals.

As a rule, when quinolones are administered orally, their absorption from the gastrointestinal tract is rapid and almost complete, but food in the stomach delays their absorption. In unweaned calves, fluoroquinolones are often given in the milk replacer, but oral bioavailability is slightly reduced compared with the oral drench (139). On the other hand, fermentation in the rumen of mature ruminants precludes the oral use of fluoroquinolones. Injectable solutions are also available for systemic therapy of large animals and turkeys.

Serum concentrations of fluoroquinolones tend generally to be lower than those of the first-generation quinolones. Most fluoroquinolones are characterized by a great availability in all monogastric animals, a large volume of distribution, and a low binding to plasma proteins. These pharmacokinetic characteristics allow them to cross membranes and reach the most remote parts of the body. Kidney, liver, and bile are the body parts presenting the highest concentrations after systemic administration of fluoroquinolones. Fluoroquinolones are partially metabolized in the liver and excreted in the urine where they can reach 100–300 times higher concentrations than in serum.

Danofloxacin is a fluoroquinolone antibacterial developed specifically for use in veterinary medicine (140). It has been studied for use in cattle, swine, chickens, and turkeys for the control of respiratory and enteric bacterial infections (141). Danofloxacin can be administered via drinking water to broiler chickens and replacement chicks at a dosage of 5 mg/kg bw for 3 days, and via the intramuscular route to calves, beef, and nonlactating cattle at a dosage of 1.25 mg/kg bw/day for 3 days.

In chickens, danofloxacin is rapidly absorbed after oral administration and rapidly distributed in tissues. In cattle, danofloxacin exhibits similar bioavailability by the intramuscular, intravenous, and subcutaneous routes of administration. The oral bioavailability in pigs is around 89%. In all species, tissue residues are highest in the liver and consist mostly of the parent drug and the N-desmethyl metabolite (142).

After oral administration of radiolabeled danofloxacin to chickens or intramuscular administration to cattle, residues of total residues in all tissues declined rapidly with time. In both species, total residues were highest in liver at all time points. Unmetabolized danofloxacin was the major component in chicken liver and constituted 47–61% of total residues at 6–24 h after treatment. Residues of N-desmethyl danofloxacin over the same period were 14–20% of the total liver residues. Residues in cattle consisted of 14–32% danofloxacin. Residues of N-desmethyl danofloxacin declined from 30–40% of the total residues at 12 h to 14% at 72 h.

Residue depletion studies in chickens showed that residues of danofloxacin in muscle declined from 36–90 ppb at 6 h to less than 25 ppb at 18 h after withdrawal of treatment. Residues of the N-desmethyl metabolite were less than 25 ppb at all time points. Residues of danofloxacin in liver declined from 157–319 ppb at 6 h to 18–66 ppb at 36 h after withdrawal of treatment. Residues of the N-desmethyl metabolite were 35–193 ppb and less than 10 ppb over the same time points.

In a residue depletion study in cattle given the normal therapeutic treatment, residues of danofloxacin in liver declined from 372 ppb at 12 h after the last dose to 13 ppb at 5 days after the last dose. Over the same time period, residues at the injection site, kidney, and muscle declined from 669 ppb to less than 10 ppb, from 426 ppb to 5 ppb, and from 112 ppb to less than 10 ppb, respectively. Residues in most fat samples were below 10 ppb.

The metabolism of danofloxacin does not differ in swine. When five daily intramuscular injections of 1.25 mg radiolabeled danofloxacin/kg bw were given to pigs, the parent drug accounted for 72–81% of the radioactivity excreted in feces and urine over the 5- day dosing period (143). In feces, 5–7% of the radioactivity was identified as N-desmethyl danofloxacin. In urine, 2–3% was N-desmethyl danofloxacin, 10–14% danofloxacin-N-oxide, and 3% danofloxacin glucuronide.

Residue depletion studies in pigs given three daily intramuscular injections of 1.25 mg danofloxacin/kg bw showed that residues of the parent drug in liver were 27 ppb at 2 days after the last dose and below 10 ppb at later time points. Mean danofloxacin concentrations in kidney declined from 36 ppb at 2 days after the last dose to 5.5 ppb at 6 days after the last dose and to below 5 ppb at later time points. Two days after the last dose, mean danofloxacin concentrations in muscle, fat, and at the injection site were 15 ppb, below 5 ppb, and 17 ppb, respectively; at later time points residues could not be detected. Residues of N-desmethyl danofloxacin could be found only in liver and declined from 622 ppb at 2 days to 221 ppb at 6 days and to 79 ppb at 18 days after the last dose.

Difloxacin is another fluoroquinolone antibacterial developed for administration via the drinking water to chickens and turkeys. When male and female broiler chickens and turkeys were administered radiolabeled difloxacin at 10 mg/ kg bw for 5 consecutive days, liver was the tissue with the highest level of total radioactive residues: 1878 and 2660 ppb of difloxacin equivalents, respectively, at 6 h after last dosing (144). Within 12 h following the last dose, total radioactivity in all edible tissues of chickens and turkeys fell well below their maximum residue limit settings (145). No gender-related differences were observed in the residue levels found in all edible tissues. It was found that in both species difloxacin could be glucuronidated or sulfated, demethylated into sarafloxacin, or oxidized into N-oxide-difloxacin. Nevertheless, the main metabolites detected were identified as hydrolyzable conjugates of difloxacin.

Enrofloxacin is another fluoroquinolone antibacterial developed exclusively for animals (146). It is administered either by parenteral route to cattle, swine, sheep and rabbits, or by the oral route to cattle, swine, rabbits, chickens, and turkeys (147). Although it is not allowed for use in dairy cows, enrofloxacin is also used in some countries for treatment of coliform mastitis in lactating cows. In addition, enrofloxacin has received growing attention during the last years for its potential against several fish pathogens (148).

Following oral administration to animals, enrofloxacin is well absorbed and widely distributed to all tissues, with highest concentrations in liver and kidney. Elimination is rapid via both urine and feces. Total enrofloxacin-related residues in urine are mainly composed of enrofloxacin, enrofloxacin amide, and ciprofloxacin and, to a lesser extent, from oxociprofloxacin, dioxociprofloxacin, desethylene ciprofloxacin, desethylene enrofloxacin, N-formyl ciprofloxacin, oxoenrofloxacin, and hydroxy oxoenrofloxacin.

Since ciprofloxacin, the major metabolite of enrofloxacin, exhibits biological activity similar to that of the parent compound, it is also used as an individual fluoroquinolone drug. In this case, ciprofloxacin is metabolized mainly to oxociprofloxacin and desethylene ciprofloxacin (149). After oral administration to broiler chickens, ciprofloxacin was rapidly and efficiently absorbed, its metabolism being similar to that observed in other animal species. It has been reported that the mean tissue concentrations of ciprofloxacin and its metabolites that ranged between 5 and 26 ppb persisted in chickens up to 12 days after treatment (149).

Residue depletion studies in chickens and turkeys orally dosed with 10 mg enrofloxacin/kg bw for 7 days showed that the sum of enrofloxacin and ciprofloxacin, which has been designated as the market residue for regulatory purposes, in the chicken liver declined from 42 ppb at 3 day withdrawal to 11 ppb at 15 day withdrawal; in turkeys, the level of the marker residue in liver declined from 1250 ppb at 1 day withdrawal to less than 10 ppb at 7 day withdrawal.

When chickens were treated orally with 7 mg/kg bw enrofloxacin, residues in muscle, liver, and kidney were 99 ppb, 88 ppb, and 154 ppb, respectively, at 1 day after the treatment (150). Eggs from breeder turkeys orally dosed with enrofloxacin were also found by a microbiological assay to contain residues by the day 11 postmedication (151).

Studies in pigs treated intramuscularly with enrofloxacin at a dosage of 2.5 mg/kg bw for 3 days showed that the parent compound was absorbed and efficiently distributed in tissues; the concentrations of enrofloxacin detected in muscle, liver, kidney, and fat tissues at 10 days after treatment were 15, 26, 20, and 29 ppb, respectively (152).

When cattle were subcutaneously injected with a single dose of 7.5 mg enrofloxacin/kg bw, the levels of the marker residue in liver, kidney, muscle, and fat fell rapidly from about 30 ppb, 20 ppb, less than 10 ppb, and less than 10 ppb, respectively, at day 3 after dosing to less than 10 ppb in all tissues at 7 day withdrawal. When enrofloxacin was injected intravenously to cows, ciprofloxacin could be detected at higher concentrations and for a longer period than the parent enrofloxacin (153). When enrofloxacin was administered parenterally to dairy cows at 5 mg/kg bw, the levels of the marker residue in milk remained above 30 ppb at day 4 after the last treatment of experimentally induced *E. coli* mastitis (154, 155). Significant concentrations of ciprofloxacin could also be found in milk of rabbits after intravenous administration of enrofloxacin (156).

The pharmacokinetics of enrofloxacin and its active metabolite, ciprofloxacin, have been further extensively studied in sea bass after treatment by oral gavage or water, at a temperature of 15°C (157). Enrofloxacin was absorbed and eliminated slowly after oral administration to the sea bass. Following bath treatment, enrofloxacin efficiently penetrated fish tissues but it was poorly metabolized compared with mammals. On the other hand, ciprofloxacin was generally detected in very low concentrations (less than 0.02 ppm) in plasma samples after both oral and bath treatment. Liver levels of ciprofloxacin were found to be 0.12 ppm after a 5 ppm bathing for 24 h, 0.06 ppm after a 10 ppm bathing for 8 h, and 0.33 ppm after a 50 ppm bathing for 4 h, suggestive of hepatic metabolism of enrofloxacin.

Flumequine is used in food-producing animals and fish for treatment and prevention of several bacterial infections. In aquaculture, the substance is administered preferably in the form of commercially available medicated feed pellets.

Its bioavailability to fish is favorable in comparison with other antibacterials such as oxytetracycline, which was used extensively in European aquaculture during the 1980s. The bioavailability of flumequine to Atlantic salmon was determined to be 40–45%, while that of oxytetracycline was only 1–5% when both compounds were administered orally to fish (158–161).

In rat, dog, and calves (162, 163), flumequine is glucuronidated and, to a lesser extent, is hydroxylated to 7-hydroxyflumequine (164). In sheep, flumequine is widely distributed in edible tissues; after a single intravenous injection of 12 mg/kg bw, residues in kidney were higher than those in liver and muscle at 24 h after drug administration (165).

Studies on flumequine administered to laying hens at a dosage of 200 mg/L water for 5 consecutive days showed that residues in eggs were present from day 2 of treatment to day 11 after the end of treatment (166). Higher accumulation of residues occurred in egg white than in the yolk. Concentrations in egg white increased with a tendency to plateau during the treatment, but in the yolk it dropped before the end of treatment (167). The slopes of those depletion curves were more pronounced for egg white than yolk; 4 days after the end of treatment, the ratio of the residue levels in those egg fractions became inverted, to proceed threafter in parallel lines.

The persistence of flumequine residues in eel plasma and tissues was also determined for a 44 day period following a single intramuscular injection (168). The time to reach maximum concentrations of flumequine in tissues (48–192 h) was comparable to that in plasma (96 h). Mean maximum concentrations in tissues ranged from 725 ppb in bone to 121,000 ppb in fat. These concentrations declined with time in all tissues to reach, 44 days after administration, the values of 769, 427, 238, 213, 197, 153, 89, and 85 ppb in liver, fat, muscle, plasma, spleen, skin, bone, and kidney, respectively.

In search of possible reservoirs of flumequine and oxolinic acid in fish, several tissues of salmon treated with the drugs were analyzed (169). The results showed that residues of these drugs were present in the fish tissues for prolonged periods after the end of treatment. It was found, however, that even when residues in muscle and liver were at the low ppb level, there were still quite high residues left in bone and skin. Residues of oxolinic acid were especially bound to bone and skin, whereas flumequine was bound to bone.

Another pertinent study (170) also showed that residues of quinolones could be present in certain tissues for a prolonged period after the end of medication. In this study, oxolinic acid and flumequine were especially entrapped in bone, enrofloxacin in skin, and sarafloxacin in both skin and bone. When salmon was treated with flumequine and oxolinic acid, highest residue levels of flumequine found in the backbone averaged 465 ppb and were detectable for 70 days posttreatment (171). Residues were also present in skin, back fat, and liver for 70 days posttreatment, but no residues could be found in muscle from fish sampled 48 days after treatment.

Following oral administration of 6 and 12 mg flumequine/kg/day for 5 days to trout at a temperature of 12°C, flumequine residues could be detected in muscle/skin by 2 days after the last treatment (172). The elimination was found to be temperature dependent. At 16°C, residues of the parent compound could be detected by the day 4 (0.083 ppm) after the last treatment, while at 7°C by the day 7 (0.084 ppm) after the last treatment. In trout, the hydroxylated metabolite of flumequine could not be found in any tissue (173).

The residue depletion profile of flumequine in trout seems to be quite similar to that in the sea bass (174). When flumequine was administered to seabass as a mixture with the feed at a dosage of 12 mg/kg bw for 5 days, residues of flumequine in muscle tissue could be detected by 36 h after the last treatment. The relatively high temperature of the sea water (21–25.3°C) in this study was suggested as the primary factor determining the rapid depletion of residues from the fish tissue. In another study (175), flumequine disappeared from muscle of sea bream at 240 h after the end of treatment, but showed a longer depletion rate from skin and vertebrae that behaved in fact as reservoir tissues. Much slower depletion profiles have been reported in studies carried out with Atlantic salmon (158, 170, 176), rainbow trout (177), and some wild fish caught in the vicinity of fish farms such as saithe and cod (178).

Marbofloxacin is a new fluoroquinolone intended for treatment of bovine respiratory disease by the oral or parenteral route, and for treatment of the masti-tis–metritis–agalactia syndrome in pigs by the parenteral route. The proposed dosage rate is 2 mg/kg bw/day for up to 5 days.

Marbofloxacin is well absorbed after oral or parenteral administration, and widely distributed to the tissues of several species (179, 180). In pigs, marbofloxa-cin is weakly bound to plasma proteins (<10%), whereas in calves binding in-creases to around 30%. It is excreted mostly unchanged in the urine. The extent of biotransformation is very limited and there are no significant species differ-ences in metabolism. The unmetabolized drug is the major component of the total residues found in both tissues and excreta, but some marbofloxacin conjugates are also present with small amounts of the desmethyl- and N-oxide metabolites.

When pigs and calves were subcutaneously given marbofloxacin, residues persisted in liver and kidney for up to 4 days posttreatment. Almost all of the residues detected in muscle and fat were due to the parent drug, whereas residues in liver and kidney were also due to drug-related metabolites as well. Residue depletion studies in dairy cows similarly treated showed that a proportion of 73–89% of the total residues in the milk was due to the parent marbofloxacin.

Nalidixic acid is a first-generation quinolone that exhibits antibacterial activity against various gram-negative bacteria. It has been used exclusively in Japan for treatment of vibriosis and furunculoses of plasmonids.

The pharmacokinetics and tissue levels of nalidixic acid were determined after oral administration of a single dose of 40 mg drug/kg bw to cultured rainbow trout and amago salmon held at 15°C (181). The absorption rate of the drug was found to be nearly equal for the two species and was completed within 48 h. Nalidixic acid could be detected in all tissues of both species at as early as 0.5 h after dosing.

In rainbow trout, maximum levels of the parent drug were observed in serum, liver, and kidney at 12 h after administration, whereas in muscle and bile these were observed at 24 and 48 h, respectively. In amago salmon, maximum levels of the parent drug occurred in serum, muscle, liver, and kidney at 24 h postdosing and in bile at 12 h. At their highest levels, the concentrations of nalidixic acid for both species were bile > liver > kidney > serum > muscle. Residues of the parent drug were present in all tissues of both species at 7 days after administration. At 10 days, residue levels in muscle, liver, and kidney were as low as 0.06, 0.14, and 0.09 ppm for trout and 0.13, 0.43, and 0.31 ppm for salmon, respectively. However, relatively high levels of the parent drug could still be detected in the bile of both species.

The glucuronide conjugate of nalidixic acid could be also seen in all tissues of both species. At 7 days postdosing, its levels in muscle, liver, and kidney were 0.07, 0.39, and 1.60 ppm for trout, and 0.14, 1.53, and 6.56 ppm for salmon, respectively. Considerable amounts of conjugated nalidixic acid were also observed in bile of both species even after 7 days postdosing.

Norfloxacin is a new water-soluble fluoroquinolone registered for veterinary use in several countries. It is commercially available as a dry powder for medication of drinking water and as a sterile injectable solution (182).

When norfloxacin was given to turkeys by oral, intramuscular, or intravenous routes, bioavailability was highest with the intramuscular route and lowest with the oral route (183). At the end of a 72 h medication with drinking water, mean tissue concentrations of norfloxacin were 0.48 ppm in the serum, 0.56 ppm in lungs, 3.2 ppm in liver, 0.68 ppm in kidney, 0.34 ppm in muscle, 0.40 ppm in spleen, 0.52 ppm in skin, 0.32 ppm in fat, and 50 ppm in feces. Residues of norfloxacin were not detected in any tissue sampled 72 h after the end of water medication.

When norfloxacin was administered orally or intravenously to healthy and *E. coli*-infected chickens, residues could be detected in tissues of both healthy and infected birds (184). Residual levels in infected birds were higher than those of healthy birds and remained longer in bile for 4 days after multiple administration. Bile, kidney, and liver accumulated the highest concentration of the drug.

When norfloxacin was given to broilers and laying hens, the highest residue concentrations were measured in tissues on day 5 of drug administration and on day 0 after the end of treatment (185). Concentrations were highest in liver at 4867 ppb and 4496 ppb on day 5 and day 0, respectively. On day 1 after the end of treatment, the level of norfloxacin decreased, with highest concentrations measured in the liver (76 ppb) and lowest in heart (17.5 ppb). By day 3, concentrations had fallen to 13 ppb in liver and 21.3 ppb in muscle. No residues were measured in tissues on days 6, 7, and 9 after the end of treatment except in muscle where 7.5 ppb was detected on day 9. The concentrations of norfloxacin measured in eggs increased steadily over the treatment period. Concentrations at days 3 and 4 of treatment were lower than those measured at day 1 after the end of treatment, with highest concentrations (103.5 ppb) detected in the egg yolk. Residual concentrations decreased steadily for the first 4 days after the end of treatment. By day 6, the concentrations measured were 12.2 ppb in yolk and 3.5 ppb in the egg white.

When norfloxacin was intramuscularly administered to calves, tissue concentrations were higher in kidney, liver, and muscle tissues at 4 h after the last dose (186). In body fluids other than bile and urine, norfloxacin concentration was lower than that in serum. None of the tissues sampled exceeded 1 ppm 24 h after the last administration; at 72 h and 120 h after the last administration, highest concentrations in liver were 60 and 80 ppb, respectively. Norfloxacin could not be detected in muscle at 120 h postmedication.

Oxolinic acid, a first-generation quinolone, has been authorized for use in fin fish, calves, swine, and poultry by the oral route. It may be given with the feed, the drinking water, or as a bolus. In 1991, 11.4 tons of oxolinic acid in addition to 5.7 tons of flumequine were used by the Norwegian aquaculture industry (187).

Oxolinic acid is quickly absorbed after oral administration, but its absorption is variable and dependent on animal species, drug formulation, diet, and disease status. After an oral dose of 10 mg/kg bw, bioavailability was approximately 82% in healthy chickens, but around 100% in diseased chickens. Oral bioavailability was also higher in swine and calves, but lower in fin fish and Atlantic salmon. The bioavailability of oxolinic acid given as medicated feed at a single dose 9–26 mg/kg bw to Atlantic salmon kept in seawater at 7.5–9°C was estimated to be 20–21% (188, 189).

When broiler chickens were given a single dose of 15 mg oxolinic acid/kg bw orally, mean residues in liver declined from 2160 ppb, 1 day after dosing, to 490 and 50 ppb at 3 and 6 days after dosing. Over the same time period, mean residues in kidney declined from 2380 ppb to 910 ppb and to 160 ppb, whereas residues in muscle decreased from 1460 ppb to 570 ppb and to 20 ppb. When laying hens were given oral doses of 15 mg oxolinic acid/kg bw/day for 5 days, mean residue in eggs were 5610 ppb 1 day after the cessation of treatment, and depleted to 1240 ppb at 3 days, 80 ppb at 6 days, and below 10 ppb at 9 day withdrawal.

When piglets were given feed containing oxolinic acid at a dosage equivalent to 15 mg/kg bw/day for 7 days, mean residues in liver, kidney, and muscle were 1080, 1350, and 1500 ppb, respectively, 1 day after the cessation of treatment, declining to below 25 ppb in all tissues at 3 day withdrawal.

In aquaculture, the salinity of the surrounding water appears to affect the pharmacodynamics of oxolinic acid in fish. Thus, the residue depletion profile of oxolinic acid in seawater coho salmon was similar to that observed in various seawater fish such as Japanese mackerel, red sea bream, yellowtail, and flounder

(190). However, tissue concentrations of the parent drug in the seawater rainbow trout decreased to undetectable levels by 72 h, whereas in the freshwater rainbow trout peaked at 48 h and were detectable for at least 244 h (191, 192). Both groups of trout metabolized oxolinic acid by the same pathway; oxolinic acid and the glucuronides of oxolinic acid, 7-hydroxy-oxolinic acid, and 6-hydroxy-oxolinic acid were the residues detected in the bile.

Residue depletion studies (193) in rainbow trout kept at a water temperature of 9–10°C and given feed containing oxolinic acid at a dosage equivalent to 12 mg/kg bw/day for 7 days showed that mean residues in muscle/skin depleted from 1970 ppb at day 1 after the end of treatment to 930 ppb at 2 day, 90 ppb at 4 day, and 50 ppb at 6 day withdrawal. When rainbow trout were given feed containing oxolinic acid at a dosage equivalent to 20 mg/kg bw/day for 5 days, mean residues in muscle at day 1 after the end of treatment were 1990 ppb for trout kept at a water temperature of 8.5–11.5°C and depleted to 540 ppb at 3 day, 40 ppb at 5 day, and 20 ppb at 7 day withdrawal. For trout kept at a water temperature of 17.1–19.6°C, mean residues in muscle at day 1 after the end of treatment were 2090 ppb, and depleted to 340 ppb at 3 day, 70 ppb at 5 day, and 60 ppb at 7 day withdrawal.

In a study in which rainbow trout were administered oxolinic acid for 7 days at a dosage of 12 mg/kg bw/day, drug level in muscle tissue was 0.03 ppm at 10 days withdrawal (194). In amago salmon held at 15°C and given a single oral dose of 40 mg/kg bw, oxolinic acid concentrations of 0.02 ppm could still be detected in muscle tissue at day 30 after administration (195). In yellowtail held at 24.5°C and administered oxolinic acid at a dose of 50 mg/kg bw, concentrations of 0.09 ppm and 0.17 ppm were recorded in muscle and kidney tissues, respectively, at day 8 posttreatment (196).

When rainbow trout were administered a single dose of 75 mg oxolinic acid/kg bw at 5, 10, and 16°C, the elimination was faster at higher water temperatures (197). Drug concentrations in muscle tissue declined to the detection limit of 0.01 ppm within 10 days at 16°C; at this temperature, however, the levels in kidney and liver persisted for 25 days. At 10°C, oxolinic acid was eliminated within 45 days postdosing, but at 5°C levels of 0.1–0.3 ppm were still present at day 55 after drug administration.

Different tissues of salmon treated with oxolinic acid in addition to flumequine were also analyzed in search of possible reservoirs of the drug (187). Results showed that low residue levels of oxolinic acid were present in muscle and liver for 2 months posttreatment. After that period, there were still quite high residues left in bone and skin. More than 6 months after the end of treatment, levels as high as 164 ppb were still present in the backbone and 35 ppb in the skin.

Sarafloxacin is another fluoroquinolone administered with the drinking water to poultry for treatment of bacterial diseases, or incorporated in fish feed at a dosage equivalent to 10 mg/kg bw for treatment of diseases such as furunculosis, vibriosis, and enteric redmouth.

Infeed treatments of Atlantic salmon held at 9–13°C with sarafloxacin at 10 mg/kg bw for 10 days or at 20 mg/kg bw for 5 days showed that the highest average concentrations of the parent drug in plasma, muscle, and liver were 0.14 ppm, 0.39 ppm, and 0.88 ppm, respectively, for the former treatment, and 0.40 ppm, 0.61 ppm, and 1.56 ppm, respectively, for the latter treatment (198). After withdrawal of the treatment, sarafloxacin concentrations in plasma and tissues declined rapidly. Sarafloxacin could not be detected in any plasma sample taken 6 days after the end of the medication. The corresponding time figures for muscle, skin, and liver tissues were 14 days, 20 days, and 22 days, respectively. The half-lives of sarafloxacin varied in the different tissues, being shortest in plasma and higher in ascending order in muscle, liver, and skin.

The distribution and elimination of radiolabeled sarafloxacin have been thoroughly examined in juvenile channel catfish orally dosed at 10 mg/kg bw for 5 consecutive days (199). At 3 h after the last dose, relative sarafloxacin concentration was greatest in the liver (4.06 ppm equivalents) and least in the residual carcass (1.13 ppm equivalents). Intermediate levels were found in the kidney (2.04 ppm equivalents), skinless fillet (1.71 ppm equivalents), and skin (1.51 ppm equivalents). Concentrations in edible skinless fillet were consistently among the lowest of all tissues examined. Highest mean concentrations of parent drug in the fillet tissue were found 12 h after administration of the last dose (2.27 ppm equivalents). Sarafloxacin constituted 80–90% of the extractable radioactivity from the fillet homogenates. The concentrations of parent sarafloxacin in samples taken at 72 h declined dramatically in liver (12-fold) and skinless fillet (29-fold) from values found in fish sampled at 24 h; the decline was much less in skin (2.6-fold), kidney (3.7-fold), and residual carcass (5-fold). After 72 h, the rate of loss of radioactivity from all tissues was much reduced. Residue concentrations were nearly constant or declined only slowly from all tissues in samples analyzed between 120 and 240 h. One exception to this trend was the increase in activity among all tissues from fish sampled at 168 h. Highest tissue concentrations at 240 h were found in the skin; lowest were in the skinless fillet. Sarafloxacin-equivalent concentrations in the skinless fillet were consistently the lowest of all the tissues examined from 72 to 240 h after dosing.

The effect of water temperature on the diffusion and metabolism of sarafloxacin has been also investigated in Atlantic salmon maintained at 15 or 5°C and given 10 mg/kg bw sarafloxacin hydrochloride daily for 5 days. At 5.5 days after withdrawal, residues in muscle of fish maintained at 15°C were below 50 ppb, whereas residues up to 166 ppb were found in muscle of fish maintained at 5°C. At the same time, residues in skin were in the range of less than 50–54 ppb for fish maintained at 15°C and less than 50 ppb for fish maintained at 5°C.

3.7 SULFONAMIDES AND DIAMINOPYRIMIDINE POTENTIATORS

Sulfonamides are a group of synthetic organic compounds that have played an important role as effective chemotherapeutics in bacterial and protozoal infections in veterinary medicine. Phthalylsulfathiazole, succinylsulfathiazole, sulfabromomethazine, sulfachlorpyrazine, sulfachlorpyridazine, sulfadiazine, sulfadimethoxine, sulfamethazine (sulfadimidine), sulfadoxine, sulfaethoxypyridazine, sulfaguanidine, sulfamerazine, sulfamethoxazole, sulfamethoxydiazine, sulfamethoxypyridazine, sulfamonomethoxine, sulfapyridine, sulfaquinoxaline, sulfathiazole and sulfisoxazole have all been used in food-producing animals (Fig. 3.7). They share a common chemical nucleus that is essential for the exhibited antibacterial activity and comes from sulfanilamide, the simpler member of the sulfonamide group; in this nucleus, the sulfonamide ($-SO_2NH_2-$) nitrogen has been designated as N^1, and the amino ($-NH_2$) nitrogen as N^4. Most sulfonamides have been synthesized by chemical substitution at the N^1 position since substitution at the N^4 position results, with certain exceptions, in compounds with greatly reduced antibacterial activity compared to their unsubstituted counterparts.

Parent sulfonamides are relatively insoluble in water but their sodium salts have greater water solubility than the parents compounds and are commonly included in commercial preparations. Indications for sulfonamides are wide owing to their wide spectrum of activity. They cover infectious diseases of the digestive and respiratory tracts, secondary infections, mastitis, metritis, and foot rot. Sulfonamides are administered to animals by all known routes at dosages noticeably higher than those for antibiotics. Sometimes several sulfonamides may be combined in only one preparation to ensure a wider range of activity and to reduce toxicity. Some sulfonamides are also used to treat bacterial infections in horses, cattle, sheep, goats, pigs, poultry, and fish in the form of potentiated formulations with synthetic diaminopyrimidines such as trimethoprim, ormetoprim, or baquiloprim. Trimethoprim is usually combined with sulfadiazine or sulfadoxine, whereas ormetoprim is combined with sulfadimethoxine, and baquiloprim with sulfamethazine. These formulations are believed to act synergistically on specific targets on bacterial DNA synthesis, with the sulfonamide blocking the conversion of p-aminobenzoic acid to dihydrofolic acid and the diaminopyrimidine inhibiting the conversion of dihydrofolic acid to tetrahydrofolic acid in the folic acid pathway, thus potentiating the antibacterial effects of the sulfonamide.

They are still widely used as feed additives for treatment or prevention of coccidiosis. In ruminants, sulfaquinoxaline, sulfadimethoxine, and sulfamethoxypyridazine are the most useful coccidiostats, although sulfachlorpyrazine, sulfathiazole, and sulfamonomethoxine are also highly effective. Additional coccidiostats or adjuvants such as amprolium, chlortetracycline, and ethopabate are often combined with sulfonamides for synergistic effects in poultry.

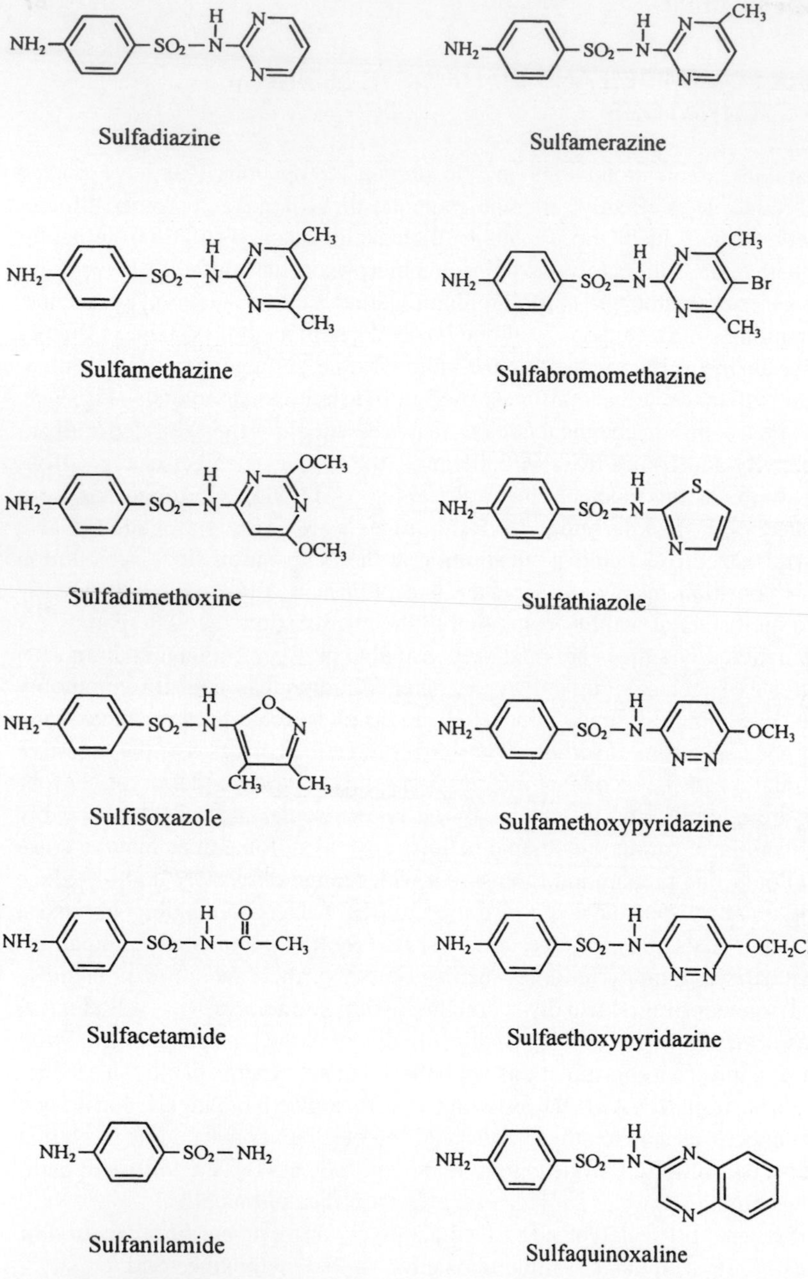

Sulfadiazine

Sulfamerazine

Sulfamethazine

Sulfabromomethazine

Sulfadimethoxine

Sulfathiazole

Sulfisoxazole

Sulfamethoxypyridazine

Sulfacetamide

Sulfaethoxypyridazine

Sulfanilamide

Sulfaquinoxaline

FIG. 3.7 Chemical structures of commonly used sulfonamides and diamino-pyrimidine potentiators.

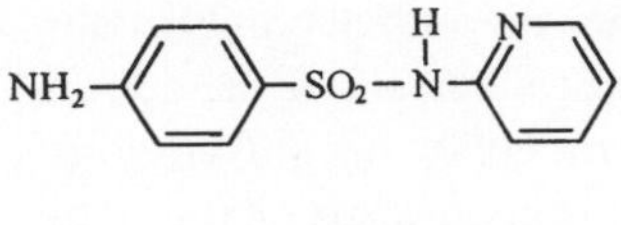

Sulfapyridine

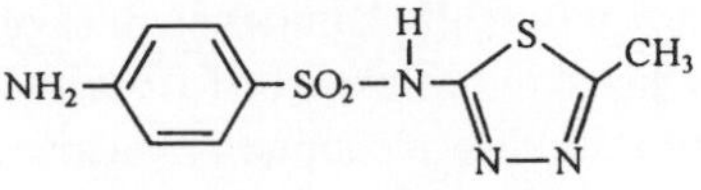

Sulfamethiazole

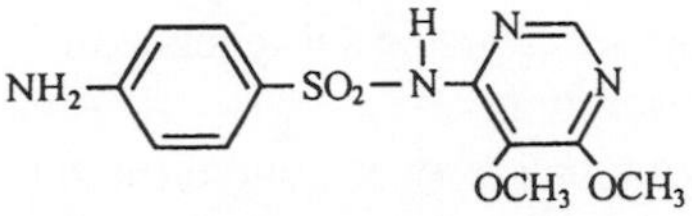

Sulfadoxine

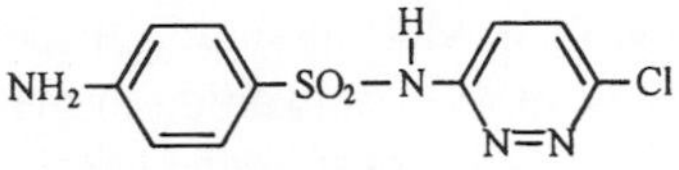

Sulfachloropyridazine

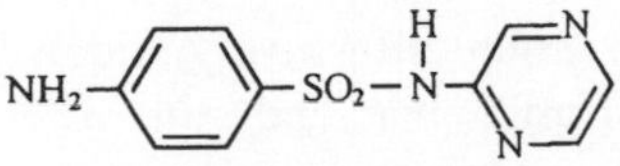

Sulfapyrazine

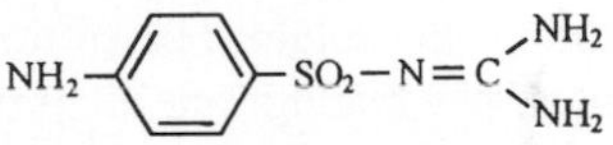

Sulfaguanidine

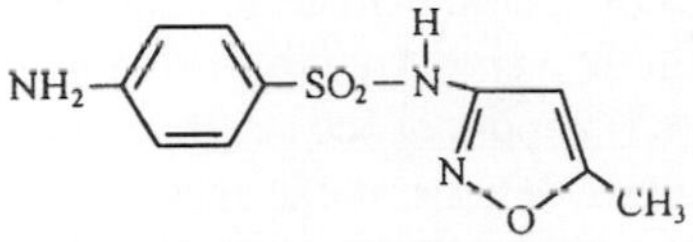

Sulfamethoxazole

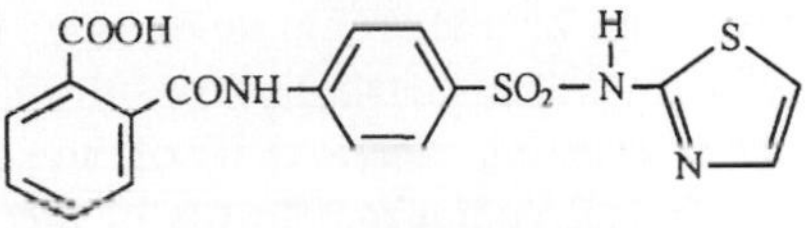

Phthalylsulfathiazole

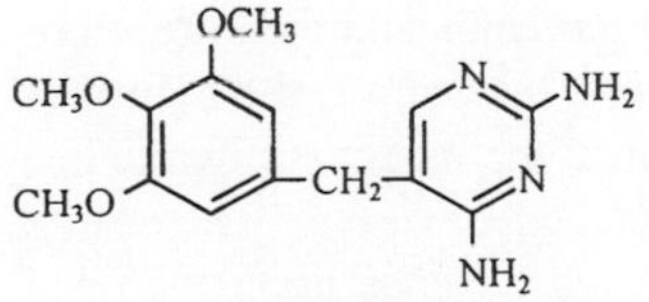

Trimethoprim

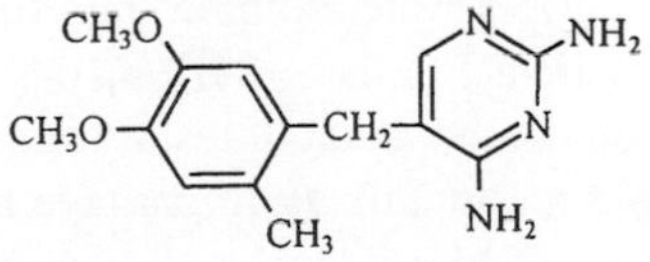

Ormetoprim

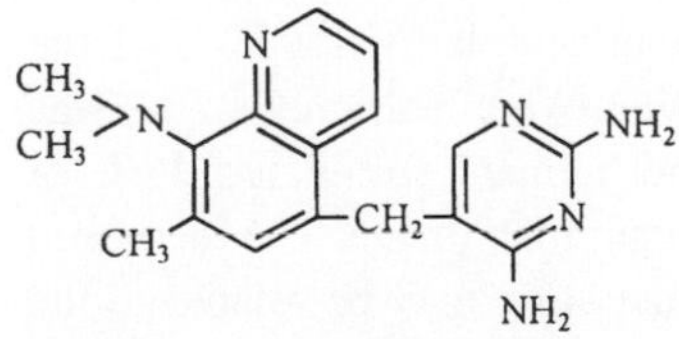

Baquiloprim

FIG. 3.7 *Continued*

Except for sulfonamides such as phthalylsulfathiazole and succinylsulfathi-azole, which are not absorbed from the intestine, most members of the sulfon-amide group follow a common pharmacological pattern. Following oral adminis-tration, absorption rates of sulfonamides are approximately proportional to their water solubility although these can vary between species. Thus, pigs and horses absorb sulfonamides move slowly than birds but better than cattle. Exceptions are sulfapyridine, which is slowly absorbed in most species, and sulfamethazine, which is second to sulfanilamide in the rate of absorption.

The absorption of sulfonamides by diseased animals may be quite different from that observed in healthy individuals of the same species. Experimental rumen stasis, produced by atropine, markedly reduced the absorption of sulfamethazine following its oral administration to sheep.

In addition, the solubilized sulfonamides as a group diffuse very widely into the tissues, penetrating into all fluids, including urine, bile, and milk. The degree of tissue penetration is influenced by several factors, including the ioniza-tion state and lipophilicity of the particular sulfonamide, the vascularity of the absorption site, and the degree of protein binding.

Metabolism of sulfonamides proceeds with acetylation, oxidation, conjuga-tion with sulfate or glucuronic acid, and cleavage at varying degrees of their heterocyclic rings. The metabolism of sulfonamides is important because it affects the antibacterial activity and toxicity of the compounds. In general, the acetylated, hydroxylated, and conjugated forms of the sulfonamides exhibit a marked de-crease in antibacterial activity compared to the parent compounds. The acetylated forms of all sulfonamides except those of sulfadiazine, sulfamerazine, and sulfa-methazine are less water-soluble than the parent compounds and thus are more likely to precipitate in the urine causing renal damage. In contrast, the hydroxy-lated and conjugated metabolites are more soluble than the parent sulfonamides, and therefore are less likely to damage renal tissues.

The extent to which a sulfonamide is acetylated depends upon the drug administered and the animal species. Acetylsulfathiazole is the principal metabo-lite found in the urine of cattle, sheep, and swine after enteral or parenteral administration of sulfathiazole. However, sheep can acetylate only 10% of the dose, while cattle can acetylate 32%, and swine 39%. When sulfamethazine was administered intravenously or orally to cattle, the animals eliminated 11% or 25% of the dose, respectively, in urine as N^4-acetylsulfamethazine. The increased acetylation that occurred following the oral administration may be related to the increased exposure of sulfamethazine to liver enzymes following its absorption into the portal circulation. The acetylation rate may also be affected by the health status of an animal. Thus, cows suffering from ketosis in cows acetylate sulfon-amides at much lower extent.

Oxidation of sulfonamide rings is another important metabolic process in certain species. Sheep eliminate 25% of an intravenous dose of sulfamethazine in the form of 4-hydroxymethyl-6-methyl-2-sulfanilamidopyrimidine, while cattle eliminate only 12% of the dose. In contrast, swine are unable to hydroxylate this drug since hydroxylated metabolites cannot not be found in urine after oral or intravenous administration of the compound. In addition, sulfonamides and their metabolites are often found in the urine in conjugated forms with glucuronic or sulfate acid, the amount of conjugation being dependent upon the individual drug and the animal species to which this is given. Conjugation commonly occurs at the N^1, N^2, or hydroxylation sites of the compounds. Ring cleavage, which also sometimes occurs, appears to be a minor metabolic pathway since only small amounts of degradation products are excreted in the urine.

Following their metabolic transformation, sulfonamides are eliminated in urine, feces, bile, and milk. However, the kidney is the organ primarily involved in the excretion of these drugs. Sulfonamide residues deplete from body tissues and fluids with widely variable velocity that depends on many factors including the nature of the compound, its formulation and the route of administration, and the animal species. Nevertheless, sulfonamide residues eliminate much earlier from liver, kidney, and milk than from muscle and fat. Withdrawal periods in meat and milk differ, therefore, for each sulfonamide.

Sulfadiazine is a relatively short-acting sulfonamide with an elimination half-life of about 3 h in cattle. The importance of this drug for control of furunculoses in fish is determined by its combined use with the potentiator trimethoprim.

When a single dose of radiolabeled sulfadiazine was administered to eels at 7°C (200), highest initial radioactivity was observed in blood, liver, kidney, and skin, with a tendency for accumulation in bile and skin. In another pharmacokinetic study (201) on sea-water rainbow trout fed a combination of sulfadiazine–trimethoprim, the elimination process for both sulfadiazine and trimethoprim rapidly reached a point at which only a small but persistent residue was left; at 8°C as opposed to 10°C, sulfadiazine was the more potent residue promoter, still being detected at 90 days posttreatment. This was suggested to be a result of the greater binding ability of sulfadiazine as a weak electrolyte. The authors proposed a withdrawal period for sulfadiazine–trimethoprim of 60 days at water temperatures above 10°C for tabled-size fish, and a prohibition on its use below 10°C for such fish.

Another study (202) of sulfadiazine pharmacokinetics in carp treated by the intraperitoneal route showed an elimination half-life of 17.5 h at 20°C. Both acetylation and hydroxylation metabolic pathways appeared to occur, but they only represented 2% and 0.41% of the dose, respectively. This is in strong contrast to the metabolism profile of sulfadiazine in mammals, where hydroxylation is much more important.

When sulfadiazine in addition with trimethoprim was fed to pigs, the absorption of trimethoprim from the gastrointestinal tract was faster than the absorption of sulfadiazine, whereas the elimination of trimethoprim was slower than that of sulfadiazine (203). One day after the last multiple-dose administration, the maximum tissue concentration of trimethoprim was 0.29 ppb and detected in liver, while the maximum tissue concentration of sulfadiazine was 0.23 ppb and detected in kidneys. Neither drug could be detected in any tissue at day 8 posttreatment.

Sulfamethazine (sulfadimidine) is perhaps one of the most widely used sulfonamides. It is employed largely in mass medication of pigs to control atrophic rhinitis and other infections, although it is also used in other species such as cattle. Beyond its therapeutic applications, sulfamethazine is widely used to promote growth in food-producing animals, although it is not approved for use in lactating dairy cows. This drug has been shown to be a thyroid nongenotoxic carcinogen in rodents.

Pharmacokinetic studies indicate that sulfamethazine is rapidly absorbed and excreted in farm animal species. The elimination is generally more rapid when the drug is injected than when it is administered orally with the feed or drinking water.

Sulfamethazine is metabolized by hydroxylation at the 5 and 6 positions of the pyrimidine ring and by acetylation–deacetylation pathways. After hydroxylation, the metabolites may become glucuronidated and also acetylated (204). In cows and calves (205), sulfamethazine is extensively metabolized into hydroxyl derivatives and, to a lesser extent, acetylated into N^4-acetylsulfamethazine. Hydroxylation of the 6-methyl group to form 6-hydroxymethylsulfamethazine dominates hydroxylation at the 5 position.

Sulfamethazine concentrations in plasma exceed those in muscle, kidney, or liver tissue, but run parallel to those in milk. The N^4-acetylsulfamethazine concentrations in muscle, kidney, and liver are always below those of the parent compound. In contrast, the 6-hydroxymethylsulfamethazine concentration in the kidney exceeds that of sulfamethazine.

Residue depletion studies (206) with lactating cows orally or intravenously dosed with 220 mg radiolabeled sulfamethazine/kg bw showed that the milk collected within 0–48 h after dosing accounted for 1.1–2.0% of the administered radioactivity. Besides the parent compound, milk was found to contain two metabolites: the N^4-lactose conjugate of sulfamethazine and the N^4-acetylsulfamethazine. A small amount of N^4-acetylsulfamethazine was also present in all of the tissues at 48 h postdosing. The parent compound was the major residue in blood, skeletal muscle, and adipose tissues. Liver and kidney were also found to contain a series of more polar metabolites similar to those isolated in the urine. They were characterized as products of various metabolic processes including oxidation of the methyl group to hydroxymethyl group followed by sulfate ester or hexuronic acid conjugation, conjugation at the N^1-position with an hexoze or hexuronic acid, hydroxylation at the 3-position of the benzene ring followed by hexuronic acid conjugation, and cleavage of the N^1-C bond to yield sulfanilamide.

When lactating cows were dosed orally or intravenously with sulfamethazine for 5 consecutive days (207), average concentrations of parent drug in the milk of the orally dosed cows were higher than in the milk of intravenously dosed cows during all stages of the withdrawal period. However, for both treatment groups, the concentration of the parent drug in milk decreased to less than 10 ppb at day 4 after the last dose. In addition, the concentrations of the N^4-lactose- and N^4-acetylsulfamethazine decreased to less than 10 ppb in the milk at day 3 posttreatment.

In swine, the acetylation pathway of sulfamethazine is predominant; the 6-hydroxymethylsulfamethazine metabolite could not be detected in plasma, edible tissues, and urine because it was also excreted in the form of the acetylated metabolite (205). The N^4-acetylsulfamethazine percentage in plasma and edible tissues of swine was relatively higher than that in calves, but its distribution pattern was similar in these two species. Other metabolites formed in swine were identified as the sulfamethazine-N^4-glucocide and desamino-sulfamethazine metabolites (208). The highest N^4-sulfamethazine concentrations were found in plasma, kidney, muscle, and liver tissue. Elimination of the parent drug and the N^4-acetylsulfamethazine metabolite from swine organs and tissues was rapid when plasma levels were high (10–14 h half-life), but much slower at lower plasma levels (3–9 days half-life); a withdrawal period of approximately 18 days was considered appropriate to meet the generally accepted tolerance level of 0.1 ppm for sulfonamide residues (209).

Laying hens eliminate sulfamethazine rapidly by metabolic pathways that include both hydroxylation and acetylation (205). Within 3 days of the last sulfamethazine administration, plasma concentrations of the drug and its metabolites fell below the level of 0.02 ppm. In eggs, increase of sulfamethazine in egg white and yolk occurs during the whole medication period. Residues of the parent drug could be detected in the eggs laid 7 days after the cessation of the administration (210). Traces of N^4-acetylsulfamethazine and hydroxyl metabolites were also detectable up to day 3 after drug withdrawal.

When sheep were injected intravenously with a single dose of 107 mg sulfamethazine/kg bw, total residues in muscle, liver, kidney, and fat declined rapidly to reach, after 5 days of withdrawal, a value of less than 0.1 ppm (211). In fish, the main metabolite is N^4-acetylsulfamethazine, although sulfamethazine is hydroxylated and acetylated only to a small degree.

Sulfadimethoxine is a low-dose, rapidly absorbed, long-acting sulfonamide that is effective in reducing mortality due to bacterial infections and coccidiosis in poultry and ruminants (212, 213). The drug is highly protein-bound (80–85%) and this probably contributes to its slow excretion.

After oral administration of sulfadimethoxine to poultry at a dosage of 100 mg/kg bw for 5 days, the drug was slowly eliminated causing accumulation in plasma and particularly in liver and kidney (212). Sulfadimethoxine residues could be reduced, however, to 0.1 ppm or less by day 8 after treatment in all chicken tissues, except kidney where they persist longer. This depletion profile is in line with that observed in another pertinent study (214). Following oral administration of the drug to young hens and turkeys, residues in tissues were undetectable at days 6 and 8 days, respectively (215). Significant levels of the N^4-acetylsulfadimethoxine metabolite could also be found in plasma, tissues, and feces, the maximum percentage of acetylation being attained within 7 days after drug withdrawal.

When sulfadimethoxine was orally administered to laying hens at doses of 1.0 or 0.5 g/L water for 5 days, drug residues accumulated in eggs to a large extent (216). This was attributed to the longer time period over which albumen formation occurs (217). Maximum concentrations in egg white and yolk could reach levels of more than 30 ppm and 9 ppm, respectively, during such a medication, but could also decline to below 0.1 ppm at day 4–6 or 7 posttreatment for egg white and yolk, respectively.

When sulfadimethoxine in addition to ormethoprim was administered through feed to Atlantic salmon for 5 consecutive days, plasma and tissue levels of both drugs reached steady-state levels between 3 and 8 days following initiation of medication (218). The highest average concentrations of sulfadimethoxine in plasma, muscle, liver, and kidney were 14.3, 17.7, 7.4, and 6.8 ppm, respectively, whereas the corresponding elimination half-lives were 20, 19, 62, and 45 h, respectively. On the other hand, the highest average concentrations of ormethoprim in plasma, muscle, liver, and kidney were 1.5, 3.7, 9.1, and 166.0 ppm, respectively, whereas the corresponding elimination half-lives were estimated at 63, 143, 95, and 410 h, respectively.

Sulfaquinoxaline, although largely superseded by more potent drugs, is still used for prevention and treatment of coccidiosis in turkeys, chickens, rabbits, and cattle. It is available as a powder for adding to drinking water or as a premix for inclusion in the feed for growth promotion purposes.

Feeding trials with rabbits orally administered 100 mg/kg bw sulfaquinoxaline twice daily for 5 days showed that the drug was preferentially accumulated in kidney and liver (219). The highest residue concentrations were observed 4 days after the start of drug feeding, whereas a posttreatment period of 7–8 days was required to reach 0.1 ppm in liver, kidneys, and plasma.

Sulfathiazole is available for oral use and is also included in some parenteral formulations in combination with other sulfonamides. It is also used as a feed additive for growth promotion purposes. It is more toxic than sulfamethazine and sulfadimethoxine but is safe when used as the phthalyl derivative.

Sulfathiazole has electrostatic properties similar to sulfamethazine, so that there is a tendency for nonmedicated feed to be contaminated during milling and on animal premises. These properties of the drug also make its use for treatment of foul brood in bees likely to contribute to the contamination of honey with sulfathiazole residues, especially if it is used during the months when honey production is in progress.

Sulfathiazole is rapidly absorbed from the gut, and rapidly excreted in the urine of animals. It is readily metabolized and residues of acetylsulfathiazole, small amounts of other unidentified polar metabolites, and the parent drug were all detected in plasma and urine of ruminants following administration (220).

Baquiloprim is a diaminopyrimidine derivative acting synergistically with sulfonamides (221). In cattle, it is used orally, intravenously, or intramuscularly for treatment of mastitis and infections of the respiratory and gastrointestinal tract, whereas, in swine, it is administered intramuscularly for treatment of the mastitis–metritis–agalactia syndrome and infections of the respiratory and gastro-intestinal tract.

Baquiloprim has a high oral bioavailability in animals where it is widely distributed in the body and slowly eliminated (222,223). In cattle, baquiloprim was reported to have a much longer half-life and a larger volume of distribution than trimethoprim (223). Both urine and bile are important routes of elimination.

Baquiloprim is extensively metabolized in the target animals to a variety of metabolites including desmethylbaquiloprim, bis-desmethylbaquiloprim, ba-quiloprim-1-N-oxide, baquiloprim-3-N-oxide, and 6-hydroxybaquiloprim. A high percentage of the total residues in liver, kidney, and injection site is covalently bound.

Baquiloprim residue depletion studies in cattle treated by oral and parenteral route and in swine treated by parenteral route showed that 14–42 days after administration, the parent compound amounted to a very small proportion of the total residues in liver, kidney, and at the injection site. This was also the case with all identified metabolites. The concentrations of the residues in fat and normal muscle were too low to permit examination of their presence. However, pig skin contained a relatively high proportion of the parent compound. Pigs generally showed a faster degradation and elimination profile than cattle at comparable times after administration, resulting in lower total and parent drug residue levels.

Trimethoprim, a structural analogue of the pteridine portion of dihydro-folic acid, is also a diaminopyrimidine derivative used extensively in food animal production for treatment of respiratory and alimentary tract infections. Although the half-life of trimethoprim is short in most species, when combined with a sulfonamide, particularly sulfadiazine or sulfadoxine, at a concentration ratio of 1:5, a pronounced clinical synergy is evident. Trimethoprim formulations are administered orally as a bolus, paste, or in the drinking water or in feed for calves, pigs, poultry, and fish at a dosage of 5 mg/kg bw. Parenteral formulations are also available for treatment of pigs, cattle, sheep, and goats at a dosage of up 3.8 mg/kg bw.

In all target species, trimethoprim is rapidly and almost completely absorbed, and widely distributed throughout the body after oral administration. A significant proportion of the residues in tissues consists of unmetabolized trimethoprim, but several metabolites including the 1-N-oxide, 3-N-oxide, 3-hydroxy, 4-hydroxy, and the α-hydroxy metabolites are also present, each metabolite comprising less than 5% of the total residues.

In gilts and hogs administered a single intramuscular injection at either the label or twice the label dose (224), no residues of trimethoprim were detected in any of the tissues of the market-ready hogs at day 3 or 10 after drug administration. In pigs fed medicated feed containing the equivalent of 5 mg trimethoprim/kg bw for 10 days, residues of the drug were detectable (limit of detection 15 ppb) only in one muscle sample (34 ppb) taken at day 3 after the end of treatment, and two samples of skin/fat taken at day 5 (31 ppb) and day 10 (27 ppb) after the end of treatment.

In calves given oral, intramuscular or intramammary doses of trimethoprim, total residues in all edible tissues fell well below 100 ppb by the 7 day after the last dose. In lactating cows intramammary infusions of 40 mg trimethoprim/quarter for three consecutive milkings resulted in mean residue concentrations in milk of 4749 ppb at 6 h after the first infusion, which declined to 215 ppb at 12 h after the first infusion. Twelve h after the second infusion, mean residue concentrations were 70 ppb. Six h after the last infusion, mean residue concentrations in milk were 2805 ppb whereas 18 h later, mean residue concentrations were 32 ppb. In goats given a single intravenous injection of 13 mg trimethoprim/kg bw, mean residue concentrations in muscle, liver, and kidney were 1100, 800, and 2100 ppb 3 h later.

In sheep given a single intramuscular injection of 5 mg trimethoprim/kg bw, mean residue concentrations in liver, muscle, and fat were 400, 30, and 40 ppb, respectively, 7 days after treatment. In broilers given oral doses of 7.5 mg radiolabeled trimethoprim/kg bw/day for 5 days, mean total residue concentrations in kidney, liver, muscle, fat, and skin declined from 1000, 1340, 110, 90, and 210 ppb at 1 day after the end of treatment to 60, 30, <10, <10, and 30 ppb at 7 days postdosing.

In fish, rates of absorption and elimination of trimethoprim are greatly dependent on water temperature. Rainbow trout given 220 mg radiolabeled trimethoprim/kg bw orally showed detectable residues in plasma within 6 h after dosing when kept at 15°C, but undetectable residues when kept at 7°C, even within 12 h after dosing. Higher residue concentrations were present in kidney than in skin, which, however, contained higher residue levels than blood. Biliary excretion was shown to be a major excretory pathway in rainbow trout, while excretion through the gill was of minor importance.

In another experiment with rainbow trout given oral trimethoprim at different dosage levels, the elimination half-life in plasma was found to be approximately 24 h (225). At 72 h, the average plasma residue levels ranged between 0.02 and 0.18 ppm. Trimethoprim concentration in plasma was two to three times lower than in muscle tissue. The highest trimethoprim concentrations at zero withdrawal time were observed in the kidney tissue.

In Atlantic salmon given feed containing trimethoprim at a dosage equivalent to 30 mg/kg bw/day for 10 days, residue concentrations in plasma peaked at around 12 ppm from day 7 to 10. Mean residue concentration in muscle was 10,740 ppb immediately after the end of treatment and declined to 100 ppb and 10 ppb after 300° and 400° days, respectively.

3.8 TETRACYCLINES

Tetracyclines are broad-spectrum antibiotics widely used in animal husbandry both for prevention and treatment of disease and as feed additives to promote growth. Three naturally occurring tetracyclines—chlortetracycline, oxytetracycline, and demeclocycline—have been isolated from fungi, and several others such as doxycycline, methacycline, minocycline, rolitetracycline, and tetracycline have been prepared semisynthetically by chemical manipulation of the basic hydronaphthacene ring of the tetracycline nucleus (Fig. 3.8). The objectives of these chemical manipulations have been to improve gastrointestinal absorption, increase tissue distribution, and prolong retention in the body. Currently, the only tetracyclines of routine use in cattle, pigs, sheep, goats, poultry, and fish are oxytetracycline, chlortetracycline, tetracycline, and doxycycline.

In food-producing animals, tetracyclines can be administered orally through feed or drinking water, parenterally, or by intramammary infusion. However, oral administration suppresses initially the ruminal fermentation of plant fiber. The absorption of tetracyclines can be further adversely affected by the presence of metallic ions in the gastrointestinal tract. All tetracyclines have an affinity for metallic ions and should not be administered with milk or high calcium levels in feed unless an upward adjustment in the dosage is made (226–228).

Tetracyclines are rapidly but moderately absorbed from the gastrointestinal tract. The degree of oral absorption of the various tetracyclines is also a function of the lipophilicity of the particular compound. The least lipophilic oxytetracycline is the least well absorbed and the most lipophilic doxycycline is the best absorbed, whereas the absorption of the other tetracyclines falls between these two extremes.

Some of the administered dosage is concentrated in liver, excreted in bile, and reabsorbed from the intestines so that a small amount may persist in the blood for a long time after administration, due to enterohepatic circulation. The persistence of tetracyclines in the blood following absorption is a surprising contrast to other antibiotics that are eliminated more rapidly. Some absorption of tetracyclines into the bloodstream may also occur following intramammary infusion.

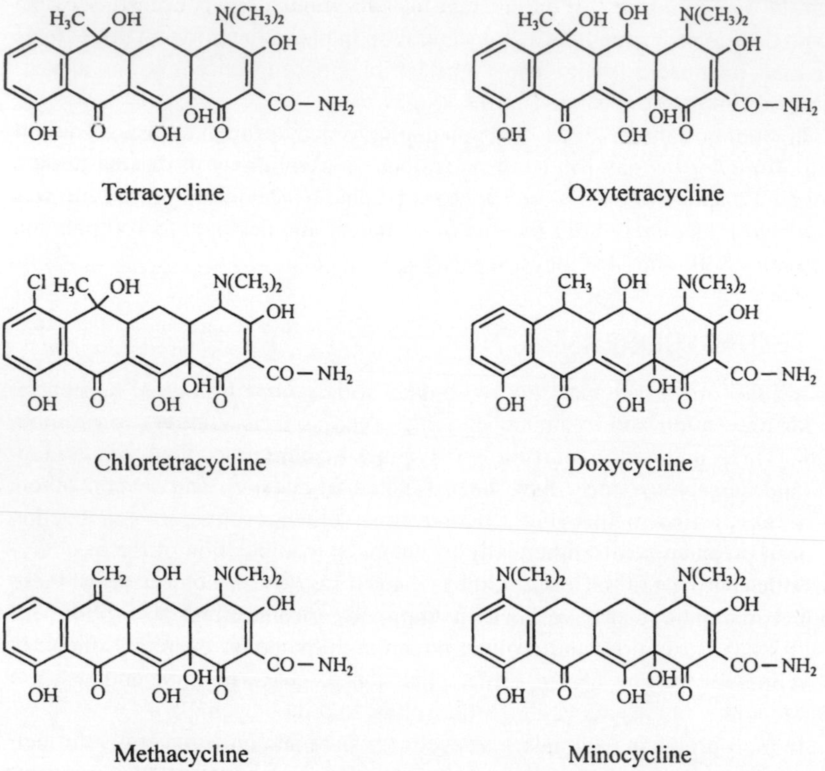

Tetracycline

Oxytetracycline

Chlortetracycline

Doxycycline

Methacycline

Minocycline

FIG. 3.8 Chemical structures of commonly used tetracyclines.

Following absorption through various routes of administration, the tetracyclines are widely distributed in the body, with highest levels in kidney and liver tissues. Because of their generally low lipophilicity, tetracyclines are not detectable in fat to any great extent. These antibiotics, owing to their affinity for calcium, also accumulate in poultry, swine, cattle, and fish bone tissue where residues have been detected following even subtherapeutic dosages (229–231). The tetracyclines can also be incorporated in egg shells. Hen and turkey eggs contained chlortetracycline for 3 days following oral or parenteral administration (232).

They undergo minimal or no metabolism and they are excreted in urine and feces either unchanged or in a microbiologically inactive form. Although there have been differences among individual tetracyclines as to their urinary and fecal excretion, these differences are not substantial. Tetracyclines are also eliminated in milk (233), attaining approximately 50–60% of the plasma concentration, the levels being often higher in mastitis milk. Peak concentrations occurred in milk 6 h after a parenteral dose, and traces were still present up to 48 h.

Oxytetracycline has a long history in human and veterinary medicine for the treatment and control of a wide variety of bacterial infections, and for its growth-promoting properties. It may be administered by any of the normal routes. It is readily absorbed from the intestine by most mammals but intestinal absorption in poultry is restricted. Oxytetracycline is most useful in that it readily disperses throughout the body, attaining therapeutic levels in most tissues and fluids within a short time.

Residue depletion studies in cattle, swine, sheep, chickens, and turkeys given oral forms of oxytetracycline including feed premixes, soluble powders, and tablets showed that residues in all edible tissues, with the exception of kidney, were cleared of detectable amounts of oxytetracycline within 5 days postdose. Injectable forms of oxytetracycline yielded higher residue levels that persisted longer than the oral forms, while long-acting formulations of oxytetracycline required extended withdrawal periods (234).

Following intramuscular injection of a long-acting oxytetracycline formulation, all sheep tissue residues were below the US tolerance of 0.1 ppm by 14 days after treatment (235). After intramuscular administration to a dairy cow of a single dose of 5 mg oxytetracycline/kg bw, residues were present in milk for as long as 4 days after dosing at concentrations ranging from 370 ppb at day 1 posttreatment to 10 ppb at day 4 posttreatment (233).

Oxytetracycline is particularly employed in swine production to treat animals for intestinal and respiratory bacterial diseases. In pigs given oxytetracycline orally at a dosage of 40 mg/kg bw/day for 5 days, residual oxytetracycline levels in all edible tissues of pigs were below 0.04 ppm within 4 days after withdrawal (236). Unlike with pigs, calves showed oxytetracycline concentrations of 0.40, 0.20, 0.060, and 0.027 ppm in kidney, liver, muscle, and fat, respectively, 5 days after cessation of the medication. When higher dosages (800–1600 ppm) were administered, oxytetracycline residues persisted in all edible tissues of pigs and calves for more than 7 days posttreatment.

Following medication via drinking water to laying hens for 7 days, oxytetracycline residues reached a maximum concentration in egg white faster than in yolk, although residues in yolk persisted longer (237). Thus, oxytetracycline residues could be detected in egg white and yolk for up to 13 days in both.

Oxytetracycline is also one of the most frequently used antibiotics in fish farming. Oxytetracycline residues exceeding the 0.1 ppm tolerance level were detected in raw catfish fillets 18 h after oral administration at a dosage of 37.5, 75, or 150 mg/kg fish for 10 days (238). Residues were highest in liver, followed by muscle, plasma, and kidney. Drug excretion was temperature dependent: higher residue levels could be detected at lower temperatures. In rainbow trout muscle, oxytetracycline residues were detectable for up to 28 days at 6–7°C, 15 days at 9–10°C, and 10 days at 12–13°C. In rainbow trout liver, residues could be detected for 28–35 days at 6–7°C and 15–21 days at 12–13°C (239).

Following a single intramuscular injection of oxytetracycline to European eels at a dosage of 60 mg/kg bw, maximum plasma oxytetracycline concentration (113 ppm) were achieved between 8 and 16 h after administration (240). At 3 weeks after drug administration, highest residue concentrations were in liver (21.7 ppb) and bones (30.2 ppb), whereas kidney, spleen, and muscle contained 6.0, 5.5, and 3.6 ppb. This experiment demonstrated that the pharmacokinetic profile of intramuscularly injected oxytetracycline to eel differed largely from those in rainbow trout, carp, and catfish (241).

When rainbow trout were kept at 5–10°C, oxytetracycline residues in muscle could be found for 29 days after intraperitoneal injection (4.2 mg/kg bw), for 23 days after continuous oral therapy (75 mg/kg bw/day for 14 days), and for 11 days after treatment with a single overdose (10.5 mg/kg bw) (242). Withdrawal periods of 60 days or 100 days have been proposed for fish treated with up to 75 mg/kg bw orally for no more that 10 days and kept at temperatures above 10°C or at 7–10°C, respectively (243,244).

Residual concentrations in tissues of cultured eel and ayu orally treated with oxytetracycline were found to be in the order of bone>liver>skin>muscle>serum for eel kept at 28°C, and in the order of liver>bone>skin>muscle>serum for ayu kept at 18°C (245). Although the elimination times from serum, muscle, and liver were calculated to be 4, 5, and 25 days for eel, and 10, 14, and 24 days for ayu, respectively, no elimination phase could be recognized up to 30 days for skin and bones of both fish.

Chlortetracycline has, in many respects, a pharmacological profile similar to that of oxytetracycline. Similarly to other tetracyclines, the main excretory routes are through the urinary system, biliary system, and intestine. Its higher biliary excretion rate makes chlortetracycline a better choice than oxytetracycline for liver infections.

Investigation of the metabolic fate of chlortetracycline in rats and dogs following oral, intravenous, or intraperitoneal administration showed that excreta from both species contained two main components—chlortetracycline and 4-epichlortetracycline—and a very small amount of isochlortetracycline (246). In spite of the finding of the 4-epi- and iso- isomers, it was concluded that chlortetracycline was not metabolized to any significant degree by rats and dogs. The presence of the chlortetracycline isomers in the excreta of those animals was ascribed to instability of the drug in the urine and feces rather than to metabolic transformation of the parent drug.

Tetracycline has activity similar but not identical to that of oxytetracycline and chlortetracycline. It may be administered by all the usual routes but absorption from the gastrointestinal tract is better than from intramuscular injection. Blood levels are higher and are maintained longer than those following equal doses of oxytetracycline and chlortetracycline.

Metabolism studies in dogs and rats with radiolabeled tetracycline showed that with the exception of metal–chelate formation, tetracycline was chemically unaltered by the rat (247). Organ extracts from dosed animals were not found to contain metabolic products of tetracycline. Dog urine also contained unchanged drug, indicating that metabolic transformation of tetracycline had not occurred.

After a single oral or intravenous administration of tetracycline to chickens at dosage rates of 100 mg/kg or 20 mg/kg bw, respectively, residue concentrations in muscle, kidney, and liver tissues were 0.03, 0.13, and 0.05 ppm, respectively, at 5 days posttreatment (248). Following intramuscular injection of tetracycline and oxytetracycline to goats at a dosage of 15 mg/kg bw at 24 h intervals for 4 days, residual levels of both drugs could be found in milk by day 4 after the last administration (249). The concentration of tetracycline at this time was 0.913 ppm, while that of oxytetracycline was 0.459 ppm in the milk.

Doxycycline tends to be more active against some bacteria than other tetracyclines. This is probably due to its slower excretion rather than to enhanced oral absorption. Doxycycline is used in cases where cost is unimportant. It is a very lipophilic drug that shows a high bioavailability, being almost completely absorbed after oral administration to different animal species except chickens (250, 251).

After oral administration, doxycycline is rapidly and well absorbed from the gastrointestinal tract. It has a half-life of 15–22 h, which is longer than that of other tetracyclines. Following administration by various routes, doxycycline is widely distributed in the body, with highest levels in kidney and liver, besides bones and dentine. Doxycycline may be metabolized for up to 40%, and is largely excreted in feces via bile and intestinal secretion.

From residue data with pigs, poultry, and cattle after oral administration, and with cattle after intravenous administration, it appears that the distribution profile of doxycycline in these animals is roughly comparable to that of oxytetracycline. Highest residue concentrations are found in kidney, followed by liver, skin, fat, and muscle. Tissue depletion studies in pigs treated intramuscularly with doxycycline at a 10 mg/kg bw dose for 4 days showed that the parent compound was absorbed and efficiently distributed in tissues (252). The concentrations of doxycycline detected in lung, muscle, liver, and kidney tissues at day 6 after treatment were 0.067, 0.047, 0.18, and 0.47 ppb, respectively; detectable doxycycline residues were not present in fat at that withdrawal time.

Residue studies (253) performed on calves after oral administration at a dosage of 10 mg/kg bw/day for 5 days showed that residues of the drug could remain in kidney and liver tissues for more than 14 days after cessation of the medication. Following a single oral or intravenous administration of doxycycline to chickens at dosage rates of 100 mg/kg or 20 mg/kg bw, respectively, residue concentrations in muscle, kidney, and liver tissues were 0.06, 0.17, and 0.12 ppm, respectively, at day 5 posttreatment (254).

3.9 MISCELLANEOUS

Novobiocin (Fig. 3.9) is a narrow-spectrum antibiotic with antibacterial activity against many gram-positive pathogens. It is frequently used, in combination with penicillin, for treatment of bovine mastitis by intramammary infusion of 200 mg/quarter in two quarters, and to control fowl cholera and staphylococcal infections in chickens and turkeys at a level of 200–350 g/ton in feed.

Upon intramammary administration to cattle, novobiocin is rapidly absorbed and excreted through milk, feces, and urine. Detectable residues are present in milk for a few days after intramammary infusion, the elimination being highly depended on dosage and formulation. One day after treatment, the concentrations of microbiologically active residues in the liver, kidney, and udder tissue were in the range 1–4 ppm, whereas concentrations in muscle and fat were below 0.1 ppm.

Polymyxin B and colistin (polymyxin E) (Fig. 3.9) are the least toxic of the five polymyxin antibiotics designated alphabetically A–E. Both polymyxin B and colistin are complex polypeptide compounds with specialized activity against gram-negative organisms but they are both nephrotoxic. Topical application and oral administration are more commonly used routes. Polymyxin B is used widely in ointments for topical applications and may be effective in case of mastitis, but it seldom is administered parenterally because of the possibility of renal toxicity.

Colistin is used primarily for oral treatment of *E. coli* infections in calves and pigs. Commercial formulations of colistin consist of two main components: colistin A and colistin B. The ratio between these two components is not constant, while small amounts of other related components are also present as minor constituents. Both polymyxin B and colistin have been frequently used orally in combination with bacitracin or neomycin.

Absorption of polymyxins from the gastrointestinal tract is slow and limited so that the usual oral dosage do not produce detectable plasma concentrations. However, polymyxins are readily absorbed when injected intramuscularly or subcutaneously. Almost the whole of any oral dose is destroyed in the intestine and only small amounts are recovered from the feces in an active form.

In chickens, residues in serum were detectable for up to 6 h after administration in the drinking water. In contrast, residues of colistin were detectable in serum for up to 24 h after intramuscular or intravenous administration to calves and dairy cows. In calves, bioavailability approached 100% after intramuscular administration.

Polymyxins are eliminated primarily through kidneys and, therefore, there is a tendency for tissue accumulation in case of renal insufficiency. Renal elimina-

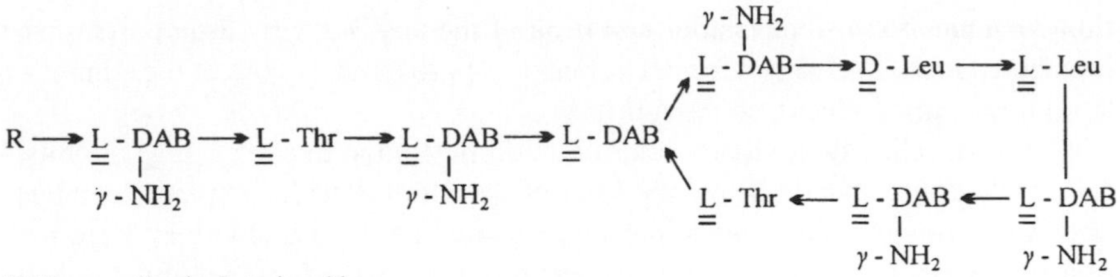

$$\gamma - NH_2$$
$$|$$
$$L - DAB \longrightarrow D - Leu \longrightarrow L - Leu$$

$$R \longrightarrow L - DAB \longrightarrow L - Thr \longrightarrow L - DAB \longrightarrow L - DAB$$
$$\underset{\gamma - NH_2}{|} \qquad \underset{\gamma - NH_2}{|}$$

$$L - Thr \longleftarrow L - DAB \longleftarrow L - DAB$$
$$\underset{\gamma - NH_2}{|} \qquad \underset{\gamma - NH_2}{|}$$

DAB = α,γ-diaminobutyric acid

Colistin

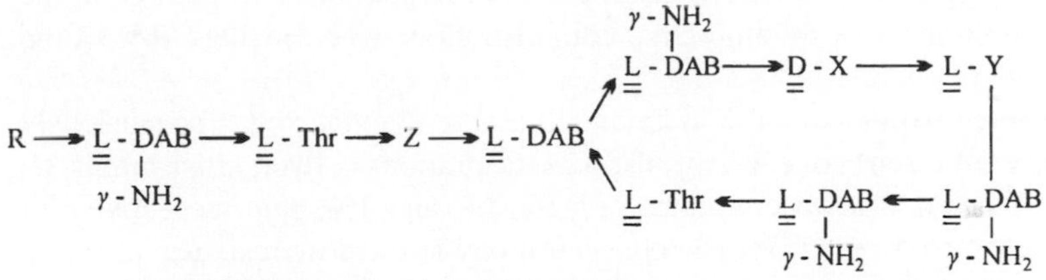

$$\gamma - NH_2$$
$$|$$
$$L - DAB \longrightarrow D - X \longrightarrow L - Y$$

$$R \longrightarrow L - DAB \longrightarrow L - Thr \longrightarrow Z \longrightarrow L - DAB$$
$$\underset{\gamma - NH_2}{|}$$

$$L - Thr \longleftarrow L - DAB \longleftarrow L - DAB$$
$$\underset{\gamma - NH_2}{|} \qquad \underset{\gamma - NH_2}{|}$$

DAB = α,γ-diaminobutyric acid

Polymyxin

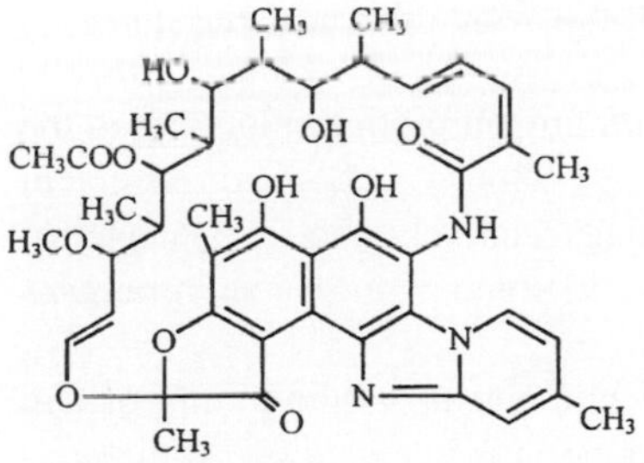

Rifaximin

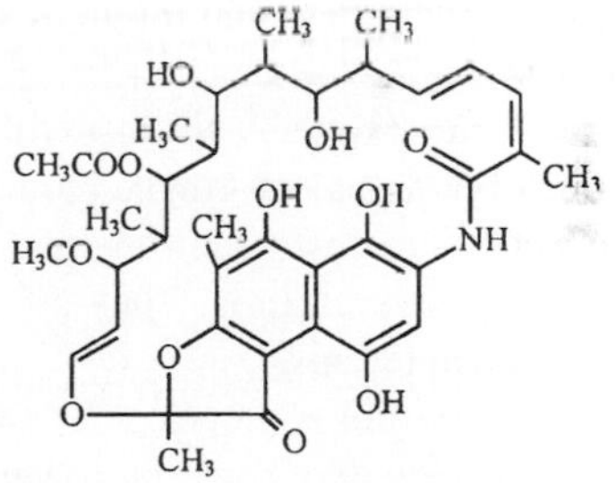

Rifamycin SV

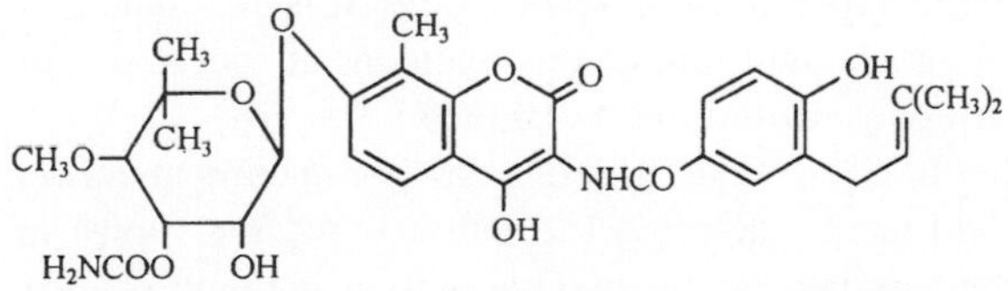

Novobiocin

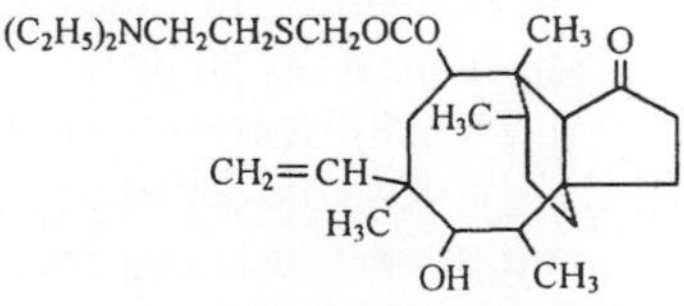

Tiamulin

Fig. 3.9 Chemical structures of colistin, polymyxin, rifaximin, rifamycin SV, novobiocin, and tiamulin.

tion continues for 1–3 days after cessation of therapy, but very little polymyxin is excreted in the unchanged form. Ultimately, approximately 60% of the administered dose can be recovered from urine.

Residues in edible tissues after oral administration to calves, pigs, rabbits, and chickens are usually below the limit of detection. Residue depletion studies in calves following intravenous injection showed that liver and kidney were the tissues containing the highest residue concentrations, in the form mainly of bound residues. Residues in milk following intramuscular administration to dairy cows were detectable for the first two to six milkings after treatment. Residues after intramammary infusion were significantly higher but undetectable by the seventh milking after treatment. In sheep milk, peak concentrations of 2 ppm could be attained within 2 h after intramuscular administration; approximately 10% of the residues were bound.

When colistin in addition to amoxicillin was administered subcutaneously to turkeys for 4 consecutive days, colistin concentrations in liver, kidney, muscle, and subcutaneous tissue were about 117, 92, 67, and 100 ppb, respectively, 1 day after the final dose (255). The concentrations of the drug residues increased by the 9th–14th day to decline slowly thereafter. However, the drug was still present at low concentrations in the kidneys of all birds and in the livers of 2 birds 30 days after the end of treatment. Residues in eggs from hens given colistin sulfate in the drinking water were below the limit of detection, whereas significant residues could be found for up to 8 days in eggs following intramuscular injection to hens.

Rifamycin SV, rifampicin, and rifaximin are antibiotics belonging to the group of naphthalene-ringed ansamycins (Fig. 3.9). Rifamycin SV and rifampicin are active against gram-positive bacteria, being relatively ineffective against gram-negative bacteria. They are both available in some countries as intramammary formulations.

Rifaximin possesses a broad spectrum of action against both gram-positive and gram-negative bacteria. In veterinary medicine, it is intended for administration by intramammary and intrauterine route in cattle, for treatment and prevention of mastitis during the dry period (100 mg rifaximin per quarter), and for treatment of postpartum metritis (50–200 mg per animal), respectively. It is also intended for topical use in cattle, sheep, goats, and rabbits for treatment of foot and skin bacterial diseases (0.34–2.44 mg/kg bw/day for 5–10 days).

Residue depletion studies of rifaximin in lactating cows or in cows at drying off showed that the drug could not be detected (detection limit, 0.01 ppm) in plasma or milk following intramammary treatment. Oral or topical administration of rifaximin also led to a negligible systemic absorption of the active ingredient.

Rifaximin could not be detected in plasma of pigs, cattle, and rabbits during and after repeated dermal applications. In addition, rifaximin could not be detected in milk after topical application. Due to its physicochemical properties, rifaximin, which is a lipophilic compound, is ionized in plasma so that its ability to circulate through the membranes and to penetrate in edible tissues is negligible.

Tiamulin (Fig. 3.9) is a semisynthetic derivative of the diterpene antibiotic pleuromutilin (255). Its antibacterial profile is poor, but it is active against gram-positive organisms and mycoplasmas. Tiamulin is used for treatment of swine dysentery and pneumonia, naturally occurring mycoplasmosis in poultry and swine, and for growth-promotion purposes (256). It is used as a hydrogen fumarate salt for administration in drinking water, or as a premix for addition to feeds at a dosage rate of 8.8 mg/kg bw/day. It is also available for parenteral administration at a dosage of 10–15 mg/kg bw.

The incompatibility of tiamulin with monensin, narasin, and salinomycin in chickens and turkeys is well documented. The toxicity of this combination in poultry may be due to interference produced by tiamulin to the metabolism of these polyether anticoccidials (257, 258).

Tiamulin is well absorbed when given orally, and is excreted mainly in bile within 28 h. The withdrawal period after oral administration to pigs is 5 days, to allow for excretion of metabolites. However, when tiamulin is administered in combination with oxytetracycline, the elimination of tiamulin residues from tissues is slightly prolonged, thus maintenance of a withdrawal period of 2 weeks is required from the public health point of view, based on an analysis of the elimination profile (259).

When tiamulin was given to farm animals by injection, mean elimination half-lives were 3, 3.3, 4.6, and 3.6 h in cattle, buffalo, sheep, and goats, respectively (260, 261). Tiamulin could not be detected at 24 h posttreatment.

REFERENCES

1. N.A. Botsoglou, and D.J. Fletouris, in Handbook of Food Analysis (L.M.L. Nollet, Ed.), Marcel Dekker, New York, p. 1171 (1996).

2. M.A. Sande, and G.L. Mandell, in The Pharmacological Basis of Therapeutics (A.G. Gilman, L.S. Goodman, T.W. Rall and F. Murad, Eds.), MacMillan Publishing Co., London, p. 1151 (1985).

3. J.E.F. Reynolds, Martindale, The Extra Pharmacopeia (J.E.F. Reynolds, Ed.), 30th Edition, The Pharmaceutical Press, London, p. 113 (1993).

4. S. Soback, and N. Isoherranen, J. Vet. Pharmacol. Ther., 20:295 (1997).

5. A.M. Ristuccia, in Antimicrobial Therapy (A.M. Ristuccia and B.A. Cunha, Eds.), Raven Press, New York, p. 305 (1984).

6. J.R. Lockyer, A. Bucknall, and I.C. Shaw, in Residues of Veterinary Drugs in Food, Proc. Euroresidue Conf., Noordwijkerhout, May 21–23, 1990 (N. Haagsma, A. Ruiter, and P.B. Czedik-Eysenberg, Eds.), Fac. Vet. Med., Univ. Utrecht, The Netherlands, p. 254 (1990).

7. T.B. Barragry, in Veterinary Drug Therapy (T.B. Barragry, Ed.), Lea & Febiger, PA (1994).

8. H. Umezawa and S. Kondo, in Aminoglycoside Antibiotics (H. Umezawa and I.R. Hooper, Eds.), Springer-Verlag, New York, p. 267 (1982).
9. G. Ziv, B. Kurtz, R. Risenberg, and A. Glickman, J. Vet. Pharmacol. Ther., 18: 346 (1995).
10. A. Vlietstra, D. Masman, and O. Steijger, in Residues of Veterinary Drugs in Food, Proc. Euroresidue II Conf., Veldhoven, May 3–5, 1993 (N. Haagsma, A. Ruiter and P.B. Czedik-Eysenberg, Eds.), Fac. Vet. Med., Univ. Utrecht, The Netherlands, p. 670 (1993).
11. R. Aerts, P. Storm, S. Hensen, G. de Snayer, J. Verbeek, G. Bongaerts, and U. Schnorf, Proc. of the 6th EAVPT Inter. Congress (P. Lees, Ed.), European Association for Veterinary Pharmacology and Therapeutics, Blackwell Scientific Publications, Edinburgh, UK, p. 217 (1994).
12. W.M. Pedersoli, J. Jackson, and R.A. Frobish, J. Vet. Pharmacol. Ther., 18:457 (1995).
13. J.E. Riviere, A.L. Craigmill, and S.F. Sundlof, in Handbook of Comparative Pharmacokinetics and Residues of Veterinary Antimicrobials (J.E. Riviere, A.L. Craigmill, and S.F. Sundlof, Eds.), CRC Press, Inc., Boca Raton, FL, p. 532 (1991).
14. G. Andreini, and P. Pignattelli, Veterinaria, 21:51 (1972).
15. G.C. Brander, D.M. Pugh, R.J. Bywater, and W.L. Jenkins, in Veterinary Applied Pharmacology and Therapeutics (G.C. Brander, D.M. Pugh, R.J. Bywater, and W.L. Jenkins, Eds.), 5th Edition, Balliere Tindall, London, UK (1991).
16. World Health Organization, in Residues of Some Veterinary Drugs in Animals and Foods, Forty-second Meeting of the Joint FAO/WHO Expert Committee on Food Additives, Food and Agriculture Organization of the United Nations, FAO Food and Nutrition Paper No 41/6, Geneva (1994).
17. R.E. Hornish, R.D. Roof, J.R. Wiest, T.S. Arnold, T.J. Gilbertson, and H.A. Deluyker, in Residues of Veterinary Drugs in Food, Proc. Euroresidue III Conf., Veldhoven, 1996 (N. Haagsma, and A. Ruiter, Eds.), Fac. Vet. Med., Univ. Utrecht, The Netherlands, p. 516 (1996).
18. R.H. Teske, L.D. Rollins, and G.G. Carter, J. Am. Vet. Med. Assoc., 160:873 (1972).
19. P.B. Hammond, J. Am. Vet. Med. Assoc., 122:203 (1953).
20. C.D.C. Salisburry, in Chemical Analysis for Antibiotics Used in Agriculture (H. Oka, H. Nakazawa, K.-I. Harada, and J.D. MacNeil, Eds.), AOAC International, Arlington, p. 310 (1995).
21. H.P. Lambert, and F.W. O'Gray, in Antibiotic and Chemotherapy (H.P. Lambert, and F.W. O'Gray, Eds.), 6th Edition, Churchill Livingstone, Edimburgh, UK, p. 136 (1992).
22. A.M. Baradat, J. Alary, and J.P. Cravedi, in Residues of Veterinary Drugs in Food, Proc. Euroresidue II Conf., Veldhoven, May 3–5, 1993 (N. Haagsma, A. Ruiter and P.B. Czedik-Eysenberg, Eds.), Fac. Vet. Med., Univ. Utrecht, The Netherlands, p. 160 (1993).
23. A.A. Yunis, Adv. Intern. Med., 15:357 (1969).
24. Official Journal of the European Communities, No. L287, Brussels, p. 1 (1994).
25. Code of Federal Regulations, Title 21, Office of the Federal Register, National Archives and Records Administration, US Government Printing Office, Washington, DC, Sec. 530.41 (1997).

26. B. Yohannes, K.H. Korfer, J. Schad, and I. Ulbtich, Arch. Lebensmittelhyg., 34:1 (1983).
27. H.J. Keukens, W.M. Beek, and M.M.L. Aerts, J. Chromatogr., 352:445 (1986).
28. P. Sanders, P. Guillot, M. Laurentie, M. Dagorn, J. Manceau, and C. Gaudiche, in Residues of Veterinary Drugs in Food, Proc. Euroresidue II Conf., Veldhoven, May 3–5, 1993 (N. Haagsma, A. Ruiter and P.B. Czedik-Eysenberg, Eds.), Fac. Vet. Med., Univ. Utrecht, The Netherlands, p. 611 (1993).
29. M.P. Laurentie, J. Manceau, and P. Sanders, Proc. of the 6th EAVPT Inter. Congress (P. Lees, Ed.), European Association for Veterinary Pharmacology and Therapeutics, Blackwell Scientific Publications, Edinburgh, UK, p. 219 (1994).
30. A.J. Glasko, W.H. Edgerton, W.A. Dill, and W.R. Lenz, Antib. Chemother., 5:234 (1952).
31. C.D.C. Salisbury, J.R. Patterson, and J.D. MacNeil, Can. J. Vet. Res., 52:15 (1988).
32. O.N. Mestorino, M.C. Alt, J.A. Speroni, and J.O. Errecalde, Proc. of the 6th EAVPT Inter. Congress (P. Lees, Ed.), European Association for Veterinary Pharmacology and Therapeutics, Blackwell Scientific Publications, Edinburgh, UK, p. 218 (1994).
33. M.H. Costa, M.E. Soares, J.O. Fernandes, M.L. Bastos, and M. Ferreira, in Residues of Veterinary Drugs in Food, Proc. Euroresidue II Conf., Veldhoven, May 3–5, 1993 (N. Haagsma, A. Ruiter, and P.B. Czedik-Eysenberg, Eds.), Fac. Vet. Med., Univ. Utrecht, The Netherlands, p. 246 (1993).
34. J.P. Cravedi, G. Heuillet, J-C. Peleran, and J-M. Wal, Xenobiotica, 15:115 (1985).
35. J.P. Cravedi, and M. Baradat, Comp. Biochem. Physiol, 100C:649 (1991).
36. G. Barba, F. Bruno, and G. Frigerio, Min. Med., 62:336 (1971).
37. D. van Beers, E. Schoutens, M.P. Vanderlinden, and E. Yourassowsky, Chemotherapy, 21:73 (1975).
38. G. Della Rocca, P. Anfossi, L. Tomas, and J. Malvisi, J. Vet. Pharmacol. Ther., 20:316 (1997).
39. Food and Drug Administration, in Compliance Program Guidance Manual, National Drug Residue Milk Monitoring Program, Food and Drug Administration, Rockville, MD, Sec. 7303.039 (1997).
40. E. Lavy, G. Ziv, S. Soback, A. Glickman, and M. Winkler, Acta Vet. Scand., 87: 133 (1991).
41. R.D. Lobell, K.J. Varma, J.C. Johnson, R.A. Saams, and D.F. Gerken, J. Vet. Pharmacol. Ther., 17:253 (1994).
42. A. Rios, M.R. Martinez-Larranaga, and A. Anadon, J. Vet. Pharmacol. Ther., 20: 182 (1997).
43. H. Fukui, Y. Fujihara, and T. Kano, Fish Pathology, 22:201 (1987).
44. B. Martinsen, T.E. Horsberg, K.J. Varma, and R. Sams, Aquaculture, 112:1 (1993).
45. K.J. Varma, I. Sutherland, T.E. Horsberg, B. Martinsen, R. Nordmo, and R. Sams, Proc. of the 6th EAVPT Inter. Congress (P. Lees, Ed.), European Association for Veterinary Pharmacology and Therapeutics, Blackwell Scientific Publications, Edinburgh, UK, p. 220 (1994).
46. L.P. Pinault, L.K. Millot, and P.J. Sanders, J. Vet. Pharmacol. Ther., 20:297 (1997).
47. H.T. Clarke, J.R. Johnson, and R. Robinson, in The Chemistry of Penicillin (H.T. Clarke, J.R. Johnson, and R. Robinson, Eds.), Princeton University Press, Princeton, NJ (1949).

48. F.P. Doyle, and J.H.C. Nayler, in Penicillins and Related Structures. Advances in Drug Research, Vol. 1 (N.J. Harper, and A.B. Simmonds, Eds.), Academic Press, NY (1964).

49. J.P. Hou, and J.W. Poole, J. Pharm. Sci., 60:503 (1971).

50. D.J. Tipper, in β-Lactam Antibiotics for Clinical Use (S.F. Queener, J.A. Webber, and S.W. Queener, Eds.), Marcel Dekker, New York (1986).

51. D. Mercer, H.F. Righter, and G.C. Carter, J. Am. Vet. Med. Assoc., 159:61 (1971).

52. W.A. Moats, E.W. Harris, and N.C. Steele, J. Agric. Food Chem., 34:452 (1986).

53. W. Jaksch, Dtsch. Tieraertzl. Wochenschr., 68:466 (1961).

54. P.B. English, Vet. Rec., 77:810 (1965).

55. J.F.M. Nouws, Ann. Res. Vet., 21:145S (1990).

56. B. Moreno, and A. Calles, An. Bromatol., 32:22 (1980).

57. World Health Organization, in Residues of Some Veterinary Drugs in Animals and Foods, Thirty-sixth Meeting of the Joint FAO/WHO Expert Committee on Food Additives, Food and Agriculture Organization of the United Nations, FAO Food and Nutrition Paper No 41/3, Rome, p. 1 (1990).

58. J.P. Moretain, and J. Boisseau, Food Add. Contam., 1:349 (1984).

59. D.J. Fletouris, J.E. Psomas and A.J. Mantis, J. Agric. Food Chem., 40:617 (1992).

60. J.P. Moretain, and J. Boisseau, Food Add. Contam., 6:79 (1989).

61. H.D. Mercer, L.D. Rollins, M.A. Garth, and G.G. Carter, J. Am. Vet. Med. Assoc., 158:776 (1971).

62. G.O. Korsud, J.O. Boison, M.G. Papich, W.D.G. Yates, J.D. Macneil, E.D. Janzen, R.D.H. Cohen, J.J. Mckinnon, D.A. Landry, G. Lambert, M.S. Yong, J.R. Messiert, and L. Ritters, in Residues of Veterinary Drugs in Food, Proc. Euroresidue II Conf., Veldhoven, May 3–5, 1993 (N. Haagsma, A. Ruiter and P.B. Czedik-Eysenberg, Eds.), Fac. Vet. Med., Univ. Utrecht, The Netherlands, p. 419 (1993).

63. G.O. Korsud, C.D.C. Salisbury, C.S. Rhodes, M.G. Papich, W.D.G. Yates, W.S. Bulmer, J.D. Macneil, D.A. Landry, G. Lambert, M.S. Yong, and L. Ritters, Food Addit. Contam., 15:421 (1998).

64. C. Nakajima, A. Okayama, T. Sakogawa, A. Nakamura, and T. Hayama, J. Vet. Med. Sci., 59:765 (1997).

65. S. Wetzlich, and A.L. Craigmill, J. Vet. Pharmacol. Ther., 20:310 (1997).

66. L. Tomasi, L. Giovannetti, A. Rondolotti, G. Dellarocca, and G.L. Stracciari, Vet. Res. Commun., 20:175 (1996).

67. R. Aerts, F. Verheijen, J. Lohuis, and J. Pasman, Proc. of the 6th EAVPT Inter. Congress (P. Lees, Ed.), European Association for Veterinary Pharmacology and Therapeutics, Blackwell Scientific Publications, Edinburgh, UK, p. 197 (1994).

68. R. Aerts, and P. Herben, Proc. of the 6th EAVPT Inter. Congress (P. Lees, Ed.), European Association for Veterinary Pharmacology and Therapeutics, Blackwell Scientific Publications, Edinburgh, UK, p. 80 (1994).

69. B. Perez, C. Prats, and M. Arboix, J. Vet. Pharmacol. Ther., 20:308 (1997).

70. European Agency for the Evaluation of Medicinal Products (EMEA), in Nafcillin, Summary Report, Committee for Veterinary Medicinal Products, EMEA/MRL/147/96-Final, London, UK (1997).

71. K.A. Caprile, J. Pharmacol. Ther., 11:1 (1988).

72. D.M. Goldberg, Med. Clin. North. Am., 71:1113 (1987).

73. European Agency for the Evaluation of Medicinal Products (EMEA), in Cephapirin, Summary Report, Committee for Veterinary Medicinal Products, EMEA/MRL/ 0128/96-Final, London, UK (1996).

74. B.I. Cabana, D.R. van Harken, and G.M. Hottendort, Antimicrob. Agents & Chemotherapy, 10:307 (1976).

75. R.N. Jones, and R.R. Parker, Diagn. Microb. Infect. Dis., 2:65 (1984).

76. K.I. Tyczkowska, R.D. Voyksner, and A.L. Aronson, J. Vet. Pharmacol. Ther., 14: 51 (1991).

77. European Agency for the Evaluation of Medicinal Products (EMEA), in Cefazolin, Summary Report, Committee for Veterinary Medicinal Products, EMEA/MRL/ 0126/96-Final, London, UK (1996).

78. European Agency for the Evaluation of Medicinal Products (EMEA), in Cefazolin, Summary Report, Committee for Veterinary Medicinal Products, EMEA/MRL/257/ 97-Final, London, UK (1997).

79. M.B. Regazzi, G. Chirico, D. Cristiani, G. Rondini, and R. Rondanelli, Eur. J. Clin. Pharm., 25:507 (1983).

80. L. Conte, M. Patergnani, M. Travaglini, P. Marino, S. Seifert, and M.A. Lacono, G. Chir., 10:117 (1989).

81. J.O. Errecalde, A.L. Soraci, O.N. Mestorino, and J.A. Speroni, Proc. of the 6th EAVPT Inter. Congress (P. Lees, Ed.), European Association for Veterinary Pharmacology and Therapeutics, Blackwell Scientific Publications, Edinburgh, UK, p. 199 (1994).

82. P.S. Jaglan, M.F. Kubicek, T.S. Arnold, B.L. Cox, R.H. Robins, D.B. Johnson, and T.J. Gilbertson, J. Agric. Food Chem., 37:1112 (1989).

83. European Agency for the Evaluation of Medicinal Products (EMEA), in Ceftiofur, Summary Report, Committee for Veterinary Medicinal Products, EMEA/MRL/498/ 98-Final, London, UK (1999).

84. M.G. Beconi-Barker, E.B. Smith, F.M. Kausche, E.J. Robb, T.V. Vidmar, and T.J. Gilbetson, in Residues of Veterinary Drugs in Food, Proc. Euroresidue III Conf., Veldhoven, 1996 (N. Haagsma and A. Ruiter, Eds.), Fac. Vet. Med., Univ. Utrecht, The Netherlands, p. 233 (1996).

85. F.M. Kausche, E.J. Robb, G. Alaniz, J.W. Hallberg, A.P. Belschner, and S.T. Chester, J. Vet. Pharmacol. Ther., 20:294 (1997).

86. S.A. Barker, L.C. Kappel, and C.R. Short, in Residues of Veterinary Drugs in Food, Proc. Euroresidue II Conf., Veldhoven, May 3–5, 1993 (N. Haagsma, A. Ruiter and P.B. Czedik-Eysenberg, Eds.), Fac. Vet. Med., Univ. Utrecht, The Netherlands, p. 165 (1993).

87. European Agency for the Evaluation of Medicinal Products (EMEA), in Cefquinome, Summary Report, Committee for Veterinary Medicinal Products, EMEA/ MRL/005/95-Final, London, UK (1995).

88. C. Carceles, E. Escudero, J.M. Serrano, and J.D. Baggot, Proc. of the 6th EAVPT Inter. Congress (P. Lees, Ed.), European Association for Veterinary Pharmacology and Therapeutics, Blackwell Scientific Publications, Edinburgh, UK, p. 211 (1994).

89. M. Horie, in Chemical Analysis for Antibiotics Used in Agriculture (H. Oka, H. Nakazawa, K.-I. Harada, and J.D. Macneil, Eds.), AOAC International, Arlington, p. 168 (1995).

90. S. Omura, Y. Hironaka, and T. Hata, J. Antibiot., 23:511 (1970).
91. M. Debono, K.E. Willard, H.A. Kirst, J.A. Wind, G.D. Crouse, E.V. Tao, J.T. Vicenzi, F.T. Counter, J.L. Ott, E.E. Ose, and S. Omura, J. Antibiot., 42:1253 (1989).
92. S. Satio, N. Muto, M. Hayashi, T. Fujii, and M. Otani, J. Antibiot., 33:364 (1980).
93. S. Harada, E. Higaside, and T. Kishi, Tetrahedron Lett., 1969:2239 (1969).
94. W. Chan, G.C. Gerhardt, and C.D.C. Salisbury, J. AOAC Int., 77:331 (1994).
95. World Health Organization, in Evaluation of Certain Veterinary Drug Residues in Food, Thirty-eighth Report of the Joint FAO/WHO Expert Committee on Food Additives, Technical Report Series 815, World Health Organization, Geneva (1991).
96. W.A. Moats, E.W. Harris, and N.C. Steele, J. Assoc. Off. Anal. Chem., 68:413 (1985).
97. M.G. Lauridsen, C. Lund, and M. Jacobsen, J. Assoc. Off. Anal. Chem., 71:921 (1988).
98. Kline, and W.P. Waitt, J. Assoc. Off. Anal. Chem., 54:112 (1971).
99. E. Dudrikova, and J. Lehotsky, Milchwissenschaft, 53:90 (1998).
100. Code of Federal Regulations, Title 21, Office of the Federal Register, National Archives and Records Administration, US Government Printing Office, Washington, DC, Sec. 522.2471 (1994).
101. E.E. Ose, and L.V. Tonkinson, Veterinary Record, 123:367 (1988).
102. A.L. Donoho, T.D. Thomson, and D.D. Giera, in Xenobiotics and Food-Producing Animals (D.H. Hutson, D.R. Hawkins, G.D. Paulson, and C.B. Struble, Eds.), American Chemical Society, Washington, DC, p. 159 (1992).
103. G. Ziv, M. Shemtov, A. Glickman, M. Winkler, and A. Saran, J. Vet. Pharmacol. Ther., 18:340 (1995).
104. S.L. Helton-Groce, T.D. Thompson, and R.S. Readnour, Can. Vet. J., 34:619 (1993).
105. R.M. Parker, R.K.P. Patel, I.M. McLaren, and P.G. Francis, Proc. of the 6th EAVPT Inter. Congress (P. Lees, Ed.), European Association for Veterinary Pharmacology and Therapeutics, Blackwell Scientific Publications, Edinburgh, UK, p. 227 (1994).
106. J. Okada, and S. Kondo, J. Assoc. Off. Anal. Chem., 70:818 (1987).
107. S. Omura, in Macrolide Antibiotics: Chemistry, Biology, and Practice (S. Omura, Ed.), Academic Press, Orlando, FL, p. 261 (1984).
108. S. Omura, in Macrolide Antibiotics: Chemistry, Biology, and Practice (S. Omura, Ed.), Academic Press, Orlando, FL, p. 301 (1984).
109. H. Takahira, Jap. J. Antibiot., 23:424 (1970).
110. L. Renard, P. Henry, P. Sanders, M. Laurentie, and J.M. Delmas, J. Chromatogr., 657:219 (1994).
111. T.B. Barragry, in Veterinary Drug Therapy (T.B. Barragry, Ed.), Lea & Febiger, PA (1994).
112. F.F. Sun, J. Pharm. Sci., 62:1657 (1973).
113. J. Yancey, M.L. Kinney, C.W. Ford, J. Antimicrob. Chemother., 15:219 (1985).
114. Food and Drug Administration, Fed. Reg., 58:58486 (1993).
115. R.D. Birkenmeyer, S.J. Kroll, C. Lewis, K.F. Stern, and G.E. Zurenko, J. Med. Chem. 27:216 (1984).

116. R.E. Hornish, T.S. Arnold, L. Baczynskyj, S.T. Chester, T.D. Cox, T.F. Flook, R.L. Janose, D.A. Kloosterman, J.M. Nappier, D.R. Reeves, F.S. Yein, and M.J. Zaya, in Xenobiotics and Food-Producing Animals (D.H. Hutson, D.R. Hawkins, G.D. Paulson, and C.B. Struble, Eds.), American Chemical Society, Washington, DC, p. 132 (1992).

117. A.D. Argoudelis, and J.H. Coats, J. Am. Chem. Soc., 93:534 (1971).

118. V.P. Marshall, T.E. Patt, and A.D. Argoudelis, J. Ind. Microbiol., 1:17 (1986).

119. A. Brisson-Noel, P. Delrieu, D. Samain, and P. Courvalin, J. Biol. Chem., 263: 15880 (1988).

120. R.M. Parker, A.M. Walker, and H.T. Hassanali, in Residues of Veterinary Drugs in Food, Proc. Euroresidue II Conf., Veldhoven, May 3–5, 1993 (N. Haagsma, A. Ruiter and P.B. Czedik-Eysenberg, Eds.), Fac. Vet. Med., Univ. Utrecht, The Netherlands, p. 523 (1993).

121. S. Swaminathan, and G.M. lower, in Carcinogenesis, Vol. 4 (S. Swaminathan, and G.M. Lower, Eds.), Raven Press, New York, p. 59 (1978).

122. Food and Drug Administration, Fed. Reg., 41:19906 (1976).

123. World Health Organization, in Evaluation of Certain Veterinary Drug Residues in Food, Fortieth Report of the Joint FAO/WHO Expert Committee on Food Additives, Technical Report Series 832, World Health Organization, Geneva (1993).

124. European Agency for the Evaluation of Medicinal Products (EMEA), in Furazoli done, Summary Report, Committee for Veterinary Medicinal Products, EMEA/ MRL, London, UK (1997).

125. K. Tatsumi, H. Nakabeppu, Y. Takahashi, and S. Kitamura, Arch. Biochem. Biophys., 234:112 (1984).

126. W. Winterlin, C. Mourer, G. Hall, F. Kratzer, G.L.H. Weaver, L.F. Tribble, and S.M. Kim, J. Environ. Sci. Health, B19:209 (1984).

127. L.H. Vroomen, M.C.J. Berghmanns, T.D.B. van Der Struijs, P.H.U. DeVries, and H.A. Kuiper, Food Addit. Contam., 4:331 (1986).

128. G. Carignan, A.I. MacIntosh, and S. Sved, J. Agric. Food Chem., 38:716 (1990).

129. M. Petz, in Residues of Veterinary Drugs in Food, Proc. Euroresidue II Conf., Veldhoven, May 3–5, 1993 (N. Haagsma, A. Ruiter and P.B. Czedik-Eysenberg, Eds.), Fac. Vet. Med., Univ. Utrecht, The Netherlands, p. 528 (1993).

130. N.A. Botsoglou, D. Koufidis, A.B. Spais, and V.N. Vassilopoulos, Arch. Geflugelk., 53:163 (1989).

131. L.H. Heaton, and G. Post, Prog. Fish-Culturist, 30:208 (1968).

132. D.W. Gottschall, and R. Wang, J. Agric. Food Chem., 43:2520 (1995).

133. A. Oeser, and M. Petz, in Residues of Veterinary Drugs in Food, Proc. Euroresidue III Conf., Veldhoven, 1996 (N. Haagsma, and A. Ruiter, Eds.), Fac. Vet. Med., Univ. Utrecht, The Netherlands, p. 765 (1996).

134. P.H. Acchimbault, G. Ambroggi, and J. Nicolas, Ann. Rech. Vet., 19:39 (1988).

135. M. Ynvestad, in Residues of Veterinary Drugs in Food, Proc. Euroresidue III Conf., Veldhoven, 1996 (N. Haagsma, and A. Ruiter, Eds.), Fac. Vet. Med., Univ. Utrecht, The Netherlands, p. 115 (1996).

136. L. Kaartinen, M. Salonen, L. Alli, and S. Pyorala, J. Vet. Pharmacol. Ther., 18: 357 (1995).

137. Food and Drug Administration, Fed. Reg., 60:50097 (1995).
138. P. Hammer, and W. Heeschen, Milchwissenschaft, 50:513 (1995).
139. G. Ziv, Proc. of the 6th EAVPT Inter. Congress (P. Lees, Ed.), European Association for Veterinary Pharmacology and Therapeutics, Blackwell Scientific Publications, Edinburgh, UK, p. 194 (1994).
140. P.R. McGuirk, M.R. Jefson, D.D. Mann, T.R. Shryock, and T.K. Schaaf, J. Med. Chem., 35:611 (1992).
141. C.J. Giles, R.A. Magonigle, W.R. Grimshaw, A.C. Tanner, J.E. Risk, M.J. Lynch, and J.R. Rice, J. Vet. Pharmacol. Ther., 14:400 (1991).
142. T.J. Strelevitz, and M.C. Linhares, in Residues of Veterinary Drugs in Food, Proc. Euroresidue III Conf., Veldhoven, 1996 (N. Haagsma, and A. Ruiter, Eds.), Fac. Vet. Med., Univ. Utrecht, The Netherlands, p. 908 (1996).
143. World Health Organization, in Residues of Some Veterinary Drugs in Animals and Foods, Forty-Eighth Meeting of the Joint FAO/WHO Expert Committee on Food Additives, Food and Agriculture Organization of the United Nations, FAO Food and Nutrition Paper No 41/10, Geneva (1998).
144. J.W. Dijkstra, J. Vet. Pharmacol. Therap., 20:297 (1997).
145. European Agency for the Evaluation of Medicinal Products (EMEA), in Difloxacin, Opinion of the Committee for Veterinary Medicinal Products on the Establishment of MRLs, EMEA/CVMP/164/96, London, UK (1996).
146. R. Bauditz, Vet. Med. Rev., 2:122 (1987).
147. P.M. Vancutsem, J.G. Babish, and W.S. Schwark, Cornell Vet., 80:173 (1990).
148. L. Dalsgaard, and J. Bjerregaard, Acta Vet. Scand. Suppl., 37:300 (1991).
149. J. Iturbe, M.R. Martinez-Larranaga, and A. Anadon, J. Vet. Pharmacol. Ther., 20: 296 (1997).
150. B. Hrvacic, Z. Kelneric, D. Sakar, J. Zivkovic, and M.D. Kramaric, J. Vet. Pharmacol. Ther., 20:316 (1997).
151. J. Delaporte, R. Froyman, J.P. Ganiere, and J.M. Florent, Proc. of the 6th EAVPT Inter. Congress (P. Lees, Ed.), European Association for Veterinary Pharmacology and Therapeutics, Blackwell Scientific Publications, Edinburgh, UK, p. 194 (1994).
152. A. Anadon, M.R. Martinez-Larranaga, M.J. Diaz, M.L. Fernandez-Cruz, M.C. Fernandez, M.A. Martinez, and J. Iturbe, in Residues of Veterinary Drugs in Food, Proc. Euroresidue III Conf., Veldhoven, 1996 (N. Haagsma, and A. Ruiter, Eds.), Fac. Vet. Med., Univ. Utrecht, The Netherlands, p. 198 (1996).
153. K.L. Tyczkowsa, R.D. Voyksner, K.L. Anderson, and M.G. Papich, J. Chromatogr., 658:341 (1994).
154. K.L. Saraste, A. Niemi, S. Pyorala, and T. Honkanen-Buzalski, in Residues of Veterinary Drugs in Food, Proc. Euroresidue III Conf., Veldhoven, 1996 (N. Haagsma, and A. Ruiter, Eds.), Fac. Vet. Med., Univ. Utrecht, The Netherlands, p. 839 (1996).
155. L. Kaartinen, M. Salonen, L. Ali, and S. Pyorala, J. Vet. Pharmacol. Ther., 18:357 (1995).
156. G. Ziv, S. Soback, A. Saran, B. Kurtz, A. Glickman, and M. Winkler, Isr. J. Vet. Med., 45:209 (1990).
157. L. Intorre, S. Cecchini, A.M. Cognetti Varriale, S. Bertini, G. Mengozzi, and G. Soldani, in Residues of Veterinary Drugs in Food, Proc. Euroresidue III Conf.,

Veldhoven, 1996 (N. Haagsma, and A. Ruiter, Eds.), Fac. Vet. Med., Univ. Utrecht, The Netherlands, p. 559 (1996).

158. A. Rogstad, O.F. Ellingsen, and C. Syvertsen, Aquaculture, 110:207 (1993).

159. A. Rogstad, V. Hormazabal, O.F. Ellingsen, and K.E. Rasmussen, Aquaculture, 96:219 (1991).

160. J.I. Grondel, J.F.M. Nouws, M. de Jong, A.R. Schutte, and F. Driessens, J. Fish Dis., 10:153 (1987).

161. M.O. Elema, K.A. Hoff, and H.G. Kristensen, Aquaculture, 136:209 (1995).

162. D.J. Mevius, H.J. Breukink, P.J.M. Guelen, T. Jansen, and B. de Greve, J. Vet. Pharmacol. Ther., 13:159 (1990).

163. L.I. Harrison, D. Schuppan, S.R. Rohlfing, A.R. Hansen, J.F. Gerster, C.S. Hansen, M.L. Funk, and R.E. Ober, Drug Metab. Dispos., 14:555 (1986).

164. T.B. Vree, E.W.J. van Ewijk-Beneken Kolmer, and J.F.M. Nouws, J. Chromatogr., 579:131 (1992).

165. P. Sanders, and J.M. Delmas, in Residues of Veterinary Drugs in Food, Proc. Euroresidue III Conf., Veldhoven, 1996 (N. Haagsma, and A. Ruiter, Eds.), Fac. Vet. Med., Univ. Utrecht, The Netherlands, p. 835 (1996).

166. A. Riberzani, G. Fedrizzi, and S. Espositi, in Residues of Veterinary Drugs in Food, Proc. Euroresidue II Conf., Veldhoven, May 3–5, 1993 (N. Haagsma, A. Ruiter, and P.B. Czedik-Eysenberg, Eds.), Fac. Vet. Med., Univ. Utrecht, The Netherlands, p. 576 (1993).

167. B. Ruodaut, and J. Boisseau, in Residues of Veterinary Drugs in Food, Proc. Euroresidue Conf., Noordwijkerhout, May 21–23, 1990 (N. Haagsma, A. Ruiter, and P.B. Czedik-Eysenberg, Eds.), Fac. Vet. Med., Univ. Utrecht, The Netherlands, p. 331 (1990).

168. M.H.T. van der Heijden, J.H. Boon, J.F.M. Nouws, and M.J.B. Mengelers, in Residues of Veterinary Drugs in Food, Proc. Euroresidue II Conf., Veldhoven, May 3–5, 1993 (N. Haagsma, A. Ruiter and P.B. Czedik-Eysenberg, Eds.), Fac. Vet. Med., Univ. Utrecht, The Netherlands, p. 357 (1993).

169. I. Steffenak, V. Hormazabal, and M. Yndestad, in Residues of Veterinary Drugs in Food, Proc. Euroresidue Conf., Noordwijkerhout, May 21–23, 1990 (N. Haagsma, A. Ruiter, and P.B. Czedik-Eysenberg, Eds.), Fac. Vet. Med., Univ. Utrecht, The Netherlands, p. 646 (1990).

170. I. Steffenak, V. Hormazabal, and M. Yndestad, Food Addit. Contam., 8:777 (1991).

171. I. Steffenak, V. Hormazabal, and M. Yndestad, Acta Vet. Scand., 35:299 (1994).

172. R. Chevalier, J.P. Gerard, and C. Michel, Revue Med. Vet., 132:831 (1981).

173. J. Guyonnet, R. le Gouvello, D. Choubert, P. Caizergues, M. Bromet-Petit, F. Spavone, and D. Thibaud, in Residues of Veterinary Drugs in Food, Proc. Euroresidue III Conf., Veldhoven, 1996 (N. Haagsma, and A. Ruiter, Eds.), Fac. Vet. Med., Univ. Utrecht, The Netherlands, p. 446 (1996).

174. U. Luzzana, V. Maria Moretti, M. Scolari, T. Mentasti, and F. Valfre, in Residues of Veterinary Drugs in Food, Proc. Euroresidue III Conf., Veldhoven, 1996 (N. Haagsma, and A. Ruiter, Eds.), Fac. Vet. Med., Univ. Utrecht, The Netherlands, p. 659 (1996).

175. J. Malvisi, G. Dellarocca, P. Anfossi, and G. Giorgetti, Aquaculture, 157:197 (1997).

176. M.O. Elema, K.A. Hoff, and H.G. Kristensen, Aquaculture, 128:1 (1994).
177. J.M. Degroodt, B. Wyhowski, and S. Srebrnik, J. Liquid Chromatogr., 17:1785 (1994).
178. A. Ervik, B. Thorsen, V. Eriksen, B.T. Lunastad, and O.B. Samuelsen, Dis. Aquat. Org., 18:45 (1994).
179. M. Schneider, V. Thomas, B. Boisrame, and J. Deleforge, J. Vet. Pharmacol. Ther., 19:56 (1996).
180. J.P. Fillastre, and E. Singlas, Clin. Pharmacokin., 20:293 (1991).
181. K. Uno, M. Kato, T. Aoki, S.S. Kubota, and R. Ueno, Aquaculture, 102:297 (1992).
182. S.A. Anadon, and R.M. Martinez-Larranga, Am. J. Vet. Res., 53:2084 (1992).
183. A. Gulkarov, and G. Ziv, Proc. of the 6th EAVPT Inter. Congress (P. Lees, Ed.), European Association for Veterinary Pharmacology and Therapeutics, Blackwell Scientific Publications, Edinburgh, UK, p. 235 (1994).
184. A. Ramadan, N.A. Afifi, and M. Atef, Proc. of the 6th EAVPT Inter. Congress (P. Lees, Ed.), European Association for Veterinary Pharmacology and Therapeutics, Blackwell Scientific Publications, Edinburgh, UK, p. 237 (1994).
185. Z. Olinski, C. Kowalski, and P. Wlaz, J. Vet. Pharmacol. Ther., 20:201 (1997).
186. M. Gips, S. Barel, and S. Soback, Proc. of the 6th EAVPT Inter. Congress (P. Lees, Ed.), European Association for Veterinary Pharmacology and Therapeutics, Blackwell Scientific Publications, Edinburgh, UK, p. 77 (1994).
187. I. Nafstad, Nor. Vet. Tidsskr., 104:215 (1992).
188. S.O. Hustvedt, R. Salte, O. Kvendset, and V. Vassvik, Aquaculture, 305:310(1991).
189. N. Ishida, Nippon Suisan Gakkaishi, 56:281 (1990).
190. S.O. Hustvedt, R. Salte, and V. Vassvik, Aquaculture, 95:193 (1991).
191. N. Ishida, Aquaculture, 102:9 (1992).
192. S.O. Hustvedt, and R. Salte, Aquaculture, 92:297 (1991).
193. Y. Kasuga, A. Sugitani, F. Yamada, M. Arai, and S. Morikawa, J. Food Hyg. Soc. Jpn., 25:512 (1984).
194. P. Archimbault, G. Ambroggi, and S. Nicolas, Ann. Rech. Vet., 19:39 (1988).
195. R. Ueno, M. Okumura, Y. Horiguchi, and S. Kubota, Nippon Suisan Gakkaishi, 54:485 (1988).
196. R. Ueno, Y. Horiguchi, and S. Kubota, Nippon Suisan Gakkaishi, 54:479 (1988).
197. H.V. Bjorklund, A. Eriksson, and G. Bylund, Aquaculture, 102:17 (1992).
198. B. Martinsen, T.E. Horsberg, and M. Burke, J. Fish Dis., 17:111 (1994).
199. W.H. Gingerich, J.R. Meinertz, V.K. Dawson, J.E. Gofus, L.J. Delaney, and P.R. Bunnell, Aquaculture, 131:23 (1995).
200. T. Bergsjo, I. Nafstad, and K. Ingebrigtsen, Acta Vet. Scand., 20:25 (1979).
201. R. Salte, and K. Leistol, Acta Vet. Scand., 24:418 (1983).
202. J.I. Grondel, J.F.M. Nouws, and O.L.M. Haenen, Vet. Immunol. Immunopathol., 12:281 (1986).
203. S. Garwacki, J. Lewicki, M. Wiechetek, S. Grys, J. Rutkowski, and M. Zaremba, J. Vet. Pharmacol. Therap., 19:423 (1996).
204. T.B. Vree, M. Tijhuis, M. Baakman, and Y.A. Hekster, Biomed. Mass Spectrom., 10:144 (1983).
205. J.F.M. Nouws, T.B. Vree, R. Aerts, and J. Grondel, in Agricultural Uses of Antibiotics (W.A. Moats, Ed.), American Chemical Society, Washington, DC, p. 168 (1986).

206. G.D. Paulson, V.J. Feil, P.J. Sommer, C.H. Lamoureux, in Xenobiotics and Food-Producing Animals (D.H. Hutson, D.R. Hawkins, G.D. Paulson, and C.B. Struble, Eds.), American Chemical Society, Washington, DC, p. 190 (1992).

207. G.D. Paulson, V.J. Feil, R.G. Zaylskie, and J.M. Giddings, J. AOAC Int., 77:895 (1994).

208. L.J. Fischer, A.J. Thulin, M.E. Zabic, A.M. Booren, R.H. Poppenga, and K.J. Chapman, J. Agric. Food Chem., 40:1677 (1992).

209. H.A. Kuiper, R.M.L. Aerts, N. Haagsma, and H. van Gogh, J. Agric. Food Chem., 36:822 (1988).

210. J.W. Pensabene, W. Fiddler, and D.J. Donoghue, J. Food Sci., 63:25 (1998).

211. World Health Organization, in Evaluation of Certain Veterinary Drug Residues in Food, Thirty-fourth Report of the Joint FAO/WHO Expert Committee on Food Additives, Technical Report Series 788, World Health Organization, Geneva, p. 32 (1989).

212. S.A.H. Youssef, M. Atef, H.A. El-Banna, M.S.M. Hanafy, M. Abornorge, and Y.A. El Katan, in Residues of Veterinary Drugs in Food, Proc. Euroresidue II Conf., Veldhoven, May 3–5, 1993 (N. Haagsma, A. Ruiter and P.B. Czedik-Eysenberg, Eds.), Fac. Vet. Med., Univ. Utrecht, The Netherlands, p. 696 (1993).

213. G. Weiss, H.J. Laurencot, A. Macdonald, P.D. Duke, K. Misra, G.M. Horton, S.E. Katz, and M.S. Brady, J. AOAC Int., 78:358 (1995).

214. H.F. Righter, J.M. Worthington, and H.D. Mercer, Am. J. Vet. Res., 32:1003 (1971).

215. H.J. Laurencot, A. Schlosser, and J.L. Hompstead, Poultry Sci., 15:1181 (1972).

216. B. Roudaut, in Residues of Veterinary Drugs in Food, Proc. Euroresidue II Conf., Veldhoven, May 3–5, 1993 (N. Haagsma, A. Ruiter and P.B. Czedik-Eysenberg, Eds.), Fac. Vet. Med., Univ. Utrecht, The Netherlands, p. 591 (1993).

217. N. Furusawa, T. Mukai, and H. Ohori, Br. Poultry Sci., 37:435 (1996).

218. O.B. Samuelsen, L. Pursell, P. Smith, and A. Ervik, Aquaculture, 152:13 (1996).

219. M. Atef, S.A.H. Youssef, N.A. Afifi, A. Ramadan, and A.A. Muity, in Residues of Veterinary Drugs in Food, Proc. Euroresidue II Conf., Veldhoven, May 3–5, 1993 (N. Haagsma, A. Ruiter and P.B. Czedik-Eysenberg, Eds.), Fac. Vet. Med., Univ. Utrecht, The Netherlands, p. 149 (1993).

220. World Health Organization, in Evaluation of Certain Veterinary Drug Residues in Food, Thirty-fourth Report of the Joint FAO/WHO Expert Committee on Food Additives, Technical Report Series 788, World Health Organization, Geneva, p. 37 (1989).

221. J.M. Ensink, B. van Klingeren, D.L. Houwers, Equine Vet. J. 25, 309, 1993.

222. N.W. Knoppert, S.M. Nijmeijer, C.T.M. van Duin, C. Korstanje, H. van Gogh, A.S.J.P.A.M. van Miert, J. Vet. Pharmacol. Ther. 11, 135, 1988.

223. G. White, S.M. Daluge, G.W. Sigel, R. Ferone, and H.R. Wilson, Res. Vet. Sci., 54:372 (1993).

224. J.O. Boison, P. Nachilobe, R. Cassidy, L. Keng, P.A. Thacker, A. Peacock, A.C. Fesser, S. Lee, G.O. Korsud, and W. Bulmer, in Residues of Veterinary Drugs in Food, Proc. Euroresidue III Conf., Veldhoven, 1996 (N. Haagsma, and A. Ruiter, Eds.), Fac. Vet. Med., Univ. Utrecht, The Netherlands, p. 273 (1996).

225. L. Intorre, H.J. Keukens, W.M.J. Beek, M.J.B. Mengelers, M.W.T. Tanck, and J.H. Boon, in Residues of Veterinary Drugs in Food, Proc. Euroresidue III Conf.,

Veldhoven, 1996 (N. Haagsma and A. Ruiter, Eds.), Fac. Vet. Med., Univ. Utrecht, The Netherlands, p. 563 (1996).

226. S. Banerjee, J. Pharm. Pharmacol., 28:133 (1976).

227. G. Gotroni, Acta Med. Scand., 191:409 (1972).

228. H.C. Heinrich, Klin, Wochenschr., 52:493 (1974).

229. J.F.M. Nouws, J.H. Boon, F. Driessens, M.J.B. Mengelers, G.H.R. Booms, and M.H.T. van der Heijden, in Residues of Veterinary Drugs in Food, Proc. Euroresidue II Conf., Veldhoven, May 3–5, 1993 (N. Haagsma, A. Ruiter and P.B. Czedik-Eysenberg, Eds.), Fac. Vet. Med., Univ. Utrecht, The Netherlands, p. 514 (1993).

230. M. Kuhne, and A. Ebrecht, in Residues of Veterinary Drugs in Food, Proc. Euroresidue II Conf., Veldhoven, May 3–5, 1993 (N. Haagsma, A. Ruiter and P.B. Czedik-Eysenberg, Eds.), Fac. Vet. Med., Univ. Utrecht, The Netherlands, p. 429 (1993).

231. U. Wolwer-Rieck, E. Blankvoort, N. Haagsma, and H. Buning-Pfaue, in Residues of Veterinary Drugs in Food, Proc. Euroresidue II Conf., Veldhoven, May 3–5, 1993 (N. Haagsma, A. Ruiter and P.B. Czedik-Eysenberg, Eds.), Fac. Vet. Med., Univ. Utrecht, The Netherlands, p. 685 (1993).

232. T.N. Ferguson, E.B. Smith, and J.R. Couch, Fed. Proc., 25:688 (1966).

233. D.J. Fletouris, J.E. Psomas, and N.A. Botsoglou, J. Agric. Food Chem., 38:1913 (1990).

234. World Health Organization, in Residues of Some Veterinary Drugs in Animals and Foods, Thirty-sixth Meeting of the Joint FAO/WHO Expert Committee on Food Additives, Food and Agriculture Organization of the United Nations, FAO Food and Nutrition Paper No 41/3, Rome, p. 97 (1990).

235. T. Arndt, D. Robinson, R.E. Holland, S. Wetzlich, and A.L. Craigmill, J. Vet. Pharmacol. Ther., 20:314 (1997).

236. E.W. van Dongen, and J.F.M. Nouws, in Residues of Veterinary Drugs in Food, Proc. Euroresidue II Conf., Veldhoven, May 3–5, 1993 (N. Haagsma, A. Ruiter and P.B. Czedik-Eysenberg, Eds.), Fac. Vet. Med., Univ. Utrecht, The Netherlands, p. 272 (1993).

237. B. Omija, E.S. Mitema, and T.E. Maitho, Food Addit. Contam., 11:641 (1994).

238. T.S. Huang, W.X. Du, M.R. Marshall, and C.I. Wei, J. Agric. Food Chem., 45: 2602 (1997).

239. R.L. Herman, D. Collis, and G. Bullock, US Fish and Wildlife Service, Tech. Paper, 37:1 (1969).

240. J.F.M. Nouws, J.H. Boon, F. Driessens, M.J.B. Mengelers, G.H.R. Booms, and M.H.T. van der Heijden, in Residues of Veterinary Drugs in Food, Proc. Euroresidue II Conf., Veldhoven, May 3–5, 1993 (N. Haagsma, A. Ruiter and P.B. Czedik-Eysenberg, Eds.), Fac. Vet. Med., Univ. Utrecht, The Netherlands, p. 514 (1993).

241. J.F.M. Nouws, J.L. Grondel, J.H. Boon, and V.J.Th van Ginneken, in Chemotherapy in Aquaculture: From Theory to Practice, Office International des Epizooties, Paris, p. 437 (1992).

242. A. McCracken, S. Fidgeon, J.J. O'Brien, and D. Anderson, J. Appl. Bacteriol., 40: 61 (1976).

243. R. Salte, Acta Vet. Scand., 23:150 (1982).

244. R. Salte, and K. Leistol, Acta Vet. Scand., 24:418 (1983).

245. M. Ryoko, and U. Kazuaki, J. Food Hyg. Soc. Jpn., 38:425 (1997).

246. H.J. Eisner, and R.J. Wulf, J. Pharmacol. Exp. Ther., 142:122 (1963).

247. R.G. Kelly, and D.A. Buyske, J. Pharmacol. Exp. Ther., 130:144 (1960).

248. A. Anadon, M.R. Martinez-Larranaga, M.J. Diaz, P. Bringas, M.L. Fernandez-Cruz, M.C. Fernandez, J. Iturbe, and M.A. Martinez, in Residues of Veterinary Drugs in Food, Proc. Euroresidue II Conf., Veldhoven, May 3–5, 1993 (N. Haagsma, A. Ruiter and P.B. Czedik-Eysenberg, Eds.), Fac. Vet. Med., Univ. Utrecht, The Netherlands, p. 138 (1993).

249. A. Reja, R. Gonzalez, J.M. Serrano, D. Santiago, M.E. Guimera, and M. Cano, Proc. of the 6th EAVPT Inter. Congress (P. Lees, Ed.), European Association for Veterinary Pharmacology and Therapeutics, Blackwell Scientific Publications, Edinburgh, UK, p. 82 (1994).

250. A. Anadon, M.R. Martinez-Larranaga, M.J. Diaz, P. Bringas, M.C. Fernandez, M.L. Fernandez-Cruz, J. Iturbe, and M.A. Martinez, Avian Pathol., 23:79 (1994).

251. C. Espigol, C. Artigas, J. Palmada, and A. Pages, J. Vet. Pharmacol. Ther., 20:192 (1997).

252. A. Anadon, M.R. Martinez-Larranaga, M.L. Fernandez-Cruz, M.J. Diaz, M.C. Fernandez, B. Sevil, and R. Anton, in Residues of Veterinary Drugs in Food, Proc. Euroresidue III Conf., Veldhoven, 1996 (N. Haagsma, and A. Ruiter, Eds.), Fac. Vet. Med., Univ. Utrecht, The Netherlands, p. 203 (1996).

253. E.W. van Dongen, and J.F.M. Nouws, in Residues of Veterinary Drugs in Food, Proc. Euroresidue II Conf., Veldhoven, May 3–5, 1993 (N. Haagsma, A. Ruiter and P.B. Czedik-Eysenberg, Eds.), Fac. Vet. Med., Univ. Utrecht, The Netherlands, p. 272 (1993).

254. A. Anadon, M.R. Martinez-Larranaga, M.J. Diaz, P. Bringas, M.L. Fernandez-Cruz, M.C. Fernandez, J. Iturbe, and M.A. Martinez, in Residues of Veterinary Drugs in Food, Proc. Euroresidue II Conf., Veldhoven, May 3–5, 1993 (N. Haagsma, A. Ruiter and P.B. Czedik-Eysenberg, Eds.), Fac. Vet. Med., Univ. Utrecht, The Netherlands, p. 138 (1993).

255. L. Tomasi, L. Giovannetti, A. Rondolotti, G. Dellarocca, and G.L. Stracciari, Vet. Res. Commun., 20:175 (1996).

256. G.C. Brander, D.M. Pugh, R.J. Bywater, and W.L. Jenkins, in Veterinary Applied Pharmacology and Therapeutics (G.C. Brander, D.M. Pugh, R.J. Bywater, and W.L. Jenkins, Eds.), 5th Edition, Balliere Tindall, London (1991).

257. N.E. Horrox, Vet. Rec., 3:278 (1980).

258. T. Unemura, H. Nakamura, M.M. Goryo, and C. Itakura, Avian Pathol., 13:459 (1984).

259. F. Simon, A. Romvary, and L. Acsne Kovacsics, Magy. Allatorv. Lapja, 47:459 (1992).

260. V.V. Ranade, M.M. Gatne, P.C. Badole, A.P. Somkuvar, and S. Jagadish, Proc. of the 6th EAVPT Inter. Congress (P. Lees, Ed.), European Association for Veterinary Pharmacology and Therapeutics, Blackwell Scientific Publications, Edinburgh, UK, p. 223 (1994).

261. G. Laber, J. Vet. Pharmacol. Ther., 11:45 (1988).

4

Anthelminthic Drugs

Anthelminthic is derived from the Greek words *anti* and *helminth*. Anthelminthics are therefore drugs that act against internal parasites of animals collectively called helminths.

Farm animals ingest material from the ground, soil, or pasture that has been contaminated with feces containing eggs and larvae of helminths. Hence, they readily become infected and without a satisfactory treatment regimen, the cycle of expulsion and reinfection is perpetuated. Reinfection can occur within hours following treatment.

Epidemics are most likely to occur when the climate provides the optimum combination of temperature and humidity or when animals are kept under crowded, damp conditions. The impact of a parasitic infection varies considerably according to the species of the worm involved. Adult tapeworms are relatively harmless, but certain blood- or tissue-feeding species of nematodes are highly pathogenic. More often than not, however, it is the invasion of the larvae rather than the adult parasites that is responsible for outbreaks of clinical disease.

Including in this group of drugs are the benzimidazoles, imidazothiazoles, and tetrahydropyrimidines that are primarily used against roundworms (nematodes) that parasitize the abomasum, intestines and lungs. Salicylanilides, substituted phenols, and sulfonamide derivatives are also anthelminthic drugs used mainly to combat flukes (trematodes) that parasitize the liver. Several drugs within the groups mentioned are further active against tapeworms (cestodes) that parasitize the intestines. The term *endectocide* has evolved to describe certain drugs such as the macrocyclic lactones that have activity both against internal parasites (endoparasites) and external parasites (ectoparasites) of animals. The use of pesticides against external parasites such as arthropods is not covered in this book.

117

Anthelminthics are used most frequently in spring and would not be given immediately prior to slaughter, thus reducing the likelihood of residues in edible animal products. Animals less than 1 year old are more susceptible to parasitic infections than adults and are treated more frequently than adults. Residues are most likely to be found in milk when the withdrawal periods have not been strictly observed or in the liver since this organ is the target tissue for the metabolism of anthelminthics.

4.1 BENZIMIDAZOLES

The benzimidazole group of anthelminthics is derived from the simple benzimidazole nucleus and includes the thiabendazole analogues and the benzimidazole carbamates. Substitution of side chains and radicals on the benzimidazole nucleus gives rise to the individual members of this group (Fig. 4.1).

Early benzimidazoles, such as thiabendazole, are quite soluble and quickly eliminated from the body. Newer benzimidazoles, such as albendazole, fenbendazole, febantel, and netobimin, are less-soluble compounds that exhibit much slower rates of elimination because they remain as solid precipitates within the gut for extended periods, increasing their efficacy against immature and arrested larvae and adult nematodes.

A number of benzimidazoles exist as prodrugs; their anthelminthic activity is due to the fact that they are metabolized in the animal body to the biologically active benzimidazole carbamate nucleus. Due to their relatively slower excretion rates, the newer insoluble benzimidazoles have fairly long withdrawal periods for edible tissues and milk in contrast to the less effective and more rapidly excreted thiabendazole analogues. Strict compliance with withdrawal periods is always necessary because of the potentially toxic and teratogenic effects of some of the benzimidazoles and their metabolites.

Thiabendazole is a broad-spectrum anthelminthic used in the form of wettable powders or suspensions in sheep, cattle, horses, and swine at dosages in the range 50–100 mg/kg bw, and in poultry at a dosage of 1000 mg/kg bw. It is also used as a food preservative or an agricultural fungicide (1), although recent research has shown to be teratogenic and nephrotoxic in mice (2, 3). However, only the unchanged thiabendazole has been implicated in embryotoxic and teratogenic effects.

Following oral administration, thiabendazole is rapidly absorbed from the digestive tract. Highest concentrations in blood appear within 3–7 h after treatment. Plasma concentrations are species dependent, being higher in sheep than in cattle and goats. This may reflect a reduced capacity for oxidative metabolism in sheep; the parent drug occurs in the urine of sheep at a proportion higher than the major 5-hydroxy metabolite, although not in cattle (1).

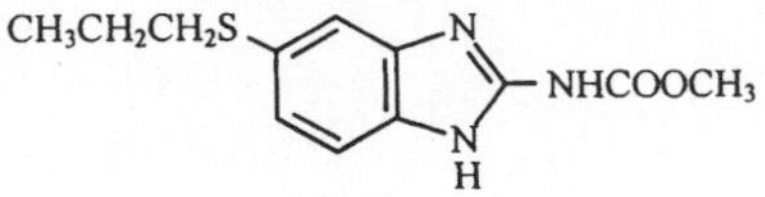

Albendazole

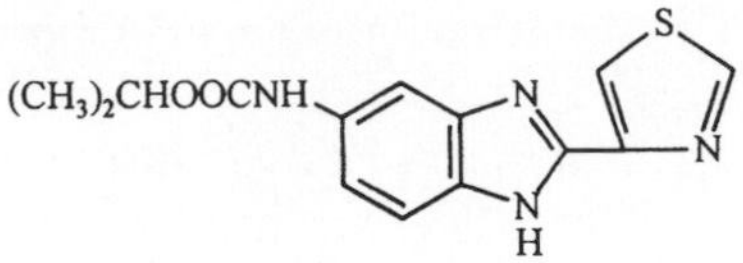

Cambendazole

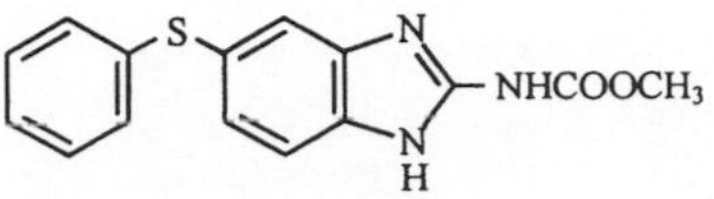

Fenbendazole

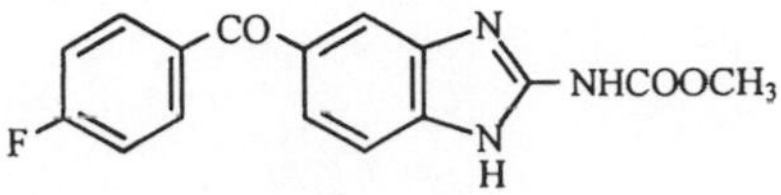

Flubendazole

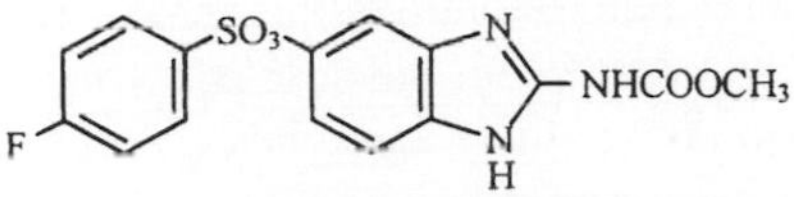

Luxabendazole

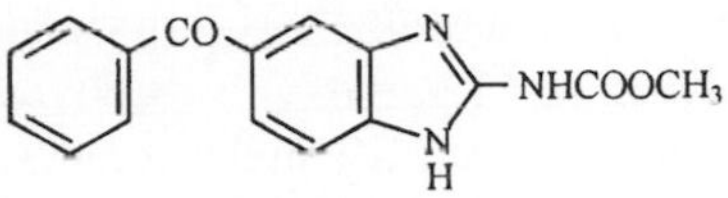

Mebendazole

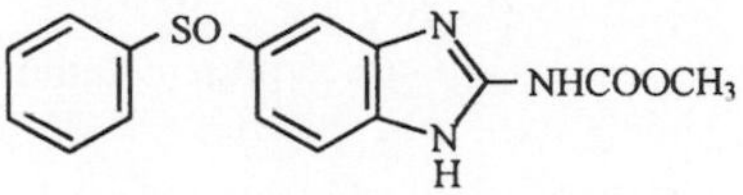

Oxfendazole

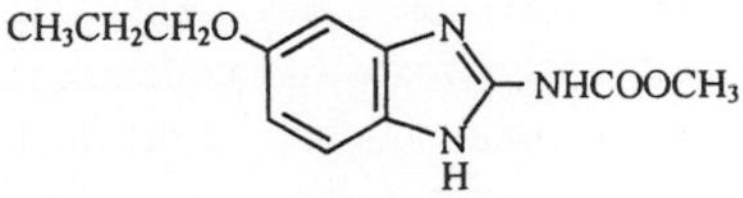

Oxibendazole

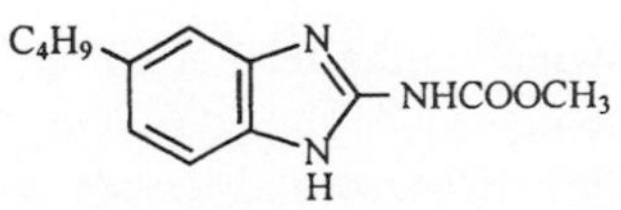

Parbendazole

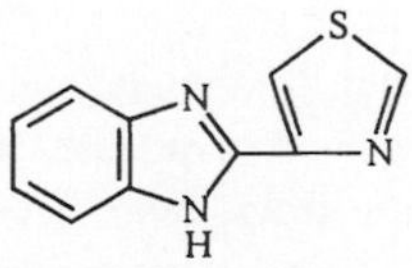

Thiabendazole

FIG. 4.1 Chemical structures of commonly used benzimidazoles.

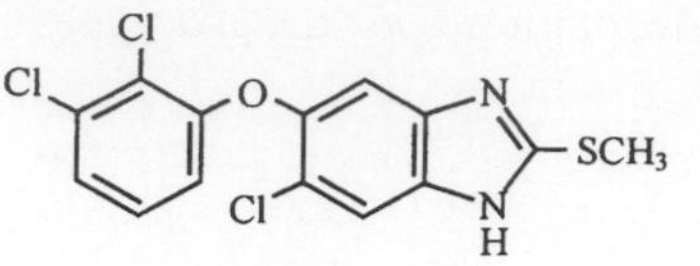

Triclabendazole

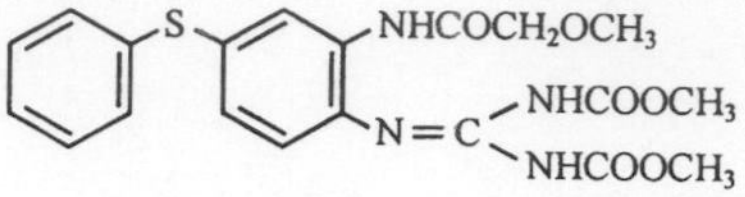

Febantel

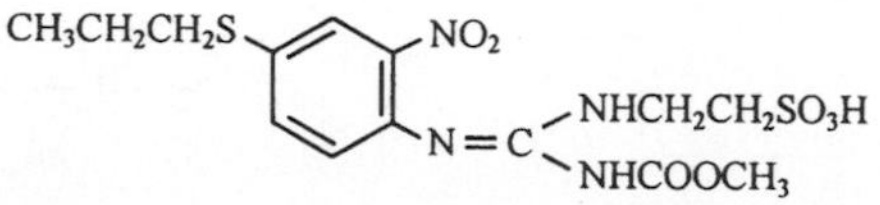

Netobimin

FIG. 4.1   Continued

Thiabendazole is rapidly metabolized in the liver of mammals to 5-hydroxy-thiabendazole, 5-hydroxy-thiabendazole-glucuronide, 5-hydroxy-thiabendazole-sulfate, and 4-hydroxy-thiabendazole (4, 5). Almost 90% of the dose is excreted in the urine, and 5% in the feces mostly in form of various metabolites; less than 1% of administered the dose corresponds to the parent compound (6).

In calves, the highest thiabendazole concentrations are found in kidney soon after dosing, but residual concentrations persist for longer in the liver (7). One day after dosing, the concentrations of thiabendazole and 5-hydroxythiabendazole in kidney and liver were 57 and 581 ppb, and 153 and 319 ppb, respectively. However, 6 days after dosing only liver contained detectable concentrations of 5-hydroxy-thiabendazole (63 ppb). Muscle and fat contained undetectable levels of thiabendazole at all time points, but detectable levels (54 and 64 ppb, respectively) of 5-hydroxy-thiabendazole were present 1 day after dosing.

In lactating cattle, mean residue levels of thiabendazole and 5-hydroxy-thiabendazole in milk were found to be 5007 and 168 ppb, respectively, 12 h after dosing, decreasing to 20 and 25 ppb at 84 h after dosing. In sheep, 7 days after oral administration of thiabendazole, no residues of the drug were found to be present in muscle, liver, and kidney tissues.

When thiabendazole was administered to swine via the feed at 40 mg/kg bw for 2 weeks, muscle, liver, kidney, and fat contained 0, 120, 190, and 170 ppb of the drug, respectively, at 2 day withdrawal. However, all tissues were found to be free of residues of the parent drug and its metabolites at 7 day withdrawal (4).

Cambendazole is a substituted thiabendazole analogue used against gastro-intestinal parasites and lungworms of sheep, cattle, swine, and horses. It is administered orally in form of drenching suspension, paste, or infeed powder at dosages of 20–40 mg/kg bw.

Following administration, the drug is rapidly metabolized into a large number of degradation products. The largest proportion of the drug and its metabolites is excreted in the feces, whereas the remainder (25%) is excreted in the urine (6). Less than 5% of the excreted drug is actually intact cambendazole. When radiolabeled cambendazole was administered to cattle, liver radioactivity was detectable for 30 days after administration, and a fraction of this was in the bound form (8).

Cambendazole has been implicated in teratogenic effects in pregnant ewes. Hence, long slaughter clearance times of 21 and 28 days have been recommended for treated cattle and sheep, respectively.

Thiophanate is a synthetic antinematodal pro-benzimidazole drug intended for oral administration in form of a feed additive, drench, or bolus to cattle, sheep, swine, and goats. Recommended dosages are either 6–7 mg/kg bw/day for at least 14 days in the feed or 50–60 mg/kg bw as a single oral dose. Thiophanate is considered a nontoxic benzimidazole.

In the gut lumen of the target animals, thiophanate undergoes cyclization, forming 2-ethoxycarbonylamino-benzimidazole, which is also known as lobendazole. The extent of thiophanate metabolism to lobendazole in cattle has been estimated at approximately 57%.

In sheep orally dosed with 40 mg/kg bw radiolabeled thiophanate, only the parent drug and its major metabolite lobendazole could be detected in plasma for 65 h after dosing. In sheep liver, thiophanate was metabolized to lobendazole at a rate of approximately 34%. Other metabolites included 2-aminobenzimidazole, low molecular-weight aliphatic acids, and limited amounts of the glucuronide and sulfate conjugates.

In goats orally dosed with 11 mg/kg bw radiolabeled thiophanate, the extent of thiophanate metabolism was about 52% in plasma (9). The major metabolites found in milk and urine at 24 h postdosing were 5-hydroxylobendazole and 2-aminobenzimidazole, each metabolite accounting for about 30% of the administered dose.

In swine orally dosed with thiophanate, the major metabolic product in the urine was 2-aminobenzimidazole, the parent drug being present only in trace amounts. Lower levels of the 2-aminobenzimidazole glucuronide conjugate and the lobendazole metabolite were also detected. Trace amounts of thiophanate were also present in the feces, which further contained lobendazole and its 5-hydroxylated metabolite. Kidney and liver tissues were found to contain 4 metabolites, two of which were identified as the 1,2,-(phenylene-bisiminocarbonothioyl)-biscarbamic acid O-ethyl-O-(1-hydroxyethyl)ester and the (phenylene-(bisimino-carbonothioyl)) biscarbamic acid O-ethyl-O-vinyl ester.

Following therapeutic treatment, thiophanate residues are higher in liver, with significant levels also being present in kidney; relatively lower concentrations are detected in the other edible tissues (9). Residue depletion studies in sheep given a single oral dose of 100 mg thiophanate/kg bw showed that the mean thiophanate residue concentrations in liver, kidney, muscle, and fat were 930, 1,060, 670, and 2930 ppb, respectively, after 1 day, and below 100 ppb on days 3 and 7 after dosing.

Calves given a single oral dose of 100 mg thiophanate/kg bw also showed thiophanate concentrations below 100 ppb in liver, kidney, and muscle, and below 200 ppb in fat at 7 days after dosing.

Residue depletion studies in swine given an infeed medication of 75 mg thiophanate/kg bw/day showed mean thiophanate concentrations in liver, kidney, muscle, and skin/fat of 5550, 6600, 2600, and 16,200 ppb, respectively, at 1 day after dosing, and 180, 100, less than 100, and 250 ppb, respectively, at 3 days after dosing. However, residue concentrations were below 100 ppb in all tissues at 7 day withdrawal.

Residue depletion studies in lactating cows given a single oral dose of 100 mg thiophanate/kg bw showed mean thiophanate residue concentrations of 440, 320, and 140 ppb in the milk collected at 6 h, 20 h, and 30 h milkings, respectively (9). However, milk collected at 44 h and thereafter was not found to contain detectable (detection limit 50 ppb) residue concentrations.

Fenbendazole is a benzimidazole anthelminthic metabolized in mammals to a series of other benzimidazole derivatives including oxfendazole. Fenbendazole, although not teratogenic per se, gives rise to the teratogenic metabolite, oxfendazole. It is administered orally to cattle, sheep, pigs, and goats for treatment and control of gastrointestinal roundworms, lung worms, and tapeworms at dosages from 3 to 10 mg/kg bw.

Absorption of fenbendazole is slow in ruminants but more rapid in monogastric animals. Maximum concentrations in blood are achieved at about 8 h in rats and rabbits, 24 h in dogs, and 2–3 days in sheep. Elimination of fenbendazole is predominantly by the fecal route. The metabolic pathway of fenbendazole is similar in rats, rabbits, dogs, sheep, cattle, goats, and chickens. It is rapidly metabolized to fenbendazole sulfoxide (oxfendazole), fenbendazole sulfone, fenbendazole 2-aminosulfone, and other minor metabolites detected in plasma.

In a study on pigs treated with fenbendazole at 5 mg/kg bw, a concentration of 0.28 ppm of the parent drug was found in the liver at 7 day withdrawal; other tissues were free of detectable fenbendazole residues. Residue depletion studies in fenbendazole-treated cattle at 10 mg/kg bw showed the presence of 8.4 ppm of the parent drug in liver, 1.04 ppm in kidney, 0.47 ppm in muscle, and 0.95 ppm in fat at 2 day withdrawal; however, at 7 day withdrawal, only liver was found to contain residues at a level of 0.67 ppm (10).

Another study with cattle treated with 7.5 mg/kg bw fenbendazole showed that liver contained 1.29, 1.92, and 0.08 ppm fenbendazole, oxfendazole, and fenbendazole sulfone, respectively, at 7 day withdrawal. Unlike with cattle, oxfendazole levels in sheep liver can reach figures almost twice those of fenbendazole and 10 times those of the fenbendazole sulfone at 7 day withdrawal.

When radiolabeled fenbendazole was given orally to lactating cows at 10 mg/kg bw, highest fenbendazole residues in milk appeared at the 12 h and 24 h milking declining to less than 100 ppb at 7 day after administration (10). Oxfendazole concentrations generally exceeded that of fenbendazole, whereas concentrations of the sulfone metabolite were comparable to the lower levels found for fenbendazole and oxfendazole. Total radioactive residues were found to be equally distributed in the fat and aqueous portions of the milk (11).

When unlabeled fenbendazole was orally administered to dairy cows, the parent drug showed its highest concentrations in milk 12–24 h after dosing, whereas it declined below detectable levels (<5 ppb) 60 h after dosing (12, 13). It was observed that fenbendazole was readily oxidized to the sulfoxide metabolite since the latter was already at its highest concentration 12 h after dosing. The sulfoxide metabolite declined rapidly thereafter to reach nondetectable levels at 96 h, while the sulfone metabolite, which is the end-product of the oxidation of fenbendazole, attained its highest level more slowly (48 h) but also disappeared at 96 h.

The somewhat delayed appearance of the highest level of the sulfone metabolite could be accounted for by its two-step oxidization process that required production of the fenbendazole sulfoxide as an intermediate substrate (14). This elimination profile indicated that the predominant metabolite in the milk collected by 36 h was the fenbendazole sulfoxide, whereas in the milk collected from 48–84 h the sulfone metabolite predominated. The p-hydroxy metabolite occurred at trace residue levels only in the milk collected at 12 h.

A residue depletion study (15) in rainbow trout given both oral and bath treatments of fenbendazole, at a water temperature of 12°C, showed that the drug was partly metabolized to fenbendazole sulfoxide. Both fenbendazole and fenbendazole sulfoxide were found to accumulate in fish skin. However, both the parent drug and its metabolite were largely depleted within 96 and 24 h, respectively, posttreatment. Formation of the sulfone metabolite was not detected in any fish tissue.

Oxfendazole may be administered orally or intraruminally to cattle and sheep for treatment and control of roundworms and tapeworms at a dosage of 4.5 mg/kg bw. Oxfendazole, although teratogenic per se in sheep, does not produce teratogenic metabolites.

Pharmacokinetic data have demonstrated very good absorption of the orally administered oxfendazole to cattle and sheep. After administration of the drug, the plasma metabolite pool is composed of oxfendazole, fenbendazole sulfone, and fenbendazole, a finding suggesting that oxfendazole and fenbendazole are metabolically interconvertible *in vivo*. Most of the drug and its metabolites are excreted in the feces within 2 days of treatment.

For cattle and sheep, liver is the tissue with the highest concentration of drug-related residues. Liver is also the tissue that exhibits the slowest rate of residue depletion. The extractable portion of the residue present in liver consists of oxfendazole, fenbendazole sulfone, and fenbendazole. A large portion of the residue present in liver is not extractable and this proportion increases with time after dosing. Evidence has been presented that bound oxfendazole residues have low bioavailability (10).

Residue depletion studies in cattle showed that liver residue concentrations declined gradually from 55.5 ppb at 10 day postdosing to below 10 ppb by 18 days after treatment (10). Residue depletion studies in sheep showed that liver residue concentrations declined gradually from 476 ppb at 10 day post-dosing to 12 ppb by 24 days after treatment.

When lactating cows were given a dose of 2.5 mg radiolabeled oxfendazole/ kg bw by gavage, the concentration of residues in milk was highest at 1 day after dosing (0.49 ppm), declining to below 0.005 ppm at 8 days after dosing. The principal metabolite in the 48–72 h milk pool was identified as fenbendazole sulfone.

Febantel is a prodrug anthelminthic metabolized *in vivo* to fenbendazole and thereafter to oxfendazole. It is administered to cattle, sheep, and swine for treatment and control of gastrointestinal nematodes at dosages of 5–7.5 mg/kg bw. Fenbendazole, although not teratogenic *per se,* gives rise to the teratogenic oxfendazole.

Intestinal absorption of febantel is quicker than oxfendazole or fenbenda-zole, peak levels in blood reaching a maximum within a few hours of dosing. Absorption of febantel is moderate in the rat, with around 25–30% of the oral dose excreted in the urine; however, the approximately 70% biliary excretion suggests a higher initial absorption in this species. In sheep, about 20% of the administered febantel is excreted in the urine during the next 4 days.

The main route of metabolism of febantel in rats, sheep, and cattle appears to be cyclization to yield fenbendazole. Oxidation at the sulfur atom can also occur to yield febantel sulfoxide, which then undergoes cyclization to give oxfen-dazole. Both fenbendazole and oxfendazole can then undergo further metabolism.

At 18 h after dosing cattle with febantel, 90% of the residues in liver were readily extractable; expressed as percentage of total residues, fenbendazole accounted for 30–41% in liver, oxfendazole 4–19%, oxfendazole sulfone 14–15%, and febantel 3–6%. Traces of the amine metabolite of fenbendazole, oxfendazole, and oxfendazole sulfone could be also detected. When residues in bovine liver were measured at 10 day withdrawal, a much lower proportion of total residues extractable, and a proportion of about 75% was identified as bound residues (10).

Residue depletion studies in rats, sheep, cattle, and pigs showed that liver contains the highest levels of residues; slightly lower amounts of residues occur in kidney and much less in muscle and fat. Seven days after febantel administration to cattle, residue concentrations in liver, fat, kidney, and muscle tissues were found to be 115, 19, less than 6, and less than 5 ppb, respectively. Following application of a similar treatment protocol to sheep, residue concentrations in liver, fat, kidney, and muscle tissues were found to be 4617, 133, 199, and 40 ppb, respectively, at 7 day postadministration. At 21 days after dosing, only the liver contained detectable residues that amounted to 123 ppb, whereas at 28 days after dosing all tissues had residue concentrations below the detection limit of 5 ppb. In pigs, residue concentrations in liver were found to reach 10-fold concentrations of those in other tissues: levels as high as 402, 245, and 57 ppb could be detected at 12 day, 20 day, and 34 day after dosing, respectively (10).

Albendazole is widely used in sheep and cattle for treating roundworms and flukes at oral dosages that range from 5 to 10 mg/kg bw. Albendazole and its sulfoxide metabolite exhibit teratogenic effects in animals.

In ruminants, oral doses of albendazole are readily absorbed from the gut. Following absorption, albendazole undergoes extensive metabolism by rapid first-pass oxidation of its sulfoxide group to form albendazole sulfoxide, then further oxidation to form albendazole sulfone, and by deacetylation of the carbamate group to form albendazole-2-aminosulfone. Albendazole sulfoxide, albendazole sulfone, and albendazole-2-aminosulfone are the main metabolites found in tissues, whereas other minor metabolites have been also detected at much lower concentrations.

In cattle given radiolabeled albendazole as a single dosage of 15 mg/kg bw, total residues were highest and more persistent in liver (16). One day after dosing, total radioactive residues in liver were more than 20 ppm, but depleted to around 6 ppm and 1.2 ppm at 4-day and 20-day, respectively, after dosing. Kidney was the tissue with the next highest and more persistent residues, while levels in muscle and fat were much lower and depleted rapidly. Muscle contained 5 ppm, 64 ppb, and 20 ppb at 1 day, 4 day, and 20 day, respectively, after dosing.

In sheep given a dose of 15 mg/kg bw, a depletion pattern similar to cattle was observed, but total residues in all tissues were lower at all time points, depleting in liver from around 16 ppm 1 day after dosing to 700 and 170 ppb 4 and 20 days after dosing, respectively. In lactating cattle, total residues in milk were nearly 5 ppm 11 h after administration of a 15 mg/kg bw dose, reducing to 640 and 35 ppb after 35 and 72 h, respectively.

When an oral suspension of albendazole was given via the drinking water to laying hens, both the parent compound and the sulfoxide and sulfone metabolites were rapidly eliminated from the tissues. At 96 h after treatment, liver contained 50 ppb total residues whereas muscle, skin, and adipose tissues contained 10 ppb (17). Both the sulfoxide and sulfone metabolites were also found to be present in the white and yolk fractions of the eggs laid by 3 days and 7 days posttreatment. Unlike the albendazole metabolites, the parent compound was never detected in the eggs laid.

Residue depletion studies in dairy cattle and sheep showed that the proportions of the major sulfoxide, sulfone, and 2-aminosulfone metabolites of albendazole change dramatically over a period of days in the case of tissues or hours in the case of milk, with albendazole sulfoxide predominating at early time points and albendazole sulfone and albendazole-2-aminosulfone appearing later (16). From day 4 onwards, more than 95% of the residues in bovine liver and kidney was in the bound form, but tissue binding in sheep tissues was less extensive.

When dairy cows were orally administered 10 mg albendazole/kg bw, the sulfoxide metabolite, which is the product of the primary oxidation of the sulfide moiety of albendazole, arrived its maximum 12 h after dosing and declined below detectable levels by 36 h (18–20). The sulfone metabolite, which is the end-product of the 2-step oxidation of albendazole, attained its highest level more slowly (24 h) and disappeared also more slowly (156 h). The N-deacetylation product of the albendazole sulfone, which is the 2-aminosulfone metabolite, was present at low concentration in the milk obtained at the 12 h milking, and arrived its maximum at the 36 h milking (36 h after dosing) to disappear slowly by the 180 h milking. Four other unidentified fluorescent metabolites could be also seen in the chromatograms of most milk samples analyzed; the earliest eluted of these unknown metabolites reached its maximum at the 12 h milking and declined below detectable levels by the 48 h milking. The others attained their maximum level 24 h after dosing to disappear slowly by the 156 h milking.

Netobimin is an albendazole prodrug intended for use in sheep and cattle. An oral dosage of 7.5 mg/kg bw is recommended for treatment of gastrointestinal infestations by roundworms and tapeworms, and 20 mg/kg bw for type II ostertagiosis and adult flukes. Netobimin exhibits teratogenic effects in animals.

In order to be pharmacologically active, netobimin needs to be converted within the body to albendazole by splitting off the side chain and formation of the benzimidazole nucleus. This is achieved naturally by the gut microflora, where albendazole is further converted to the sulfoxide metabolite. The absorbed albendazole sulfoxide is subsequently oxidized in the liver to the corresponding sulfone. The degree of absorption of the unchanged netobimin is minimal and, therefore, only traces have been detected in tissues and milk from treated animals. Hence, albendazole sulfoxide, albendazole sulfone, and albendazole-2-aminosulfone are the main metabolites found in tissues irrespective of whether the animals have been dosed with netobimin or albendazole. However, no information is available on the metabolic fate of the side-chain ($NHCH_2CH_2SO_3H$) that splits off from the netobimin molecule when albendazole is formed.

After subcutaneous or intramuscular injection of netobimin into cattle, absorption was rapid but plasma levels of radioactivity were lower than those achieved following oral administration. This indicates that absorption occurred prior to the conversion to albendazole since high levels of parent drug were found in plasma and milk soon after the injection. On the other hand, at 12 h after the injection the parent drug could not be detected at the injection site or in liver.

Excretion of orally administered netobimin takes place through urine and feces. In adult cattle and sheep, the percentage of administered dose excreted via urine was 45% in cattle and 48% in sheep, whereas that excreted via feces was 37% in cattle and 40% in sheep. In calves, however, the percentage of the administered dose excreted in the urine was less (31%) than that in feces (46%).

When a single oral dose of 20 mg radiolabeled netobimin/kg bw was given to calves, total residues were highest and most persistent in liver at 10 h, depleting to around 3500 ppb at 10 days posttreatment (21). Levels in kidney were around 22000 ppb at 10 h but depleted rapidly, reaching at 620 ppb at 10 days posttreatment. Residues in muscle and fat were much lower at all time points and depleted to 43 and 97 ppb, respectively, by 10 days. Residue levels in adult cattle receiving the same dose were rather higher, whereas total residues in milk from dairy cows were more than 5000 ppb at 8 h posttreatment, dropping to 60 ppb after 71 h.

When sheep were similarly treated with an oral dose of netobimin, total residues in all tissues except milk were generally lower than those in cattle. Albendazole, albendazole sulfoxide, albendazole sulfone, and albendazole-2-aminosulfone accounted for nearly all the residues in muscle and fat tissues at time points ranging from 18 h to 20 days. In liver and kidney, however, these metabolites accounted for a lower proportion of the total residues as time progressed, indicating the presence of bound residues.

Mebendazole is an antinematodal drug for use in horses, sheep, swine, and poultry at dosages of 5–15 mg/kg bw. It is also used extensively in eel culture for the control of gill infections by *Pseudodactylogyrus* spp. (22, 23). Mebendazole, although not teratogenic per se, gives rise to teratogenic metabolites.

Owing to its low water solubility, mebendazole is poorly absorbed from the gastrointestinal tract. Nevertheless, the absorption rate is generally rapid, peak plasma levels occurring within 2–4 h after dosing. Mebendazole is also poorly metabolized and, therefore, most is excreted unchanged in feces within 24–48 h, whereas 5–10% is excreted in urine. Only a small portion of the administered dose is excreted as the decarboxylated amino metabolite.

In vitro biotransformation studies in pig, rat, and dog liver revealed that hydroxyl mebendazole and amino mebendazole are the main metabolites of mebendazole (24). To verify the formation in vivo of the expected metabolites in eel, wild European eels were subjected to 6, 24, and 48 h treatments (25). The results clearly indicated that mebendazole given to eels via the water was absorbed and metabolized into the hydroxyl and amino metabolites, as was also the case with the other animal species. The amino metabolite was found to be the main meben-dazole metabolite in eels. In most eel tissues, the levels of the parent drug and its hydroxyl and amino metabolites increased with increasing treatment time.

Low tissue levels of mebendazole have been detected in lambs given radio-labeled mebendazole. Residue levels in liver were very persistent, total radioactivity in this organ being detectable by 15 days postdosing. In another experiment (26), the maximum level of mebendazole-related metabolites was found in liver and kidney tissues. In contrast, fat was found to contain the highest level of the parent drug. Skin exhibited the highest levels for both the parent drug and its metabolites compared with the muscle tissue samples. Mebendazole and its hydroxyl metabolite were eliminated within 5 days from muscle and skin, while the hydroxyl metabolite could be still detected in fat at 14 days posttreatment.

Parbendazole is an old anthelminthic that has been widely used against gastrointestinal nematodes and lungworms in cattle, sheep, and swine at dosages in the range 15–50 mg/kg bw. It is the drug in which the teratogenic effects of benzimidazoles were first identified.

After oral dosing to sheep, parbendazole was rapidly absorbed and peak plasma levels were reached within about 6 h. Plasma levels decreased gradually thereafter to reach a level lower than 1 ppm by 48 h. In sheep urine, seven metabolites have been identified. In liver, total residue levels of parbendazole corresponded to 1.41 ppm equivalents at 16 days posttreatment (8).

Oxibendazole is a broad-spectrum anthelminthic used for treatment of intestinal nematodes in various animal species including pigs, cattle, sheep, and horses. It is given as a single oral dose of 5–15 mg/kg bw or incorporated in feed at a dosage of 40 mg/kg feed/day for 10 days. Oxibendazole and its metabolites are not teratogenic.

Administered orally, oxibendazole is rapidly absorbed from the gastrointestinal tract. In sheep, the maximum plasma content is reached within 6 h. Much of the dose administered to cattle is eliminated in urine.

Metabolism studies have indicated that oxibendazole is readily metabolized in the liver (27). Hence, a significant portion of the total radioactivity found in liver and kidneys does not bear any structural relation to the parent drug, which can nevertheless serve as a marker residue in tissues. In liver, the ratio of the unchanged oxibendazole to the total radioactivity was estimated at 1% at 2 days postdosing. In kidney, this ratio was of the same magnitude but in muscle the unchanged drug represented the majority of the residues.

Residue depletion studies in cattle, sheep, swine, and horses showed that residue levels in tissues rapidly decreased with time (27). Total residue levels in muscle and fat, although higher than in liver and kidneys, were generally lower than 0.1 ppm at 4 days postdosing. Levels of extractable residues were also lower than 0.1 ppm at 7 days after treatment.

When pigs were orally dosed with radiolabeled oxibendazole, total residues were highest in liver and kidneys (24 ppm) after 24 h withdrawal and depleted relatively slowly to reach approximately 1.8 ppm at 7 day withdrawal (28). Extractable residues decreased from 35% to 11% over the same period. Milk from treated cows also showed that total radioactive residues were rapidly eliminated following drug withdrawal.

Flubendazole is used against gastrointestinal nematodes and lungworms in swine and poultry at dosages of 5 mg/kg bw or 30 ppm in the feed. This anthelminthic is poorly absorbed from the gut and, therefore, exhibits low toxicity.

Unlike mebendazole, flubendazole which is its halogenated analogue, produces only one-tenth of the plasma levels attained with mebendazole. When swine or poultry are treated with flubendazole, the tissue with the highest residues concentration and the slowest depletion rate is the liver. Residues in swine liver are primarily composed of the (2-amino-1H-benzimidazol-5-yl)-4-fluorophenyl-methanone metabolite, which is generally found at a much higher concentration than the parent drug.

Residue depletion studies in sows receiving 30 mg flubendazole/kg bw in the feed for 10 days showed that the mean concentrations of the unchanged flubendazole in liver, kidney, muscle, and fat were 59, 67, 13, and 33 ppb, respectively, 7 days after cessation of the treatment (4).

When hens were given feed containing 60 mg/kg flubendazole for 7 days, muscle, kidney, and liver tissues contained 79, 173, and 198 ppb of unchanged flubendazole at zero withdrawal. Flubendazole could not be detected in any tissue by 6 and 7 days after withdrawal. In contrast, residues of the parent drug could be detected at the level of 19 ppb in the yolks of the eggs laid at 11 days after the end of the treatment. Residues in eggs were generally higher and more persistent in the yolk than in the white fraction.

Triclabendazole is a very potent anthelminthic used against all stages of liver flukes in sheep, goats, and cattle at dosages of 10–12 mg/kg bw. This drug does not exhibit nematocidal activity and is not teratogenic.

Following oral administration to animals, triclabendazole is satisfactorily absorbed from the gastrointestinal tract. Peak plasma levels are generally achieved within 8 h, with more than 95% of the administered dose being eliminated in feces, about 2% in urine, and less than 1% in the milk.

Triclabendazole is rapidly and extensively degraded in cattle, buffalo, rabbits, dogs and humans, with the sulfoxide and sulfone being the main metabolites found in plasma (4, 29, 30). In addition to these oxidation products, rat excreta also contain the 4-hydroxytriclabendazole and 2-benzimidazolone metabolites. As with several other benzimidazoles, the use of triclabendazole in food-producing animals results in a large portion of total residues bound to endogenous tissue components. The proportion of bound residues to total residues increases with increasing withdrawal periods.

The marker residue for triclabendazole is 5-chloro-6-(2′,3′-dichlorophe-noxy)-benzimidazole-2-one, a compound formed when common fragments of triclabendazole-related residues are hydrolyzed under alkaline conditions at 90–100°C. Since the marker residue does not represent total residues, the marker residue levels are converted to triclabendazole equivalents using a conversion factor of 1.09 (31).

Residue depletion studies in cattle showed that liver, kidney, muscle, and fat contained 109, 103, 104, and 40 ppb of the marker residue at 28 day withdrawal. Residue depletion studies in sheep showed that liver, kidney, muscle, and fat contained 440, 260, 180, and 40 ppb of the marker residue at 10 day withdrawal.

Luxabendazole is a novel broad-spectrum benzimidazole for use in sheep against nematodes, cestodes, and trematodes at dosages of 7.5–10 mg/kg bw. Luxabendazole has no mutagenic or teratogenic effects.

Following oral administration, approximately 95% of the absorbed drug is bound to serum proteins. About 71% of the dose is excreted in feces as parent luxabendazole, a further 12% occurring in form of various metabolites. A portion of 13% is detected in the urine, 5% of which is attributed to the unchanged drug (32).

4.2   IMIDAZOTHIAZOLES

The racemic DL-tetramisole and its levo-isomer, levamisole, constitute the best-known members within this group of drugs (Fig. 4.2). Since the anthelminthic activity of tetramisole, which was first marketed in 1966, resides almost entirely in its levo-isomer, levamisole rather than the parent tetramisole is the drug currently used in most countries.

Levamisole possesses a broad spectrum of activity against lung and gut nematodes, but it has no activity against cestodes, trematodes, and arthropods. It is commonly used in swine, nonlactating dairy cattle, beef cattle, sheep, goats, and poultry in the forms of "pour-on," bolus, drench, feed additive, or injectable

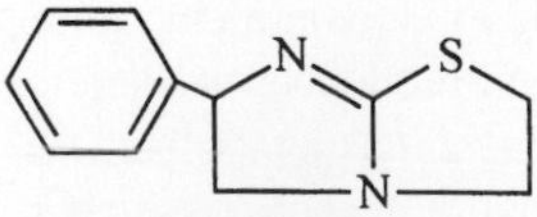

Levamisole

FIG. 4.2   Chemical structure of levamisole.

solution. The usual maximum dose rate of levamisole for cattle, sheep, swine, and goats is 8 mg/kg bw, while for poultry it is 25–50 mg/kg bw.

Following either oral or parenteral administration, levamisole is rapidly absorbed, but the parenteral route produces higher blood levels (6). When given intramuscularly, peak plasma levels are almost twice those attained by oral administration of the same dose. After subcutaneous administration, peak plasma levels of levamisole occur within 30 min, with 90% of the total dose being excreted in 24 h, mainly in the urine.

Following oral or subcutaneous administration to cattle, levamisole residues were detected in muscle, fat, liver, and kidney at 2 h postdosing, declining to below 100 ppb at 2 day after oral treatment, and at 7 or 8 days after parenteral treatment; highest residue levels appeared in liver.

Following a single oral administration to sows, residues in muscle and fat were below 100 ppb at 3 day withdrawal, whereas residues in kidney and liver were below 100 ppb and 310 ppb, respectively, at 5 day withdrawal. When different levamisole formulations including drench, pellets, bolus, and injectable solutions were administered to lactating cows at the same dosage, residues in milk averaged 500, 550, 580, and 320 ppb, respectively, 12 h after the cessation of treatment, declining to below 10 ppb at 48 h after the treatment with drench and at 60 h after the treatment with the other three formulations (8).

Literature data on the depletion of levamisole residues from edible animal products concern only the parent drug (33). It appears, however, that the metabolism of levamisole in food-producing animals is qualitatively similar to that in rats, since limited data from swine (34) and goats (35) are generally consistent with those observed for rats. Metabolism studies in rats using radiolabeled levamisole showed extensive metabolism of levamisole, with at least 50 metabolites identified in some samples of urine from treated rats.

Four major metabolic pathways have been proposed to account for many of these metabolites (36). The most important pathway appears to be an oxidative introduction of a double bond into the imidazoline ring followed by parahydroxylation of the phenyl ring and oxidation of the sulfur atom to the sulfoxide and sulfone metabolites. Hydroxylation of the thiazole ring may initiate a second pathway, where the thiolactone formed is hydrolyzed either to a thiohydantoic acid or to the hydantoic acid metabolite. Formation of parahydroxylevamisole followed by formation of conjugates may be another metabolic pathway, whereas opening of the thiazole ring followed by oxidation or methylation of the sulfydrylic group appears to constitute the quantitatively least important pathway.

The toxic effects of levamisole, for which no safety threshold can be set, to induce idiosyncratic organulocytosis in some individuals have caused concern. The identified metabolites of levamisole are, however, much less toxic than the parent compound. Hence, the parent compound is sought in analysis of tissue samples.

4.3 ORGANOPHOSPHATES

A number of organophosphates originally employed as broad-spectrum parasiticides against both nematodes and insects have come to be used as alternatives
for treating benzimidazole-resistant nematodes in recent years (Fig. 4.3). Organophosphates tend to be labile to alkaline media and may therefore be partially
hydrolyzed and inactivated in the alkaline region of the small intestine. As a result,
oral dosage rates are severalfold higher than those parenterally administered in
sheep, cattle, and swine. Organophosphates are usually rapidly oxidized and inactivated in the liver, but their safety margin is generally less than that of benzimidazoles.

Haloxon is probably the safest of the organophosphate anthelminthics (37).
It is approved by the Food and Drug Administration (FDA) for use in sheep,
cattle, and goats at a dosage of 30–50 mg/kg bw. It is not intended for use in
swine and poultry, although certain parasites can be very effectively controlled
by the drug in these hosts. It is usually administered orally in the form of a paste,
bolus, drench, or liquid suspension, and as a feed premix for poultry.

Haloxon is rapidly absorbed from the gut, metabolized extensively in the
liver to nontoxic metabolites, and excreted in the urine. In sheep, the rapidity of
hydrolysis of haloxon varies widely among individual animals and is genetically
determined by the presence or absence of the enzyme A-esterase (6). Residues
of haloxon are present in the milk of treated animals and, therefore, the drug
should not be used for treating dairy cattle or goats of breeding age or older.

Coumaphos, like other organophosphates, was originally developed as a
pesticide for treatment of external parasites of animals, but later came to be used

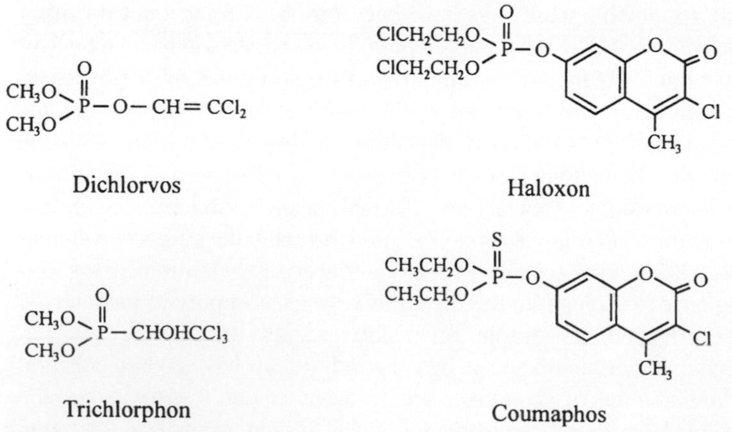

Dichlorvos

Haloxon

Trichlorphon

Coumaphos

FIG. 4.3 Chemical structures of commonly used organophosphates.

as an anthelminthic. Unlike haloxon, coumaphos can be used in lactating animals without requiring the milk to be discarded after treatment.

Drenching is the common means of administering coumaphos to beef cattle and swine in Europe at a dosage of 8–15 mg/kg bw. Coumaphos is also administered to beef and dairy cattle as a top dressing or a feed premix at a rate of 2 mg/kg bw/day for 6 days. Coumaphos is further prepared as a feed premix for use in replacement pullets older than 8 weeks and in laying flocks at a dosage of 30–40 ppm in the feed for 10–14 days.

Dichlorvos is a particularly versatile organophosphate since it can be incorporated as a plasticizer into polyvinyl chloride resin pellets and can be released slowly from the undigestible pellets as they pass through the digestive tract. This allows for a therapeutic concentration against parasites all along the digestive tract.

It is used in swine in a single oral administration with feed at a dosage of 7.5–35 mg/kg bw for control of internal and external parasites. Although its anthelminthic spectrum is acceptable in cattle (38) and sheep (39), dichlorvos does not have FDA approval for use in ruminants due to its narrow safety margin. Also, dichlorvos cannot be used in poultry because birds accumulate the resin pellets in their gizzard. Dichlorvos is generally toxic to animals, and it is less toxic via the dermal and oral routes than by parenteral routes. Moreover, dichlorvos is a suspect carcinogen.

Following oral administration to animals, dichlorvos is rapidly absorbed from the digestive tract and extensively metabolized in the liver. The metabolism of dichlorvos has not been clearly elucidated because almost none of its potential metabolites has been yet unequivocally identified due mainly to its very rapid biotransformation rate (6). It appears, however, that the initial hydrolysis of dichlorvos, which occurs in all species, leads presumably to dichloroacetaldehyde (40), which is further metabolized by reduction to dichloroethanol or oxidation to dichloroacetic acid. In addition, dealkylation to desmethyldichlorvos appears to be another minor route of biotransformation, except in the mouse where desmethyldichlorvos constitutes at least 18% of the administered radioactivity. The metabolites of dichlorvos do not persist in tissues, whereas only trace levels occur in the milk of lactating mammals (41). There is no evidence that the metabolites of dichlorvos are toxic.

Trichlorphon is a precursor of dichlorvos used in swine and horses against gastrointestinal nematodes at dosages of 40–50 mg/kg bw. It is metabolized rapidly to dichlorvos, which is responsible for its therapeutic efficacy. The toxicity of trichlorphon is similar to that of dichlorvos.

4.4 TETRAHYDROPYRIMIDINES

Pyrantel and its methyl analogue, morantel, constitute the group of the tetrahydropyrimidine anthelminthics currently used in food-producing animals. Both

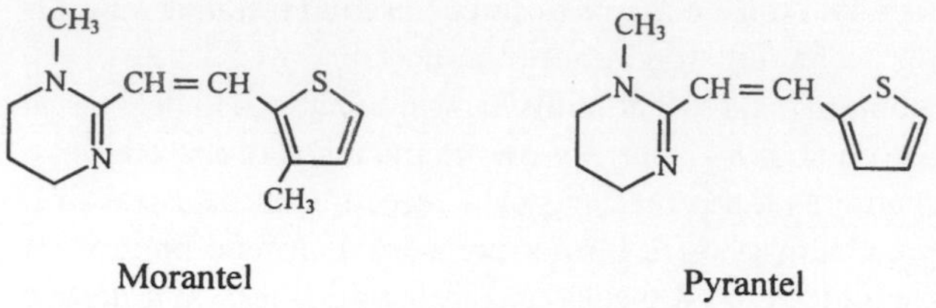

Morantel   Pyrantel

FIG. 4.4   Chemical structures of commonly used tetrahydropyrimidines.

drugs are commercially available for veterinary use in the form of tartrate salts (Fig. 4.4), whereas morantel is also available as a fumarate salt and pyrantel as a pamoate salt.

Morantel tartrate is used in cattle for eradication and control of mature gastrointestinal nematode infections. It is administered orally either as a bolus containing 11.8 g of the drug or as an aqueous solution at a dosage of 6–7.5 mg/ kg bw, and in swine and sheep as a single oral dosage of 5–7.5 mg/kg bw. The fumarate salt is also used in sheep at a dosage of 12.5 mg/kg bw. Morantel exhibits no teratogenicity.

In all species, morantel is mostly unabsorbed and excreted in the feces. Only a small proportion of the administered dose is rapidly absorbed, producing peak blood levels within 4–6 h. The drug is quickly metabolized, presumably in the liver, and 17% of the administered dose is excreted in the urine of sheep in the form of metabolites within 4 days after administration (1). In cattle, less than 20% of the administered dose is recovered in the urine over 4 days after administration, whereas in swine 45% of the administered dose is excreted in urine within 24 h.

Metabolism of morantel proceeds via three main routes involving oxidation of the thiophene, oxidation of the tetrapyrimidine ring, and conjugation with glutathione. Oxidation of thiophene in urine leads to acidic metabolites including 4-ketohept-2-eneldioic acid, levulinic acid, 4-ketopimimelic acid, and α-ketoglutaric acid, which are all highly polar. This acidic residue fraction can represent from 3% for sheep to 25.7% for dogs of the total urinary radioactivity. A proportion of around 57% for dog and pig to 86% for rats of the total urinary radioactivity, accounts for metabolites that contain the tetrahydropyrimidine ring and are convertible to N-methyl-1,3-propanediamine.

Due to the extensive metabolism of morantel in vivo, total morantel-related residues in edible animal products are usually determined after their conversion to either N-methyl-1,3-propanediamine through alkaline hydrolysis or to 3-(3-methyl-2-thienyl)acrylic acid through digestion with hydrochloric acid.

When calves were given orally a single dose of 5.9 mg radiolabeled morantel tartrate/kg bw, kidney contained 60 ppb, fat 20 ppb, and muscle less than 10 ppb of morantel equivalents at 7 days after dosing. In liver, the amounts of radioactivity were 495, 250, and 140 ppb morantel equivalents at 7, 14, and 28 day after dosing, respectively. Following conversion of residues to N-methyl-1,3-propanediamine, the proportion of this compound in total residues in liver was found to be 59%, 54%, and 40% at 7, 14, and 28 day after dosing, respectively.

When ruminating calves were given an intraruminal bolus containing 12 g morantel, the concentrations of morantel residues, after their conversion into 3-(3-methyl-2-thienyl)acrylic acid, in muscle, kidney, and liver, were 15, 40, and 150 ppb morantel equivalents, respectively, at 7 days after dosing.

When pigs were orally treated with a single dose of 15 mg radiolabeled morantel/kg bw, the amounts of radioactivity in muscle, skin, fat, liver, and kidney were 50, 100, 50, 826, and 150 ppb morantel equivalents, respectively, at 14-day after dosing.

When sheep were given a single oral dose of 9 mg radiolabeled morantel/kg bw, the amounts of radioactivity in muscle, fat, liver, and kidney, were 20, 20, 1130, and 190 ppb morantel equivalents, respectively, at 7 day after dosing. At 14 days, radioactivity levels were still high in liver and kidney, amounting to 1050 and 80 ppb, respectively.

When dairy cows were treated with a single oral dose of 5 mg radiolabeled morantel/kg bw, total radioactivity in milk peaked at 84 ppb at the second milking to decline thereafter to 49 ppb and 19 ppb at the fourth and sixth milking, respectively.

Pyrantel, the parent compound of morantel, is used against gastrointestinal parasites of sheep, goats, pigs, cattle, and deer at dosages in the range 15–20 mg/kg bw. Its tartrate salt is administered orally to animals in forms of a feed premix, pellets, or drench.

Pyrantel exhibits absorption, distribution, biotransformation, and elimination profiles similar to those of morantel. Pyrantel tartrate is well absorbed with peak plasma levels occurring 2–3 h after dosing. In ruminants, urinary excretion accounts for about 25% of the administered dose, while much of the remainder passes unchanged in feces. However, the pamoate salt is very poorly absorbed, most of the dose being excreted in feces.

Pyrantel is quickly metabolized in the body, a small proportion remaining intact by the time it is excreted. Individual metabolites of pyrantel have not been yet identified. Nevertheless, it is known that at least half of them contain the N-methyl-1,3-propanediamine structure of the tetrahydropyrimidyl ring, which is more resistant to the metabolic attack than the thiophene ring (6).

In swine, residues of pyrantel depleted most slowly from the liver. Metabolism of pyrantel was rapid in this species, with no residues of the unchanged drug being detected in liver at 4 days after treatment. In swine liver, 40–50% of the total residues were convertible to *N*-methyl-1,3-propanediamine, at 4–42 days after treatment. In ovine and bovine liver, these figures amounted to approximately 30–60% and 86–99%, respectively.

4.5 SALICYLANILIDES

Closantel, niclosamide, oxyclozanide, rafoxanide, dibromsalan, and tribromsalan are the better-known members of the salicylanilides group of anthelminthics (Fig. 4.5). They are all used to control primarily liver flukes in animals. On absorption, most salicylanilides are bound strongly to plasma proteins, with the exception of the tapeworm remedy niclosamide. These drugs are not soluble in water; nevertheless, solutions have been formulated that enable closantel and rafoxanide to be administered parenterally.

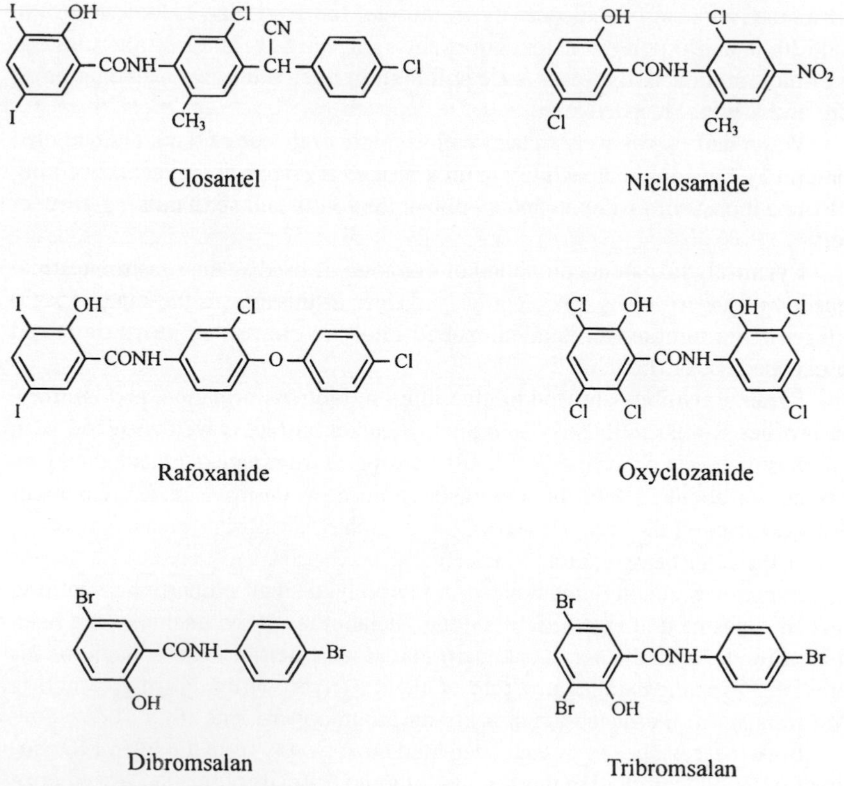

Closantel

Niclosamide

Rafoxanide

Oxyclozanide

Dibromsalan

Tribromsalan

Fɪɢ. 4.5 Chemical structures of commonly used salicylanilides.

Closantel is used primarily in cattle and sheep for treatment of mature and immature liver flukes, hematophagous nematodes, and larval stages of some arthropods. It is administered orally or parenterally at dosages of 5–15 or 2.5–7.5 mg/kg bw, respectively. Closantel does not exhibit carcinogenic, teratogenic, or embryotoxic activities.

Closantel is well absorbed, achieving peak plasma levels within 24 h after its oral administration. With parenteral treatment, peak plasma levels are reached within 24–48 h. The primary route of metabolism of closantel is reductive deiodination leading to monoiodoclosantel metabolites (42). Although complete deiodination is possible, no evidence for deiodinated closantel has been yet presented.

Metabolism studies in sheep with radiolabeled closantel showed that the parent drug accounted for nearly all the radioactivity in muscle, fat, and kidney. In contrast to tissues in which no metabolism occurred, liver contained two closantel metabolites, 3-monoiodoclosantel and 5-monoiodoclosantel, besides the parent drug. The same metabolites were also identified in feces, although 80–90% of the total radioactivity was due to the parent drug. While amide hydrolysis would also appear to be an alternative metabolism pathway, metabolites that would result from this pathway, such as 3,5-diiodosalicylic acid, have not yet been identified. It might well be that steric hindrance around the amide bonds prevents their hydrolysis (42).

The residue depletion profiles of closantel in cattle and swine are almost similar. Highest concentrations of closantel are seen in kidney, whereas the depletion of closantel from all edible tissues is very slow over the first 28 days of withdrawal. Within animal species, the parenteral and the oral routes of administration yield comparable residue concentrations provided that the oral dose is twice the parenteral dose. A dose linearity is also observed for residue concentrations in tissues; doubling the dose for a particular route of administration doubles the residue level.

In tissues of sheep treated orally with a single dose of 5 mg/kg bw, residue levels of closantel were 0.06–0.09 ppm in fat and muscle and up to 0.47 ppm in kidney and liver at 56 day withdrawal; at 84 days, residues could not be detected in fat and muscle, whereas liver and kidney contained levels as low as 0.06–0.17 ppm (43).

In treated cattle, highest concentrations of closantel were found in kidney; they ranged from 3.29 ppm at 14 days to 0.11 ppm at 42 days. In muscle, closantel concentrations ranged from 0.58 ppm at 14 days to less than 0.1 ppm at 42 days, whereas in liver they ranged from a maximum at 1.55 ppm at 14 days to less than 0.1 ppm at 42 days (44).

In milk from dairy cows treated intramuscularly with closantel, mean concentrations of residues peaked at about 1 ppm from 4 days to 7 days, to decline thereafter to 0.22 ppm at 35 days postdosing (43). All depletion studies suggest that closantel residues occur in bound form in incurred samples.

Niclosamide is an oral teniacidal drug administered to ruminants in the form of drench at a dosage of 50 mg/kg bw for cattle and 100 mg/kg bw for sheep and goats. It is also administered to ruminants for convenience with the feed at a dosage of 70 mg/kg bw.

Niclosamide is poorly absorbed from the gastrointestinal tract. Unlike other salicylanilides, niclosamide is very rapidly excreted. The small amount absorbed is transformed into the inactive metabolite, aminoniclosamide (32).

Oxyclozanide possesses activity against only adult flukes, but at elevated dosage levels some activity against the later parenchyma stages (flukes of more than 4 weeks of age), may be obtained. In sheep and cattle, recommended oral dosages are 10–15 mg/kg bw. It is frequently combined with levamisole or oxibendazole for combined treatment of gastrointestinal nematodes and liver fluke infections.

Following absorption, oxyclozanide reaches its highest concentrations in liver, kidney, and intestines, and is excreted into the bile in form of an active glucuronide metabolite. Oxyclozanide has a terminal half-life in sheep of 6.4 days. This long half-life is related to its high protein-binding tendency and, therefore, residues in liver are detectable for extended periods after administration (32). Since detectable amounts of oxyclozanide can pass into milk, treatment of lactating animals with this drug is contraindicated.

Rafoxanide is a halogenated salicylanilide that is commercially formulated for use in sheep and cattle in the form of bolus or drenching suspension at a dosage of 7.5 mg/kg bw. It is also administered subcutaneously to cattle at a dosage of 3 mg/kg bw. It is highly effective against adult flukes and the later parenchyma stages. Rafoxanide is frequently combined with thiabendazole for combined treatment of gastrointestinal nematodes and liver fluke infections.

Following oral dosing, rafoxanide is well absorbed, reaching peak plasma levels between 24 and 48 h, but it is slowly excreted. In sheep, its biological half-life ranges from 5 to 10 days due mainly to its high protein-binding tendency (32).

In cattle and sheep, rafoxanide is not metabolized to any detectable degree and residues in liver are detectable for weeks after its administration. Residue depletion studies in cattle given a single oral dose of 15 mg rafoxanide/kg bw showed that edible tissues are free of drug residues at 28 days postdosing.

Dibromsalan and **tribromsalan** are both closely related salicylanilides are commercially available as a mixture for treatment of adult and juvenile fluke infections in sheep at oral dosages of 30 and 60 mg/kg bw, respectively.

4.6   SUBSTITUTED PHENOLS

A wide range of substituted phenols has been used for treatment of liver flukes and tapeworms in animals. Most drugs within this group have a low safety index

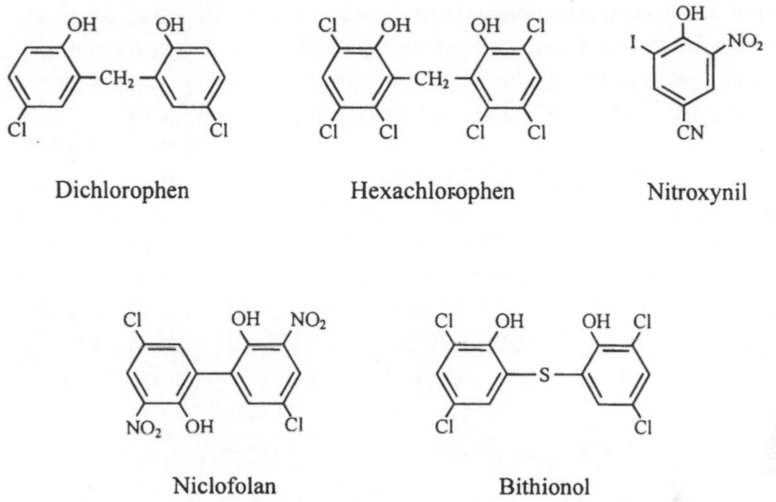

FIG. 4.6 Chemical structures of commonly used substituted phenols.

and, thus, have been largely superseded by less toxic and more effective drugs. Nevertheless, a range of substituted phenols including nitroxynil, dichlorophen, hexachlorophen, niclofolan, and bithionol are still used as anthelminthics (Fig. 4.6).

Nitroxynil is one of the few injectable flukicides available and possesses activity not only against adult flukes but also against flukes of more than 4 weeks of age. Nitroxynil also displays a stunting effect against early immature larvae and, hence, reduces pasture contamination by suppressing egg output. It is used in cattle and sheep subcutaneously at a dosage of 10 mg/kg bw, but is contraindicated for use in lactating cows. It is also administered orally although with less success, because its nitro group is reduced to an inactive metabolite by the rumen microorganisms (32).

Nitroxynil is well absorbed after oral administration, with peak plasma levels being achieved within 5 h after dosing. In cows, sheep, and rabbits, nitroxynil is highly bound to plasma proteins. In all species, residues in plasma are higher than in tissues and consist almost entirely of the unchanged drug. Nitroxynil is extensively metabolized, 4-cyano-2-nitrophenol and 3-iodo-4-hyroxyaminobenzamide being identified as the metabolites of the greatest concern.

Studies on the composition of nitroxynil-related residues in calves and sheep after subcutaneous treatment showed that the unchanged nitroxynil was the major component of the residues in calf kidney, muscle, and fat, accounting for around 56%, 69%, and 78% of the total residues, respectively. The 4-cyano-

2-nitrophenol was the major component of the residues in calf liver with unmetabolized nitroxynil composing only 2% of the residues. In sheep, nitroxynil was the major component of the residues in kidney, muscle, and fat, accounting for 45–56%, 90–100%, and 64–100% of the extractable residues, respectively, at 5-day withdrawal. In sheep liver, most of the residues were in the form of 3-iodo-4-hydroxy-aminobenzamide, while 4% was unchanged nitroxynil.

Nitroxynil has a tendency to bind strongly to proteins and therefore is retained in animal tissues and milk for long periods after its administration (8). Residue depletion studies in cattle subcutaneously treated with nitroxynil showed that kidney contained 252, 107, and <90 ppb, muscle 149–587, 89–131, and <50, and the injection site 90–504, <90–207, and <90 ppb of the parent drug at 30, 45, and 60 days, respectively, after withdrawal of the treatment. In sheep, residues of nitroxynil in kidney were 382, 208, and <102 ppb, and at the injection site 161–508, 102–189, and <90 ppb at 30, 45, and 60 days, respectively, after withdrawal of treatment.

Dichlorophen is a safe, narrow-spectrum drug that, in addition to its bactericidal and fungicidal properties, has been used as a teniacide in veterinary medicine for many years. It is administered to sheep as a tablet or suspension at a dosage of 0.5g/2.5 kg bw. The insolubility of dichlorophen in water limits its absorption from the gastrointestinal tract and probably accounts for its low toxicity. Worms are killed in the gut where they disintegrate prior to expulsion in the feces.

Hexachlorophen is a very efficient drug against mature flukes in sheep and cattle, but is not effective in removing immature flukes from the liver parenchyma. This is due, at least in part, to the protein-binding tendency of the drug in blood and the consequent reduced availability to the immature flukes, which are bathed in blood.

Hexachlorophen is excreted into the animal bile in the form of its glucuronide metabolite, which has high activity against the adult flukes occupying the bile ducts (6). Although the principal anthelminthic use of hexachlorophen is for liver flukes in sheep and cattle, it has also limited use as an anticestodal drug in these species and in poultry. The main anticestodal use of hexachlorophen in the United States has been for the control of chicken tapeworms, when administered at an oral dosage of 30–60 mg/kg bw.

Niclofolan is a nitrosubstituted analogue of hexachlorophen. It is highly effective against adult flukes in sheep, cattle, and swine at dosages of 3–5 mg/kg bw. Toxicity can occur at two times the recommended dosage rate. Although niclofolan can be administered subcutaneously in sheep, it is usually administered orally as a drench or in bolus forms.

Following its oral administration, niclofolan is metabolized to some degree in the rumen of cattle (45). Niclofolan passes into the milk of cattle at concentrations not exceeding 100 ppb and remains at detectable levels for up to 5–8 days posttreatment.

Bithionol is used for the treatment of tapeworm infections in poultry, and tapeworm and rumen fluke infections in sheep, cattle, and goats. An oral dose of approximately 200 mg/kg bw is used in sheep and goats, whereas two treatments, 4 days apart, of 200 mg/kg bw are used for chickens. The drug is administered to poultry with the feed, whereas to other animals it is administered in the form of gelatin capsules, tablets, or boluses.

Bithionol is absorbed to a limited degree from the digestive tract of the host and is detected in blood and particularly in the bile. Peak concentrations of bithionol are found in the bile within 2 h following treatment. Blood concentrations of the drug are significantly lower than those found in bile (6).

4.7 MACROCYCLIC LACTONES

Macrocyclic lactones are active against a variety of nematodes but lack activity toward cestodes and trematodes. They are also active against a wide variety of insects and other arthropods, including mites, ticks, and lice. Since these compounds encompass activity against both endo- and ectoparasites, they are also called ectendocides.

Included in this group are avermectins and milbemycins, which are fermentation products possessing a 16-member cyclic lactone, a spirochetal moiety, and a disaccharide unit. Abamycin, ivermectin, doramectin, and eprinomectin are major avermectins available for anthelminthic treatment of livestock, whereas moxidectin is a milbemycin with worldwide acclaim as a cattle anthelminthic (Fig. 4.7).

Abamectin is a specific mixture of two components: avermectin B_{1a} and avermectin B_{1b}. Both of these components possess a double bond between C_{22} and C_{23} and differ by a methylene group in the side-chain substituents on C_{25}. The mixture containing not less than 80% avermectin B_{1a} and not more than 20% avermectin B_{1b} is known as abamectin. Abamectin has a broad spectrum of activity against nematodes, but is primarily used in agriculture as an acaricide and insecticide (46).

Following subcutaneous administration of 0.3 mg radiolabeled abamectin/kg bw to cattle, a mean peak plasma radioactivity level of 0.09 ppm equivalents was detected. Depletion half-life rates for liver, kidney, muscle, fat, and plasma were estimated at 4.6, 5.7, 5.6, 8.1, and 4.7 days, respectively. About 70% of radioactivity was detected in feces, and 1–2% in the urine, within 7 days of treatment.

Residue depletion studies in cattle following subcutaneous treatment with a single dose of 0.3 mg radiolabeled abamectin/kg bw showed total residues in liver and fat to be significantly higher than those in kidney and muscle at any

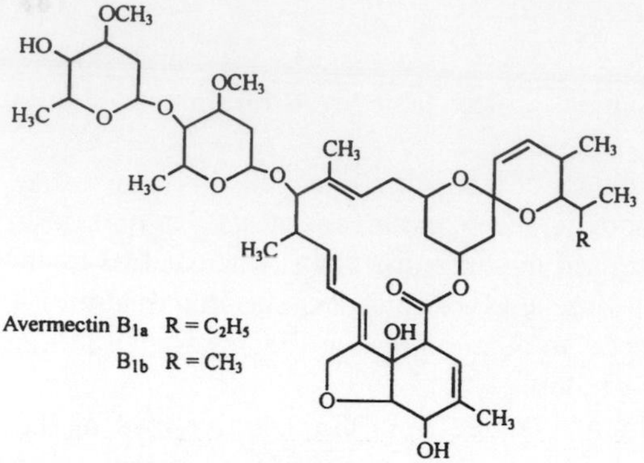

Avermectin B₁ₐ R = C₂H₅
        B₁ᵦ R = CH₃

Abamectin

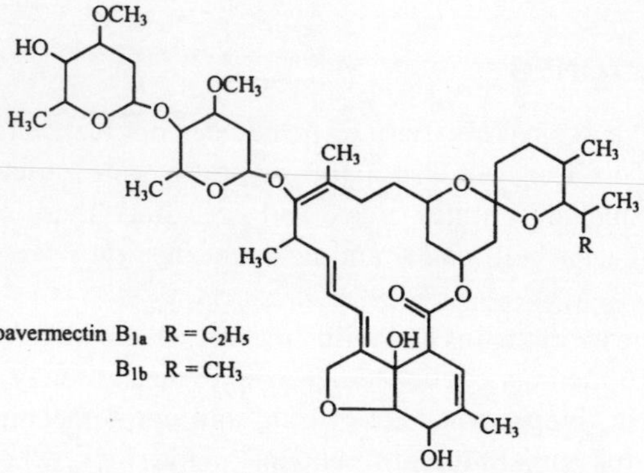

Dihydroavermectin B₁ₐ R = C₂H₅
               B₁ᵦ R = CH₃

Dihydroavermectin

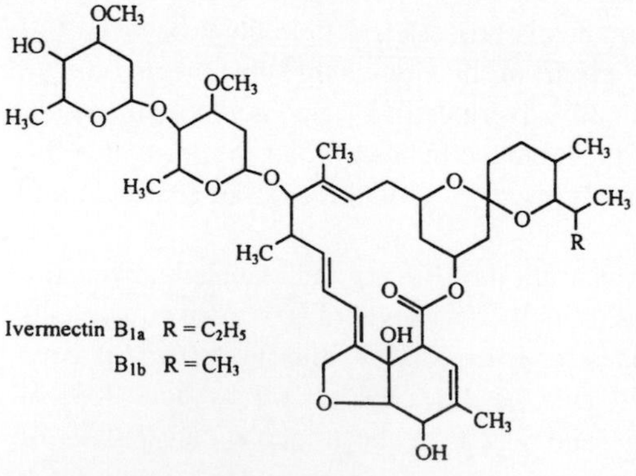

Ivermectin B₁ₐ R = C₂H₅
         B₁ᵦ R = CH₃

Ivermectin

FIG. 4.7 Chemical structures of commonly used macrocyclic lactones.

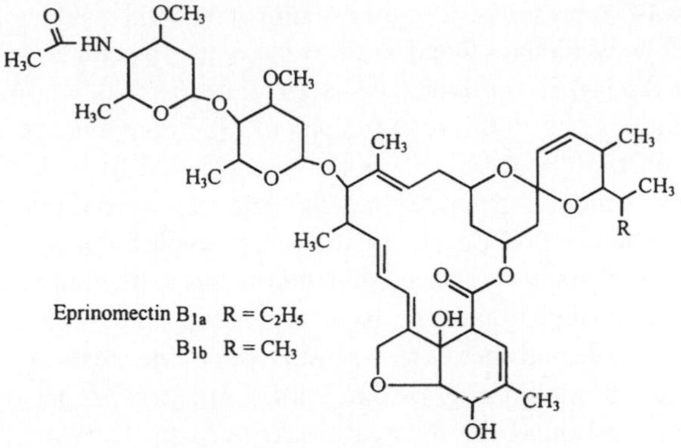

Eprinomectin B$_{1a}$ R = C$_2$H$_5$
         B$_{1b}$ R = CH$_3$

Eprinomectin

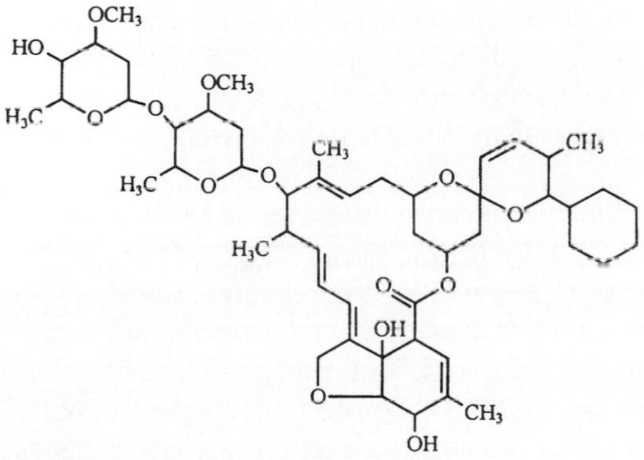

Doramectin

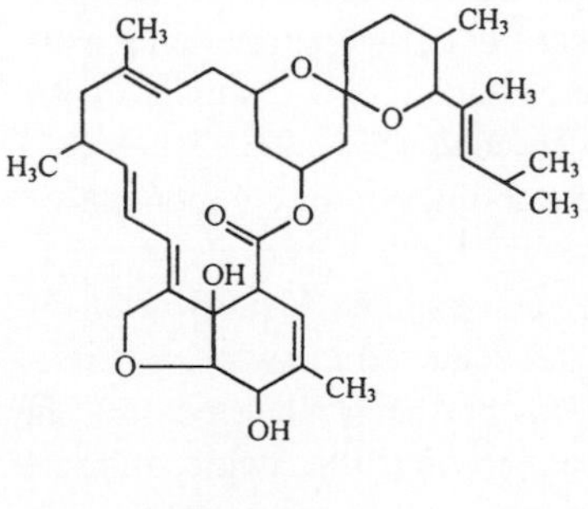

Moxidectin

Fig. 4.7   Continued

time after dosing. Avermectin B_{1a} represented a major fraction of the total residues in all edible tissues examined; between days 7 and 21, the ratio of avermectin B_{1a}/ total residues was in the range 0.55–0.36 for liver, 0.65–0.20 for fat, 0.74–0.51 for muscle, and 0.48–0.24 for kidney. In addition to the parent drug components, the 24-hydroxymethylavermectin B_{1a} metabolite was also identified in liver and fat (47). Hydroxylation of the 24-methyl group appeared to be a major metabolic pathway in cattle and goats, whereas 3-O-desmethylation also occured but at a limited extent. Unlike in cattle and goats, 3-O-desmethylation seems to be a major metabolic pathway in rats and hydroxylation of the 24-methyl group a minor one.

Consistent with results in cattle and sheep are the results of pertinent experiments in fish (48). Abamectin did not strongly bioconcentrate in aquatic organisms and would not be expected to biomagnify. Nine days after a 28 day exposure of bluegill sunfish to radiolabeled abamectin in water, samples of whole fish, fillets, and viscera were found to contain 0.32, 0.27, and 0.53 ppm abamectin equivalents, respectively.

Ivermectin is produced from abamectin by reduction of the double bond at the C_{22}–C_{23} position, a process that leads to formation of dihydroavermectin B_{1a} and dihydroavermectin B_{1b}. The reaction product that contains no less than 80% dihydroavermectin B_{1a} and no more than 20% dihydroavermectin B_{1b} constitutes ivermectin.

Ivermectin is exceptionally effective in very low dosages against nematodes and arthropod parasites in cattle and has been widely used for treatment of endo- and ectoparasites in cattle, sheep, goats, and swine (49). It is administered orally, parenterally, or as a pour-on preparation at dosages ranging from 0.2 to 0.6 mg/ kg bw. Ivermectin exhibits teratogenic effects in rat, rabbit, and mouse.

The pharmacokinetics of ivermectin differ with the animal species, formulation, and the route of administration (50). When goats were given a subcutaneous administration of 0.2 mg ivermectin /kg bw, the mean concentrations of ivermectin in plasma and milk increased initially to reach at 2.8 day the maximum levels of 6.12 and 7.26 ppb, respectively (51). The drug could be detected in milk for 25 days postdosing, the total drug amount recovered over this period being estimated at 0.6% of the administered dose. This percentage is low compared with the 4% level determined in sheep (52) and 5.6% in cows (53).

Metabolism studies showed that the major metabolites of the components of ivermectin in cattle, sheep, and rats were 24-hydroxymethyl compounds, whereas major metabolites in swine were 3-O-desmethyl compounds. Identification of the 24-hydroxymethyl metabolites has not been yet achieved in swine, whereas identification of the 3-O-desmethyl metabolites has not been made possible in cattle or sheep (54, 55). Recent metabolism studies (56) in cattle, swine, and rats have indicated, however, that the metabolism of avermectins was qualitatively similar for all three species. There were quantitative differences both between species and between compounds for a given species, but all three species produced either 24-hydroxymethyl- or 3-O-desmethyl-compounds as the major metabolites, other drug-related compounds being of minor importance.

Depletion studies showed that the parent drug could account for the major proportion of total residues in the edible tissues of cattle, sheep, and swine. In addition, a relatively nonpolar fraction but more polar than the parent drug could account for 26–55% of the total residues in fat. This fraction in fat was found to be composed of acyl esters of major ivermectin metabolites. Their deposition in fat probably explains the high concentrations and the persistence of ivermectin residues in fat (57). The slow excretion rate together with the long half-lives in the peripheral tissues, especially fat, and the short residing time of the drug at the site of administration suggest that the drug is rapidly absorbed into the peripheral circulation from which it is taken up into secondary depots. Ivermectin and its metabolites are probably released gradually into the peripheral circulation, metabolized in the liver, and excreted into the bile and pass into feces.

Residue depletion studies in cattle, sheep, and swine revealed that drug residue levels are higher in liver and fat, with much lower values in kidney and muscle (57). Following subcutaneous or oral administration of ivermectin to cattle at a dosage of 0.3 mg/kg bw, residual levels of ivermectin B_{1a} in muscle, liver, kidney, and fat tissues were 37, 244, 62, and 201 ppb at 7 day post dosing, and 0, 11, 1 and 4 ppb at 28 day post dosing. Milk also contained residues of ivermectin B_{1a} that peaked at about 28 ppb at 2–3 days postdosing and declined thereafter to 2 ppb at 21 days postdosing. Swine and sheep exhibited a residue depletion profile analogous to that of cattle.

Doramectin, unlike ivermectin components, possesses a double bond between C_{22} and C_{23} and a cyclohexyl ring on C_{25}. This novel avermectin is intended for use in cattle and sheep in the form of a single subcutaneous injection at a dosage of 0.2 mg/kg bw, or in pigs in the form of a single intramuscular injection at a dosage of 0.3 mg/kg bw (58).

Pharmacokinetic studies (59) in cattle treated with the recommended dosage showed that the drug was well dispersed from the injection site, with less than 1% of the dose remaining at 21 day withdrawal. By 14 days, 87% of the dose was excreted via the bile and feces whereas less than 1% was eliminated via urine. Mean plasma half-life was found to be 6.2 days for the parent compound and 5.9 days for total drug-related residues.

Concentrations of total residues were highest at the injection site, liver, and fat. Much lower concentrations were present in muscle and kidney tissues. In all samples, unchanged doramectin represented a major fraction of the total residues, the remaining being composed of the major metabolite, 3″-O-desmethyldoramectin, and two minor metabolites, 24-hydroxymethyldoramectin and 24-hydroxymethyl-3″-O-desmethyldoramectin. Another metabolite identified as the 2-epimer of doramectin was also detected in fat. Residue depletion studies showed that mean levels of the parent drug in fat, liver, muscle, kidney, and injection site declined from 493, 319, 33, 96.2, and 2530 ppb at 7 days after treatment to 16.7, 13.2, less than 2.1, 3.1, and 18 ppb at 42 days posttreatment, respectively.

Residue depletion studies (60) in swine given a single intramuscular injection of doramectin at a dosage of 375 mg/kg bw showed that residues of the parent drug were always higher at the injection site and declined from 9000 ppb at 7 days after treatment to 70 ppb at 35 days after treatment. Residues in back fat declined from 470 ppb at 7 days after treatment to 50 ppb at 35 days after treatment. Residues in liver declined from 160 ppb at 7 days after treatment to 18 ppb at 35 days after treatment. Residues in kidney and muscle declined from 80 and 40 ppb, respectively, at 7 days after treatment to 18 and 11 ppb, respectively, at 21 days after treatment.

Metabolism studies in sheep given a single subcutaneous injection of 0.3 mg radiolabeled doramectin/kg bw showed that unmetabolized doramectin made up 92%, 75%, 73%, and 67% of the total radioactivity present in muscle, liver, kidney and fat, respectively, at 14 days after treatment. The metabolite 3″-O-desmethyldoramectin was found to be a minor component in all edible tissues of sheep except muscle. A metabolite tentatively identified as the 2-epimer of doramectin was also found to constitute a minor component in sheep fat. The metabolites 24-hydroxymethyldoramectin and 24-hydroxymethyl-3″-O-desmethyldoramectin were found in sheep feces but not in tissues. Mean residue levels of the parent drug in pooled renal and omental fat declined from 62.8 ppb at 14 days after treatment to less than 4.5 ppb at 35 days after treatment. Mean levels in liver were 47.5 ppb at 14 days after treatment, and were below 2.5 ppb in three of the four sheep slaughtered at 35 days after treatment. Residues in kidney and muscle were 17.9 ppb and 13.5 ppb, respectively, at 14 days after treatment, and were below 2.5 ppb in all samples at 35 days after treatment. Residue levels at the injection site were variable, declining from a mean of 2554 ppb at 14 days after treatment to 365 ppb at 35 days after treatment. Fifty-six days after the treatment, residues at the injection site were still present at levels below 113 ppb.

Eprinomectin is derived from the natural product abamectin by conversion of the 4″-hydroxy group to the 4″-*epi*-N-acetyl substituent. Like abamectin, eprinomectin is a mixture of two active constituents that contain more than 90% 4″-deoxy-4″-(*epi*-acetylamino)avermectin B_{1a} and less than 10% 4″-deoxy-4″-(*epi*-acetylamino)avermectin B_{1b}. It is indicated for treatment of internal and external parasites in beef and dairy cattle at a dosage of 0.5 mg/kg bw and is applied along the midline of the animal's back (61).

Following topical application to cattle, only 29% of the dose was absorbed through the skin. Most of the absorption occurred within 7–10 days postdosing, after an initial time lag of about 24 h, and continued for 17–21 days postdosing, but to a minor extent. Metabolism studies (62) in calves treated with the recommended dosage showed that only 0.35% of the applied dose was present in urine over 28 days, while 17–19.8% was present in feces. In feces, the eprinomectin

B_{1a} was the most abundant residue representing 78.3% of the total residues, the eprinomectin B_{1b} 8.3%, the 24a-hydroxymethyl metabolite 7.4%, whereas the sum of the minor 24a-hydroxy-, 26a-hydroxymethyl-, and N-deacetylated metabolites represented less than 1.6%. The metabolism profile also indicated that eprinomectin B_{1a} was the major residue in all edible tissues, the eprinomectin B_{1b} representing 7.2–9.3%, whereas five to seven minor metabolites represented only 1–2% of the total radioactivity. In muscle, however, the N-deacetylated metabolite accounted for as much as 3.9% of the total residues. Eprinomectin B_{1a} was also found to be a major metabolite, accounting for 80–85.6% of the total extractable radioactivity in milk. In this matrix, the 24a-hydroxymethyl metabolite represented less than 2%, the N-deacetylated metabolite 0.7–2.5%, whereas the contribution by the other metabolites was negligible.

In a radiometric depletion study (62) carried out in cattle, the concentrations of eprinomectin B_{1a} residues in muscle, injection site, fat, liver, and kidney were 6, 17, 30, 807, and 161 ppb, respectively, at 7 days postdosing, and declined to 3, 14, 14, 369, and 54 ppb, respectively, at 21 days after the treatment. In a nonradiometric study with dairy cows dosed topically with 0.5–0.55 mg eprinomectin/kg bw, 5 ppb was the highest concentration of eprinomectin B_{1a} residues observed in milk obtained at the fifth to sixth milking postdosing; residues in milk declined to 0.5 ppb by the 13th milking.

Moxidectin is a semisynthetic milbemycin intended for treatment of endectoparasites in cattle, sheep, and horses. It is administered by oral or subcutaneous routes at a dosage of 0.2 mg/kg bw in cattle and sheep, and 0.4 mg/kg bw in horses.

After a single oral administration of 0.4 mg radiolabeled moxidectin/kg bw to horses, a mean peak serum concentration of 0.134 ppm moxidectin equivalents was attained at 6 h postdose (63). Oral availability was estimated at 40%, while the terminal elimination half-life was approximately 80 h. Within 168 h, 77% of the total radioactivity was excreted mostly by the fecal route. In feces, the parent drug represented approximately 70% of the fecal radioactivity, whereas a fraction of 0.28–3.45% was due to four minor metabolites resulting from oxidation mainly on C_{14}, C_{24}, and/or C_{28} positions.

At 168 h postadministration, the parent drug represented 48% of the total radioactivity in muscle, 87% in fat, 61% in liver, and 78% in kidney. In a pertinent radiometric depletion study (64) carried out in horse, moxidectin residues in fat were found to be 221, 165, 130, and 131 ppb at 28, 35, 42, and 49 days, respectively. In all other edible tissues, residue concentrations were below 10 ppb even at the first sampling.

In cattle and sheep, parent moxidectin represented 40% of the total radioactivity in liver, 50% in muscle, 60–75% in kidney, and 90% in fat. When moxidectin was given subcutaneously to steers, both the parent drug and at least seven metabolites could be detected in extracts of tissues, feces, and bile (65). The parent drug accounted for 36–91% (4–275 ppb) of the residues in fat, tissues, and the injection site, and 26% of the residue in feces collected at 2 days. At 28 day withdrawal, residue levels of metabolites in tissues were as low as 2 ppb. Two major metabolites accounting for 9% and 11% of the total residues monitored in liver at 7 days, or for 25% and 9% of the total residues monitored in feces at 7 days, were isolated and identified as the C_{29}–C_{30} hydroxymethyl metabolite and the C_{14} hydroxylated metabolite.

When moxidectin was administered orally to lambs, residue levels in liver, muscle, fat, and kidney were 35, 17.5, 259, and 35 ppb, respectively, at 7 day withdrawal; at 28 day withdrawal, the levels in the same tissues changed to 3.0, 10, 70.4, and 5.6 ppb, respectively (66). This depletion profile is in good agreement with biotransformation studies of radiolabeled moxidectin (67).

4.8   PIPERAZINE DERIVATIVES

Included in this group are the anthelminthics piperazine and diethylcarbamazine (Fig. 4.8). They are both safe drugs available in the form of simple salts, mainly citrates.

Piperazine is a diethylenediamine used extensively in swine and chickens, but seldom in cattle and sheep. Piperazine preparations can be administered via either the feed or drinking water at a dosage of 275–440 mg/kg bw to pigs and 250 mg/kg bw to chickens.

Piperazine and its salts are readily absorbed from the gastrointestinal tract, but nitrosation may occur in the stomach (32). The major portion of the absorbed drug is metabolized in tissues and the remainder, which is about 30–40%, is excreted in the urine. Piperazine is detectable in the urine as early as 0.5 h after drug administration. Although there is a wide variation in the rates at which piperazine is excreted by different animal species, urinary excretion is practically complete within 24 h.

Diethylcarbamazine has long been used in sheep and especially in cattle for treatment of lungworm infections. Intramuscular injection is the routine

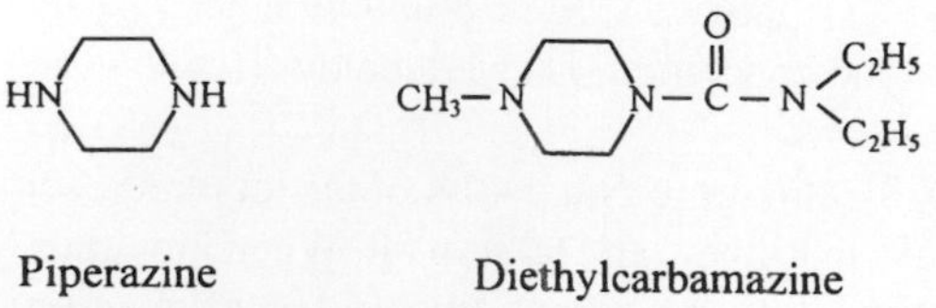

Piperazine   Diethylcarbamazine

FIG. 4.8   Chemical structures of commonly used piperazine derivatives.

method of administration, but results of equal efficacy can be obtained when an initial intramuscular injection is followed by two orally administered doses.

Diethylcarbamazine is rapidly absorbed from the gastrointestinal tract. Peak concentration in the blood occurs at about 3 h after oral administration and falls to zero within 48 h. The drug is distributed almost equally throughout all body compartments, with the exception of the fat, and there is little tendency for accumulation with repeated doses. Excretion occurs almost entirely through the urine, with most of the drug appearing in form of metabolites.

4.9 MISCELLANEOUS

Clorsulon (Fig. 4.9) is a benzenesulphonamide derivative recommended for treatment and control of adult and immature liver flukes in cattle and sheep (68). It is administered orally or subcutaneously at a dosage of 7 or 2 mg/kg bw, respectively, in association, frequently, with ivermectin.

Following subcutaneous administration of 2 mg radiolabeled clorsuron/kg bw to cattle, a maximum peak plasma level of about 1.3 ppm was attained at about 6 h, declining to 0.01 ppm at 7 days after injection. Following intraruminal administration of 10 mg radiolabeled clorsuron/kg bw to cattle, a maximum peak plasma level of about 3 ppm occurred at about 24 h, declining to 0.014 ppm by 21 days postdosing. In the same study (69), the ratios of the unchanged clorsulon to total residues in kidney, liver, and muscle were estimated at about 75%, 55%, and 41%, respectively. About 80% of the radioactivity in kidney and liver was extractable by organic solvents. Acid hydrolysis of liver extracts revealed the presence of 10 metabolites less polar and 3 metabolites more polar than the parent drug, none of the metabolites accounting for more than 5% of the total residues. In kidney, major component of the total residues was the parent drug, whereas five less polar and three more polar metabolites could be also detected.

Residue depletion studies in cattle administered 3 mg clorsulon/kg bw by the subcutaneous route showed that kidney and liver were the tissues with the highest residue concentrations containing 3.3 and 2.2 ppm of parent clorsulon, respectively, at 1 day posttreatment and 0.1 and 0.04 ppm, respectively, at 7 days post treatment. When steers were dosed intraruminally with radiolabeled clorsulon at 10 mg/kg bw, edible tissues contained 100–400 ppb clorsulon equivalents at 7 days after dosing (70). A major part of the radioactive residues found in the liver and kidney tissues was attributed to the unchanged drug.

When cows were dosed singly with an oral suspension of radiolabeled clorsulon at 7 mg/kg bw, average milk residue levels decreased from 0.54 ppm at 0.9 days posttreatment to 0.004 ppm at 6.9 day is posttreatment, with a half-life of 0.81 days (71). The unchanged drug was identified as the major residue component in the milk collected by the 4 day postdosing, and accounted for

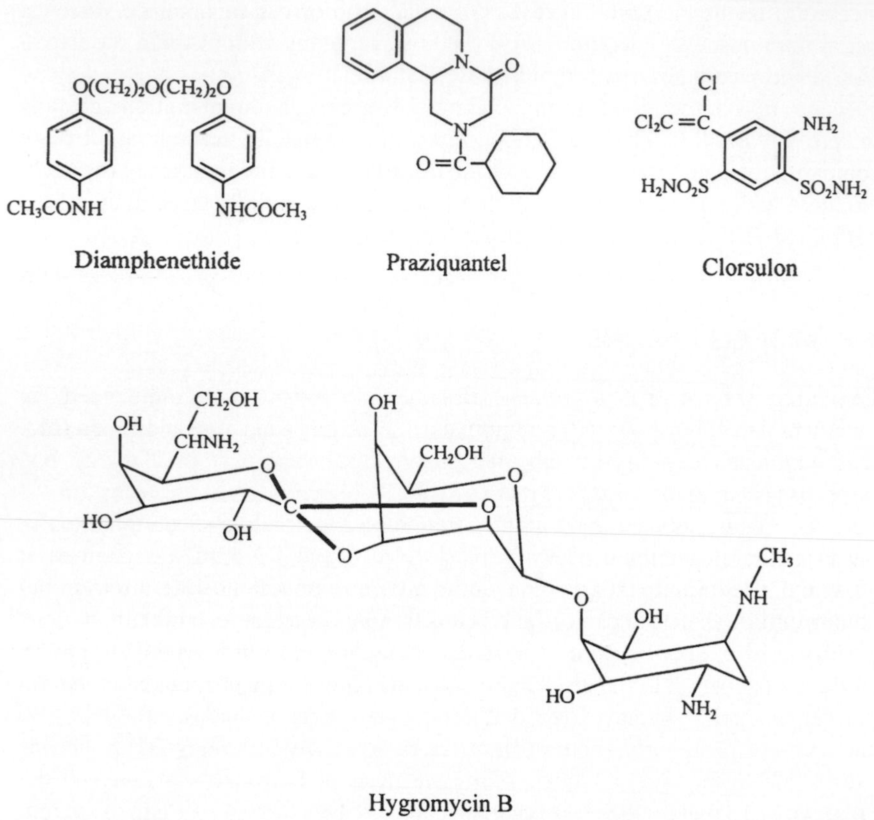

Diamphenethide   Praziquantel   Clorsulon

Hygromycin B

FIG. 4.9 Chemical structures of diamphenethide, praziquantel, clorsulon, and hygromycin B.

56–99% of the total radioactivity. About 0.7% of the dose could be recovered in the milk during the 6.9 day period.

Praziquantel (Fig. 4.9), a racemate derivative of pyrazino-isoquinoline, is effective against many species of cestodes and trematodes. It is indicated for use in nonlactating sheep in form of a single oral dose of 3.75 mg/kg bw.

Pharmacokinetic studies with sheep treated with the recommended dosage showed that praziquantel was rapidly absorbed, peak plasma concentration being reached within 2 h of dosing (72). A half-life of 4.2 h was determined and excretion from plasma was rapid, 98% being excreted within 72 h. At 8 h posttreatment, the maximum levels present in liver, kidneys, muscle, and fat were 2.87, 2.55, 0.19, and 0.13 ppb, respectively, of praziquantel equivalents. At 24 h posttreatment, levels in muscle and fat were 0.02 ppb of praziquantel equivalents. Metabolism studies in a variety of animal species indicated rapid and almost total biotransformation of the drug in the liver (32).

Diamphenethide, an aromatic amide (Fig. 4.9), is effective against young flukes and, hence, is indicated against acute fascioliosis. The drug is available commercially as a ready-to-use suspension for oral administration to sheep in a single dose of 100 mg/kg bw. The high anthelminthic efficacy of this compound in sheep, is due to the deacetylated metabolite formed locally in the host liver. This metabolite is also responsible for the activity exhibited against liver parenchyma stages.

Following oral administration, diamphenethide is absorbed into the blood and distributed throughout the animal body. At 3 days postdosing, its concentration is highest in liver and gallbladder. At 7 days postdosing, concentrations of the drug in these tissues were reduced approximately 10-fold to a range of 0.1–0.5 ppm, while low concentrations in the musculature were about 0.02 ppm.

Hygromycin B (Fig. 4.9) is an antibiotic that exhibits anthelminthic properties. Although it is also active against both Gram-positive and Gram-negative bacteria, its antibacterial activity is too poor to be therapeutically useful. However, its anthelminthic activity has been confirmed in poultry and swine. It is used as feed additive in swine and poultry, for consumption over periods of several weeks. A dosage of 12 g hygromycin B/ton of total ration is recommended for swine, while a dosage of 8 g hygromycin B/ton of total ration is recommended for chickens.

REFERENCES

1. R.V. Arenas, and N.A. Johnson, J. AOAC Int., 77:741 (1994).
2. A. Ogata, H. Ando, Y. Kubo, and K. Hiraga, Food Chem. Toxicol., 22:509 (1984).
3. T. Mizutani, K. Ito, H. Nomura, and K. Nakanishi, Food Chem. Toxicol., 28:169 (1990).
4. World Health Organization, in Evaluation of Certain Veterinary Drug Residues in Food, Fortieth Meeting of the Joint FAO/WHO Expert Committee on Food Additives, Food and Agriculture Organization of the United Nations, Geneva, (1992).
5. J.A. Gardiner, J.J. Kirkland, H.L. Klopping, and H. Sherman, J. Agric. Food Chem., 22:419 (1974).
6. E.L. Roberson, in Veterinary Pharmacology and Therapeutics (L. Meyer Jones, N.H. Booth, and L.E. McDonald, Eds.), 4th Edition, The Iowa State University Press, Ames, IA (1977).
7. European Agency for the Evaluation of Medicinal Products (EMEA), in Thiabendazole, Summary Report, Committee for Veterinary Medicinal Products, EMEA/MRL/269/97-Final, London, UK (1997).
8. T.B. Barragry, in Veterinary Drug Therapy (T.B. Barragry, Ed.), Lea & Febiger, PA (1994).

9. European Agency for the Evaluation of Medicinal Products (EMEA), in Thiophanate, Summary Report, Committee for Veterinary Medicinal Products, EMEA/MRL, London, UK (1998).
10. World Health Organization, in Evaluation of Certain Veterinary Drug Residues in Food, Thirty-eighth Report of the Joint FAO/WHO Expert Committee on Food Additives, Technical Report Series 815, World Health Organization, Geneva, p. 13 (1991).
11. L.C. Kappel, and S.A. Barker, J. Vet. Pharmacol. Ther., 19:416 (1996).
12. D.J. Fletouris, N.A. Botsoglou, I.E. Psomas, and A.I. Mantis, Analyst, 119:2801 (1994).
13. D.J. Fletouris, N.A. Botsoglou, I.E. Psomas, and A.I. Mantis, J. Agric. Food Chem., 44:3882 (1996).
14. C.R. Short, S.A. Barker, L.C. Hsieh, S.-P. Ou, L.E. Davis, G. Koritz, C.A. Neff-Davis, R.F. Bevill, I.J. Munsiff, and G.C. Sharma, Am. J. Vet. Res., 48:811 (1987).
15. E.G. Iosifidou, N. Haagsma, M.W.T. Tanck, J.H. Boon, and M. Olling, Aquaculture, 154:191 (1997).
16. European Agency for the Evaluation of Medicinal Products (EMEA), in Albendazole, Summary Report, Committee for Veterinary Medicinal Products, EMEA/MRL/247/97-Final, London, UK (1997).
17. G. Csiko, G. Banhidi, G. Semjen, J. Fekete, P. Laczay, and J. Lehel, Magyar Allatorvosok Lapja, 50:867 (1995).
18. D.J. Fletouris, N.A. Botsoglou, I.E. Psomas, and A.I. Mantis, J. AOAC Int., 79:1281 (1996).
19. D.J. Fletouris, N.A. Botsoglou, I.E. Psomas, and A.I. Mantis, J. Chromatogr. B, 687: 427 (1996).
20. D.J. Fletouris, N.A. Botsoglou, I.E. Psomas, and A.I. Mantis, Anal. Chim. Acta, 345:111 (1997).
21. European Agency for the Evaluation of Medicinal Products (EMEA), in Netobimin, Summary Report, Committee for Veterinary Medicinal Products, EMEA/MRL/97-Final, London, UK (1997).
22. K. Buchmann, A. Poepstorff, and P.J. Waller, J. Fish Dis., 15:393 (1992).
23. J.G. Steenbaar, C.A.J. Hajee, and N. Haagsma, J. Chromatogr., 615:186 (1993).
24. W.E.G. Meuldermans, R.M.A. Hurkmans, W.F.J. Lauwers, and J.J.P. Heykants, Eur. J. Drug Metab. Pharmacokinet., 1:35 (1976).
25. C.A.J. Hajee, M. Olling, and N. Haagsma, in Residues of Veterinary Drugs in Food, Proc. Euroresidue III Conf., Veldhoven, 1996 (N. Haagsma, and A. Ruiter, Eds.), Fac. Vet. Med., Univ. Utrecht,, The Netherlands, p. 466 (1996).
26. E.G. Iosifidou, N. Haagsma, M. Olling, J.H. Boon, and M.W.T. Tanck, in Residues of Veterinary Drugs in Food, Proc. Euroresidue III Conf., Veldhoven, 1996 (N. Haagsma, and A. Ruiter, Eds.), Fac. Vet. Med., Univ. Utrecht, The Netherlands, p. 568 (1996).
27. European Agency for the Evaluation of Medicinal Products (EMEA), in Oxibendazole, Summary Report, Committee for Veterinary Medicinal Products, EMEA/MRL/268/97-Final, London, UK (1997).
28. D.W. Gottschall, and R. Wang, Vet. Parasitol., 64:83 (1996).
29. P.K. Sanyal, J. Vet. Pharmacol. Ther., 18:370 (1995).

30. P.K. Sanyal, J. Vet. Pharmacol. Ther., 20:127 (1997).
31. World Health Organization, in Evaluation of Certain Veterinary Drug Residues in Food, Fortieth Report of the Joint FAO/WHO Expert Committee on Food Additives, Technical Report Series 832, World Health Organization, Geneva (1993).
32. G.C. Brander, D.M. Pugh, R.J. Bywaters, and W.L. Jenkins, in Veterinary Applied Pharmacology and Therapeutics (G.C. Brander, D.M. Pugh, R.J. Bywaters, and W.L. Jenkins, Eds.), 5th Edition, Bailliere Tindall, London (1991).
33. World Health Organization, in Residues of Some Veterinary Drugs in Animals and Foods, Thirty-sixth Meeting of the Joint FAO/WHO Expert Committee on Food Additives, Food and Agriculture Organization of the United Nations, FAO Food and Nutrition Paper No 41/3, Rome, p. 65 (1990).
34. P. Galtier, L. Escoula, and M. Alvinerie, Am. J. Vet. Res., 44:583 (1983).
35. P. Nielsen, and F. Rasmussen, Pharmacol. Toxicol. Vet., 8:431 (1982).
36. G. Graziani, and G.L. De Martin, Drugs Exp. Clin. Res., 2:221 (1977).
37. J.D. Malone, Res. Vet. Sci., 5:17 (1964).
38. G.P. Poeschel, and A.C. Todd, Am. J. Vet. Res., 33:1071 (1972).
39. A.C. Todd, Vet. Med., 57:322 (1962).
40. L.R. Robinson, and R.L. Ziegler, Lab. Anim. Care, 18:50 (1968).
41. J.E. Casida, L. McBride, and R.P. Niedermeir, J. Agric. Food Chem., 10:370 (1962).
42. M. Michiels, W. Meuldermans, and J. Heykants, Drug Metab. Rev., 18:235 (1987).
43. World Health Organization, in Residues of Some Veterinary Drugs in Animals and Foods, Thirty-sixth Meeting of the Joint FAO/WHO Expert Committee on Food Additives, Food and Agriculture Organization of the United Nations, FAO Food and Nutrition Paper No 41/3, Rome, p. 32 (1990).
44. World Health Organization, in Evaluation of Certain Veterinary Drug Residues in Food, Fortieth Meeting of the Joint FAO/WHO Expert Committee on Food Additives, Food and Agriculture Organization of the United Nations, Geneva, p. 19 (1992).
45. E. Zarnowski, Acta Parasitol. Pol., 15:1 (1967).
46. N.C. Cambell, and G.W. Benz, J. Vet. Pharmacol. Ther., 7:1 (1984).
47. P.K.A. Lo, D.W. Fink, J.B. Williams, and J. Blodinger, Vet. Res. Commun., 9:251 (1985).
48. W.J.A. Vandenheuvel, A.D. Forbis, B.A. Halley, C.C. Ku, T.A. Jacob, and P.G. Wislocki, Environ. Toxicol. Chem., 15:2266 (1996).
49. M. Alvinerie, J.F. Sutra, and P. Galtier, in Residues of Veterinary Drugs in Food, Proc. Euroresidue II Conf., Veldhoven, May 3–5, 1993 (N. Haagsma, A. Ruiter and P.B. Czedik-Eysenberg, Eds.), Fac. Vet. Med., Univ. Utrecht, The Netherlands, p. 134 (1993).
50. S.E. Marriner, I. McKinnon, and J.A. Bogan, J. Vet. Pharmacol. Therap., 10:175 (1987).
51. P.L. Toutain, M. Campan, P. Galtier, and M. Alvinerie, J. Vet. Pharmacol. Ther., 11:288 (1988).
52. World Health Organization, in Residues of Some Veterinary Drugs in Animals and Foods, Thirty-sixth Meeting of the Joint FAO/WHO Expert Committee on Food Additives, Food and Agriculture Organization of the United Nations, FAO Food and Nutrition Paper No 41/3, Rome, p. 45 (1990).
53. W.C. Cambell, in Ivermectin and Abamectin (W.C. Cambell, Ed.), Springer-Verlag, NY (1989).

54. S.H.L. Chiu, R. Taub, E. Sestokas, A.Y.H. Lu, and T.A. Jacob, Drug Metab. Dispos., 18:289 (1987).
55. M.S. Maynard, B.A. Halley, M. Green-Erwin, R. Alvaro, V.F. Gruber, S.C. Hwang, B.W. Bennett, and P.G. Wislocki, J. Agric. Food Chem., 38:864 (1990).
56. B.A. Halley, N.I. Narasimhan, K. Venkataraman, R.T. Taub, M.L.G. Erwin, N.W. Andrew, and P.G. Wislocki, in Xenobiotics and Food-Producing Animals (D.H. Hutson, D.R. Hawkins, G.D. Paulson, and C.B. Struble, Eds.), American Chemical Society, Washington, DC, p. 203 (1992).
57. S.H.L. Chiu, E. Sestokas, R. Taub, R.P. Buhs, M. Green, R. Sestokas, W.J.A. Van den Heuvel, B.H. Arison, and T.A. Jacob, Drug Metab. Dispos., 14:590 (1986).
58. P.P. Niutta, E. Giudice, D. Britti, and A. Pugliese, J. Vet. Pharmacol. Ther., 20:159 (1997).
59. European Agency for the Evaluation of Medicinal Products (EMEA), in Doramectin, Summary Report, Committee for Veterinary Medicinal Products, EMEA/MRL/136/96-Final, London, UK (1997).
60. European Agency for the Evaluation of Medicinal Products (EMEA), in Doramectin, Summary Report, Committee for Veterinary Medicinal Products, EMEA/MRL/186/97-Final, London, UK (1997).
61. J.M. Ballard, L.D. Payne, R.S. Egan, T.A. Wehner, G.S. Rahn, and S. Tom, J. Agric. Food Chem., 45:3507 (1997).
62. European Agency for the Evaluation of Medicinal Products (EMEA), in Eprinomectin, Summary Report, Committee for Veterinary Medicinal Products, EMEA/MRL/114/96-Final, London, UK (1997).
63. J. Azfal, A.B. Burke, P.L. Batten, R.L. Delay, and P. Miller, J. Agric. Food Chem., 45:3627 (1997).
64. European Agency for the Evaluation of Medicinal Products (EMEA), in Moxidectin, Summary Report, Committee for Veterinary Medicinal Products, EMEA/MRL/250/97-Final, London, UK (1997).
65. J. Zulalian, S.J. Stout, A.R. Dacunha, T. Garces, and P. Miller, Proc. of the 6th EAVPT Inter. Congress (P. Lees, Ed.), European Association for Veterinary Pharmacology and Therapeutics, Blackwell Scientific Publications, Edinburgh, UK, p. 275 (1994).
66. A. Fernandez Suarez, M. Alvinerie, J.F. Sutra, and P. Galtier, J. Vet. Pharmacol. Ther., 20:314 (1997).
67. J. Azfal, S. Stout, and P. Miller, J. Agric. Food Chem., 42:1767 (1994).
68. H.H. Mrozik, Merck & Co., Substituted benzenedisulfonamide, German Patent DE 2556122, June 24 (1976).
69. European Agency for the Evaluation of Medicinal Products (EMEA), in Clorsulon, Summary Report, Committee for Veterinary Medicinal Products, EMEA/MRL/037/95-Rev. 1, London, UK (1997).
70. S.H.L. Chiu, E. Sestokas, R. Raub, R. Walker, and A.Y.H. Lu, Drug Metab. Disp., 13:374 (1985).
71. S.H.L. Chiu, F.P. Baylis, R. Raub, M. Green, B.A. Halley, and R.M. Bodden, J. Agric. Food Chem., 37:819 (1989).
72. European Agency for the Evaluation of Medicinal Products (EMEA), in Praziquantel, Summary Report, Committee for Veterinary Medicinal Products, EMEA/MRL/141/96-Final, London, UK (1996).

5

Anticoccidial and Other Antiprotozoal Drugs

High-intensity rearing systems, particularly in the poultry industry, have resulted in a dependence on anticoccidial feed additives to provide prophylactic control against protozoal infections caused by pathogenic species of *Eimeria* (1). Nine species of coccidia belonging to the genus *Eimeria* are known to infect poultry that are most susceptible, due to the warm humid environment created in intensive rearing units on modern farms. The degree of pathogenesis caused by each species of *Eimeria* varies. The most pathogenic species in chickens are *Eimeria tenella, Eimeria necatrix,* and *Eimeria brunetti,* which can give rise to spectacular outbreaks of disease. In addition to poultry, coccidiosis also affects pigs, cattle, and sheep. However, the disease is usually less than a problem in food-producing animals other than chickens since pigs, cattle, and sheep are reared less intensively with less chance of infection.

In general, protozoa are transmitted through feces contaminated with coccidial oocysts. When oocysts are swallowed, the membrane is damaged, releasing sporozoites that penetrate the epithelial cells and multiply rapidly in both asexual and sexual cycles. Some also enter the bloodstream and are transmitted to the liver and kidney. During the reproductive cycle, which takes 7–10 days to be completed, the parasites multiply 100,000-fold before being excreted with the feces. The effects of coccidial infestation in animals vary from poor weight gain and reduced egg production to hemorrhage, destruction of cells on a massive scale, and, very often, death.

A closely related disease, particularly in turkeys, is known as histomoniasis or blackhead, in which the liver is badly damaged by the attack of a protozoan parasite, *Histomonas meleagridis* and, unless properly treated, rapidly results in death. Parasitic protozoa are also responsible for a wide range of diseases of worldwide importance but that are difficult to eliminate since they are frequently transmitted by ticks, flies, and tabanids. Trypanosomiasis, piroplasmosis, and anaplasmosis caused by *Trypanosoma, Babesia* and *Anaplasma* species, respectively, are severe hemotrophic diseases of cattle that have hampered, to a large extent, the development of the livestock industry in tropical and subtropical areas of the world.

Parasitic diseases pose an ever-present threat to any intensive poultry or livestock rearing unit but can be controlled by addition of low levels of drugs to the daily ration. In good veterinary practice, the drugs used to control coccidiosis and other protozoal diseases are used at levels that do not allow resistant strains to be developed and are selected to be rapidly metabolized to keep residues in edible tissues to a minimum. The residue problem could be controlled using mandatory withdrawal periods, but under practical farming conditions such restrictions are not always observed. On the other hand, since so many coccidiostats are available, many farmers switch from one compound to another to prevent the development of drug resistance over the years. Hence, most poultry are given feeds containing drugs for the whole or the majority of their lives.

The major anticoccidial and other antiprotozoal drugs have no common chemical structure and therefore no group tests can be used to screen for residues in animal-derived foods. This is in complete contrast to the antibacterials previously discussed, which can be detected, although not identified, on the basis of their biological activity.

Some drugs, including sulfaquinoxaline, sulfadimethoxine, sulfamethoxypyridazine, sulfachlorpyrazine, sulfamethazine, sulfaguanidine, furazolidone, nitrofurazone, tetracycline, and chlortetracycline, in addition to their role as coccidiostats, are also used as antibacterials. These drugs will not be discussed in this chapter since they have been discussed previously. On the other hand, other compounds such as roxarsone, are classified as growth promoters and therefore will be described in the corresponding chapter. This chapter is limited to compounds whose primary function and use are as antiprotozoals.

5.1 BENZAMIDES

Aklomide, nitromide, and **dinitolmide** are the major drugs used within this group (Fig. 5.1). Subsequent to their initial marketing, each of these drugs has appeared in formulations with roxarsone and sulfanitran or roxarsone alone. All three drugs, but especially dinitolmide, have been used worldwide as chicken coccidiostats. Dinitolmide, also known as zoalene, has moderate to good activity against chicken coccidia. It is added to animal feeds at 125 ppm for chickens and at 125–187 ppm for turkeys but is not intending for laying hens.

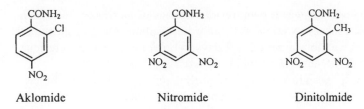

Aklomide   Nitromide   Dinitolmide

FIG. 5.1 Chemical structures of commonly used benzamides.

Following administration to poultry, dinitolmide is mainly metabolized to 3-amino-5-nitro-*o*-toluamide and 5-amino-3-nitro-*o*-toluamide metabolites that are bound to tissues. Residue depletion studies of dinitolmide in chicken, also showed the formation in chicken liver of an acid-labile conjugate of the 5-amino-3-nitro-*o*-toluamide metabolite, presumably the *N*5-glucoside conjugate (2). However, no evidence was presented for the formation of the corresponding 3-amino-5-nitro-*o*-toluamide conjugate in chicken tissues.

5.2 CARBANILIDES

Nicarbazin and **imidocarb** represent the major drugs within this group (Fig. 5.2). Nicarbazin constitutes an equimolar mixture of 4-4'-dinitrocarbanilide and 2-hydroxy-4,6-dimethylpyrimidine. Its activity is predominantly coccidiocidal, but it also exhibits coccidiostatic properties. It is used as a feed additive at 125 ppm for prevention rather than treatment of intestinal and cecal coccidiosis in chickens. However, it is not intended for use in breeding or laying hens because egg production and hatchability may be reduced because of its use.

Following administration, the two moieties of the nicarbazin molecule are absorbed separately from the digestive tract of the chicken. Metabolism studies have shown that the 2-hydroxy-4,6-dimethylpyrimidine moiety of nicarbazin is absorbed and excreted or metabolized more rapidly than the 4,4'-dinitrocarbani-

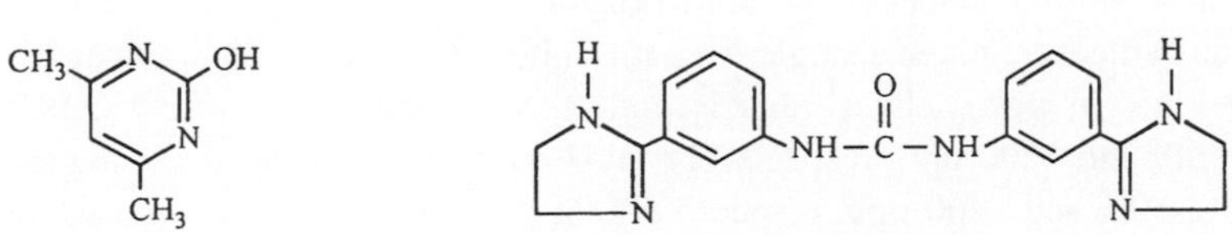

Nicarbazin   Imidocarb

FIG. 5.2 Chemical structures of commonly used carbanilides.

lide moiety (3). Since this was shown, residue studies of nicarbazin have been carried out almost exclusively on the 4,4'-dinitrocarbanilide moiety of the molecule. The required withdrawal period is 9 days in order not to exceed a residue level of 0.2 ppm of 4,4'-dinitrocarbanilide in liver.

Imidocarb is a carbanilide used for treatment and prophylaxis of piroplasmosis and anaplasmosis. It can be administered by subcutaneous or intramuscular injection to cattle, sheep, and horse at dosages of 1.2–3.4 mg/kg bw.

Although its mode of action is uncertain, two mechanisms, one involving interference with the production and/or utilization of polyamines and the other preventing the entry of inositol into the erythrocyte that contains the parasite, have been proposed. It is a compound with low safety margin since administration of as low as 10 mg/kg bw to cattle can cause death. By now, its withdrawal periods in edible animal products are under review by the licensing authorities and, in some cases, a 90-day withdrawal period may be required (4).

In cattle, imidocarb is well absorbed and distributed throughout the body. After subcutaneous administration to calves of 3 mg radiolabeled imidocarb/kg bw, absorption of the drug was rapid with mean peak plasma concentrations of 1316 ppb equivalents occurring 1 h after dosing. The level of radioactivity remained constant for up to 4 h after dosing but declined to 279 ppb equivalents 24 h after dosing. More than 70% of the radioactivity was found to be bound to plasma proteins. Most of the administered radioactivity was excreted in feces, with smaller amounts in the urine. The major component of both urine and feces was identified as the unchanged imidocarb.

In sheep treated intramuscularly with radiolabeled imidocarb, there was also no evidence for formation of imidocarb metabolites in urine, bile, liver, or kidney tissues, although the drug was widely distributed to all tissues and remained detectable in most tissues by 32 days after dosing. Residue depletion studies in sheep given two intramuscular doses of 1.2 mg imidocarb/kg bw, 7 days apart, showed that residues in kidney, liver, and muscle were in the range of 22,600–121,200, 5700–14,300, and 1100–1200 ppb, respectively, at 7 days after the last dose, declining to 5600–9600, 900–3100, and <100–400 ppb, respectively, at 28 days after the last dose. In lactating sheep given an intramuscular injection of 4.5 imidocarb/kg bw, residues in milk were found to be 4500 and 5300 ppb at 4 and 6 h, respectively, after dosing.

When cattle were given a single intramuscular injection of 3 mg imidocarb/kg bw, residues in kidney, liver, muscle and at the injection site were 13,600, 16,300, 1500, and 4200 ppb, respectively, at 7 days after dosing, declining to 3200, 3700, 500, and 1700 ppb, respectively, at 28 days after the last dose. In lactating cows given two injections of 3 mg imidocarb/kg bw, 28 days apart, residues in milk were in the range of 604–793 ppb 1 day after the first treatment and these declined to below 10 ppb at 7 days after treatment.

5.3 NITROIMIDAZOLES

Ronidazole, dimetridazole, metronidazole, and ipronidazole are all nitroimidazole drugs that have been extensively used as growth promoters and therapeutic anti-bacterial and antiprotozoal agents in food-producing animals (Fig. 5.3). Since they are mutagens and suspect carcinogens, a number of nitroimidazoles have been already banned even for therapeutic purposes within the European Union. Use of ronidazole has been banned by Council Regulations 3426/93/EEC (5), whereas use of dimetridazole is banned by Council Regulations 1798/95/EEC (6).

Their antibacterial and mutagenic activity is closely related to the reduction of the 5-nitro group, which is common to all nitroimidazole drugs, and the subse-quent formation of reactive metabolites that bind to bacterial DNA, inhibiting DNA and protein synthesis in the microorganisms. Metabolism of 5-nitroimidaz-oles in mammals usually leads to covalently bound residues with a persistent imidazole structure.

Dimetridazole has been traditionally used for treatment and prevention of histomoniasis in turkeys and chickens, trichomoniasis in cattle, and dysentery in swine. Concentrations of 125–500 ppm are satisfactory feed levels for turkeys, 75–500 ppm for chickens, and 1000 ppm for pigs. The drug has also been used as a feed or water additive in pigs for growth-promoting purposes. A 5-day withdrawal period is required to ensure absence of residues in edible tissues.

Orally administered dimetridazole is well absorbed from the gastrointestinal tract (7). Approximately 88% of the administered dose is eliminated within 3 days in turkeys, whereas around 76% is eliminated within 7 days in pigs. In

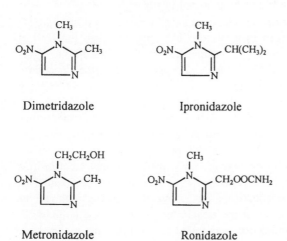

Dimetridazole   Ipronidazole

Metronidazole   Ronidazole

FIG. 5.3 Chemical structures of commonly used nitroimidazoles.

laying hens, turkeys, and pigs, 2-hydroxymethyl-1-methyl-5-nitroimidazole has been identified as the predominant metabolite (8). Additional ring-intact, nitro-containing metabolites including 1-methyl-5-nitroimidazole-2-carboxylic acid and the sulfate and glucuronide conjugates of 2-hydroxymethyl-1-methyl-5-nitro-imidazole have been also identified. Apart of these metabolites, several other metabolites presumably formed through reduction of the nitro group, fragmentation of the imidazole ring, and generation of covalently bound residues have been also reported but not identified.

When pigs were given a single oral dose of radiolabeled dimetridazole, the concentrations of total residues in muscle, liver, kidney, and fat were found to be 8.6, 15.4, 36.1, and 3.6 ppm, respectively, at 0 withdrawal time, declining to 0.32, 0.91, 0.81, and 0.37 ppm, respectively, 7 days after dosing.

Other residue depletion studies of dimetridazole in chickens, turkeys, and swine generally showed that the concentrations of dimetridazole residues decreased to less than 0.1 ppm in the edible tissues of chickens at 1 day withdrawal, and to less than 2 ppm in the edible tissues of turkeys and swine at 2-day withdrawal (9, 10).

When laying hens were given feed containing dimetridazole at dosages of 0.5, 1.0 and 1.5 mg/kg for 21 days (11), residue levels in eggs from all feed levels rose rapidly, reaching a plateau at 5 days after the treatment. Residue levels in eggs showed a good dose–response relation to the levels of the drug in the diet. The sum of the parent compound and the 2-hydroxy metabolite was found to be higher in egg white than in yolk, the metabolite accounting for some 75–80% of the total residues. After feed withdrawal, residue levels in eggs declined below the limit of detection within 5 days. Glucuronidated conjugates of the parent compound or its metabolite could not be detected in the eggs laid.

Ipronidazole and **ronidazole** are very similar in structure to dimetridazole and, thus, have several properties in common. They are added to the feed at dosages of 50–200 mg/kg for treatment and prevention of histomoniasis in turkeys, treatment of trichomoniasis in cattle, and treatment of swine dysentery. They have been also used as weight-gain and feed-efficiency improvers. A 4 day withdrawal period is recommended for both of these compounds.

Residue depletion studies in turkeys orally treated with radiolabeled ipronidazole showed that the total residue concentrations in muscle, liver, kidney, fat, and skin were 71.2, 285.4, 257.7, 24.8, and 92.9 ppb of of ipronidazole equivalents, respectively, at 5 days after dosing. In similarly treated pigs, total residue concentrations in muscle, liver, kidney, and fat were 41.1, 192.7, 189.5, and 20.6 ppb ipronidazole equivalents, respectively, at 5 days after dosing. Among the total residues present in the tissues of the treated turkeys and pigs, 1-methyl-2-(2'-hydroxyisopropyl)-5-nitroimidazole was found to constitute the major drug-related residue besides the parent drug.

Ronidazole is absorbed well from the gastrointestinal tract and is widely distributed throughout the body (12–14). The parent compound accounts for part of the urinary excretion whereas it is almost absent from feces, which contain only metabolized ronidazole. In turkeys administered radiolabeled ronidazole at the normal feed level for 4 days (11), total residue concentrations in muscle, kidney, and liver averaged 3, 4.7, and 4.5 ppm of ronidazole equivalents, respectively, at 0 withdrawal; concentrations fell to 0.26, 0.14, and 0.05 ppm, respectively, at 10 days after treatment.

In swine given radiolabeled ronidazole at the normal feed level for 3 days, total residue concentrations in muscle, kidney, liver, and fat were 8.6, 12.3, 11.9, and 2.5 ppm ronidazole equivalents, respectively, at 0 withdrawal. Total residues persisted in edible tissues by 42 days of withdrawal, at which time muscle contained 130 ppb, whereas liver, kidney, and fat contained 50–60 ppb. Nevertheless, the concentration of the parent drug in the edible tissues was less than 2 ppb at 2 days withdrawal. Ring-intact metabolites including 2-hydroxymethyl-1-methyl-5-nitroimidazole, 1-methyl-2-hydroxymethyl-5-acetamidoimidazole, and 1-methyl-2-carbamoyloxymethyl-5-acetamidoimidazole were found to constitute part of the total residues monitored in the tissues of both animal species.

Metronidazole is used for treatment of bovine trichomoniasis by topical application or intravenous injection of 75 mg/kg bw. It is also used for treatment of swine dysentery at a dosage of 25 mg/kg bw/day for 4 days, whereas, for eradication of the disease in herds, treatment for 7 days followed, after 3–4 weeks, by a second treatment for 5 days in indicated. Metronidazole is a genotoxic carcinogen in animals.

Like other nitroimidazoles, metronidazole is rapidly metabolized in the body. Oxidation of the two side-chains and formation of the corresponding metabolites followed by conjugation of the unchanged drug and its metabolites appears to be the major metabolic pathway of this compound. Another important metabolic pathway appears to be the degradation of the compound via reduction of the nitro group and cleavage of the imidazole ring. Acetamide and N-(2-hydroxyethyl) oxamic acid are produced as final metabolites.

In humans, hydroxymetronidazole was identified as the main metabolite, accounting for 40–50% of the total residues. In rats, 97% of the radioactivity that excreted in urine was attributed to the parent drug.

Residue depletion studies are very limited for metronidazole. After intra-uterine treatment of cows with metronidazole at the recommended dosage, residues of metronidazole and its main metabolite hydroxymetronidazole could be detected in the milk collected at 2 and 6 h after dosing; residues declined to below the limit of detection at 43 h postdosing.

5.4 POLYETHER IONOPHORE ANTIBIOTICS

Among the anticoccidials, polyether antibiotics constitute the most widely used agents by the poultry industry over the last two decades. They provide excellent disease control and are refractory to development of resistance (15).

Monensin, narasin, lasalocid, salinomycin, maduramicin, and semdura-micin are all polyether antibiotics produced by various actinomyces, mostly *Strep-tomyces* species. Chemically, they are all organic acids with fairly complex mole-cules consisting of an array of heterocyclic ether-containing rings (Fig. 5.4). Biologically, the polyether antibiotics are compounds that are able to form lipid-soluble, reversible complexes with cations thus participating in the transport and

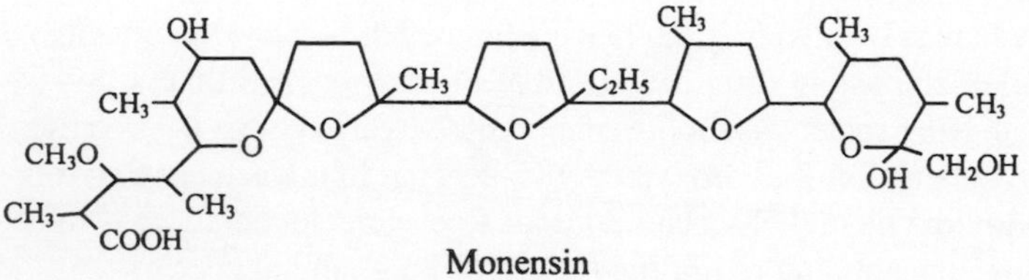

Monensin

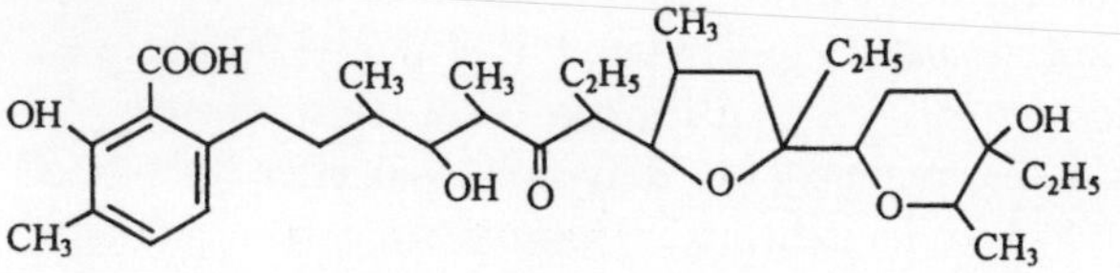

Lasalocid

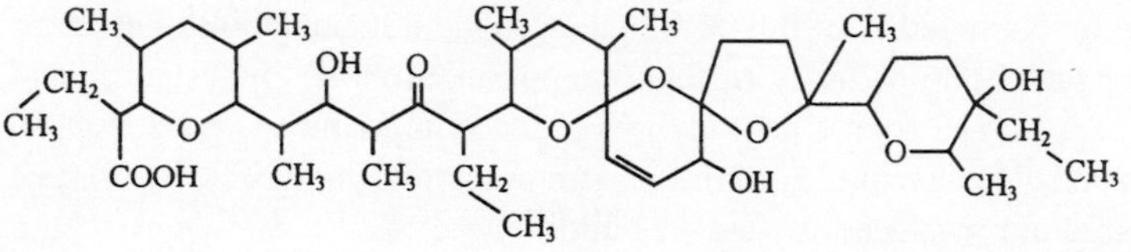

Narasin

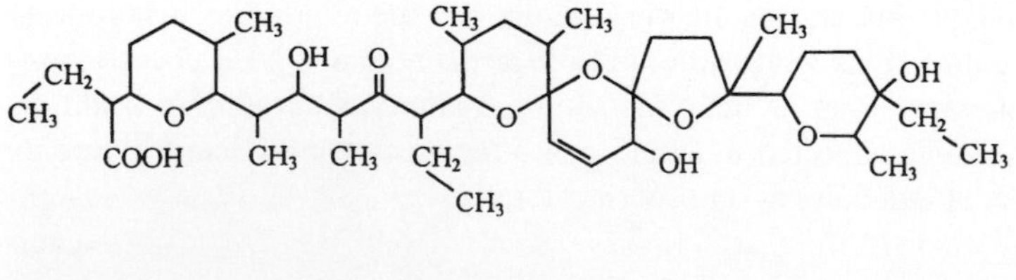

Salinomycin

FIG. 5.4   Chemical structures of commonly used polyether ionophore antibi-otics.

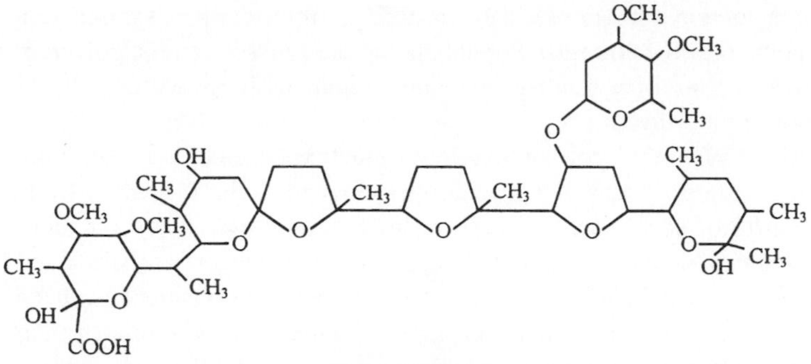

Maduramicin

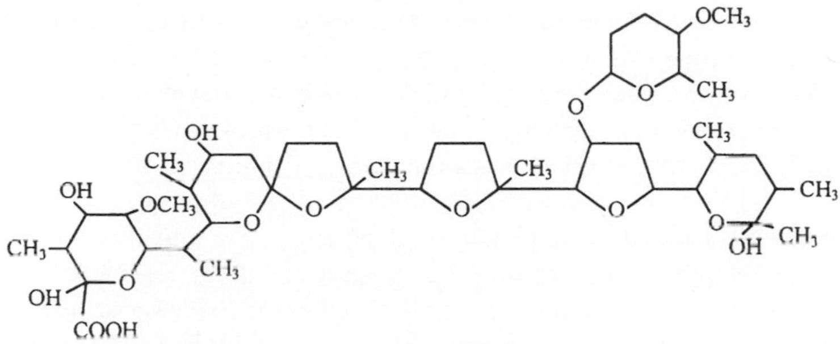

Semduramicin

FIG. 5.4 Continued

exchange of these cations across the biological membranes (16). The result of this transport is an alteration in the levels of cations and anions inside the cell and its subcellular components, which influences the regulation of the body functions.

Although the polyether antibiotics do not exhibit a similar tendency for cation complexation, with the exception of lasalocid that binds only divalent cations, all other members of this group of drugs from complexes mainly with monovalent cations (17). Due to these functional properties, the polyether antibiotics are frequently also called ionophores. The name ionophore comes from the Greek language, *ion* meaning something that goes and *phore* meaning carrier.

Oral administration of polyether antibiotics allows, initially, for regulation of the body function at the site of digestion by positively affecting feed conversion efficiency and negatively affecting the developmental stage of coccidia. Since their activity is directed particularly towards sporozoites and merozoites, the polyethers must be fed continuously to be fully effective but are not recommended for treating established infections. They have a low therapeutic index and may be very toxic in certain species (18, 19). In turkeys, for example, salinomycin and narasin can be fatally toxic (20). For enhancing their effectiveness, polyether antibiotics are often used in poultry in combinations with roxarsone, virginiamycin, and/or bambermycin.

Monensin plays a dual role in veterinary practice because it is used both as a coccidiostat in poultry and as a growth promotant in cattle. It is also efficacious in the control of coccidiosis in lambs and calves, can treat ketosis in dairy cows, and can control bloat in pastured dairy cattle. It is administered incorporated in poultry feeds as a coccidiostat at a dose up to 120 ppm, and in cattle and sheep feeds at a dose of 11–33 ppm. Monensin is not recommended for administration to laying hens, while a 3 day withdrawal period is required for chicken meat.

Following oral administration to cattle, it is absorbed from the gastrointestinal tract, rapidly distributed, metabolized, excreted in the bile, and eliminated in the feces. Residues in liver averaged 0.4 ppm at 12 h after the last dose, whereas residues detected in other tissues were negligible (21). When radiolabeled monensin was administered to steers, essentially all radioactivity was eventually excreted in the feces after conversion to many metabolites that accumulated in the liver (22).

A residue depletion study with radiolabeled monensin given to chickens at a concentration of 120 ppm in the feed for 2 weeks, showed highest residue levels of 495 ppb equivalents in liver samples during the feeding period; residue levels of 106 and 50 ppb monensin equivalents could be still detectable in liver and fat, respectively, at 5 days posttreatment (23). Other workers found lower concentrations of monensin residues in liver than in fat and muscle tissues when chickens were withdrawn at 0, 1, 2, 3, and 26 days after following a standard therapeutic scheme for 30 days (24). In this study, residual levels of monensin persisted in all edible chicken tissues postwithdrawal far longer than the putative fall in plasma levels would indicate. When monensin was fed to laying hens, low residue levels (<4.0 ppb) in eggs were detected even in cases in which the diet contained monensin at a level of 13 ppm (25).

Monensin has been shown to form within the body more than 50 metabolites, among which the glucoside metabolite is also active as a coccidiostat (26). Clear evidence of the extensive monensin metabolism has been provided by another study based on the administration of radiolabeled monensin to chickens (21). Chromatographic analysis of the incurred livers showed how many metabolites were present in the analyzed extracts. It was found that only 7% of the radioactivity detected in liver and 70% of that in fat were due to the presence of the parent monensin. The rapid metabolism and depletion of the unchanged monensin were attributed to O-demethylation and oxidation at various positions along the carbon backbone of its molecule.

Maduramicin, unlike other polyether anticoccidials produced by *Streptomyces* species, is a fermentation product of *Actinomadura yumaense*. The compound should not be confused with maduramycin ($C_{28}H_{22}O_{10}$) produced by *Actinomadura rubra*. Maduramicin exhibits a 12–24-fold greater anticoccidial potency than other polyether antibiotics and as such it is administered to broilers at a level of 5 ppm continuously with the feed (27–29). However, its use is prohibited within 7 days before slaughter.

Metabolism of maduramicin in various animal species seems to proceed in a manner similar to monensin. Selective *O*-demethylation of one or two methoxy groups has been reported as the major biotransformation route in chickens and rats (30), whereas *O*-demethylation of one or more methoxy groups followed by hydroxylation is the major biotransformation route in turkey excreta (31). Conjugation with glucuronic acid also occurs but it is of minor metabolic importance.

Residue depletion studies (32) in chickens fed 5 ppm maduramicin for 2 weeks showed residue levels of 106 and 28 ppb in liver and muscle, respectively, at zero withdrawal, declining to 20 and 3 ppb, respectively, at 3 days after withdrawal.

Salinomycin is used in broiler chickens for prophylaxis of coccidiosis at a dose of 50–70 ppm continuously in the feed; a 5 day withdrawal period is required before slaughter (33). Salinomycin also constitutes the first licensed growth promoting polyether antibiotic for use in swine. Its unique mode of action ensures disruption of the growth and reproduction of certain intestinal bacteria. This particular mechanism also helps to counteract bacterial resistance, so salinomycin continues to improve growth performance in the long term. Inclusion rates for pigs range from 50 ppm in starter rations to 25 ppm in finisher rations.

Pharmacokinetic studies have shown that most salinomycin appears in feces in the form of an inactive metabolite that is subsequently degraded with a half-life of less than 50 h. Residue depletion studies in chickens showed wide variation in the concentrations of residues appearing in edible tissues. Some workers have reported levels of salinomycin residues as high as 1100 ppb in liver of chickens at 0 withdrawal (34, 35). In contrast, other workers reported residue levels as low as 3 ppb in the same tissue under similar experimental conditions (36).

All depletion studies carried out by now in poultry have clearly shown that at 1 day of withdrawal the concentrations present in edible tissues are very low and barely detectable (37–40). For example, after administration of feed containing salinomycin at 60 mg/kg, levels of 0.08, 0.14, and 0.08 ppm were found in muscle, liver, and fat, respectively, of nonwithdrawn birds (37), whereas levels in muscle and liver decreased to below 0.05 ppm at 1 day withdrawal. Levels in fat decreased to 0.05 ppm at 1 day withdrawal and to below 0.05 ppm at 2 day withdrawal.

Other pertinent studies have also demonstrated levels of 0.05–0.09 ppm parent salinomycin in livers of nonwithdrawn birds fed salinomycin at 75 ppm (39). However, this accounted for only 3% of the total salinomycin-related residues in liver.

When day-old broilers were fed a ration containing 66, 90, or 120 ppm salinomycin sodium for 6 weeks, concentrations of salinomycin at 0 withdrawal time in breast skin/fat, thigh skin/fat, and abdominal fat increased as the level of the drug in the ration also increased; after 6 h of withdrawal, salinomycin concentrations in tissues were decreased, whereas after 24 h of withdrawal, salinomycin could not be detected in any tissue. It appears that salinomycin residues are concentrated in the more fatty tissues, such as subcutaneous fat, and follow the order liver>kidney>thigh>breast muscles (40).

Studies in laying hens have shown that salinomycin has the tendency to accumulate in the egg yolk (41). When laying hens were fed a ration containing 60 ppm salinomycin sodium for 5 days, considerable concentrations of salinomycin were found in the produced eggs (42). Residues in the egg yolk persisted for 8 days, while residues in the egg white were negligible.

Semduramicin is a relatively new polyether antibiotic that exhibits potent antimicrobial and anticoccidial activities. It is intended for use in broilers at a dosage of 25 ppm in the feed for 7 consecutive days.

The absorption profile of semduramicin is characterized by low levels in plasma, muscle, kidney, fat, and skin, but higher levels in the bile and liver (43). Liver constitutes the edible tissue with the highest total residues at all withdrawal times. Over a 5 day withdrawal period, total residues in each of liver, kidney, muscle, fat, and skin/fat tissues were depleted to 0.057, 0.022, 0.015, 0.011, and 0.009 ppm semduramicin, respectively. The consistently low plasma concentrations and relatively higher residue concentrations found in bile and excreta were consistent with the metabolic clearance and the efficient hepatic route of drug elimination.

Residues in liver of poultry sacrificed at 6 h after withdrawal, were comprised of unchanged semduramicin at a percentage of 45%, whereas an array of more polar, low-level (<0.1 ppm) metabolites could be also detected. Using bile as a source of major semduramicin metabolites, the metabolism of semduramicin was spectrometrically determined to proceed by O-demethylation of the methoxy groups in the "A" and "G" rings, as it has been also described for maduramicin (30, 31) and monensin (21, 44).

Since the unchanged semduramicin represented a significant portion of the residues in liver, use of the parent drug as a marker residue has been recommended. The utility of determining unchanged semduramicin levels in poultry liver to monitor drug elimination substantially differentiates this compound from the other polyether antibiotics. While relatively high concentrations of total residues have been reported for monensin (44, 45), and salinomycin (46) in poultry liver, total residues of these compounds were generally characterized by lower participation of the parent drugs. Only in fat, where total residues of monensin was generally low, was it possible to detect a higher percentage of the parent drug.

Lasalocid is the more disruptive polyether antibiotic to biological systems. This is due to its high tendency to dimerize and form complexes with biologically important divalent ions such as Ca^{++} and Mg^{++}. Lasalocid exhibits a wide range of complexation affinities and transport capabilities, encompassing not only inorganic polyvalent ions but also primary amines and catecholamines (22).

Lasalocid is widely used for controlling poultry coccidiosis since it is very efficient against all species of *Eimeria* at the optimal dose of 90 ppm in the feed. It is licensed for use in broilers and hens up to 16 weeks from hatching but is not licensed for use in laying hens. It has been also used as a growth promoter in cattle.

Following administration, lasalocid is rapidly metabolized in animals. Residue depletion studies in chickens fed 90 ppm lasalocid for 2 weeks showed residue levels of 450 and 1 ppb in liver and muscle, respectively, at 0 withdrawal; residues declined to 10 and 1 ppb, respectively, at 3 day withdrawal (36). Lasalocid concentrations in liver were approximately 10 ppb at 7 days posttreatment.

When lasalocid was fed to layer hens at a dosage of 5 ppm, considerable accumulation of drug residues in eggs occurred (25); the highest mean egg lasalocid concentration in eggs was found to be in excess of 400 ppb after the medication period.

Narasin is effective against all intestinal and cecal coccidia if administered continuously in the feed. It is used for treatment of *Eimeria* species in broiler chickens at a dosage of 60–80 ppm in the feed. Narasin has been also used as a growth-promoting agent. However, it should not be given to laying hens or to other species of birds or animals to which it is toxic.

After administration to chickens, edible tissues of muscle, liver, or fat from nonwithdrawn birds did not contain detectable levels of the parent drug (37). Nevertheless, a withdrawal period of 5 days is required to be observed before slaughter.

5.5 QUINOLONE DERIVATIVES

Although hundreds of different quinolone derivatives have been synthesized, only buquinolate, decoquinate, and methylbenzoquate have shown good efficacy against all species of chicken coccidia (Fig. 5.5). Their activity is essential coccidiostatic against the invading sporozoites; as a result, if treatment is delayed after animals have become infected, anticoccidial activity is not effective. All quinolones are virtually insoluble in water and very poorly absorbed and, as a consequence, are nontoxic and result in low residue levels in the tissues of treated animals.

Buquinolate is used at a level of 82–110 ppm in the feed, often in association with arsenicals or antibiotics, for prevention of coccidiosis in chickens. Their minimal absorption by the host probably accounts for the remarkable freedom

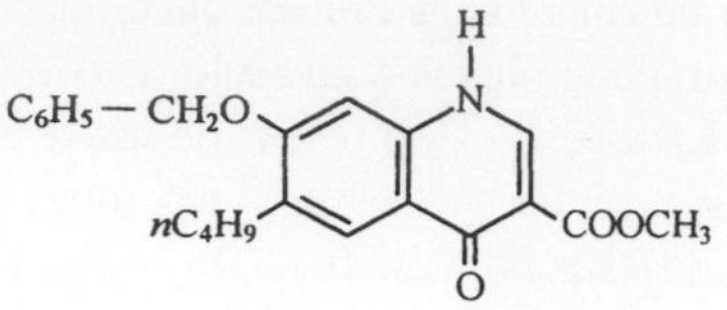

Methylbenzoquate 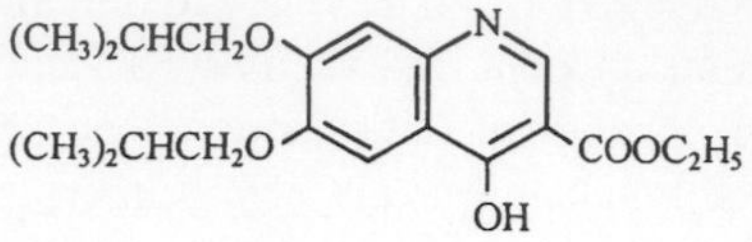   Buquinolate

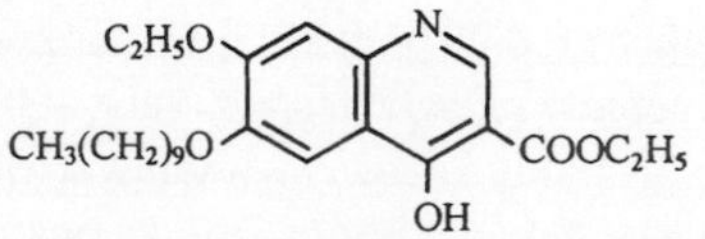

Decoquinate

FIG. 5.5   Chemical structures of commonly used quinolone derivatives.

of toxicity. At 0 withdrawal period, residues in tissues are as low as 0.1 ppm in muscle and 0.4 ppm in liver.

Decoquinate is another quinolone derivative also incorporated in the feed. It is administered at a level of 20–40 ppm in the feed continuously for prevention of coccidiosis in broiler chickens, at 100 ppm for 28 days for prevention of coccidiosis in ewes and lambs, and at 500 ppm for at least 28 days for prevention of coccidiosis in cattle. Many feedlot farmers also use a 28 day feeding program for all incoming cattle to guard against costly disease that can destroy a feedlot. It is an approved feed additive in Europe, as defined by Directive 70/524/EEC (47).

Little is known about the absorption of orally administered decoquinate. It is assumed, however, that some decoquinate must be absorbed since drug-related residues are consistently found in tissues (47). Most decoquinate is rapidly excreted in feces, whereas some is excreted via the urine.

The highest levels of decoquinate are found in liver and kidney with variable amounts in fat. Low levels are usually found in muscle, whereas residues in all edible tissues reach a plateau after 3 days of administration. Most of the residues (at least 50% of the total residues) appear to be in the form of the parent compound. Decoquinate is a low-toxicity compound requiring a 3-day withdrawal period for meat.

Methylbenzoquate is probably the most potent among the anticoccidial quinolone derivatives. It is often used at 8.35 ppm in the feed in conjunction with other coccidiostats, especially clopidol, for prophylaxis of coccidiosis in chickens and turkeys.

5.6 TRIAZINES

Major drugs within this group of compounds are clazuril, diclazuril, and toltrazuril. They are all triazine derivatives used for prevention and treatment of coccidiosis in avian species (Fig. 5.6).

Clazuril is intended for oral use in pigeons at a dosage of 2.5 mg/pigeon/month. Pigeons given clazuril at the recommended dosage showed a maximum concentration of 14,700 ppb of the parent drug in plasma within 5 h following treatment. At both 8 and 24 h time points after treatment, muscle contained a maximum of 4600 ppb clazuril. The maximum concentration in liver (13,200 ppb) appeared at 24 h after treatment.

Diclazuril is recommended for broilers, turkeys, and rabbits at a dosage of 1 ppm in the feed. Broiler chickens given a single oral dose of 1 mg radiolabeled diclazuril/kg bw showed peak plasma concentrations of 1.5 and 2 μg diclazuril equivalents/ml, respectively, within 6 h after dosing (48). All radioactivity in plasma for up to 72 h after dosing was found to be due to the parent diclazuril.

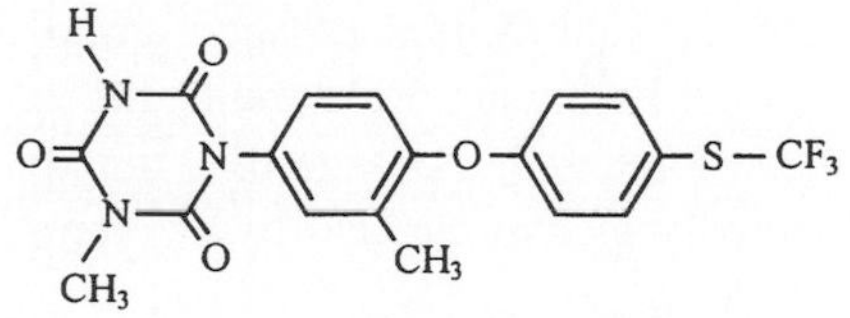

Toltrazuril 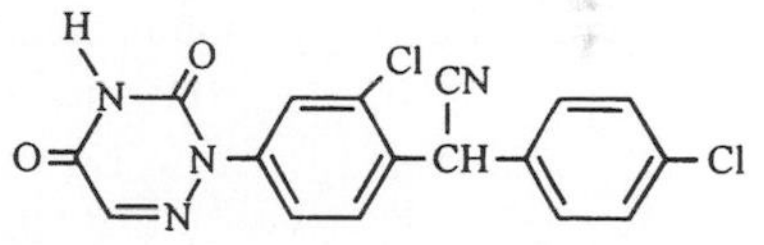   Clazuril

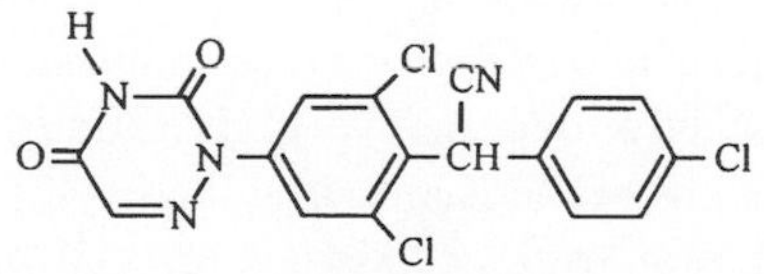

Diclazuril

Fig. 5.6 Chemical structures of commonly used triazines.

Plasma concentrations were about 2–10 times higher than tissue concentrations. Liver and kidney contained the highest levels of residual radioactivity, while muscle and skin/fat contained much less. In liver, the parent drug accounted for more than 90% of the residual radioactivity. About half of the radioactivity was excreted within 24 h, almost exclusively as parent diclazuril. At longer time points, several transformation products were recovered in the excreta. In turkeys similarly treated, liver and kidney showed a maximum of 1400 and 1090 μg diclazuril equivalents/kg, respectively, at 6 h after dosing. The parent drug accounted for about 98% and 85% of the radioactivity in liver at 6 and 48 h, respectively, after dosing.

When diets containing 1 ppm of diclazuril were fed to laying hens for 32 days, the maximum level of the parent drug in the egg yolks was 322 ppb at 3 day withdrawal. In egg white, 82 ppb of parent diclazuril were detected at both 14 and 29 days of treatment (49). However, withdrawal of the treatment could result in a rapid decrease of diclazuril in the egg white (below 50 ppb at 4 day after withdrawal) but a slower decrease in the yolk (below 50 ppb at 15 day withdrawal). The steady-state concentrations of diclazuril in the eggs laid when hens were given a 5 ppm diet were found to be very close to those observed for the 1 ppm diet; in this case, the maximum values reached in yolk amounted to 1280 ppb at 4 day withdrawal, and to 325 ppb in the egg white at 26 day withdrawal. The depletion of residues was slower, however, in the eggs laid from the highly dosed birds, lasting up to 10 days of withdrawal in the egg white and still longer in the yolk, where residues could be detected even at 20 h day withdrawal.

Toltrazuril is administered with drinking water at a concentration of 10–25 ppm for treating coccidiosis in turkey, chicken, and rabbits. It is a suspect teratogen so an extended withdrawal period is required. Following oral administration of radiolabeled tortrazuril to chickens at the recommended dosage of 7 mg/kg bw/day for 2 days, 50% of the total radioactivity was eliminated by 4.5 days after the last dose, increasing to 90% at 15.5 days.

Nine drug-related metabolites could be isolated from chicken feces, with the parent drug and its major sulfoxide and sulfone metabolites accounting for 33.1%, 15%, and 16.4%, respectively, of the fecal radioactivity measured at 1 day after the end of the treatment.

Toltrazuril residue depletion studies in chickens orally given 14.1 mg/kg bw/day for 2 consecutive days per week, three times at a week interval, showed that the concentrations of the parent drug were 342, 1845, 870, 1332, and 1077 ppb in muscle, fat, skin, liver, and kidney, respectively, 1 day after the cessation of treatment. These concentrations declined thereafter to reach, at 6 days after dosing, <10, 81, 33, 22, and 15 ppb in muscle, fat, skin, liver, and kidney, respectively. At 10 days postdosing, 24 ppb were found in fat and 11 ppb in skin, whereas other tissues did not contain detectable residue levels.

One day after the cessation of treatment, the residues of toltrazuril sulfoxide were found to be 773, 1268, 1030, 3416, and 4411 ppb in muscle, fat, skin, liver, and kidney, respectively. These levels declined thereafter to reach, at 6 days postdosing, 10 ppb in muscle, fat, and skin tissues; however, concentrations of 54 and 95 ppb could be still measured in liver and kidney, respectively. Ten days after dosing, the sulfoxide metabolite could only be detected in the liver (16 ppb) and kidney (36 ppb).

The concentrations of the sulfone metabolite were much higher: at 1 day after the cessation of treatment, the levels were 4742, 13,267, 7931, 21,275, and 17,084 ppb in muscle, fat, skin, liver, and kidney, respectively. At 16 days postdosing, concentrations of 38, 104, 97, 225, and 152 ppb were still present in muscle, fat, skin, liver, and kidney tissues, respectively. At 20 days postdosing, 117 and 152 ppb could be still detected in liver and kidney, respectively, whereas other tissues contained low residue levels in the range of 30–85 ppb. The profile of toltrazuril depletion in edible tissues of chickens is similar to that observed in turkeys.

5.7 MISCELLANEOUS

Aminonitrothiazole and **nithiazide** are both nitrothiazole derivatives (Fig. 5.7) used against histomoniasis by the poultry industry. Aminonitrothiazole is used both therapeutically and prophylactically against blackhead in turkeys; treatment is achieved by administering feed medicated with aminonitrothiazole at the level of 0.1% for 14 days, and then reducing the level to 0.05% and continue feeding for a further 18 weeks.

Nithiazide is used for prevention and treatment of histomoniasis and hexamitiasis in fowls and turkeys also by feed medication; treatment is achieved by administering feed medicated at the level of 0.04% for 7 days, and subsequently decreasing the level to the prophylactic dosage of 0.025%, which is continued for a further 2 weeks.

Amprolium (Fig. 5.7) is a vitamin B_1 analogue. It is a competitive antagonist of the thiamine transport mechanism. Amprolium has been used as a coccidiostat mainly in chickens, laying hens, turkeys, and ruminants. It is available as a soluble powder for addition to drinking water (60–240 mg/L) or as a premix, usually in combination with ethopabate and/or sulfaquinoxaline, for mixing with the feed (125–500 mg/kg feed). A withdrawal period of 3 days is required for chickens.

Pharmacokinetic studies in chickens orally dosed with 12 or 20 mg amprolium/kg bw showed that maximum blood concentrations of 9.5 and 26 ppm, respectively, were achieved at 4 h after dosing. At 8 h after dosing, residue concentrations in kidney and cecum were 18 and 46 ppm, respectively, for the low-dose group, and 36 and 74 ppm, respectively, for the high-dose group.

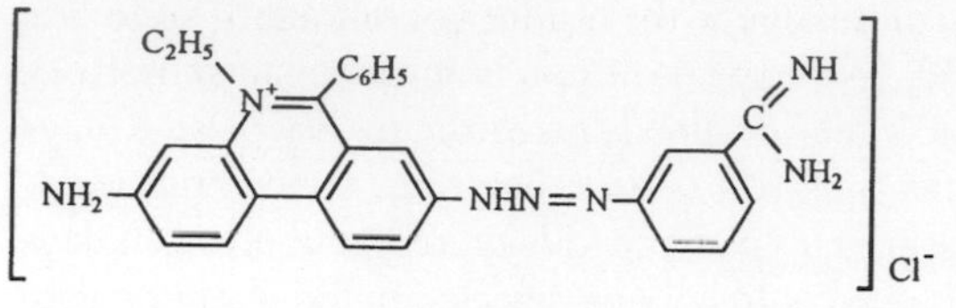

Isometamidium

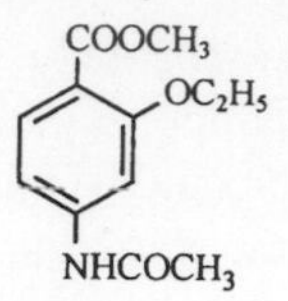

Ethopabate

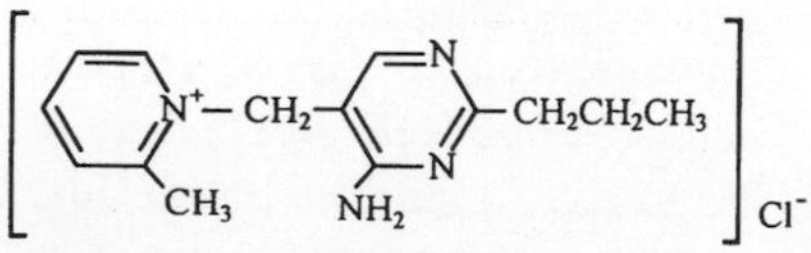

Amprolium

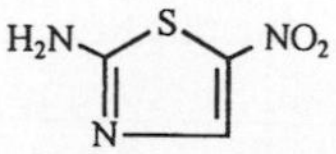

Aminonitrothiazole

Quinuronium

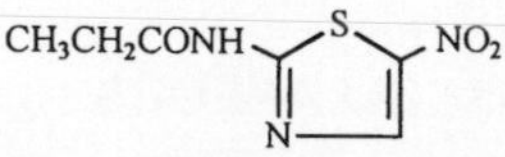

Nithiazide

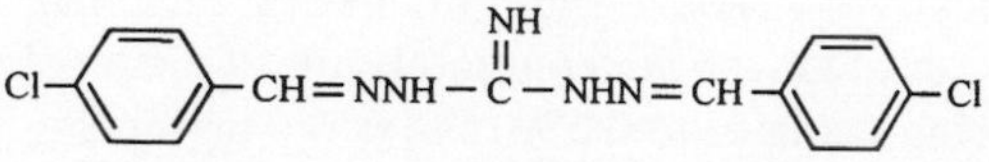

Robenidine

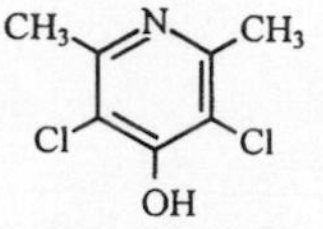

Clopidol

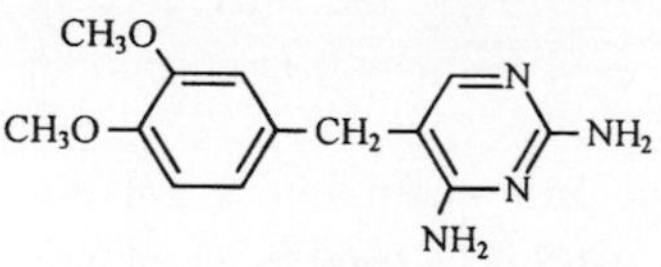

Diaveridine

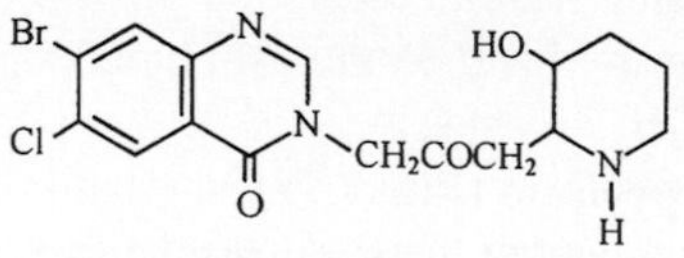

Halofuginone

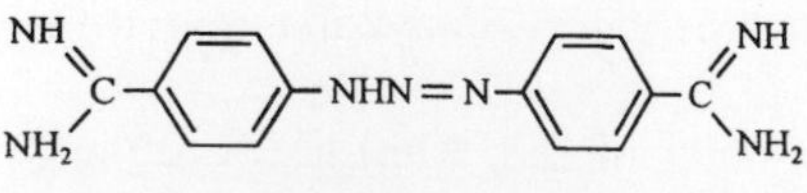

Diminazene

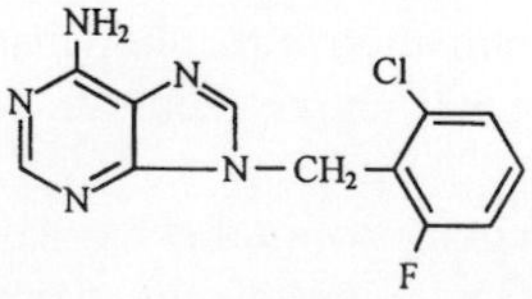

Arprinocid

FIG. 5.7 Chemical structures of various anticoccidial drugs.

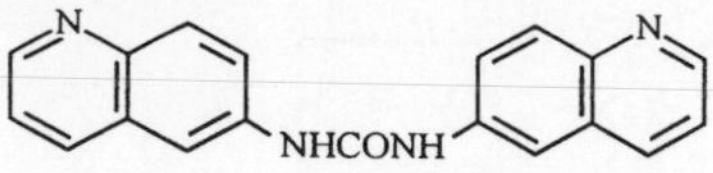

Residue depletion studies in chicks given a diet containing 150 or 250 mg amprolium/kg feed from day 1 to day 32 of age showed that amprolium concentrations at 0 day and 2 day withdrawal from the high-dose diet were 90 and less than 10 ppb, respectively, in muscle, 410 and less than 20 ppb, respectively, in liver, 380 and less than 40 ppb, respectively, in kidney, and 420 and less than 20 ppb, respectively, in skin/fat. With the low-dose diet, the corresponding concentrations found were 90 and less than 10 ppb, respectively, in muscle, 420 and less than 20 ppb, respectively, in liver, 350 and less than 10 ppb, respectively, in kidney, and 160 and less than 10 ppb, respectively, in skin/fat.

When hens were fed diets containing 5 or 250 mg amprolium/kg feed for 21 days, the concentrations of the parent drug in the egg yolks plateaued at 200 and 2000 ppb, respectively. Concentrations in the egg whites were 7 and 50 ppb, respectively. Following withdrawal of the medications, a linear decline in the concentrations of amprolium residues in yolks was observed; at 10 days after the cessation of treatments, concentrations in the egg yolks were lower that 5 ppb.

Arprinocid (Fig. 5.7) is a benzyl purine derivative shown to be effective against all species of turkey and chicken coccidia. It is administered continuously with the feed at a dose of 60 ppm for chickens and 90–120 ppm for turkeys.

Following administration, the drug is rapidly metabolized to arprinocid-1-N-oxide, which is the major metabolite excreted in the urine. In chicken, arprinocid-1-N-oxide is thought to affect microsomal metabolism and DNA synthesis in the coccidia.

Clopidol (Fig. 5.7), also called meticlorpindol or clopindol, is the only member of the pyridinol group of anticoccidials that has been commercially successful. It is most active against the sporozoite stage of *Eimeria,* and represents one of the few drugs used to control the disease in rabbits.

It is administered continuously with the feed at a dose of 200 ppm for rabbits and 125 ppm for chickens. A mixture with methylbenzoquate is also available for prevention of coccidiosis in chickens and turkeys. Clopidol is more coccidiostatic than coccidiocidal. Its coccidiostatic activity may hold the sporozoite undeveloped in the host cell for as long as 60 days; if the drug is withdrawn during this static phase, latent coccidiosis may appear as the parasite resumes development. For clopidol, a withdrawal period of 5 days has been set for all animal species.

Diaveridine, a pyrimidine derivative (Fig. 5.7), is a compound used primarily as a synergist with sulfaquinoxaline or other sulfonamide drugs.

Diminazene, an aromatic diamidine (Fig. 5.7), is a veterinary drug employed for the treatment of piroplasmosis and trypanosomiasis. A combination product consisting of 44.5% diminazene and 55.5% phenazone is authorized for use in cattle, sheep, and horses at an intramuscular dosage of 3.5 mg/kg bw. Diminazene acts against *Babesia* by affecting the fine structure and function of the cell membranes. It also acts against trypanosomes by binding to DNA and blocking kinetoplast DNA replication.

In rats and monkeys, moderate absorption of diminazene has been reported following its oral administration. In studies with rabbits given the combination product at 3.5 mg/kg bw intramuscularly, maximum blood levels at 15 min and 3 h were 1.3 and 0.116 ppm, respectively. Tissue levels at 7 days after treatment were highest in the liver (40 ppm), brain (2.5 ppm), and kidney (3 ppm), whereas 40–50% of the administered was eliminated in the urine and 8–20% in the feces.

Following intramuscular administration of 3.5 mg radiolabeled diminazene/kg bw in cattle, the metabolites *p*-aminobenzamidine and *p*-aminobenzamide were found in the urine besides the parent drug; these metabolites constituted 22% and 4% of the total radioactivity, respectively. Liver, kidney, and muscle tissues were found to contain total residue levels of 75, 55, and 2.5 ppm diminazene equivalents, respectively, at 7 days postdosing, declining to 24, 12, and 1 ppm, respectively, at 20 day postdosing.

When dairy cows were administered 3.5 mg diminazene/kg bw, highest residue levels in milk were found at 6 h postdosing, declining to below 0.07 ppm at 48 h post dosing (50).

Ethopabate (Fig. 5.7) is a substituted benzoic acid having anticoccidial activity against a number of *Eimeria* species. It is always used in combination with amprolium.

Halofuginone, a quinazoline derivative (Fig. 5.7), is a potent anticoccidial drug for chickens and turkeys since it requires incorporation of only 3 ppm in the feed (51). Because of its steep dose–response curve, which allows little deviation from the therapeutic dosage before the onset of drug toxicity, difficulties have arisen in ensuring even distribution of halofuginone in the diet. When given in high dosages, halofuginone is a growth depressant, it impairs feed utilization, and reduces feed intake whereas in rats it causes alopecia. Whether similar problems could occur in humans consuming products with residues of halofuginone is still unknown. To protect consumer health, a withdrawal period of 7 days has been set for turkeys and of 5 days for broilers.

Results from a feeding trial in which chickens were fed a commercial feed containing 3 ppm halofuginone showed that liver could contain about 0.2 ppm, kidney 0.15 ppm, whereas muscle and fat residue levels lower than 0.02 ppm.

Isometamidium, a phenanthridium derivative (Fig. 5.7), is a veterinary drug effective for the treatment of trypanosomiasis in cattle, horses, buffaloes, and camels. It is administered by intramuscular injection at dosages in the range 0.5–2 mg/kg bw.

In rats, isometamidium is poorly absorbed from the gastrointestinal tract, approximately 99% of an oral dose being excreted in the feces. A similar absorption/excretion profile is exhibited by homidium, one of the four major impurities of the commercial product that normally contains about 70% of pure isometamidium. Available information on calves, dairy cows, and goats indicates that high levels of residues of isometamidium occur at the injection site, liver, and kidneys after intramuscular administration. Reported levels at the injection site exceeded 1000 ppm, whereas levels in kidney and liver stayed in the range of 2–7 ppm several days after dosing.

Quinuronium is a complex urea compound (Fig. 5.7) widely used in *Babesia* infections in horses, cattle, sheep, and swine. The drug is administered only subcutaneously at dosages of 0.3–0.5 mg/kg bw in horses and 0.5 mg/kg bw in cattle, sheep and swine.

Robenidine, a guanidine derivative (Fig. 5.7), is suitable for the effective control of all intestinal coccidia affecting turkey, chicken, and rabbits. Early formulations of robenidine were administered to poultry at 66 ppm and had no withdrawal requirements. Complaints of adverse flavoring of meat and eggs from metabolites of the drug were answered by decreasing the incorporation level to 33 ppm and by enforcing a 5 day withdrawal period. It is now administered during the risky period by continuous medication in the feed at a dosage of 33 ppm for broilers and turkeys and 55–66 ppm for rabbits.

REFERENCES

1. M.A. Fernando, in The Biology of Coccidia (P.I. Long, Ed.), University Park Press, Baltimore, MD, p. 287 (1982).
2. O.W. Parks, J. Assoc. Off. Anal. Chem., 67:566 (1984).
3. C.C. Porter, and J.L. Gilfillan, Poultry Sci., 34:995 (1955).
4. G.C. Brander, D.M. Pugh, R.J. Bywater, and W.L. Jenkins, in Veterinary Applied Pharmacology and Therapeutics (G.C. Brander, D.M. Pugh, R.J. Bywater, and W.L. Jenkins, Eds.), 5th Edition, Balliere Tindall, London (1991).
5. Official Journal of the European Communities, No. L312, Brussels, p. 15 (1993).
6. Official Journal of the European Communities, No. L174, Brussels, p. 20 (1995).
7. European Agency for the Evaluation of Medicinal Products (EMEA), in Dimetridazole, Summary Report, Committee for Veterinary Medicinal Products, EMEA/MRL, London, UK (1993).
8. M.M.L. Aerts, I.A. Egberink, C.A. Kan, H.J. Keykens, and W.M.J. Beek, J. Assoc. Off. Anal. Chem., 74:46 (1991).
9. C.A. Kan, H.J. Keukens, and W.M.J. Beek, in Residues of Veterinary Drugs in Food, Proc. Euroresidue III Conf., Veldhoven, 1996 (N. Haagsma, and A. Ruiter, Eds.), Fac. Vet. Med., Univ. Utrecht, The Netherlands, p. 586 (1996).
10. A. Posyniak, S. Semeniuk, J. Zmudzki, J. Niedzielska, and B. Biernacki, Food Addit. Contam., 13:871 (1996).
11. World Health Organization, in Evaluation of Certain Veterinary Drug Residues in Food, Thirty-fourth Report of the Joint FAO/WHO Expert Committee on Food Additives, Technical Report Series 788, World Health Organization, Geneva (1989).

12. European Agency for the Evaluation of Medicinal Products (EMEA), in Ronidazole, Summary Report, Committee for Veterinary Medicinal Products, EMEA/MRL, London, UK (1993).

13. F.J. Wolf, F.P. Baylis, G.E. Smith, C. Rosenblum, H.T. Meriwether, R.F. Alvaro, D.E. Wolf, F.R. Koniuszy, and T.A. Jacob, J. Agric. Food Chem., 31:559 (1983).

14. F.J. Wolf, R.F. Alvaro, J.J. Steffens, D.E. Wolf, F.R. Koniuszy, M.L. Green, and T.A. Jacob, J. Agric. Food Chem., 32:717 (1984).

15. L.R. McDougald, In The Biology of Coccidia (P.L. Long, Ed.), University Park Press, Baltimore, MD, p. 373 (1982).

16. W. Brand, in Use of Drugs in Food Animal Medicine, Proc. of 10th Annual Food Animal Medicine Conf., (J.D. Powers, and T.E. Powers, Eds.), Ohio State University Press, p. 281 (1984).

17. T.S. Rumsey, J. Anim. Sci., 58:1461 (1984).

18. V.P. Simpson, Vet. Rec., 114:434 (1984).

19. D.J.S. Miller, Vet. Rec., 108:317 (1981).

20. J. Weissinger, in Animal Drugs and Human Health (L.M. Crawford, and D.A. Franco, Eds.), Technomic Publishing Co, Lancaster, PE, p. 113 (1994).

21. A.L. Donoho, R.J. Herberg, L.L. Zornes, and Van-Duyn, J. Agric. Food Chem., 30: 909 (1982).

22. B.B. Pressman, and M. Fahim, Ann. Rev. Pharmacol. Toxicol., 22:465 (1982).

23. A.L. Donoho, J. Anim. Sci., 58:1528 (1982).

24. M.A.J. Godfrey, M.F. Luckey, and P. Kwasowski, Food Addit. Contam., 14:281 (1997).

25. D.G. Kennedy, W.J. Blanchflower, P.J. Hughes, W.J. McCaughey, in Residues of Veterinary Drugs in Food, Proc. Euroresidue III Conf., Veldhoven, 1996 (N. Haagsma and A. Ruiter, Eds.), Fac. Vet. Med., Univ. Utrecht, The Netherlands, p. 601 (1996).

26. J.W. Westley, in Applied Microbiology (D. Perlman, Ed.), Academic Press, New York, p. 177 (1969).

27. S. Kantor, and R.H. Shenkel, Poultry Sci., 63:1497 (1984).

28. S. Kantor, R.H. Shenkel, and R.L. Kennet, Poultry Sci., 63:1506 (1984).

29. B. Donev, A. Vladimirova, and E. Kodjuharov, J. Vet. Pharmacol. Ther., 20:177 (1997).

30. M.A. Brown, and S. Rajan, J. Agric. Food Chem., 34:470 (1986).

31. S.J. Stout, J. Wu, A.R. DaCunha, K.G. King, and A. Lee, J. Agric. Food Chem., 39:386 (1991).

32. D.G. Kennedy, W.J. Blanchflower, and B.C. Odornan, Food Addit. Contam., 14:27 (1995).

33. G.O. Korsrud, C.D.C. Salisbury, V.K. Martz, J.D. MacNeil, and G. Royan, in Residues of Veterinary Drugs in Food, Proc. Euroresidue III Conf., Veldhoven, 1996 (N. Haagsma and A. Ruiter, Eds.), Fac. Vet. Med., Univ. Utrecht, The Netherlands, p. 625 (1996).

34. M. Atef, A. Ramadan, and K. Abo-El-Sooud, Br. Poutry Sci., 34:195 (1993).

35. M. Atef, A. Ramadan, S.A.H. Youssef, and K. Abo-El-Sooud, Res. Vet. Sci., 54: 179 (1993).

36. D.G. Kennedy, W.J. Blanchflower, and B.C. Odornan, Food Addit. Contam., 12:83 (1995).

37. J.A. Tarbin, S. Chapman, W.H.H. Farrington, A.L. Patey, and G. Shearer, in Residues of Veterinary Drugs in Food, Proc. Euroresidue II Conf., Veldhoven, May 3–5, 1993 (N. Haagsma, A Ruiter, and P.B. Czedik-Eysenberg, Eds.), Fac. Vet. Med., Univ. Utrecht, The Netherlands, p. 655 (1993).

38. D.G. Kennedy, W.J. Blanchflower, and B.C. Odornan, Food Addit. Contam., 12:93 (1995).

39. G.P. Dimenna, F.S. Lyon, F.M. Thompson, J.A. Creegan, and G.J. Wright, J. Agric. Food Chem., 37:668 (1989).

40. M.H. Akhtar, K.A. El-Sooud, and M.A.A. Shehata, Food Addit. Contam., 13:897 (1996).

41. K. Sinigoj-Gacnik, in Residues of Veterinary Drugs in Food, Proc. Euroresidue III Conf., Veldhoven, 1996 (N. Haagsma and A. Ruiter, Eds.), Fac. Vet. Med., Univ. Utrecht, The Netherlands, p. 859 (1996).

42. K. Sinigoj-Gacnik, in Residues of Veterinary Drugs in Food, Proc. Euroresidue Conf., Noordwijkerhout, May 21–23, 1990 (N. Haagsma, A. Ruiter, and P.B. Czedik-Eysenberg, Eds.), Fac. Vet. Med., Univ. Utrecht, The Netherlands, p. 859 (1990).

43. M.J. Lynch, G.M. Frame, J.F. Ericson, E.F. Illyes, and M.A. Nowakowski, in Xenobiotics and Food-Producing Animals (D.H. Hutson, D.R. Hawkins, G.D. Paulson, and C.B. Struble, Eds.), American Chemical Society, Washington, DC, p. 49 (1992).

44. A.L. Donoho, J. Manthey, J. Accolowitz, and L. Zornes, J. Agric. Food Chem., 26: 1090 (1978).

45. K.L. Davidson, J. Agric. Food Chem., 32:1273 (1984).

46. G.P. Dimmena, F.S. Lyon, F.M. Thompson, J.A. Creegan, and G.J. Wright, J. Agric. Food Chem., 37:668 (1989).

47. European Agency for the Evaluation of Medicinal Products (EMEA), in Decoquinate, Summary Report, Committee for Veterinary Medicinal Products, EMEA/MRL/017/95-Final, London, UK (1995).

48. European Agency for the Evaluation of Medicinal Products (EMEA), in Diclazuril, Summary Report, Committee for Veterinary Medicinal Products, EMEA/MRL/086/96-Final, London, UK (1996).

49. Scientific Committee for Animal Nutrition, in Extension of Use of Diclazuril to the Feedingstuffs for Chickens Reared for Laying, Report of the Scientific Committee for Animal Nutrition, Directorate General XXIV, The European Commission, November (1997).

50. World Health Organization, in Evaluation of Certain Veterinary Drug Residues in Food, Thirty-fourth Report of the Joint FAO/WHO Expert Committee on Food Additives, Technical Report Series 788, World Health Organization, Geneva, p. 43 (1989).

51. Y. Debuf, in The Veterinary Formulary (Y. Debuf, Ed.), The Pharmaceutical Press, London (1991).

6

Antimicrobial Growth Promoters

Antimicrobial growth promoters are substances that, when added to feeds at subtherapeutic dosages for an extended period of time, produce improvements in growth rate and feed conversion efficiency, mortality, and morbidity.

The era of antimicrobial growth promoters began in the late 1940's when scientists found that chicks fed a dried fermentation mash of *Streptomyces aureofaciens* grew faster and to a greater final weight than those fed a diet supplemented with liver extract. The component of the fermentation mash responsible for the stimulation of growth was identified as chlortetracycline. Soon after the ability of chlortetracycline to enhance growth was confirmed in turkeys and swine, several other drugs were added to the list of the compounds that could enhance growth and improve feed efficiency when used at levels ranging from 2 to 50 ppm in feed. Since the process by which farm animals convert feed protein into edible protein for the consumer is not particularly efficient, the extensive and continuous use of antimicrobial growth promoters as feed additives was rapidly become a major feature in modern intensive livestock production systems.

In nonruminating animals, antimicrobial growth promoters act primarily in the digestive tract, exerting a beneficial effect on the composition of microorganisms inhabiting the gut. It has long been known that a well-balanced intestinal flora obstructs the way to pathogens trying to enter the body. Antimicrobials also act to slow down bacterial metabolism, thus reducing, the rate at which the intestinal flora break down feed proteins to substances such as ammonia and biogenic amines, which are toxic to the animals and interfere with the absorption of nutrients through the intestinal wall. Antimicrobials help to increase, therefore, the availability of nutrients and improve intestinal absorption. At the same time, they also exert a positive effect on metabolism, increasing the rate at which animals lay down protein, thus improving weight gain and feed efficiency.

In ruminants, the extent or importance of changes in the small intestine similar to those observed in nonruminants has not, so far, been documented. In the case of ruminants, however, the beneficial effects of antimicrobial growth promoters lies more clearly in their ability to influence the balance of microbial species inhabiting the rumen. A higher level of rumen propionate is produced in treated animals at the expense of acetate and sometimes of butyrate production, and there are significant reductions in energy losses due to the ruminal production of methane. The total effect is to make rumen fermentation more efficient, thus increasing the metabolizable energy content available for lean meat production.

In the United States, permitted antimicrobial growth promoters include several antibiotic and synthetic antibacterial agents. The former group is composed of three aminoglycoside antibiotics including neomycin, streptomycin, and bambermycin; three macrolide antibiotics including erythromycin, oleandomycin, and tylosin; three polyether ionophore antibiotics including lasalocid, monensin, and salinomycin; two tetracycline antibiotics including chlortetracycline and oxytetracycline; three peptide antibiotics including avoparcin, bacitracin, and virginiamycin; and a series of miscellaneous antibiotics including lincomycin, penicillin procaine, avilamycin, and tiamulin. Within the latter group, several compounds such as arsenical compounds, nitrofurans including furazolidone and nitrofurazone, sulfonamides including sulfamethazine, nitrofurans including furazolidone and nitrofurazone, sulfonamides including sulfamethazine, sulfathiazole and sulfaquinoxaline, and quinoxaline-1,4-dioxides are included.

In the European Union, significant changes in use of the permitted antimicrobial growth promoters have occurred during the last decade. Currently, only four antibiotics including monensin, salinomycin, bambermycin, and avilamycin, and two synthetic antibacterials including carbadox and olaquindox, and authorized. It is important to note that continued use of the antimicrobial growth promoters is constantly under review throughout the world because of consumer discontent.

Since many of the above-mentioned compounds possess major anti-infectious activity in addition to their role as growth promoters, their application in animal farming has already been discussed in previous chapters. Hence, this chapter concentrates on the remaining compounds within this group, namely the organic arsenicals, peptide antibiotics, quinoxaline-1,4-dioxides, and miscellaneous substances.

6.1 ORGANIC ARSENICALS

Certain organic arsenicals are incorporated in pig and broiler feeds to improve weight gain and feed efficiency and to combat enteric infections. Arsanilic acid

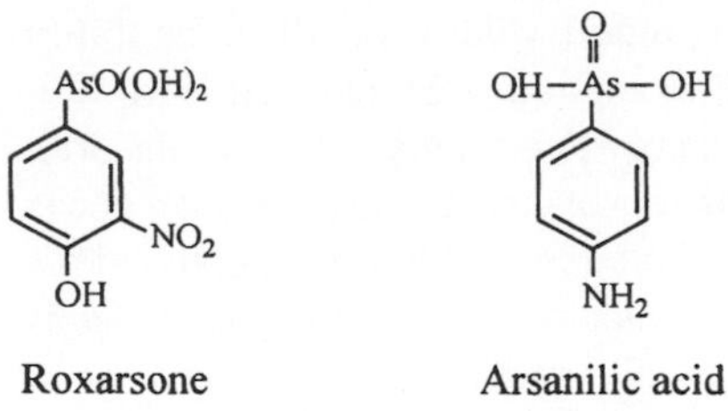

FIG. 6.1 Chemical structures of commonly used organic arsenicals.

and its sodium salt are most commonly used, particularly in pigs, whereas roxarsone and the related compound 4-nitro-phenylarsonic acid are used mainly in broilers (Fig. 6.1). The exact mode of action of these compounds is not yet understood but it is assumed that it is associated with their antibacterial activity. They are also efficacious in the egg-producing industry and were previously approved for use in laying hens, although presently these drugs are no longer approved for this purpose. However, their use in animals is, generally, rather limited and the risk–benefit ratio is questionable because these drugs can produce toxicosis known as peripheral nerve demyelination.

Organic arsenicals are poorly absorbed from the gastrointestinal tract and are excreted mainly in feces (1). After their absorption, organic arsenicals are distributed throughout the body and rapidly excreted in the urine without being metabolized to a great extent. Elimination of the parenterally administered compounds is nearly complete within 24–48 h, while several days are required for elimination of the compounds from the gut.

When animals do not have constant access to organic arsenicals, there is a high possibility that significant levels of arsenic residues will not appear in tissues. However, excessive feeding of these compounds can result in arsenic concentrations as high as 3–10 ppm in liver and kidney and 1–2 ppm in blood (1). Feeding organic arsenicals to laying hens also produces a substantial increase in arsenic residues in eggs, especially in the yolk. It is interesting to note that arsenic residue concentrations in incurred tissues increase in a dose-dependent manner and, therefore, a maximum limit of arsenic transfer is not normally reached (2).

Arsanilic acid is added to swine and poultry feeds at a dosage rate of up to 100 ppm for growth-promoting purposes. It is also effective for prophylaxis and treatment of many outbreaks associated with *E. coli* infections in swine. To treat scour in swine, arsanilic acid is administered in the feed, at a level of 250 ppm for up to 3 weeks. Arsanilic acid may also be administered to poultry for treatment of coliform septicemia at a level of 250 ppm in the feed for 5–8 days.

Roxarsone has been used by the poultry industry due primarily to its ability to improve growth, feed conversion, and pigmentation to broilers. At least 50% of the poultry industry has used roxarsone as a growth promoter, although the drug also exhibits anticoccidial activity similar to that of arsanilic acid (3). Roxarsone is not approved for use as anticoccidial in the United States, but it is approved for use in chicken and turkey feeds as a growth promoter. It is added in poultry feeds at a rate of 50 ppm and in swine feeds at 25–37.5 ppm.

When diets that contained 11–88 mg/kg arsenic originating from the incorporated roxarsone were fed to layer hens for 4 weeks, arsenic residues in liver, eggs, and the excreta significantly increased with increasing arsenic levels in feeds (4).

6.2   PEPTIDE ANTIBIOTICS

Peptide antibiotics are compounds containing amino acids that are covalently linked to other chemical entities and consist of more than one component. In contrast to naturally occurring proteins that are built up from L-amino acids only, peptide antibiotics usually contain D-amino acids. Avoparcin, bacitracin, efrotomycin, enramycin, thiopeptin, and virginiamycin constitute the main members within this group of drugs (Fig. 6.2). They usually added to animal feeds at low concentrations, and produce residues in tissues at very low or undetectable levels. Unfortunately, the metabolic pathways of most peptide antibiotics have not been still elucidated. Within the European Union, these antibiotics are regulated under a separate legislation (Directive 70/524/EEC).

Avoparcin is a narrow-spectrum glycopeptide antibiotic composed of two components. It is used solely for growth-promoting purposes, although it is also primarily active against gram-positive bacteria. Avoparcin is administered as a feed additive to improve the rate of weight gain in chickens, turkeys, pigs, and calves, and to enhance milk production in lactating cattle (5). It is also recommended at dosages of 15–40 ppm in the feed for beef cattle to improve live weight gain by 5–15%.

In ruminants, avoparcin has a dual action. It acts in the rumen by enhancing fermentation, and in the intestine by improving the absorption of nutrients. Following feeding to animals, avoparcin is virtually unabsorbed from the gastrointestinal tract and is rapidly eliminated in the form of the parent compound. As a result, no withdrawal period is required.

Bacitracin is a linear-ring peptide antibiotic produced by *Bacillus subtilis* and *Bacillus licheniformis*. Commercial formulations of bacitracin comprise a mixture of many closely related compounds classified into bacitracin A, B, C, D, E, F, and G (5). The main components are bacitracin A, B_1, and B_2, constituting 57%, 22%, and 13%, respectively, of the mixture, whereas bacitracin F constitutes less than 2%. Bacitracin F is actually a degradation product of bacitracin A that

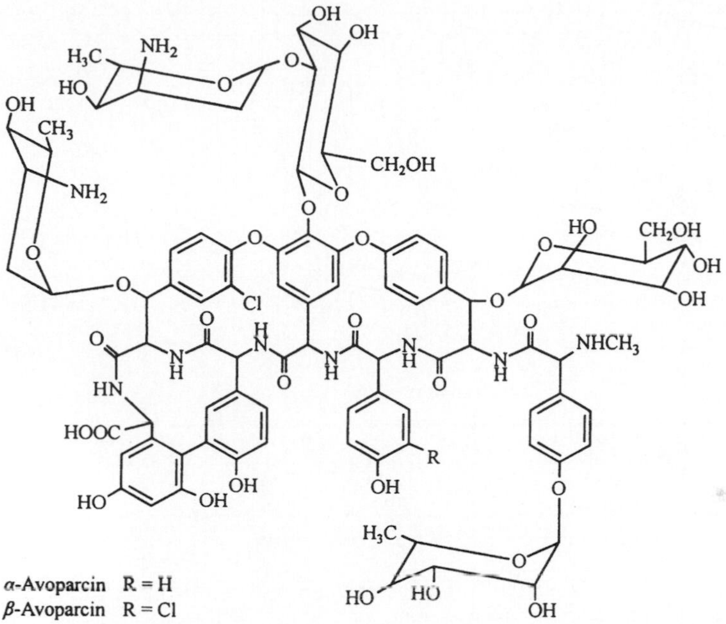

α-Avoparcin R = H
β-Avoparcin R = Cl

Avoparcin

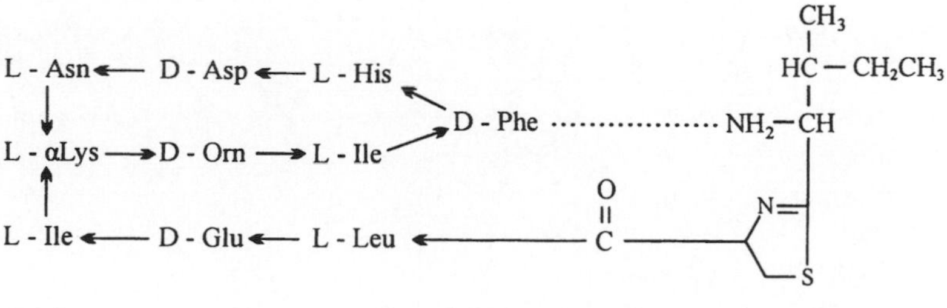

Bacitracin A

FIG. 6.2 Chemical structures of commonly used peptide antibiotics.

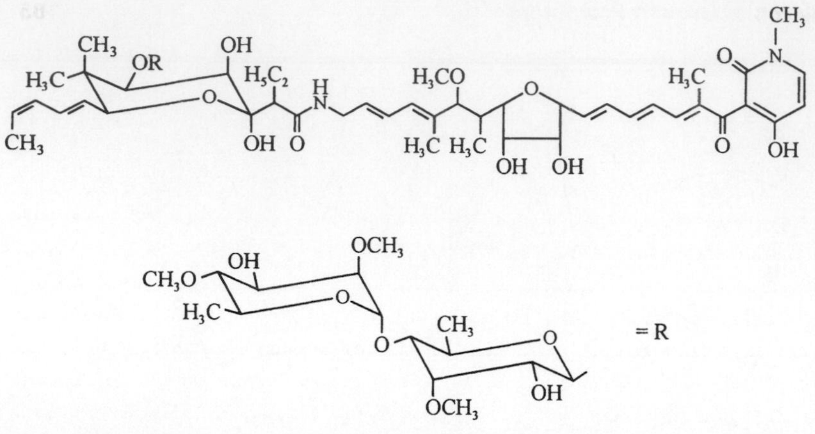

Efrotomycin

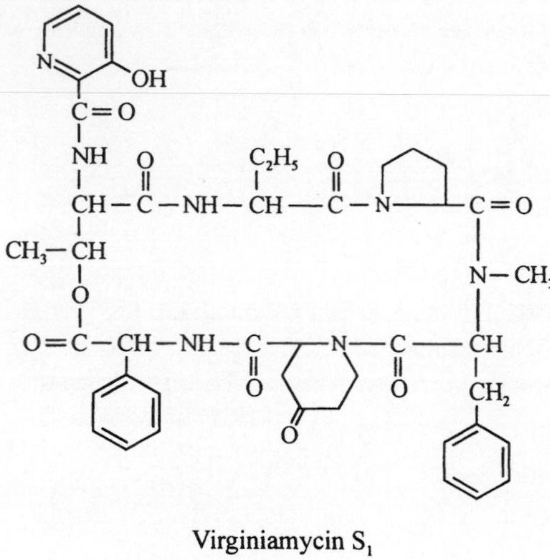

Virginiamycin S₁

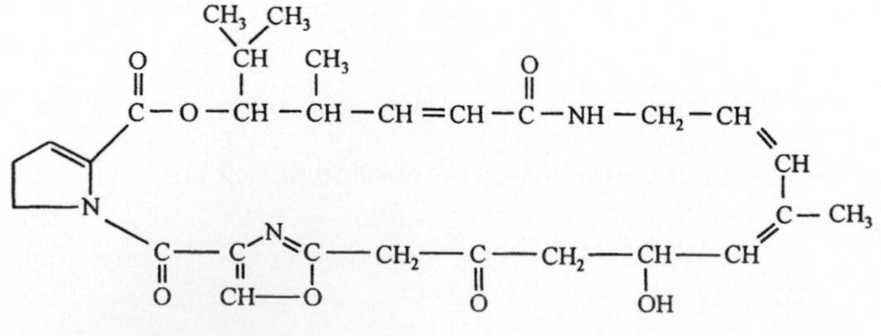

Virginiamycin M₁

Fig. 6.2 *Continued*

184

shows nephrotoxic activity. Except for bacitracin A and F, which have known molecular structures, the chemical formulas of other existing bacitracin forms have not been yet elucidated.

Although the A, B, and C forms are microbiologically active, bacitracin F exhibits no activity. The bacitracin mixture is active against gram-positive organisms, and is usually added to feeds in the form of the zinc salt to promote growth and enhance egg production. Zinc bacitracin is indicated as a growth-promoting agent for calves, lambs, swine, and turkeys at a dose of 5–50 ppm and for rabbits at 5–20 ppm in the feed. It is further used for treatment of mastitis in cows by the intramammary route. No withdrawal period is required, but the compound should not be used as a feed additive for adult breeding stock or lactating cattle. Manganese and sodium salts of bacitracin are also commercially available but have never gained extensive use.

After oral application, bacitracin is hardly absorbed by the gastrointestinal tract and, therefore, its distribution in tissues is considered negligible (6). Approximately 95% of an orally administered dose is excreted via feces, and only 3% or less via urine. Bacitracin is primarily metabolized to desamidobacitracin and further to smaller peptides and amino acids. Main metabolites identified in feces are bacitracin A, B_1, B_2, F, desamidobacitracin, and catabolic peptides. In urine and bile, only hydrolytic cleavage products such as small peptides are present.

Intramammary use of bacitracin resulted in residues in milk, but not in plasma, udder, or any other tissue. Residue depletion studies in cows given intramammary bacitracin treatment showed that muscle, liver, kidney, fat, udder, and milk from untreated quarters did not contain detectable residues (<0.003–0.005 IU/ml) after the end of treatment. In milk from treated quarters, however, residues of bacitracin could be detected during treatment, declining to around 0.04 IU/ml at the sixth milking after treatment.

Efrotomycin is a peptide antibiotic produced by *Streptomyces lactamdurans* (7). It is used as a growth stimulant for swine by incorporation at a minimum level of 4 ppm and a maximum of 8 ppm in the feeds.

Enramycin is also a linear-ring peptide antibiotic produced by *Streptomyces fungicidicus*. Enramycin consists of two main components called enramycin A and enramycin B. It is active against gram-positive and acid-fast bacteria and is an approved growth promoter for poultry and swine. Enramycin is usually incorporated in feeds in the form of its monohydrochloride form.

Thiopeptin is a sulfur-containing peptide antibiotic complex produced by *Streptomyces tateyamensis*. It is composed of five closely related components, the thiopeptins A_1, A_2, A_3, A_4, and B (8). Commercially available thiopeptin is primarily composed of thiopeptins B. This antibiotic is active against gram-positive bacteria and is used exclusively as a feed additive for pigs.

Virginiamycin is a mixture of macrocyclic lactones with a peptide part, collectively called peptolides, that is produced by cultures of *Streptomyces virgin-*

iae. These peptolides are classified into the components M_1 and M_2 that constitute the so-called factor M, and the components S_1, S_2, S_3, S_4, and S_5 that make up the so-called factor S. These two types of microbiologically active factors show a natural synergism.

Commercially available virginiamycin is prepared by mixing the isolated components M_1 and S_1 at a ratio of 4 : 1. Virginiamycin is primarily effective against gram-positive bacteria, and has been used as a growth-promoting agent in nonruminating animals. It can also increase egg production in laying hens (9), and is effective against necrotic enteritis in broilers and against dysentery in pigs. Virginiamycin is added to broiler feeds at a dosage rate of 20 ppm, to swine and calves feeds at 20–50 ppm, and to turkey feeds up to 20 ppm.

Pharmacokinetic studies (10) showed that virginiamycin is not significantly absorbed and is eliminated mostly in the feces. Following administration of radio-labeled virginiamycin to rats, turkeys, and cattle, metabolites of the drug appeared in liver of all animals. Most of these metabolites were covalently bound to tissues, whereas the extractable metabolites could not be identified. No residues of virgin-iamycin could be detected in edible tissues and consequently no withdrawal period has been set up.

When laying hens were fed a diet supplemented with 10 or 40 ppm radiola-beled virginiamycin, about 0.05% of the ingested dose was recovered in eggs (11). Radiolabeled residues expressed in terms of virginiamycin equivalents were found to be 5.1 ppb in the albumen and 31.8 ppb in the egg yolk from hens fed the 10 ppm diet. However, antibacterial activity could not be detected in these eggs. Tentative identification showed that about 17% of the total radiolabeled residues in the albumen behaved chromatographically like the parent drug, while about 18% was associated with ovalbumin. In the yolk, 31% of the radioactivity was associated with proteins, 58% with fatty acids, and 4% with nonsaponifiable matter.

6.3 QUINOXALINE-1,4-DIOXIDES

The importance of quinoxaline-1,4-dioxides to swine was recognized many years ago, when quindoxin was first marketed as an antibacterial growth-promoting agent. However, quindoxin caused persistent photocontact dermatitis in several agricultural workers and, as a result, it was rapidly withdrawn from use. A number of analogues including carbadox and olaquindox were subsequently introduced in the market (Fig. 6.3).

The growing concern of consumer groups and of policymakers in drug regulatory agencies regarding the mutagenic and carcinogenic potency of the quinoxaline-1,4-dioxides and their possible residues in edible animal products has caused much debate. Carbadox was initially the main drug in use, but suspicion as to its safety arose because this compound exhibited both genotoxic and mutagenic

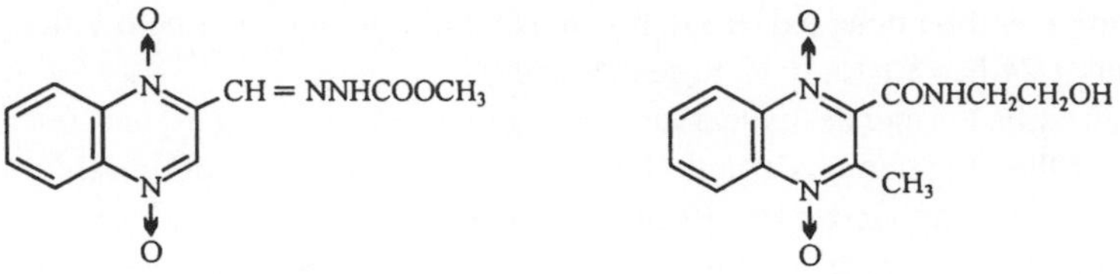

Carbadox   Olaquindox

FIG. 6.3   Chemical structures of commonly used quinoxaline-1,4-dioxides.

activity. Its mutagenic activity appeared to be connected with the mechanism of antibacterial action, thereby indicating that quinoxaline-1,4-dioxides with antibacterial activity will also inevitably show mutagenic activity to some extent (12). Olaquindox is also a strongly mutagenic agent but seemingly devoid of carcinogenic activity.

Carbadox is an antimicrobial agent used in swine feeds for growth promotion, improved feed efficiency, increased rate of weight gain, and control of swine dysentery and bacterial swine enteritis (13). The product is sold for use in starters and/or grower rations but not in finisher rations. In most areas of the world it is fed to pigs at 50 ppm in the feed and may be used in animals up to 4 months of age, with a 4 week withdrawal period before slaughter. In the United States, it is approved for use in feed at 55 ppm for pigs up to 35 kg bw with a 70 day withdrawal period.

In swine, carbadox is metabolized rapidly to quinoxaline-2-carboxylic acid, with the intermediary formation of the aldehyde and the desoxy metabolite of the parent compound. Metabolism studies with radiolabeled carbadox showed that the parent compound and its three metabolites are present in plasma within hours after drug administration, but all four compounds can disappear within 24 h postdosing. The major urinary metabolite was shown to be the quinoxaline-2-carboxylic acid, which was also excreted in the conjugated form. N-oxides were not found in urine. Feces also contained some quinoxaline-2-carboxylic acid but no unchanged carbadox (14).

Residue depletion studies in young pigs fed carbadox-supplemented rations for 1 week showed the parent compound to be present at 20 ppb in blood, and at 26 ppb in muscle tissue at 24 h withdrawal; residues were reduced to less than 2 ppb at 48 h, and eliminated at 72 h (15). Desoxycarbadox, although not detected in blood, could be detected in muscle at the 17 ppb level at 24 h withdrawal to be reduced, subsequently, to 9 ppb at 48 h and to below the detection limit at 72 h. Whereas only traces of carbadox were found in kidney at 24 h withdrawal, desoxycarbadox could be detected in kidney at 186 ppb, 34 ppb, and below the detection limit at 24 h, 48 h, and 72 h, respectively.

Although carbadox and desoxycarbadox are suspected carcinogens, the conditions of use of the drug and its depletion patterns lessen the human food safety concerns from these compounds (16). Residues of carbadox in the animal carcass can be monitored by analyzing liver for the noncarcinogenic quinoxaline-2-carboxylic acid. Unlike carbadox and its desoxy metabolite, quinoxaline-2-carboxylic acid persisted in liver although not in kidney, muscle, and fat of pigs fed 55 ppm carbadox for 5 days; average levels of 18.9 ppb at 30 day, 5.5 ppb at 45 day, and 1.3 ppb at 70 day withdrawal were reported (14). In another study, alkaline hydrolysis of liver and muscle samples of swine treated with carbadox showed that the concentration of quinoxaline-2-carboxylic acid ranged from less that 3 ppb to 45.3 ppb for liver and to 10.8 ppb for muscle (17).

Olaquindox is an antibacterial also used as a growth promoter for swine at an incorporation rate in feeds of 25–100 ppm. In swine, olaquindox is metabolized either by oxidation of the alcohol group on the side chain or removal of one or both of the N-oxide groups at the positions 1 and 4 on the quinoxaline ring.

Metabolism studies in swine with radiolabeled olaquindox showed that the drug was rapidly absorbed from the gut, more than 90% of the dose being excreted in urine within 48 h after administration (18). In urine, the parent drug constituted more than 60% of the original dose, whereas the remainder was due to five metabolites identified as metabolites II, III, IV, V, and VI. Less than 0.1% of the dose was excreted in the feces within 48 h.

Radiolabeled residue depletion studies in swine also showed that the maximum concentrations of total olaquindox residues at 2 days after its oral administration occurred in the kidney (110 ppb) and liver (52 ppb); much lower concentrations could be seen in the plasma (10 ppb) and muscle (9 ppb), whereas fat did not contain detectable residues (7). These residue levels declined with time so that at 28 days postdosing they were negligible in kidney (1 ppb) and liver (2 ppb) and nondetectable in muscle and fat.

Feeding low levels of olaquindox (2.0 and 6.0 ppm in feed) to laying hens for 21 days, resulted in residues in eggs that reached a plateau after some 10 days of medication (19). The sum of residues of the parent compound and the N^4-monooxy metabolite, which was the only metabolite observed, was higher in egg white than in yolk, the amount of the metabolite accounting for 15–20% of the total residues. After cessation of the medication, the residues in both yolk and white declined below 2 ppb in about 5 days.

6.4 MISCELLANEOUS

Avilamycin is a polyether antibiotic of the orthosomycin family that consists of a six-member oligosaccharide, dichloroisoeverninic acid, and methyl eurekanate

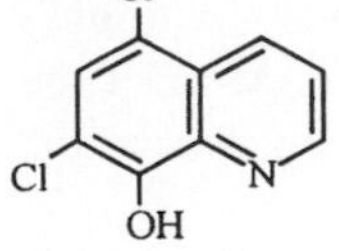

Halquinol

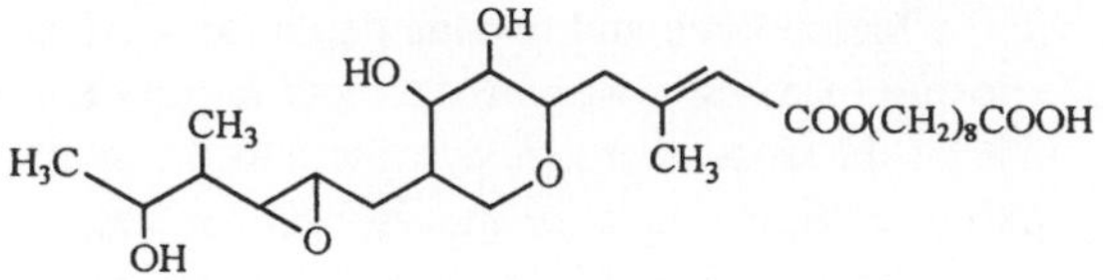

Mupirocin

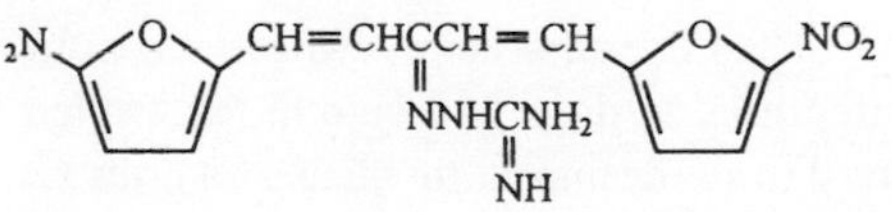

Nitrovin

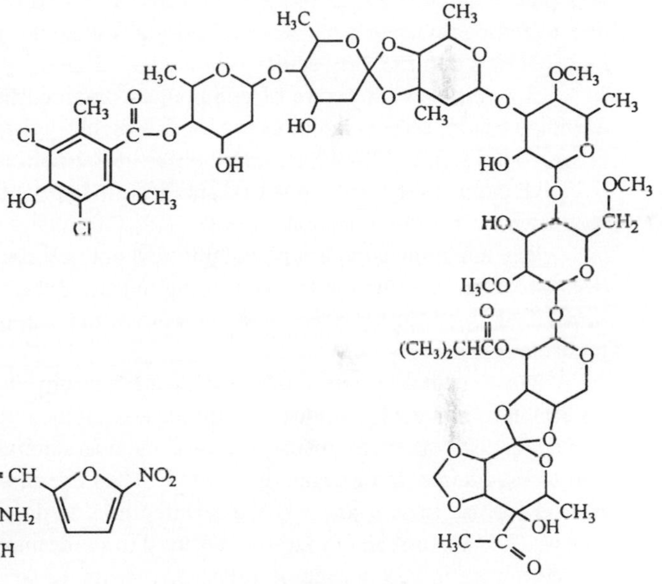

Avilamycin A

Fig. 6.4 Chemical structures of avilamycin A, halquinol, mupirocin, and nitrovin.

(Fig. 6.4). The avilamycin complex is produced by *Streptomyces viridochromogenes* and is composed of factor A as the major component with several other minor components (20). It is used as a feed additive for swine at a level of 20–40 ppm for animals up to 4 months of age and at 10–20 ppm for animals of 4–6 months of age (21, 22). When fed to swine, avilamycin causes an increase in gain rate and efficiency of feed utilization.

Metabolism and residue depletion studies of avilamycin in swine and rats showed that oral doses are excreted rapidly and nearly quantitatively, with only 5% of the dose excreted in urine and the remainder in feces (23). Most of the parent compounds were metabolized or degraded, since only about 8% of the total residues in feces was parent avilamycin.

Pigs dosed with radiolabeled avilamycin produced three unidentified fecal metabolites derived from the oligosaccharide and/or the eurekanate moieties. However, the primary metabolite in feces and liver was flambic acid. Mean total residues in muscle were all below 0.2 ppm, whereas residues in other edible tissues were all below 1 ppm. Most of tissue residues were derived from the oligosaccharide and/or the eurekanate portion of avilamycin, whereas very little was parent avilamycin. In fat, the avilamycin related residues was found to be due to radioactivity that had entered normal metabolic pathways and had been incorporated into the fatty acids.

Halquinol is a mixture of compounds obtained by the chlorination of 8-quinolinol (Fig. 6.4). It is composed of 5,7-dichloro-8-quinolinol (57–74%), 5-chloro-8-quinolinol (23–40%), and 7-chloro-8-quinolinol (up to 3%). Halquinol is active against both gram-positive and gram-negative bacteria, fungi, and protozoa.

When administered orally, halquinol is not absorbed by the gastrointestinal tract and, thus, is effective for controlling intestinal tract infections in swine and poultry. It is added to swine feeds at a level of 100–600 ppm and to poultry feeds at 30 ppm.

Mupirocin is an antibiotic complex produced by *Pseudomonas fluorescens*. Its structure contains a unique 9-hydroxy-nonanoic acid moiety (Fig. 6.4). It is active against both gram-positive bacteria such as staphylococci and streptococci and against some gram-negative bacteria of lesser importance. Mupirocin is licensed for use in skin and soft tissue infections in dogs and cats in the United States. The calcium salt of mupirocin is used in swine and cattle feeds as a growth-promoting agent at a dosage of 120–300 mg/day (24).

Nitrovin (Fig. 6.4) is a nitrofuran used as a growth promoter in animal feeds for chickens, turkeys, swine, and calves at concentrations varying from 10 to 40 ppm in the feed. The compound has been withdrawn in the European Union.

REFERENCES

1. W.B. Buck, G.D. Osweiler, and G.A. van Gelder, in Clinical and Diagnostic Veterinary Toxicology (W.B. Buck, G.D. Osweiler, and G.A. van Gelder, Eds.), Kendall/Hunt, Dubuque, IA (1973).
2. D.J. Donoghue, H. Hairston, M.J. Bartholomew, and D.D. Wagner, in Residues of Veterinary Drugs in Food, Proc. Euroresidue II Conf., Veldhoven, May 3–5, 1993

(N. Haagsma, A. Ruiter and P.B. Czedik-Eysenberg, Eds.), Fac. Vet. Med., Univ. Utrecht, The Netherlands, p. 276 (1993).'

3. W.M. Reid, Am. J. Vet Res., 36:593 (1975).
4. P.W.S. Chiou, K.L. Chen, and B. Yu, J. Sci. Food Agric., 74:229 (1997).
5. Y. Ikai, in Chemical Analysis of Antibiotics Used in Agriculture (H. Oka, H. Nakazawa, K. Harada, and J.D. MacNeil, Eds.), AOAC International, Arlington, VA, p. 407 (1995).
6. J. Donoso, G.O. Craig, and R.S. Baldwin, Toxicol. Appl. Pharmacol., 17:366 (1970).
7. E. Higashiide, K. Hatano, M. Shibata, and K. Nakazawa, J. Antibiot., 21:126 (1968).
8. O.D. Hensens, and G. Albers-Schonberg, Tetrahedron Letters, 36:49 (1978).
9. R.D. Miles, D.M. Janky, and R.H. Harms, Poultry Sci., 64:139 (1985).
10. D.W. Gottschall, C. Gombatz, and R. Wang, J. Agri. Food Chem., 35:366 (1970).
11. D.E. Corpet, M. Baradat, and G.F. Bories, J. Agric. Food Chem., 36:837 (1988).
12. T.B. Barragry, in Veterinary Drug Therapy (T.B. Barragry, Ed.), Lea & Febiger, Philadelphia, p. 649 (1994).
13. G.C. Brander, D.M. Pugh, R.J. Bywater, and W.L. Jenkins, in Veterinary Applied Pharmacology and Therapeutics (G.C. Brander, D.M. Pugh, R.J. Bywater, and W.L. Jenkins, Eds.), 5th Edition, Balliere Tindall, London (1991).
14. World Health Organization, in Residues of Some Veterinary Drugs in Animals and Foods, Thirty-sixth Meeting of the Joint FAO/WHO Expert Committee on Food Additives, Food and Agriculture Organization of the United Nations, FAO Food and Nutrition Paper No 41/3, Rome, p. 19 (1990).
15. A.I. MacIntosh, G. Lauriault, and G.A. Neville, J. Assoc. Off. Anal. Chem., 68:665 (1985).
16. R.F. Bevill, in Veterinary Pharmacology and Therapeutics (N.H. Booth, and L.E. McDonald, Eds.), Iowa State University Press, Ames, IA p. 785 (1988).
17. M. Rutalj, D. Bazulic, J. Sapunarpostruznik, J. Zivkovic, and I. Ljubicic, Food Addit. Contam., 13:879 (1996).
18. World Health Organization, in Residues of Some Veterinary Drugs in Animals and Foods, Thirty-sixth Meeting of the Joint FAO/WHO Expert Committee on Food Additives, Food and Agriculture Organization of the United Nations, FAO Food and Nutrition Paper No 41/3, Rome, p. 85 (1990).
19. H.J. Keukens, C.A. Kan, and M.J.H. Tomassen, in Residues of Veterinary Drugs in Food, Proc. Euroresidue III Conf., Veldhoven, 1996 (N. Haagsma, and A. Ruiter, Eds.), Fac. Vet. Med., Univ. Utrecht, The Netherlands, p. 611 (1996).
20. J.L. Mertz, J.S. Peloso, B.J. Barker, G.E. Babbitt, J.L. Occolowitz, V.L. Simson, and R.M. Kline, J. Antibiot., 39:877 (1986).
21. D.J. Jones, D.H. Mowrey, D.B. Anderson, and R.H. Wellenreiter, J. Anim. Sci., 65: 881 (1987).
22. L.E. Watkins, D.H. Mowrey, D.B. Anderson, L.J. Camp, D.L. Feller, H.P. Greuter, D.J. Jones, J.A. Miyat, and R.D. Olson, J. Anim. Sci., 65:313 (1987).
23. J.D. Magnussen, J.E. Dalidowicz, T.D. Thomson, and A.L. Donoho, J. Agric. Food Chem., 39:306 (1991).
24. A. Kaukas, and M. Hinton, Br. Vet. J., 144:302 (1988).

7

Anabolic Hormonal-Type Growth Promoters

It has long been established that the sexual status of an animal controls and coordinates its growth rate and speed of fattening. Bulls grow faster and lay down more lean meat in the carcass than steers, whereas steers grow faster with a higher feed conversion efficiency than cows. These beneficial effects on animal performance are due to the sex steroids produced in the testes.

The decreased level of androgens in castrated male cattle as a result of testicular removal leads to production of a carcass that is intermediate between that of an intact male and a female. Since the increased proportion of fat in such a carcass makes it less valuable for the health-conscious consumer, extensive research has been directed towards replacing the loss of carcass quality resulting from castration, by administration to the animals of various natural and synthetic hormonal substances, collectively called anabolic hormonal-type growth promoters. These compounds can substantially increase growth rate and improve feed efficiency and carcass composition in a process that may be highly profitable for the animal feeders.

These beneficial effects, which are on the order of 10–40%, are achieved predominantly in ruminants. It has been estimated that use of hormonal implants can improve farmers' margins by up to £30 a head for steers and £15 a head for heifers. Applications in other food-producing animals such as sheep, swine, and poultry occur to a lesser extent and, thus, are of limited importance.

The use of anabolic hormonal-type growth promoters in ruminants can create a hormonal situation in castrates, females, and young stock that may be similar to that found in intact males and pregnant females. Accordingly, the

193

greatest benefits are seen in cows treated with androgens, bulls treated with estrogens, and castrates treated with combined formulations of androgens and estrogens. Beyond their hormonal estrogenic, androgenic, and gestagenic activity, the anabolic hormonal-type growth promoters can be classified according to their chemical structure or origin into endogenous sex steroids, steroidal compounds not occurring naturally, nonsteroidal compounds not occurring naturally, and polypeptide hormones.

For all these hormonal substances to exert their desired effect, the method of administration to the animal is most important. They can be administered to animals by intramuscular injections but some compounds can be also administered incorporated into the feeds. However, the best method is one in which they are administered in form of a subcutaneous implant in the ear. This allows for a controlled slow release of the active ingredients, exposing the animal to a constant stimulating effect of the anabolic agent.

The overall rate of absorption of an anabolic agent from an implant can be influenced by a number of factors, including the technique of administration, total dosage given, integrity of the implant, presence of a second anabolic in the implant, implant size, shape, and hardness. Since at the end of the withdrawal period, up to 10% of the initial dose may still be found at the site of implantation, care should always be taken to discard this area at slaughter.

Unlike in the United States where some anabolic hormonal-type growth promoters are permitted, use of these compounds, either natural or synthetic, as growth promoters in meat-producing animals has not been allowed in the European Union since 1988, due to potential adverse effects to human health. Nevertheless, many anabolic hormonal-type growth promoters are still used illegally in the European Union.

The distribution of residues of anabolic hormonal-type growth promoters in animal tissues depends on their mode of metabolism and excretion. Residues are commonly found in muscle, fat, liver, kidney, and milk, as well as in urine, bile, and feces. In general, residue concentrations tend to be higher in the excreta than in tissues. Control of the abuse of these compounds is usually carried out through the analysis of edible tissues, injection sites, kidney, fat, urine, or even feces. In recent years, use of fecal samples has become of increasing importance because of their ease of collection in intensive livestock farming.

7.1 ENDOGENOUS SEX STEROIDS

Two female sex hormones, estradiol-17β and progesterone, and one male sex hormone, testosterone, are used as growth promoters on beef cattle (Fig. 7.1). By nature, they are all endogenous products playing an important role in controlling reproductive functions in humans and animals. When applied exogenously they will enter the same metabolic pathways as the endogenously produced molecules.

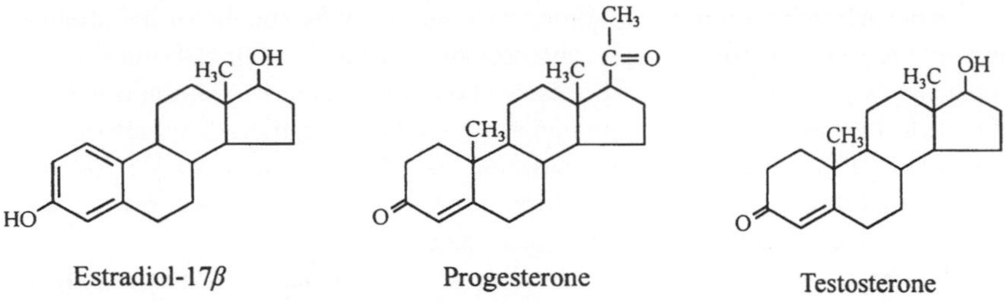

Estradiol-17β   Progesterone   Testosterone

FIG. 7.1   Chemical structures of commonly used endogenous sex steroids.

Metabolism leads to their rapid deactivation in the body and, hence, these compounds exhibit little oral activity. Thus, they have to be given parenterally. Most of the catabolism of these compounds occurs in liver, and enterohepatic circulation may then occur, with the metabolites exerting little if any biological activity. In cattle, most of these compounds are eliminated in feces where 60–90% of the metabolites are found in the free form. In contrast, metabolites occurring in urine are predominantly in conjugated forms.

Residue depletion studies in animals have generally indicated that administration of natural sex steroids resulted in residues in the edible tissues orders of magnitude lower than those naturally occurring in mature males, females, and pregnant females. Thus, in order to define such residues after exogenous administration, it is necessary to establish previously the physiologically occurring range of values. Ever since people started to use animals as a source of food, they have been exposed to such levels of endogenous sex steroids.

Estradiol-17β is given to animals in form of a subcutaneous implant in the ear, alone or in combination with other hormonally active compounds such as progesterone or trenbolone acetate. Estradiol-17β is used in steers, to best advantage, but also exhibits some anabolic effects in heifers and veal calves. It works best in lambs in conjunction with androgens, but is not effective as an anabolic agent in pigs. It has been used in many forms in the past including the benzoate, dipropionate, hemisuccinate, heptanoate, propionate, undecanoate, and valerate esters.

Estradiol-17β derived from an implant is indistinguishable from the endogenous estradiol-17β in the circulatory animal's system. Following administration of radiolabeled estradiol-17β to calves, radioactivity in urine was mainly due to estradiol-17α, with much lower amounts of estrone. Apart of the free forms, both compounds were present as conjugates as well. Radioactivity in feces was primarily due to estradiol-17α and to estradiol-17β and estrone, each compound occurring in the nonconjugated form (1).

After administration of estradiol benzoate to calves, the major metabolites found in muscle were estradiol-17α and estrone. The pattern of metabolites occurring in fat was similar to that in muscle. Highest residue concentrations were found in kidney and liver, the major metabolites being identified in kidney including estradiol-17α, estradiol-17α-glucuronide, estradiol-17β, and estrone. In liver, major metabolites could not be identified but estradiol-17β, estrone, estriol, and glucuronides accounted for the remaining radioactivity (2).

Unlike in calves, the nature of the major liver metabolites was identified in steers; the β-D-glucopyranoside of estradiol-17α was found to be a major metabolite, whereas the 3-β-D-glucosiduronate of estradiol-17α and other 17-glucosides of estradiol-17α and estradiol-17β were found to be minor ones (3). Residue depletion studies in steers implanted for 70–180 days with controlled-release implants containing 24 mg estradiol-17β showed that 24 h after implant removal the concentrations of residual estradiol-17β and estrone were 4.0 and 4.0 ppt in muscle, 5.0 and 4.7 ppt in liver, 7.5 and 7.1 ppt in kidney, and 7.1 and 14.3 ppt in the fat, respectively. These concentrations of residual estradiol-17β and estrone in the incurred samples were very close to those in the control tissues, which accounted for 5.8 and 4.8 ppt in muscle, 4.0 and 6.5 ppt in liver, 6.7 and 7.9 ppt in kidney, and 6.8 and 10.5 ppt in the fat, respectively.

Progesterone is used primarily as a growth promotant in cattle in combination with estradiol or its esters. Administration is carried out by subcutaneous implant in the ear, which is subsequently discarded at slaughter. When administered exogenously, progesterone enters the same metabolic pathways and is indistinguishable from the endogenously produced compound.

In the liver of treated steers and calves, the major metabolites of progesterone were identified as the 3-α-hydroxy-5β-pregnan-20-one and 5β-pregnan-3α,20β-diol. In kidney, the major metabolites were identified as the 20β-hydroxypregn-4-en-3-one, 3α-hydroxy-5α-pregnan-20-one, 3β-hydroxy-5α-pregnan-20-one, and 5α-pregnan-3β,20β-diol, whereas about 15% of the total residues was due to the unchanged progesterone. In muscle and fat, there was also evidence of hydroxylated metabolites that constituted minor fractions and possessed greatly diminished biological activity compared with the parent compound. The observed residues in these tissues were primarily composed of the parent compound and its glucuronide conjugate (4).

Similarly to other endogenous sex steroids, residue levels of progesterone in edible tissues of treated animals were very low. Residue depletion studies (5) in steers showed progesterone levels of 0.4 ppb in muscle, liver, and kidney, and 3.5 ppb in fat; these levels compare well with the normal levels amounting to approximately 0.2 ppb in muscle, liver, and kidney and about 2.5 ppb in fat from untreated animals.

Testosterone is used for growth-promoting purposes in cattle as an subcutaneous implant in the ear, in combination with estradiol or its esters. It is usually administered in the form of its acetate, propionate, or isobutyrate esters.

When administered exogenously, testosterone enters the same metabolic pathways and is indistinguishable from the endogenously produced molecule. Since testosterone is normally produced in all mammalian species, it is always present in plasma of untreated animals but in a wide range of concentrations. The testosterone levels determined in plasma of the male calf are related to its age but are higher than those in immature and mature females. Compared to bull calves, slightly higher values for testosterone were determined in male piglets. As determined in veal calves, the percentage of conjugated testosterone was found to vary in the range 20–55% (6).

In all species, metabolism of testosterone leads to its biological deactivation. In sheep and cattle, this biological deactivation leads mainly to formation of epitestosterone, whereas in nonruminants it leads to androsterone, etiocholanolone, and dehydroepiandrosterone (7–9). Residues of endogenous testosterone are usually highest in the kidneys of animals such as heifers with a low testosterone production rate, and highest in fat of animals such as bulls, with a high production rate.

Residue depletion studies (10) with nonpregnant heifers showed that at 30 days after implantation of testosterone and estradiol-17β, mean levels of testosterone in fat increased from 26 to 340 ppt, in muscle from 20 to 100 ppt, in liver from 13 to 34 ppt, and in kidney from 190 to 450 ppt. These levels were progressively decreased to reach the concentrations expected for the endogenous hormone levels at 130 days. The maximum levels of testosterone in all tissues of treated heifers were less than the levels found, in the untreated pregnant heifers. In kidney, this difference was of the order of three-to eightfold, depending on the length of pregnancy. Similar differences were seen in kidneys of treated heifers and untreated bulls; however, the difference in the fat of treated heifers and untreated bulls was found as high as 30-fold.

7.2 STEROIDAL COMPOUNDS NOT OCCURRING NATURALLY

Synthetic steroidal compounds currently in use in many countries as officially licensed anabolic agents for food-producing animals include trenbolone acetate and melengestrol acetate (Fig. 7.2). In addition, a great variety of other synthetic steroidal compounds that may be used illegally for growth-promoting purposes are also available. Examples of such compounds that are approved only for therapy of behavior and reproductive disorders in non-food-producing animals are boldenone, chlormadinone acetate, ethylenestrol, fluoxymesterone, medroxyprogesterone acetate, megestrol acetate, methandienone, methylboldenone, methyltestosterone, drostanolone, norethandrolone, norgestomet, norgestrel, nortestosterone (nandrolone), nortestosterone decanoate, oxymetholone, and stanozolol (Fig. 7.2).

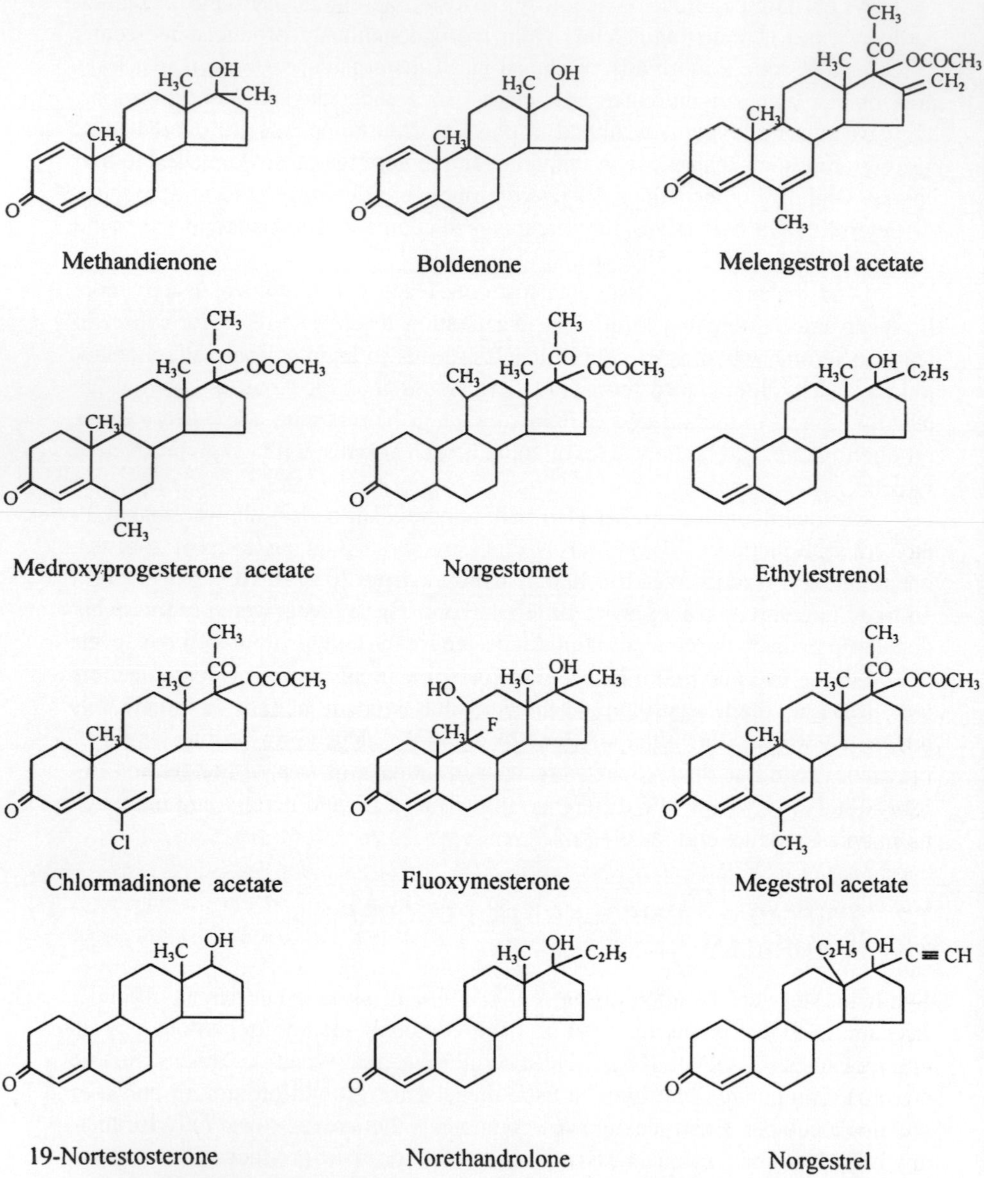

Methandienone

Boldenone

Melengestrol acetate

Medroxyprogesterone acetate

Norgestomet

Ethylestrenol

Chlormadinone acetate

Fluoxymesterone

Megestrol acetate

19-Nortestosterone

Norethandrolone

Norgestrel

FIG. 7.2 Chemical structures of commonly used steroidal compounds not occurring naturally.

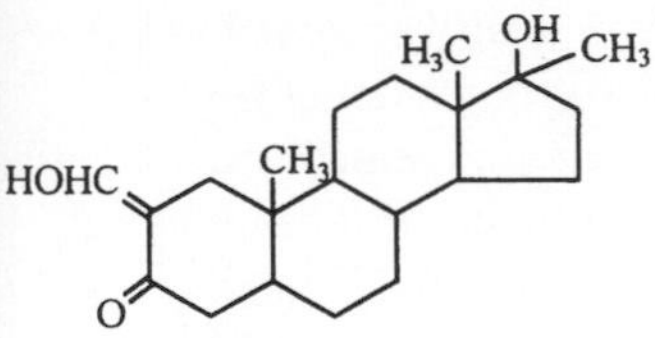

Oxymetholone 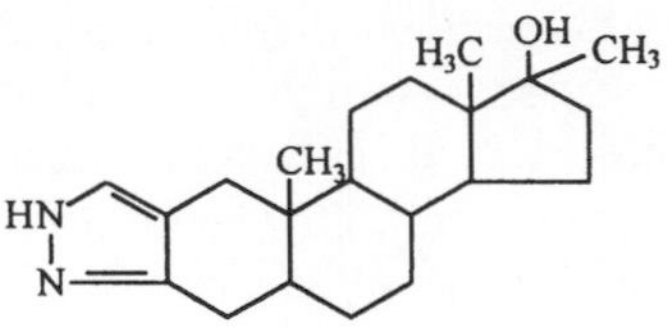   Stanozolol 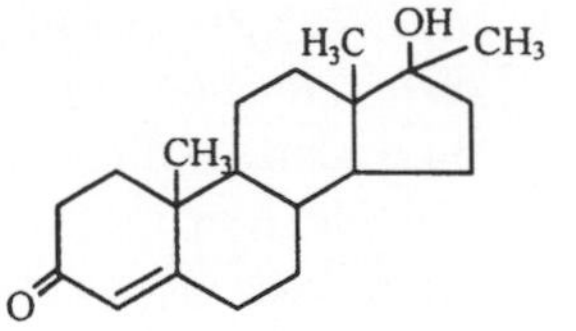   17-Methyltestosterone

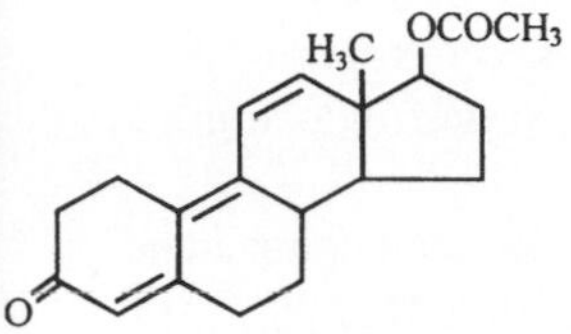

Trenbolone acetate 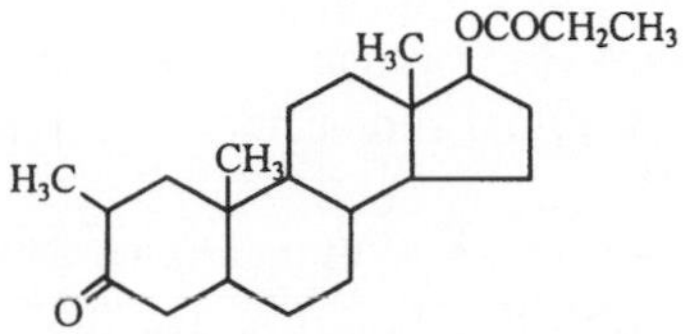   Drostanolone propionate

FIG. 7.2 Continued

Boldenone (17β-boldenone) is an androgenic steroid with known anabolic properties. As the oxidation of 17-ol to 17-one steroids is a recurring pathway both in vivo and in vitro, boldenone studies in cattle liver microsomes performed in vitro showed that the most prominent metabolite formed was androst-1,4-diene-3,17-dione (11). Not long ago, it was assumed that the presence of boldenone or its main metabolite in the urine implied illegal administration of this steroid to the animal. Evidence has been recently presented that the presence of only the boldenone metabolite in urine cannot be taken as a proof of the illegal use of this compound because boldenone is a naturally occurring steroid in urine of cattle (12). Nevertheless, the presence of 17β-boldenone in urine at levels above 1–2 μg/L seems to be clear proof of its illegal use, although clear cut-off levels have not been yet assessed.

Chlormadinone acetate is a synthetic progestagen used to prevent or suppress ovulation. Injection of chlormadinone acetate intramuscularly at a level of 200 mg in the neck of a veal calf results in relatively high residue concentrations in the urine of the treated animal (13). Levels of chlormadinone acetate residues in the urine of calves were found to range between 6 and 18 ppm.

Chlortestosterone is a steroid that is biotransformed in cattle to various metabolites. Urine analysis showed that the major metabolites were represented by the compounds 4-chlorandrost-4-ene-3,17-dione, 4-chlorandrost-4-ene-3α, 17β-diol, and 4-chlorandrost-4-ene-3-ol-17-one (14).

Ethylenestrol, a 17α-methylated steroid, represents a further step from testosterone towards an estrogen, given the removal of an oxygen atom at the C-3 position. In disagreement with the commonly occurring oxidative pathway of steroids from 17-ol to 17-one forms, ethylenestrol cannot produce a dione analogue, both in vivo and in vitro, possibly due to shielding of the 17-OH function by an alkyl group. However, norethandrolone has been clearly identified as a major metabolic product of ethylenestrol.

Medroxyprogesterone acetate is a synthetic long-acting progestagen closely related to progesterone, although it is 20–30 times more potent in suppressing ovulation in animals. In veterinary medicine, medroxyprogesterone acetate is used at a dosage of 60 mg/animal for synchronization and induction of estrus in sheep.

In sheep treated intravaginally with medroxyprogesterone acetate, residues were highest and more persistent in fat; lower residue levels were found in liver and muscle. Mean residue concentrations in fat were higher than 20 ppb at 2 h posttreatment, declining to 14 ppb at 2 days and to approximately 7.5 ppb at 5 days posttreatment. Residues in liver and muscle were 2 ppb at 2 h and 1 ppb at 2 days posttreatment, respectively, declining to less than 1 ppb at 5 days posttreatment. In kidney, residue levels were less than 1 ppb at all time points.

Studies on the excretion of medroxyprogesterone acetate in veal calves following intramuscular injection of a "hormone cocktail" containing 24 mg medroxyprogesterone acetate, 100 mg estradiol-17β benzoate, and 200 mg nortestosterone decanoate, showed that residue levels in plasma were about 1 ppb at 2 day postdosing, declining rapidly thereafter to reach 30 ppt at 14 days postdosing (15). Urinary medroxyprogesterone acetate could be detected for only a few days after injection, reaching 37 ppt at 14 days postdosing; residue levels in kidney fat were much higher and, thus, this tissue was suggested to serve as target tissue.

Melengestrol acetate, a synthetic progestagen, is an effective agent in promoting growth and improving feed efficiency in feedlot heifers. The progestagenic activity of melengestrol acetate is approximately 125 times greater than that of progesterone. Since it is orally active, this steroid is usually administered as a feed supplement at a dosage of 0.25–0.5 mg/day for 140–185 days.

Pharmacokinetic data with radiolabeled melengestrol acetate showed that the parent compound and/or its metabolites are primarily eliminated with the feces (16). At 6 h postdosing, total radioactivity in heifer liver, fat, kidney, and muscle tissues was 9–15 ppb, 7–8 ppb, 1.2–1.8 ppb, and 0.5–1 ppb of melengestrol acetate equivalents, respectively. In fat, most of this radioactivity (80%) was found to be due to the parent drug, while in liver, kidney, and muscle tissues the parent drug represented about 37%, 30%, and 45% of the total residues, respectively.

Residue depletion studies (1) using melengestrol acetate as marker residue and fat as marker tissue have demonstrated that residues in fat remained well below the level of 25 ppb, even when animals were still consuming the drug. A 48-h withdrawal period has been established by the US Food and Drug Administration. Although widely used in the United States, melengestrol acetate is not approved for use in the European Union.

Norgestomet, a synthetic derivative of progesterone, has been widely used for synchronization of estrous in cattle. It is administered with an intramuscular injection in combination with a subcutaneous ear implant that contains 3 mg norgestomet and is removed after 9–10 days.

Pharmacokinetic studies in heifers showed that plasma peak levels of norgestomet were reached within 2–6 h after dosing. Plasma elimination half-lives were estimated at 4.3–9.5 days after removal of the implant. Elimination occurred mainly via feces within 18 days after treatment.

In heifers and cows, norgestomet was extensively metabolized into several polar metabolites. Besides the parent compound, three metabolites including a norgestomet metabolite with a degraded pregnane chain, a norgestomet metabolite with a hydrolyzed 17α-acetyl chain, and a norgestomet metabolite with a hydrolyzed 17α-acetyl chain reduced at the C-20 position were identified in plasma, urine, and bile of heifers. However, the greater part of the total polar metabolites, a small fraction of which corresponded to glucuronides or sulfates, could not be identified.

Immediately after removal of norgestomet implants from cows, highest mean residue levels were found in fat (0.37 ppb), followed by the injection site (0.09 ppb), kidney (0.07 ppb), and liver (0.05 ppb). Norgestomet levels in liver and fat declined rapidly to below 0.03 and 0.07 ppb, respectively, at 2 days withdrawal. Norgestomet levels in kidney declined more gradually from 0.05 ppb at 2 days to below 0.03 ppb at 5 and 8 day withdrawal. In the injection site, norgestomet levels showed no apparent decline: the levels were in the range 0.07–0.15 ppb from 2 day to 8 day withdrawal. Lactating cows similarly treated showed highest mean norgestomet concentration in milk (0.138 ppb) at 2 days postdosing, declining gradually to 0.008 ppb upon removal of the implant.

Nortestosterone and its derivatives are banned for use in livestock production within the European Union, but have been abused as growth promoters in cattle (17). Abuse can be detected by finding injection sites at slaughter and also by monitoring bile and urine for 17β-19-nortestosterone and/or its 17α-epimer, the major metabolite in cattle (18, 19). However, it is known that 17α-19-nortestosterone occurs naturally in pregnant cows (20), and 17β-19-nortestosterone is produced in boars (21) and stallions (22). To evade detection of injection sites at slaughter, some producers have used either multiple injections of small volumes at obscure sites or pour-on formulations.

The pharmacokinetics and residue excretion profiles of differing formulations/administration routes of nortestosterone esters were examined in beef heifers (23). Differences were not found in the pharmacokinetic parameters

between single and multiple treatments for either nortestosterone phenylpropionate or nortestosterone laurate. Relative bioavailability of pour-on formulations
was 8.2% and 9.8% for multiple and single nortestosterone phenylpropionate
treatments, and 31.9% and 24.6% for multiple and single nortestosterone laurate
treatments, respectively, whereas 17α-19-nortestosterone was the only biliary
metabolite detected in animals receiving injections. Both 17α- and 17β-19-nortes-
tosterone were detected in animals given pour-on formulations, but 17α-19-nort-
estosterone was the only one found for a short period following withdrawal.
Apart from these major metabolites, several other minor metabolites that were
hydroxylated degradation products of nortestosterone could be detected (18).

Following injection of nortestosterone esters in veal calves, residues were
detectable, even after a long waiting period of 73 days, in fat, whereas in urine
residues were below 1 ppb (24). Elevated dosages and shorter waiting periods
resulted in an almost proportional increase in the residue levels in both fat and
urine. In contrast, nortestosterone given orally did not cause residue formation
in the fat but nortestosterone was present in urine.

These residue patterns may be explained on the basis of the different metabolic routes by which nortestosterone reaches blood circulation. Nortestosterone
esters that come from the injection site are hydrolyzed and partly oxidized within
the blood, and then 17β-19-nortestosterone and norandrostendione migrate into
fat and muscle. After epimerization and conjugation to 17α-19-nortestosterone
glucuronide, this metabolite also enters the circulation and is excreted via bile
and urine. Following oral uptake, nortestosterone is transported to the liver by
the portal vein, and is almost completely metabolized to 17α-19-nortestosterone
glucuronide during the first passage of the liver. Predominantly this metabolite
enters the circulation prior to excretion; hence residues of 17β-19-nortestosterone
or norandrostendione remain below the detection limit

Stanozolol is an androgenic anabolic steroid used in cases of deficiency in
protein synthesis and osteoporosis. In spite of its prohibition by the International
Olympic Committee since 1974, this compound has been often abused by athletes
and in horse-races to enhance performance (25). In recent times, the discovery
of stanozolol at injection sites revealed its illegal use as a growth promoter in
breeding, despite the ban in the European Union in effect since 1988 (26).

Metabolism studies of stanozolol in cattle showed the presence in urine of
treated animals of the parent stanozolol and its 16-hydroxystanozolol metabolite
in case of oral administration, or the presence of the two hydroxylated metabolites,
16-hydroxystanozolol and 4,16-dihydroxystanozolol, in case of subcutaneous administration (27).

Trenbolone acetate is a synthetic steroid with hormonal activity similar
to testosterone but with greater anabolic activity. After administration to cattle,
trenbolone acetate is rapidly hydrolyzed to its free hydroxylated form (28). The
17β-OH epimer is the major metabolite occurring in the excreta, bile, and liver,

while the 17α-OH epimer that has one-tenth of the hormonal activity of the 17β-OH epimer, is the major metabolite occurring in muscle (29). A number of other metabolites have been also identified in the bile, but only trendione seems to occur in some quantitative amounts. The major route of elimination is via the bile and feces, whereas elimination with the bile and urine occurs following conjugation, predominantly to glucuronic acid (30).

Following implantation of 200 mg of radiolabeled trenbolone acetate in calves and heifers, maximum levels of residues in tissues occurred at about 30 days postimplantation (31). The highest total drug-related residues expressed as trenbolone equivalents were approximately 50 and 3 ppb in liver and muscle, respectively. Only 25% and 10% of those residues could be extracted by ether or ethyl acetate from glucuronidase-treated liver and muscle samples, respectively. The majority of trenbolone residues were not extractable by organic solvents, a finding suggesting that they were covalently bound to tissues (32).

Additional studies demonstrated that the ratio of 17β- to 17α-OH epimers in liver and kidney was about 1:5 and 1:2.5, respectively, while it was the reverse in muscle and fat (33). The levels of the conjugated 17β- and 17α-OH epimers in liver were two- to fourfold than those in free form, while there were about equal or double amounts of conjugated trenbolone residues in kidney. Levels of conjugated trenbolone were found to be very close to the detection limits in muscle and fat (34).

7.3 NONSTEROIDAL COMPOUNDS NOT OCCURRING NATURALLY

Zeranol and stilbene estrogens are the two major types of compounds included in this class of anabolics (Fig. 7.3). Major members of group of stilbene estrogens are diethylstilbestrol, hexestrol, and dienestrol.

Zeranol (α-zearalanol) is a semisynthetic estrogen prepared industrially by reduction of zearalenone, which is one of three closely related toxins produced by *Fusarium* spp. fungi. The isomeric β-zearalanol is called taleranol. Only zeranol from these resorcyclic acid lactones is used as a growth promoter. Administration is performed by a subcutaneous ear implant at a dose of 36 mg for suckling, weaned, growing, and finishing cattle, and at 12 mg for sheep, with a duration of activity of 90–120 days. The implant is used alone or with another hormonally active ingredient to increase weight gain and improve feed efficiency. Unlike in the United States, the administration of zeranol to fatten animals is prohibited in the European Union.

The metabolism of zeranol has been studied in many species, including cattle, sheep, and rabbits. In all mammals, zeranol was metabolized in liver mainly to zearalanone and taleranol (35). The ratios of zeranol to zearalanone to taleranol in tissues and excreta varied with the animal species. In cattle, taleranol has been

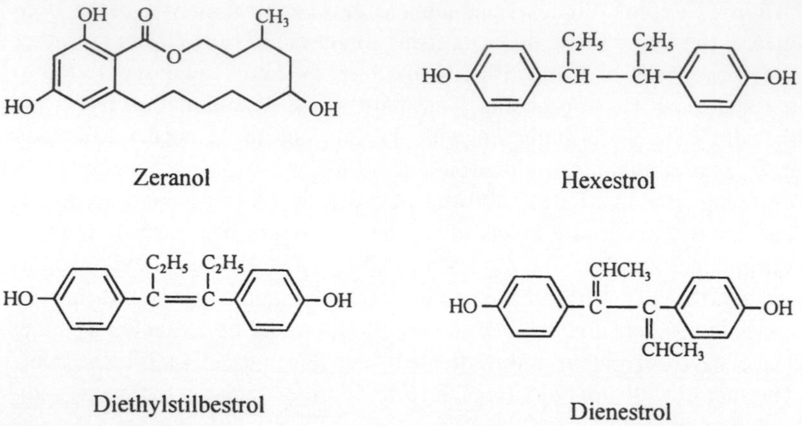

Fig. 7.3 Chemical structures of commonly used nonsteroidal compounds not occurring naturally.

identified as a major metabolite (36). Additional minor metabolites of unidentified structure that demonstrated polar characteristics were observed in urine, liver, and feces from cattle treated with radiolabeled zeranol (37). Since the concentrations of these metabolites were reduced but not eliminated after prolonged incubation with either β-glucuronidase or sulfatase enzyme preparations, it was speculated that there might be multiple conjugates of zeranol and its metabolites.

In all animal species except rabbits, zeranol and its metabolites were excreted through the bile to feces both as free compounds and glucuronidated and/ or sulfated conjugates. Elimination with urine could also be monitored over an extended period of time following implantation at the recommended dosage (29). Concentrations in urine of sheep were generally higher than in cattle, due presumably to the lower dose per unit of body weight in cattle than in sheep. In rabbits, zeranol and its metabolites were excreted primarily through urine.

Total tissue residues resulting from ear implantation of radiolabeled zeranol to cattle at the recommended dosage peaked from 5 days to 15 days, decreasing slowly thereafter as the implantation time increased (38). At 65 days, approximately 60% of the initial dose remained at the implant site, 12–18% was recovered in the urine, and 21–34% in the feces. Total residue levels in edible tissues at all times postimplantation were generally very low. Highest residue concentrations occurred in liver but never exceeded the level of 10 ppb. Residue concentrations in muscle, kidney, and fat were below 0.2, 2 and 0.3 ppb, respectively, at any time postimplantation.

Following implantation of radiolabeled zeranol and trenbolone acetate to pigs, a considerable biliary excretion occurred that presumed the existence of an intense enterohepatic circulation (39). Free zeranol, zearalanone, and taleranol as well as the corresponding glucuronated and sulfated conjugates were identified in the urine, bile, and feces. Glucuronated conjugates were the major metabolites found, and zearalanone was the major aglycon (39–41). Liver was the target tissue, and most of the residual radioactivity corresponded to similar quantities of zeranol and its conjugated metabolites.

Diethylstilbestrol, hexestrol, and **dienestrol** are all stilbene estrogens currently banned worldwide for use in food-producing animals. They are genotoxic, not easily metabolized compounds, which are considered capable of irreversibly initiating the carcinogenic process even at small residue concentrations.

Diethylstilbestrol and hexestrol have been legally permitted for use as anabolics for quite some time in many countries, while the use of dienestrol, which is a metabolite of diethylstilbestrol, was restricted to illegal practice. Since all stilbene estrogens have high oral activity, both oral and parenteral formulations have been in use in cattle and, to a lesser extent, in sheep and swine.

Pharmacokinetic studies, particularly with diethylstilbestrol, showed that 70–80% of the dose administered to ruminants was eliminated through the feces, whereas less than 50% of the dose administered to pigs was excreted in urine (42, 43). At 1 day after oral administration of radiolabeled diethylstilbestrol to cattle, approximately 1% of the initial dose was found in organs and muscle tissue, the value decreasing to 0.29% and 0.01% at 2 days and 5 days postdosing, respectively. Therefore, in spite of enterohepatic circulation and binding to plasma proteins, the overall elimination of diethylstilbestrol from muscle and organs was rather rapid. At least for cattle, more than 60% of the diethylstilbestrol given was eliminated in the glucuronated form with bile and urine. Hence, in liver and kidney the concentrations of the conjugated diethylstilbestrol and dienestrol exceeded by far those occurring in the free form.

In the living organism, the conjugated diethylstilbestrol reaching the gut with the bile is hydrolyzed by intestinal enzymes and then is available for enterohepatic circulation. Metabolism of diethylstilbestrol is similar among species: a major part of the administered dose is eliminated as unchanged diethylstilbestrol, but it is different in respect to the type of the metabolites formed.

In rodents, some of the urinary metabolites were identified as dienestrol, and as hydroxy- and methoxy-derivatives of dienestrol and diethylstilbestrol. When diethylstilbestrol was given orally to ostriches, parent compound and the metabolite dienestrol could be detected in urine (44). Diethylstilbestrol was rapidly excreted, its concentration being above 2 ppb for only 4 days although it could be detected by 18 days. The concentration of dienestrol was just above 2 ppb for 1 day only and could be detected for 3 days only.

In cattle feces, 64% of the total residues was identified as diethylstilbestrol, 23% as 3-(p-hydroxyphenyl)-2-hexene-4-one, and less than 1% as 4'-hydroxypropiophenone (43). The identification of 4'-hydroxypropiophenone as a metabolite of diethylstilbestrol implies that dienestrol is formed through an epoxide-diol pathway and that these metabolites show electrophilic reactivity (45). These observations have to be seen in connection with the mutagenic and carcinogenic activity of diethylstilbestrol and possibly also the other stilbene estrogens.

7.4 POLYPEPTIDE HORMONES

The most common polypeptide compound affecting growth is a natural hormone known as somatotropin. It is a single-chain polypeptide of 191 amino acids with two intrachain disulfide bridges, its precise structure being species-specific. Thus, the specific somatotropin found in cows, also called bovine somatotropin, exhibits maximal biological activity in cattle, but it is inactive in humans or other species. Somatotropins, in general, have a short half-life of 20–30 min, they are not orally active, and are rapidly metabolized and excreted by gut, liver, and kidney. Kidney constitutes the major site of degradation and clearance of somatotropins and other polypeptide hormones such as insulin, corticotrophin, and somatomedins. Although natural somatotropins substantially improve carcass composition, production efficiency, and lactation in farm animals, their only source until recently was that extracted in small quantities from the pituitary gland of slaughtered animals. With the development, however, of genetic engineering techniques it has recently become possible to produce large quantities of some somatotropins at relatively low cost, using recombinant DNA technology (46).

Long-term administration of somatotropins to growing pigs, lambs, heifers, and steers has been shown to increase live weight gain, an increase typically associated with increased protein accumulation, decreased fat content, and improved feed conversion efficiency (47, 48). Experiments with cattle showed that live weight responses to the administration of somatotropins were generally lower than those normally observed with steroid implants. In contrast, somatotropins were potent stimulators of milk production, increasing the milk yield by 20–40% in dairy cows (49, 50). It should be emphasized that, in this case, the effect of somatotropins was to increase the efficiency of milk production, not milk yield per se, by improving feed efficiency (51).

Bovine somatotropin in the form of several recombinant DNA-derived analogues, such as sometribone, somagrebone, somidobone, and somavubone, is used to increase milk production in lactating dairy cows. There is available a great variety of commercial formulations including daily formulations as well as 7 day-, 14 day-, and 28 day-prolonged-release formulations. The daily formulations are based on homology with natural bovine somatotropin, whereas the 14 day and 28 day formulations are based on methionyl bovine somatotropin (sometribone). The recombinantly derived somatotropins differ structurally from the pituitary bovine somatotropin by about 0.5–5% in the amino acid sequence at the terminal end of the molecule.

Somatotropins, including recombinantly derived somatotropin, are degraded by enzymes of the gastrointestinal tract and are therefore inactive when administered orally. Thus, they must be injected rather than fed to animals. Treatment of lactating dairy cows with recombinantly derived somatotropin causes an increase in plasma bovine somatotropin concentrations physiologically indistinguishable from the changes induced with pituitary-derived bovine somatotropin. The major metabolite identified in the serum was the same as the bovine somatotropin fragment cleaved by thrombin, occurring between amino acid 132 and 133. The analytical methods used to determine the concentration of bovine somatotropin in plasma, milk, or tissues do not differentiate between recombinantly derived somatotropin and endogenous bovine somatotropin. Thus, when concentrations are given, they actually represent total bovine somatotropin concentrations.

Milk residue studies demonstrated that use of recombinantly derived somatotropin, even at exaggerated doses, did not lead to concentrations of bovine somatotropin in milk above those normally present in the untreated cows (0.9–1.6 ppb) (52, 53). Bovine somatotropin occurs naturally in cow milk at variable levels generally less than 2 ppb, but they may occasionally range up to 10 ppb.

There tends to be more prolonged debate however, about the effects of bovine insulin-like growth factor-I levels in milk. Insulin-like growth factor-I (IGF-I), also called somatomedin, is produced mainly in liver in response to somatotropin, and is probably involved in mediating the action of somatotropin on milk production. Relevant studies demonstrated that IGF-I concentrations in plasma and milk were slightly elevated in somatotropin-treated cows. Although IGF-I is a single-chain peptide containing 70 amino acids and is therefore digested in the gastrointestinal tract into its constituents, it might be important to establish that these elevated concentrations do not affect the human gut epithelium before digestion.

In regard to tissue residue data, recombinantly derived somatotropin treatment of cows leads, at most, to a doubling of bovine somatotropin concentrations to levels of 4.2 ppb in muscle and 25 ppb in liver. Cows treated with recombinantly derived somatotropin further show an up to doubling in IGF-I levels in muscle and liver.

Porcine somatotropin and **poultry somatotropin** are both under development for use in swine and poultry. Recombinantly produced porcine somatotropin has been found to enhance performance dramatically. Increases in protein deposition, decreases in fat deposition, and depression of voluntary feed intake after injections of recombinant porcine somatotropin have been found across breeds, nutritional levels, genders, and various management systems in different parts of the world.

REFERENCES

1. G.W. Ivie, R.J. Christopher, C.E. Munger, and C.E. Coppock, J. Anim. Sci., 62:681 (1986).
2. T.G. Dunn, C.C. Kaltenbach, D.R. Koritnik, D.L. Turner, and G.D. Niswender, J. Anim. Sci., 46:659 (1977).
3. P.N. Rao, R.H. Purdy, M.C. Williams, P.H. Moore, J.W. Goldzieher, and D.S. Layne, J. Steriod Biochem., 10:179 (1979).
4. R.H. Purdy, C.K. Durocher, P.H. Moor, and P.N. Rao, J. Steroid Biochem., 13:1307 (1980).
5. World Health Organization, in Residues of Some Veterinary Drugs in Animals and Foods, Thirty-second Meeting of the Joint FAO/WHO Expert Committee on Food Additives, Food and Agriculture Organization of the United Nations, FAO Food and Nutrition Paper, Rome, p. 18 (1987).
6. B. Hoffmann, and E. Rattenberger, J. Anim. Sci., 46:635 (1977).
7. P.R. Martin, Endocrinology, 78:907 (1966).
8. W. Velle, in Environmental Quality and Safety, Anabolic Agents in Animal Production, Suppl. Vol. V (F. Coulston, and F. Corte, Eds.), Thime, Stuttgart, p. 159 (1976).
9. A.G. Rico, V. Burgat-Sacaze, J.P. Brown, and P. Bernard, in Anabolic Agents in Beef Veal Production, Proc. EEC-Workshop, Brussels, p. 45 (1981).
10. World Health Organization, in Residues of Some Veterinary Drugs in Animals and Foods, Thirty-second Meeting of the Joint FAO/WHO Expert Committee on Food Additives, Food and Agriculture Organization of the United Nations, FAO Food and Nutrition Paper, Rome, p. 24 (1987).
11. M. van Puymbroeck, E. Royackers, R.F. Witkamp, L. Leyssens, A.S. van Miert, J. Gelan, D. Vanderzande, and J. Raus, in Residues of Veterinary Drugs in Food, Proc. Euroresidue III Conf., Veldhoven, 1996 (N. Haagsma, and A. Ruiter, Eds.), Fac. Vet. Med., Univ. Utrecht, The Netherlands, p. 808 (1996).
12. C.J.M. Arts, R. Schilt, M. Schreurs, and L.A. van Ginkel, in Residues of Veterinary Drugs in Food, Proc. Euroresidue III Conf., Veldhoven, 1996 (N. Haagsma and A. Ruiter, Eds.), Fac. Vet. Med., Univ. Utrecht, The Netherlands, p. 212 (1996).
13. H. Hooijerink, R. Schilt, E.O. van Bennekom, B. Brouwer, and P.L.M. Berende, in Residues of Veterinary Drugs in Food, Proc. Euroresidue III Conf., Veldhoven, 1996 (N. Haagsma and A. Ruiter, Eds.), Fac. Vet. Med., Univ. Utrecht, The Netherlands, p. 505 (1996).
14. L. Leyssens, E. Royackers, B. Gielen, M. Missotten, J. Schoofs, J. Czech, J.P. Noben, L. Hendriks, and J. Raus, J. Chromatogr., 654:43 (1994).
15. M. Rapp, and H.H.D. Meyer, Food Addit. Contam., 6:59 (1989).
16. A.W. Neff, in Anabolics in Animal Production, Proc. Symp. OIE, Paris, p. 457 (1983).
17. K. Vanoosthuyze, E. Daeseleire, A. Vanoverbeke, C. van Peteghem, and A. Ermens, Analyst, 119:2655 (1994).

18. E. Benoit, J.L. Guyot, D. Courtot, and P. Delatour, Annals Rech. Vet., 20:485 (1989).
19. J.D.G. McEvoy, C.E. McVeich, W.J. McCaughey, D.G. Kennedy, and B.M. McCartan, J. Vet. Pharmacol. Ther., 20:307 (1997).
20. H.H.D. Meyer, D. Falckenberg, T. Janowski, M. Rapp, E.F. Rosel, L. van Look, and H. Karg, Acta Endocrinol. 126:369 (1992).
21. G. Mafhuin-Rogister, A. Bosseloire, P. Gaspar, C. Dasnois, and G. Pelzer, Ann. Med. Vet., 132:437 (1988).
22. E. Benoit, F. Garnier, D. Courtot, and P. Delatour, Ann. Rech. Vet., 16:379 (1985).
23. J.D.G. McEvoy, C. McVeigh, D.G. Kennedy, and W.J. McCaughey, in Residues of Veterinary Drugs in Food, Proc. Euroresidue III Conf., Veldhoven, 1996 (N. Haagsma, and A. Ruiter, Eds.), Fac. Vet. Med., Univ. Utrecht, The Netherlands, p. 690 (1996).
24. M. Rapp, and H.H.D. Meyer, J. Chromatogr., 489:181 (1989).
25. W.M. Muck, and J.D. Xenion, Biomed. Environ. Mass Spectrom., 19:37 (1990).
26. Official Journal of the European Communities, No. L222, Brussels, p. 32 (1981).
27. V. Ferchaud, B. Lebizec, M.P. Montrade, D. Maume, F. Monteau, and F. Andre, J. Chromatogr., 695:269 (1997).
28. J. Pottier, C. Cousty, R.J. Heitzman, and A. Reynolds, Xenobiotica, 11:489 (1981).
29. S.N. Dixon, and R.J. Heitzman, in Anabolics in Animal Production, Proc. Symp. OIE, Paris, p. 381 (1983).
30. J. Pottier, M. Busigny, and J.A. Grandadam, J. Anim. Sci., 41:962 (1975).
31. World Health Organization, in Residues of Some Veterinary Drugs in Animals and Foods, Thirty-second Meeting of the Joint FAO/WHO Expert Committee on Food Additives, Food and Agriculture Organization of the United Nations, FAO Food and Nutrition Paper, Rome, p. 29 (1987).
32. B. Hoffmann, D. Schopper, and H. Karg, Food Addit. Contam., 1:253 (1984).
33. R.J. Heitzman, A. Carter, S.N. Dixon, D.J. Harwood, and M. Plillips, in Manipulation of Growth in Farm Animals, Proc. SEC-Semin., Brussels, p. 1 (1984).
34. B. Hoffmann, and G. Oettel, Steroids, 27:509 (1976).
35. C.K. Parekh, M.K. Terry, and R.D. Williams, in Anabolics in Animal Production, Proc. Symp. OIE Paris, p. 307 (1983).
36. D.G. Lindsay, Food Chem. Toxicol., 23:767 (1985).
37. B.H. Migdalof, H.A. Dugger, J.G. Heider, R.A. Coonbs, and M.K. Terry, Xenobiotica, 13:209 (1983).
38. World Health Organization, in Residues of Some Veterinary Drugs in Animals and Foods, Thirty-second Meeting of the Joint FAO/WHO Expert Committee on Food Additives, Food and Agriculture Organization of the United Nations, FAO Food and Nutrition Paper, Rome, p. 38 (1987).
39. G.F. Bories, J.-F.P. Sutra, and J.E. Tulliez, J. Agric. Food Chem., 40:284 (1992).
40. G.F. Bories, and A. Fernandez-Suarez, J. Chromatogr., 489:191 (1989).
41. G.F. Bories, E. Perdu, J.-F. Sutra, and J.E. Tulliez, Drug Metab. Dispos., 19:140 (1991).
42. P.W. Aschbacher, and E.J. Thacker, J. Anim. Sci., 39:1185 (1974).
43. P.W. Aschbacher, J. Toxicol. Environ. Health, Suppl. 1:45 (1976).
44. P.J. van Der Merwe, A. Pretorius, and W. Burger, in Residues of Veterinary Drugs in Food, Proc. Euroresidue III Conf., Veldhoven, 1996 (N. Haagsma, and A. Ruiter, Eds.), Fac. Vet. Med., Univ. Utrecht, The Netherlands, p. 695 (1996).

45. M. Metzler, J. Toxicol. Environ. Health, Suppl. 1:21 (1976).
46. G.S.G. Spencer, Reprod. Nutr. Dev., 27:581 (1987).
47. T.D. Etherton, J.P. Wiggins, C.M. Evock, C.S. Chung, J.F. Rebhun, P.E. Walton, and N.C. Steele, J. Anim. Sci., 64:433 (1987).
48. L.D. Sandles, and C.J. Peel, Anim. Prod. 44:21 (1987).
49. P.J. Eppard, D.E. Bauman, C.R. Curtis, H.N. Erb, G.M. Lanza, and M.J. de Geeter, J. Dairy Sci., 70:582 (1987).
50. D.E. Bauman, P.J. Eppard, M.J. de Geeter, and G.M. Lanza, J. Dairy Sci., 68:1352 (1985).
51. W. Chalupa, B. Veechiarelli, P.L. Schneider, and R.G. Eggert, in Residues of Veterinary Drugs in Food, Proc. Euroresidue Conf., Noordwijkerhout, May 21–23, 1990 (N. Haagsma, A. Ruiter, and P.B. Czedik-Eysenberg, Eds.), Fac. Vet. Med., Univ. Utrecht, The Netherlands, p. 134 (1990).
52. World Health Organization, in Evaluation of Certain Veterinary Drug Residues in Food, Fortieth Meeting of the Joint FAO/WHO Expert Committee on Food Additives, Food and Agriculture Organization of the United Nations, Geneva, p. 62 (1992).
53. M.R. Coleman, H.W. Smith, C.M. Zwickl, C.H. Marsden, P.H. Bick, M.L. Heiman, F.C. Tinsley, J. Saunders, and J. Wilkinson, in Residues of Veterinary Drugs in Food, Proc. Euroresidue Conf., Noordwijkerhout, May 21–23, 1990 (N. Haagsma, A. Ruiter, and P.B. Czedik-Eysenberg, Eds.), Fac. Vet. Med., Univ. Utrecht, The Netherlands, p. 134 (1990).

8

Other Drug Classes

8.1 ANTIFUNGAL DRUGS

Drugs grouped as antifungals either destroy parasitic fungi, in which case they are called fungicides, or prevent growth and multiplication of fungi and are called fungistatics. Antifungal drugs may also be grouped according to their intended application as local or systemic.

Antifungals applied topically are used to treat dermatophytic infections caused by *Trichophyton* and *Microsporum* species. Ringworm is the most common and widely known of such fungal skin diseases of animals and birds. In recent years, a number of reports have appeared drawing attention to the high incidence of human ringworm caused by fungi from animals. The public health aspects of the disease is of considerable importance, whereas the economic impact to the farmer is yet not clearly defined.

On the other hand, systemic administration of antifungal drugs offers opportunities for treating not only systemic mycoses such as histoplasmosis and aspergillosis but also dermatophytic mycoses. Amphotericin B, natamycin, nystatin, and griseofulvin are all widely used drugs for the management of antifungal infections in animals (Fig. 8.1).

Amphotericin B, a polyene antibiotic, is the most suitable remedy, despite the nephrotoxicity that may occur, for treating systemic mycoses such as coccidiomycoses, histoplasmosis, and blastomycosis in animals. It is not effective against dermatophytes and has no activity against bacteria. It is only available in form of a colloidal dispersion for intravenous injection since its poor absorption from the gastrointestinal tract obviates oral administration.

Data on tissue distribution and possible pathways of drug metabolism are very limited. It is probable that most of the antibiotic is bound to sterol-containing

211

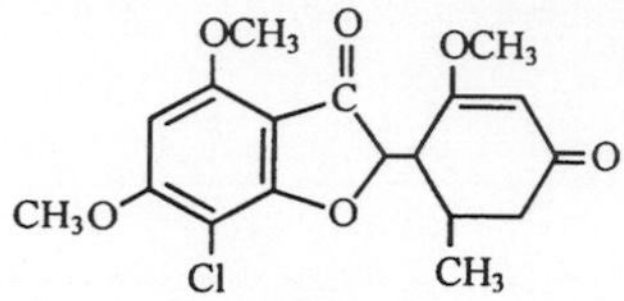

Griseofulvin

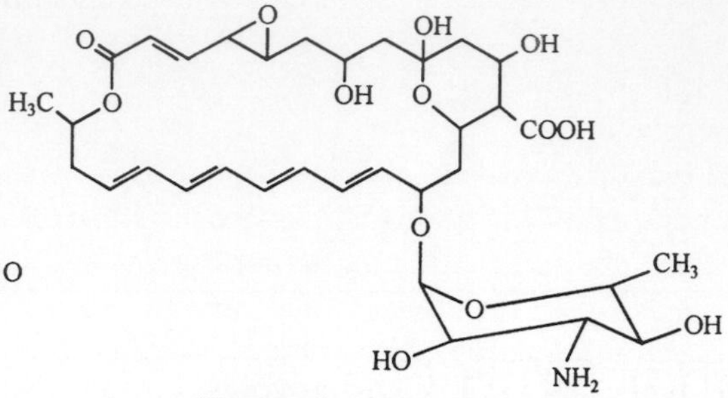

Natamycin

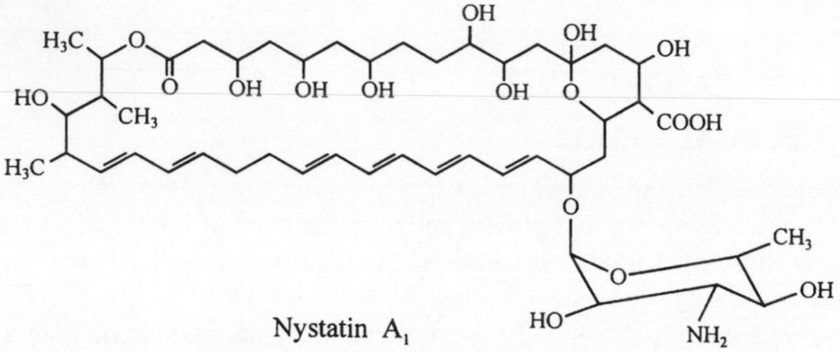

Nystatin A_1

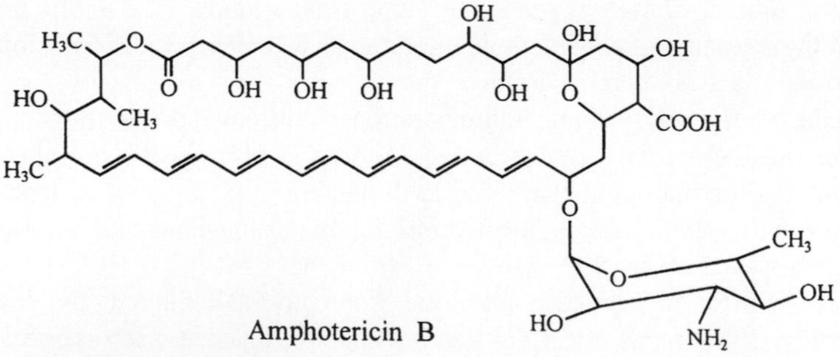

Amphotericin B

FIG. 8.1 Chemical structures of commonly used antifungal drugs.

membranes in many different tissues. Amphotericin B is excreted very slowly in urine, whereas only a small fraction of a given dose is excreted in active form. The parent drug can be detected in the urine for at least 7–8 weeks after a treatment (1).

Natamycin is another polyene antibiotic effective against dermatophytes. The name originally proposed for the compound was pimaricin, which has been used in some of the earlier literature studies and reports. It has been used as topical therapeutic in animals and humans for over 30 years, and it is also used as an antifungal agent in food processing.

It is administered topically to skin or mucous membranes for treatment of ringworm in cattle and horses. It is usually applied in form of a suspension that contains 0.1 mg natamycin/ml. Natamycin is not toxic.

Studies on the absorption of natamycin through the skin and the gastrointestinal tract of rats and cows suggested that if percutaneous or gastrointestinal absorption occurs at all, it does so at a very low level (2). Treated cattle absorb negligible amounts of natamycin through the skin, whereas they absorb less than 2 mg natamycin via the gastrointestinal tract. A maximum theoretical level of 0.1 ppm for milk contamination would occur if all of the absorbed natamycin were to be excreted into the milk over a short period of time; this would only occur if all of the absorbed natamycin from a single treatment could be excreted into the milk collected at a single milking.

Nystatin, a polyene antibiotic with fungicidal and fungistatic action against yeast and yeastlike fungi, is mainly used to treat candidiasis. It is not effective against dermatophytes and is inactive against bacteria. It is an heterogenous complex of polyene compounds consisting mainly of three biologically active components designated nystatin A_1, A_2, and A_3.

Nystatin is available as an ointment for topical applications and as a suspension or tablet for oral administration. It is approved for oral administration at 100,000 IU/day for 7 days in chickens and turkeys by the Food and Drug Administration (FDA), but it is also used in cattle for treatment of genital mycoses. Nystatin is remarkably low in toxicity when given orally, but it is much more toxic after parenteral administration.

Absorption of nystatin from the gastrointestinal tract is negligible, and the drug appears in feces. In turkeys and chickens, dietary dosing with nystatin resulted in residue concentrations below 2,500 ppb in muscle, liver, kidney, fat, and skin, and below 500 ppb in blood. In laying hens, dietary dosing with nystatin resulted in residue concentrations in eggs below 500 ppb of the parent compound.

Griseofulvin is a fungistatic antibiotic with no antibacterial activity. It is highly effective against dermatophytes and has therefore been used orally for treatment of ringworm in a variety of animals. For calves and horses, it is mainly used as a feed additive at dosages of 10–30 mg/kg bw/day for 7–35 days.

After oral administration, griseofulvin is absorbed from the gastrointestinal tract and deposited in new epithelial cells that make up skin, hair, claws, and nails. The drug has a greater affinity for diseased skin than for normal skin. Increasing the surface area of the griseofulvin particles and the dietary fat intake also increases drug absorption.

Most of orally ingested griseofulvin is eliminated in unchanged form in feces. Less than 1% of an oral dose is excreted in urine. Griseofulvin is mainly metabolized to 6-dimethylgriseofulvin and its glucuronated conjugate (1).

8.2 β-ADRENERGIC AGONISTS

Following the ban of stilbene and other hormonal-type growth promoters, interest has focused on alternative compounds for promoting live weight gain in food-producing animals. The β-adrenergic agonists constitute such group of compounds. Including in this group are certain synthetically produced phenethanolamines such as bambuterol, bromobuterol, carbuterol, cimaterol, clenbuterol, dobutamine, fenoterol, isoproterenol, mabuterol, mapenterol, metaproterenol, pirbuterol, ractopamine, reproterol, rimiterol, ritodrine, salbutamol, salmeterol, terbutaline, and tulobuterol (Fig. 8.2).

β-Agonists, in addition to their therapeutic role in veterinary medicine as bronchodilatory and tocolytic agents, are able to enhance growth rate and improve feed efficiency and lean-meat content of beef cattle, sheep, pigs, and poultry. These compounds, are also referred to as repartitioning agents, because their effect on carcass composition is to increase the deposition of protein while reducing fat accretion, but the organoleptic quality of meat may be adversely affected.

The dose level of β-agonists affects the response obtained, the optimum dose often varies for the different production parameters measured. The mode of action of β-agonists is poorly understood, but their interaction with membrane-bound receptors increases lipolysis in adipose cells and stimulates hypertrophy in muscle fibers. Although β-agonists are known to stimulate the secretion of growth hormone and insulin, there is no direct evidence that these hormones mediate the tissue responses to the drug.

Although most β-agonists are well absorbed, they are not equally available to target tissues after absorption (3). Following oral administration of radiolabeled β-agonists, the quantity of the parent compounds, in general, in plasma or urine is less than 50% of the total radioactivity measured. For phenethanolamine β-agonists of the catechol-type such as isoproterenol and dobutamine, phenol-type such as ractopamine and ritodrine, resorcinol-type such as fenoterol and terbutaline, and saligenin-type such as salbutamol and salmeterol, the level of the parent compound accounts for 25% or less of the urinary radioactivity in cattle, with the exception of salbutamol. The halogenated drugs exhibited greater percentages of unchanged drug in plasma or urine after their oral administration. However,

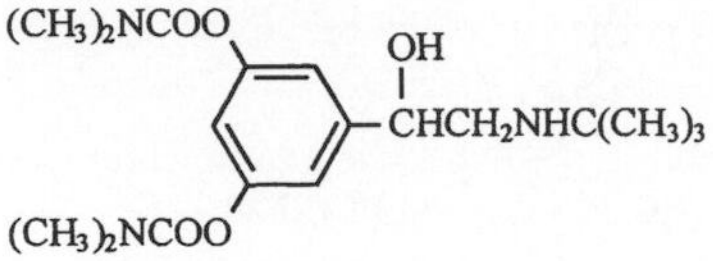

Bambuterol

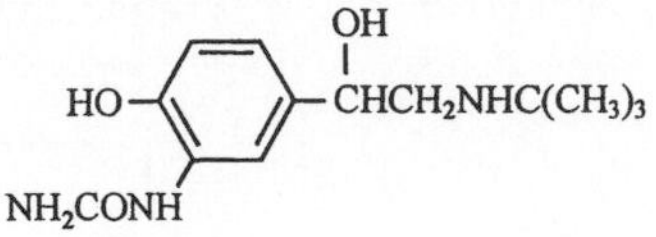

Carbuterol

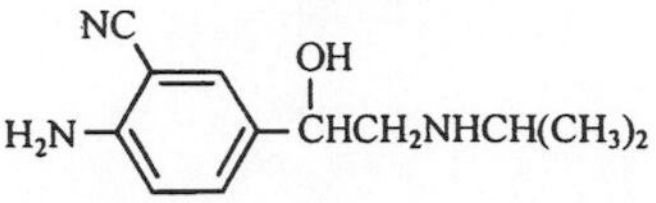

Cimaterol

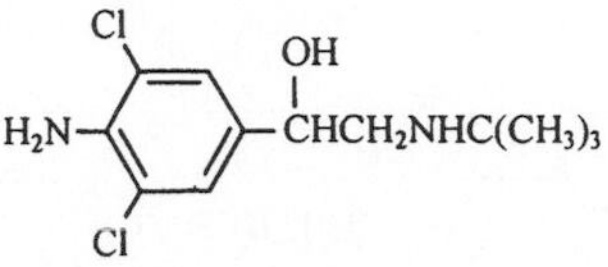

Clenbuterol

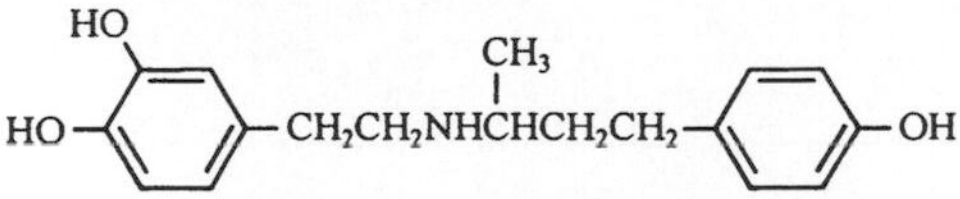

Dobutamine

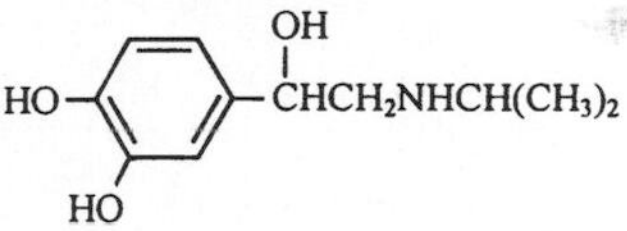

Isoprotenerol

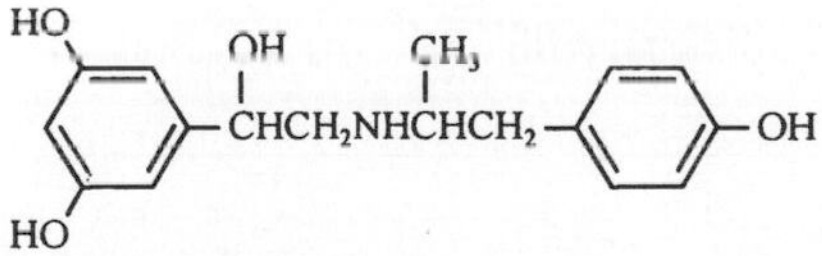

Fenoterol

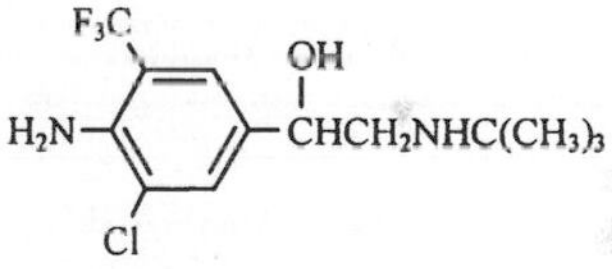

Mabuterol

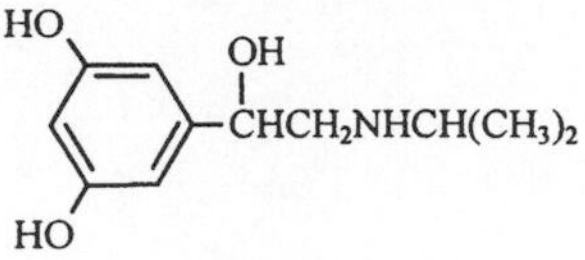

Metaproterenol

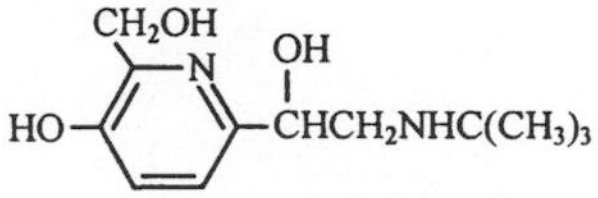

Pirbuterol

Fig. 8.2 Chemical structures of commonly used β-adrenergic agonists.

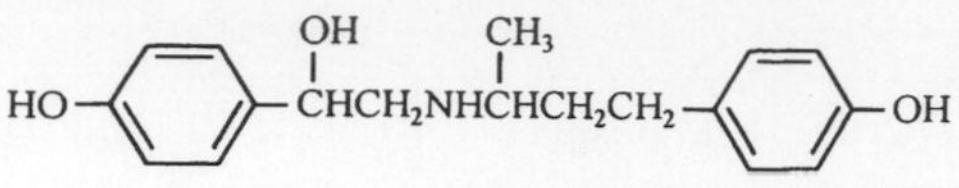

Ractopamine

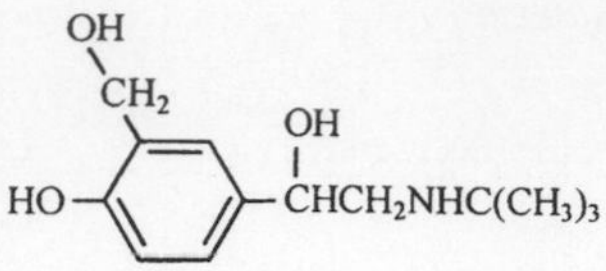

Salbutamol

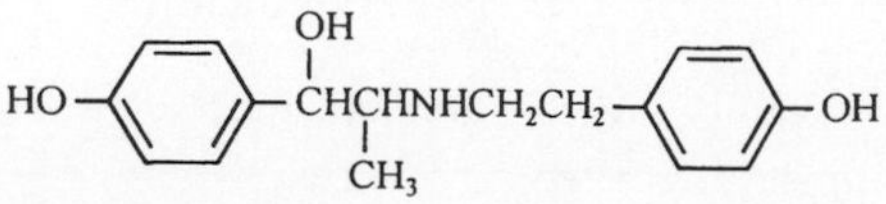

Ritodrine

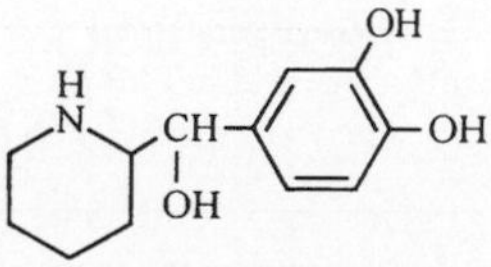

Rimiterol

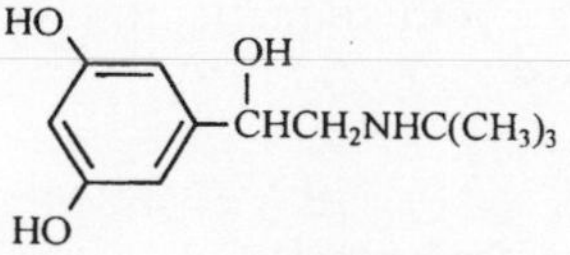

Terbutaline

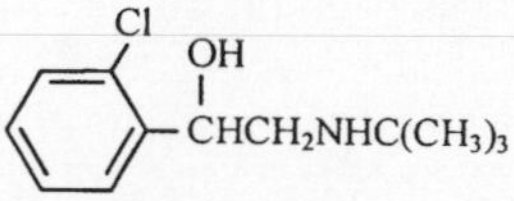

Tulobuterol

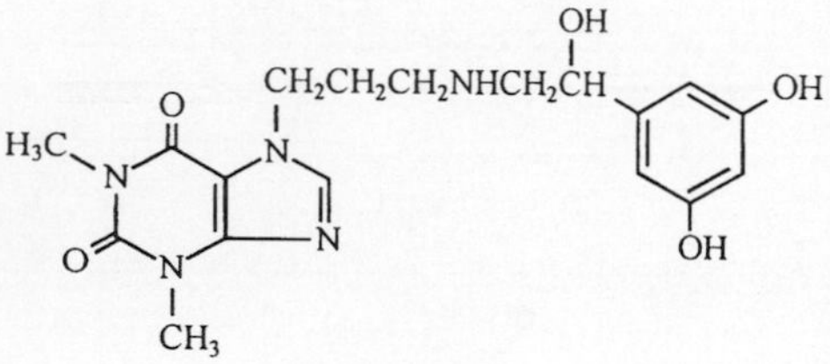

Reproterol

FIG. 8.2 Continued

regardless of the structure of the compound, intravenous administration resulted in proportion of the parent drug in urine of animals higher than after oral administration. These data indicate that intestine and liver may play an important role in the biotransformation of the β-agonists after oral administration (4).

β-Agonists are generally rapidly excreted from the animal body. Hence, when used therapeutically at the recommended low dosing and allowing the toxicologically established withdrawal period for elimination, no major risk would exist. For use in lean meat production, however, dosages of 5–15 times greater than the therapeutic dosage would be required, together with a more prolonged period of infeed administration, which is often quite near to slaughter, to obviate the elimination problem. Such a use would result in significant residue levels of these compounds in edible tissues of treated animals, which might, in turn, exert adverse effects on the cardiovascular and central nervous system of consumers (5).

Pharmacokinetic studies have shown that β-agonists with halogenated aromatic ring systems are metabolized by oxidative and conjugative pathways and have longer plasma half-lives than the compounds with hydroxyl groups on their aromatic rings and that are metabolized solely by conjugation (4). β-Agonists having high oral bioavailabilities, long plasma half-lives, and relatively slow rates of elimination have high oral potencies in humans. Residues of such illegally used compounds in edible tissues of livestock may represent a genuine risk to consumers.

Despite the proven beneficial effects on animal performance that β-agonists have achieved, there are a number of well-documented cases in which the illegal use of such compounds has resulted in human food poisoning (6). Although without exception these incidents have all been caused by the toxicity of clenbuterol, the entire group of β-agonists are now treated with great suspicion by regulatory authorities and are unlikely ever to be accepted as licensed growth promoters in the European Union in the foreseeable future. To protect public health, use of all β-agonists in farm animals for growth-promoting purposes has been prohibited by regulatory agencies in Europe, Asia, and the Americas. In spite of that, veterinary use of some β-agonists such as clenbuterol, cimaterol, and ractopamine is licensed in several parts of the world for therapeutic purposes.

However, β-agonists are being used illegally in parts of Europe and United States by some livestock producers (7, 8). This use has given rise to much concern in recent years, not least because of the high pharmacological potency of such drugs and reports of food poisoning associated with residues in liver (9, 10). As a result, clenbuterol has been banned by the FDA for any animal application in the United States, whereas it is highly likely to be banned even for therapeutic use in the European Union in the near future.

In the illegal practice of application of growth-promoting β-agonists in cattle raising, new analogues are regularly and continuously introduced, often with deviating structural properties but with a common pattern of biological activity (11). As a result, specific knowledge of the target residues appropriate to surveillance is very limited for many of the β-agonists that have potential black-market use. Thus, continuous improvement of detection methods is necessary to keep pace with the rapid development of these new, unknown β-agonists used for growth-promoting purposes.

Clenbuterol is known to be illegally used orally in the feed or drinking water to improve carcass characteristics and productivity in animals (12). After administration at anabolically effective levels, clenbuterol residues are present in most tissues of treated animals, particularly in liver, even after long periods of withdrawal (13). Massive human toxicity has been related to consumption of liver and meat from such illegally treated animals (5).

Clenbuterol absorption by calves is rapid. Radioactivity in the blood averaged 160 ppb clenbuterol equivalents within 1 h of an oral dose of 3 mg/kg bw. By 48 h after dosing, less than 50% of the total dose administered was excreted in urine and less than 2% in feces. Rabbits excreted in the urine within a 72 h period 92% of the radioactivity present in a 2.5 mg/kg bw oral dose of radiolabeled clenbuterol; 83% of the administered radioactivity was excreted during the first 24 h (14).

Following administration to rat, dog, rabbit, and cow, clenbuterol was rapidly eliminated, being largely excreted in urine in the form of the parent drug (15). Following a 4 day treatment of cattle at the therapeutic dosage (0.8 μg/kg bw) and a 7 day withdrawal, concentrations of clenbuterol in liver were at the level of 0.35 ppb or below, whereas concentrations in urine were approximately one-tenth of the levels in liver (16). Administration. on the other hand, of a single oral dose of radiolabeled clenbuterol to cattle showed that 40% of the urinary radioactivity was due to the parent compound. The urinary half-life of clenbuterol in cattle, estimated from the urinary excretion of the parent compound, was approximately 36 h (17).

Studies on the metabolic fate of radiolabeled clenbuterol in rats and bovine showed that several metabolites were present in urine and feces of both species (18–20). Clenbuterol arylhydroxylamine was the major metabolite found in urine, whereas clenbuterol arylsulfamate was the major one in the feces. The corresponding nitro- and hydroxylated derivatives of clenbuterol were identified in rat urine.

Residue depletion studies (21) in calves orally given a single dose of 3 mg/kg bw radiolabeled clenbuterol showed that total urinary, fecal, and carcass radioactivity averaged 41.5%, 2.4%, and 52.3% of the dose, respectively. Radioactive residues detected in carcass at 2 days postdosing averaged 0.6 ppm in blood, 1.4 ppm in heart, 8.4 ppm in lungs, 2.6 ppm in spleen, 5.0 ppm in liver, 5.9 ppm in kidney, 1.9 ppm in brain, 1.0 ppm in skeletal muscle, 12.5 ppm in bile, 0.7 ppm in white skin, and 4.0 ppm in black skin. Ocular residues were 13.5 ppm in cornea, 255.8 ppm in iris, and 84.5 ppm in retina/choroid. Mean concentrations of parent clenbuterol were 6.8 ppm in lungs, 3.7 ppm in kidney, and 0.9 ppm in heart. Parent clenbuterol corresponded to about 43.9% of the total residues in liver and 81.2% in lungs.

Other pertinent studies also indicated that melanin-containing tissues, such as retina and hair, could accumulate clenbuterol (22, 23). In cattle orally treated with clenbuterol at a therapeutic dosage, the only tissue containing detectable residues beyond 14 days of drug withdrawal was the eye, with a mean level of 6.3 ppb at 42 days after treatment (24).

In black hair of male veal calves orally treated with clenbuterol at 0.8 mg/ kg bw twice daily for 10 days, residues could be detected at 60 days after treatment. This was also the case for fair-colored hair, although at much lower levels. Once incorporated into the hair, no depletion of clenbuterol occurred, making hair a promising matrix to monitor for abuse in live animals. Such accumulation is not unusual since it occurs also for drugs such as phenothiazine (25), chloroquine (26), rifampicin (27), and epinephrine and norepinephrine (28), and has been associated with an intense affinity for melanin-containing tissues.

Clenbuterol is secreted into the milk of dairy cows. Following administration of 10 mg/kg bw, concentrations of parent clenbuterol in bovine milk were in the range of 5.5–22.5 ppb. Following treatment with 5 mg/kg bw twice daily, concentrations of parent clenbuterol in bovine milk were in the range of 3–9 ppb. The levels of the parent drug in milk can be directly related to plasma levels, but it is unknown whether metabolites of the drug are also excreted into milk.

For inspection at slaughterhouses liver has been suggested as appropriate target tissue, because residues of clenbuterol persisted longer in this tissue after repartitioning treatment of calves (29) and sheep (30). Sheep orally treated with clenbuterol displayed a tissue distribution profile similar to that observed in calves (30). The accumulation of clenbuterol in liver and kidney was dosage- and time-dependent (24, 31).

In cattle, the accumulation of clenbuterol in liver reached a maximum after 15 days of treatment (31). Parent clenbuterol depleted fairly rapidly from liver and kidney during the first 48 h after withdrawal, but depleted more slowly after the first 48 h (32). Liver residues of clenbuterol remained at the ppb range from 16 to 39 days after the termination of treatment, and at the ppt range by 56 days withdrawal (33).

In broilers, the concentrations of clenbuterol after 1 day withdrawal were 1.1, 2.7, 6.8, 22.6, and 4.6 ppb in meat, kidney, liver, cecum, and gizzard, respectively (34). Therefore, liver seems again to be the most suitable target tissue for control of clenbuterol residues in poultry.

In rainbow trout, clenbuterol residues were at levels as high as 24 ppb in liver at 30 day withdrawal (35). The relatively high dose of 5 ppm dietary clenbuterol used in this study undoubtedly contributed to these high level residues in liver. Sheep fed 3.1 ppm dietary clenbuterol for 14 days showed clenbuterol residues in liver at the mean level of 3.6 ppb following a 15 day withdrawal. Since residues in sheep liver were 35-fold lower than residues in trout liver, it was concluded that trout eliminates clenbuterol more slowly than terrestrial animal species.

Salbutamol studies in cattle showed that plasma levels of the parent drug peaked at levels similar to those of clenbuterol, even though the dosage of the administered salbutamol in these studies was several times higher than that of clenbuterol (36). Unlike with other species, salbutamol has a relatively high oral bioavailability in cattle. Peak salbutamol concentrations in cattle plasma were 4.8 and 4.0 ppb within 3–4 h after an oral dose of 78 μg/kg bw at 1 day and 10 days of dosing, respectively. In lactating dairy cows that received orally 50 μg salbutamol/kg bw twice daily, plasma salbutamol levels peaked at approximately 6 ppb, whereas there was no evidence for residue accumulation in plasma with repeated dosing.

A study employing oral administration of nonradioactive salbutamol in cattle at a dosage rate of 1 mg/kg bw showed 40–70% of the dose to be excreted into urine as parent drug (37). Oxidative biotransformation of salbutamol has been suggested in this study, but definitive evidence for this metabolic route was not presented. Salbutamol has also been shown to be glucuronidated by intestinal tissues at rates that could limit bioavailability (38). The parent salbutamol was secreted into the milk of treated dairy cows, but it is unknown whether drug-related metabolites could also excrete into milk (39). Nevertheless, the extensive biliary elimination of salbutamol in form of conjugates in laboratory animals suggests that liver should play a major role in the formation of such conjugates (9).

Melanin-binding studies have shown that the affinity of salbutamol for melanin-containing tissues should be lower than that of clenbuterol (40, 23). A residue depletion study in calves orally treated with 1 mg salbutamol/kg bw/day for 7 days showed that liver residues of salbutamol were almost 4 ppm at 0 withdrawal, falling to about 0.11 ppb after a 7 day withdrawal period (37).

In broiler chickens fed 10 ppm salbutamol for 14 consecutive days, the concentrations of terbutaline residues in the liver, kidney, and eye of the treated birds were found to be 334 ppb, 110 ppb, and 85 ppb, respectively, at 0 withdrawal, declining to less than 1 ppb in the liver and kidney and to 4 ppb in the eye 43 days after withdrawal.

Terbutaline residues can appear in blood after oral administration of the compound to dairy cattle and chickens (32). In dairy cows dosed twice daily with 50 μg terbutaline/kg bw, residue concentrations in plasma ranged from below 0.5 ppb to about 4 ppb during the course of a 6 day treatment period.

In broiler chickens fed 10 ppm terbutaline for 14 consecutive days, plasma residues at 0 withdrawal averaged 42.8 ppb. The concentrations of terbutaline residues in the liver, kidney, and eye of the treated birds were found to be 165 ppb, 55 ppb, and 22 ppb, respectively, at 0 withdrawal, declining to 7 ppb in the liver and to less than 2 ppb in the kidney and eye at 14 day withdrawal. Terbutaline has been shown to be glucuronidated by intestinal tissues at rates that could limit its bioavailability (38).

Ractopamine is another β-agonist that increases nitrogen retention and protein synthesis, enhances lipolysis, suppresses lipogenesis, and increases the rate of weight gain and feed conversion when given with feed to farm animals (41–43).

Studies with radiolabeled ractopamine in several species have indicated a rapid absorption following oral administration (44). When calves were treated orally with ractopamine at 0.1 mg/kg body mass for 17 days, high residue concentrations were found in urine throughout the medication period; residue levels could be detected in urine for several days following removal of the drug from the diet (45). Ractopamine residues could not be detected in urine at only 14 days withdrawal. Ractopamine residues were excreted mainly in form of glucuronides that could be deconjugated using *Helix pomatia* and *Escherichia coli* as sources of the enzyme β-glucuronidase.

Ractopamine is extensively and rapidly absorbed in turkeys and swine. In swine, radiolabeled ractopamine was excreted at a rate of 88% in urine and 9% in feces. The parent compound accounted for 4–16% of the total urinary radioactivity following a single oral dose of ractopamine, but this could increase to 36–85% after repeated dosing (46). In turkeys, only 8% of an oral dose of ractopamine was excreted unchanged in the urine (47). Biliary excretion was observed to be of major importance in turkeys treated with ractopamine, but it was of less importance in swine in which 88% of the oral dose was eliminated in the urine.

Residue and metabolism studies in swine fed diets containing 20 or 30 ppm of radiolabeled ractopamine for 4–10 days indicated that the elimination of ractopamine was very rapid, resulting in relatively low tissue concentrations of residues (46). Two days after diet withdrawal, total radioactive residues levels in liver and kidney were less than 90 ppb. Most of this radioactivity was found to be due to ractopamine metabolites rather than the parent compound whose concentration in both liver and kidney was less than 10 ppb. Liver, kidney, and urine were each found to contain the same three monoglucuronidated and one diglucuronidated metabolites of ractopamine. Muscle and fat did not contain any detectable residues of ractopamine.

8.3 CORTICOSTEROIDS

Evidence has been presented recently that the already large number of the illegal anabolic growth promoters has been further expanded with another group of synthetic glucocorticosteroids derived from endogenous cortisol and cortisone. Included in this group of compounds are betamethasone, dexamethasone, flumethasone, isoflupredone, methylprednisolone, prednisolone, prednisone, and triamcinolone. They are all frequently used therapeutic drugs in veterinary practice for treatment of bovine ketosis, inflammatory diseases, and induction of parturition.

Although their use in farm animals is not allowed for growth-promoting purposes, some of the glucocorticosteroids are known to be illegally used as feed additives in livestock production, often in combination with β-agonists, to improve live weight gain. Dexamethasone is frequently encountered in feeding stuffs, urine, and feces of cattle (48). Although little information is available on the dosages of the glucocorticosteroids illegally used for fattening purposes, effective concentrations in feed and premixes are estimated to be in the sub-ppm level. Residues of these compounds in edible animal products are hazardous since they may have pharmacological and toxicological effects for the consumer.

Glucocorticosteroids, in general, predominantly affect carbohydrate, fat, and protein metabolism, and exert an anti-inflammatory effect. They can also exert effects on the endocrine and hematopoietic system, growth, and wound healing. In general, glucocorticosteroids have weak mineralocorticosteroid effects influencing water and electrolyte metabolism. They act through binding to specific receptors found in most mammalian tissues.

Glucocorticosteroids are readily absorbed after oral and parenteral administration, being extensively but reversibly bound to plasma proteins, mainly to transcortin or corticosteroid-binding globulin and less to albumin. Only the unbound fraction exerts its pharmacological effects and is metabolized. The synthetic corticosteroids bind less extensively to plasma proteins than cortisol, and their metabolism is slower, resulting in longer half-lives. Corticosteroids are metabolized mainly in the liver but also in kidney and mammary glands, giving rise to inactive, water-soluble conjugates excreted in urine (75%) and feces (25%). It has long been recognized that large dosages of synthetic glucocorticosteroids reduce growth rates and lead to muscle atrophy. On the other hand, low dosages resulted in increased live weight gain and reduced feed conversion ratio and nitrogen retention; the proportions of the adipose and muscle tissues in the carcass remained unchanged, while water retention and muscle fat were increased in the longissimus dorsi (49). These are indications that combinations of corticosteroids with β-agonists might lead to enhanced growth promotion, due to effects at the receptor level (50).

The well-known effect of appetite stimulation and the generally better feeling could also be responsible for the stimulation of growth. Being a group of compounds with hormonal action, the corticosteroids exert a variety of effects on tissues in terms of endocrinology and metabolism and can therefore be regarded as growth promoters according to EU and US legislation. Comparing the status within the European Union member states, it appears that there is no uniform approach as far as the control of the anabolic use of corticosteroids is concerned. In Belgium, for example, corticosteroids cannot be used in fattening animals, whereas in The Netherlands corticosteroids are not specifically excluded. Prednisolone, as another example, is included in 11 veterinary drugs registered for use in the German market (51).

Dexamethasone (Fig. 8.3) is used for treatment of metabolic diseases in ruminants and for inflammatory diseases in a number of animal species. It is

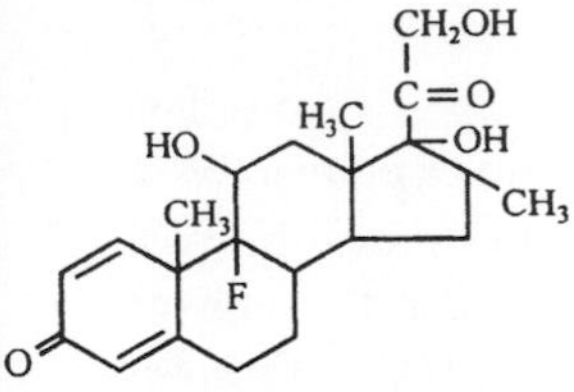

Betamethasone

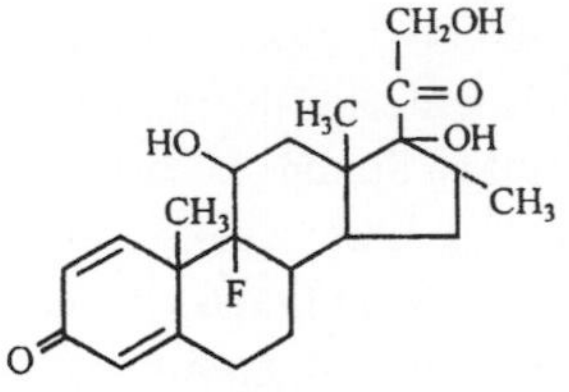

Dexamethasone

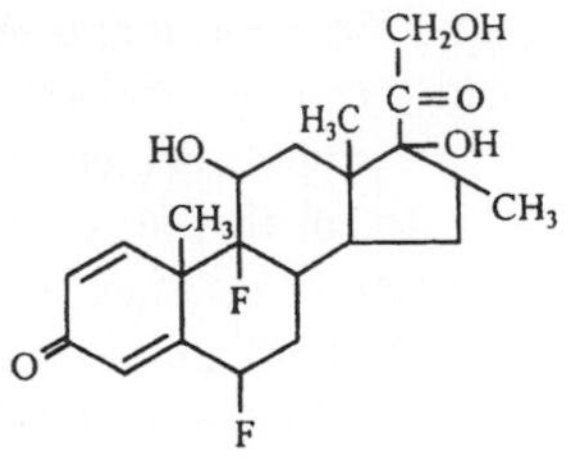

Flumethasone

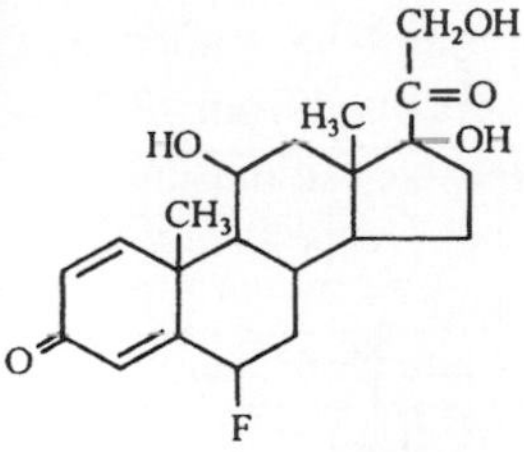

Fluprednisolone

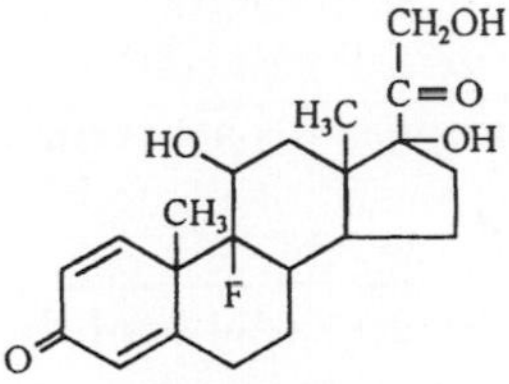

Isoflupredone

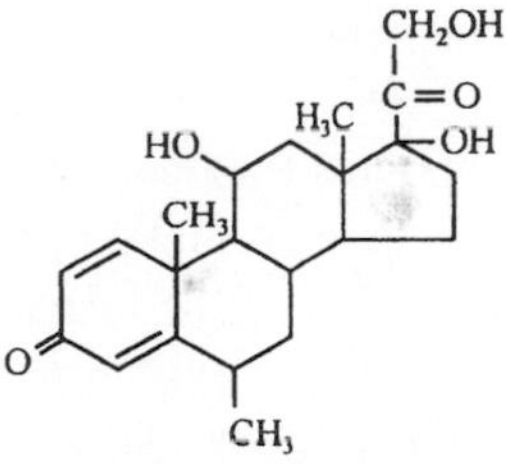

Methylprednisolone

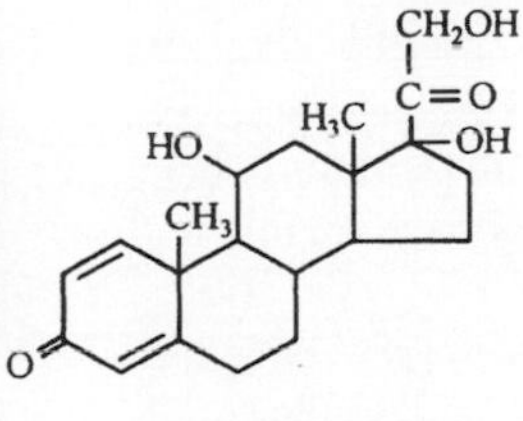

Prednisolone

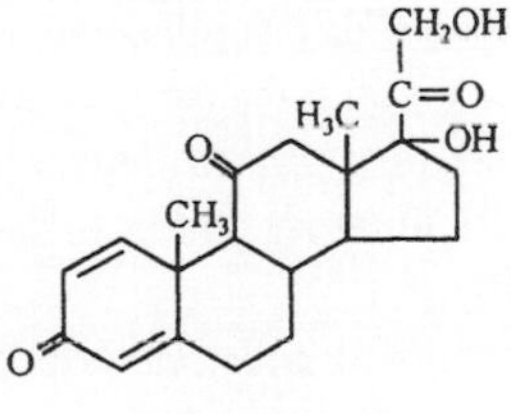

Prednisone

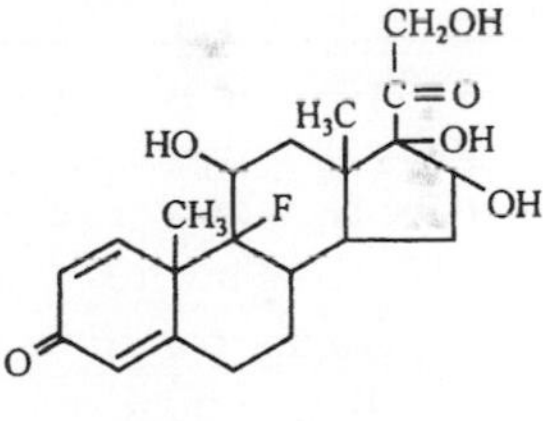

Triamcinolone

FIG. 8.3 Chemical structures of commonly used corticosteroids.

usually administered intramuscularly or intravenously at dosages equivalent to 60 μg/kg bw to cattle, pigs and horses.

Pharmacokinetic studies revealed rapid systemic absorption after intramuscular administration of dexamethasone, with peak plasma levels attained at 0.5 h and 6 h in dogs and rats, respectively. It is rapidly excreted in urine and feces. Its biotransformation profile is comparable in rats and humans and mainly involves hydroxylation to 6-hydroxy- and 2-dihydroxy-derivatives followed by conjugation. These metabolic pathways lead to rapid and extensive loss of corticosteroid activity.

Residue depletion studies indicated that different formulations led to different dexamethasone depletion rates. Studies in cattle and pigs indicated that dexamethasone residues were quickly eliminated from muscle and milk of cows. Residues did not occur in the free form in fat, whereas the depletion rate in liver was the slowest. Following intramuscular administration of 60 μg/kg bw to cows, mean dexamethasone levels in milk declined from 8.4 ppb at the first milking after treatment to below 1 ppb at the sixth milking after treatment (52).

Following dexamethasone treatment of heifers and young bulls with 60 μg/kg bw, mean dexamethasone levels in liver declined from 127 ppb at 1 day after treatment to 16 ppb at 2 days after treatment to below 2.6 ppb at 4 days after treatment. Over the same time period, mean residues in kidney declined from 78 ppb to 13 ppb and finally to less than 0.9 ppb, respectively. Residues in muscle declined from 3.3 ppb to 0.75 ppb and finally to less than 0.5 ppb, respectively. Residues at the injection site declined from 8 ppb to 3.7 ppb and finally to 2.2 ppb, respectively. However, residues could not be detected in fat. Unlike with cattle, residues could not be detected in pigs given 60 μg dexamethasone/kg bw intramuscularly.

Betamethasone has a chemical structure similar to that of dexamethasone (Fig. 8.3), except for the conformation of the 16-methyl group that projects above the plane of the steroid moiety in the betamethasone molecule forming the 16β-epimer and below the plane in the dexamethasone molecule forming the 16α-epimer. For therapeutic purposes, betamethasone is administered to cattle, sheep, goats, pigs, and turkeys intravenously or intramuscularly at a maximum dosage of 80 μg/kg bw for treating inflammatory conditions, shock, and acetonemia and for inducing parturition in cattle.

Betamethasone is well absorbed after oral administration to be extensively bound to plasma proteins in humans, dogs, cows, and rats. Its metabolism does not differ of the other corticosteroids, involving oxidation of the 11β-hydroxyl group to ketone, reduction of the ketone group at the position C-20 to give the corresponding alcohol, and hydroxylation at the C-6 position and loss of the C-17 side chain to give 17-oxosteroids.

Residue depletion studies in cattle given a single intramuscular injection of 80 μg betamethasone/kg bw showed that the concentrations of the parent drug in liver of 2 animals were 5.4 and 7.8 ppb at 2 days post dosing. Residues in liver from one of the animals slaughtered at 8 days postdosing were 10.9 ppb, whereas residues in kidney, muscle, and fat were below 2.3, 3.9, and 4.4 ppb, respectively. In similarly treated pigs, residues of the parent drug could be detected in only one muscle sample at the 3.9 ppb level and in two samples from the injection sites at the levels of 6.9 and 13.8 ppb at 4 days post dosing.

Residue depletion studies in lactating cattle given a single intramuscular injection of 1 μg betamethasone/kg bw showed that the concentrations of the parent drug in milk were in the range 3.82–38.22 nmol/L at the first milking, and lower than 1.6 ppb at the seventh milking.

Flumethasone (Fig. 8.3) is primarily indicated for treatment of inflammatory diseases, dermatosis, shock, and primary cattle ketosis. It is administered parenterally at dosages of 2.5–40 μg/kg bw.

Pharmacokinetic data after intravenous, intraruminal, or subcutaneous administration of 0.25–0.5 mg flumethasone/kg bw/day for 8 days in sheep showed that maximum plasma levels were reached within 48 h postdosing. The metabolic clearance was estimated at about one-quarter to three-quarters of that found for cortisol in sheep.

When 13.5 μg flumethasone/kg bw was injected intramuscularly in lactating dairy cows, residues in milk were below the detection limit of 0.23 ppb at 2 days after administration (52). However, urine was found to contain 5–50-fold higher concentrations than the corresponding milk samples.

8.4 DIURETIC DRUGS

Diuretics are drugs used in certain pathological conditions to eliminate somatic fluids by promoting renal excretion of water and salts (53). Chemically, they are heterogenous compounds that present different pharmacological properties and, accordingly, are classified into several different groups. The groups of loop diuretics and thiazide diuretics are the most important in veterinary practice (54). The former group includes three compounds (furosemide, ethacrynic acid, and bumetadine), but only furosemide has been approved for use in cattle (55). Included in the latter group are chlorothiazide, hydrochlorothiazide, and trichlormethiazide.

Furosemide and thiazide diuretics (Fig. 8.4) have been approved for use in dairy cattle for treatment of postparturient edema of the mammary gland and associated structures (56). Furosemide and hydrochlorothiazide are administered intramuscularly or intravenously at a dosage of 500 and 125–250 mg/animal, respectively. Chlorothiazide and trichlormethiazide are administered orally at dosage of 2000 and 200 mg/animal, respectively.

Unauthorized use of these diuretics, or the failure to follow label indications for approved use in the cattle, could lead to unacceptable residues in meat and milk destined for human consumption. While there are no official tolerances for these drugs in milk, the Food and Drug Administration (FDA) has established safe levels that range from 7 ppb for trichlormethiazide, to 10 ppb for furosemide, and 67 ppb for the other thiazides (56). Administration of diuretics is associated with potential toxic effects such as bone marrow depression, hyperbilirubinemia,

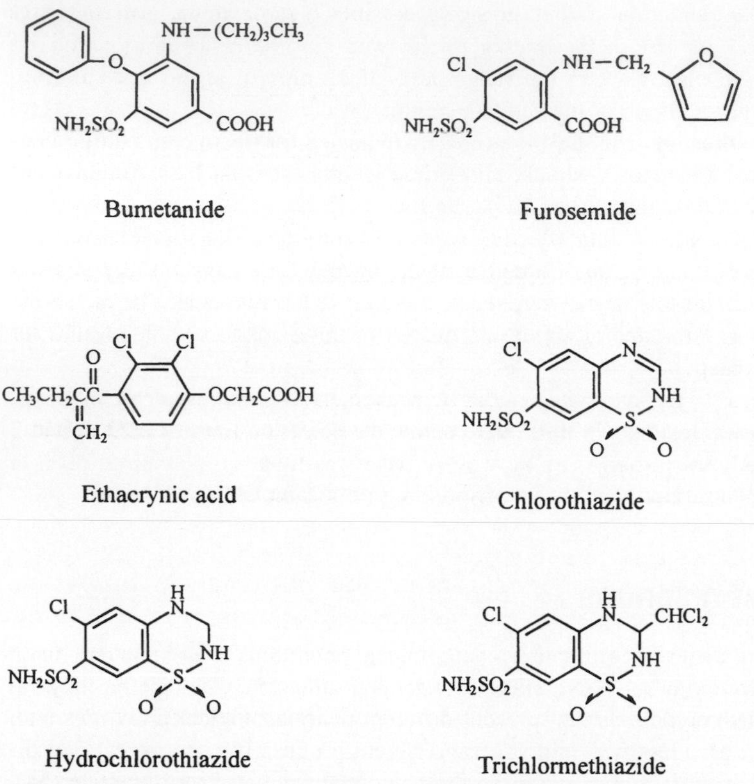

FIG. 8.4   Chemical structures of commonly used diuretic drugs.

altered carbohydrate metabolism, and elevated levels of urea, uric acid, and sugar (57).

Furosemide is a strongly acidic *o*-chlorosulfonamide compound that includes an additional carboxyl group that differentiates it from the weakly acidic thiazides.

Pharmacokinetic studies showed that 30 min after oral administration of 20 mg furosemide/kg bw in dogs, 22.73 ppb was the maximum plasma concentration attained. The oral bioavailability of the compound was estimated at approximately 77%. Furosemide is extensively bound to plasma proteins (91%). In dogs, the elimination half-life of furosemide was found to be 1.42 h after oral dosing, and 1.13 h after intravenous dosing. Excretion of furosemide was rapid and proceeded primarily through kidney, mostly in form of the parent drug.

Following oral administration of radiolabeled furosemide, excretion was reported to be almost complete within 3 days in rats (96–98%) and dogs (98–99%). Rat urine contained 40–50% of the parent drug, 30% 4-chloro-5-sulfamoyl-anthranilic acid, and four unidentified metabolites that accounted for the rest of the administered radioactivity. In contrast, urine of dog and monkey contained 85% unmetabolized furosemide, 7% 4-chloro-5-sulfamoyl-anthranilic acid, and the remainder was due to unidentified metabolites. Following intramuscular injection of 5 mg furosemide/kg bw in cattle, the half-life for plasma elimination was estimated at 4.3 h. In contrast, the half-life of furosemide in cattle was reported to be less than 1 h following intravenous administration.

Residue depletion studies in lactating cows given an intramuscular injection of 5 mg furosemide/kg bw showed that residues could be detected in milk for at least 24 h after treatment. The half-life in milk was estimated to be 3 h. When cows were administered three intramuscular injections of 1.5 mg furosemide/kg bw per day, milk contained 660 ppb at 7 h after dosing.

Trichlormethiazide is often given in combination with dexamethasone because in this way effects can be achieved with a minimum dosage of trichlormethiazide, since the two drugs are complementary in their action. Studies in humans and experimental animals have shown that trichlormethiazide presents a favorable pattern of lower potassium excretion than the other thiazides. The clinically determined saluretic potency of trichlormethiazide was estimated to be 10–20 times lower than that of hydrochlorothiazide and 100–200 times lower than that of chlorothiazide; this results in decrease in the incidence of hypokalemic manifestations.

Milk from a lactating cow treated with 200 mg trichlormethiazide and 5 mg dexamethasone for 3 days was found to contain 6 ppb trichlormethiazide residues at 8 h after the last dose, and no detectable residues at the 24 h milking (58). Hence, milk taken from dairy animals during trichlormethiazide treatment and for 72 h after the last treatment must not be used for consumption by humans (59).

8.5 DYE DRUGS

Dyes are used for numerous purposes including treatment of diseases. Dyes used as therapeutic agents can be classified in terms of their chemical structure into several groups—the triphenylmethane, phenothiazine, and acridine groups—that are all of interest to animal husbandry and aquaculture (Fig. 8.5).

The first group includes a series of dyes including gentian violet and malachite green that are active in basic medium against gram-positive bacteria. The second group includes dyes such as methylene blue and toluidine blue O that do not exhibit antibacterial activity but are useful for certain medical situations. Methylene blue is valuable as an antidote in cyanide and nitrate poisoning,

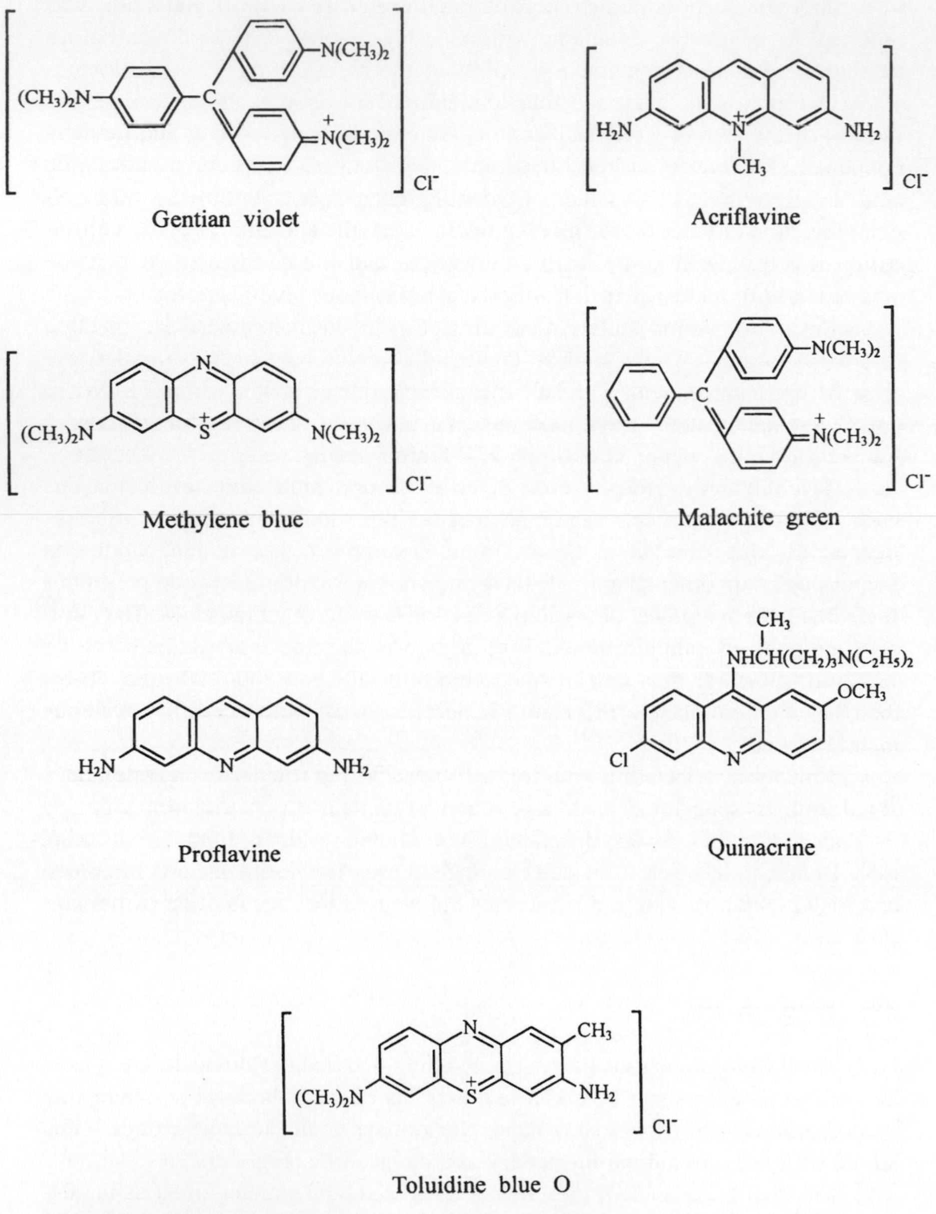

Gentian violet

Acriflavine

Methylene blue

Malachite green

Proflavine

Quinacrine

Toluidine blue O

FIG. 8.5 Chemical structures of commonly used dye drugs.

whereas toluidine blue O has been used clinically as an antiheparin agent to control idiopathic uterine bleeding. Acriflavine, proflavine, and quinacrine are major drugs within the third group that have a demonstrated utility for bactericidal action. Acriflavine has been shown to be an effective treatment for bovine mastitis and local and urinary infections. Proflavine is particularly effective against enterobacterial infections, whereas quinacrine is an effective antiprotozoal/teniacide agent (60).

Gentian violet has been utilized in the past as a feed additive for inhibiting mold and fungal growth in poultry feeds at a level of up to 8 ppm. The authorization of this dye as a feed additive was withdrawn in 1991, because evidence was presented that gentian violet had a tumorigenic effect in several organs of mice (61).

Metabolism studies in chickens showed that residues of this drug in carcass were very persistent, remaining at a level of 20.9 ppb in liver at 240 h after final administration (62). Additional residue studies in chickens demonstrated that the biotransformation of gentian violet resulted in several demethylated tabolites besides the parent drug (63, 64). Pentamethylpararosaniline, N,N,N',N'-1-tetramethylpararosaniline, N,N,N',N'-2-tetramethyl-pararosaniline, and the completely reduced form, leucogentian violet, were the metabolites that could be identified in thigh and breast muscle. Leucogentian violet was in the range of 2.1–4.6 ppb and 0.4–3.7 ppb in thigh and breast, respectively. Leucogentian violet was also the major metabolite found in fat. Liver contained an average total residue of 105 ppb composed of gentian violet and its pentamethyl and tetramethyl metabolites with mean individual values of 31.2, 34.2, and 39.6 ppb, respectively, with no leucogentian violet detected. The metabolic profile of gentian violet was not found to differ among mice, rat, hamster, guinea pig, and chickens (65).

Malachite green has been used for treatment of external fungal, protozoal, and bacterial infections in farmed fish for more than 50 years (66). It is normally administered as a flush at the 1 ppm level. Although this dye is not approved by the FDA for use in aquaculture because of its potential carcinogenic activity (67), it has a high probability of abuse due to its effectiveness for treating fungal infections in aquatic species. Unfortunately, no equally effective alternative for malachite green has been found to date.

The metabolism of malachite green has been well studied in trout and catfish (68–70). It is rapidly absorbed through the gill to be partially reduced to leucomalachite green and deposited in the fatty fish tissue. Trout excretes the parent drug relatively rapidly, but the leucomalachite green metabolite slowly. Average concentrations of malachite green and leucomalachite green in the 24 h depuration catfish tissue were 73.4 and 289 ppb, respectively. The half-life of leucomalachite green was estimated at about 40 days. It was observed that fat content influenced the excretion rate: the higher the content, the greater the deposition of leucomalachite green. This effect was found to be cumulative with repeated treatments. No evidence of systematic demethylation was observed in aquatic species.

In other studies in which channel catfish were exposed to radiolabeled malachite green, the parent compound was rapidly eliminated from plasma with extensive biotransformation to leucomalachite green (71, 72). Malachite green and leucomalachite green concentrations in plasma of fish sampled immediately after the exposure period were 2632 and 2208 ppb, respectively. At 24 h, the concentration of malachite green approached the limit of detection (10 ppb). Extensive metabolism of malachite green to leucomalachite green was also observed in the muscle tissue of catfish. At 336 h postdosing, the concentration of malachite green in muscle approached the limit of detection (5 ppb), whereas the concentration of leucomalachite green in the same tissue was approximately 50-fold higher.

Methylene blue is primarily employed for treatment of ruminant poisoning. Although not regulated for use with edible fish, methylene blue has been also shown to be effective for the control of infections by *Ichthyophthirius multifiliis*, a protozoal parasite affecting freshwater fish, at concentrations of 2 ppm in water (73). Therefore, a potential exists that this dye could become an alternative to malachite green as an antifungal and antiparasitic agent in aquaculture.

Residues of methylene blue in edible animal tissues are of public health concern because this dye and its metabolites are mutagenic (74). Metabolism studies in cattle have indicated that methylene blue can be eliminated in urine partly unchanged, partly metabolized to leucomethylene blue, or demethylated to N-methyl homologues of thionin, the completely demethylated metabolite of methylene blue, or reduced in vivo and subsequently eliminated in its leuco-form or in one or more "chromogenic" substances (75).

Although the leucometabolite of methylene blue has been repeatedly detected (75, 76), recent research (77) cannot confirm its presence in milk; various metabolites at different stages of demethylation, in addition to a methylene blue complex, are found instead. Among these metabolites, a trimethyl derivative called azure A, a dimethyl derivative called azure B, a monomethyl derivative called azure C, and completely demethylated thionin have been positively identified. Further investigation demonstrated that the methylene blue complex was a protein–thionin conjugate, whereas thionin was the residue with the longest residence time in milk (78).

Little is known about the fate of methylene blue in fish. Absorption of methylene blue appears to be low in fish. Thus, methylene blue could not be detected (<100 ppb) in muscle of eel after exposure of the fish to 3 ppm drug in water for 1–3 h (79). Analysis of catfish exposed to 5 ppm methylene blue bath treatment for 1 h showed that muscle tissue contained 10–20 ppb drug (80).

Acriflavine and proflavine have historically been used as topical antiseptics in human and veterinary medicine. In aquatic species, acriflavine has been used to treat external parasitic and fungal infections and to reduce transport mortality, particularly in tropical fish. It is also of value in monosex aquaculture since it exhibits sex-manipulating activity in fish (81).

Commercially available acriflavine is a mixture of acriflavine and proflavine, in which proflavine forms 30–35% of the total dye. For treatment of fish, commercial acriflavine is usually administered in a bath solution at various levels, depending on treatment duration (82). Acriflavine is not regulated for use in food fish aquaculture in the United States.

Following exposure of channel catfish to commercial acriflavine (10 ppm total dye in the water for 4 h), proflavine levels in muscle were consistently higher than those of acriflavine, although the concentration ratio of these dyes in the dosing solution was 1:2 (83). Immediately after dosing, acriflavine and proflavine levels in muscle were 9.8 and 14.4 ppb, respectively. Acriflavine and proflavine concentrations in muscle increased for up to 12 h after dosing, possibly due to redistribution of residues from other tissues such as skin. The skin of catfish was noticeably stained during waterborne exposure, but staining diminished during the elimination period. From 12 to 72 h after dosing, acriflavine and proflavine concentrations in muscle declined with half-lives of approximately 108 and 66 h, respectively. At 168 h, acriflavine and proflavine levels were below 5 ppb. No metabolites of acriflavine and proflavine were observed in this study.

When channel catfish were intravascularly dosed with radiolabeled acriflavine or proflavine, total residue equivalent concentrations were highest in the excretory organs and lowest in muscle, fat, and plasma (84). In proflavine-dosed fish, residues in liver and trunk kidney were composed primarily of glucuronosyl and acetyl conjugates of proflavine; residues in muscle were composed mostly of the parent drug. In acriflavine-dosed fish, the parent compound made up 90% of the to' ıl residues in all tissues examined.

8.6 NONSTEROIDAL ANTI-INFLAMMATORY DRUGS

Nonsteroidal anti-inflammatory drugs are widely used in veterinary practice and are, therefore, of growing interest to the residue control of animal-derived food. Veterinarians are seeing an increased use of anti-inflammatory agents, administered with or without antibiotics, for treatment of mastitis because of the increase in efficiency of these agents over antibiotics alone.

Little information is available regarding tissue distribution or metabolic products of nonsteroidal anti-inflammatory drugs in cattle. The early synthetic compounds were simple derivatives either of salicylic acid such as acetylsalicylic acid and methylsalicylic acid, or of pyrazolone such as metamizole, oxyphenbutazone, phenylbutazone, propylphenazone, and suxibuzone. Modern nonsteroidal anti-inflammatory drugs are derivatives either of anthranilic acid such as diclofenac, flunixin, and tolfenamic acid; or of arylpropionic acid such as ketoprofen and naproxen; and of indene such as indomethacin (Fig. 8.6).

Acetylsalicylic acid is readily absorbed from the gastrointestinal tract in dogs, cats, and swine due to its ionization suppression by the stomach acid. In the more alkaline small intestine, the large surface area for absorption makes up for the increased ionization of the drug and rapid absorption continues. In contrast, absorption is slower from the rumen in cattle.

The plasma half-life of acetylsalicylic acid varies from 0.8 h in the ruminant to 37.5 h in the cat. This is due partly to the very short elimination in cattle, which is 10 times more rapid in cattle than in most other animals. The clearance is also very high in cattle.

Metabolism of acetylsalicylic acid is similar among all animal species and involves hydrolysis in the plasma, liver, and some other organs to salicylic acid followed by formation of salicyluric acid, salicyluric glucuronide, salicyl ester glucuronide, salicyl phenol glucuronide, gentisic acid, and gentisuric acid. Orally administered methylsalicylate is nearly completely hydrolyzed to salicylate within 1 h in rats and dogs. The liver is the main site of methylsalicylate hydrolysis in rats, rabbits, and dogs.

Methylsalicylic acid, unlike acetylsalicylic acid, is nearly exclusively used as an external rubifacient drug for painful muscles or joints and distributed as ointments or liniments due to their irritating effects on the gastrointestinal mucosa. Absorption through intact skin is possible and has led to prosecution following detection in race-horse urine.

Metamizole, also known as dipyrone, is a pyrazolone derivative. Metamizole is administered by intramuscular or intravenous routes to cattle, pigs, sheep, and goats at dosages in the range 15–50 mg/kg bw as an adjunct to therapy in many inflammatory conditions of the musculoskeletal and locomotor systems.

It is rapidly and almost completely absorbed after oral administration to humans and laboratory animals. It is extensively metabolized to a variety of metabolites, none of which is significantly bound to plasma proteins. After intravenous administration to humans, unmetabolized metamizole is rapidly undetectable in plasma, the majority of the administered dose being excreted in urine. Pharmacological studies in rats showed that 4-methylaminoantipyrin, 4-aminoantipyrin, 4-formylaminoantipyrin, and 4-acetylaminoantipyrin constitute all major metabolites of metamizole.

Following administration of metamizole to pigs, cattle, and lactating cows at or above the recommended therapeutic dosages, all muscle, liver and kidney samples contained residues of the 4-methylaminoantipyrin metabolite well below the detection limit of 100 ppb at all time points.

Suxibuzone, another pyrazolone derivative, is intended for the treatment of inflammatory conditions of the musculoskeletal and locomotor systems in

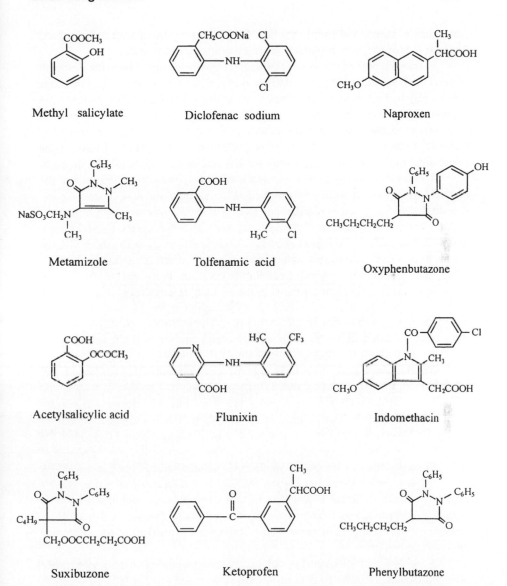

Methyl salicylate

Diclofenac sodium

Naproxen

Metamizole

Tolfenamic acid

Oxyphenbutazone

Acetylsalicylic acid

Flunixin

Indomethacin

Suxibuzone

Ketoprofen

Phenylbutazone

FIG. 8.6 Chemical structures of commonly used nonsteroidal anti-inflammatory drugs.

horse, cattle, sheep, and swine (85, 86). The dosage recommended for cattle and swine is 7.5 mg/kg bw administered either orally or intramuscularly.

Following oral treatment, suxibuzone is slowly absorbed from the gastrointestinal tract, but is very rapidly distributed in the body. In all species, suxibuzone was rapidly metabolized to phenylbutazone, which subsequently was metabolized to oxyphenbutazone and γ-hydroxyphenylbutazone. Animals treated with suxibuzone exhibited lower plasma concentrations of the parent drug than the phenylbutazone metabolite. Available data on phenylbutazone, the principal suxibuzone metabolite, indicated that phenylbutazone has carcinogenic potential for animals.

Species differences in peak plasma levels or in urine concentrations of the respective metabolites were also observed. After a single oral dose of suxibuzone, the suxibuzone half-life in plasma was approximately 8 min in rats, 3 h in dogs, and 4 h in rabbits, while that of phenylbutazone was 5–6 h in rats, 6–7 h in dogs, and 4–8 h in rabbits. Following intramuscular treatment in cattle, the half-lives for phenylbutazone and oxyphenbutazone were estimated at 48–53 h and 56–70 h, respectively. After intravenous treatment of horse, the half-lives for phenylbutazone and oxyphenbutazone were 6–9 h and 11 h, respectively. After repeated oral treatment of suxibuzone, the half-life of phenylbutazone was lower, however, at approximately 3 h in rats and 2.5 h in dogs. The plasma levels of phenylbutazone after repeated treatment with either suxibuzone or phenylbutazone were much lower than those obtained after a single treatment in several species.

Residue depletion studies in pigs treated intramuscularly with 15 mg suxibuzone/kg bw for 3 days showed that suxibuzone was present in muscle and at the injection site only at 1 day after the last dose. Phenylbutazone was present in muscle tissue up to 3 days, in liver up to 6 days, and at the injection site up to day 10. Oxyphenbutazone was also present in all tissues up to 3 days after the last dose.

Phenylbutazone, the major suxibuzone metabolite, has been approved by the FDA for use in dogs and horses (87). It is not licensed in cattle but its properties make it useful in this species for the treatment of musculoskeletal conditions, mastitis, endotoxemia, and castration. Since there is evidence of extralabel use for treatment of mastitis in lactating cows, residues of this drug may be found in bovine milk.

After oral administration to calves, the bioavailability of phenylbutazone was approximately 66%; peak concentrations occurred at 12 h (88). In contrast, the concentration of its active metabolite, oxyphenbutazone, was very low or undetectable in plasma.

Diclofenac, an indolacetic acid derivative, is considered to be one of the strongest nonsteroidal antiphlogistics. It is administered intramuscularly in cattle and swine at a dosage of 2.5 mg/kg bw/day for 7–21 days.

The pharmacokinetics of diclofenac have been investigated in calves and swine. In the former species, plasma levels were 5.4 ppm at 15 min postdosing and attained a maximum of 8.5 ppm at 60 min, whereas in the latter species levels were 3.7 ppm at 15 min postdosing and attained a maximum of 5.8 ppm at 45 min.

Biotransformation and excretion of diclofenac appear to be species-specific. In the bile of rats and dogs, glucuronated conjugates dominated although these conjugates did not occur in human bile. In rat and human urine, diclofenac conjugates were predominant, but in dog urine nonconjugated metabolites were mainly present. The sum of the excreted residues in urine and bile accounted for more than 100% of the administered dose, indicating enterohepatic circulation.

Diclofenac undergoes hepatic methylation and oxidation, creating (6 metabolites that are all susceptible to conjugation by glucuronidation and sulfation. A major metabolite of diclofenac is considered to be its hydroxylated derivative, 4-hydroxydiclofenac.

Flunixin is registered or is under development in many countries for use in horses, cattle, and swine for treatment of equine colic, musculoskeletal disorders, acute endotoxin-induced mastitis in cattle, and respiratory disease (89–91). It is administered orally or parenterally for a maximum of 5 successive days (92). Flunixin is a genotoxic but not carcinogenic compound. Its mechanism of action is believed to be via the inhibition of cycloxygenase to reduce the presence of arachidonic acid metabolites produced during inflammation (93).

Following single daily intravenous injections of radiolabeled flunixin in cattle at the rate of 2.2 mg/kg bw for 3 consecutive days, the parent compound accounted for 50% of the extractable tissue radioactivity, composing the major residue in liver and kidney (94). Three metabolites were also present in both liver and kidney samples: 4-hydroxyflunixin was present at higher levels, whereas 5-hydroxyflunixin and 2-methylhydroxyflunixin occurred at lower levels.

These results indicated that the primary routes of metabolism of flunixin were through oxidation of the pyridine and the phenyl ring systems, and oxidation of the methyl substituent on the phenyl moiety. The mean concentrations of flunixin in the liver were 389 ppb at 12 h postdosing, 53 ppb at 24 h, 13 ppb at 48 h, and less than 8 ppb at 72 h of withdrawal.

Following intravenous dosing of lactating cows with 2.2 mg flunixin/kg bw, residues in milk ranged from 7.3 ppb at 16 h postdosing to 1.7 ppb at 24 h postdosing (95).

Tolfenamic acid is used as an injectable formulation in cattle and swine. In rats and target animals, tolfenamic acid is metabolized by hydroxylation either of the methyl or the methylchlorophenyl group producing two metabolites; further oxidation of the hydroxymethyl group to the corresponding aldehyde or carboxylic acid can produce two additional metabolites. The two hydroxylated metabolites of tolfenamic acid, N-(2-hydroxymethyl-3-chlorophenyl)-anthranilic acid and N-(2-hydroxymethyl-3-chloro-4-hydroxyphenyl)-anthranilic acid, are much less potent than the parent compound in terms of anti-inflammatory and analgesic activities. In cattle and swine, the major elimination route is through the urine, the parent drug representing the major excreted component.

Intravenous administration followed by intramuscular administration 24 h later of radiolabeled tolfenamic acid in dairy cattle at a dosage of 4 mg/kg bw or two intramuscular administrations of 2 mg/kg bw showed that at 8 days after the cessation of treatment, the concentrations of residues in liver, kidney, and injection site were 0.07, 0.09, and 39.6 ppm tolfenamic acid equivalent. The proportion of the parent drug relative to total residues was 51% in liver, 56.7% in kidney, and 78% at the injection site. Residues of tolfenamic acid could not be detected in milk at 24-h, following intravenous and intramuscular administrations.

Ketoprofen is an arylpropionic acid derivative that contains a single asymmetrical carbon atom and therefore exists in two enantiomeric forms that differ in their pharmacokinetic and pharmacodynamic properties (96). It is available for veterinary use in products containing the racemic mixture, and is indicated for treatment of respiratory infections in sheep and mastitis–metritis–agalactia syndrome in the sow. The recommended dosage is 3 mg/kg bw in a single injection (97).

Following a single intravenous administration of ketoprofen at the recommended dosage rate in swine, the parent compound was poorly distributed. Its principal metabolic pathway consisted of reduction of its carbonyl group. Following three repeated intramuscular injections of 3 mg/kg bw in pigs at 12 h intervals, the concentrations of the parent drug in all edible tissues were below 50 ppb at 4 days after the last dose, while those of its reduced metabolite were below 100 ppb in all tissues even at 1 day postdosing.

Indomethacin is a useful drug for the relief of symptoms of rheumatoid arthritis in humans (98). In veterinary medicine, it is effective in the treatment of inflammatory processes related to infectious diseases. The drug is usually administered orally with drinking water.

Pharmacokinetic studies of intravenously administered indomethacin in cattle showed a wide extravascular distribution as suggested by the high volume of distribution and the long elimination half-life observed (99). Similar kinetic behavior of indomethacin was noticed after intramuscular administration in sheep (100). These results suggested that indomethacin could induce high residue levels in tissues.

Following oral administration of indomethacin to chickens at a dosage of 2 mg/kg bw, significant levels of indomethacin residues were detected in liver, muscle, and fat of treated birds (101). However, 24 h after administration, tissue concentrations declined to very low levels and even undetectable in some animals.

8.7   SEDATIVES AND β-BLOCKERS

Meat-producing animals, especially pigs, do not have enough capacity in adapting to stress situations such as those that occur during the transportation of animals to the slaughterhouse. The main consequence of this syndrome is the possible death of the animals during transportation, as a result of a heart attack. In addition, this circumstance may generate some metabolic changes in the muscle that brings about undesirable modifications on the postmortem process, leading to production of the so-called pale soft exudative (PSE) meat. To avoid this, as well as making animals more manageable when loading trucks, sedatives and β-blockers are used.

On the basis of the type of the effect produced, sedatives can be differentiated into the tranquilizer–sedatives and the classic sedatives. On the basis of their chemical structure, further subdivisions within the two general groups of sedatives can be made. Major members of the group of tranquilizer–sedatives are the phenothiazine-type drugs such as acepromazine, chlorpromazine, merazine, promazine, promethazine, and propiopromazine, and the butyrophenone-type drugs such as azaperone (Fig. 8.7). Major members of the group of the classical sedatives are the thiazine-type drugs such as xylazine and detomidine, and the benzodiazepine-type drugs such as brotizolam, diazepam, temazepam, and triazolam (Fig. 8.7).

The drugs in the former group exert quieting, calming effects on animals, lessening anxiety and sometimes reducing fear and aggression in animal species with naturally nervous temperaments. These drugs do not produce loss of consciousness even at high dosages. Drugs in the latter group can depress the central nervous system sufficiently to cause lethargy, drowsiness, and indifference to surroundings. They decrease locomotor activity, fear, and apprehension, and may produce loss of consciousness when high dosages are used.

Among the β-adrenergic receptor-blocking agents used in food-producing animals for the prevention of shipment stress caused by transportation and formation of new herds, carazolol and propranolol are the best-known representatives (Fig. 8.7).

The health hazard presented by the use of these veterinary drugs in farm animals is even more crucial than that of other drugs since sedatives and β-blockers are frequently injected just a few hours before slaughter. As a result, high levels of active residues may be present in edible animal tissues. Furthermore, administration by injection is known to create a local area of high concentration of the drug, which, in part, is likely to be present at the time of slaughter and, if in edible tissue, is a potential hazard to the consumer.

Acepromazine is used in cattle, swine, sheep, and goats by parenteral routes at dosages of 0.01–0.22 mg/kg bw. In contrast to some other phenothiazine derivatives such as chlorpromazine and promazine, acepromazine is not used in human therapy.

Little is known about the pharmacokinetics and biotransformation of acepromazine in food-producing animals. After intramuscular injection of 0.1 mg/kg bw to horses, the unchanged acepromazine was detectable in plasma 1.5–3 h

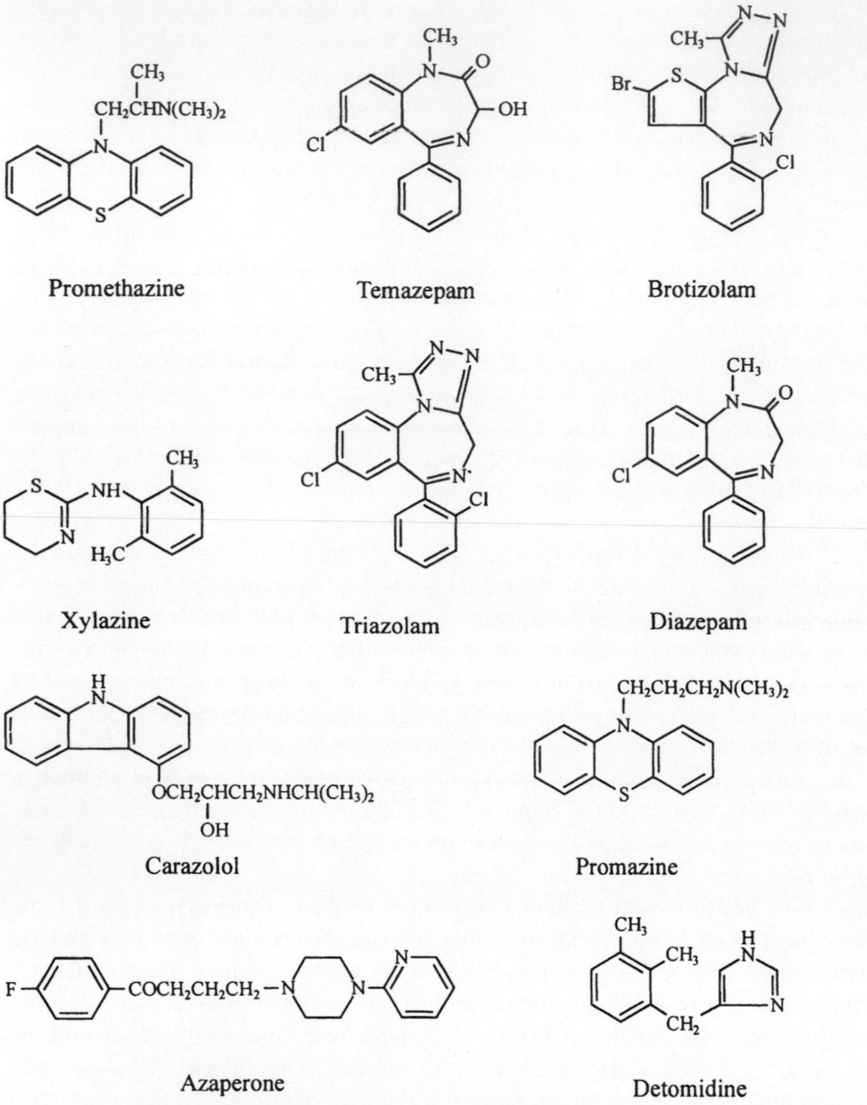

FIG. 8.7 Chemical structures of commonly used sedatives and β-blockers.

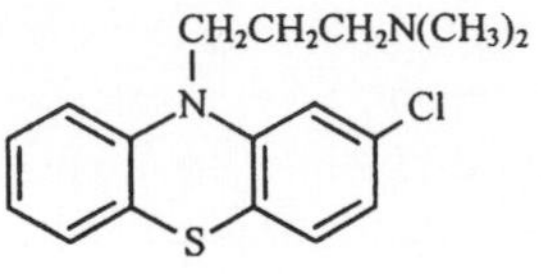

$CH_2CH_2CH_2N(CH_3)_2$

Chlorpromazine

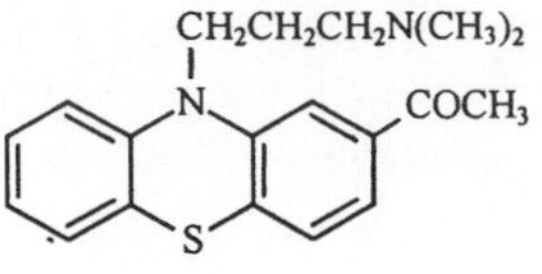

$CH_2CH_2CH_2N(CH_3)_2$

Acepromazine

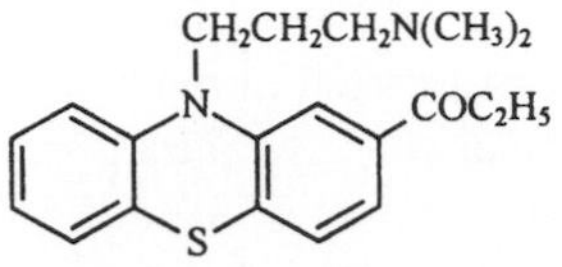

$CH_2CH_2CH_2N(CH_3)_2$

Propiopromazine

$OCH_2CH(OH)CH_2NHCH(CH_3)_2$

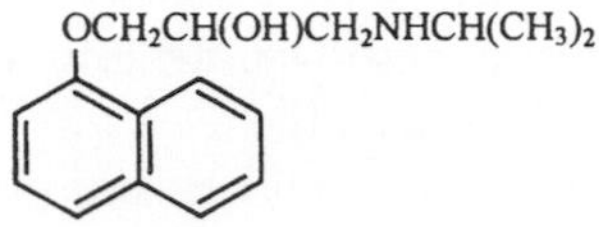

Propranolol

FIG. 8.7   Continued

after injection. Elimination in the urine began at 6 h after injection and was completed after 24 h. Following an oral dose of 105 mg acepromazine to horse, the parent drug was detectable in plasma up to 24 h, with a peak level between 1.5 and 3 h. Elimination in feces started 12 h after injection and was maximum at 24 h, this excretion route being more important than urine.

Acepromazine is rapidly metabolized, and it is eliminated mainly in the urine in form of the sulfoxide metabolite. Following oral administration of 1 mg acepromazine/kg bw to the horse, the maximum rate of residues excretion was achieved within 8 h. However, after intramuscular injection of 0.5 mg acepromazine/kg bw to the horse, the maximum rate was not obtained until 8–16 h. Metabolites were no longer detectable in the urine by 40 h after administration. The nonconjugated residues fraction consisted mainly of promazine sulfoxide. Glucuronidated and sulfated conjugates were found only in trace amounts after intramuscular injection, but accounted for approximately 20% and 27%, respectively, of the total residues recovered after oral administration. After intravenous injection with doses between 5 and 50 mg acepromazine, a single nonconjugated metabolite, 2-(1-hydroxyethyl)promazine sulfoxide, and 2 conjugated metabolites, 2-(1-hydroxyethyl)-7-hydroxypromazine and (7-hydroxyacetylethyl)promazine, were isolated.

Following intramuscular injection of 0.1 mg acepromazine/kg bw in the horse, the parent acepromazine was present only in the kidney at a level of 43 ppb. At the injection site, both acepromazine and its sulfoxide metabolite were present at concentrations of 65 and 36 ppb, respectively.

Chlorpromazine is a tranquilizing and antiemetic agent that may cause a number of side effects in the circulatory and nervous system and adverse effects on blood cells, skin, and the eye. Recent studies suggest a possible genotoxic activity for chlorpromazine, whereas it has been established that certain reactive metabolic intermediates are capable of binding with macromolecules including DNA.

Chlorpromazine appears to be variably absorbed and is metabolized in the gut as well as in the liver, where it can accelerate its own hepatic metabolism or conjugation. After being absorbed, the drug was widely distributed in the body and its lipophilicity allowed it to achieve sufficient intramembrane concentrations to influence the stability or fluidity of cell membranes.

In blood more than 90% of the drug was plasma-protein bound. Oxidation, demethylation, and hydroxylation together with conjugation with glucuronic acid were its major metabolic pathways. These led to formation of a sulfoxide metabolite with about one-eighth of the sedative action of the parent drug in the dog. N-oxide metabolites, on the other hand, underwent significant reduction back to the parent drug in a number of species including humans, in whom chlorpromazine and its metabolites could be detected in urine for 6–18 months after the cessation of treatment (102).

Propiopromazine has been used in all the domesticated animals. Although very limited information is available on the absorption, distribution, metabolism, and elimination of propiopromazine in animals, several studies (103) have reported the presence of propiopromazine in pig kidney collected from abattoirs, so that human exposure should therefore be presumed. Both pigs and horses are able to metabolize propiopromazine, at least in part. The drug binds extensively to tissue proteins, and also accumulates in fatty tissues.

Following injection to horse, the drug was rapidly absorbed, with plasma levels peaked at 30-min after dosing. Propiopromazine was extensively metabolized in horse to form numerous metabolites, four of which have been identified in the urine.

Following intramuscular injection of 0.5 mg propiopromazine/kg bw in swine, the parent drug decreased in kidney from 215 to 53 ppb between 2 and 24 h postdosing, although not in the liver where it remained at about 200 ppb. The concentrations of propiopromazine at the injection site also decreased with time, being 22, 19, and 6 ppm at 2, 8, and 24 h, respectively (103).

Azaperone is a widely used sedative drug in pigs. Available pharmacokinetic studies are insufficient to determine the extent of absorption of azaperone from the gastrointestinal tract. However, by comparison with the excretion profile following parenteral dosing, absorption after oral dosing is probably high. Distribution within the body of rats was extensive, and excretion was primarily in the feces (81%), with lesser amounts in urine (16%) (104).

Metabolism studies in swine showed that the drug was extensively and rapidly metabolized to at least 11 metabolites (105). The three major metabolic pathways elucidated primarily through in vitro studies were reduction of the ketone group to yield azaperol and other reduced compounds, oxidative N-deacetylation, and hydroxylation of the pyridine ring. Apart form swine, these primary pathways were also observed in rats but there were quantitative differences between these species.

Metabolism studies in female adult pigs administered with each of azaperone, acepromazine, and propiopromazine showed that urine contained several metabolites, besides the parent compounds, during the first day following administration (104, 106). The administration of azaperone led to formation of both a hydroxylated (phenolic) metabolite and a biotransformation product formed by reduction of the ketonic function. The metabolic pathway of acepromazine was close to that found for azaperone, with similar hydroxylation processes on the aromatic ring that did not carry the short side-chain. Propiopromazine was also biotransformed through hydroxylation reactions occurring independently on both short and long side chains, leading to formation of an alcoholic function on both the methyl and ethyl group, respectively. In addition, reduction of the ketone group with formation of the corresponding alcoholic group was observed. In all urine specimens, the consecutive hydroxylated products were highly conjugated with glucuronic acid, generating thus hydrophilic compounds that were rapidly eliminated with urine. These metabolic profiles observed in pigs were close to those noticed in other species for the same drugs (107–111).

Following intramuscular administration of radiolabeled azaperone in swine at a dosage of 4 mg/kg bw, total radioactivity decreased rapidly in all edible tissues reaching at 48 h postdosing very low levels in muscle, plasma, skin, and fat, but higher levels in liver and kidney (105). Although kidney was the tissue with the highest total residue concentration at 2 h postdosing, residue levels in liver at 24, 48, and 72 h after dosing were the highest among all edible tissues: 0.698, 0.441, and 0.228 ppm, respectively. In contrast, the levels of total residues in muscle were the lowest among all tissues: 0.041, 0.020, and 0.013 ppm at 24, 48, and 72 h postdosing, respectively. Determination of both the parent drug and its reduced metabolite, azaperol, in all incurred tissue samples, showed that azaperol was at much higher concentrations than azaperone at all withdrawal times.

Xylazine is widely used in veterinary practice for its potent sedative, analgesic, and myorelaxant properties. It may be administered intramuscularly or intravenously to all animal species, although not to pigs due to the very high dose rates required.

Pharmacokinetic studies in horses, cattle, sheep, and dogs have shown that the differences between the four species were remarkably small (112). After intravenous administration of xylazine, systemic half-lives ranged from 22 min for sheep to 50 min for horse. The distribution phase was transient with half-lives ranging from 1.2 min for cattle to 5.9 min for horse. After intramuscular administration, peak levels in plasma of all species were reached within 12–14 min.

Following intramuscular administration to sheep of 1 mg xylazine/kg bw, two-thirds of the injected dose could be absorbed within 10 min (113). The drug was rapidly distributed to different tissues, and rapidly eliminated. The rapid elimination of xylazine in sheep is probably related to its intense metabolism rather than to its rapid renal excretion. This hypothesis was supported by the lack of significant amounts of the intact drug in urine samples collected every 10 min from treated sheep.

Experiments using radiolabeled xylazine in rats have clearly demonstrated the rapid metabolism of the drug since about 20 unidentified end-products have been detected (114). In the urine of cattle injected with 0.2 mg xylazine/kg bw, less than 1% of the unchanged drug was eliminated during the first 2 h, with an apparent half-life of 40 min (113). In this study, peak excretion of xylazine metabolites occurred between 2 and 4 h after the administration of the drug, a finding confirming the extensive metabolism of xylazine.

Because of its relatively short excretion time, xylazine produces residue concentrations below 0.1 ppm in all edible tissues of sheep and cows except the injection site, liver, and kidney, at 20 h after intramuscular administration (115). In addition, xylazine is not excreted with cow milk. Hence, only 2 days are recommended in Norway between treatment and slaughter of cattle or the delivery of milk for human consumption. However, liver and kidney should be discarded if slaughter has taken place less than 4 days after medication.

Brotizolam, diazepam, temazepam, and **triazolam** are all classic benzodiazepine-type sedative drugs that exhibit antihypertensive and myorelaxant properties, and further act as feed-intake and weight-gain promoters.

In field conditions, benzodiazepines can be illegally administered to food-producing animals, apart from any therapeutic purpose, in order to tranquillize animals during the transport to slaughterhouse, and also to counteract the side effects of β-agonist drugs on the central nervous system, such as muscular tremors, nervousness, and depression in feed intake during long-term treatment. At present, however, only brotizolam, a short-acting benzodiazepine, is licensed as an antianorexic drug in food-producing animals.

Benzodiazepines undergo extensive and complex metabolism. They are excreted mainly in the urine, largely in the form of several metabolites. Biotransformation processes include mainly hydroxylation and N-dealkylation reactions, whereas the end-products include both free and conjugated compounds (116). Chlordiazepoxide, for example, is metabolized to oxazepam and other metabolites and, depending on its dosage, urine may contain significant concentrations of oxazepam (117).

Carazolol, a major β-adrenergic receptor-blocking agent used in food-producing animals, is indicated for use in swine by the intramuscular route to prevent sudden death due to stress during transport. It is also intended for use in cattle, at a single intramuscular or intravenous dosage of 0.01 mg/kg bw, for prevention of the shipment stress caused by transportation and formation of new herds, for the facilitation of parturition and expulsion of the placenta, to increase fertility, and for training to mechanical milking (118–121).

In cattle given a single intramuscular injection of 0.02 mg carazolol/kg bw, the drug was rapidly absorbed reaching a maximum concentration of 6.9 ppb in plasma within 30 min after injection. Thereafter, carazolol concentrations declined rapidly, being detectable in only one animal at 8 h after dosing. Plasma was found to contain, besides the parent compound, several carazolol-related metabolites including carazolol lactate, carazolol diol, carazolol glucuronide, and 4-hydroxycarazolol, among which carazolol diol persisted longer and at higher levels. In contrast, urine did not contain the diol and hydroxylated metabolites, but contained carazolol acetate instead. The relative concentrations of the metabolites in urine were similar to those observed in swine and dogs after intramuscular or intravenous injections and the same metabolites were also found in urine from humans after oral administration. It can therefore be concluded that carazolol follows the same metabolic pathways in most animal species.

When pigs were intramuscularly administered 10 mg radiolabeled carazolol/kg bw, highest residual concentrations were detected in liver, kidney, and lungs, with generally much lower levels in muscle, fat, and brain (122). Residues were present in all tissues at 16 h after dosing. Although the identity of the residues was not examined, data from one pig suggested that residues in muscle corresponded to the parent drug. In liver and kidney, the parent drug accounted for about 15% and 20%, respectively, of the total residues.

Carazolol dosing of cattle by intramuscular or intravenous injections gave distribution patterns similar to those seen in pigs. In cattle given a single intramuscular injection of 0.01 mg carazolol/kg bw, residues in tissues depleted to below 1.5 ppb within 24 h after dosing. At 8 h postdosing, carazolol residues could be detected only in liver, kidney, and injection site. In dairy cattle, carazolol residues could be detected in milk from treated animals during the first milking only.

8.8 THYREOSTATIC DRUGS

Thyreostatics, also known as antihormones, are drugs capable of inhibiting the production of thyroid hormones (123). One side effect of their use is the build up of water in muscle tissues and this property has led to their illegal use in some sections of the livestock industry to increase meat yield.

When thyreostatic drugs are given to animals, the decreased production of thyroid hormones reduces basal metabolism, lowers gastrointestinal motility, and favors extracellular water retention (124, 125). Therefore, the mass gain obtained with thyreostatics is due mainly to an increased filling of the gastrointestinal tract and increased water retention by the animal (126).

The result of the abuse of the thyreostatic drugs in animal production is not only the potential risk to human health of drug residues but also production of inferior quality meat. Furthermore, the consumer is deceived since water is sold for the price of meat. Consequently, a worldwide agreement has been promulgated prohibiting the use of these drugs in animal breeding (127).

The group of thyreostatic drugs includes compounds that are either thiouracil analogues, such as thiouracil, methylthiouracil, phenylthiouracil, and propylthiouracil; or mercaptoimidazole analogues, such as tapazole (Fig. 8.8). These drugs can be administered to animals orally by mixing with feed or dissolving in drinking water (128).

Thyreostatics are generally excreted in urine in the form of both the parent and conjugated compound (129). Excretion studies in cows showed that methylthiouracil can be detected as a free unchanged compound, for several weeks after oral administration (130). However, the highest concentration of thyreostatics occur in the thyroid drug when these compounds are distributed to farm animals as illegal feed additives. In regulatory control at the farm, plasma, urine, and/or feces may be sampled. At the retail level or in the case of import/export, sampling is restricted to tissue only, whereas at the slaughterhouse tissue as well as excreta can be sampled.

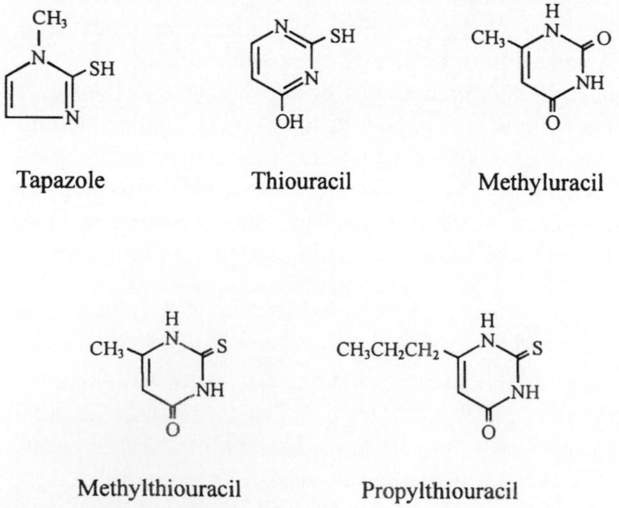

Tapazole   Thiouracil   Methyluracil

Methylthiouracil   Propylthiouracil

FIG. 8.8 Chemical structures of commonly used thyreostatic drugs.

REFERENCES

1. L. Weinstein, in The Pharmacological Basis of Therapeutics (L.S Goodman, and A. Gilman, Eds.), 5th Edition, MacMillan Publishing Co., Inc., New York, N.Y. (1975).
2. European Agency for the Evaluation of Medicinal Products (EMEA), in Natamycin, Summary Report, Committee for Veterinary Medicinal Products, EMEA/MRL/342/98-Final, London, UK (1998).
3. M. Gibaldi, in Biopharmaceutics and Clinical Pharmacokinetics (M. Gibaldi, Ed.), 4th Edition, Lea & Febiger, Philadelphia, PA (1991).
4. D.J. Smith, J. Anim. Sci., 76:173 (1998).
5. J.F. Martinez-Navarro, Lancet, 336:1311 (1990).
6. C. Pulse, D. Lamison, F. Keck, J. Nocoles, and J. Descotes, Vet. Hum. Toxicol., 33:80 (1991).
7. H.A. Kuiper, M.Y. Noordam, M.M.H. van Dooren-Flipsen, R. Schilt, and A.H. Roos, J. Anim. Sci., 76:195 (1998).
8. G.A. Michell, and G. Dunnavan, J. Anim. Sci., 76:208 (1998).
9. L.E. Martin, J.C. Hobson, J.A. Page, and C. Harrison, Eur. J. Pharmacol., 14:183 (1971).
10. G.R. Manchee, A. Barrow, S. Kulkarni, E. Palmer, J. Oxford, P.V. Colthrup, J.G. Maconochie, and M.H. Tarbit, Drug Metab. Disp., 93:2106 (1993).
11. D. Courtheyn, V. Bakeroot, F. de Volder, and J. Vercammen, Food & Agric. Immunol. 6:131 (1994).
12. J.P. Hanrahan, in β-Agonists and Their Effects on Growth and Carcass Quality (J.P. Hanrahan, Ed.), Elsevier Applied Science, New York (1987).
13. J.M. Degroodt, B. Wyhowsky, D. Bukanski, J. de Groof, and H. Beernaert, Z. Lebensm. Unters. Forsch., 192:430 (1991).
14. V.A. Zimmer, Arzneim.-Forsch., 26:1442 (1976).
15. M.C. Saux, J. Girault, S. Bouquet, J.B. Fourtillan, and P. Courtois, J. Pharmacol., 17:692 (1986).
16. M.J. Sauer, R.J.H. Pickett, and A.L. MacKenzie, Anal. Chim. Acta, 275:195 (1993).
17. H. Hooijerink, R. Schilt, W. Haasnoot, and D. Courtheijn, J. Pharm. Biomed. Anal., 9:485 (1991).
18. D. Zalko, G. Bories, and J. Tulliez, in Residues of Veterinary Drugs in Food, Proc. Euroreside III Conf., Veldhoven, 1996 (N. Haagsma, and A. Ruiter, Eds.), Fac. Vet. Med., Univ. Utrecht, The Netherlands, p. 993 (1996).
19. D. Zalko, G. Bories, and J. Tulliez, J. Agric. Food Chem., 46:1935 (1998).
20. L. Debrauwer, D. Zalko, and J. Tulliez, in Residues of Veterinary Drugs in Food, Proc. Euroresidue III Conf., Veldhoven, 1996 (N. Haagsma, and A. Ruiter, Eds.), Fac. Vet. Med., Univ. Utrecht, The Netherlands, p. 367 (1996).
21. D.J. Smith, and G.D. Paulson, J. Anim. Sci., 75:454 (1997).
22. C.T. Elliott, J.D.G. McEvoy, W.J. McCaughey, S.R.H. Crooks, and S.A. Hewitt, Vet. Rec., 132:301 (1993).
23. M.J. Sauer, and S.P.L. Anderson, Analyst, 119:2553 (1994).
24. C.T. Elliott, W.J. McCaughey, S.R.H. Crooks, J.D.G. McEvoy, and D.G. Kennedy, Vet. Q., 17:100 (1995).

25. A.M. Potts, Trans. Am. Ophthalmol. Soc., 60:517 (1962).

26. N.J. Zvaifler, H. Bernstein, and M. Rubin, Arthritis Rheum., 5:667 (1962).

27. G. Boman, Acta Pharmacol. Toxicol., 36:267 (1975).

28. N.G. Lindquist, Acta Radiol. Suppl., 325:1 (1973).

29. M.J. Sauer, R.J.H. Pickett, S. Limer, and S.N. Dixon, J. Vet. Pharmacol. Ther., 18: 81 (1995).

30. C.T. Elliott, W.J. McCaughey, and H.D. Shortt, Food Addit. Contam., 10:231 (1993).

31. C.T. Elliott, S.R.H. Crooks, J.D.G. McEvoy, W.J. McCaughey, S.A. Hewitt, D. Patterson, and D. Kilpatrick, Vet. Res. Commun., 17:459 (1993).

32. A. Malucelli, F. Ellendorff, and H.H.D. Meyer, J. Anim. Sci., 72:1555 (1994).

33. C.T. Elliott, J.D.G. McEvoy, W.J. McCaughey, H.D. Shortt, and S.R.H. Crooks, Analyst, 118:447 (1993).

34. W. Haasnoot, A.R.M. Hamers, R. Schilt, and C.A. Kan, in Food Safety and Quality Assurance: Applications of Immunoassay Systems (M.R.A. Morgan, C.J. Smith, and P.A. Williams, Eds.), Elsevier Applied Science, London, p. 185 (1992).

35. G. Brambilla, A. Bocca, M. Delise, and E. Guandalini, Vet. Res. Commun., 18:37 (1994).

36. K. Pou, A. Adam, P. Lamothe, P. Cravel, J. Messier, A. Cravel, and H. Ong, Can. Vet. J., 33:467 (1992).

37. M.P. Montrade, B. Lebizec, F. Monteau, and F. Andre, Food Addit. Contam., 12: 625 (1995).

38. A.S. Koster, A.C. Frankhuijzen-Sierevogel, and J. Noordhoek, Drug Metab. Dispos., 13:464 (1985).

39. B. Stoffel, and H.H.D. Meyer, J. Anim. Sci., 71:1875 (1993).

40. L. Howells, M. Godfrey, and M.J. Sauer, Analyst, 119:2691 (1994).

41. R.A. Merkel, P.S. Dickerson, S.E. Johnson, R.L. Burkett, A.L. Burnett, W.G. Bergen, and D.B. Anderson, Fed. Proc., 46:1177 (1987).

42. W.G. Bergen, S.E. Johnson, D.M. Skjaerlund, A.S. Babiker, N.K. Ames, R.A. Merkel, and D.B. Anderson, J. Anim. Sci., 67:2255 (1989).

43. E.L. Veenhuizen, K.K. Schmiegel, W.P. Waitt, and D.B. Anderson, J. Anim. Sci., 65:130 (1987).

44. World Health Organization, in Evaluation of Certain Veterinary Drug Residues in Food, Fortieth Meeting of the Joint FAO/WHO Expert Committee on Food Additives, Food and Agriculture Organization of the United Nations, Geneva, p. 63 (1992).

45. C.T. Elliott, C.S. Thompson, Cor. J.M. Arts, S.R.H. Crooks, M.J. van Baak, E.R. Verheij, and G.A. Baxter, Analyst, 123:1103 (1998).

46. J.E. Dalidowicz, T.D. Thomson, and G.E. Babbitt, in Xenobiotics and Food-Producing Animals (D.H. Hutson, D.R. Hawkins, G.D. Paulson, and C.B. Struble, Eds.), American Chemical Society, Washington, DC, p. 234 (1992).

47. D.J. Smith, V.J. Feil, J.K. Huve, and G.D. Paulson, Drug Metab. Dispos., 21:624 (1993).

48. D. Courtheyn, N. Verheye, V. Bakeroot, V. Dal, R. Schilt, H. Hooijerink, E.O. van Bennekom, W. Haasnoot, P. Stouten, and F.A. Huf, in Residues of Veterinary Drugs

in Food, Proc. Euroresidue II Conf., Veldhoven, May 3–5, 1993 (N. Haagsma, A. Ruiter and P.B. Czedik-Eysenberg, Eds.), Fac. Vet. Med., Univ. Utrecht, The Netherlands, p. 251 (1993).

49. L. Istasse, V. de Haan, C. van Eenaeme, B. Buts, P. Baldwin, M. Gielen, D. Demeyer, and J.M. Bienfait, J. Anim. Physiol. Anim. Nutr., 62:150 (1989).

50. M.L.J. Rijckaert, and H.P.J. Vlemmix, in Benelux Working Group on Hormones and Antihormones, SP/Lab/, p. 6 (1992).

51. M. Groot, R. Schilt, W. Haasnoot, P.L.M. Berende, V. Ramazza, D. Courtheyn, J. Vercammen, and M. Logghe, in Residues of Veterinary Drugs in Food, Proc. Euroresidue III Conf., Veldhoven, 1996 (N. Haagsma and A. Ruiter, Eds.), Fac. Vet. Med., Univ. Utrecht, The Netherlands, p. 440 (1996).

52. J. Reding, A. Sahin, J. Schlatter, and H. Naegeli, J. Vet. Pharmacol. Ther., 20:198 (1997).

53. R. Herraez-Hernandez, P. Campins-Falco, and A. Sevillano-Cabeza, Chromatographia, 33:177 (1992).

54. S.F. Cooper, R. Masse, and J. Dugal, J. Chromatogr., 489:65 (1989).

55. D.R. Gross, in Veterinary Pharmacology and Therapeutics (N.H. Booth and L.E. McDonald, Eds.), The Iowa State University Press, Ames, IA, p. 551 (1988).

56. Code of Federal Regulations, Title 21, Office of the Federal Register, National Archives and Records Administration, US Government Printing Office, Washington, DC, Sec. 520.420, 520.1010, 522.1010, 522.1150 (1993).

57. M.W. Werthmann, Jr., and S.V. Krees, J. Pediatrics, 81:781 (1972).

58. B. Shaikh, and N. Rummel, J. Chromatogr., 709.137 (1998).

59. B. Shaikh, in Veterinary Drug Residues (W.A. Moats and M.B. Medine, Eds.), ACS Symposium Series 636, American Chemical Society, Washington, DC, p. 161 (1992).

60. T. Sollmann, in A Manual of Pharmacology (T. Sollmann, Ed.), 8th Edition, W.B. Saunders, Philadelphia, PA, p. 570 (1964).

61. N.A. Littlefield, in Chronic Toxicity and Carcinogenicity Studies of Gentian Violet in Mice, NCTR Technical Report for Experiment No. 304 (1984).

62. J.J. McDonald, in Metabolism of Gentian Violet in Chickens, NCTR Technical Report for Experiment No. 6040 (1985).

63. R.K. Munns, J.E. Roybal, J.A. Hurlbut, and W. Shimoda, J. Assoc. Off. Anal. Chem., 73:705 (1990).

64. J.E. Roybal, R.K. Munns, J.A. Hurlbut, and W. Shimoda, J. Assoc. Off. Anal. Chem., 73:940 (1990).

65. J.J. McDonald, C.R. Breeden, B.M. North, and R.W. Roth, J. Agric. Food Chem., 32:596 (1984).

66. R.A. Schnick, Prog. Fish Cult., 50:190 (1988).

67. S.J. Culp, in Malachite Green: A Literature Review, Reviewed for the NCTR/TSSRC/NTP, Jefferson, AK (1994).

68. D.J. Alderman, and R.S. Clifton-Hadley, J. Fish Dis., 16:297 (1993).

69. K. Bauer, H. Dangschat, H.O. Knoeppler, and J. Neudegger, Arch. Lebensmittelhyg., 39:97 (1988).

70. J.E. Roybal, A.P. Pfenning, R.K. Munns, D.C. Holland, J.A. Hurlbut, and A.R. Long, J. AOAC Int., 78:453 (1995).

71. S.M. Plakas, K.R. El Said, G.R. Stehly, and J.E. Roybal, J. A.O.A.C. Int., 78:1388 (1995).
72. S.M. Plakas, K.R. El Said, G.R. Stehly, W.H. Gingerich, and J.L. Allen, Can. J. Fish. Aquat. Sci., 53:1427 (1996).
73. J. Antychowicz, Bull. Inst. Pulawy, 21:35 (1977).
74. K.-T. Chung, G.E. Fulk, and A.W. Andrews, Appl. Environ. Microbiol., 42:641 (1981).
75. A.R. DiSanto, and J.C. Wagner, J. Pharm. Sci., 61:598 (1972).
76. J. Watanabe, and R. Fujita, Chem. Pharm. Bull., 25:2561 (1977).
77. R.K. Munns, D.C. Holland, J.E. Roybal, J.G. Meyer, J.A. Hurlbut, and A.R. Long, J. AOAC Int., 75:796 (1992).
78. J.E. Roybal, R.K. Munns, D.C. Holland, J.A. Hurlbut, and A.R. Long, in Residues of Veterinary Drugs in Food, Proc. Euroresidue II Conf., Veldhoven, May 3–5, 1993 (N. Haagsma, A. Ruiter, and P.B. Czedik-Eysenberg, Eds.), Fac. Vet. Med., Univ. Utrecht, The Netherlands, p. 601 (1993).
79. M. Nakagawa, K. Murata, T. Shimodawa, T. Honda, S. Kojima, and M. Uchiyama, Eisei Kagaku, 30:301 (1984).
80. S.B. Turnipseed, J.E. Roybal, S.M. Plakas, A.P. Pfenning, J.A. Hurlbut, and A.R. Long, J. AOAC Int., 80:31 (1997).
81. G.A. Hines, and S.A. Watts, J. World Aquacult. Soc., 26:98 (1995).
82. C.L. Goh, Contact Derm., 17:256 (1987).
83. S.M. Plakas, K.R. El Said, E.L.E. Jester, and F.A. Bencsath, J. A.O.A.C. Int., 80:486 (1997).
84. S.M. Plakas, K.R. El Said, F.A. Bencsath, S.M. Musser, and W.L. Hayton, Xenobiotica, 28:605 (1998).
85. D. Sabate, J. Homedes, and I. Mayos, J. Vet. Pharmacol. Ther., 20:162 (1997).
86. J.M. Denoix, and I. Delannoy, Rec. Med. Vet., 168:679 (1992).
87. Code of Federal Regulations, Title 21, Office of the Federal Register, National Archives and Records Administration, US Government Printing Office, Washington, DC, Sec. 520.1720 and 522.1720 (1991).
88. A. Kadir, and P. Lees, J. Vet. Pharmacol. Ther., 20:164 (1997).
89. A.K. Singh, Y. Jang, U. Mishra, and K. Granley, J. Chromatogr., 568:351 (1991).
90. P. Jaussaud, D. Courtot, and J.L. Guyot, J. Chromatogr., 423:123 (1987).
91. K.L. Anderson, A.R. Smith, R.D. Shanks, H.L. Whitmore, L.E. Davis, and B.K. Gustafsson, Am. J. Vet. Res., 47:2405 (1986).
92. Q.A. Mckellar, S.A. May, and P. Lees, Small Anim. Pract., 32:225 (1991).
93. K.L. Anderson, H. Kindahl, A.R. Smith, L.E. Davis, and B.K. Gustafsson, Am. J. Vet. Res., 47:1373 (1986).
94. R.P. Clement, R.D. Simmons, R.J. Christopher, S.F. Charles, C.N. Casciano, C.B. McCullough, J.F. Lamendola, and M.N. Cayen, in Xenobiotics and Food-Producing Animals (D.H. Hutson, D.R. Hawkins, G.D. Paulson, and C.B. Struble, Eds.), American Chemical Society, Washington, DC, p. 37 (1992).
95. H.S. Rupp, D.C. Holland, R.K. Munns, S.B. Turnipseed, and A.R. Long, J. AOAC Int., 78:959 (1995).
96. A. Abas, and P. Meffin, J. Vet. Pharmacol. Ther., 9:204 (1986).

97. A. Kadir, and P. Lees, J. Vet. Pharmacol. Ther., 20:166 (1997).

98. L. Hellenberg, Clin. Pharmacokin., 6:245 (1981).

99. C. Cristofol, J.E. Valladares, C. Franquelo, G. Marti, and M. Arboix, J. Vet. Pharmacol. Ther., 19:72 (1996).

100. M.E. Vinagre, C. Ballesteros, C. Rodriguez, J.M. Ros, F. Gonzalez, J.C. Baggio, T. Encinas, and M.D. San Andres, J. Vet. Pharmacol. Ther., 20:84 (1997).

101. C. Cristofol, B. Perez, M. Pons, J.E. Valladares, G. Marti, and M. Arboix, J. Chromatogr., 709:310 (1998).

102. World Health Organization, in Evaluation of Certain Veterinary Drug Residues in Food, Thirty-eighth Report of the Joint FAO/WHO Expert Committee on Food Additives, Technical Report Series 815, World Health Organization, Geneva, p. 45 (1991).

103. World Health Organization, in Evaluation of Certain Veterinary Drug Residues in Food, Thirty-eighth Report of the Joint FAO/WHO Expert Committee on Food Additives, Technical Report Series 815, World Health Organization, Geneva, p. 47 (1991).

104. World Health Organization, in Evaluation of Certain Veterinary Drug Residues in Food, Thirty-eighth Report of the Joint FAO/WHO Expert Committee on Food Additives, Technical Report Series 815, World Health Organization, Geneva, p. 40 (1991).

105. World Health Organization, in Evaluation of Certain Veterinary Drug Residues in Food, Thirty-eighth Report of the Joint FAO/WHO Expert Committee on Food Additives, Technical Report Series 815, World Health Organization, Geneva, p. 43 (1991).

106. J. De Graeve, and P. Kremers, in Residues of Veterinary Drugs in Food, Proc. Euroresidue III Conf., Veldhoven, 1996 (N. Haagsma and A. Ruiter, Eds.), Fac. Vet. Med., Univ. Utrecht, The Netherlands, p. 436 (1996).

107. E.A. Dewey, G.A. Maylin, J.G. Ebel, and J.D. Henion, Drug Metab. Dispos., 9:30 (1981).

108. J.J. Weir, and J. Sanford, J. Pharm. Pharmacol., 21:169 (1969).

109. J. Park, O.Y. Shin, and P.H-Y. Choo, J. Chromatogr., 489:313 (1989).

110. M. van Boven, and P. Daenens, J. Anal. Toxicol., 16:33 (1992).

111. P.H-Y. Choo, O.Y. Shin, and J. Park, J. Anal. Toxicol., 14:116 (1990).

112. R. Garcia-Villar, P.L. Toutain, M. Alvinerie, and Y. Ruckebusch, J. Vet. Pharmacol. Ther., 4:87 (1981).

113. J. Putter, and G. Sagner, Vet. Med. Nachr., 133 (1973).

114. B. Duhm, W. Maul, M. Medenwald, K. Patzschke, and L.A. Wagner, Munch. Tierarztl. Wochenschr. 82:104 (1969).

115. A.P. Knight, J. Am. Vet. Med. Assoc., 176:454 (1980).

116. D. Laurie, A.J. Mason, N.H. Piggot, F.J. Rowell, J. Seviour, D. Strachan, and J.D. Tyson, Analyst, 121:951 (1996).

117. S. Caccia, and S. Garattini, Clin. Pharmacokinet., 18:434 (1990).

118. E.K. Fiebiger, K.J. Nitz, K. Vollers, and W. Bartsch, Tierarztl. Umsch., 33:531 (1978).

119. G. Ballarini, and F. Guizzardi, Tierarztl. Umsch., 36:171 (1981).

120. H. Bostedt, and P.R. Rudloff, Theriogenology, 20:191 (1983).
121. A.G. Rauws, Tijdschr. Diergeneeskd., 10:659 (1983).
122. World Health Organization, in Evaluation of Certain Veterinary Drug Residues in Food, Thirty-eighth Report of the Joint FAO/WHO Expert Committee on Food Additives, Technical Report Series 815, World Health Organization, Geneva, p. 10 (1991).
123. R. Verbeke, H.F. de Brabander, and A. Ermens, Proc. of the 30th European Meeting of Meat Research Workers, Bristol, p. 385 (1984).
124. H.F. de Brabander, and R. Verbeke, J. Chromatogr., 252:225 (1982).
125. T.J. Wisser, and E. van Over Meeren-Kaptein, Biochim. Biophys. Acta, 658:202 (1981).
126. G. Terplan, L. Kotter, B. Rolle, and H. Geist, Fleischwirtschaft, 44:457 (1964).
127. W. Wohlbier, and W. Schneider, Z. Tierphysiol., 21:34 (1966).
128. Official Journal of the European Communities, No. L275, Brussels, p. 36 (1986).
129. H.F. de Brabander, PhD Thesis, University of Ghent, Ghent (1984).
130. H.F. de Brabander, and R. Verbeke, Trends Anal. Chem., 3:162 (1984).

9

Benefits and Risks of Drug Usage

Like humans, food-producing animals fall sick, suffer accidents, and need protection from disease. As a result, a whole range of drugs have been developed and used to help the veterinarian and the food animal producer to prevent and cure diseases. Drugs are also used at subtherapeutic levels in order to improve the efficiency of feed utilization and to promote growth of healthy animals so they can produce more meat, eggs, or milk on less feed. Drug usage in food-producing animals, however valuable for increasing livestock productivity it may be, is of particular concern because of the possible impact on human health. Benefit and risk analysis of drug usage has therefore become a topic of great importance to food animal producers, consumers, veterinarians, pharmaceutical firms, and regulatory agencies.

9.1 BENEFITS TO ANIMALS, HUMANS, AND THE ENVIRONMENT

Whenever health safety issues in food-producing animals are considered, benefits versus possible risks of drug usage are always evaluated. The antithesis is that the benefits of using versus the risks of not using these drugs in food-producing animals are rarely addressed although they are equally if not more important to consider.

Never before in human history has our planet been so densely populated: nearly 6 billion people now live on Earth and, even though birth rates are decreasing in some developing countries, others are experiencing constant birth rates at a higher level (1–4). In the aggregate, the population of the developing countries that constitute about 80% of the global total continues to increase at record levels. With an increase of 56 million per year, Asia has the highest absolute growth, whereas Africa has the steepest rate with 2.8% population growth per year. World population is now increasing at about 1.7% per year, corresponding to a doubling time of 40 years (5). With the current annual increase in the world human population of 100 or more million people, food problems will become increasingly severe. According to the World Bank and the Food and Agricultural Organization of the United Nations, 1–2 billion people, the largest number of hungry humans ever recorded in history, are currently malnourished.

In the early 1960s, most nations were self-sufficient in food, but now only a few are. In the period 1950–1984, the introduction of high-yield crops and energy-intensive agriculture ushered in the Green Revolution, leading to increased crop production. Except for parts of Africa, world grain output in this period expanded at an annual rate of 2.8% compared with a 2.6% increase in the population. Since then, the world grain reserves have steadily declined (6, 7) and, it appears, are unlikely to be resumed although some countries in Asia and Latin America are still gaining total annual increases in grain yield (8). Factors such as adverse weather conditions, enhanced soil erosion, fuel and resource shortages, and socioeconomic instability have been contributing to the decline of food production (9–14). In the United States, which has one of the best records with corn, the rate of increase from 1945 to 1990 was about 3% per year. Since 1980, this rate has slowed. With wheat, however, the record is not as good, the increase in world grain yield being less than 2% per year.

A major difficulty arises simply from the rate with which food supplies would have to be expanded to keep pace with or exceed population growth rates in countries experiencing high growth rates. To stay even with population growth, it will be necessary to expand food supplies, globally, by the rate of population increase. For many countries, the rate of population expansion is in the range of 2–3% per year. As an example, in order to achieve an increase of 50% in the per capita food production, by the end of a population doubling, the rate of expansion of agricultural production must be appropriately larger. If the population grows at 2% per year, the food production must increase at 3.2% per year; if it is 3% per year, the food production must grow at 4.8% per year. This will result in an increased demand for foods of animal origin and a concomitant decrease in a surplus of food crops to be used in their production. If a deficit in cereal grains develops as anticipated, because of an increasing world population, greater diversion of cereals directly into the human diet will be necessary. This means that the supply of cereal grains for use in composite feeds for animals will decline. Such a decline will adversely affect the pork and poultry industries to a greater extent than the production of ruminants. Ruminants such as cattle, sheep, and goats have the ability to survive on land of varying topography and vegetation as well as to convert grass and shrub forages, which are unsuitable for human food, into milk and meat for use by humans.

Ruminant livestock currently graze about half of the earth's total land area, an area that does not lend itself to cereal crop production (15). Plant or crop production provides the basis for any subsequent consumption by livestock or humans. Theoretically, humans in the position of primary consumers should produce the greatest efficiency, but the relationship is complex and not always rational. Most crops are grown primarily because some part of the plant can be consumed directly by people. Under many conditions, however, much of the plant material cannot be used because it is indigestible by humans. Ruminants, other herbivorous animals such as horses and camels, and some omnivores, such as ducks, geese, and pigs, possess specially modified digestive systems that can extract substantial amounts of nutrients from plant material that is not suited for human food. These species have the digestive ability to satisfy much of their requirements for both maintenance and some production through grazing on marginal land and consumption of the considerable byproducts left over after extraction of plant components that can be used directly in human diets. However, faster growth or higher yields can be obtained whenever herbivores or omnivores receive better-quality feeds such as cereal grains that are also suited for direct consumption by humans.

Critics of intensive livestock production allege that when consuming grains, domesticated animals compete directly with humans and are responsible for considerable malnutrition in lesser developed countries. Such simplistic arguments are naive since almost all intensively managed animal units operate in affluent, industrialized countries where cereal grains grow in surplus rather than deficit amounts. Farmers often find they cannot dispose of surplus cereals for even the cost of production, and so they cycle the crops through animals to obtain value-added products.

Approximately one-quarter of the worlds cropland is devoted to producing grains and other feed for livestock. About 38% of the world's grain production is now fed to livestock (15). In the United States, for example, this amounts about 135 million tons of grain/year, of a total production of 312 million tons/year, sufficient to feed a population of 400 million on a vegetarian diet. With greater deficits in the production of cereal crops, animal production will need to become more efficient than it is now (16). Improved feed efficiency of livestock and poultry is necessary or more cereal grains may be directed to the diet of human beings. Improved efficiency decreases the amount of feed to produce meat as well as the time animals spend in the feedlot or poultry batteries prior to slaughter.

Increased animal productivity and improved feed efficiency cannot occur without the benefits derived from the use of drugs. Drug are administered in relatively large dosages to treat sick animals and in lower dosages to prevent disease in exposed animals. Without drugs, diseases that could lead to reduced productivity and finally to direct losses through death of food-producing animals would not be controlled. It has been estimated for example, that, even using drugs, the annual loss per cow caused by mastitis in the United States totals $181. In addition, diseased animals take much longer to reach marketable weight and some must be even be shipped in poor condition. Even if they pass the quality inspection within the slaughterhouse, these older or emaciated carcasses are generally used for processed products rather than for the more profitable meat trade. Organs or regions showing any evidence of infection or injury cannot be used for human consumption. The portions removed by inspectors during carcass examination cost producers many million of dollars each year.

Some critics of current intensive animal production methods suggest that drugs are necessary only because of the stressful rearing conditions and that the return to more extensive rearing systems would obviate the need for drugs. However, returning to the extensive animal rearing systems would result in exposure to greater environmental extremes and increase the exposure to internal parasites and the associated susceptibility to diseases. Hence this would increase rather than decrease the response to drugs. People have largely forgotten such episodes as, in 1950, when bloody diarrhea caused obvious suffering and death in young pigs, when chickens died in thousands suffocated by air-sac disease, and baby calves perished from scours. These various forms of acute distress were rapidly alleviated by antibiotics.

Growth hormones are also used by livestock producers for different profitable purposes. US farmers and feedlots generally raise steers (i.e., castrated bulls) instead of bulls. Bulls are much more aggressive and difficult to manage. Meat from steers is considered more desirable than bull meat, which is usually less tender, less marbled, and of a darker red color. Castration results in lower androgen hormone production. Androgen supplementation allows steers to achieve the higher growth rates more typical of bulls.

The use of hormones in heifers, (i.e., young cows) stimulates growth rates and feed efficiency. The treated animal converts the feed better into meat; thus a treated animal needs less feed to gain weight than an animal that has not been treated. In this way, the farmer is making a considerable saving of costs in his or her food supply. Treated animals also gain weight more quickly than untreated animals. This means that the treated animals needs less time to reach its slaughtering weight, allowing the farmer savings in work, loans, and standing charges. Some growth hormones allow the feed to be converted in meat without fat. This fat-reducing effect is positive for the livestock breeder, as it increases the trade and value of the animal since consumers are asking for more fat-freemeat.

Other hormones are used for increasing the milk production and efficiency of lactating dairy cows. In the United States an estimated 63% of all cattle and about 90% of feedlot animals are implanted with growth hormones. Beef and sheep may be also implanted but not swine. When implants are used in young cattle, they will improve body weight gain by 8–20% and feed conversion efficiency by 6–10%. Growth implants reduce the total cost of beef production by $50–80 per steer. If implants were banned, the average retail price of all cuts of beef would increase by 10–15%, or about 20–30¢ per pound.

In current veterinary practice, small amounts of antimicrobial drugs are added to animal feeds to prevent or reduce diseases and to improve feed efficiency and growth. The value of these feed additives in improving the rate and efficiency of growth has been well documented by many researchers. A comprehensive summary involving 937 experiments and more than 20,000 pigs showed that the magnitude of the response was greater for the younger animals and declined as the animal matured (17). The improvement attained by the use of feed additives was found to be in the range 16.9–28.4% for daily gain and 7.0–14.5% for feed conversion factor (18). Similar results were presented for chicks, turkeys, and cattle. It is estimated, that, with the help of feed additives and advances in genetic selection of animals that are more efficient in the production of meat, milk, and eggs, the broiler feed conversion factor was reduced to 1.7 lb of feed/lb of broiler from 2 lb in 1975. Egg production reached 273 eggs/hen/year compared to the 220 eggs produced annually in 1975. Feed conversion in beef animals has declined to a ratio of 6:1 from the levels of 8:1 or 9:1, and daily weight gains in the feedlot have attained an average of 3.5 lb compared to 2.75 lb in 1975 (19).

Drug usage has also reduced the amount of animal waste per animal and hence alleviated the problem of environmental pollution. For competitive reasons, the stimulus to improve efficiency in the production of animals is also beneficial to the consumer in the reduction of food costs. The total aggregate of these benefits to all of animal agriculture is very substantial; it has been estimated at as much as $3.5 billion per year reduction in food costs to the US consuming public in 1981 (20). The future role of drugs in this endeavor will be more important than in the past in providing a wholesome and ample food supply.

Some livestock diseases, in addition to causing a reduction in the supply of edible animal products, may also affect human health directly or indirectly. Many disease organisms are pathogenic in both humans and animals. Infections commonly known as zoonoses, could be spread by direct contact or through consumption of contaminated animal products, such as unpasteurized milk and dairy products, causing public health and socioeconomic problems of considerable magnitude. Zoonotic diseases such as salmonellosis cannot be efficiently controlled or eliminated if prevention and control activities are not carried out through the use of suitable drugs.

Improved animal performance and reduced mortality are definite benefits. It would not be difficult to hypothesize on the problems that would arise if no drug medication were available. Large numbers of farm animals would die, chronic bacterial disease would be commonplace, and the consequent losses both of life and productivity would drastically inflate the cost of food of animal origin and lead to the economic death and disappearance of many livestock producers.

9.2 RISKS RELATED TO FOOD CONTAMINATION AND BACTERIAL RESISTANCE

Human health risks from drug usage in food-producing animals, whether real or perceived, are generally topics of intense debate. An issue that has gained world-wide attention as a potential health hazard is connected with the potential contamination of the food supply by the drugs used in animal farming. Another issue rapidly moving to the forefront of public health is associated with bacterial resistance and the effects on human health from the use of antibacterials in livestock and poultry production.

9.2.1 Food Contamination

When drugs are administered to food-producing animals, residues may appear in edible tissues, milk, or eggs. Violative drug residues in animal products can be avoided by using prescribed treatment protocols and allowing sufficient withdrawal periods after treatment for the compounds to be depleted from the animals. There is nonetheless a potential for abuse from failure to adhere to prescribed dosages and withdrawal periods, and use of unproved compounds. Violative drug residues are of concern because they may produce toxicological, pharmacological, microbiological, immunological, and enzyme perturbation hazards which are discussed exhaustively in Part II.

9.2.2 Bacterial Resistance

Veterinary drugs constitute a class of compounds with diverse usefulness. Not only we have to rely on these agents to maintain a cost efficient food supply through their growth-promoting and anticoccidial benefits, but we also expect them to protect human health from lethal diseases. These uses increase the total selective pressure exerted on microorganisms to adapt or die and favor the emergence of bacterial resistance.

Development of resistance in bacterial populations is an extremely complex subject (21). The origin of drug resistance may be nongenetic because inherent resistance to some antibacterials is always present in the population. However, most drug-resistant bacteria emerge as a result of genetic change and subsequent selection processes by the drugs.

Chromosomal resistance develops as a result of spontaneous mutation in a locus that controls susceptibility to a given antimicrobial drug; the presence of the drug serves as a selecting mechanism to suppress susceptible organisms and favor the growth of drug-resistant mutants. In addition, extrachromosomal resistance develops by transduction, transformation, conjugation, and transposition transfer of the so-called R factors between bacterial isolates, species, and even genera.

The R factors constitute a class of plasmids that are extrachromosomal genetic elements that carry genes for resistance to one or several antibacterial drugs. These shared genetic elements may encode for multiple resistance, enabling the use of one antibacterial to select for resistance to multiple antibacterials. Such a possibility exists mainly between drugs that are closely related chemically (e.g., polymyxin B–colistin, erythromycin–oleandomycin, neomycin–kanamycin), but it may also exist between unrelated chemicals (erythromycin–lincomycin). In certain classes of drugs such as tetracyclines and cephalosporins, the active nucleus of the compound is so similar among many congeners that extensive cross-resistance is to be expected. Other antibacterials, such as the fluoroquinolones, have been shown to select only for resistance derived from chromosome-coded resistance, and are not known to be subject to plasmid-mediated resistance (22). Conditions favoring the development and selection of bacteria carrying resistance factors are thought to be associated with repeated or long-term exposure to antibacterials, and low-level dosing (22).

It is widely believed that the phenomenon of bacterial resistance is a problem created by human intervention through the discovery of antibiotics. It is not very well known that, soon after the discovery of penicillin, resistant strains were isolated in cultures of bacteria that had been laid down in the preantibiotic era. Since then, resistant isolates have been obtained from sources of great antiquity. Since the first emergence of life on earth, its lower forms have been involved in a continual form of biochemical war; each species sought to defend and extend its ecological niche. When molds came into conflict with bacteria, there were strong evolutionary pressures for the molds to develop antibacterial weapons and for the bacteria to defend themselves, a common feature of the constant competition for the recycling of biological matter.

Antibiotic resistance in bacteria is not a fixed property, and the degree of resistance detectable in the laboratory probably bears little relationship to the resistance of the organism when growing in the intestinal tract of animals. The types of resistance that bacteria may develop to the action of antibiotics involve two distinct mechanisms: mutation and inheritance. The former mechanism affects DNA sequence and results in the synthesis of a protein or macromolecule by the bacterial chromosome that differs from the original chemical entity, with the ability to interfere with the antibiotic activity. Because an antibiotic hinders a bacterium only after it has entered or crossed the cell wall and has bound to a target site, resistance can develop directly if the mutation has so altered the characteristics of the protein or macromolecule that the cell wall, receptor site, or transport mechanism is no longer "friendly" to the antibiotic.

Resistance can also develop indirectly if the altered protein blocks a bio-chemical pathway used by the antibiotics. In the simplest terms, a sensitive popu-lation of bacteria can be changed into a resistant population by the selection pressure created by the presence of an antibiotic. Resistance can derive from mutation of a single pre-existing gene or from new mutants or variants that may appear during multiplication. Mutants remain unrecognized until the sensitive organisms are eliminated. This occurs when antibiotic is present in excess of the minimum inhibitory concentration (MIC). Hence, it is the high-level therapeutic use of antibiotics and not the low-level growth-promotion use that exerts selection pressure in favor of the mutants. Selection pressure can thus occur both in human and in veterinary medicine.

In human medicine, selection pressure is at its most intense in hospitals, where antibiotics are extensively used. The major cause of problems of antimicro-bial resistance in humans arises from overuse of antimicrobials at therapeutic levels in humans. It is generally accepted that drug resistance that develops in a bacterium as a result of mutation is only of importance within the individual host and a single bacterial strain. Because the determinant is chromosomal, the resistance cannot be transferred between different bacterial species and genera. In addition, the mutationally resistant microorganism is not usually as viable as the wild ones; hence once the selective antibiotic is removed from the environ-ment, the proportions of the mutant decrease. If exposure to the antibiotic contin-ues, however, the mutants can become life-threatening to the patient. It should be understood that the antibiotic does not induce the mutation. The mutant simply takes advantage of its fortuitous spontaneous appearance to flourish in the pres-ence of a selected antibiotic.

The mechanism of inherited resistance proceeds through R-plasmids, which, like chromosomes, are also collections of DNA representing genes capable of coding and inducing the production of new proteins in the bacterial cell. In this fashion, the plasmid can provide the cell with a greater chance of survival and propagation.

A number of characteristics of plasmids are significant in relation to the development of bacterial resistance. These include the encoding of resistance capability for as many as six unrelated antibiotics in the same DNA material, the capacity to transfer from one cell to another and thus disseminate the resistance, and the mobilization by which ordinarily nontransferable gene fragments can be transferred by the plasmid from one bacterial cell to others. Plasmids are of varying size and have been identified in most bacteria. Their majority carries resistance determinants for two or more antibiotics not of the same chemical class. It appears that two identical plasmids cannot coexist in one cell, but plasmids of different groups can occur, increasing even further the possibilities for resistance spread. The transfer or acquisition of other plasmid-mediated characteristics, such as virulence and enterotoxin production, in gram-negative bacteria is facilitated by the presence of resistance plasmids.

The transfer of resistance can be achieved by conjugation, transduction, and transformation. There is also a phenomenon of transposition by which resistance determinants pass from one plasmid to another or to a chromosome or to a bacteriophage, thus allowing construction of new plasmids under the pressure of new antibiotic exposure.

Inherited resistance in bacteria is accepted as the most important type from the standpoint of the community and the environment. Studies of isolated microorganisms of animal and human origin have demonstrated that plasmids from both sorts of isolates were practically identical. In terms of the dissemination of resistance determinants of R-plasmids, one must regard the problem as involving both humans and animals as vectors. Presence of a large reservoir of antibiotic-resistant organisms in animals has been demonstrated in the United States.

R-plasmid-mediated resistance is almost invariably associated with cross-resistance to a number of related and unrelated antibiotics. The reasons for the association lie in the resistance mechanism to related compounds that have been coded, the usual presence of more than one R determinant in the same plasmid, and the frequent coexistence of several different plasmids in the same bacterial cell. As a result, use of any antibiotic can lead to development of resistance to itself and to other related and unrelated antibiotics. If, for example, a plasmid is encoded for resistance to ampicillin, tetracycline, sulfonamide, and streptomycin, exposure to any of these antibiotics results in resistance to all the others, whereas the use of a β-lactamase-containing strain results in resistance to other members of this group.

If resistant organisms are selected due to the use of an antibiotic, they do not only show resistance to this particular substance, but also resistance to many other antimicrobial agents. This principle became even clearer when molecular biologists and geneticists examined the structure of R factors in more detail. They found a further fundamental component of the "infectious antibiotic resistance": the transposons or "jumping genes." A characteristic of transposons is that they are capable of jumping from one DNA molecule to another, for example, from plasmid to plasmid, plasmid to chromosome, plasmid to bacteriophage, and vice versa, thus giving rise to another effective mode for the spread of resistance genes.

In short, the spreading of R factors and transposons as a consequence of the uptake of antimicrobial agents represents the major risks for human health. In turn, this spreading results in development and an increasing incidence of organisms such as *Salmonella, Escherichia coli, Campylobacter, Vibrio cholerae, Yersinia pestis, Shigella, Proteus,* and *Pseudomonas aeruginosa* that are not accessible to therapy. These organisms may be the causative agents of diseases such as typhoid fever, infantile gastroenteritis, pyelitis, plague, and cholera. A number of pertinent reports have increasingly appeared showing an alarming rise in the incidence of organisms resistant to the usual antibiotics.

9.2.3 Impact of Resistance on Human Health

Bacteria of animal origin that are resistant to a particular antibacterial may make the agent ineffective for controlling human infections with pathogens bearing the kind of resistance as a consequence of the pathogenic properties of the animal bacteria as such, or the transference of the resistance to other bacteria that may be human pathogens. The transfer may occur in animals as well as in humans via direct contact with animals or through consumption of contaminated food or water. Adverse consequences of such a transfer include increase in the incidence of human infections caused by resistant pathogens, and potential therapeutic failures in animals and humans. In some cases, resistance may render an infection immune to any drug available. More often, bacterial resistance increases therapeutic costs because more diagnostics are required, more costly and sometimes more toxic drugs are needed, and hospitalization may be extended.

The impact of transmissible drug resistance on public health has been a point of great debate since the early days of the use of antimicrobials in animal farming. There has been great concern that the feeding of low levels of antibiotics that are also used in human medicine can lead to serious human health problems. In intensive livestock production, animals are mass-medicated with growth-promoting antibiotics for much of their life at levels considered too low to inhibit the growth of most pathogens but are more than ideal for development of bacterial resistance. If resistance factors carried in animal isolates are transmitted to humans by ingestion or contact, it is not clear how much effect on human therapy is enough to outweigh the benefits gained by the use of antibiotics in animal feed to maintain a cost-effective food supply.

In contrast to the risk associated with low-level, long-term use of antibacterials for growth promotion, the risk of the development of resistance due to therapeutic use in animals has been deemed within acceptable limits. With therapeutic usage, the dosages administered are considered sufficient to eliminate pathogens, the periods of drug exposure are generally limited to days, and the number of animals undergoing treatment is relatively small compared to those receiving growth-promoting agents. However, as veterinary medicine expands its therapeutic armamentarium into more powerful antimicrobials, including those considered secondary human therapeutics such as fluoroquinolones, and concern over human drug resistance increases, physicians and microbiologists are voicing concern. The willingness to accept risks associated with therapeutic use, particularly in mass-medication practices, of newer antibiotics in animals is lessening. Fortunately, since resistance factors have not yet been demonstrated to transfer beyond mutations passed to progeny, the human health effects of bacterial resistance are limited to zoonotic bacterial pathogens such as *Salmonella, Campylobacter, Enterococci,* and *Escherichia* species that occur in animal reservoirs that serve as sources of human exposure.

9.2.3.1 Salmonella

Numerous episodes have occurred in which humans have developed drug-resistant nontyphoid *Salmonella* infections that have been traced to animal sources (23). These bacteria can be transmitted to humans in food or through direct contact with animals. Antimicrobial resistance limits the therapeutic options available to veterinarians and physicians for the subset of clinical cases of nontyphoid *Salmonella* that require treatment. A recent example is a clone of *Salmonella typhimurium* DT 104 with chromosomally encoded resistance to ampicillin, tetracycline, streptomycin, chloramphenicol and sulfonamides, which has become increasingly common in humans in England and Wales since 1990 (24). Since 1992, only *Salmonella enteritidis* has accounted for more cases of human salmonellosis than *Salmonella typhimurium* DT 104 (25, 26). Multiresistant DT 104 has currently emerged in several European countries (27–29); outbreaks have been also reported in the United States in both cattle (30) and humans (31).

There is little doubt that the persistence of *Salmonella typhimurium* DT 104 in food animals has been enhanced by the use of antibiotics in animal husbandry for the treatment of sick animals and also for prophylactic purposes. Although there is no microbiologically proven link between antibiotic resistance and virulence for humans in zoonotic *Salmonella,* increased rates of hospitalization have been reported for patients with infections with multiresistant *Salmonella typhimurium* DT 104. The World Health Organization Scientific Working Group on Monitoring and Management of Bacterial Resistance to Antimicrobial Agents has discouraged the unnecessary use of antibiotics for prophylaxis or for hygiene purposes in animal husbandry (32).

It has been reported that common serotypes of *Salmonella* were found responsible for human bacteremia in 0.5–2.5% of culture-confirmed salmonellosis cases in the United Kingdom and in fewer than 6% in the United States. Untreated or ineffectively treated *Salmonella* bacteremia in humans can be fatal. There has been only one published case of a nonfatal infection by a *Salmonella typhimurium* DT204c resistant strain of animal origin that failed to respond to fluoroquinolone therapy (33).

Subsequent to the introduction in 1988 of the use of fluoroquinolones for livestock production in Germany, an emergence of fluoroquinolone-resistant variants of the multiresistant *Salmonella typhimurium* clone DT 204c was observed; resistance reached a prevalence of 50% in isolates from calves in a defined area of this country (33). In following years, the prevalence of such resistant strains diminished. Unfortunately, epidemiological data associating this change in prevalence with changes in fluoroquinolone usage have never been available. Hence, there is uncertainty about the relative contribution of direct selective pressure versus the spread of resistant strains in the presence or absence of quinolone use to the emergence and dissemination of quinolone-resistant *Salmonella*.

There has been, however, a temporal association between the introduction of fluoroquinolones in food-producing animals and the emergence of reduced susceptibility to ciprofloxacin in *Salmonella typhimurium* DT 104 in the United Kingdom. Indications of reduced susceptibility to ciprofloxacin in human isolates of a variety of zoonotic salmonellae following the introduction of fluoroquinolones into food-producing animals have been reported in the United States and Denmark (33). Although correlations between quinolone usage in general and the emergence of resistance are hard to be made, there is concern that zoonotic salmonellae with decreased susceptibility to fluoroquinolones are increasing and that a small proportion of these will cause invasive infections that require treatment, possibly with a fluoroquinolone, and that treatment failure could occur. While fluoroquinolones are not used as growth promoters, they are currently used for treatment of animal disease in many countries, and, in some regions, they are also used for preventive purposes.

9.2.3.2 *Campylobacter*

Following the use of fluoroquinolones by the poultry industry, there has been a dramatic rise in the prevalence of the fluoroquinolone-resistant *Campylobacter jejuni* isolated in poultry muscle and liver, and in infected humans (34). Prior to the use of fluoroquinolones in poultry, no resistant strains were reported in individuals with no previous exposure to these drugs. In the past, some studies based on molecular markers showed a link between human and animal isolates of susceptible *Campylobacter*. Similar links of fluoroquinolone-resistant strains of *Campylobacter jejuni* with therapeutic failures in humans have recently been confirmed (34).

Campylobacter species are most commonly responsible for outbreaks of bacterial gastroenteritis in developed countries. The majority of the gastrointestinal *Campylobacter* infections do not require antibiotic treatment and are self-limiting. Where treatment is required, erythromycin is usually recommended. However, fluoroquinolones are often also used pending laboratory results, because they can cover additional bacterial pathogens and are better tolerated than erythromycin.

The effect of fluoroquinolone-resistance in *Campylobacter* on the clinical outcome of treatment with a fluoroquinolone is not yet clear. There are conflicting data on whether resistant *Campylobacter* can cause more severe disease. Although there has been little documented impact of this resistance on human health, current concern about the potential human health consequences if resistance were to increase and spread, is high. Thus, further research and data-gathering are essential to quantify this potential. In addition to quinolone resistance, coresistance with other antibiotics such as macrolides has been also observed in Spain and Thailand. High resistance to erythromycin and streptomycin has been also found in swine isolates in Portugal (35).

9.2.3.3 *Enterococci*

The use of avoparcin as a growth-promoting feed additive in animal husbandry has contributed to a reservoir of transferable resistance genes to glycopeptides, including vancomycin, in the commensal enterococci of animals. Glycopeptide-resistant enterococci from animals may reach humans via the food chain. Although glycopeptide resistance genes have been shown (34) to be widely disseminated, the extent to which the gene pool in animals contributes to the prevalence of glycopeptide-resistant commensal enterococci in humans has not been yet quantified. Glycopeptide-resistant enterococci have caused serious infections in hospitalized immune-impaired patients. In this setting, these organisms contribute to increased morbidity and mortality, in part because of limited therapeutic options. This medical impact may be greater in countries where vancomycin is used intensively (34).

There is concern that there will be increased dissemination of glycopeptide-resistance genes to *Enterococcus faecalis* and their spread to other gram-positive organisms, particularly to multiresistant *Staphylococcus aureus* for which vancomycin is the drug of last resort. Due to the limited number of agents available for treatment of glycopeptide-resistant enterococci, antimicrobial agents not previously used in humans are being sought, including drugs from groups currently used as growth promoters in animals. However, the selection of further resistance in enterococci, such as streptogramin resistance due to use of virginiamycin as a feed additive in animals, is undesirable.

9.2.3.4 *Escherichia*

Multiresistant *Escherichia coli* have been selected by the use of broad-spectrum antimicrobials in both livestock and humans (36). The development of antimicrobial resistance in *Escherichia coli* creates problems due to the high propensity of these bacteria to disseminate antimicrobial resistance genes. Resistance genes have been traced from *Escherichia coli* in animals to *Escherichia coli* in humans. *Escherichia coli* O157:H7 has been recently recognized as an important human pathogen (37). The mode of its transmission is primarily through the food, but person-to-person transmission has been also identified in some day-care center and nursing home outbreaks (38).

9.2.4 Magnitude of the Resistance Transfer to Humans

In recent years, antimicrobial-resistant pathogens have been emerging in human medicine and spreading more rapidly than in previous decades. Treatment of resistant-infections is increasingly hampered due either to the prohibitive cost of existing new-generation drugs or to a total lack of effective antimicrobial agents on the market. Antimicrobial resistance has become a global problem, affecting developed and developing countries, and it is rapidly spreading between continents through international travel (39). There is no question that bacteria develop resistance to antibacterials, and that they can transfer their resistance to other bacteria, even of other species. However, the extent to which the administration of antibacterials to animals has contributed to the human health problem is still unclear and a source of great controversy.

Prior to the use of antibacterials to control infectious diseases, the frequency of resistance to these agents in human pathogenic species was probably low (40). Surveys in the early 1970s demonstrated that their use resulted in a rise in the frequencies of resistant strains and, with respect to some agents and in some species, this rise was rapid and to high levels (41–43). In later years, significant frequencies of resistance were encountered in human pathogens, but there was no rise. A survey conducted on almost 6 billion strains from 242 hospitals in the United States in the period 1971–1984 showed that, with respect to the most pathogens, the frequencies of resistance to 16 most commonly used antibiotics remained stable during this period (36). However, a survey on *Salmonella* isolates in the United States showed significant decreases in the frequency of resistance during almost the same period (44). A study carried out in the same period in central Europe also failed to detect any increase in the overall levels of resistance (45). A more recent survey of 86,000 strains isolated in a district general hospital in the United Kingdom between 1984 and 1991 provided no evidence that this situation has changed with time (46).

In contrast to these large-scale surveys that failed to identify significant rises in resistance, a plethora of articles have appeared in recent literature reporting increasing resistance as a major problem in the therapy of infections in hospitals (47–50). Some studies suggested that this apparent conflicting evidence was because most outbreaks of bacterial resistance are usually localized and the increases in the resistance frequency in human pathogens were determined in specific niches in specific hospitals (51, 52). An epidemiological study (53) of antibiotic resistance in hospitals identified the specific niches in hospitals where increased resistance was a problem; these were units where patients were immunocompromised and subject to invasive procedures, or obliged to remain for a long time. This would suggest that the selective pressure for the emergence of resistant strains was internal to the hospital environment. Hence, problems encountered in antimicrobial therapy of infections in hospitals might primarily be those related to the pathogens acquired in these hospitals where resistance is a function of the antimicrobial agent used there.

In general, there is little doubt that treatment problems in humans associated with resistant bacteria are primarily due to the prescribing practices of health workers and to medication-taking practices of patients. The liberal availability of antimicrobials in some countries can also contribute to the basic problem of bacterial resistance. A recent analysis (54) of the frequency of multiresistant strains in community-acquired and nosocomial infections lends support to this conclusion, since the data collected could not support the hypothesis that such strains were selected by veterinary use of drugs.

In 1987, the US National Institutes of Health reviewed existing worldwide data on the prevalence of antibiotic resistance (51). They concluded that resistance to antibiotics was not solely a function of usage, but might result from the inevitable process of bacterial evolution. Other phenomena, including increased human resistance to antibiotics never used in animals and the prevalence of antibiotic resistance in developing countries where use of animal antibiotics is uncommon, led the experts to support that human antibiotic resistance should primarily be due to a variety of factors other than animal antibiotics.

Additional studies, such as those conducted by the US Institute of Medicine Report (IOM) in 1988, also attempted to determine the impact of drug usage in food-producing animals on antimicrobial resistance of human pathogens, using penicillin and tetracycline on *Salmonella* as a model. The authors of this study attempted to describe the extent to which transfer of resistance factors occurred between human and animals and to define whether the risk to human therapy was enough to outweight the benefits of a cost-effective food supply. The result of the IOM Report was that the information available to answer the question was insufficient.

Reasons for the magnitude of the problem being unknown are manifold, but are related to the paucity of national and regional information on antimicrobial drugs use and resistance trends in hospitals and the community. Scarcity of pertinent data complicates attempts to quantify the proportion of resistance problems in humans caused by antimicrobial use in livestock production. Data are even more limited on antimicrobial consumption, antimicrobial use in agriculture, and the prevalence of antimicrobial-resistant zoonotic bacteria in animals and animal-derived food.

Despite the uncertainty there is enough evidence, however, to cause concern. Microbiological and clinical evidence that resistant bacteria or resistance determinants might be passed from animals to humans is mounting (55–67). Therefore, continuous close monitoring is needed in order to determine the magnitude and trends of the resistance and to define the relative importance of different contributing factors such as therapeutic, behavioral, economic, social, and health system factors, and/or veterinary and agricultural misuse.

Based on this understanding, it might be possible to develop effective methods to contain antimicrobial resistance in different settings. This will require close cooperation between sectors involved in food hygiene, prevention and control of diseases transmitted from animals to humans, hospital infection control, resistance monitoring, and prudent use of antimicrobials in humans and animals. The animal production sector shares with other sectors the responsibility for the provision of safe and wholesome food for human consumption. Among other things, this sector must ensure that animals are healthy and are not a reservoir for antimicrobial-resistant bacteria.

REFERENCES

1. World Population Data Sheet 1996, Population Reference Bureau, Washington, DC (1996).
2. United Nations Population Fund, in Population, Resources and the Environment, United Nations, New York, NY (1991).
3. United Nations Population Fund, in The State of World Population, United Nations, New York, NY (1991).
4. T.F. Homer-Dixon, Inter. Sec., 16:76 (1991).
5. D. Pimentel, R. Harman, M. Pacenza, J. Pecarsky, and M. Pimentel, Population and Environment, 15:347 (1994).
6. A.S. Moffat, Science, 256:1140 (1992).
7. H.W. Kendall, and D. Pimentel, Ambio, 23:198 (1994).
8. N.E. Borlaug, in Water and Water policy in World Food Supplies, Proc. of the Conf., May 26–30, Texas University, Texas A&M University Press, College Station, Texas (1985).
9. D. Pimentel, C. Harvey, P. Resosudarmo, K. Sinclair, D. Kurz, M. McNair, S. Crist, L. Sphpritz, L. Fitton, R. Saffouri, and R. Blair, Science, 267:1117 (1995).
10. K.A. Dahlberg, in Beyond the Green Revolution: The Ecology and Politics of Global Agricultural Development (K.A. Dahlberg, Ed.), Plenum Press, New York, NY (1979).
11. K.A. Dahlberg, in Environment and the Global Arena: Actors Values, Policies (K.A. Dahlberg, Ed.), Duke University Press, Durham, NC (1985).
12. M.K. Tolba, Bioscience, 39:725 (1989).
13. R.A. Kerr, Science, 256:1138 (1991).
14. A.H. Teramura, and J.H. Sullivan, in Preparing for Climate Change: A Cooperative Approach, Proc. of the 2nd North American Conf., p. 203 (1989).
15. A.T. Durning, and H.B. Brough, in State of the World (L.R. Brown, Ed.), W.W. Norton & Co., New York, NY, p. 66 (1992).
16. A.W.A. Burt, J. Sci. Food Agric., 24:493 (1973).
17. V.W. Hays, in Agricultural Uses of Antibiotics (W.A. Moats, Ed.), American Chemical Society, Washington, DC, p. 74 (1986).
18. V.W. Hays, in Effectiveness of Feed Additive Usage of Antibacterial Agents in Swine and Poultry Production, Rachelle Lab., Long Beach, CA (1977).
19. E.C. Naber, Poult. Meat, 25:62 (1974).
20. CAST, in Antibiotics in Animal Feeds, Council for Agricultural Science and Technology, Ames, IA, Report No. 88 (1981).

21. E. Jawetz, J.L. Melnick, and E.A. Adelberg, in Review of Medical Microbiology (E. Jawetz, J.L. Melnick, and E.A. Adelberg, Eds.), 17th Edition, Appleton & Lange, Norwalk, CT, p. 133 (1987).

22. P. Smith, M.P. Hiney, and O.B. Samuelsen, Ann. Rev. Fish Dis., 4:273 (1994).

23. S.B. Levy, in the Antibiotic Paradox (S.B. Levy, Ed.), Plenum Press, New York, NY (1992).

24. E.J. Threlfall, J.A. Frost, L.R. Ward, and B. Rowe, Vet. Rec., 134:577 (1995).

25. Threlfall EJ, Frost JA, Ward LR, Rowe B. Lancet, 347:1053 (1996).

26. N. Limpitakis, A. Abrahim, A. Kansouzidou, V.D. Daniilidis, C. Genigeorgis, in Epidemiology and Control of Salmonella in Pork, Proc. 3rd Inter. Symp., August 5–7 (P.B. Bahnson, Ed.), Washington, D.C., p. 257 (1999).

27. A. Brisabois, I. Cazin, J. Breuil, and E. Collatz, Eurosurveillance, 2:19 (1997).

28. H. Kohn, and H. Tschope, in Salmonellosen des Menschen (H. Kohn, and H. Tschope, Eds.), Berlin, RKI Schriften (1996).

29. I.S.T. Fisher, Eurosurveillance, 2:4 (1997).

30. T.E. Besser, C.C. Gay, J.M. Gay, D.D. Hancock, D. Rice, and L.C. Pritchett, Vet. Rec., 140:75 (1997).

31. CDC, in Multidrug-Resistant Salmonella Serotype Typhimurium—United States, 1996. MMWR Morbid. Mortal. Wkly Rep., 46:308 (1997).

32. World Health Organization, in Bacterial, Viral Diseases and Immunology, Scientific Working Group on Monitoring and Management of Bacterial Resistance to Antimicrobial Agents, WHO/CDS/BVI/95.7, World Health Organization, Geneva (1994).

33. World Health Organization, in Use of Quinolones in Food Animals and Potential Impact, Report of a WHO Meeting, World Health Organization, Geneva (1998).

34. World Health Organization, in The Medical Impact of the Use of Antimicrobials in Food Animals, Report of a WHO Meeting, World Health Organization, Berlin (1998).

35. J. Gabrita, J. Rodrigues, F. Braganca, C. Morgado, I. Pires, and A. Penha Goncalves, J. Appl. Bacteriol., 73:279 (1992).

36. B.A. Atkinson, and V. Lorian, J. Clin. Microbiol., 2:791 (1984).

37. L.W. Riley, R.S. Remis, S.D. Helgerson, H.B. McGee, J.G. Wells, B.R. Davis, R.J. Herbert, E.S. Olcott, L.M. Johnson, N.T. Hargrett, P.A. Blake, and M.L. Cohen, N. Engl. J. Med., 308:681 (1983).

38. N.V. Padhye, and M.P. Doyle, J. Food Prot., 55:555 (1992).

39. World Health Organization, Weekly Epidemiol. Rec. 72:333 (1997).

40. V.M. Huges, and N. Datta, Nature, 302:725 (1983).

41. R.J. Bulger, C.E. Roberts, and J.C. Sherris, Antimicrob. Agents Chemother., 11: 1966 (1967).

42. N. Datta, Ann. N. Y. Acad. Sci., 182:59 (1971).

43. M. Finland, Ann. N. Y. Acad. Sci., 182:5 (1971).

44. V. Lorian, J. Clin. Microbiol., 23:826 (1986).

45. M. Kresken, and B. Wiedemann, J. Antimicrob. Chemother., 18:235 (1986).

46. A.P. MacGowan, N.M. Brown, H.A. Holt, A.M. Lovering, S.Y. McCulloch, and D.S. Reeveds, J. Antimicrob. Chemother., 31:543 (1993).

47. M.L. Cohen, Science, 257:1050 (1992).

48. B. Murray, J. Infect. Dis., 163:1185 (1991).

49. H.C. Neu, Science, 257:1064 (1992).
50. D. Shales, S. Levy, and G. Archer, ASM News, 57:455 (1991).
51. T.F. O'Brien, Members of the Task Force 2, Rev. Infect. Dis., 244 (1987).
52. M.J. Blaser, in Bacterial Infections of Humans (A.S. Evans, and H.A. Feldman, Eds.), Plenum Medical Book Co., New York, p. 137 (1982).
53. K.H. Mayer, J. Antimicrob. Chemother., 18:223 (1986).
54. P.M. Shah, V. Schaffer, and H. Knothe, Vet. Microbiol., 35:269 (1993).
55. A.H. Linton, J. Antimicrob. Chemother., 18:189 (1986).
56. E. Chaslus-Dancla, in Chemotherapy in Aquaculture: From Theory to Reality (C. Michel, and D. Alderman, Eds.), Office International des Epizooties, Paris, p. 243 (1992).
57. S.D. Holmberg, J.G. Wells, and M.J. Cohen, Science, 225:833 (1984).
58. T.F. O'Brien, J.D. Hopkins, E.S. Gilleece, A.A. Medeiros, R.L. Kent, B.O. Blackburn, M.B. Holmes, J.P. Reardon, J.M. Vergeront, W.L. Schell, E. Christenson, M.L. Bissett, and E.V. Morse, N. Engl. J. Med., 307:1 (1982).
59. B. Rowe, and E.J. Threlfall, PHLS Microbiol. Digest., 3:23 (1986).
60. J.S. Spika, S.H. Waterman, G.W. Soo Hoo, M.E. St. Louis, R.E. Pacer, S.M. James, M.L. Bissett, L.W. Mayer, J.Y. Chiu, B. Hall, K. Greene, M.E. Potter, M.L. Cohen, and P.A. Blake, N. Engl. J. Med., 316:565 (1987).
61. E.J. Threlfall, J. Appl. Bact., 73:96S (1992).
62. H.P. Endtz, G.J. Ruijs, B. van Klingeren, W.H. Jansen, T. van der Reuden, and R.P. Mouton, J. Antimicrob. Chemother., 27:199 (1991).
63. E. Perez-Trallero, C. Zigorraga, C. Cilla, P. Idigoras, C. Lopez Lopategui, and L. Solaun, Scand. J. Infect. Dis., 20:573 (1988).
64. M.F. DeFlaun, and S.B. Levy, in Gene Transfer in the Environment (S.B. Levy, and R.V. Miller, Eds.), McGraw-Hill Inc., New York, p. 1 (1989).
65. S.B. Levy, and B.M. Marshall, in The Release of Genetically-Engineered Microorganisms (M. Susman, C.H. Collins, F.A. Skinner, and D.E. Stewart-Tull, Eds., Academic Press, New York, p. 61 (1988).
66. N.B. Shoemaker, G.-R. Wang, and A.A. Salyers, Appl. Environ. Microbiol., 58: 1313 (1992).
67. R.V. Tauxe, S.D. Holmberg, and M.L. Cohen, in Gene Transfer in the Environment (S.B. Levy and R.V. Miller, Eds.), McGraw-Hill Inc., New York, p. 377 (1989).

10

Drug Residues and Public Health

The most serious objections to the presence of drug residues in food intended for human consumption arise as a consequence of human health considerations. With the extensive use of drugs in animal production, residues of the parent drugs and/or metabolites have a high potential to be present in the edible animal products. The public health significance of such adulteration of the food supply is determined mainly by the level of the residues and the individual drugs they are originated from.

Drug residues normally appear in meat, milk, eggs, and honey at very low concentrations and, therefore, risks for public health are practically excluded. Exceptions are some non-dose-related side effects, such as allergic reactions that may arise from β-lactam residues in sensitized consumers. In instances, however, of extralabel use or noncompliance with withdrawal periods, much higher residue levels may appear in the edible animal products. Such residues in food constitute a variety of public health hazards including toxicological, microbiological, immunological, pharmacological, and other hazards.

Health hazards from drug residues in food depend on the frequency and degree of human exposure. Increase in the degree of human exposure occurs when injection sites are accidentally consumed. Continuous exposure is more probable when a side or quarter of a contaminated food animal is purchased by a consumer for deep-freeze use. Basic antibiotics such as chloramphenicol, erythromycin, tylosin, and oleandomycin, are more likely to accumulate in tissue at a higher concentration than in plasma due both to ion trapping, which results from a pH difference between blood and tissue, and to the innate lipid solubility of the compounds (1). A factor with the potential to reduce the drug residues intake is that most animal tissues are cooked before eating, which may decrease the degree of food contamination by several types of residues including penicillins and tetracyclines.

Proper assessment of public health hazards is a complicated task and has become one of the most vexing problems. The diverse opinions associated with defining exactly what constitutes a hazard to human health have further perplexed existing mechanisms to determine whether human health is affected or not by the therapeutic or subtherapeutic use of drugs in food-producing animals. In spite of the obvious limitations, the attitude of drug residues will be approached in this chapter from the public health perspective, since the requirement for safe food is of utmost importance as far as consumer health is concerned. Existing evidence for specific health hazards of certain groups of drugs will be described and the risks associated with the consumption of residues of these drugs in edible animal products will be explained. The focus will be on the possible health consequences that may occur as a result of acute exposure to illegal residues, but long-term chronic effects will be also considered.

10.1 TYPES OF RESIDUES AND THEIR TOXICOLOGICAL SIGNIFICANCE

There has been an increasing worldwide public outcry to know what residues and contaminants are in the food supply, and a demand that food be free of residues that could have an impact on the public health. A simplistic but often voiced concept is that edible animal products should be only consumed when all administered drugs and drug-related residues have been totally eliminated. For some time in the past, this concept seemed to guarantee the highest degree of food safety as animal products destined for human consumption were found to be free of drug residues by the analytical methods applied at that time.

However, as the sensitivity of the analytical methodology increased with time, this concept had to be abandoned because animal-derived food formerly believed to be free of residues was found to be contaminated after all. With the current extensive use of drugs in treatment of disease and as feed additives for food-producing animals, it is highly probable that drug-related residues will always be present, most often at practically nonmeasurable concentrations, in the edible products of the treated animals. It is now realized that the goal of producing food free of residues in absolute terms is, to all practical purposes, impossible to achieve (2). Such a target could theoretically be attained by entirely abandoning the use of veterinary drugs, but this is an unacceptable option in modern animal farming (3). On the other hand, drug residues at any level or form in food are not necessarily toxic.

In general, safety evaluation is primarily based on the toxicological testing of the parent drug. However, consumers of edible animal products are also exposed to many other products of drug metabolism, including free metabolites of

TABLE 10.1   Compounds Described Under the Concept of "Total
Residues"

Parent compound
Free metabolites produced by addition, cleavage, oxidation and reduction bio-
   transformations of the parent compound
Conjugates to small molecules (glucuronides, glutathione, etc.)
Conjugates to macromolecules (proteins, nucleic acids, etc.)
Covalently bound metabolites
Drug fragments incorporated into endogenous cellular components (amino
   acids, proteins, lipids, etc.)

---

the parent drug, conjugates to small molecules and macromolecules, and covalently bound metabolites, which are all described under the concept of "total
residues" (Table 10.1). It is very possible that some metabolites are devoid of
the toxicity of the parent drug, but others may be equally or more responsible
for the exhibited toxicity. According to the Food and Drug Administration (FDA),
the concept of "total residues" should apply to any compound from the use of
the drug in the target animal resulting in the edible tissues. Compounds would
include the parent compound, its metabolites, and any other substances formed
in or on the food because of the use of the drug (4).

The amount of total residues is generally determined by study with radiolabeled drugs and is expressed as the parent drug equivalent in milligrams per
kilogram of the food. Bound metabolites can be measured as the difference between the total and extractable residue. Microbiological assays measure the parent
molecule and its bioactive metabolites; immunochemical assays measure the parent molecule and closely chemically related metabolites.

Regulatory requirements in the field of drug residues analysis are limited,
in most cases, to the identification of only the major metabolites. Quantitative
selection of major over minor metabolites is certainly devoid of rational biological
ground, since several studies have shown that the toxic metabolites are usually
transitory and often present in small quantities. However, isolation and identification of all these metabolites are difficult and proper assessment of the toxicity
of drug residues is still a real challenge.

Metabolic activation of drugs forming highly reactive intermediates that
react with tissue macromolecules can be an important mechanism for drug toxicity, although not necessarily the most important one (5–7). Reactive intermediates, such as electrophiles, free radical, and active oxygen species, have the potential to initiate toxicity by interacting with critical macromolecules or by generating
propagate oxidative mechanism that lead to both structural and functional altera-

tions. Covalent binding of such intermediates to macromolecules is the first effect in an organism receiving drug therapy.

From the standpoint of consumer safety, reactive intermediates are of little, if any, toxicological significance. There is little chance of finding reactive intermediates in edible animal products because of their high reactivity and very short half-life. Free radical intermediates may be formed by one-electron oxidation, one-electron reduction, or homolytic cleavage of many compounds, including nitrofurans, amines, phenols, quinones, and halogenated derivatives. These toxic intermediates may induce protein and lipid alkylation, and peroxidation of membranes, which is considered as a primary event in the toxicity of several drugs. Electrophilic intermediates, on the other hand, may be produced by metabolic oxidative or reductive processes leading to formation of epoxides and oxiranes, which are very unstable and rarely identified. These compounds may interact with various cellular components causing alkylation of cellular molecules and subsequent damage but leading also to deactivation of reactive intermediates.

In contrast, all free metabolites potentially present in animal products are stable chemical species with defined toxic potential for which safety margins can be determined, and, thus, are of toxicological concern. The biological activities serving as criteria for determining their toxicity are those most relevant to humans, primarily the teratogenic and the mutagenic activity. Apart from free metabolites, their conjugates to small molecules and macromolecules present also the potential of toxicological concern. Such residue forms can be deconjugated into the human organism after ingestion of the contaminated food. This leads to formation of new electrophilic derivatives that may readily react with human macromolecules. This process is defined as secondary bioavailability since it represents the beginning of a second passage of the drug through the mammalian organism (8, 9).

Covalently bound drug residues in edible animal products are not necessarily toxic because this type of binding is normally not cleaved during digestive processes. By definition, a residue is designated as bound if it cannot be released from the macromolecular fraction after mild but exhaustive extraction procedures. The nonextractable material may include two different residue fractions that cannot be differentiated by this experimental approach. One fraction may consist of certain elements of the drug that have been incorporated by normal metabolic pathways into endogenous components, such as amino acids, proteins, or nucleotides, and is of no more toxicological significance. The other fraction may contain metabolites covalently bound to cellular macromolecules and is considered to be of toxicological concern. This concern must be considered equal to that of the parent compound unless proven otherwise. This level of toxicological concern may be a conservative assumption, but it is impossible to establish the concern as zero or any other value without scientific information (10, 11).

The extremely complex chemistry of bound residues contributes to the difficulty in assessing their safety in food. Reactive intermediates can bind with numerous naturally occurring compounds, yielding a plethora of derivatives, most of which are likely to be present in extremely low concentrations. As a consequence, the structural determination of the bound residue is difficult, if not impossible, in many cases. It is extremely difficult to differentiate analytically between a drug metabolite chemically bound in nonextractable form to tissue macromolecules such as proteins, lipids, nucleic acids, or glycogen, and extensively metabolized drug fragments that have entered the metabolic pool, becoming incorporated into the same macromolecules. Although the portion of the bound residue shown to be due to endogenous incorporation can be discounted from the total residue of toxicological concern, such an incorporation may be widespread in some instances and makes an accurate quantification very difficult.

A concept that is critical in the complex evaluation of bound residues is the adduct residue. The concept of adduct residue can be applied to any metabolite covalently linked to an endogenous component. Hydrolysis of the macromolecular bound residue, whether by enzymatic or chemical means, may lead to lower-molecular-weight adduct residues, free residues, and residue fragments. Since bound residues are derived from reactive metabolites, the reversibility of adduct formation to yield reactive compounds may be a key factor in the safety assessment of bound residues.

For example, the macromolecule to which the metabolite is bound may undergo digestion to peptide or amino acid adducts that may themselves be toxic or may be chemically or enzymatically transformed into an active species, as in the case of certain cysteine adducts shown to be activated through subsequent metabolism in the kidney (12), thereby eliciting toxicity. A demonstration that the reactive metabolite cannot be regenerated under various conditions, such as mild acid or enzymatic digestion, would lessen the concern for the toxicological significance of the bound residue. Tissue-bound residues liberated by hydrolysis or enzymatic procedures are likely to be in a highly oxidized or polar state, and, in general, may be expected to have reduced toxic potential (13).

Because differentiating among drug-related residues and drug fragments that have entered the normal metabolic pool is difficult, alternative indirect methods are employed to gain further insight into the toxicological potential of bound residues. The most straightforward approach is the so-called relay toxicity method (14). This procedure provides a useful means of equating test animals and human exposure. Target tissue from farm animals receiving the drug is mixed with normal feed and fed to laboratory animals for varying periods. The animals are then sacrificed and observed for signs of toxicity. The technique is attractive because it simulates experimentally the exposure of humans to tissue residues by ensuring that the test animal (i.e., the rat) is exposed to the same mixture of metabolites as humans. It is a relatively inexpensive test because it is not necessary to characterize the residues present in the target animal tissues. The residue containing the parent drug and its metabolites is present in the proportions to which humans might be exposed.

Any positive response in a relay toxicity test is indicative of a serious toxicological residue hazard that cannot be ignored. It is argued, however, that negative results are inconclusive since the animals are not exposed to high enough concentrations of residues. Even when the tissues containing the incurred residues are used as the only dietary source in order to reach the highest concentration possible, the total residue concentration given to rats will still be orders of magnitude lower than the lowest concentration of the parent drug that would give a positive carcinogenic or toxicological response. At a minimum, levels at least as high as those for which a carcinogenic or toxicological end point are observed would be needed.

When, for example, relay embryotoxicity studies were used to study the total residues of cambendazole and albendazole, no toxicity was detected when livers incurred with residues were fed to pregnant rats (15, 16). However, for extrapolation to humans, these studies did not allow the demonstration of a wide safety margin because of the low residue levels present in the tested edible tissue. To eliminate this major drawback, Galer and Monro (17) have made some recommendations including treatment of the target species at a dose level three- to fivefold higher than normal, killing of experimental animals several days earlier than the projected withdrawal period, and administration of the tissues containing the artificially high-level residues to laboratory animals for conventional toxicological evaluation.

Due to the obvious limitations of other methods, the relay bioavailability method is more widely used. The method of relay bioavailability endeavors to provide information about the degree of absorption of residues by establishing a ratio between the absorbed and unabsorbed fractions. This involves feeding residue-containing tissues from treated target animals to rodent pseudoconsumers that have been used in the overall toxicological assessment of the drug. These target animal tissues contain the metabolites to which humans are exposed. Relay bioavailability can be carried out by feeding freeze-dried tissues from target animals treated with radiolabeled drug to laboratory animals. A bile-canulated rat model similar to that developed by Gallo-Torres is often used (18). After sacrificing the animals, the radioactivity of the liver and kidney is measured. An approximate estimate of the proportion of radioactivity absorbed can be made by summing the radioactivity found in the bile and urine.

The experimental design of the relay bioavailability method allows the toxicological assessment of bound residues by comparing their relative bioavailability to that of the parent compound, and deducing the amount of the nonbioavailable bound residues from the total residue of toxicological concern. This has been found to be true for several drugs including cambendazole and albendazole where total residue bioavailabilities were low compared with the parent drugs

(15, 19). In the cambendazole study, the bioavailability of the parent drug in rats was determined at 50%, but when rats were given total residues of cambendazole through the ingestion of liver of calves treated with the drug, only 15% of the total radioactivity was absorbed. Thus, on the same withdrawal day, the amount of residues found in the rats used as pseudoconsumers was 30 times less than that in the rats fed the parent drug. It appears that, despite bioactivation processes, total residues do not account for a higher toxic risk than the parent drug.

The US Food and Drug Administration (FDA) has recently proposed an approach to the safety assessment of bound residues derived from carcinogenic drugs thought to be both scientifically valid and reasonably capable of being accomplished (20, 21). This approach is based on the data collected from a combination of both in vitro and in vivo tests in the areas of the bioavailability and toxicological potential of bound residues, the reversibility of adduct formation, and the mechanism of bound residue formation.

Although the human food safety assessment has long challenged regulatory agencies and extensive research on the issue of bound residues has been carried out, the scientific knowledge about the real chemical nature, bioavailability, and coherent toxicity as well as on the release of fragments during digestive degradation of tissues containing bound residues is still very limited. Real progress in finding answers to these questions and establishing a rational basis for risk assessment can only be achieved with a more detailed analysis of the chemical nature of such residues.

10.2 TOXICOLOGICAL HAZARDS

Drug residues in contaminated foodstuffs have the potential to produce direct toxic effects. However, the residue concentrations in food are generally so low that direct toxic effects are improbable. Next to direct toxicity, possible toxicological hazards with respect to the presence of drug residues in food may be of carcinogenic, mutagenic, and/or teratogenic nature. Long-term low-level mutagenic or carcinogenic effects, if any, are far more relevant from a public health point of view. However, the greatest hazard from the human health safety point of view may be the unrecognizable exposure to possible teratogens.

10.2.1 Direct Toxic Effects

The likelihood of acute toxicity from drugs or their metabolites in edible animal products is extremely low, a fact confirmed by the lack of documented scientific reports in the pertinent literature (22, 23). This lack can be best exemplified in two cases of premature thelarche outbreaks The first of these outbreaks of breast development before the age of 8 years occurred in children attending an Italian school, the second in Puerto Rico. In both outbreaks, meat containing estrogenic substances was implicated as the cause of precocious sexual development (24).

More significant by far in terms of the number of infants and children affected was the outbreak that occurred in Puerto Rico. In 1980 through 1981 pediatric endocrinologists in Puerto Rico reported a threefold increase in the number of premature thelarche cases compared with 1978. The outbreak was originally alleged to be caused by consumption of poultry or meat containing residues of naturally occurring or synthetic hormonal substances (24). Beef and pork meat, milk, drinking water, and blood and urine samples from affected and unaffected children were analyzed for synthetic and naturally occurring hormones, but no underlying cause for the increase in premature thelarche cases could be determined (25). It was finally concluded that the increased number of cases might be attributed to better diagnosis and reporting of premature thelarche by physicians, or to the presence of entirely new, unexpected factors, but not to drug residues in food (26).

Among all groups of drugs used in food animal production, none has evoked greater emotional response in the public than the hormonal growth-promoting drugs. One event more than others may have been responsible for precipitating the present consumer attitudes. In 1980, high concentrations of diethylstilbestrol were found in baby food in Europe (27). Although it was later surmised that the extreme concentration of diethylstilbestrol in the baby food could have only resulted from severe misuse or intentional and malicious adulteration, the incident implanted in the public a fear of all hormonal growth-promoting drugs.

Despite public apprehensions concerning the use of the hormonal growth-promoting drugs, numerous scientific studies have demonstrated that when these drugs are used in accordance with good husbandry practices, residual concentrations in meat remain within the normal physiological range established for untreated cattle of the same age and gender. Based on these facts, the FDA has concluded that no harmful effects will occur in persons who daily consume animal tissues that contain an incremental increase of endogenous hormone equal to 1% or less of the amount produced daily by the segment of the population with the lowest daily production rate. Prepubertal boys synthesize the least estradiol and progesterone, whereas prepubertal girls synthesize the least amount of testosterone per day. Prepubertal boys produce, on average per day, 100–3,000 times the amount of estradiol and more than 500 times the amount of progesterone that would be expected to occur in 500 g meat from treated animals. Prepubertal girls likewise produce 600–900 times the amount of testosterone that would be expected to be present in 500 g meat from treated animals (27, 28).

Unlike the naturally occurring hormones for which human food safety assessment is based on a ratio of their amount consumed in food compared to their amount produced endogenously by the consumer, safety assessment for the synthetic trenbolone acetate and zeranol hormones is based on alternative strategies. Considerable research has gone into assessing the risk of cancer to the consumer from use of synthetic hormones in food-producing animals. The establishment of hormonal no-effect levels as a basis for assessing human food safety and setting tolerances for residues is scientifically sound: the hormonally active compounds cause no increased incidence of tumors when administered to laboratory animals in amounts below those required to produce detectable hormonal activity (29). The major impediment to establishing safe tissue concentrations of the synthetic hormones results primarily from their ability to produce tumors in laboratory animals when these compounds are fed at high concentrations. These tumors occur only in endocrine-sensitive tissues and are similar to those produced by high doses of the naturally occurring hormones. On the other hand, the newest members of the anabolic hormonal growth-promoting drugs, bovine somatotropin, or porcine somatotropin do not leave hazard residues in meat or milk.

Exceptions, however, to this situation may occur for some drugs, particularly those possessing inherent properties that can threaten human health. One such example is chloramphenicol, which has been implicated as the causative agent in many cases of fatal aplastic anemia, a condition reported to be non-dose related and potentially could be induced by even extremely low levels of this antibiotic in food (30). Thus, the establishment of a safe level in chloramphenicol residue exposure from food animal tissues can be precluded.

Aplastic anemia in humans represents an idiosyncratic reaction affecting 1:20,000–50,000 patients receiving a typical course of chloramphenicol therapy. The mechanism of chloramphenicol-induced aplastic anemia is uncertain, but bone narrow stem cells are believed to be involved. Thiamphenicol, an analogue of chloramphenicol lacking the p-nitro group, although sharing many of the clinical antibacterial and toxicological properties of chloramphenicol, has not been implicated to date in the aplastic anemia syndrome. As a result, it has been postulated that a nitroso reduction product of the p-nitro group of chloramphenicol can irreversibly inhibit the growth of bone marrow precursor cells. Considerable controversy still exists as to whether chloramphenicol-associated bone marrow depression is a toxigenic or allergenic effect.

The resulting disease is fatal in approximately 70% of the cases and those who recover experience a high incidence of acute leukemia (31). It has been reported that a 6-year-old girl died after receiving only 2 g chloramphenicol (32), while a 73-year-old woman died following an estimated total dose of only 82 mg chloramphenicol received as an ophthalmic drug (33). These total dosages have the potential to be present in human food: it has been confirmed in a report in which chloramphenicol residues were found in 13 of 3020 calves tested (31). Ten muscle samples had levels above 1 ppm, while one was reported to contain about 12 ppm chloramphenicol.

Although there have been no reported cases of aplastic anemia attributable to consumption of chloramphenicol residues through food, the possibility of such an event is not remote. Use of chloramphenicol in cattle is thought to be responsible for the death of a Kansas rancher. The rancher was diagnosed as having aplastic anemia 4 months after he began treating his cattle with chloramphenicol (31).

In the past, chloramphenicol was approved for use in food-producing animals in Canada and Europe (31). In the United States it has never been approved for such use although it was approved for use in dogs. However, chloramphenicol has gained wide popularity among food animal veterinary practitioners in the United States because of its effectiveness in treating bacterial infections. By 1985, FDA had accumulated enough data to establish that most chloramphenicol oral solution marketed for use in dogs was being used to treat food-producing animals, usually by injection or infusion. Since the labeling directions for use had not been followed in practice and were not likely to be followed in the future, the FDA withdrew approval of all oral solutions containing chloramphenicol (34).

Although in 1983 approximately 0.5% of all calves in the United States contained residues of chloramphenicol, by 1984 the violation rate declined to 0.09% as a result of chloramphenicol withdrawal and no violations were detected under the US Department of Agriculture Food Safety Inspection Service (FSIS) monitoring program in 1985 or 1986 (35–38). Veterinarians were forbidden from using chloramphenicol for any purpose that would result in the presence of residues in food for consumption by humans. Use of chloramphenicol in food-producing animals was also specifically restricted in the Extra-Label Drug Use policy of the FDA (39), and FDA has prosecuted veterinarians who have disregarded this policy.

Clenbuterol has been also implicated as the causative agent in many cases of human poisoning. This β-agonist has been illegally incorporated into animal feeds in a number of European countries and Canada for the purpose of enhancing animal growth rates. Its administration in feedlots can constitute a severe risk for animal welfare and exposes consumers to involuntary drug consumption at pharmacologically active concentrations. Most reported poisoning episodes have been associated with the consumption of beef liver, in which clenbuterol residues particularly accumulate.

In Spain, a foodborne clenbuterol poisoning outbreak occurred in the central part of the country between October, 1989, and July, 1990, affecting 135 persons (40). Epidemiologists located the cases using the pharmacological profile of clenbuterol and the appearance of symptoms 30 min to 6 h after ingestion, lasting for approximately 40 h. Consumption of liver containing clenbuterol in the range 160–291 ppb was identified as the common point in the 43 families affected, while symptoms were observed in 97% of all family members who consumed liver (41).

Between January and April, 1992, another outbreak occurred in the northern part of Spain, affecting 232 persons (42). Clinical signs of poisoning in more than half of the patients included muscle tremors and tachycardia frequently accompanied by nervousness, headaches, and myalgia. Intervals between exposure and onset of symptoms ranged from 15 min to 6 h and the duration varied from 90 min to 6 days. Clenbuterol levels in the urine of the patients were found to range from 11 to 486 ppb, but clenbuterol could not be detected in serum. Based on food consumption data obtained from the patients, the origin of the contaminated foodstuffs was determined (43). A total of 61 of those afflicted had eaten at either the same restaurant or company canteen, whereas all patients had consumed veal liver, veal tongue, or cannelloni before the onset of symptoms.

In addition, an incident of food poisoning by residues of clenbuterol in veal liver occurred in the fall of 1990 in the cities of Roanne and Clermont-Ferrand, France (44). A total of 22 persons from eight families were affected. Symptoms appeared 1–3 h after consuming veal liver meals, and all patients recovered within 1–3 days. A woman with a prior heart disease developed marked palpitations but her son, who consumed the same meal, did not, indicating that heart conditions can make a person more susceptible. In two of the liver samples originated from a slaughterhouse in Roanne, relatively high concentrations of clenbuterol, reaching 375 and 500 ppb, were determined.

Two farmers in Ireland were also reported to have died while preparing clenbuterol for feeding to livestock (45). In August 1996, 62 persons asked for medical help at the emergency rooms of two hospitals near the city of Caserta, Italy (46). Their clinical profile was characteristic of previously occurring clenbuterol intoxication, including superventricular extrasystoles and atrial fibrillation. All patients had consumed beef meat 10–30 min to 2–3 h before symptoms developed. Definitive confirmation of clenbuterol and determination of the drug content in meat samples was obtained by gas chromatography–mass spectrometry, using two different derivatization procedures. Clenbuterol levels in the meat ranged from 0.8 to 7.4 ppm. This case demonstrates that clenbuterol poisoning can also occur after consumption of beef meat other than liver.

All intoxication cases described above demonstrate clearly that safety evaluation of pharmacologically active compounds to which consumers are exposed as residues in food must be based on both toxicological and pharmacological criteria. Consumption of 100 g liver containing clenbuterol in concentration levels as determined in liver samples contaminated with 160–500 ppb, would exceed the pharmacological effect level of 5 µg per person (47).

The thyreostat methimazole has been reported to be illegally added to cattle feeds along with clenbuterol to increase animal weight and water retention (48). Maternal use during pregnancy for the treatment of hyperthyroidism is associated with a high incidence of congenital aplasia cutis, which is a characteristic scalp defect in children. In Spain, there has been a significant increasing trend in the prevalence of aplasia cutis from 1984 to 1991. This trend has not been related to maternal treatment of hyperthyroidism but it is closely associated with outbreaks of clenbuterol poisoning. Thus, it was eventually postulated that the increase in congenital scalp defects in Spain was caused by consumption of beef containing illegal residues of methimazole.

10.2.2 Carcinogenicity

The major concern as far as the potential carcinogenicity of veterinary drugs is concerned is directed toward their residues in edible animal products (49). The number of chemicals shown to be carcinogenic in animals has increased enormously over the past decade. They represent a wide spectrum of unrelated chemical structures, including many that are apparently nongenotoxic in most test systems.

Cell damage induced by chemical carcinogens involves the conversion in the body of a proximate carcinogen (inert) to the ultimate carcinogen that is a reactive electrophilic compound. This ultimate carcinogen may then interact or, more frequently, combine covalently with intracellular components, such as DNA, RNA, phospholipids, or glutathione.

In terms of molecular activity, the precise mechanism of carcinogenesis has not been fully elucidated. Many general mechanisms underlie induction of carcinogenic changes. Alone or in combination, these may initiate neoplastic alterations. Formation of chemically reactive metabolites or ultimate carcinogens may occur by a complicated, varied process of biological mechanisms. A number of metabolites may exist in the free radical form or the epoxide form, which then complex with cellular macromolecules, initiating structural, functional, or chemical change, especially in informational proteins. Reactive metabolites can give rise to various types of toxicity, including carcinogenesis, mutagenesis, teratogenesis, cellular necrosis, blood dyscrasias, and immunological effects. Mechanisms underlying these toxic manifestations are largely unknown.

Carcinogens can be subdivided into two major types: genotoxic and epigenetic compounds. Genotoxic carcinogens are compounds that either in their parent form or after metabolism in the body possess direct biological capability to damage DNA. Genetic toxicity tests reveal such carcinogens. They pose a major hazard because they can be effective after a single exposure. Aromatic and heterocyclic amines, nitrofurans, azo and N-nitroso compounds, and carbamates are included in this class.

Epigenetic carcinogens do not directly damage DNA. They operate indirectly by a variety of mechanisms, including hormonal effects, immunosuppression, and cocarcinogenic effects. Carcinogenic effects occur with high or sustained levels of exposure, which in turn can lead to physiological imbalances, hormonal dysfunction, or tissue injury. Included in this category are promotional agents, cytotoxic agents, and hormone modifiers.

The distinction between different types of carcinogens is extremely important in the area of food toxicology. The characteristics of genotoxic carcinogens make them qualitative hazards, but with epigenetic agents a safe threshold of exposure may be delineated. DNA reactive chemicals represent significant health hazards. They have the potential to produce toxicity, birth defects, genetic disease, and cancer. A drug that is not genotoxic in hepatocyte cultures in vitro but that can induce this effect in vivo is suggestive of epigenetic mechanisms of activity by conversion to electrophilic metabolites in the body.

Diethylstilbestrol (DES), which has been used as a feed additive growth promoter, possesses a stilbene double bond and therefore has been suggested to be capable of interacting with DNA through formation of a reactive species. With chronic exposure in adult mice, DES produces tumors only in mice carrying the mammary tumor virus. Thus, its effect is a promotional type. After high exposure to DES in neonates, tissue changes are likewise induced in the hormonally sensitive target tissues, such as the vagina. Neoplasia occurs later in life only when endocrine changes occur in the female reproductive system. DES then would be mechanistically classed as an epigenetic carcinogen and therefore requires a different evaluation from "straightforward" genotoxic in vitro carcinogens. This classification, however, is currently under review. DES may be a genotoxic carcinogen.

Quinoxaline compounds are commonly used agents for growth promotion or enteric disease therapy in swine. Therefore two closely related veterinary compounds, carbadox and olaquindox, were evaluated in the *Salmonella*/microsome test (Ames test) and the hepatocyte/DNA repair test (Williams test). Both were positive. Thus, not only are they potentially genotoxic and mutagenic, but also should be considered potential carcinogens. Not only do they share a common structural similarity, but they are also deemed to be a hazard at any level of exposure because of their in vitro genotoxic activity. In short, nongenotoxic or epignetic carcinogens may represent only quantitative human hazards because of their dependence on mammalian activation systems of variable intensities. Thus, safe levels of exposures of these types of agents could be at least theoretically defined. Conversely, human exposure to direct genotoxic carcinogenic veterinary drugs must be minimized.

Lengthy toxicological studies are required when carcinogenicity is suspected because of the drug's chemical similarity to known carcinogens or mutagens. The procedure is to treat animals for their lifespan and to determine the differences between control and treated groups with regard to tumor time of appearance, number, and type. Differences in susceptibility to carcinogens, however, can be seen between different strains of laboratory animals. For example, Fischer rats are relatively resistant to the induction of extrahepatic neoplasms by aromatic amines, whereas these compounds can cause increased occurrence of mammary tumors in Sprague-Dawley rats.

Other known carcinogens in humans may not necessarily act as carcinogens in rats. Susceptibility of animals to carcinogens is influenced not only by the potency or toxicity of the chemical agent but also by many additional factors, including diet, species, period of exposure, strain, organ sensitivity, transplacental exposure, gender, endocrine balance, stress, disease, and exposure to secondary compounds that suppress or induce drug-metabolizing enzymes. Exposure to minute amounts of carcinogens raises many difficult questions. This is important to regulatory agencies that must decide whether any degree of exposure to a carcinogen can be permitted.

The biological reactivity of ultimate carcinogens is nonetheless causing increased concern. Induced conformational changes in DNA can affect replication transcription and translation processes within the cell. In many cases, the lag period for carcinogenesis can be 20 years in humans, and so it is extremely difficult not only to design effective toxicity tests for drugs whose residues have carcinogenic potential but also to interpret mechanisms of activation and to define interpretive and predictive criteria. The rodent is used in assessment for carcinogenic potential of drugs or chemicals because its 2–3.5 year lifespan is shorter than that of humans.

Accumulation of DNA damage over a period of years can contribute to carcinogenesis by way of somatic mutagenesis. Mammalian cells possess an enzymatic mechanism for the removal of certain carcinogens bound to DNA. Not only is repair a natural process, but also spontaneous depurination of DNA is a naturally occurring phenomenon, albeit at a low rate constant. Exposure to carcinogens can increase the rate of depurination with a significant increase in the number of apurinic sites. This creates vast capability for miscoding potential, especially if DNA repair is not complete. DNA repair errors induced by chemical exposure is another mechanism of action of carcinogens leading to mutations or carcinogenesis.

The FDA has chosen to define "no residue" operationally based on quantitative carcinogenicity testing of residues and the extrapolation of animal test data to arrive at a concentration of residue that presents an insignificant risk to humans. The virtually safe level of exposure is determined by this linear-extrapolation model for each test compound, expressed as a fraction of the total diet fed to the test animal, calculated for a maximum lifetime risk that is essentially zero but never expected to exceed 1 : 1,000,000. The lowest of all calculated acceptable levels for the parent drug or its metabolites is designated as the required sensitivity of the method for the tissue assay. The 1 : 1,000,000 level of risk used in the FDA guidelines does not mean that 1 : 1,000,000 people will develop cancer as a result of the regulation of an animal drug carcinogen. Rather it represents 1 : 1,000,000 increase of risk over the normal risk of death and also represents a lifetime but not an annual risk.

10.2.3 Mutagenicity

Mutagenesis is the induction of changes in the genetic component of the cell. In many cases, mutagens also cause cancer in laboratory animals. Because of this, an added benefit of mutagenicity studies is to provide short-term predictive tests of carcinogenicity potential. Mutagenic compounds may react with a base in DNA and modify it chemically. At the next replication, the modified base may pair with a new base partner. Subsequent replication ensures completion of the mutational process. The sequence of base pairs determines the corresponding sequence of base pairs in DNA, which determines the corresponding sequence of bases in RNA. When DNA base pairings are changed by mutational mechanisms, during replication and transcription, because a new genetic code has now been established, formation of a different amino acid may be specified. This may be quite deleterious to cellular function.

The *Salmonella*/microsome assay, referred to as the Ames test, is currently the most widely used short-term assay for mutagenic compounds. Although the Ames test possesses good routine predictive value, it is often criticized on grounds of selectivity of chemicals tested, the occurrence of false-negative results, and for various chemicals inherently toxic to bacteria. A major disadvantage of the test system has been the failure to detect mutagenicity attributable to drug or chemical metabolites. Incorporation of a mammalian metabolic activation system or various microsomal tissues facilitates increased reliability by detecting mutagenic effects induced by metabolites. Without this addition, the performance of the Ames test would be limited exclusively to direct-acting agents that do not require metabolic activation.

Because most carcinogens are not carcinogenic themselves but are active only after metabolism, the compounds are tested in the Ames test in the presence of a mammalian metabolizing system as well as directly. Such an artificially created bacterial in vitro system does not truly mimic the mammalian system as exemplified by humans or animals. Despite these limitations, the Ames test, although controversial, still remains one of the primary assay systems for quick screening and detection of possible mutagens and is of importance as a predictive test for carcinogens. The question arises whether the Ames test is the appropriate tool with which to investigate mutagenicity of anabolic drugs. Although steroids are proven carcinogens in several animal models, they are not mutagenic in the bacterial test system.

10.2.4 Teratogenicity

The greatest problem from the human health safety point of view is inadvertent or accidental exposure to possible teratogens. This invisible exposure poses the greatest risk, especially in the context of drug residues from food animals. A teratogen is a chemical agent that can affect the somatic cells of a developing fetus such that defective development of organ systems occurs. During the embryonic stages, organogenesis is taking place and at this stage the conceptus is particularly sensitive to the toxic effects of drugs. Because the rate of cellular turnover is high in the first trimester of gestation, agents that interfere with the cellular proliferation can be embryotoxic, giving rise to a variety of developmental abnormalities. For teratogenic effects to occur, all that is required is transient exposure to a potentially embryotoxic agent during a critical period of early pregnancy.

During early fetal development, there are critical or sensitive periods when malformations are most likely to be induced. These critical periods are short windows of time during the phase of organogenesis. Teratological calendars have been drawn up for humans, laboratory animals, and target animals identifying the critical time periods.

Teratogenicity is essentially a "one hit" phenomenon; that is, it is really a form of acute toxicity, and it can appear after only a single exposure to the drug or chemical. Level of exposure and dosage are important because although certain fetal concentrations may be teratogenic, higher levels may actually kill a fetus and are not necessarily teratogenic for the survivors.

Many agents that are mutagenic and carcinogenic also display teratogenic activity. Induction of mutational or chromosomal abnormality can cause abnormal fetal development. Teratogenicity and congenital abnormalities, however, are not necessarily associated with obvious chromosomal abnormalities, and so the malformations are not heritable. This is in contrast to mutagens and carcinogens, in which a heritable alteration in a cell line is a prerequisite.

In laboratory animals, teratogenic effects have been demonstrated for antithyroid substances, alkylating agents, antifolate agents, hormonal excesses, and some antibacterial sulfonamides. A number of organophosphates and carbamate insecticides, and certain corticosteroids are also teratogenic in a number of laboratory animals. During the later stages of pregnancy, the urogenital system is susceptible to the action of steroid hormones. Progesterone and progestagens given to the dam can produce masculinization of female fetuses; androgens and anabolic steroids may induce female pseudohermaphroditism. In the bitch, dexamethasone may result in birth of pups with deformed limbs. Griseofulvin, a fungistatic antibiotic, is teratogenic in cats but not in dogs.

Many of the benzimidazole drugs also exhibit teratogenic properties. This was first recorded with parbendazole, which is teratogenic in sheep and rats but not in pigs, cattle, or rabbits. Species sensitivities can thus be quite dissimilar. In the well-documented case of parbendazole in sheep, dosing of the pregnant ewe is associated with congenital abnormalities in the offspring. The anomalies are primarily those of the bones and joints affecting the pelvis, long bones, and digits. Exposure at different times of early pregnancy give rise to different mani-

festations of abnormality, for example, day 12 exencephaly, day 16 fused vertebrae, and day 24 arthrogryposis.

Oxfendazole, on the other hand, is teratogenic in sheep but not in cattle.
Albendazole administered on day 12 in sheep causes exencephaly and on day 17
causes skeletal abnormalities. In sheep, head and face abnormalities tend to occur
following exposure from day 12 to 17, spinal column defects from day 16 to 21,
and limb distortion from day 22 to 25.

Depending on the species, parbendazole, mebendazole, albendazole, oxfendazole, cambendazole, and febantel can be teratogenic in the parent form or
indirectly from metabolite formation. Oxibendazole and fenbendazole in parent
form are not teratogenic, although one of the metabolites of fenbendazole, a
sulfoxide found in the milk of cows treated with fenbendazole, is teratogenic in
the rat and sheep. Albendazole displays similar biotransformation pathways in
cattle as it does in sheep, yet the bovine animal is refractory to its teratogenic
effect at normal dosage rates.

With many of the benzimidazoles, the critical exposure time span of early
pregnancy is important as well as the dosage rate. Many label instructions accom-
panying these anthelminthics draw attention of the necessity to avoid suprathera
peutic dosages in early pregnancy. The general pharmacological principles for
species variation in the metabolism of drugs in the liver and to a lesser extent in the
placenta may be an important underlying factor in explaining this refractoriness of
some species to teratogenic drugs. Even when identical active metabolites for
teratogenic drugs are present in different species, other factors, such as placental
transfer, ion trapping in fetal tissues, mechanism of action, the critical exposure
period, and the different rates and patterns of organogenesis and morphological
differentiation, may determine the presence or absence of a congenital abnormality effect.

Although voluntary medication during human pregnancy is best avoided,
the risks inherent from the possible intake of teratogenic compounds in foodstuffs
during pregnancy always exist. One of the dilemmas of this accidental human
exposure to teratogens is knowing whether pregnancy can be recognized early
enough so that exposure can be avoided. Experiments for teratogenic effects in
laboratory animals are conducted under highly artificial conditions: the precise
time of mating is established and so the crucial dates of early pregnancy are
known and identified. This obviously does not mirror the human situation. For
a woman with irregular cycles, it takes longer for a missed cycle to be noted and
therefore for the woman to consider herself pregnant. By that time, however,
drug effects on the developing fetus through inadvertent exposure to a possible
teratogen may already be taking place. Potentially a large population of women
of childbearing age could unknowingly expose their embryos to the risks of
malformation before their pregnancies are recognized.

10.3 PHARMACOLOGICAL HAZARDS

Also of concern are drug residues whose presence in food could result in a pharmacological effect in the consumer in the absence of conventional toxicological effects. A few reports have suggested that prolonged ingestion of tetracyclines from any source, including food, has detrimental effects on teeth and bones in growing children. In addition, reactivation of signs of chloramphenicol toxicity have been reported after consumption of meat, milk, or eggs containing chloramphenicol residues (50). The quantities that could be ingested by such means, however, scarcely approach the therapeutic range and do not reach the levels ordinarily required to produce toxicity, which are usually 100 times the therapeutic dosage.

A pharmacological effect may be observed only when food contains elevated concentrations of potent therapeutics, as in the case of the β-blocker carazolol whose residues in tissues caused sedation; residues of the β-agonist clenbuterol that produced bronchodilatory action; and residues of the anthelminthic ivermectin that produced antiparasitic activity (51).

10.4 MICROBIOLOGICAL HAZARDS

The question of whether residues of veterinary drugs in food can, upon ingestion, exert a selective pressure on the bacterial population of the human gut, thereby favoring the development of resistant bacteria, still is controversial. The same holds for the influence of antibiotic residues on the perturbation of human intestinal microflora. These aspects are increasingly believed not to be a high risk to public health, certainly if compared with the risk of multiple-drug resistance of pathogens, resulting from both the therapeutic and growth-promoting use of antimicrobials.

10.4.1 Perturbation of Human Intestinal Microflora

Therapeutic dosages of antibiotics can cause adverse effects on the ecology of human intestinal microflora. Such adverse effects are a concern because of the important role that the intestinal microflora play in maintaining human health. The bacteria of the human intestine ingest nutrients and intestinal secretions but also play a major role in the metabolism of endogenous substrates such as estrogens, vitamins, cholesterol, and bile acids (52). They contribute to the health of the host due to their inherent colonization resistance property, a natural defense system of the microflora in the gut against colonization of pathogens (53).

The bacterial composition of the intestinal microflora is relatively stable; however, the metabolic activity of the organisms can be easily altered (54). Any metabolic alteration caused by perturbation of the intestinal microflora may affect the metabolism of endogenous compounds and also compromise the effectiveness of other drug therapies, particularly with agents undergoing enterohepatic circulation and, thereby, adversely affect public health.

Most studies of antimicrobial drugs and their effects on human intestinal microflora have been performed at therapeutic drug levels. As an example (55), antibiotics such as tetracycline or erythromycin can greatly decrease the ability of *Eubacterium lentum,* a specific intestinal microorganism, to metabolize the antiarythmic drug digoxin. In individuals taking therapeutic levels of antibiotics, serum digoxin levels were reported to rise by 30–100%. Elevation of serum digoxin levels can result in serious digitalis toxicity.

Another example of concern is the effect of antibiotic therapy on the efficiency of the synthetic and semisynthetic steroids used by more than 50 million women as contraceptive agents. Since 1973, many antibiotics such as ampicillin, amoxycillin, chloramphenicol, and sulfonamides have been shown to cause failures of oral contraceptives due to perturbation of intestinal microflora (56, 57).

In contrast to the well-documented negative effects of therapeutic dosages of antibiotics, the effect of low levels of antibiotics on perturbing the intestinal microflora is not well defined. It is generally anticipated that the effects of antibiotics on the colonic bacteria are commonly minimized by the large number and slow growth rate of these cells. In addition, the infrequency of exposure to residues further decreases the potential for antibiotic drug residues to have any adverse effects on the intestinal microflora. However, it cannot be excluded that low dosages of antimicrobial drugs, such as those found as residues in foods, may alter the intestinal enzyme activity and, thus, have an effect on certain hormones and drugs.

In order to eliminate the potential hazard from the effect of antimicrobial residues on human intestinal microflora, regulatory agencies have determined a maximum safe concentration of 1 ppm in a total diet of 1.5 kg as the level of total antimicrobial residues in food that would produce no effects on the intestinal microflora. All studies on antibiotics performed to date support 1 ppm as being below the effect level for humans (58).

10.4.2   Bacterial Resistance

There has been considerable debate over the role of antimicrobial residues as factors contributing to the relatively high levels of resistance found in human enteric bacterial populations. Whether the relatively high levels of antimicrobial resistance found among enteric bacterial populations arise from medical use, from selection due to exposure to antimicrobial residues, from colonization by antibiotic-resistant organisms related to food production, or from transient colonization of antibiotic-resistant species and transfer of resistance to indigenous populations is undefined (59–62).

The emergence of resistant strains of microorganisms usually follows the prolonged use of drugs at therapeutic levels; however, low levels of drugs may also lead in the development of resistance. Enteric organisms can become resistant to antibiotics at the relatively low exposure rate of 2 ppm antibiotic/day (63). Therefore, any discussion in dealing with residues of antimicrobial agents in food must always address itself to the possibility of induced antibiotic resistance in the consumer. It is important to consider whether residues of antimicrobial agents ingested in food of animal origin constitute a hazard to human health by exerting a selective pressure on the intestinal flora, thereby favoring the growth of microorganisms with natural or acquired resistance. As an alternative, the possibilities of giving rise directly or indirectly to the development of acquired resistance in the pathogenic Enterobacteriaceae cannot be ignored.

By now, it has not been made possible to determine the levels of antimicrobials that can cause an increase of primarily resistant Enterobacteriaceae in the gut of the consumer. As a result, measuring the microbial significance of antimicrobial residues continues to be the subject of considerable discussion. Much of the discussion involves the development of model systems that will reflect the effects of residue levels of antimicrobials on human intestinal microbial populations. The consensus of opinion at a recent symposium is that no such single system is available (64). The human intestine is a very complex microbial ecosystem, about which little is known of the effects of antimicrobial residues on the population dynamics and biochemical responses (65).

In evaluating the effect of residues of antimicrobial drugs on the human gut flora, the characteristics of the flora should be taken into account. There are approximately 10^{11} microbes/g feces, more than 90% of which are anaerobic bacteria. The flora is stable and specific for human individuals, meaning that the bacterial ecology generates important barrier effects that tend to prevent intrusion by foreign microbes (66). Given these characteristics, the establishment of the minimal exposure time or the minimum antimicrobial concentration in the human digestive tract should be based on data obtained from in vivo experiments that take into account the barrier effects and pertain to the identification of bacteria that constitute the human gut flora and to bacteria representative of the whole flora. For this possibility to arise, there is undoubtedly a considerable degree of variation between the susceptibility of individual consumers to such induced bacterial resistance following residue intake.

At present, human epidemiological studies are not able to provide adequate information in this area, given the variations in resistant bacterial flora due to human drug therapy. Nevertheless, published data have suggested that experimentation in human volunteers may be an appropriate methodology.

If human data are not available, other data on experiments in animals may be considered. However, models that involve feeding of low levels of antimicrobials to animals to determine the effects on intestinal bacterial populations are generally complicated by the high percentages of drug-resistant intestinal organisms usually present in the intestinal tract of animals (67). Because of the ubiquitousness and extremely high numbers of antibiotic-resistant organisms in the intestinal populations of animals, nonanimal systems are normally required to evaluate the potential for antimicrobials at residue levels to select for resistant populations, unless special animal models such as holoxenic rodents implanted with human gut flora are used.

Using either animal or human subjects requires keeping exacting records of exposure to antimicrobials, frequently examining fecal samples, studying antimicrobial resistance patterns, and following the molecular biology of the bacteria and plasmids used as indicators over an extended time (68). Regardless of the care taken, conclusions concerning the ecological sequence of events in the processes of selection, development, and transfer of resistance between genera and species would be limited (69).

The fact that an accurate animal model does not exist has not precluded the use of other systems to make estimates of the potential of residues to select for resistance. In the absence of in vivo data, in vitro data such as the minimum inhibitory concentrations (MIC) may be used, on a temporary basis, for safety evaluations. The MIC has been defined as the minimum concentration of an antimicrobial drug giving complete inhibition of growth of a particular microorganism, as judged by the naked eye after a given period of incubation.

The current approach to antimicrobial residue control is based on in vitro experimentation and analysis. Indicator organisms can be representative of target populations or can represent a specific response to a phenomenon. There is always the potential for criticism of the use of an organism whose normal environment is not the intestinal tract. Strains of enterobacteria (*Escherichia coli*) as representatives of the normal gut flora are being increasingly used as test organisms in microbiological assay systems (70). This approach has the advantage of taking into account the relevance of antibiotic residues to organisms of direct significance in human health. The successful growth of the organisms in the presence of animal tissue extracts is conventionally interpreted as an indication of no detectable antimicrobial residues.

Although microbiological in vitro assays are the currently accepted international detection methods, many problems surround their usefulness. Test strains of microorganisms differ widely, as also does their susceptibility to antimicrobial inhibition. A negative result generated from one particular assay technique may yield a positive result when a different test organism is used.

The predictive value of such microbiological tests is also open to question since the site of action is the agar plate and not the human colon, under the conditions of those systems. Using gram-positive and/or gram-negative microorganisms, some authors reported recently a few data on the significance of individual and multiple antimicrobial residues in the development/selection for resistant

populations. Since these data suggested that the safe levels of antimicrobial residues have a strong potential for selecting for resistant populations of bacteria,
the authors further recommended that greater emphasis should be placed on keeping the food supply residue-free rather than reliance on maintaining the working
residue levels suggested by the term "safe levels" (65, 69–71).

The question is not whether there may be in vitro evidence but whether
residue levels, singly or in combination, can select for resistant populations in
vivo experiments. Under in vivo conditions, an antimicrobial residue that is stable
to cooking processes would have to move through the stomach and the intestine,
would then be metabolized during the passage or would be absorbed and excreted.
A portion of it will not occur in the colon, the site of this specific action. Only
a small portion of the ingested dose will reach the colon and remain there for a
certain time, since many conditions have an influence upon the final concentration
at the site of action in the colon.

10.4.3   Effects on the Food Processing Industry

Apart from public health impacts, residual antimicrobials in animal products can
bring about technoeconomic losses in the food processing industry. It has long
been known that the presence of some antimicrobial compounds in milk can
dramatically affect the production of fermented dairy products such as yogurt,
cheese, buttermilk and sour cream (72, 73). As shown in Table 10.2, even minute
concentrations of antibiotics in milk can cause inhibition of the growth of commonly used dairy starter cultures (74).

Table 10.2 further shows that the minimum inhibitory concentration may,
for some antibiotics and some cultures, be lower than the corresponding detection

TABLE 10.2   Minimum Inhibitory Concentrations of Antibiotics for Common Dairy
Starter Cultures and *Bacillus stearothermophilus*

Culture	Chloramphenicol (mg/ml)	Chlortetracycline (mg/ml)	Oxytetracycline (mg/ml)	Penicillin (IU/ml)	Streptomycin (μg/ml)
B. stearothermophilus var. *calidolactis*	1.0	0.6–1.0	1.0	0.001–0.008	0.6–1 .0
Butter starter	0.1–0.2	0.01–0.10	0.01–0.10	0.017–0.170	0.1–0.2
Cheese starter	0.04	0.02–0.25	0.01	0.05–0.20	0.04
Lactobacillus bulgaricus	0.5–5.0	—	—	0.3–0.6	—
Streptococcus cremoris	—	—	—	0.05–0.10	—
Streptococcus thermophilus	0.05–0.10	0.001–0.010	0.001–0.010	0.0017–0.170	0.5–5.0

Source: From Ref. 74.

limit of the commonly used assay microorganism *Bacillus stearothermophilus* var. *calidolactis*. Moreover, residue levels lower than the MIC are sometimes capable of affecting the flavor and texture properties of the dairy products (73, 75) while promoting the growth of undesirable antibiotic resistant coliforms (73, 76). Therefore, routine application of adequately sensitive test kits is required to avoid major losses due to presence of undetected but fermentation-inhibiting residues in milk.

Among the antimicrobial residues giving rise to such technological problems in the manufacture of dairy products, residues of penicillin G in particular have been determined as most important. This is the reason why measures to reduce the presence of penicillin G residues in milk were originally taken: to prevent economic loss and not due to public health concerns.

The technological consequences of the presence of drug residues in meat should not be neglected. Fermentation failure in the production of dry sausages was recently demonstrated to be caused by the presence of residues of antimicrobial drugs such as penicillin and tetracycline in the raw material (77). The concentrations involved were about 0.9 and 1.6 IU penicillin and about 4 and 1.9 μg tetracycline/g sausage.

10.5 IMMUNOLOGICAL HAZARDS

Drug residues in animal-derived food are sometimes incriminated in human allergic reactions as well. There are not many reported cases of humans exhibiting an allergic reaction that can be definitely traced to a drug residue source, and the overwhelming majority of these pertain to allergic reactions to penicillin. It is supported, however, that the observations made in the field actually represent a small percentage of the food intolerance problem. Most reactions of this type, of known cause, are mainly attributed to normal food constituents (78). The inherent complexity of retrospective-case epidemiological studies, which is confounded with the perplexity of marketing, processing, and distribution practices of most animal products, is considered the major cause of the existing debate.

Antibiotic allergy in humans is a complex subject. For a drug to produce an allergic reaction, a prior sensitizing contact is required either with the same drug or with one closely related. Exposure to the drug, which is the primary eliciting contact, results in an antigen–antibody interaction that provokes the typical manifestation of allergy (79).

For small molecules to stimulate an immunological hypersensitivity response, covalent binding with macromolecules such as proteins or polysaccharides should occur (80). The resultant immunological response will be specific for the drug portion of the conjugate, and antibody precursor cells will respond by producing immunoglobulins (IgE) antibodies. The first step in an acute allergic reaction is the fixation of IgE antibody to blood basophilic or tissue mast cells. The dosage of a drug necessary to produce this primary sensitization is considerably higher than that required to elicit an allergic response. When a drug appears again in the body as a result of ingestion of food contaminated with residues, the IgE antibodies attached to the surface of the sensitized basophilic bind to the antigenic form of the drug. The sensitized tissue mast cells and blood basophilics release histamine, leukotrienes, and other mediators with the ability to act on smooth muscle and other end-organs to produce a variety of hypersensitive allergic responses including anaphylaxis, urticaria, and angioedema.

The reactive antigenic fraction for many veterinary drugs is a cleavage metabolite. In the case of penicillin G, the major reactive product is the penicilloyl moiety that forms more than 95% of the penicillin conjugates. This determinant can combine with a carrier protein through opening of the β-lactam ring. Since all penicillins share the basic 6-amino-penicillinic acid nucleus, they can form the benzyl penicilloyl metabolite following opening of the β-lactam ring. This derivative is responsible for the cross-allergenicity demonstrated to other β-lactams such as cephalosporins and the semisynthetic penicillins such as carbenicillin or ampicillin.

Animal drug residues are unlikely to play a role as sensitizing agents but could trigger an allergic response in sensitized persons. Although reports of allergic reactions following ingestion of antibiotic residues in food have been uncommon, the risk to already sensitive individuals cannot be discounted. The majority of the few reported cases implicate penicillin as the offending agent (81–86) and the source of penicillin residues originated mostly from intramammary infusions (87) or from minced meat taken from an injection site (88). In all instances, the patients reported a history of penicillin allergy or skin disease unrelated to penicillin therapy.

For penicillin, primary sensitization usually follows parenteral administration (80) and seldom oral therapy (89). Therefore, development of primary sensitization following consumption of foodborne residues is a negligible risk. The probability of eliciting an allergic response in an individual who has consumed penicillin residues and has been previously sensitized depends on the threshold dosage necessary to elicit a reaction. It has still not been determined if repeated ingestion of subthreshold dosage could subsequently produce allergic symptoms.

Foodborne allergic reactions to other drugs have been documented only in a single report of a 14-year-old girl who experienced anaphylaxis on four separate occasions. Before each attack, the girl, who had positive skin test reactions and evidence of antibodies to streptomycin, had eaten a meal containing ground beef. Although the meat was not available for testing, the girl had eaten beef before with no problem. Thus, while this case is highly suggestive of streptomycin involvement, there was only presumptive evidence of food contamination (90).

Besides β-lactams and streptomycin, many other drugs including sulfon-amides, and to a lesser extent neomycin, nitrofurans, erythromycin, spiramycin, novobiocin, and the tetracyclines, are known to cause allergic reactions in sensitive persons (80, 91). However, such reactions in humans are variable and are mostly related to therapeutic use.

The scarcity of reported allergic problems due to antimicrobial drug residues in food is surprising in light of the estimate that high proportions of the population are allergic to these drugs. Numerous surveys carried out on both the general population and patients attending hospital clinics have indicated that the incidence of antibiotic allergies in the population is 10% for penicillins including ampicillin, 5% for cephalosporins, 0.5% for erythromycin, 13% for sulfonamides, 5% for tetracyclines, and 3% for trimethoprim (92). Possibly, the reason that few cases are documented is that many may be masked by other health conditions, particularly in elderly populations, and/or by the inclination of humans to develop allergic sensitivity to milk proteins, by the variable nature and extent of penicillin allergy, and possibly by the likely exposure to penicillin-like molecules in molds in the environment. However, the low number of reports might equally well be attributed to insufficient amounts or absence of drug residues in foods. In a total of 252 patients with chronic recurrent urticaria, 70 (27.8%) were determined to be allergic to penicillin (93). When 52 of the positive-reacting patients were placed on a milk-free diet, 30 (58%) experienced remission of symptoms. Conversely, changing to a milk-free diet caused remission of symptoms in only 2 patients of a group of 40 (5%) with chronic urticaria but with negative results of tests for allergies to penicillin.

Because of the paucity of valid predictive tests for assessing the allergenic potential of veterinary drug residues (16), the lowest practical tolerance levels must be set for drugs for which high allergenic potential is likely. For example, 10 IU benzyl penicillin has been regarded as safe for oral ingestion in sensitized individuals (81, 94). Microbiological assays capable of detecting 0.005 ppm of this antibiotic should accordingly be adequate to guard against the likely induction of allergy in sensitized individuals. Nonetheless, some extremely sensitive individuals may experience adverse reactions to lower levels of penicillin, even to levels undetectable by standard analytical methods. Because of the limitations of current knowledge on the role of low drug concentrations in hypersensitivity reactions, there are few clinical experimental or epidemiological data from which to estimate the risk to humans from consumption of food products containing antibiotic residues.

10.6 ENZYME PERTURBATION HAZARDS

Some other hazards that have not been still widely considered concern the effect drug residues in edible animal products may have on consumers' enzyme systems.

Although it is difficult to assess whether induction or inhibition of hepatic micro-somal enzyme systems will have any practical bearing on the health of humans, such hazards cannot be excluded.

Due to detoxification and sequestration mechanisms inherent in any living organism, humans have an apparent unlimited capacity to adapt to contact with xenobiotic compounds, provided that this contact is on a low scale. However, this potential for detoxification may be insufficient at certain stages of the human lifespan. This is especially true for the embryo in the uterus, the newly born infant, the elderly, or the individual with dysfunction of the liver or kidney. In such instances, severe toxic reactions to the intake of drugs can be manifested in a most severe fashion. Such groups may also be at most risk from ingestion of residue-contaminated food. What may be considered an acceptable risk for a healthy adult may not be so for an infant with a partly developed drug-metaboliz-ing enzyme capacity. Therefore, a substance with an established lack of safety should obviously not be used, whereas a substance with a potential for human health hazard must be assessed under the circumstances of its use and toxicologi-cal potential.

Enzymes responsible for the bioactivation of drugs to chemically reactive metabolites constitute the microsomal P-450 mixed function enzymes. Such major drug-metabolizing enzymatic systems can be induced or inhibited after exposure to lipophilic drugs of relatively long biological half-lives with an ability to bind to cytochrome P-450 enzymes. Induction of such enzymes by secondary drugs may play a critical role, albeit an indeterminate one, in the final establishment of the ultimate toxicity of the metabolite to the body system. Enzyme induction involves an adaptive change and increase in the number of drug metabolizing enzymes in response to an enzyme-inducing agent.

Exposure, for example, of newly born rats to hormones alters their response later in life to carcinogens that are biotransformed in the liver. Diethylstilbestrol is genotoxic, but restriction of its carcinogenic effects to hormonally responsive tissues indicates the hormonal mechanisms underlying its carcinogenicity. The subsequent appearance of diethylstilbestrol tumors in the neonate suggests the development of neoplasia by the process of imprinting of enzymatic systems during exposure in the uterus.

A number of substances that are enzyme inducers are also carcinogens. Establishing a correlation between the two properties is vexing. The possibility remains, however, that enzyme induction may influence both the initiation and the promotion of experimentally induced carcinogenesis. Commonly used veterinary drugs including phenobarbital, phenylbutazone, griseofulvin, and halogenated an-esthetics are known enzyme inducers. Phenobarbital and griseofulvin have been observed to increase the incidence of hepatic neoplasms in mice.

Significant changes in drug-metabolizing activities can be detected by phar-macokinetic studies, which indicate an increased ability to stimulate the metabolism of differing substrates by a variety of biotransformation pathways. Relative changes in the amounts of multiple forms of cytochrome P-450 can be induced by exogenous or endogenous factors, such as disease states, drug intake, and perhaps drug residues in food. Polycyclic aromatic hydrocarbon produced from steroids in meat when cooked over charcoal can exert a selective inductive effect.

Enzymatic induction may result in diminished biological effect in response to increased biotransformation activity. Drug interaction can also arise after the concomitant administration of two or more drugs, either or both of which may be enzyme inducers. Increased toxicological effects by which the endogenous production of chemically reactive electrophilic metabolites can trigger a range of toxic activities by reacting covalently with essentially cellular components is another significant possibility.

Enzyme inhibition mediated via suicide enzyme inactivators and suicide enzyme inhibitors is another critical dimension of the toxicological potential of drugs. This phenomenon may induce side effects or drug interactions. Impairment of microsomal drug-metabolizing capacity can lead to reduced clearance and elevated plasma levels of other drugs or metabolites. Interactions with oral hypoglycemic agents, such as tolbutamide, can precipitate a hypoglycemic crisis from the coadministration of chloramphenicol, a known microsomal enzyme inhibitor. Chloramphenicol increases the duration of pentobarbital anesthesia significantly in dogs and cats. Steroid metabolism is impaired by drug-metabolizing enzyme inhibitors.

REFERENCES

1. A.P. Knight, J. Am. Vet. Med. Assoc., 178:309 (1981).
2. Council of Europe, in Residues of Veterinary Drugs in Food of Animal Origin, Straatsburg, p. 18 (1986).
3. Food and Agriculture Organization (FAO), in Residues of Veterinary Drugs in Food, Report of a Joint FAO/WHO Expert Consultation, No. 32, Rome (1985).
4. Food and Drug Administration, Fed. Reg, 50:45530 (1985).
5. J.R. Gillette, Biochem. Pharmacol., 23:2785 (1974).
6. J.R. Gillette, and L.R. Pohl, J. Toxicol. Environ. Health, 2:849 (1977).
7. P. Delatour, F. Garnier, E. Benoit, and C. Longin, J. Vet. Pharmacol. Ther., 7:139 (1984).
8. H. Gottmanns, R. Kroker, and F.R. Ungemach, in Residues of Veterinary Drugs in Food, Proc. Euroresidue Conf., Noordwijkerhout, May 21–23, 1990 (N. Haagsma, A. Ruiter, and P.B. Czedik-Eysenberg, Eds.), Fac. Vet. Med., Univ. Utrecht, The Netherlands, p. 196 (1990).
9. S. Klee, F.R. Ungemach, and R. Kroker, in Residues of Veterinary Drugs in Food, Proc. Euroresidue Conf., Noordwijkerhout, May 21–23, 1990 (N. Haagsma, A. Ruiter, and P.B. Czedik-Eysenberg, Eds.), Fac. Vet. Med., Univ. Utrecht, The Netherlands, p. 240 (1990).

10. N.E. Weber, J. Environ. Pathol. Toxicol., 3:35 (1980).
11. N.E. Weber, Toxicol. Eur. Res., 4:271 (1982).
12. J.L. Stevens and A. Wallin, Drug Metabol. Rev., 22:827 (1977).
13. W. Jaggi, W.K. Lutz, J. Luthy, U. Zweifel, and C. Schlatter, Food Cosmet. Toxicol., 18:257 (1980).
14. R. Truhaut, and R. Ferrando, Toxicology, 3:361 (1975).
15. J.E. Baer, T.A. Jacob, and F.J. Wolf, J. Toxicol. Environ. Health, 2:895 (1977).
16. P. Delatour, R.C. Parish, and G.J. Gyurik, Ann. Rech. Vet., 12:159 (1981).
17. D.M. Galer and A.M. Monro, Food Addit. Contam., 15:494 (1998).
18. H. Gallo-Torres, J. Toxicol. Environ. Health, 2:827 (1977).
19. G.C. Scott and S.J. DiCuollo, Int. Conf. Eur. Assoc. Vet. Pharmacol. Toxicol., Cambridge, UK (1980).
20. Food and Drug Administration, in General Principles for Evaluating the Safety of Compounds Used in Food-Producing animals, revised 1994, VIII, Center for Veterinary Medicine, Rockville, MD, USA (1994).
21. A.Y.H. Lu, S.L. Chiu, and P.G. Wislocki, Drug Metabol. Rev., 22:891 (1990).
22. W.L. Hewitt, Fed. Proc., 34:202 (1975).
23. W.D. Black, Can. J. Physiol. Pharmacol., 62:1044 (1984).
24. A.M. Bongiovanni, J. Pediatr., 103:245 (1983).
25. W.H. Hannon, R.H. Hill, J.T. Bernet, L. Haddock, G. Lebron, and J.F. Cordero, Arch. Environ. Contam. Toxicol., 16:255 (1987).
26. Food Safety and Inspection Service (FSIS), in Special Meat and Poultry Sampling Program, US Department of Agriculture, Washington, DC, p. 1 (1986).
27. B. Hoffman, in The Use of Hormones in Food-Producing Animals, Proceedings of the Health Aspects of Residues of Anabolics in Meat, Vol. 59, p. 16 (1982).
28. G.R. Foxcroft, in Drug Residues in Animals (A. Rico, Ed.), Academic Press, Orlando, FL, p. 147 (1986).
29. G.E. Lamming, Vet. Rec., 121:389 (1987).
30. B.C. Polak, P.H. Wesseling, A. Herxheimer, and L. Meyler, Acta Med. Scand., 192:409 (1972).
31. J.A. Settapani, J. Am. Vet. Med. Assoc., 184:930 (1984).
32. T.E. Cone, and S.M. Abelson, J. Pediatr., 41:340 (1952).
33. F.T. Fraunfelder, and G.C. Bagby, Jr., Am. J. Ophthalmol., 93:356 (1982).
34. Food and Drug Administration, Fed. Reg., 50:27059 (1985).
35. Food Safety and Inspection Service (FSIS), in Domestic Residue Data Book, National Residue Program 1983, US Department of Agriculture, Washington, DC, July, p. 71 (1986).
36. Food Safety and Inspection Service (FSIS), in Domestic Residue Data Book, National Residue Program 1984, US Department of Agriculture, Washington, DC, October, p. 70 (1986).
37. Food Safety and Inspection Service (FSIS), in Domestic Residue Data Book, National Residue Program 1985, US Department of Agriculture, Washington, DC, May, p. 53 (1987).
38. Food Safety and Inspection Service (FSIS), in Domestic Residue Data Book, National Residue Program 1986, US Department of Agriculture, Washington, DC, October, p. 69 (1987).

39. Food and Drug Administration, in Extra-Label Use of New Animal Drugs in Food-Producing Animals, Compliance Policy Guide 7126.06, Food and Drug Administration, Rockville, M.D. (1986).
40. Anonymous, Weekly Epidemiol. Rec., 37:279 (1992).
41. J.F. Martinez-Navarro, Lancet, 336:1131 (1990).
42. Anonymous, Ned. Tijdschr. Geneeskd., 136:2144 (1992).
43. L. Salleras, A. Dominguez, E. Mata, J.L. Taberner, I. Moro, and P. Salva, Public Health Rep., 110:338 (1995).
44. C. Pulce, D. Lamaison, G. Keck, C. Bostvirnnois, J. Nokolas, and J. Descotes, Vet. Human Toxicol., 33:480 (1991).
45. W.C. Keller, FDA Veterinarian, 6:9 (1991).
46. V. Sporano, L. Grasso, M.E. Chem, G.O. Chem, G. Brambilla, and A. Loizo, Vet. Human Toxicol., 40:141 (1998).
47. H.A. Kuiper, M.Y. Noordam, M.M.H. van Dooren-Flipsen, R. Schilt, and A.H. Roos, J. Anim. Sci., 76:195 (1998).
48. M.L. Martinez-Frias, A. Cereijo, E. Rodriquez-Pinilla, and M. Urioste, Lancet, 339: 742 (1992).
49. A.R.M. Kidd, Pig Vet. Soc. Proc., 16:82 (1986).
50. T.B. Barragry, in Veterinary Drug Therapy (T.B. Barragry, Ed.), Lea & Febiger, Philadelphia, p. 336 (1994).
51. F.X.R. van Leeuwen, Proceedings of PAON-course on Veterinary Drugs and Vaccins, 14–15 November, Zeist, The Netherlands, 1989
52. G.L. Simon, and S.L. Gorbach, Dig. Dis. Sci., 1:475 (1986).
53. L. Tollefson, Reg. Toxicol. Pharmacol., 13:150 (1991).
54. S.L. Gorbach, Vet. Hum. Toxicol., 35:15 (1993).
55. R.J. Carmen, R.L. Van Tassell, and R.D. Willens, Vet. Hum. Toxicol., 35:11 (1993).
56. J. Lindenbaum, D.L. Rund, and V.P. Butler, N. Engl. J. Med., 305:789 (1981).
57. M.J. Tikkanen, H. Adlercreutz, and M.O. Pulkkinen, Br. Med. J., 2:369 (1973).
58. J.C. Paige, L. Tollefson, and M. Miller, Vet. Hum. Toxicol., 39:162 (1997).
59. K.A. Bettleheim, F.M. Bushrod, M.E. Chandler, E.M. Cooke, S. O'Farrell, and R.A. Shooter, J. Hyg., 73:467 (1974).
60. S.B. Levy, G.B. Fitzgerald, and A.B. Macone, Nature, 260:40 (1976).
61. A.H. Linton, K. Howe, P.M. Bennett, M.H. Richmond, and E.J. Whiteside, J. Appl. Bacteriol., 43:465 (1977).
62. D.C. Hirsh, and N. Wigner, J. Anim. Sci., 46:1437 (1978).
63. W.G. Huber, Adv. Vet. Sci. Comp. Med., 15:101 (1971).
64. Food and Drug Administration, in Microbiological Significance of Drug Residues in Foods, Symp., June 8, Food and Drug Administration, Animal Health Institute and Center for Veterinary Medicine, Rockville, MD (1992).
65. M.S. Brady, N. White, and S.E. Katz, J. Food Prot., 56:229 (1993).
66. World Health Organization, in Evaluation of Certain Veterinary Drug Residues in Food, Thirty-sixth Report of the Joint FAO/WHO Expert Committee on Food Additives, Technical Report Series 799, World Health Organization, Geneva, p. 13 (1990).
67. S.W. Mamber, and S.E. Katz, Appl. Environ. Microbiol., 50:638 (1985).
68. M.W. Richmond, in The Evolution of Antibiotic Resistance, Squibb Institute for Medical Research, New Brunswick, NJ (1980).

69. M.S. Brady, and S.E. Katz, J. Assoc. Off. Anal. Chem., 71:299 (1988).
70. M.S. Brady, R.J. Strobel, and S.E. Katz, J. Assoc. Off. Anal. Chem., 71:295 (1988).
71. M.S. Brady, and S.E. Katz, J. AOAC Int., 75:738 (1992).
72. A. Kilara, in Safety of Foods (H.D. Graham, Ed.), The Avi Publishing Company, Westport, CT, p. 536 (1982).
73. H. Mol, in Antibiotics in Milk, Thesis, Utrecht, Rotterdam (1975).
74. International Dairy Federation, Chemical Residues in Milk and Milk Products, Document 113, International Dairy Federation, Brussels, Belgium (1979).
75. G.J.E. Hunter, J. Dairy Res., 16:235 (1949).
76. P. Kastli, Schweiz. Arch. Tierheilk., 90:685 (1948).
77. K. Koenen-Dierick and J. van Hoof, Vlaams Diergeneeskd. Tijdschr., 57:109 (1988).
78. V. Burgat-Sacaze, A. Rico, and J.-C. Panisset, in Drug Residues in Animals (A.G. Rico, Ed.), Academic Press, Inc., Orlando, FL, p. 1 (1986).
79. R.R.A. Coombs, and P.G.M. Gell, in Clinical Aspects of Immunology (PGM Gell, Ed.), Blackwell Scientific, Oxford, p. 761 (1975).
80. W.G. Huber, in Drug Residues in Animals (A.G. Rico, Ed.), Academic Press, Inc., Orlando, FL, p. 33 (1986).
81. P. Borrie, and J. Barrett, Br. J. Med., 2:1267 (1961).
82. D. Erskine, Lancet, 1:431 (1958).
83. H.R. Vickers, L. Bagratuni, and S. Alexander, Lancet, 1:351 (1958).
84. H.R. Vickers, Proc. R. Soc. Med., 57:1091 (1964).
85. K. Wicher, R.E. Reisman, and C.E. Abresman, JAMA, 208:143 (1969).
86. I. Tscheuchner, Z. Haut. Gescl., 47:591 (1972).
87. B. Siegel, Bull. WHO, 21:703 (1959).
88. R.C. Wilson, in Animal Drugs and Human Health (L.M. Crawford, and D.A. Franco, Eds.), Technomic Publishing Co., Lancaster, PA, p. 63 (1994).
89. J.P. Girard, Helv. Med. Acta, 36:3 (1972).
90. D.G. Tinkleman, and S.A. Bock, Ann. Allergy, 53:243 (1984).
91. L.E. Schindel, Antibiot. Chemother., 13:300 (1965).
92. J.R. Algird, Conn. Med., 30:878 (1966).
93. W.J. Boonk, and W.G. van Ketel, Br. J. Dermatol. 106:183 (1982).
94. H. Lindemayr, R. Knobler, D. Kraft, and W. Baumgartner, Allergy, 36:471 (1981).

11

Safety Assessment and Control of Residues

A large variety of active ingredients and increasingly sophisticated formulations are now available in the market for the animal industry. When these drugs are administered to food-producing animals, the main area of concern is undoubtedly consumer safety arising from the presence of residues. Because it is perceived as a food safety issue, the topic of drug residues in food is a highly emotive one and can elicit a strong public reaction that can adversely influence both domestic and international markets.

As human food safety from drug residues is of utmost importance, a large amount of information is required to be presented by the pharmaceutical industry before marketing authorization for a particular drug can be granted. No veterinary drug can be marketed in a country before having received approval of the competent national authority. Different regulatory authorities have differing requirements; thus, it would be impracticable to try to describe the various procedures established by regulatory authorities throughout the world. Instead, a general overview of those procedures will be given below. Pertinent legislation giving the frame of adequate handling of drugs in intensive livestock farming is now available in most developed countries and is also briefly outlined below.

11.1 GENERAL OVERVIEW

To evaluate the safety aspects of a drug intended for use in food-producing animals, multistep procedures have to be applied. A major portion of these procedures refer to toxicity studies. Over the last 30 years, a broadly accepted package of toxicity studies conducted in laboratory animals has emerged for assessing drug toxicity.

Although the need to conduct a particular toxicity study may depend on the results of another, most regulatory authorities generally request a package of toxicity studies including an acute toxicity study, a 28 day or 90 day short-term toxicity study, and long-term studies on genotoxicity, carcinogenicity, teratogenicity, and reproductive performance. The major goal is to identify a dosage level that will have no effect on the most sensitive animal species, assuming that long-term toxicological studies have not shown adverse manifestations such as genotoxic carcinogenicity but some toxicity has been identified (1). This dosage is what is called the "no-observed effect level" (NOEL).

For a genotoxic carcinogen—an agent that causes cancer by a direct effect on the genetic material of a cell—a NOEL cannot be established. Current scientific knowledge indicates that it is unacceptable to be faced with the possibility of residues of genotoxic carcinogens in edible animal products. However, a few genotoxic carcinogens are biotransformed to nonactive metabolites after their administration to food-producing animals. This is the case with carbadox, a growth promoter for swine, which produces nontoxic residues although the drug itself is both mutagenic and carcinogenic in laboratory studies (2). For such compounds, alternative risk assessment is possible and residues may be viewed as more acceptable.

Once a NOEL has been established, an acceptable daily intake (ADI), which is the quantity that can be taken by the consumer without the likelihood of being harmful, can be calculated using a suitable safety factor (3, 4). There has been considerable debate over the magnitude of this safety factor but the one usually chosen is 100. If toxic effects in laboratory species are not observed but some minor adverse reactions in humans are identified, a smaller factor, usually 10, may be employed instead. When severe forms of toxicity are noted or there is some degree of uncertainty about the performance of the toxicity studies, a larger factor may be chosen and a temporary ADI can be adopted (5, 6). An ADI can also be calculated for a nongenotoxic carcinogen, if the mechanism of carcinogenicity is known. Sulfamethazine and steroid hormones are examples of such nongenotoxic compounds for which a NOEL and an ADI can be determined in suitable experimental models (7, 8).

After an ADI has been determined, it is essential that a maximum residue limit (MRL) in each particular edible animal product be specified so that its consumption by humans will not result in a residue intake exceeding the ADI. The elaboration of MRLs depends on a number of food intake factors including the likely degree of consumption of the edible animal product in question and the normal dietary habits among the population. Currently, there is much debate over these factors and their realistic evaluation for the commodities involved.

Residues at the MRL in a food commodity usually result in intakes well below the ADI. As a result, residues above the MRL do not represent any immediate risk to a consumer. A residue will need to be many times greater than the MRL in a food before the ADI is approached by the consumer. However, in the face of strict trade requirements, a residue above the MRL could mean failure to meet specifications and loss of access to export markets.

Once MRLs have been established, it is next essential to ensure that the edible products of the treated animals do not exceed these values. This is not as simple as it might appear at first (9). The requirements of therapy dictate that numerous formulations administered by various routes be used even for a single active ingredient. Therefore, the depletion profile of a particular drug in the living animal will not be constant but will vary according to the formulation given and the route of administration. Moreover, the species, or more correctly the metabolism in that species, will determine the rate of residue depletion. This means that residue depletion studies are generally required by regulatory authorities for each species using each formulation and route of administration.

Drug residue studies usually involve treating the animal in question with the intended formulation under the intended route of administration, usually at the highest recommended dosage and the maximum duration of administration. Animals are then serially slaughtered so that residues depletion can be studied and the time taken to achieve levels below the MRL can be established. These studies should, if conducted properly, show the residue depletion profile of the formulation under study and will reveal any reemergence of residues because, for example, of enterohepatic recirculation. The time taken for the residues to be depleted to below the MRL for each of the tissues of interest is then usually defined as the withdrawal period for that formulation. Usually the studies must be conducted in each of the indicated species, although simpler and cheaper bioequivalence studies, in which pharmacokinetic profiles are examined and compared, may be used to evaluate the withdrawal period in other food-producing species.

Withdrawal periods can be a cause for argument between pharmaceutical companies and regulatory authorities, often for competitive marketing reasons. If two similar pharmaceutical products are available for a particular therapeutic purpose, the veterinarian or farmer will usually choose the one with the shorter withdrawal periods so that, if necessary, the animal can be sent to slaughter at the earliest possible time after therapy. These considerations are extremely important for milk and eggs because animals can be retained from slaughter using a suitable withdrawal time until drug residues decay to below the MRLs, but residues in the milk and eggs collected during drug administration do not deplete with time. Consequently, it is necessary to discard these products until levels fall to or below the MRL Similar considerations can be applied to honey. When bees are treated for disease conditions, the drug accumulates in the honey (10, 11), and, if it slowly changes to nonbiologically active residues, the honey may be consumed. If it persists, the honey will need to be discarded until treatment has finished (12, 13).

Determining MRLs in fish presents particular problems because the metabolic rates of drugs are partly governed by fish body temperature, which is, in turn, dependent upon the ambient temperature of the water in which they live: the cooler the water, the longer residue depletion takes. For this reason, residue depletion studies in fish are usually conducted at several temperatures chosen to represent the range of temperatures to which they will be exposed under normal farming conditions. Withdrawal periods are then quoted in degree days, a unit that is a function of both time and temperature.

Present regulatory standards require that drugs be regulated on the basis of total residues. Total residues resulting from drug administration to an animal consist of the parent drug and all metabolites, conjugates, and residues bound to endogenous macromolecules. To ensure compliance with the withdrawal period, an assay is needed to monitor total residues in the edible tissues. However, it would be impractical to subject all known metabolites of a drug to analysis, since some drugs can give rise to numerous metabolites. The anthelminthic levamisole, for example, affords over 50 metabolites in the rat (14).

Because it is impractical to develop assays for each residue in each of the edible tissues, the concepts of the "marker residue" and the "target tissue" have been introduced. Marker residue is a selected analyte whose level in a particular tissue has a known relationship to the level of the total residue of toxicological concern in all edible tissues. Therefore, it can be taken as a measure of the total residue of interest in the target animal. Information obtained from studies on the depletion of radiolabeled total residue can be used to calculate a level of the marker residue that must not be exceeded in a selected in a selected tissue, (the target tissue) if the total residue of toxicological concern in the edible tissues of the target animal is not to exceed its safe concentration.

Questions are often raised for bound residues because their impact on the ADI must be assessed as well. Such an assessment raises the question of the degree of bioavailability of bound residues and their biological activity (15). In most cases, this question has no simple answers. Of course a drug may be metabolized to carbon dioxide or some other simple precursor of normal endogenous biochemicals. If these arise from a radiolabeled portion of the molecule, measurements of residues simply as incorporated radiolabel will lead the investigator to suspect bound residues when in fact there are only normal bodily constituents containing incorporated isotope. The complexity of the problem can easily be seen in the case of ronidazole (16). Ronidazole itself is mutagenic but its bound residues are devoid of genotoxic potential and so do not offer a risk to the consumer. Bound residues of carbadox, cambendazole and furazolidone have been also shown to be devoid of toxicological concern (17–19). In contrast, reactive metabolites have been regenerated from bound residues of trenbolone by hepatic monooxygenases in vitro, although the toxicological significance for the in vivo situation is still unclear (20).

The overall effect of regulating on total residues as opposed to the parent drug is a lowering of the MRL level. The amount by which the MRL decreases depends on the proportion of the parent drug to the sum of total residues. For some antibiotics, the parent drug may be a good approximation of total residues if the compounds are not metabolized. For other drugs, however, the parent drug may be a vanishingly small fraction of the total residues and, therefore, the parent drug would not able to serve as a marker residue for total residues; if not, the MRLs would be greatly reduced due to the low percentage of the parent drug.

Only a few of the currently regulated antibiotics would not require total residue studies to support requests for new uses. Examples include the tetracyclines, aminoglycosides, bacitracin, and bambermycin. The tetracyclines are not significantly metabolized and the parent drug is a good approximation of the total residues, since degradation to the epi-form may occur to only a small extent. The aminoglycosides undergo limited metabolism and their absorption from the gastrointestinal tract is low, whereas the lack of absorption also has been demonstrated with bacitracin and bambermycin.

Specific problems are sometimes presented by residues of drugs that exhibit pharmacological activity. The pharmacological effect that is desired for the patients is unwelcome for the consumers, particularly if they are extremely sensitive to such an effect, β-Blockers such as carazolol are examples in which the inadvertent pharmacological effect can be extremely undesirable in individuals with cardiovascular or respiratory diseases. Other examples of drugs with pharmacological activity are the tranquillizers, β-agonists, and anesthetics. Since the protective effect of most of these drugs, used to minimize preslaughter losses in pigs, is normally required right to the time of slaughter, it is highly likely that their residues will be present in animal tissues in high concentrations.

Under such circumstances, acceptable safety for the consumer would require the demonstration that these residues are not only toxicologically acceptable but also are without the possibility of pharmacological effect. Even in the case of a drug that has been allocated a zero withdrawal period, as in the case of azaperone in some countries, it is unlikely that these criteria would be met. In the case of a drug licensed for use with any longer withdrawal period, as in the case of propiopromazine, the criteria are even less likely to be met. These considerations have caused some manufacturers to remove the immediate preslaughter use from clinical indications for their products.

A controversial area of risk assessment concerns the possible effects of residues of antimicrobial drugs on the human gut flora, favoring the growth of microorganisms with natural or acquired resistance to the drug in question. Available risk assessment studies include studies in human volunteers, studies in germ-free (holoxenic) rodents, and in vitro studies with bacterial populations (16, 21). Studies in human volunteers involve examination of the human fecal flora before and after treatment with antibiotics; colonization of the gastrointestinal tract by adventitious microorganisms is also investigated.

Studies in germ-free rodents follow the same design as with human volunteers. Animals are inoculated with human gut flora and the effects of antimicrobials are then studied. In vitro studies with bacterial populations, examine the effects of varying concentrations of the drug or drugs of interest on cultures of indicator organisms. All three studies can be used to derive NOELs for toxicity towards the bacteria employed. More specifically, the minimum inhibitory concentration (MIC) values can be determined. However, applying the results of testing for antimicrobial resistance may result in very low MRLs and long withdrawal periods.

Because drug registration processes that establish MRLs are typically complex and involve lengthy procedures that require investment of considerable technical and financial resources, in countries where a particular drug is not used or needed, its registration is not normally sought by drug manufacturers. In these circumstances, regulatory authorities usually do not establish an MRL and set a default tolerance for a particular commodity/residue combination at zero. Because default tolerances are not based on a scientific evaluation of the drug concerned, they have no intrinsic food safety standing. However, they serve as a regulatory limit by which foods produced domestically or overseas must comply.

Problems sometimes can arise when an importing country has not established an MRL for a certain drug in common use in the exporting country. This does not necessarily mean that the drug has been banned but it could mean that the importing country has no need for the particular drug and has had no cause to establish an MRL. The absence of an MRL, however, has exactly the same effect as an MRL of zero, because in the absence of an MRL any detectable residue is unacceptable.

11.2 REGULATORY OUTLINE BY INTERNATIONAL ORGANIZATIONS

The global nature of the food supply and world food trade have made food quality and food safety international issues. Hence, since its inception, the World Health Organization (WHO) has been working toward the improvement of food safety. In partnership with the Food and Agriculture Organization of the United Nations (FAO), WHO provides for the Secretariat of the Codex Alimentarius Commission (CAC). The latter Commission is responsible for all matters pertaining to the implementation of the Joint FAO/WHO Food Standards Program.

The purpose of this program is to protect the health of consumers and ensure fair practices in the food trade; to promote coordination of all food-standards labor undertaken by international governmental and nongovernmental organizations; to determine priorities and to initiate and guide the preparation of draft standards through and with the aid of appropriate organizations; to finalize food standards; after acceptance by governments, to publish them in a Codex Alimentarius either as regional or worldwide standards together with international standards already finalized by other bodies; and to amend published standards after appropriate survey in the light of new research developments.

The Codex Alimentarius is a code of food standards for all nations. All members of CAC and interested international organizations are invited to comment on proposed standards, including possible implications for their economic interests. Members are encouraged to consult with interested and affected parties in their countries. Codex standards are recognized by the World Trade Organization as the international reference standards for food safety.

Development of standards, guidelines, and recommendations for veterinary drug residues in food has been delegated by CAC to its subsidiary body, the Codex Committee on Residues of Veterinary Drugs in Foods (CCRVDF), which is more routinely involved in risk management. The work of this subcommittee is mainly supported by the Joint FAO/WHO Expert Committee on Food Additives (JECFA).

JECFA is a scientific advisory body established in the 1950s, prior to the establishment of the CAC. Over the past 40 years, it has provided independent scientific advice to all FAO and WHO member countries. The traditional and current activities of JECFA are mainly in the area of risk assessment, not risk management. To some extent, however, JECFA activities also touch on risk management. Risk assessment, risk management, and risk communication constitute the three basic elements of risk analysis that are taken into account in the Codex procedure for setting MRLs of veterinary drug residues in foods (Table 11.1).

Risk assessment, a process used to evaluate potential adverse effects on health from human exposure to veterinary drug residues, involves four stages starting from hazard identification and terminating through the hazard characterization and exposure assessment stages to risk characterization.

In the hazard identification stage, all drug residues in food that are capable of causing adverse effects on human health have to be identified. The definition of veterinary drug residue adopted by the Codex Alimentarius includes both the parent drug and the sum of its biotransformation products that may be present in animal-derived food. The metabolic changes vary in magnitude depending on the substances and may in some cases be intense and rapid. In such cases, it is technically and hence economically difficult to identify all the residues resulting from the parent substance. Therefore, in the case of heavy metabolism of the substance under study, hazard identification is basically limited in practical terms to this substance and to the main residues resulting from its metabolism. Consequently, while for practical reasons the MRL values are usually expressed in

TABLE 11.1 Maximum Residue Limits (MRLs) and Acceptable Daily Intake (ADI) for Veterinary Medicinal Products in Foodstuffs of Animal Origin According to the Codex Alimentarius

Compound(s)	Residue definition	Animal species	Tissue	MRLs (μg/kg)	ADI (μg/kg b.w.)	Other provisions
ANTIBACTERIAL DRUGS						
Benzylpenicillin, procaine benzylpenicillin	Benzylpenicillin	Cattle, pig, chicken	Muscle	50	0–30	Refers to μg/ person/day
			liver	50		
			kidney	50		
		Cattle	Milk	4		
Ceftiofur	Desfuroylceftiofur	Cattle, pig	Muscle	1000	0–50	
			liver	2000		
			kidney	6000		
			fat	2000		
		Cattle	Milk	100		
Chloramphenicol	Chloramphenicol			NA	NA	
Chlortetracycline, oxytetracycline, tetracycline	Parent drugs, singly or in combination	Cattle, pig, sheep, poultry	Muscle	200	0–30	MRL for fish muscle is temporary
			liver	600		
			kidney	1200		
		Cattle, sheep	Milk	100		
		Poultry	Eggs	400		
		Fish, giant prawn	Muscle	200		
Danofloxacin	Danofloxacin	Cattle, chicken	Muscle	200	0–20	
			liver	400		
			kidney	400		
			fat	100		
		Pig	Muscle	100		
			liver	50		
			kidney	200		
			fat	100		
Dihydrostreptomycin, streptomycin	Sum of dihydrostreptomycin and streptomycin	Cattle, pig, sheep, chicken	Muscle	600	0–50	MRL for cattle milk is temporary
			liver	600		
			kidney	1000		
			fat	600		
		Cattle	Milk	200		

Compound	Species	Tissue	MRL		Notes
Flumequine	Cattle, pig, sheep, chicken	Muscle	500	0–30	MRLs for pig, sheep, chicken and trout tissues are temporary
		liver	1000		
		kidney	3000		
		fat	1000		
	Trout	Muscle/skin	500		
Gentamicin	Cattle, pig	Muscle	100	0–20	
		liver	2000		
		kidney	5000		
		fat	100		
	Cattle	Milk	200		
Neomycin	Pig, sheep, goat, chicken, turkey, duck	Muscle	500	0–60	
		liver	500		
		kidney	500		
		fat	500		
	Cattle	Muscle	500		
		liver	15000		
		kidney	20000		
		fat	500		
		milk	500		
	Chicken	Eggs	500		
Sarafloxacin	Chicken, turkey	Muscle	10	0–0.3	
		liver	80		
		kidney	80		
		fat	20		
Spectinomycin	Cattle, pig, sheep, chicken	Muscle	500	0–40	
		liver	2000		
		kidney	5000		
		fat	2000		
	Cattle	Milk	200		
	Chicken	Eggs	2000		

(continued)

TABLE 11.1 Continued

Compound(s)	Residue definition	Animal species	Tissue	MRLs (μg/kg)	ADI (μg/kg b.w.)	Other provisions
Spiramycin	Sum of spiramycin and neospiramycin	Cattle, pig,	Muscle	200	0–50	
			liver	600		
			kidney	300		
			fat	300		
		Chicken	Muscle	200		
			liver	600		
			kidney	800		
			fat	300		
		Cattle	Milk	200		
Sulfadimidine	Sulfadimidine	Not specified	Muscle	100	0–50	
			liver	100		
			kidney	100		
			fat	100		
		Cattle	Milk	25		
Thiamphenicol	Sum of thiamphenicol and thiamphenicol conjugates as free thiamphenicol	Pig	Muscle	50	0–5	Temporary MRLs
			liver	100		
			kidney	500		
			fat	50		
		Fish	Muscle	50		
Tilmicosin	Tilmicosin	Cattle, sheep	Muscle	100	0–40	MRL for sheep milk is temporary
			liver	1000		
			kidney	300		
			fat	100		
		Pig	Muscle	100		
			liver	1500		
			kidney	1000		
			fat	100		
		Sheep	Milk	50		

ANTHELMINTHIC DRUGS

Abamectin	Avermectin B_{1a}	Cattle	Liver	100	0–2
			kidney	50	
			fat	100	
Albendazole	Sum of albendazole, albendazole sulfoxide, albendazole sulfone, and albendazole 2-amino-sulfone, expressed as albendazole	Not specified	Muscle	100	0–50
			liver	5000	
			kidney	5000	
			fat	100	
			milk	100	
Closantel		Cattle	Muscle	1000	0–30
			liver	1000	
			kidney	3000	
			fat	3000	
		Sheep	Muscle	1500	
			liver	1500	
			kidney	5000	
			fat	2000	
Doramectin		Cattle	Muscle	10	0–0.5
			liver	100	
			kidney	30	
			fat	150	
		Pig	Muscle	5	
			liver	100	
			kidney	30	
			fat	150	
Eprinomectin	Eprinomectin B_{1a}	Cattle	Muscle	100	0–10
			liver	2000	
			kidney	300	
			fat	250	
			milk	20	

(continued)

TABLE 11.1 Continued

Compound(s)	Residue definition	Animal species	Tissue	MRLs (μg/kg)	ADI (μg/kg b.w.)	Other provisions
Febantel, fenbendazole, oxfendazole	Sum of fenbendazole, oxfendazole and oxfendazole sulfone expressed as oxfendazole sulfone	Cattle, pig, sheep, goat, horse	Muscle	100	0–7	
			liver	500		
			kidney	100		
			fat	100		
			Milk	100		
Flubendazole	Flubendazole	Cattle, sheep	Muscle	10	0–13	
		Pig	liver	10		
		Poultry	Muscle	200		
			liver	500		
			eggs	400		
Ivermectin	22,23-Dihydroavermectin B$_{1a}$	Cattle	Liver	100	0–0.2	
			fat	40		
		Pig, sheep	Liver	15		
			fat	20		
Levamisole	Levamisole	Cattle, pig, sheep, poultry	Muscle	10	0–6	
			liver	100		
			kidney	10		
			fat	10		
Moxidectin	Moxidectin	Cattle, deer	Muscle	20	0–2	
			liver	100		
			kidney	50		
			fat	500		
		Sheep	Muscle	50		
			liver	100		
			kidney	50		
			fat	500		

Drug	Residue definition	Species	Tissue	Value	Range	Notes
Thiabendazole	Sum of thiabendazole and 5-hydroxy-thiabendazole	Cattle, pig, sheep, goat	Muscle	100	0–100	
			liver	100		
			kidney	100		
			fat	100		
			Milk	100		
Triclabendazole	5-Chloro-6-(2,3-dichlorophenoxy)-benzimidazole-2-one	Cattle, sheep Cattle	Muscle	200	0–3	
			liver	300		
			kidney	300		
			fat	100		
		Sheep	Muscle	100		
			liver	100		
			kidney	100		
			fat	100		
ANTICOCCIDIAL AND OTHER ANTIPROTOZOAL DRUGS						
Diclazuril	Diclazuril	Sheep, rabbit, poultry	Muscle	500	0–30	
			liver	3000		
			kidney	2000		
			fat	1000		
Diminazene	Diminazene	Cattle	Muscle	500	0–100	
			liver	12000		
			kidney	6000		
			milk	150		
Imidocarb	Imidocarb	Cattle	Muscle	300	0–10	Temporary MRLs
			liver	2000		
			kidney	1500		
			fat	50		
			milk	50		
Isometamidium	Isometamidium	Cattle	Muscle	100	0–100	
			liver	500		
			kidney	1000		
			fat	100		
			milk	100		

(continued)

TABLE 11.1 Continued

Compound(s)	Residue definition	Animal species	Tissue	MRLs (μg/kg)	ADI (μg/kg b.w.)	Other provisions
Nicarbazin	N,N′-Bis-(4-nitrophenyl)urea	Chicken (broilers)	Muscle	200	0–400	
			liver	200		
			kidney	200		
			fat/skin	200		
ANTIMICROBIAL GROWTH PROMOTERS						
Carbadox	Quinoxaline-2-carboxylic acid	Pig	Muscle	5	NA	
			liver	30		
ANABOLIC HORMONAL-TYPE GROWTH PROMOTERS						
Bovine somatotropins	Not applicable	Cattle	Muscle	NS	NS	
			liver			
			kidney			
			fat			
			milk			
Porcine somatotropin	Not applicable	Pig	Muscle	NS	NS	
			liver			
			kidney			
			fat			
Estradiol-17β	Estradiol-17β	Cattle	Muscle	NS	0–0.05	
			liver			
			kidney			
			fat			
Progesterone	Progesterone	Cattle	Muscle	NS	0–30	
			liver			
			kidney			
			fat			

					Temporary MRLs
Testosterone	Testosterone	Cattle	Muscle liver kidney fat	NS	0–2
Trenbolone acetate	β-Trenbolone (muscle) α-Trenbolone (liver)	Cattle	Muscle liver	2 10	0–0.02
Zeranol	Zeranol	Cattle	Muscle liver	2 10	0–0.5
β-ADRENERGIC AGONISTS					
Clenbuterol	Clenbuterol	Cattle, horse	Muscle liver kidney fat	0.2 0.6 0.6 0.2	0–0.004
		Cattle	Milk	0.05	
SEDATIVES AND β-BLOCKERS					
Azaperone	Sum of azaperone and azaperol	Pig	Muscle liver kidney fat	60 100 100 60	0–6
Carazolol	Carazolol	Pig	Muscle liver kidney fat/skin	5 25 25 5	0–0.1
CORTICOSTEROIDS					
Dexamethasone	Dexamethasone	Cattle, pig, horse	Muscle liver kidney	0.5 2.5 0.5	0–0.015
		Cattle	Milk	0.3	

NA, not allocated.
NS, not specified (residue does not represent a health concern).
Source: From Refs. 2, 7, 8 75–82.

substance equivalent, the calculations of consumer exposure consider the full range of residues from its metabolism.

Once the adverse effects of the drug residues have been quantitatively evaluated in the hazard characterization stage, the toxic effects observed in laboratory animals have to be extrapolated to humans. The question is whether the drug residues present in the food from treated animals are likely to have the same toxic effects on the consumer as those observed in the laboratory animals. This can only be answered by comparing the metabolic profiles of the substance in the laboratory animals where the adverse effect was identified, and in the food-producing animals that will be the source of consumer exposure to the drug residues. Analogy of metabolic profiles provides the scientific basis for the results of the toxicological evaluation of the laboratory animals to be extrapolated to humans. Such metabolic information is, however, incomplete and any extrapolation from animal to human is based more on assumption than analogy of metabolic profile.

In the hazard characterization stage, the nature of the adverse effects associated with drug residues that may be present in the food is evaluated qualitatively and/or quantitatively. This difficult task requires a methodology to evaluate the results of the necessary toxicological and pharmacological tests. In this connection, WHO published the methodology for evaluating the safety of food contaminants together with a list of toxicological tests in its 1987 compendium entitled *Environmental Health Criteria.* Hazard characterization can sometimes be based on observations in humans, but is more generally carried out by means of toxicological studies on laboratory animals. It can also be done with the help of in vitro experiments.

Epidemiological studies carried out on humans are very useful because a hazard can be directly characterized without need for extrapolation. Unfortunately, the statistical power of this methodological tool is too weak to identify with the required accuracy the adverse effects of lower quantities of residues unlikely to produce acute toxic effects. The evidence of allergic effects in humans from penicillin residues is a fortunate exception. More frequently, useful information can be obtained for drugs also used in human medicine.

In these cases it is possible to observe adverse effects caused by the higher dosages used when treating humans. But it is still necessary to extrapolate the chronic risks at exposure to low dosage. Therapeutic tests carried out on humans using drugs that are also employed in veterinary medicine can provide indications of dosage associated with pharmacological effects. The difficulty, however, lies in the fact that the purpose of human medicine is to determine an effective, optimal dosage and only rarely a dose without effect, which is the point of evaluating the harmless of veterinary drug residues.

The limitations of studies conducted in vitro and on humans make animal experimentation the best source of the toxicological and pharmacological information needed to evaluate the safety of veterinary drug residues. The JECFA uses a complete battery of toxicological tests to detect general or specific toxic effects. It combines acute, subacute or chronic toxicity tests, toxic effects on reproduction, and teratogenic, mutagenic, carcinogenic, and immunotoxic effects. For ethical and economic reasons, this complex battery of toxicological tests is restricted to the parent substance and is not used to assess the toxicity of all residues resulting from its metabolism. This neglect of the specific toxic potential of each residue has given rise to the assumption that the parent substance and all its metabolites are jointly responsible for the observed toxic effects and that the toxicity of each metabolite is similar to that of the parent substance.

In each toxicological test, the laboratory animals are exposed to increasing doses of the substance, calculated to cause adverse effects to emerge. Identifying the correlation between dosage and effect is an important component of hazard characterization. The objective is to determine any relationship that might exist between degree of exposure to a chemical agent and severity and/or frequency of adverse effect on health. The joint FAO/WHO expert consultation of March, 1995, estimated that setting an ADI is the final stage of the hazard characterization process. It should therefore be inferred that, as far as veterinary drug residues are concerned, this stage concerns both the dose–response relationship that helps in determining a NOEL and the extrapolation to humans to set an ADI.

In the dose–response assessment to determine a dosage that is risk-free for human health, the JECFA has never used mathematical models to extrapolate risks at low dose and determine a "virtually safe" dose, on the grounds that the lack of validation would produce very different results. However, the JECFA could usefully address this matter in its deliberations. When progress in this area permits selection from various validated models, this exercise should no longer be solely associated with risk assessment but will also incorporate an element of risk management.

The JECFA procedure is therefore more pragmatic. It is based on determining a NOEL for the laboratory animal and a subsequent ADI for humans based on NOEL and safety factor. The value of the safety factor used to calculate an ADI from a NOEL is normally 100 and itself comprises two factors. The first is designed to offset the uncertainty of the NOEL that arises from the necessarily restricted number of animals used in the toxicological study. It also takes into account the possibility that human beings might be more sensitive to the toxic effect than the most sensitive laboratory animal. When the NOEL has been determined on the basis of undesirable effects on humans, this factor is not used.

The second factor is designed to take account of the genetic variability of consumers likely to consume these drug residues, which is much wider than the genetic variability of the laboratory animals used in the toxicological study. The safety factor value of 100 can be increased to take account of the severity of the toxic effect observed and/or to offset shortcomings in the toxicological study.

An ADI is therefore calculated for each toxicological study and the ADI with the lowest value will be the one eventually adopted.

This ADI calculation process is based on the assumption that humans are at least as sensitive as the most sensitive laboratory animal exposed to the most sensitive test. This concept is not based on any scientific evidence but is used as a precaution against the uncertainties inherent in the process of risk assessment. The ADI corresponds to the quantity of residues consumers can take each day throughout their lives without incurring any appreciable risk to their health and, as such, expresses the intention to keep the risk to public health so low as to be insignificant. Under this perspective, the setting of this value is therefore strongly influenced by the concept of risk management.

This approach has two drawbacks, one relating to the need to have a NOEL, the other concerning the standard nature of the security factor. If, for any reason, it is not possible to determine a NOEL for an animal then it is not possible to establish an ADI. In such a case, if it is still possible or desirable to set MRLs, the pragmatic approach used is an exercise in risk management. The safety factor value of 100 often used does not consider the slope of the curve expressing the relationship between dosage and frequency and/or severity of adverse health effect. It does not therefore always guarantee the same margin of safety in extrapolation from animals to humans.

In the exposure assessment stage, qualitative and quantitative evaluation of the likely intake of drug residues through food as well as exposure from other sources are performed. Estimating consumer exposure is based on the daily consumption of a particular food commodity combined with its content of veterinary drug residues.

The worst-case scenario is based on the assumption that all edible products from animals likely to have been treated with a veterinary drug are contaminated by residues at a level at most equal to the value of the MRLs set for the drug. This scenario is not a realistic reflection, because very few veterinary drugs are administered on a massive scale to all the animals, and throughout their lives, of any species. On the contrary, there are many seasonal and even occasional uses of veterinary drugs, or cases in which they are only administered to treat sick animals. Lastly, statistical methods for establishing withdrawal periods used by national authorities responsible for registering veterinary drugs strengthen the highly protective character of this scenario in relation to public health. On the other hand, the possibility of using veterinary drugs incorrectly reduces this margin of safety.

Concern for international standardization translates as the adoption of 300 g muscle, 100 g liver, 50 g kidney, 50 g fat, 100 g eggs, 1.5 L milk, and 20 g honey as daily food intake by humans. The value set for milk seems to be particularly high, but has been estimated as appropriate to ensure that infants do not consume drug residues at levels exceeding ADIs. The JECFA has considered that the potential error from using these intakes only accounts for a small proportion of the uncertainty inherent in the risk assessment procedure and that there is no need to specify these values any further. The components of this diet should, however, be reconsidered on the basis of more relevant studies of intake if the exposure assessment stage is to use the scientific approach employed in the risk assessment procedure. Because the administration of veterinary drugs to an animal takes place under strictly controlled conditions, the values of maximum residue contents in foods can be also defined in particular by establishing appropriate withdrawal periods. The MRL values are therefore established in such a way that maximum daily intake of residues is below that authorized by the corresponding ADI. Hence, the determination of MRL relates more to risk characterization than to exposure assessment.

Risk characterization, the final stage of risk assessment, sets out to provide a qualitative and/or quantitative estimate, given the uncertainties of assessment, the probability of occurrence, and the severity of known or potential adverse health effects in a given population based on hazard identification, hazard characterization, and exposure assessment. The aim is to characterize the risks to the consumer from residues possibly present in animal products on the basis of use of the substance and particularly the withdrawal period, given that the period of administration and the dosage are predetermined by the objective of effectiveness.

The conditions under which the drug is used need to be estimated as do acceptable residues linked to the level of acceptable risk to the consumer. The acceptable level of risk, which is determined in theory at the risk management stage, has already been expressed in terms of residues by the ADI under hazard characterization. Moreover, the elements considered for hazard identification, hazard characterization, and exposure assessment make it possible, for a given form of utilization of a particular substance, to establish a profile of residues in animal tissues and to associate this with a profile of consumer exposure. Comparison of this consumer profile and ADI indicates whether the mode of utilization of the substance is acceptable or not. Analysis of the different results of residue content in animal products then provides an indication of level of residues in one or several animal tissues, making it possible to differentiate between veterinary drug applications that do or do not permit compliance with the ADI.

As expressed by the 1995 joint FAO/WHO expert consultation, this risk characterization stage leads to one or several proposed MRLs associated with sound veterinary drug practices, which, on the basis of established food intake, can guarantee that ADI values will not be exceeded. The JECFA does not use rigorous mathematical models to set MRLs from a particular ADI. The MRLs are set, using available metabolism and pharmacokinetic data, at the end of a procedure heavily dependent on trial and error and strongly influenced by risk management. The few examples below illustrate the close interaction between risk assessment and risk management in setting MRLs.

Since it is difficult, in practical terms, for a monitoring plan to measure analytically a series of residues with widely differing chemical structures, control exigencies require that MRL values be expressed in terms of a single chemical entity, know as the marker residue. It is important that the contents of this marker residue evolve in the different tissues of treated animals in proportion to all targeted residues, if it is to reflect them. For obvious practical reasons, this marker residue must also satisfy two requisites: it must permit a practical dosage and must be commercially or otherwise available for the purposes of official controls.

The MRL values for muscle, liver, kidney, and fat are set in proportions that reflect the tissue distribution of the residues. To avoid producing a set of highly complex figures for different tissues and different animal species, the JECFA tries as far as possible to harmonize these values to keep their number down. When it appears that the residue contents in a given tissue are likely to be too small for the feasible control after a recommended withdrawal period of residue contents in other tissues, the JECFA likewise cannot propose any MRL for that particular tissue.

When a veterinary drug is used for both meat and dairy animals, the ADI breakdown between meat and milk is done by trial and error. This is a decision pertaining to risk management. The MRL values may be reduced to take into account the normal conditions under which a particular veterinary drug is used when these lower MRL values can always be controlled by a viable analytical method.

Even though the JECFA is not involved in setting withdrawal periods, it has to refer to a practical withdrawal period in order to establish a consistent set of MRL values. If it emerges that compliance with the MRLs requires unrealistically long withdrawal periods, the JECFA cannot recommend any MRL. This situation can arise in particular for milk and eggs. Furthermore, the JECFA presently limits its proposed MRLs to animal species for which the necessary information is already available. This strict approach raises the problem of controlling drug residues for the so-called minor animal species, for which the veterinary drug industry considers the economic market too small to justify the funding of the studies required. The whole pragmatic approach used in establishing MRLs indicates strong interlinkage between risk assessment and risk management.

Apart from risk assessment, risk management and risk communication are the other basic elements of risk analysis. Risk management is the process by which the policy options determined by risk assessment findings are weighed and any necessary control and regulation measures are instituted and put into effect. The joint FAO/WHO expert consultation that discussed this issue in January, 1997, organized risk management into risk evaluation, assessment of management options, implementation of management options, and monitoring and review stages.

Risk evaluation proceeds through identification of the public health problem, description of the problem, classification of the identified danger in terms of risk assessment and management priorities, establishment of a risk assessment policy, appointment of a body to conduct the risk assessment, and consideration of risk assessment findings. In the field of veterinary drug residues, all these actions defining risk evaluation are under the responsibility of the Codex Member Nations sitting on the CCRVDF. The first five elements of risk evaluation correspond to the work of the CCRVDF at step 1 of the Codex standard drafting procedure. At this step, the CCRVDF establishes a priority list of veterinary substances that could pose a risk to public health and submits this list to the JECFA Secretariat so that its WHO and FAO experts can assess the related risks at the step 2 of the Codex procedure.

Central element of risk evaluation is the establishment of a risk assessment policy. The 1997 FAO/WHO consultation considered that such policy should protect scientific integrity, coherence, and transparency of risk assessment. More specifically, this component of risk management should deal with identification of populations at risk, criteria for ranking hazards, and modalities for determining safety factors. The protection of scientific integrity, coherence, and transparency of risk assessment by the JECFA is crucial if confidence in the JECFA and its MRL proposals is to be total. Since the JECFA is not strictly speaking a Codex structure, the CCRVDF and FAO/WHO should discuss how this objective of risk management can be achieved. They should focus on the management of JECFA meetings by FAO and WHO and look into the modalities of selection of the experts who should complete a declaration of interest.

The 1997 consultation addressed the topic of safety factors, which is vitally important for the protection of public health. Setting MRLs is in fact based on a series of assumptions. One assumption is that humans are at least as sensitive as the most sensitive laboratory animal to a potentially toxic residue. Another assumption is that all the residues covered by the MRLs are as toxic as the parent substance. A third assumption is that residues "free" from the human gastrointestinal tract are all totally bioavailable. A fourth assumption is the safety factor used to infer an ADI from a NOEL, including the additional safety factor, generally with a value of 2, to establish a provisional ADI until further information is available to convert this into a definite ADI. Other assumptions are the overestimation of consumer exposure to drug residues and the reduction of MRL values to take account of normal conditions under which the veterinary drugs are administered.

Establishing the value of these different assumptions would seem to be a basic component of public health policy. The exercise involves decisions on the magnitude of a socially acceptable risk. This needs to be assessed in the light of observed toxic effect, quality of information on residue toxicity and content, benefit–risk trade-off assessment determined by the therapeutic or productive purpose for administering the substance in question. This is a central aspect of risk management that should be dealt with by the mandated parties.

The stage of assessment of management options has been classified by the joint FAO/WHO consultation into three parts: the identification of possible management options, selection of preferred option, and the final decision. So far, the CCRVDF has done very little in this area for which the member states have the required competence. The joint FAO/WHO consultation on risk management has insisted that decisions on acceptable levels of risk should be based on considerations of public health. It also accepted that other considerations such as economic costs, expected benefits, technical feasibility, and social choices could be considered, where these could be objectively determined. For its part, the JECFA has advised against using certain veterinary drugs with dairy cattle and laying hens when the withdrawal times needed to meet the MRLs seemed unrealistic in view of the drugs' normal conditions of use.

Implementation of management options and monitoring and review, the two last stages of risk management, are essentially under state responsibility. However, the JECFA advises states on appropriate methods of analysis to ensure compliance with the MRLs. It is important to stress that risk management goes beyond straightforward analytical study of residues in animal products and must also include the control of good practices at, and prior to, the time of drug administration. The JECFA can also make a contribution when it studies the validity of analytical methods proposed to check MRLs, specifies the statistical basis for establishing withdrawal times, and recommends the conditions of use of certain veterinary drugs in relation to MRLs set, such as in the case of tranquillizers for pigs, to reduce consumer exposure to veterinary drug residues.

One of the recommendations of the 1995 joint FAO/WHO expert consultation was to separate as far as possible the two phases of risk assessment and risk management in the risk analysis process. Examination of risk analysis and MRL-setting revealed that this recommendation has been largely followed, as the JECFA, a committee of independent experts acting in their personal capacity, worked on risk assessment. The CCRVDF, a committee of national delegations, was essentially involved in risk management. However, closer examination shows a slightly different picture and indicates that the respective roles of the CCRVDF and the JECFA in the risk analysis process need to be better defined. Since the organization and division of work were decided on before the introduction of the risk analysis concept, de facto systems have arisen that are perfectly logical in functional terms but that do not fulfill the recommendation of separate responsibilities for risk assessment and risk management. As a result, the JECFA includes elements of risk management in its risk assessment work.

JECFA utilizes certain significant risk assessment policies at specific decision points in its work. Such risk assessment policies are properly the responsibility of CCRVDF and CAC. They are, however, used by JECFA and are described in detail in relevant WHO Environmental Health Criteria documents. Examples include the reliance on animal models to establish potential human effects, use of body weight scaling for interspecies comparison, assumption that absorption in animals and humans is approximately the same, use of a 100-fold safety factor to account for likely inter- and intraspecies differences in susceptibility, decision not to assign ADIs to veterinary drugs found to be genotoxic carcinogens, and establishing of temporary ADIs for residues of veterinary drugs pending submission of requested data. In carrying out their work the experts in JECFA continually need to select and utilize various scientific assumptions. This is necessary because there are inevitable gaps in the science of risk assessment that need to be filled with default assumptions to allow for the conduct of a risk assessment. These assumptions also need to be reevaluated constantly to keep them up-to-date with scientific developments. Each of these represent risk assessment policies, and the assumptions embodied in them can significantly influence the outcome of the risk assessment. Each also represents a choice among a number of plausible alternatives.

This can be acceptable for proper Codex functioning, particularly as it echoes a pragmatic observation made by the consultation of 1995 that there might be exceptions to any hard and fast separation of responsibilities. When these aspects of risk management go to the very heart of public health protection, it would seem inappropriate for the CCRVDF not to assume its appointed risk management responsibilities. A clear example is establishing the values of the safety factors used in the different stages of risk assessment. It would be useful if, for each substance studied, the JECFA could clearly indicate the assumptions and choices made during the risk assessment process that relate to risk management, thus providing more information on its proposals. This would not be necessary for routine assumptions and decisions already announced in a general paper. Greater involvement in JECFA activities by experts put forward by consumer associations and greater transparency in the nomination of experts would greatly enhance this interactive process of risk communication.

The primary role of CCRVDF is to recommend MRLs for residues of veterinary drugs in food. CCRVDF relies on its expert committee (JECFA) to derive initial recommendations for MRLs. In this regard, CCRVDF has accepted some risk management decisionmaking by JECFA. This includes the decision to use different safety factors based on the amount and quality of data available to JECFA and the formulation of new guidelines when necessary to address new or emerging issues, such as the establishment of microbiological end-points as a safety criterion for antimicrobial drug residues. CCRVDF reviews the basis for JECFA recommendations before deciding whether to accept the proposed MRL.

CCRVDF may determine that an MRL should not be adopted because adequate methods of analysis are not available for detecting the residues in specific animal-derived foods, or because pertinent new information has been generated that was not available to JECFA when it undertook its evaluation. CCRVDF may request that JECFA reassess the recommendation for an MRL based on concerns raised by CCRVDF. On occasion, CCRVDF has chosen not to accept the recommendations of JECFA by retaining indefinitely the MRL in the Codex process. To date, however, CCRVDF has not attempted to change the numerical value of an MRL without the concurrence of JECFA.

The role of the CCRVDF in communication of risks, the third component of risk analysis, is limited to reports of meetings, which, for budgetary reasons, are increasingly succinct to the point of having little substance to communicate. The important step of drawing up priority lists of substances, which is the point of departure of the JECFA and the CCRVDF work, provides no explanation for the choices made. Even the general criteria adopted in 1986 to determine priority lists have lost their transparency. It is also important to recall that the Codex procedure for establishing MRLs only considers substances for which the JECFA has been able to propose ADIs and MRLs. Other substances, whatever the reasons for the nonexistence of ADI and MRL, are cast aside and simply ignored.

The CCRVDF should review the procedure for establishing priority lists of substances to be evaluated by the JECFA. One criterion for including a candidate substance on the priority list is that all the necessary information be made available to the JECFA, but this condition can only be met by the veterinary pharmaceutical industry because of the growing complexity of the documentation. As a result, the JECFA works on the basis of CCRVDF priorities that are heavily influenced by industry decisions.

Thought should be given to the ultimate aim of the work of the CCRVDF and JECFA and to the respective importance of public health and international trade. Without wishing to lower the importance of evaluating new substances, which are at the forefront of modern medicine and are a lifeline to the veterinary pharmaceutical industry, there is at the same time no reason to neglect older substances still in widespread use. The problem is that these substances are no longer protected by patent and therefore no longer represent an economic market sufficiently important to justify investment in the requisite studies. The unfortunate result is that the JECFA focuses especially on evaluation of new molecules, which, under constant pressure from ever-tighter technical requirements, offer increasing guarantees of safety. It perhaps does not spend enough time addressing long-established substances, some of which, although prohibited here and there, can expose public health to considerable risk. There is an urgent need to draw up a list of these substances and to agree on an appropriate methodology to identify their associated residue risks and/or provide interested parties with all relevant information.

11.3 REGULATORY OUTLINE IN THE UNITED STATES

The regulatory authority for approving veterinary drugs in the United States resides with the Food and Drug Administration (FDA) Center for Veterinary Medicine (CVM), of the Department of Health and Human Services. For gaining drug approval, the sponsor is required to furnish FDA with the necessary scientific data for demonstrating the safety and efficacy of the compound and proof that the residues in the edible products of treated animals are safe. These data must be provided from studies and procedures approved by the FDA, and must be consistent with the regulatory requirements in force at the time of registration.

To assist the animal health industry, the FDA has developed a set of general guidelines that may be used as an acceptable basis for determining drug safety (22). Included in this set are guidelines concerning metabolism studies, selection of residues for toxicological testing, toxicological testing, threshold assessment, establishing a tolerance, approval of a method of analysis for residues, establishing a withdrawal period, and guidelines for new animal drugs and food additives derived from fermentation. These guidelines describe studies that the Sponsor needs to conduct in order to meet the statutory provisions of the FDA. Although these guidelines may be followed by the Sponsors with the assurance that they describe FDA approved procedures, alternative approaches may equally well be used, provided that the sponsors have previously reviewed the appropriateness of their approach with the FDA.

11.3.1 Safety Assessment

The procedure established by FDA to regulate drugs used in food-producing animals is complex. In reviewing the historical basis for the process and the development of the scientific concepts, one finds two types of tolerances, the so-called negligible tolerance and finite tolerance, that have been used in regulating drug residues since 1966. A negligible tolerance has a maximum value of 0.1 ppm in meat and 0.01 ppm in milk and eggs. Negligible tolerances were calculated on the basis of 90-day subacute studies in rats and dogs using a safety factor of 2000. In cases where the calculated tolerance exceeded 0.1 ppm, the tolerance was arbitrarily set at 0.1 ppm. As a consequence, most tolerances set in the past were of the value of 0.1 ppm. When the drug manufacturer desired a tolerance above 0.1 ppm, additional toxicological studies were required to set exactly the value of that finite tolerance. Because of the chronic nature of these studies, the safety factor was reduced in that case from 2000 to 100, or in case of teratogenic activity from 2000 to 1,000 (23).

From the results of the toxicological studies, a NOEL for the most sensitive species could be determined. This NOEL was used in the calculation of the tolerance according to the equation

$$\text{Tolerance} = \text{NOEL (ppm/day)} \times 60 \text{ (kg)} \, / \\ \text{Safety factor} \times \text{Food factor} \times 0.5 \text{ (kg/day)}$$

where 0.5 kg is the estimated consumption of meat per day, and the food factor is an acknowledgment that tissues such as liver and kidney are not consumed to the same extent as the muscle tissue. Because of the different food factors, the tolerances in the Code of Federal Regulations (CFR) differ depending on what edible tissue is being described. However, some of the tolerances in the CFR give the same value for all edible tissues because some drugs have been regulated before the introduction of the food factors in the calculation of tolerances.

The food factors suggested by the FDA for various edible products of different animal species are given in Table 11.2 In cattle, the food factor for muscle is 1.0 but it is 0.5 for liver. Because of the halving of the food factor for liver, the tolerance in this tissue is twice the value of the tolerance in muscle. The food factor for swine liver is 0.33, indicating that swine liver si consumed less than beef liver. Poultry kidney is not given a factor because its consumption is insignificant in the human diet and it is usually removed with the viscera.

The concept of negligible tolerance is no longer used by the CVM in its approval process. Starting with the will of the Congress to permit the use of carcinogens in food-producing animals, the regulatory concept for all and drugs and feed additives has been changed. The established procedure was founded on the DES Proviso, an exception to the Delaney anticancer amendment of the Federal Food, Drug, and Cosmetic Act (24). According to this proviso, a potential carcinogen might be used in animals if it did not adversely affect the animal and if no residues of the compound could be detected by an analytical method prescribed or approved by the Secretary of Health, Education, and Welfare. The presence or absence of residues was, however, a function of the residue detection

TABLE 11.2   Food Factor Breakdown of a
1500 g Diet According to the FDA

Cattle		Swine	
Muscle	1.00	Muscle	1.00
Liver	0.50	Liver	0.33
Kidney	0.33	Kidney	0.25
Fat	0.25	Fat	0.25
Skin	a	Skin	0.25
Milk	3.00		
Sheep		Poultry	
Muscle	1.00	Muscle	1.00
Liver	0.20	Liver	0.33
Kidney	0.20	Kidney	a
Fat	0.20	Fat	0.50
Skin	a	Skin	0.50
		Eggs	1.00

a Not used for human food.

technique employed. Each time more sophisticated analytical methods were developed, the "no residue" level should be redefined because increasingly smaller amounts of residue could be detected. On account of the constant redefining of "zero," the FDA, based on the principle that once a drug is given to an animal residues will not deplete to absolute zero, followed another scientific approach to surmount the associated problems. This has become known as the sensitivity of the method (SOM) procedure because it is based on a process that determines the level (sensitivity/concentration) required for no residue (25).

The SOM procedure outlines the process for assessing the carcinogenic potential of the sponsored compounds. It uses a simple approach that involves extrapolating cancer data from animal models (usually mice or rats) from the observed natural or background incidence to a predicted increased incidence of no more than 1 tumor in 1,000,000 test animals as a result of ingesting the sponsored compound. These calculations involve the number of animals with tumors compared to the total number of animals exposed at a given dosage in their diet over a lifetime. For calculating the 1 : 1,000,000 dose, a multistage mathematical model is usually applied (26). The 1,000,000 dose becomes the permitted concentration used to calculate the no-residue level required for the method of analysis for residues in food for human consumption. Although this value is involved in the calculation, an additional calculation is needed to take into consideration total residues in the food animal before a specific value for a specific analyte can become the no-residue value by which the drug is regulated.

Although the SOM procedure was developed initially to implement the process by which carcinogenic animal drugs could be approved, it was fully integrated thereafter into the general food safety concept that the FDA applies for all animal drugs and feed additives. This unified concept applies to both carcinogens and noncarcinogens. The SOM document begins the process by subjecting the drug to a threshold assessment in order to assess its carcinogenic potential. The process initially involves a structure–activity assessment to determine whether the drug is a suspect carcinogen. The compound must also be tested in a battery of mutagenicity tests and in subchronic 90-day studies usually in the rat and dog. The carcinogenic potential of the compound may be suggested by these tests. If any of the tests signal a potential for carcinogenicity, chronic lifetime studies are usually required. When a carcinogenic potential is not seen, the level of residue in edible tissues further determines whether a drug has to undergo chronic studies. Other toxicological studies of concern are teratogenesis and multigeneration reproduction studies. These studies essentially replaced the studies required to obtain a negligible tolerance. A liberalizing aspect of the new toxicological requirements is that the safety factor for subchronic studies can be reduced from 2000 to 1000.

If the drug is not a carcinogen, a NOEL will be determined from the noncarcinogenic toxicity endpoints. The NOEL is then used in calculation of the safe concentration (SC) for total residues of the compound in each edible animal tissue. The calculation is based on the use of safety and food factors as well as a scale up factor for the body weight of humans (60 kg). With this new procedure, the safety factor is set at 100 or 1000 depending on the length of the study.

If the drug gives a carcinogenic response in the chronic bioassay, the multistage model is used to determine the level of insignificant risk, which is considered to be $1:1,000,000$ (26). The mathematically derived value is called the virtually safe dose (S_o). This value is multiplied by food factors to give the permitted concentrations for total residues of the drug in the edible animal tissues. All residues that result from administering a drug to food-producing animals are considered as potentially toxic as the parent compound unless additional studies are performed to remove this concern.

After estimating the permitted safe concentration or the virtually safe dosage, a total residue study is also required to determine a target tissue, a marker residue, and a tolerance for the marker residue in meat as well as in milk and eggs where appropriate. A total residue study generally involves 12 animals dosed with the radiolabeled drug according to label directions and slaughtered at several time points after cessation of the treatment. From this experiment, the depletion of total residues in each of the tissues can be followed. Target tissue is that in which residues having depleted to their safe concentration will ensure that all of the tissues in the animal are below their permitted safe concentration. Therefore, the food factors previously mentioned have been applied and the results plotted on a semilog graph, the last tissue to deplete to its food factor adjusted safe concentration is the target tissue. As far as the withdrawal period is concerned, this can be approximated by the point in time where the total residue curve intersects the safe concentration level, previously referred to as the tolerance, as determined by the prementioned equation.

Having determined the target tissue, the parent drug and/or one or more of the metabolites in the target tissue are chosen to be the marker residue. The proportion of the marker residue to total residues is obtained at the point on the total residue depletion curve where this line crosses its permitted safe concentration. The level of the marker residue at that point represents the tolerance since it is specified in the Code of Federal Regulations, Title 21, Part 556.

In some instances additional specialized studies may be required to assess drug-specific toxicological concerns. For example, hypersensitivity tests may be required for the β-lactam antibiotics FDA has recently been concerned with how this standard human food safety assessment process accurately determines the safe concentration of antibiotic residues based on the traditional toxicological end-points. Of particular concern was the impact of low levels of antibiotics on the intestinal microflora.

In June 1992, CVM and the Animal Health Institute sponsored a symposium on the Microbiological Significance of Drug Residues in Food to assess whether the current toxicology models were appropriate in determining the impact of low concentrations of antibiotics on the human intestinal microflora (27). After considering data from a large number of substances, including animal drugs and food additives, CVM has concluded that, based on the results of the standard toxicology tests, noncarcinogens will receive a maximum safe concentration of 1 ppm in the total diet of 1.5 kg. Therefore, the total residue limit for new animal antimicrobial products with no carcinogenic potential will be 1 ppm in the total diet unless additional microbiological testing is performed.

In instances where there are antimicrobial residues with only limited antimicrobial activity, CVM notes that all new animal antimicrobial drugs consumed as residues will have to be exposed to the metabolic activities of the target animal. Again, based on their review of the data, in most instances the metabolic action of the microflora- and drug-metabolizing enzymes of the target species will inactive the antibiotic. When the total microbiologically active residue is below 1 ppm in the total diet, no further microbiological testing will be required.

One conclusion in the proposed guidelines is that it is the sponsor's responsibility to identify comprehensively the microbiological activity of their product, to determine the appropriate microbiological end-points to be measured, and to establish the antimicrobial NOEL in an appropriate model system. These new guidelines may have a significant impact on future registration of antimicrobial animal drug products.

The tolerances permitted by the FDA typically range from 0 to 10 ppm, their value depending on the toxicity of the drug as determined by its toxicology, residue, and metabolism studies. Table 11.3 lists drugs and tolerances approved by the FDA. Action levels, although not supported by law, are used by the FDA in a discretionary manner to determine the safety of food when no tolerance exists for a compound. Where a zero tolerance is required, the Code of Federal Regulations provides a full description of the suggested analytical method, since the concept of zero tolerance is dependent on the particular method applied for the determination of the analyte.

Current regulations require that the drug sponsor further submit an analytical method suitable for determining and confirming the marker residue in the target tissue at the tolerance level that will successfully pass a multilaboratory validation study. The quantitative methods should be sensitive enough to quantitate residues at one-half the residue tolerance, and should be practical and rugged to be useful for routine surveillance monitoring of residues in US Department of Agriculture (USDA) field laboratories. On the other hand, the confirmatory methods must permit unequivocal identification of the marker residue so that the identity of a residue that exceeds the tolerance can be supported in a court of law.

All analytical methods presented to the FDA undergo a desk review and then trial by at least three government laboratories. Screening tests are not required

TABLE 11.3 Tolerances for Veterinary Medicinal Products in Foodstuffs of Animal Origin According to the US Code of Federal Regulations

Compound(s)	CFR Sec.	Residue definition	Animal species	Tissue	Safe concentration (μg/kg)	Tolerance (μg/kg)
ANTIBACTERIAL DRUGS						
Amoxycillin	556.38	Amoxycillin	Cattle	Edible tissues	—	10
			Not specified	Milk	—	10
Ampicillin	556.40	Ampicillin	Cattle, swine	Edible tissues	—	10
			Not specified	Milk	—	10
Apramycin	556.52	Apramycin (marker)	Swine	Kidney (target)	—	100
Ceftiofur	556.113	Ceftiofur	Cattle, swine, sheep, poultry	Edible tissues	—	Not required
Cephapirin	556.115	Cephapirin	Dairy cattle	Edible tissues	—	100
			Not specified	Milk	—	20
Chlortetracycline	556.150	Sum of tetracyclines residues	Beef cattle, nonlactating dairy cows, calves, swine, sheep, turkey, duck, chicken	Muscle	—	2000
				liver	—	6000
				kidney	—	12000
				fat	—	12000
			Cattle	Milk	—	300
Cloxacillin	556.165	Cloxacillin	Cattle	Edible tissues	—	10
			Not specified	Milk	—	10
Dihydrostreptomycin	556.200	Dihydrostreptomycin	Cattle, swine	Kidney	—	2000
				other edible tissues	—	500
Enrofloxacin	556.228	Enrofloxacin (marker)	Not specified	Milk	—	125
			Chicken, turkey	Muscle (target)	—	300

Drug	No.	Marker/target residue	Species	Tissue		
Erythromycin	556.230	Erythromycin	Beef cattle, swine	Edible tissues	—	100
			Chicken, turkey	Edible tissues	—	125
			Not specified	Milk	—	0
			Not specified	Eggs	—	25
Florfenicol	556.283	Total florfenicol residues	Cattle	Muscle	2000	—
				liver	6000	—
				kidney	12000	—
				fat	12000	—
		Florfenicol amine (marker)		Liver (target)	—	3700
Furazolidone	556.290	Furazolidone	Swine	Edible tissues	—	0
Gentamicin sulfate	556.300	Total gentamicin residues	Swine	Muscle	—	100
				liver	—	300
				kidney	—	400
				fat	—	400
		Gentamicin sulfate	Chicken, turkey	Edible tissues	—	100
Lincomycin	556.360	Lincomycin	Swine	Edible tissues	—	100
			Chicken	Edible tissues	—	Not required
Neomycin	556.430	Neomycin (marker)	Cattle, swine, sheep, goat	Kidney (target)	—	7200
				muscle	—	1200
				liver	—	3600
				fat	—	7200
			Not specified	Milk	—	150
Novobiocin	556.460	Novobiocin	Cattle, chicken, turkey, duck	Edible tissues	—	1000
			Dairy animals	Milk	—	100
Oleandomycin	556.480	Oleandomycin	Swine, chicken, turkey	Edible tissues	—	150

(continued)

TABLE 11.3 Continued

Compound(s)	CFR Sec.	Residue definition	Animal species	Tissue	Safe concentration (μg/kg)	Tolerance (μg/kg)
Ormetoprim	556.490	Ormetoprim	Chicken, duck, turkey, catfish, salmonids	Edible tissues	—	100
Oxytetracycline	556.500	Sum of tetracyclines residues	Cattle, beef calves nonlactating dairy cattle, dairy calves, swine, sheep, turkey, chicken, catfish, lobsters, salmonids	Muscle liver kidney fat	— — — —	2000 6000 12000 12000
Penicillin	556.510	Penicillin and its salts	Cattle Cattle Turkey Swine, sheep, chicken, quail, pheasant Not specified Not specified	Milk Edible tissues Edible tissues Edible tissues Eggs Milk	— — — — — —	300 50 10 0 0 0
Pirlimycin	556.515	Pirlimycin (marker)	Cattle Not specified	Liver (target) Milk	— —	500 400
Sarafloxacin	556.594	Sarafloxacin	Chicken (broiler), turkey	Edible tissues	—	Not required

Spectinomycin	556.600	Spectinomycin	Chicken, turkey	Edible tissues	—	100
Streptomycin	556.610	Streptomycin	Calves, swine, chicken	Kidney	—	2000
				other edible tissues	—	500
Sulfabromomethazine sodium	556.620	Sulfabromomethazine sodium	Cattle	Edible tissues	—	100
Sodium sulfachloropyrazine monohydrate	556.625	Sodium sulfachloropyrazine monohydrate	Not specified	Milk	—	10
			Chicken	Edible tissues	—	0
Sulfachlorpyridazine	556.630	Sulfachlorpyridazine	Calves, swine	Edible tissues	—	100
Sulfadimethoxine	556.640	Sulfadimethoxine	Cattle, turkey, chicken, duck, salmonids, catfish	Edible tissues	—	100
Sulfaethoxypyridazine	556.650	Sulfaethoxypyridazine	Not specified	Milk	—	10
			Cattle	Edible tissues	—	100
			Swine	Edible tissues	—	0
Sulfamerazine	556.660	Sulfamerazine	Not specified	Milk	—	0
Sulfamethazine	556.670	Sulfamethazine	Trout	Edible tissues	—	0
			Cattle, swine, chicken, turkey	Edible tissues	—	100
Sulfanitran	556.680	Sulfanitran and its metabolites	Chicken	Edible tissues	—	0
Sulfaquinoxaline	556.685	Sulfaquinoxaline	Cattle, calves, chicken, turkey	Edible tissues	—	100
Sulfathiazole	556.690	Sulfathiazole	Swine	Edible issues	—	100
Sulfomyxin	556.700	Sulfomyxin	Chicken, turkey	Edible tissues	—	0
Tetracycline	556.720	Sum of tetracyclines residues	Calves, swine, sheep, chicken, turkey	Muscle	—	2000
				liver		6000
				kidney		12000
				fat		12000
			Cattle	Milk	—	300

(continued)

TABLE 11.3 Continued

Compound(s)	CFR Sec.	Residue definition	Animal species	Tissue	Safe concentration (μg/kg)	Tolerance (μg/kg)
Tiamulin	556.738	8-alpha-hydroxymutilin (marker)	Swine	Liver (target)	—	600
Tilmicosin	556.735	Tilmicosin (marker)	Cattle	Liver (target)	—	1200
			Swine	Liver (target)	—	7500
Tylosin	556.740	Tylosin	Cattle, swine, chicken, turkey	Muscle	—	200
				liver	—	200
				kidney	—	200
				fat	—	200
			Not specified	Milk	—	50
			Not specified	Eggs	—	200
ANTHELMINTHIC DRUGS						
Albendazole	556.34	Albendazole 2-amino-sulfone (marker)	Cattle	Liver (target)	—	200
			Sheep	Liver (target)	—	250
Clorsulon	556.163	Total clorsulon residues	Cattle	Muscle	1000	—
				liver	2000	—
				kidney	3000	—
				fat	4000	—
				Kidney (target)	—	1000
Dichlorvos	556.180	2,2-dichlorovinyl dimethyl phosphate	Swine	Edible tissues	—	100
Doramectin	556.225	Doramectin (marker)	Cattle	Liver (target)	—	100
			Swine	Liver (target)	—	160
Eprinomectin	556.227	Eprinomectin B_{1a} (marker)	Not specified	Liver (target)	—	4800
			Not specified	Milk	—	12

Drug	No.	Marker residue	Animal species	Target tissue		
Ethylenediamine	556.270	Ethylenediamine	Not specified	Milk	—	0
Fenbendazole	556.275	Total fenbendazole residues	Cattle	Milk	1670	—
		Fenbendazole (marker)	Cattle, goat	Liver (target)	—	800
			Swine	Not specified	—	Not required
		Fenbendazole sulfoxide (marker)	Cattle	Milk	—	600
Haloxon	556.310	Haloxon	Cattle	Edible tissues	—	100
Hygromycin B	556.330	Hygromycin B	Swine, poultry	Edible tissues	—	0
			Not specified	Eggs	—	0
Ivermectin	556.344	22,23-dihydroavermectin B$_{1a}$ (marker)	Cattle	Liver (target)	—	100
			Swine	Liver (target)	—	20
			Sheep	Liver (target)	—	30
			Reindeer, American bison	Liver (target)	—	15
Levamisole hydrochloride	556.350	Levamisole hydrochloride	Cattle, swine, sheep	Edible tissues	—	100
Morantel tartrate	556.425	N-methyl-1,3-propanediamine (marker)	Cattle, goat	Liver (target)	—	700
			Not specified	Milk	—	Not required
Moxidectin	556.426	Moxidectin	Cattle	Muscle	—	50
				liver	—	200
Oxfendazole	556.495	Total oxfendazole residues	Cattle	Muscle	840	—
				liver	1700	—
				kidney	2500	—
				fat	3300	—
		Fenbendazole (marker)		Liver (target)	—	800

(continued)

TABLE 11.3 Continued

Compound(s)	CFR Sec.	Residue definition	Animal species	Tissue	Safe concentration (µg/kg)	Tolerance (µg/kg)
Pyrantel tartrate	556.560	Pyrantel tartrate	Swine	Muscle	—	1000
				liver	—	10000
				kidney	—	10000
Thiabendazole	556.730	Thiabendazole	Cattle, swine, sheep, goat, pheasant	Edible tissues	—	100
			Not specified	Milk	—	50
ANTICOCCIDIAL AND OTHER ANTIPROTOZOAL DRUGS						
Aklomide	556.30	Sum of aklomide and 4-amino-2-chloro-benzamide	Chicken	Muscle	—	4500
				liver	—	4500
				skin/fat	—	3000
Amprolium	556.50	Amprolium	Chicken, turkey	Muscle	—	500
				liver	—	1000
				kidney	—	1000
				egg yolk	—	8000
				whole egg	—	4000
			Calves	Muscle	—	500
				liver	—	500
				kidney	—	500
				fat	—	2000
			Pheasant	Muscle	—	500
				liver	—	1000
Buquinolate	556.90	Buquinolate	Chicken	Muscle	—	100
				liver	—	400
				kidney	—	400
				skin/fat	—	400
				yolk	—	500
				whole egg	—	200

Compound	No.	Marker residue	Species	Tissue		
Clopidol	556.160	Clopidol	Cattle, sheep, goat	Muscle	—	200
				liver	—	1500
				kidney	—	3000
			Swine	Edible tissues	—	200
				Muscle	—	5000
				liver	—	15000
			Chicken, turkey	kidney	—	15000
				Milk	—	20
Decoquinate	556.170	Decoquinate	Not specified	Muscle	—	1000
			Cattle, goat, chicken	other edible tissues	—	2000
Ethopabate	556.260	Ethopabate converted to metaphenetidine	Chicken	Muscle	—	500
				liver	—	1500
				kidney	—	1500
Halofuginone hydrobromide	556.308	Total halofuginone hydrobromide residues	Broiler, turkey	Muscle	100	—
				liver	300	—
				skin/fat	200	—
		Halofuginone hydrobromide (marker)	Chicken (broiler)	Liver (target)	—	160
			Turkey	Liver (target)	—	130
Lasalocid	556.347	Total lasalocid residues	Cattle	Muscle	1200	—
				liver	4800	—
				kidney	3600	—
				fat	4800	—
			Sheep	Muscle	1200	—
				liver	6000	—
				kidney	6000	—
				fat	6000	—
			Chicken	Muscle	1200	—
				liver	7200	—
				skin/fat	2400	—
		Lasalocid (marker)	Cattle	Liver (target)	—	700
			Sheep	Not specified	—	Not required
			Chicken	Skin/fat (target)	—	300

(continued)

TABLE 11.3 Continued

Compound(s)	CFR Sec.	Residue definition	Animal species	Tissue	Safe concentration (μg/kg)	Tolerance (μg/kg)
Maduramicin ammonium	556.375	Total maduramicin ammonium residues	Chicken	Muscle	240	—
				liver	720	—
				skin	480	—
				fat	480	—
		Maduramicin ammonium (marker)		Fat (target)	—	380
Monensin	556.420	Total monensin residues	Chicken, turkey, quail	Muscle	1500	—
				liver	4500	—
				skin/fat	3000	—
		Monensin	Cattle, goat	Edible tissues	—	50
			Chicken, turkey, quail	Not specified	—	Not required
Narasin	556.428	Total narasin residues	Chicken	Muscle	600	—
				liver	1800	—
				skin/fat	1200	—
				fat	1200	—
		Narasin		Not specified	—	Not required
Nicarbazin	556.445	Nicarbazin	Chicken	Muscle	—	4000
				liver	—	4000
				kidney	—	4000
				skin	—	4000
Robenidine hydrochloride	556.580	Robenidine hydrochloride	Chicken	Skin	—	200
				fat	—	200
				other edible tissues	—	100

Compound	Code	Marker/definition	Species	Tissue		Value
Zoalene	556.770	Sum of zoalene and 3-amino-5-nitro-o-toluamide	Chicken	Muscle	—	3000
				liver	—	6000
				kidney	—	6000
				fat	—	2000
			Turkey	Muscle	—	3000
				liver	—	3000
ANTIMICROBIAL GROWTH PROMOTERS						
Arsenic	556.60	Total arsenic residues	Swine	Muscle	—	500
				liver	—	2000
				kidney	—	2000
				edible by-products	—	500
			Chicken, turkey	Muscle	—	500
				edible by-products	—	2000
				eggs	—	500
Bacitracin	556.70	Bacitracin	Cattle, swine, chicken, turkey, pheasant, quail	Edible tissues	—	500
			Not specified	Milk	—	500
			Not specified	Eggs	—	500
Carbadox	556.100	Quinoxaline-2-carboxylic acid (marker)	Swine	Liver (target)	—	30
Virginiamycin	556.750	Virginiamycin	Cattle	Not specified	—	Not required
			Swine	Muscle	—	100
				liver	—	300
				kidney	—	400
				fat	—	400
				skin	—	400
			Chicken (broiler)	Muscle	—	100
				liver	—	300
				kidney	—	500
				fat	—	200
				skin	—	200

(continued)

TABLE 11.3 Continued

Compound(s)	CFR Sec.	Residue definition	Animal species	Tissue	Safe concentration (μg/kg)	Tolerance (μg/kg)
ANABOLIC HORMONAL-TYPE GROWTH PROMOTERS						
Estradiol and related esters	556.240	Estradiol	Calves, steers, heifers	Muscle	—	0.12
				liver	—	0.24
				kidney	—	0.36
				fat	—	0.48
			Lambs	Muscle	—	0.12
				liver	—	0.6
				kidney	—	0.6
				fat	—	0.6
Melengestrol acetate	556.380	Melengestrol acetate	Cattle	Fat	—	25
Progesterone	556.540	Progesterone	Calves, steers	Muscle	—	3
				liver	—	6
				kidney	—	9
				fat	—	12
			Lambs	Muscle	—	3
				liver	—	15
				kidney	—	15
				fat	—	15
Testosterone propionate	556.710	Testosterone	Heifers	Muscle	—	0.64
				liver	—	1.3
				kidney	—	1.9
				fat	—	2.6

	Number	Substance	Animal	Tissue		
Trenbolone	556.739	Total trenbolone residues	Cattle	Edible tissues	—	Not required
				Muscle	50	—
				liver	100	—
				kidney	150	—
				fat	200	—
Zeranol	556.760	Total zeranol residues	Cattle	Edible tissues	—	Not required
				Muscle	150	—
				liver	300	—
				kidney	450	—
				fat	600	—
ANTIFUNGAL DRUGS						
Nystatin	556.470	Nystatin	Swine, poultry	Edible tissues	—	0
			Not specified	Eggs	—	0
Corticosteroids						
Hydrocortisone	556.320	Hydrocortisone sodium succinate or hydrocortisone acetate	Not specified	Milk	—	10
Methylprednisolone	556.400	Methylprednisolone	Not specified	Milk	—	10
Prednisolone	556.520	Prednisolone	Not specified	Milk	—	0
Prednisone	556.530	Prednisone	Not specified	Milk	—	0
NONSTEROIDAL ANTI-INFLAMMATORY DRUGS						
Salicylic acid	556.590	Salicylic acid	Not specified	Milk	—	0

PROHIBITED DRUGS FOR FOOD-PRODUCING ANIMALS

Chloramphenicol
Clenbuterol
Diethylstilbestrol (DES)
Dimetridazole
Ipronidazole
Other nitroimidazoles
Furazolidone (except approved topical use)
Nitrofurazone (except approved topical use)
Sulfonamide drugs in lactating dairy cattle (except approved use of sulfadimethoxine, sulfabromomethazine, and sulfaethoxypyridazine)
Fluoroquinolones (except approved use for chicken and turkey)
Glycopeptides

of drug sponsors as a condition of approval at this time. However, the need by USDA to screen large numbers of samples may require the development of a screening test or the inclusion of the marker residue in an existing screening procedure in the future as part of the methods package needed for approval.

11.3.2   Residue Control

Once a drug is marketed, the FDA continues, through postmarketing surveillance, to oversee the safety and efficacy of the drug. In this role, however, FDA control over the usage is reduced considerably because the regulatory authority for determining compliance of animal-derived food with established tolerances rests with the USDA Food Safety and Inspection Service (FSIS). FDA regulates and inspects foods other than meat and poultry and regulates animal feeds.

FSIS is the agency responsible for enforcing the Federal Meat Inspection Act and the Poultry Products Inspection Act. Under these laws, FSIS is responsible for ensuring that USDA-inspected meat and poultry products are safe, wholesome, free of adulterating residues, and accurately labeled. As part of this responsibility, FSIS conducts the National Residue Program (NRP) to help prevent the marketing of animals containing unacceptable (violative) residues from animal drugs, pesticides, or potentially hazardous chemicals. The specific objectives of the NRP are to assess and communicate the exposure potential from residues in the US meat and poultry supply, to prevent live animals with violative concentrations of residues in their tissues from being presented for slaughter, and to prevent edible tissues from slaughtered animals containing violative concentrations of residues from entering the food supply. There should be no impetus to livestock owners to misuse drugs.

To prevent marketing of edible animal products containing illegal drug residues, FSIS has been conducted residue testing since 1967. Sample specimens of livestock and poultry tissues are collected at both domestic slaughterhouses and ports of entry of imported products. To accomplish this, about 7000 federal inspectors and veterinarians carry out inspections in some 7200 meat and poultry plants throughout the country. This is the largest inspection force in the federal government, both in absolute numbers and in the ratio of inspectors to regulated facilities. Within the NRP, over 2 million laboratory analyses and inplant tests are performed on over 450,000 samples each year to test for the presence of unacceptable levels of drugs and other potential contaminants in food of animal origin (28).

At the point of the slaughterhouse, the NPR conducts two types of residue testing in domestic animal populations. Population sampling testing is the one used to acquire information about the occurrence of residues in the domestic food animal populations going to slaughter, whereas enforcement testing is used to minimize the potential of violative animals entering the food chain. The population sampling testing operates in three basic modes: monitoring, surveillance, exploratory (29).

In the monitoring program mode, all animals slaughtered at federally inspected plants are subject to random sampling of carcasses for residues determination. The target is to explore the occurrence of violative residues of drugs for which there are established tolerances in each healthy-appearing animal population. The data gained from analysis of these samples provide the most meaningful residue statistics, because the samples are randomly selected according to a statistical plan and, moreover, their sampling is nationwide. The number of samples chosen provides a 95% probability of detecting at least one violation, when 1% of the animal population is in violation. When a problem in a major species is suspected, a larger number of samples may be assayed.

The results from the monitoring programs, which are conducted on an annual calendar year basis, can define the profile of residues over time and highlight potential problems for which intensive testing may be necessary to protect the public health (30). They can also provide a good foundation for long-term future planning, helping the agencies to implement a fully coordinated approach to residue control and prevention. Thus, monitoring not only gathers information but also deters practices that lead to violative residues.

The surveillance programs are designed to measure the magnitude of residue problems in a population and to control the movement of potentially adulterated products when there is some prior knowledge or suspicion of a high potential for violative residues. Such knowledge comes from experience and a familiarity with agricultural production practices. Surveillance programs, however, are not nationwide in scope and not random.

Sampling is biased and is directed at particular carcasses, producers, buyers, or products in response to information of monitoring, or other information sources, or from observations during ante- or postmortem inspection indicating that adulterating concentrations of residues may be present. Inplant testing procedures may be performed by the inspector, or samples may be submitted to an FSIS laboratory for analysis. Depending upon the weight of evidence that led to the testing, products may be retained until test results indicate the appropriate regulatory disposition. Laboratory testing of surveillance samples is completed as rapidly as possible and takes precedence over monitoring samples.

The exploratory programs aim to strengthen the National Residue Program as a whole. They are conducted for a variety of reasons, but these activities, whatever their objective, have in common the fact that test results are not ordinarily used to take regulatory action or to trigger follow-up surveillance testing. Gathering information about the occurrence of residues for which no safe concentrations have yet been established, about animal species not approved for use of a particular drug, about residues being considered for inclusion in the monitoring program, or evaluating new methods and approaches to monitoring, are usually some of the targets of the exploratory programs. These programs may be nation-wide or limited to specific geographic areas. Sample collection may be random and statistically based, or biased to obtain worst-case information. Exploratory programs planned on a limited scale may be expanded if preliminary results cause greater concern and make acquiring comprehensive information more urgent.

Inplant tests are also a key part of the NRP because they provide rapid screening of residues at the plant level. The sulfa-on-site (SOS) test was implemented in April 1988 to test swine urine for sulfonamide residues. It is used in many of the largest swine slaughtering facilities but laboratory confirmation of violations is required. The calf antibiotic and sulfonamide test (CAST) is used to test bob veal calves (under 150 pounds and less than 3 weeks old). Prior to 1996, CAST did not require laboratory confirmation of the result; any violation found with CAST resulted in immediate condemnation of the calf. Beginning in 1996, any zone of inhibition measuring greater than 18 mm is sent to the laboratory for confirmation. The swab test on premises (STOP) was implemented in 1979 to detect the presence of antibiotic residues in kidney tissue. Originally developed for testing dairy cows, STOP is now used for a number of slaughter classes. Laboratory confirmation is required before the animal carcass is condemned. Certain STOP-positive samples are tested for both antibiotics and sulfonamides. Confirmed STOP-positive sample specimens with sulfonamide residues that have no established limits are considered violative in those slaughter classes for which they are not approved for use. The fast antimicrobial screen test (FAST) quickly detects both antibiotic and sulfonamide drug residues in kidneys and livers and has proved to be a suitable replacement for CAST and STOP. Though FAST is capable of detecting sulfonamides, this test is significantly less sensitive than the SOS test. FAST was implemented in pilot plants in 1995. FAST has been extended to approximately 50 of the largest cow and bob veal slaughtering plants in 1996.

Despite those extensive residue testing programs, it is, of course, not feasible for any inspection authority to monitor residues of all drugs that theoretically could contaminate meat and poultry, nor is this necessary to adequately protect public health. It is important, however, to monitor those drugs most likely to present the greatest risk. Within this concept, FSIS has included, over the last three decades, the testing of the compounds listed in Table 11.4, leaving out a plethora of other drugs. A hierarchical compound evaluation system (CES) has been used in this selection (31). This system was designed to provide FSIS with a more systematic approach to the categorization of compounds with respect to their likelihood of occurrence in meat and poultry, and their potential impact on public health.

Under the initial version of CES developed in 1985, compounds that may leave residues were ranked both for toxicity and for probability of human exposure. After several years' experience with the CES, the Agency determined that

TABLE 11.4 Drugs Included in the US National Residue Program from 1972 to 1997

Type of drug	Years	Type of drug	Years
Antibacterials		Coumaphos	1972–1976, 1978, 1980–1994
Apramycin	1983–1985, 1987–1990	Dichlorvos	1972–1976, 1978, 1980–1983, 1985–1987, 1989, 1991–1997
Chloramphenicol	1972–1997	Fenbendazole	1984–1992
Chlortetracycline	1972–1997	Ivermectin	1984–1997
Dihydrostreptomycin	1972–1997	Levamisole	1976, 1978–1979, 1984–1986, 1993–1994
Erythromycin	1972–1997	Mebendazole	1986–1989
Gentamicin	1984–1997	Morantel tartrate	1983–1985, 1993–1997
Lincomycin	1985–1987, 1990	Nicarbazin	1989–1991
Neomycin	1972–1997	Oxfendazole	1986–1992
Novobiocin	1985–1990	Pyrantel tartrate	1983–1985, 1990–1997
Oxytetracycline	1972–1997	Thiabendazole	1976–1978, 1985–1992
Penicillins	1972–1997	*Anticoccidial and other antiprotozoal drugs*	
Streptomycins	1972–1997	Buquinolate	1975–1976
Sulfabromomethazine	1973–1997	Clopidol	1975, 1977–1979, 1986
Sulfachloropyrazine	1991–1997	Dimetridazole	1978–1979
Sulfachlorpyridazine	1984–1997	Deccuinate	1975–1976, 1983–1984, 1986–1988, 1990
Sulfadiazine	1986–1997	Halofuginone	1986–1997
Sulfadimethoxine	1973–1997	Ipronidazole	1974–1978, 1984–1991
Sulfadoxine	1990	Lasalocid	1983–1985
Sulfaethoxypyridazine	1984–1997	Monensin	1974–1978, 1980–1985
Sulfamethazine	1973–1997	*Antimicrobial growth promoters*	
Sulfamethoxypyridazine	1984–1997	Arsenicals	1972–1997
Sulfanitran	1990–1997	Bacitracin	1974–1975, 1981–1990
Sulfaphenazole	1990	Carbadox	1973–1985, 1987–1994
Sulfapyridine	1973–1997	Virginiamycin	1985–1990
Sulfaquinoxaline	1973–1997	*Anabolic hormonal-type growth promoters*	
Sulfathiazole	1973–1997	Diethylstilbestrol	1972–1991
Sulfisoxazole	1990–1997	Estradiol	1987–1990
Tetracycline	1972–1997	Melengestrol acetate	1978–1983, 1987–1990
Tylosin	1984–1997	Zeranol and metabolites	1973–1974, 1977, 1985–1989
Anthelminthics		*Dyes*	
Albendazole	1984–1985, 1987–1992	Gentian violet	1990, 1993
Benomyl	1989–1992		
Cambendazole	1990		
Clorsulon	1986–1989		

additional criteria were needed in order to select chemicals for our testing program that are most likely to leave a residue. In the revised version of 1991, developed by the Residue Evaluation and Planning Division of USDA/FSIS/S&T, CES has changed to include three elements. The first element is determining if a compound produces a residue. If so, the second CES element is assessing the toxicological hazardous of the compound. This hazardous element is ranked from A (high) to D (low) and Z (unknown). The third element is assessing the potential human exposure resulting from residues occurring in meat and poultry. This exposure element is ranked from 1 (likely) to 4 (unlikely) to Z (unknown). Hence, the CES ranking or risk characterization is actually a product of both hazard and exposure.

Compound evaluation and classification is a dynamic process. Thus, additional compounds are to be considered in the system, and additional research on a drug toxicity and its potential for leaving harmful residues may affect previous rankings. The selection of drugs for monitoring is based on the compound ranking assigned, on whether a practical test method suitable for regulatory use is available, on whether the compound can be determined at low cost in a multiresidue method, and on whether monitoring or other experience shows that violative residues are present in edible animal products. As such, the CES serves as a useful guide in the planning and allocation of the NRP recourses for those residues considered to represent the greatest potential effect on public health. As Table 11.4 indicates, one of the strengths of the NRP is the dynamic nature of the FSIS residue test programs. Compounds may be rotated out of the NRP but can be added during the year if needed. Over the past 10 years, virtually all drugs for which suitable methods were available have been included in the NRP, except for compounds with especially low rankings such as tiamulin and others.

When FSIS finds levels of drugs in edible animal products that are above the set tolerances, FDA and CVM are notified so that enforcement action can be considered. Enforcement testing is conducted on individual animal carcasses or lots. Testing is performed in populations of animals known to have had problems with residues to assist in preventing carcasses with residues from entering the food supply. Testing decisions are made by FSIS employees in slaughterhouses on an individual animal basis based on clinical signs or lesions. In addition, enforcement testing may be based on herd history, or previous laboratory results to follow up on producers, and other sources identified as marketing animals with violative residues.

FSIS requires all slaughterhouses to maintain records of the ownership of animals for a 30-day period immediately preceding slaughter. When an animal leaves the rearing farm, it may be sold through a dealer to a producer and then again to another factory supplier. As a result, only 5–10% of residue violations are untraceable, particularly in poultry. In addition, FSIS has implemented a nationwide database, the Residue Violation Information System (RVIS), to handle all residue data obtained by all regulatory agencies from residue violation cases.

This includes names and addresses of sellers, producers, dealers, and the results of investigations.

In the enforcement phase of testing, FDA may also conduct follow-up investigation at the animal producer level to uncover the original source and cause of the contamination problem. This often results to seizure of animal feed or seizure and condemnation of carcasses. In accordance with the federal law, offenders may face prosecution if found guilty of contravening FDA tolerance levels. In addition, farmers harboring violative residues may find future shipments impounded unless they can clearly demonstrate compliance with residue standards.

If violative residues are demonstrated as a recurring problem on a particular premises, a surveillance program may be mounted. This intensive monitoring scheme is investigated when animals are known to belong to producers responsible for reaching illegal residue levels in the past. Such surveillance programs involve a regular, routine sampling program that continues until the residue problem is deemed to be under control. Sometimes surveillance sampling can be as broad in scope as the United States Nationwide Program since 1988 for sulfonamides in the 100 largest hog-slaughtering plants. Monitoring results have helped to trigger this program, showing unacceptable levels of sulfamethazine residues in swine over time.

Depending on the needs, enforcement testing can be of small or high scale. When an injection site is seen postmortem, an inspector-generated sample is taken. The carcass is retained until laboratory results verify the presence or absence of illegal residues. In such cases, inspection findings can trigger enforcement testing. If, for example, chloramphenicol violations are found on monitoring, all the meat products will be recalled. In addition, FDA and cooperating state agencies may make on-site visits to these firms. Typically, an educational visit by the state is the first step in attempting to correct a residues problem. If the problem is not corrected, subsequent visits made by FDA could result in enforcement action, including prosecution.

Although the demonstrated presence of drug residues in an edible tissue is a requirement for regulatory action in most cases, regulatory authorities will usually act on any proof that a food-producing animal has been exposed to a banned drug, such as chloramphenicol. In such situations, the FDA will take action even on positive urine results and the qualitative confirmatory identification of the banned drug becomes of primary importance.

In the US, the effort to reduce the incidence of antibiotic residues in the meat supply involves not only FSIS and FDA but also the farmers, their trade associations, feed manufacturers, and veterinarians. FSIS has expended considerable resources recently, investigating several antibiotic residue problems, such as sulfonamides and antibiotic residues in bob veal calves, and sulfonamides and chloramphenicol in pigs. Agency representatives advise the industry and other involved parties on the problem and provide resources such as educational materials and field tests to resolve the residue problems on the farm, before the animals are sent to market. When these efforts do not produce the desired results, FSIS implements intensive in-plant testing programs to detect the residues in the meat at slaughter and takes corresponding regulatory action against the offending producers.

11.4   REGULATORY OUTLINE IN THE EUROPEAN UNION

In common with most legislative authorities throughout the world, drug legislation in the European Union is concerned with the quality, efficacy, and safety of medicinal products from the standpoint of their effects on animals, humans, and the environment. In addition to these objectives, the European Union is further concerned with the harmonization of differing standards throughout the Member States, so permitting the free circulation of goods in the intra-Community trade

11.4.1   Safety Assessment

Unlike in the United States, veterinary drugs are regulated in the European Union as two distinct assemblies. One assembly includes drugs used for therapeutic purposes; the other comprises drugs incorporated into feeding stuffs for prophylactic, coccidiostatic, and growth-promotion purposes. The former assembly is regulated under veterinary medicines directives dealt with by the Directorate General III responsible for human and veterinary pharmaceuticals. Latter is regulated by the feed additives directives which do not cover medicinal products added to feeds for therapeutic purposes and are dealt with by the Directorate General XXIV, which is responsible for agriculture. Thus, a complex legal framework has been established within the members of the EU.

Major veterinary medicines directives within the EU are thought to be the Council Directives 81/851/EEC (32) and 81/852/EEC (33) of 28 September, 1981. Although both served to ensure that regulatory requirements of veterinary medicinal products were the same throughout the Member States, the main objective of the former, along with its amending directives 90/676/EEC (34) and 93/40/EEC (35), was to establish the Committee for Veterinary Medicinal Products (CVMP). The latter, along with its amending directives 87/20/EEC (36), 92/18/EEC (37), and 93/40/EEC, mainly targeted the laying down of analytical, pharmacological, and clinical standards and protocols regarding the testing of veterinary drugs. These directives have set out the basic rules for the assessment and authorization of drugs in the European Union.

According to these rules, Member States may, with some exceptions, make their own authorization at the national level. In this type of authorization, the drug sponsor submits an application to the regulatory authority of the country in which the drug is to be marketed. If the application is successful, the drug can be marketed only in the Member State in which the application was made.

A sponsor that has obtained an authorization in at least one Member State can further request extension of the authorization to at least five other Member States. In this type of authorization, the sponsor follows a decentralized procedure by which the application is forwarded to each of the selected Member States and to the CVMP secretariat in Brussels. The regulatory authorities of the Member States have 120 days to access the supporting data of the application and to provide objections, if any, to the CVMP, whose main role is to advise and give opinion on whether a particular veterinary drug complies with the requirements of the European Union legislation. The application and the objections are considered by the CVMP, which then issues an opinion that is not binding on Member States. If a favorable decision is given, Member States then have 30 days to decide individually on granting marketing authorization, and the CVMP is informed accordingly. This procedure applicable to the majority of conventional veterinary products operates by mutual recognition of the national marketing authorizations.

In the event of disagreement between Member States about the quality, safety, or efficacy of a medicinal product that is the subject of a decentralized authorization procedure, the matter can be resolved only by a binding Community decision within a European regulatory framework. This task has been allocated to the European Agency for the Evaluation of Medicinal Products (EMEA), which was established by Council Regulation 2309/93/EEC (38) of 22 July, 1993. The primary task of this Agency is to provide scientific advice of the highest possible quality to Community institutions and Member States for the exercise of powers conferred upon them by Community legislation in the field of authorization and supervision of medicinal products. When mutual recognition of the national marketing authorizations is not possible, the EMEA is called on to prepare a binding arbitration.

Apart from establishing the EMEA, the Regulation 2309/93/EEC offers alternative approaches for marketing authorization in the so-called centralized procedure. According to this procedure, no medicinal product containing a new active substance can be placed in the market, unless a marketing authorization has been granted by the Community. To obtain marketing authorization, the sponsor must submit an application accompanied by a complete technical dossier supplying all the information required to the EMEA. The Agency shall ensure that the opinion of the Committee is given within 210 days of the receipt of a valid application. To prepare its opinion, the Committee shall examine whether the submitted data comply with the requirements of Directives 81/851/EEC and 81/852/EEC, and whether they satisfy the conditions specified in the Regulation 2309/93/EEC for issuing a marketing authorization.

Within 30 days of receipt of the opinion, the Commission prepares a draft of the decision to be taken in respect of the application, taking account of Community law. The draft decision is be forwarded to the Member States and the applicant. Where, in the opinion of the Commission, the written observations of a Member State raise important new questions of a specific or technical nature that have not been addressed in the opinion of the Agency, the Chairman suspends the procedure and refers the application back to the Agency for further consideration. The Agency, upon request, will inform any person concerned of the final decision.

Authorization can be refused if, after verification of the submitted data, it appears that the drug is harmful under the conditions of use stated at the time of application for authorization, it has no therapeutic effect or the applicant has not provided sufficient proof of such an effect, its qualitative and quantitative composition has not been stated, or the recommended withdrawal period is not long enough to ensure that foodstuffs obtained from treated animals do not contain residues that might constitute a health hazard for consumers.

Marketing authorization granted in accordance with the centralized procedure applies throughout the EU Member States. It confers the same rights and obligations in each of the Member States as a marketing authorization granted by that Member State. Notification of marketing authorization is published in the *Official Journal of the European Communities,* quoting in particular the date of authorization and the number in the Community Register.

After authorization has been issued, the person responsible for placing the veterinary drug on the market takes account of all technical and scientific progress and make changes that may be required to enable the product to be manufactured and checked by means of generally accepted scientific methods. Where the competent authorities of any Member State are of the opinion that the sponsor is no longer fulfills the obligation laid by Directive 81/851/EEC, they forthwith inform the committee and the commission, stating their reasons in detail and indicating the course of action taken. The Commission, in consultation with the Agency, forthwith examines the reasons advanced by the Member State concerned and prepares a draft of the decisions to be taken that will be adopted. Where urgent action is essential to protect human or animal health or the environment, a Member State may suspend the use on its territory of an authorized veterinary medicinal product, informing the Commission and the other Member States no later than the following working day of the reasons for action.

In mentioned centralized procedures, the CVMP is responsible for formulating the opinion of the Agency on any question concerning the admissibility of the files submitted, the granting, variation, suspension, or withdrawal of an authorization to place a veterinary drug on the market arising in accordance with the provisions of this regulation and pharmacovigilance. To assist it in its work, the CVMP has established a number of working groups, among which the Working Group on the Safety of Residues is responsible for carrying out the safety assessment of new and existing active substances, establishing MRLs, and making recommendations to the CVMP accordingly.

Up to the end of 1991, establishing MRLs had been a very much ad hoc procedure, the priorities for MRL setting being identified by the Working Group. However, from January, 1992, Regulation 2377/90 (39) as amended by Regulations 762/92 (40), 675/92 (41), 3093/92 (42), 895/93 (43), and 2901/93 (44) requires that no Member State may authorize a new pharmacologically active substance for use in veterinary medicine unless a Union-wide MRL has been established, and that MRLs for all existing drugs must be established up to the end of 1999.

In accordance with these regulations, the Commission has published a timetable for the consideration of establishing MRLs for substances currently authorized for use in food-producing animals, including time limits for submission of the relevant information by the sponsors. Information and particulars to be included in an application for the establishment of MRLs for a pharmacologically active substance used in veterinary medicinal products are provided in the 2377/90/EEC Regulation. It is essential for this application to contain two particular documentation files: the safety and the residue files.

The safety file specifies the pharmacological, toxicological, and microbiological studies usually required to allow the construction of the toxicological profile of a pharmacologically active substance. The EU guidelines are notable in that while they indicate in some detail the types of toxicological tests required, pharmacology studies appear under the two broad headings of pharmacodynamic and pharmacokinetic studies. There is a good reason for this. Whereas toxicology studies have evolved into rigid investigations to maintain standards and ensure that chemicals are tested using similar models, pharmacodynamic, and especially pharmacokinetic, studies have remained as ad hoc experimental investigations. The design of each experiment depends very much on the nature of the chemical agent and on its interaction with the animal in which the experiments are being carried out. As a consequence, each experiment is usually designed de novo depending on the drug being tested, the effect being investigated, and the animal being used. For these reasons there are no strict pharmacological testing guidelines comparable with those developed for toxicological testing.

The overall approach to the safety evaluation of residues of veterinary medicinal products within the Community is similar to that employed by the Joint FAO/WHO Expert Committee on Food Additives (JECFA). The approach is based on the type and amount of residue considered to be without any toxicological hazard for human health as expressed by the ADI, or on a temporary ADI that uses an additional safety factor. It also takes into account other relevant public health risks as well as food technology aspects and estimated food intakes. From the toxicological data on single- and repeated-dose toxicity, reproductive effects, embryotoxicity/fetotoxicity including teratogenicity, mutagenicity, carcinogenicity, immunotoxicity, effects on the human gut flora, effects on the micro-organisms used for industrial food-processing, and observations in humans provided in the safety file a suitable NOEL can be determined. The ADI is calculated from the NOEL determined for the most sensitive parameter in the most sensitive appropriate test species, according to the equation

$$\text{ADI (mg/day)} = \text{NOEL (mg/kg body weight)}$$
$$\times \text{Standard Human Weight (kg) / Safety Factor}$$

Because the ADI is related to body weight, a 60 kg average body weight has been accepted. In addition, the safety factor takes a value of 100 when the NOEL is derived from a long-term animal study, on the assumption that humans are 10 times as sensitive as the test animals and that there is a 10-fold range of sensitivity within the human population. There have been cases, however, in which a safety factor of 100 is considered insufficient. Higher safety factors may be required when the data are incomplete, the study in which the NOEL was established is inadequate, or teratogenic and carcinogenic effects have been seen.

The objective of the Residue File is to allow the elaboration of MRLs taking into account the ADI calculated in the Safety File in conjunction with the pharmacokinetics, residues depletion data, and a knowledge of target tissues and marker residues. The individual MRLs in different tissues should be a function of the amount of the food items consumed, and should also reflect the kinetics of the depletion of the residues to be consistent with the established withdrawal periods. MRLs should be proposed in such a way that the total amount of residues ingested with 500 g meat or 500 g poultry or 300 g fish, plus 1500 g milk, plus 100 g egg, plus 20 g honey does not exceed the ADI. The EU uses the daily intake values presented in Table 11.5. After an MRL has been established for a

TABLE 11.5 Daily Food Consumption According to the European Union (g)

Large animals		Poultry		Fish	
Muscle	300	Muscle	300	Muscle/skin	300
Liver	100	Liver	100		
Kidney	50	Kidney	10		
Fat[a]	50	Fat/skin	90		
Total	500	Total	500	Total	300
Milk	1500				
Egg	100				
Honey	20				

[a] For pigs, 50 g fat and skin in natural proportions.

named marker residue, the corresponding withdrawal period must be calculated such that the concentration of this residue in the target tissue falls with reasonable statistical certainty below it.

Although the ADI is related to any residue of toxicological concern, the marker residue represents the preferable analyte for a residue assay method. The target tissue is usually, but not necessarily, the tissue with the slowest depletion rate of the residues. When a compound is to be used in lactating animals or laying birds, milk or eggs are usually target tissues in addition to the target tissue selected for residue monitoring in the edible carcass.

For residue monitoring purposes, it is frequently useful to define MRLs for a particular marker residue. A specific quantitative analytical method for measuring the concentration of the residue with the required sensitivity must be available. The MRL establishes the concentration of the marker residue permitted in the target tissue. Marker residue and target tissue are selected in such a way that total residues in each edible tissue are at or below its safe concentration if the marker residue is at or below the MRLs. For milk or eggs, it may be necessary to select a marker residue different from the marker residue selected for the target tissue representing the edible carcass.

By now, MRL values have been established for many pharmacologically active substances as shown in Table 11.6. It is expected, however, that with the start of the new century all active substances intended for use in food-producing animals will be listed in one of the Annexes I–III of the amendments of the regulation 2377/90/EEC; if not, their administration to animals will be prohibited.

Annex I contains the list of pharmacologically active substances in respect of which MRLs have been established. Entry into Annex I depends on full packages of toxicological and residue data, the analysis of which suggests no major human health concerns.

Substances included in the list of Annex II are those not thought to represent a hazard to health and, thus, establishment of an MRL value is not necessary for the protection of public health. Annex II substances include endogenous compounds, such as 17-β-estradiol, and other drugs that are either not absorbed or do not leave potentially hazardous residues such as cefazolin, detomidine, diclazuril, and dicloxacillin. It is worth mentioning that a recommendation to insert a compound in Annex II should not be interpreted as automatically implying that no withdrawal time is necessary. If there is any indication that the amount of drug derived residues in an edible portion of the carcass, including injection sites for intramuscularly or subcutaneously injected drugs, exceeds the ADI, a withdrawal period has to be set. Since no MRLs are set for Annex II compounds, withdrawal periods have to be estimated on the basis of the ADI.

Annex III is reserved for substances that do not fully meet the requirements of Annexes I and II. Sometimes this may be due to the absence of a key study or because of difficulties in interpreting the studies provided. The MRLs listed in Annex III are considered provisional because they are subject to a time limit

TABLE 11.6 Maximum Residue Limits (MRLs) for Veterinary Medicinal Products in Foodstuffs of Animal Origin According to the European Communities ANNEX I

Compound(s)	Marker residue	Animal species	Target tissues	MRLs (μg/kg)	Other provisions
ANTIBACTERIAL DRUGS					
Amoxycillin	Amoxycillin	All food producing species	Muscle	50	
			fat	50	
			liver	50	
			kidney	50	
			milk	4	
Ampicillin	Ampicillin	All food producing species	Muscle	50	
			fat	50	
			liver	50	
			kidney	50	
			milk	4	
Benzylpenicillin	Benzylpenicillin	All food producing species	Muscle	50	
			fat	50	
			liver	50	
			kidney	50	
			milk	4	
Baquiloprim	Baquiloprim	Bovine	Fat	10	
			liver	300	
			kidney	150	
			milk	30	
		Porcine	Skin/fat	40	
			liver	50	
			kidney	50	
Cefazolin	Cefazolin	Bovine, ovine, caprine	Milk	50	

		Species	Tissue	MRL	Notes
Cefquinome	Cefquinome	Bovine	Muscle	50	
			fat	50	
			liver	100	
			kidney	200	
			milk	20	
Ceftiofur	Sum of all residues retaining the β-lactam structure expressed as desfuroylceftiofur	Bovine	Muscle	1000	Not for intramammary use
			fat	2000	
			liver	2000	
			kidney	6000	
			milk	100	
		Porcine	Muscle	1000	
			fat	2000	
			liver	2000	
			kidney	6000	
Chlortetracycline	Sum of parent drug and its 4-epimer	All food-producing species	Muscle	100	
			liver	300	
			kidney	600	
			milk	100	
			eggs	200	
Cloxacillin	Cloxacillin	All food-producing species	Muscle	300	
			fat	300	
			liver	300	
			kidney	300	
			milk	30	
Danofloxacin	Danofloxacin	Bovine	Muscle	200	
			fat	100	
			liver	400	
			kidney	400	
			milk	30	
		Chicken	Muscle	200	Not for use in animals producing eggs for human consumption
			skin/fat	100	
			liver	400	
			kidney	400	

(continued)

TABLE 11.6 Continued

Compound(s)	Marker residue	Animal species	Target tissues	MRLs (µg/kg)	Other provisions
Difloxacin	Difloxacin	Chicken, turkey	Muscle	300	
			skin/fat	400	
			liver	1900	
			kidney	600	
Doxycycline	Doxycycline	Bovine	Muscle	100	
			liver	300	
			kidney	600	
		Porcine, poultry	Muscle	100	
			skin/fat	300	
			liver	300	
			kidney	600	
Enrofloxacin	Sum of enrofloxacin and ciprofloxacin	Bovine	Muscle	100	
			fat	100	
			liver	300	
			kidney	200	
			milk	100	
		Rabbits	Muscle	100	
			fat	100	
			liver	200	
			kidney	300	
		Porcine, poultry	Muscle	100	Not for use in animals producing eggs for human consumption
			skin/fat	100	
			liver	200	
			kidney	300	
Florfenicol	Sum of florfenicol and its metabolites measured as florfenicolamine	Bovine	Muscle	200	
			liver	3000	
			kidney	300	

Drug	Residue marker	Species	Tissue	Value
Lincomycin	Lincomycin	Bovine	Muscle	100
			fat	50
			liver	500
			kidney	1500
			milk	150
Oxacillin	Oxacillin	All food-producing species	Muscle	300
			fat	300
			liver	300
			kidney	300
			milk	30
Oxytetracycline	Sum of parent drug and its 4-epimer	All food-producing species	Muscle	100
			liver	300
			kidney	600
			milk	100
			eggs	200
Penethamate	Benzylpenicillin	Bovine	Muscle	50
			fat	50
			liver	50
			kidney	50
			milk	4
Sarafloxacin	Sarafloxacin	Chicken	Skin/fat	10
			liver	100
		Salmonidae	Muscle/skin	30
Spiramycin	Sum of spiramycin and neospiramycin	Bovine	Muscle	200
			fat	300
			liver	300
			kidney	300
			milk	200
		Chicken	Muscle	200
			skin/fat	300
			liver	400

(continued)

TABLE 11.6 Continued

Compound(s)	Marker residue	Animal species	Target tissues	MRLs (μg/kg)	Other provisions
Sulfonamides	Parent drugs	All food-producing species	Muscle	100	Sum of total residues of all compounds should not exceed 100 μg/kg
			fat	100	
			liver	100	
			kidney	100	
		Bovine, ovine, caprine	Milk	100	
Tetracycline	Sum of parent drug and its 4-epimer	All food-producing species	Muscle	100	
			liver	300	
			kidney	600	
			milk	100	
			eggs	200	
Thiamphenicol	Thiamphenicol	Bovine	Muscle	50	
			fat	50	
			liver	50	
			kidney	50	
			milk	50	
		Chicken	Muscle	50	Not for use in animals producing eggs for human consumption
			skin/fat	50	
			liver	50	
			kidney	50	
Tilmicosin	Tilmicosin	Bovine, ovine, porcine	Liver	1000	
			kidney	1000	
		Ovine	Milk	50	

		Animal	Tissue	Value	Remarks
Trimethoprim	Trimethoprim	Bovine	Muscle	50	
			fat	50	
			liver	50	
			kidney	50	
			milk	50	
		Porcine	Muscle	50	
			skin/fat	50	
			liver	50	
			kidney	50	
		Equidae	Muscle	100	
			fat	100	
			liver	100	
			kidney	100	
		Poultry	Muscle	50	Not for use in animals producing eggs for human consumption
			skin/fat	50	
			liver	50	
			kidney	50	
		Fin fish	Muscle and skin	50	
Tylosin	Tylosin A	Bovine	Muscle	100	
			fat	100	
			liver	100	
			kidney	100	
			milk	50	
		Porcine	Muscle	100	
			skin/fat	100	
			liver	100	
			kidney	100	
		Poultry	Muscle	100	Not for use in hens producing eggs for human consumption
			skin/fat	100	
			liver	100	
			kidney	100	

(continued)

TABLE 11.6 Continued

Compound(s)	Marker residue	Animal species	Target tissues	MRLs (μg/kg)	Other provisions
ANTHELMINTHIC DRUGS					
Abamectin	Avermectin B$_{1a}$	Bovine	Fat	10	
			liver	20	
Closantel	Closantel	Bovine	Muscle	1000	
			fat	3000	
			liver	1000	
			kidney	3000	
		Ovine	Muscle	1500	
			fat	2000	
			liver	1500	
			kidney	5000	
Doramectin	Doramectin	Bovine	Muscle	10	
			fat	150	
			liver	100	
			kidney	30	
		Porcine, ovine	Muscle	20	Not for use in ovines producing milk for human consumption
			fat	100	
			liver	50	
			kidney	30	
Eprinomectin	Eprinomectin B$_{1a}$	Bovine	Muscle	30	
			fat	30	
			liver	600	
			kidney	100	
			milk	30	
Febantel	Sum of extractable residues that may be oxidized to oxfendazole sulfone	Bovine, ovine, porcine, equidae	Muscle	50	
			fat	50	
			liver	500	
			kidney	50	
		Bovine, ovine	Milk	10	

Drug	Marker residue	Species	Tissue	MRL
Fenbendazole	Sum of extractable residues that may be oxidized to oxfendazole sulfone	Bovine, ovine, porcine, equidae	Muscle	50
			fat	50
			liver	500
			kidney	50
			Milk	10
Flubendazole	Sum of flubendazole and (2-amino 1H-benzimidazol-5-yl) (4-flurorophenyl) methanone	Bovine, ovine Porcine, chicken, game birds	Muscle	50
			skin/fat	50
			liver	400
			kidney	300
	Flubendazole	Chicken	Eggs	400
Ivermectin	22,23-Dihydroavermectin B1a	Bovine	Fat	40
			liver	100
		Porcine, ovine, equidae	Fat	20
			liver	15
		Deer, reindeer	Muscle	20
			fat	100
			liver	50
			kidney	20
Levamisole	Levamisole	Bovine, ovine, porcine, poultry	Muscle	10
			fat	10
			liver	100
			kidney	10
Moxidectin	Moxidectin	Bovine, ovine	Muscle	50
			fat	500
			liver	100
			kidney	50
Nitroxinil	Nitroxinil	Bovine, ovine	Muscle	400
			fat	200
			liver	20
			kidney	400
Oxfendazole	Sum of extractable residues that may be oxidized to oxfendazole sulfone	Bovine, ovine, porcine, equidae	Muscle	50
			fat	50
			liver	500
			kidney	50
		Bovine, ovine	Milk	10

(continued)

TABLE 11.6 Continued

Compound(s)	Marker residue	Animal species	Target tissues	MRLs (μg/kg)	Other provisions
Oxibendazole	Oxibendazole	Porcine	Muscle	100	
			skin/fat	500	
			liver	200	
			kidney	100	
Thiabendazole	Sum of thiabendazole and 5-hydroxy-thiabendazole	Bovine	Muscle	100	
			fat	100	
			liver	100	
			kidney	100	
			milk	100	
Triclabendazole	Sum of extractable residues that may be oxidized to ketotriclabendazole	Bovine, ovine	Muscle	100	Not for use in animals producing milk for human consumption
			liver	100	
			kidney	100	
SEDATIVES AND β-BLOCKERS					
Carazolol	Carazolol	Porcine	Muscle	5	
			skin/fat	5	
			liver	25	
			kidney	25	
NONSTEROIDAL ANTI-INFLAMMATORY DRUGS					
Vedaprofen	Vedaprofen	Equidae	Muscle	50	
			fat	20	
			liver	100	
			kidney	1000	
Tolfenamic acid	Tolfenamic acid	Bovine	Muscle	50	
			liver	400	
			kidney	100	
			milk	50	
		Porcine	Muscle	50	
			liver	400	
			kidney	100	

CORTICOSTEROIDS

		Milk	Other provisions
Dexamethasone	Bovine	0.3	
	Bovine, porcine, equidae	Muscle 0.75 liver 2 kidney 0.75	

ANNEX II

Compound(s)	Animal species	Other provisions
17β-Estradiol	All mammalian food-producing species	For therapeutic and zootechnical uses only
Cefacetrile	Bovine	For intramammary use only and for all tissues except milk
Cefazolin	Bovine, ovine, caprine	For intramammary use only (except if the udder may be used for human consumption)
Detomidine	Bovine, equidae	For therapeutic uses only
Diclazuril	Ovine	For oral use in lambs only
Dicloxacillin	All food-producing species	
Ketoprofen	Bovine, porcine, equidae	
Mecillinam	Bovine	For intrauterine use only
Medroxyprogesterone acetate	Ovine	For intravaginal use for zootechnical purposes only
Praziquantel	Ovine	For nonlactating sheep only
Rifaximin	Bovine	For intramammary (except if the udder may be used for human consumption) and intrauterine use only

(continued)

TABLE 11.6 Continued
ANNEX III

Compound(s)	Marker residue	Animal species	Target tissues	MRLs (μg/kg)	Other provisions
ANTIBACTERIAL DRUGS					
Aminosidine	Aminosidine	Bovine, porcine, rabbits, chicken	Muscle	500	Provisional MRLs expire July 1, 2000
			liver	1500	
			kidney	1500	
Apramycin	Apramycin	Bovine	Muscle	1000	Provisional MRLs expire July 1, 1999
			liver	1000	
			kidney	20000	Not for use in lactating cattle
		Porcine	Muscle	1000	
			skin/fat	1000	
			liver	1000	
			kidney	5000	
Bacitracin	Bacitracin	Bovine	Milk	150	Provisional MRLs expire July 1, 2001
Cefacetrile	Cefacetrile	Bovine	Milk	125	Provisional MRLs expire January 1, 2001
					For intramammary use only
Cefquinome	Cefquinome	Porcine	Muscle	50	Provisional MRLs expire January 1, 2000
			skin/fat	50	
			liver	100	
			kidney	200	
Cephapirin	Sum of cephapirin and desacetylcephapirin	Bovine	Muscle	50	Provisional MRLs expire January 1, 2001
			fat	50	
			liver	50	
			kidney	100	
			milk	10	

Marker residue	Drug	Animal species	Target tissue	MRLs (µg/kg)	Other provisions
Clavulanic acid	Clavulanic acid	Bovine, ovine, porcine	Muscle fat liver kidney Milk	200 200 200 200 50	Provisional MRLs expire July 1, 1999
Clorsulon	Clorsulon	Bovine, ovine Bovine	Muscle liver kidney	150 400	Provisional MRLs expire January 1, 2000
Colistin	Colistin	Bovine, ovine, porcine, chicken, rabbits Bovine, ovine Chicken	Muscle fat liver kidney Milk Eggs	150 150 150 200 50 300	Provisional MRLs expire July 1, 2000
Danofloxacin	Danofloxacin	Porcine	Muscle skin/fat liver kidney	100 50 200 200	Provisional MRLs expire January 1, 2000
Decoquinate	Decoquinate	Bovine, ovine	Muscle fat liver kidney	500 500 500 500	Provisional MRLs expire July 1, 2000
Difloxacin	Difloxacin	Bovine	Muscle fat liver kidney	400 100 1400 800	Provisional MRLs expire January 1, 2001
		Porcine	Muscle skin/fat liver kidney	400 100 800 800	Not for use in lactating cattle
Dihydrostreptomycin	Dihydrostreptomycin	Bovine, ovine, porcine, poultry Bovine, ovine	Muscle fat liver kidney Milk	500 500 500 1000 200	Provisional MRLs expire June 1, 2000

(continued)

TABLE 11.6 Continued

Compound(s)	Marker residue	Animal species	Target tissues	MRLs (μg/kg)	Other provisions
Enrofloxacin	Sum of enrofloxacin and ciprofloxacin	Ovine	Muscle	100	Provisional MRLs expire July 1, 1999
			fat	100	
			liver	300	
			kidney	200	
Erythromycin	Erythromycin	Bovine, ovine, porcine, poultry	Muscle	400	Provisional MRLs expire June 1, 2000, MRLs apply to all microbiological active residues expressed as erythromycin equivalent
			fat	400	
			liver	400	
			kidney	400	
		Poultry	Eggs	200	
		Bovine, ovine	Milk	40	
Florfenicol	Sum of florfenicol and its metabolites measured as florfenicolamine	Fish	Muscle and skin	1000	Provisional MRLs expire July 1, 2001
Flumequine	Flumequine	Bovine, ovine, porcine, chicken	Muscle	50	Provisional MRLs expire January 1, 2000
			skin/fat	50	
			liver	100	
			kidney	300	
		Salmonidae	Not specified	150	
Gentamicin	Gentamicin	Bovine, porcine	Muscle	100	Provisional MRLs expire June 1, 2000
			fat	100	
			liver	200	
			kidney	1000	
		Bovine	Milk	100	

Substance	Marker residue	Species	Tissue	MRL	Notes
Josamycin	Sum of microbiologically active metabolites expressed as josamycin	Porcine, chicken	Muscle	200	Provisional MRLs expire July 1, 2002
			skin/fat	200	
			liver	200	
			kidney	400	
			Eggs	200	
Lincomycin	Lincomycin	Chicken	Muscle	100	Provisional MRLs expire January 1, 2001
		Ovine	fat	50	
			liver	500	
			kidney	1500	
			milk	150	
		Porcine, chicken	Muscle	100	
			skin/fat	50	
			liver	500	
			kidney	1500	
		Chicken	Eggs	50	
Marbofloxacin	Marbofloxacin	Bovine	Muscle	150	Provisional MRLs expire July 1, 2000
			fat	50	
			liver	150	
			kidney	150	
			milk	75	
		Porcine	Muscle	150	
			skin/fat	50	
			liver	150	
			kidney	150	
Morantel	Sum of residues which may be hydrolyzed to N-Methyl-1,3-propanediamine and expressed as morantel equivalents	Bovine, ovine	Muscle	100	Provisional MRLs expire July 1, 2001
			fat	100	
			liver	800	
			kidney	200	
			milk	100	
		Porcine	Muscle	100	
			skin/fat	100	
			liver	800	
			kidney	200	

(continued)

TABLE 11.6 Continued

Compound(s)	Marker residue	Animal species	Target tissues	MRLs (µg/kg)	Other provisions
Nafcillin	Nafcillin	Bovine	Muscle	300	Provisional MRLs expire January 1, 2001
			fat	300	
			liver	300	
			kidney	300	For intramammary use only
			milk	30	
Neomycin (including framycetin)	Neomycin	Bovine, ovine, caprine, porcine, chicken, turkey, duck	Muscle	500	Provisional MRLs expire June 1, 2000
			fat	500	
			liver	500	
			kidney	5000	
		Bovine, ovine, caprine	Milk	500	
		Chicken	Eggs	500	
Oxolinic acid	Oxolinic acid	Bovine	Muscle	100	Provisional MRLs expire January 1, 2001
			fat	50	
			liver	150	
			kidney	150	
		Porcine, chicken	Muscle	100	
			skin/fat	50	
			liver	150	
			kidney	150	
		Chicken	Eggs	50	
		Fin fish	Muscle/skin	300	
Oxyclozanide	Oxyclozanide	Bovine, ovine	Muscle	20	Provisional MRLs expire July 1, 2000
			fat	20	
			liver	500	
			kidney	100	
		Bovine	Milk	10	

			Tissue	MRL	
Penethamate	Benzylpenicillin	Ovine	Muscle	150	Provisional MRLs expire January 1, 2000
			fat	150	
			liver	150	
			kidney	150	
			milk	4	
		Porcine	Muscle	50	
			fat	50	
			liver	50	
			kidney	50	
Pirlimycin	Pirlimycin	Bovine	Muscle	100	Provisional MRLs expire July 1, 2000
			fat	100	
			liver	1000	
			kidney	400	
			milk	100	
Spectinomycin	Spectinomycin	Bovine, porcine, poultry	Muscle	300	Provisional MRLs expire July 7, 2000
			fat	500	
			liver	2000	
			kidney	5000	
			Milk	200	
Streptomycin	Streptomycin	Bovine	Muscle	500	Provisional MRLs expire June 1, 2000
		Bovine, ovine porcine, poultry	fat	500	
			liver	500	
			kidney	1000	
		Bovine, ovine	Milk	200	
Thiamphenicol	Thiamphenicol	Ovine	Muscle	50	Provisional MRLs expire January 1, 2001
			fat	50	
			liver	50	
			kidney	50	
		Porcine	Muscle	50	
			skin/fat	50	
			liver	50	
			kidney	50	
		Fin fish	Muscle/skin	50	

(continued)

TABLE 11.6 Continued

Compound(s)	Marker residue	Animal species	Target tissues	MRLs (μg/kg)	Other provisions
ANTHELMINTHIC DRUGS					
Albendazole sulfoxide	Sum of albendazole, albendazole sulfoxide, albendazole sulfone, and albendazole 2-aminosulfone, expressed as albendazole	Bovine, ovine, pheasant	Muscle	100	Provisional MRLs expire January 1, 2000
			fat	100	
			liver	1000	
			kidney	500	
		Bovine, ovine	Milk	100	
Imidocarb	Imidocarb	Bovine, ovine	Muscle	300	Provisional MRLs expire January 1, 2002
			fat	50	
			liver	2000	
			kidney	1500	
			milk	50	
Moxidectin	Moxidectin	Equidae	Muscle	50	Provisional MRLs expire January 1, 2000
			fat	500	
			liver	100	
			kidney	50	
Netobimin	Sum of albendazole, albendazole sulfoxide, albendazole sulfone, and albendazole 2-aminosulfone, expressed as albendazole	Bovine, ovine, caprine	Muscle	100	Provisional MRLs expire July 31, 1999
			fat	100	
			liver	1000	
			kidney	500	
			milk	100	
ANTICOCCIDIAL AND OTHER ANTIPROTOZOAL DRUGS					
Halofuginone	Halofuginone	Bovine	Muscle	10	Provisional MRLs expire January 1, 2001
			fat	25	
			liver	30	
			kidney	30	

β-Adrenergic agonists

Clenbuterol	Species	Tissue	MRL	Remarks
Clenbuterol hydrochloride	Bovine	Muscle	0.1	Provisional MRLs expire July 1, 2000. For tocolysis in parturient cows only
		liver	0.5	
		kidney	0.5	
		milk	0.05	
	Equidae	Muscle	0.1	For locolysis and the treatment of respiratory ailments only
		liver	0.5	
		kidney	0.5	

Sedatives and β-blockers

Carazolol				
Carazolol	Bovine	Muscle	5	Provisional MRLs expire January 1, 2000
		fat	5	
		liver	15	
		kidney	15	
		milk	1	

Nonsteroidal anti-inflammatory drugs

Carprofen				
Carprofen	Bovine	Muscle	500	Provisional MRLs expire January 1, 2000
		fat	500	
		liver	1000	
		kidney	1000	
	Equidae	Muscle	50	
		fat	100	
		liver	1000	
		kidney	1000	
Meloxicam	Bovine	Muscle	25	Provisional MRLs expire January 1, 2000
		liver	60	
		kidney	35	

ANNEX IV
Compound(s)
Chloramphenicol
Chlorpromazine
Dapsone
Dimetridazole
Furazolidone
Metronidazole
Nitrofurans
Ronidazole

Source: From Refs. 83–92.

during which the sponsors should prepare their response to the questions raised, or conduct further studies that have been requested. When it appears that an MRL for a specific drug cannot be established because residues in edible animal products, at whatever level, constitute a hazard to the health of the consumer, the drug is included in Annex IV. Substances in this Annex are prohibited for use in food-producing animals and thus, after 1 January, 2000, Annex IV is becoming redundant because drugs included in Annexes I, II, and III will then be permitted for such a use.

In the European Union, the medicinal products incorporated into feeding stuffs for prophylactic, coccidiostatic, and growth-promotion purposes are not subject to the above-mentioned authorization procedures for establishing MRLs. Being regulated under Directive 70/524/EEC (45) and its major amendments, especially 84/587/EEC (46) and 96/51/EEC (47), these products do follow, however, a centralized procedure through an EU system. Although no formal MRLs have been yet established for these products, the types of toxicity and residues data mentioned above are also required (48).

Approval of feed additives is currently coordinated through Directorate General XXIV of the European Commission. To gain market authorization within the Community, a feed additive must be entered into either Annex I or Annex II of Directive 70/524/EEC. This Feed additive Directive contains a list of substances that can be incorporated into an animal feeding stuff as well as the level of this incorporation.

To be considered for Annex I entry, an applicant usually approaches its own national authority. Should the opinion on the application be considered favorable, officials then guide the application through the EU procedures which take the form of the Standing Committee for Feeding Stuffs and an EU Expert Working Group. Advice on toxicological and other specialized areas is provided by the Scientific Committee on Animal Nutrition (SCAN) and, ultimately, if all is satisfactory, Annex I entry is recommended. Inclusion in Annex I means that the compound in question must be made freely available throughout the European Union. Compounds with a less complete data package may enter into Annex II as a transitory measure pending further information. If these data are both forthcoming and satisfactory, the ingredient in question will enter Annex I, but if the data show adverse effects or are not supplied by a sponsor, the compound falls from the Annexes and effectively losses market authorization.

A number of additives have, since the original feed additives list in 1970, been withdrawn from the list of authorized additives for different reasons including their contribution to the generation of resistance to bacteria (avoparcin, tylosin, virginiamycin), and the decision to restrict certain antibiotics to therapeutic use (penicillin, streptomycin, tetracyclines). Until recently there has been an incoherence between feed additive and veterinary medicine legislation in the European Union since use of some agents such as dimetridazole and ronidazole was prohibited as veterinary drugs because of a safety risk, but they were still allowed to be used as feed additives. Presently authorized medicinal products for incorporation in feeds for prophylactic, coccidiostatic, and growth-promotion purposes (Annex I or II of 70/524/EEC) are presented in Table 11.7.

11.4.2 Residue Control

According to Directive 86/469/EEC of 16 September, 1986 (49), and its amendments, each Member State is required to test for the presence of antibiotics and other veterinary drug residues in edible animal products. Under the EU Annual National Plan (ANP) program, each Member State has to submit every year to the Commission a monitoring plan taking into account the specific national situation and setting out the national measures to be taken. The Commission examines the plans communicated by Member States to determine if they conform to the provisions laid down by Directive 86/469/EEC.

In 1987 for the first time all Member States presented a plan to the Commission to identify illegal use of hormones. In 1988 they further presented a plan for identification of other contaminants including antimicrobial substances. These plans are updated each year in search of new substances and in light of the experience gained from positive samples recorded during previous year or improvements on analytical techniques. The European Union requires the Member States to report the results of National Plans to the Commission that will possibly publish the data in the future. Countries exporting to the EU are also required to present comparable results.

According to the ANP, 0.1% of all cattle, swine, sheep, goats, and horse produced in each Member State must be sampled at the slaughterhouse for testing for drug residues. Although the percentage appears small, it actually represents enormous sample numbers for the regulatory authorities. The number of the main farm animals slaughtered annually in the European Union has been estimated at approximately 250 million, whereas only in the United Kingdom it is about 35 million.

Each country within the European Union has established its own surveillance schemes for controlling drug residues. In the United Kingdom, for example, there are the National Surveillance (NSS) and the Non-Statutory Surveillance Schemes (50). The former concerns large-scale random sampling at slaughterhouses and onfarm to determine the concentration, if present, of some 90 substances within 8 groups of compounds including hormones, antimicrobials, β-agonists, tranquilizers, and anthelminthics. In 1995 approximately 44,000 samples were scheduled for collection, and 48,000 analyses were conducted. The cost of the NSS is recovered in full from the red-meat slaughterhouse industry on the basis of a charge per head levied on each animal sent for slaughter. Follow-up action is taken on all samples that, on confirmatory analysis, show concentrations

TABLE 11.7 Veterinary Drugs Authorized as Feed Additives Within the European Union

Compound(s)	Animal species/category	Maximum age	Content in feed (mg/kg)	Withdrawal (days)
Antibacterials				
Avilamycin	Piglets	4 months	20–40	Not specified
	Slaughter pigs	4–6 months	10–20	Not specified
	Chickens	Not specified	2.5–10	Not specified
Flavophospholipol	Layers	Not specified	2–5	Not specified
(flavomycin,	Turkeys	26 weeks	1–20	Not specified
bambermycins)	Other poultry (certain species excepted)	16 weeks	1–20	Not specified
	Piglets	3 months	10–25[a]	Not specified
	Slaughter pigs	6 months	1–20	Not specified
	Calves	6 months	6–16	Not specified
	Beef	Not specified	2–10	Not specified
ANTICOCCIDIALS				
Amprolium	Poultry	From laying onwards	62.5–125	3
Amprolium/ ethopabate	Chickens for laying, turkeys, guinea fowls	From laying onwards	66.5–133	3
Arprinocid	Chickens	Not specified	60	5
	Chickens for laying	16 weeks	60	5
Decoquinate	Chickens for fattening	Not specified	20–40	3
Diclazuril	Chickens for fattening	Not specified	1	5
Dinitolmide (DOT)	Poultry	From laying onwards	62.5–125	3
Halofuginone	Chickens for fattening	Not specified	2–3	5
	Turkeys	12 weeks	2–3	5
Lasalocid	Chickens for fattening	Not specified	75–125	5
	Chickens for laying	16 weeks	75–125	Not specified
	Turkeys	12 weeks	90–125	5
Maduramicin	Chickens for fattening	Not specified	5	5

Meticlorpindol	Chickens for fattening	Not specified	125	5
	Guinea fowls	From laying onwards	125	5
	Rabbits	Not specified	125–200	5
Meticlorpindol/ methylbenzoquat	Chickens for fattening	Not specified	110	5
	Chickens for laying	16 weeks	110	Not specified
	Turkeys	12 weeks	110	5
Monensin	Beef	Not specified	10–40	Not specified
	Chickens for fattening	Not specified	100–125	3
	Chickens for laying	16 weeks	100–120	Not specified
	Turkeys	16weeks	90–100	3
Narasin	Chickens for fattening	Not specified	60–70	5
Narasin/nicarbazin	Chickens for fattening	Not specified	80–100	7
Nicarbazin	Chickens for fattening	4 weeks	100–125	9
Robenidine	Chickens for fattening	Not specified	30–36	5
	Turkeys	Not specified	30–36	5
	Rabbits	Not specified	50–66	5
Salinomycin	Chickens for fattening	Not specified	50–70	5
	Piglets	4 months	30–60	Not specified
	Slaughter pigs	6 months	15–30	Not specified
Semduramicin	Chickens for fattening	Not specified	25	5
ANTIMICROBIAL GROWTH PROMOTERS				
Carbadox	Piglets	4 months	20–50	28 days
Olaquindox	Piglets	4 months	15–50	28 days
	Piglets	4 months	50–100[a]	Not specified
OTHER VETERINARY DRUGS				
Dimetridazole	Turkeys	From laying onwards	100–200	6
	Guinea fowl	From laying onwards	125–150	6
Ipronidazole	Turkeys	From laying onwards	50–85	6
Nifursol	Turkeys	Not specified	50–75	5

[a] Milk replacements only

in excess of MRLs. Farmers are advised on the steps that need to be taken to avoid residues of veterinary medicines entering the food chain. When the follow-up visits indicate serious shortcomings, consideration is given to prosecuting the farmers concerned.

The UK Non-Statutory Surveillance Scheme of the covers animal products and veterinary medicines not included within the NSS scheme. The work is entirely funded by the Ministry of Agriculture, Fisheries and Food (MAFF) and is directed toward home-produced and imported meat and animal products. Since this is a nonstatutory scheme, legal action cannot be taken on any sample shown to contain drug residues. However, the retailers concerned are informed by the UK Veterinary Medicines Directorate of any samples purchased from their stores that, on analysis, have revealed illegal drug concentration. In 1995 approximately 4000 samples were scheduled to be collected on which up to 15,000 analyses would be conducted for a wide range of drugs including β-agonists, sulfonamides, ivermectin, and malachite green. The samples were purchased from retail outlets chosen on a random basis throughout the country and included baby food, calf and cattle kidney, cattle liver and muscle, chicken liver and muscle, eggs, honey, swine liver, kidney, muscle and pate, rabbit, salmon, sheep liver, kidney and fat, tiger prawns, trout, turkey muscle, and milk.

Within the European Union, all collected samples are analyzed for potential drug contamination in approved routine or field laboratories in each country. In case of an official sample revealing the presence of residues of prohibited drugs or quantities of authorized drugs exceeding Community or National levels, the competent authorities must ensure that investigations take place at the farm of origin without delay and must launch an inquiry into the origin of the residues. Test-positive animals are banned from human and animal consumption and additional monitoring takes place on the farm. Investigations are undertaken in all production units or holdings in the same region or locality. All necessary administrative and penal sanctions must be taken.

Recent Council Regulations have further clarified and improved procedures for the control of residues. Control has to be based primarily on targeted and unannounced inspections, with less emphasis on the system of random sampling. The monitoring plans have to be extended to poultry meat, fish, milk, and some other products including honey, rabbit meat, and eggs. Furthermore, more flexibility is given to sampling plans, according to the specific problems of each Member State.

The actions taken for positive findings vary from country to country. In some states a positive finding is sufficient to have the carcass condemned. In other states a trace back to the farm is undertaken, and verbal or written advice is given to the farmer. Animals from that farm are then targeted in future surveilance. The introduction of authorized MRLs for all drugs will change the situation because it will then be possible to take legal action against the suppliers. This should further reduce the number of infringements.

Routine or field laboratories involved in the ANP are controlled in each Member State by at least one National Reference Laboratory (NRL) designated by the National Government (51, 52). National Laboratories are in turn responsible for the standards maintained in any other laboratories in their own country that are involved in the National Sampling Plan program. National Reference laboratories coordinate standards and methods of analysis for each group of residues, and may undertake work on all or limited classes of the veterinary drug areas listed in Directive 86/469/EEC.

To oversee this surveillance, the European Union has developed a system based on four fundamental cornerstones and controlled by four Community Reference Laboratories (Decision 91/664/EEC) hierarchically linked to a series of 36 authorized National Laboratories (Decision 93/257/EEC). The four cornerstones are a program of reference materials (53), a set of regularly updated mandatory minimum quality criteria for analytical techniques (54–57), a series of Reference Manuals (58, 59), and a continuous series of laboratory workshops plus a future Peer Review Group (60).

The responsibility of the Community Reference Laboratories (CRLs) designated in 1991 within Directorate VI (61), is to support and advise the National Laboratories, and further to ensure that the methodology and the performance standards used by each of the National Laboratories are adequate for enforcement (Decision 89/187/EEC). The EU Community Reference Laboratories are hierarchically equal; however, each of them is designated for a dedicated set of compounds. The Rijksinstituut voor de Volksge-zondheid en Milicuhygiene (RIVM) in Holland is responsible for the analysis of stilbenes, thyreostats, steroids, and zeranol hormones. The Bundesgesundheitsamt (BGA) in Germany covers the β-agonists, chloramphenicol, and sulfonamides. The Laboratoire des Medicaments Veterinaires (CNEVA) in France is involved in the analysis of antibiotics, quinolones, nitrofurans, and nitroimidazoles. The Istituto Superiore di Sanita (ISS) in Italy is responsible for trace metals and pesticides.

The CRLs are currently implementing programs to monitor the performance of the National Laboratories. The powers and conditions of operation of the CRLs concerning the examination of animals and fresh meat for the presence of residues are defined by the EU Council Decision of 6 March, 1989 (62). Their major tasks and duties are as follows:

- To coordinate the application of good laboratory practices within the NRLs (63, 64).
- To provide the NRLs within the European Union and "third countries" with methods of analysis, technical advice, scientific assistance, and to promote and coordinate research into new methods (65). A series of

manuals is available and electronic databases such as the CB\METHODS with information on methods validation are continuously updated (58, 59).

- To organize comparative ring tests between NRLs. A few ring tests have been completed or are still running, such as for chloramphenicol (66), diethylstilbestrol (67), clenbuterol (68), and estradiol in bovine blood (69).
- To conduct training courses for analysts of NRLs. A continuous series of laboratory workshops have been organized, (e.g., on immunoassays, high-performance liquid chromatography, and gas chromatography–mass spectrometry). A workshop held in 1991 at RIVM focused on β-agonists whereas a workshop in March 1994 at RIVM focused on quality assurance (70).
- Last but not least, to perform the "final analysis" in case of dispute between Member States. So far, this challenge has not been met. However, discussions about the degree of reliability and the cost efficiency of such a "final analysis" are still going on.

Since residue analyses relate to both the public health and the international trade, they have to be performed quickly and reliably, based on an integrated analytical chemical approach and professional consensus within a limited budget. This requires good professional behavior (GPB) of all involved officials as well as quality assurance such as good laboratory practices (71, 72). Methods for surveillance testing may be subdivided into screening methods and confirmatory methods. In most EU countries screening and some confirmatory methods are available for monitoring drug residues.

The most relevant difference between the traditional quality assuring approach of harmonizing methods of analysis and the alternative EU approach is that no methods but quality criteria and critical control points are harmonized. Triggered by a continuous series of residue scandals with illegal "anabolic hormones" in cattle, the European Union developed instead of methods, analytical strategies for residue analysis of veterinary drugs and contaminants in food of animal origin. Thus, official methodology for routine residue testing in the European Union does not exist. Instead, certified reference materials (CRMs) that are produced on behalf of the Bureau Community Reference (BCR) can be employed to check whether the methodologies being used are effective or not (73).

A group of expert EU analysts from the have drawn up a Guideline Criteria for Reference Methods (Decision 89/610/EEC) that lists the standards such methodology ought to achieve to be considered acceptable for use. Although the criteria for hormonal substances have been separated from the criteria for other drug residues including antibiotics, the two sets are broadly similar and demand high standards of recovery, reproducibility, and repeatability for the ideal method (71).

With this EU approach, analytical strategies are applied that are defensible in Court of Justice and are complying explicitly with the objectives of the EU regulatory investigations.

11.5 REGULATORY OUTLINE IN AUSTRALIA

Management of veterinary drugs in Australia is a responsibility shared among the Commonwealth, States, and Territories, the industry, users, and the wider community. The starting point for the management arrangements is the National Registration Scheme, which became fully operational on 15 March, 1995, and replaced preexisting State and Territory systems.

11.5.1 Safety Assessment

Before drugs can be used to prevent or treat animal diseases in Australia, they must be registered by the Commonwealth National Registration Authority (NRA) for Agricultural and Veterinary Chemicals. In registering veterinary drugs, the NRA regulates their manufacture, distribution, and supply up to and including the point of retail sale.

To be registered, drugs must meet standards of safety, quality, and efficacy. They undergo a rigorous hazard and risk assessment to determine the acceptability of the proposed use in terms of potential impacts on public health, occupational health, trade and commerce, and the environment. In evaluating a drug, the NRA takes full account of the nature of the compound, the amount and completeness of the submitted data for review, and the extent of consultation required among the NRA, manufacturers, advisory agencies, and State and Territory departments.

The registration of a drug starts with an application in which the sponsor includes all data required by the NRA for evaluating new animal drugs. An outline of the required data includes:

- Data to identify the active constituent, its chemical and physical properties, formulation composition, batch analysis and stability, process chemistry, analytical methods, and quality control
- Results of acute, short-term and long-term toxicity studies, reproduction studies, developmental studies, genotoxicity studies, and studies of the toxicity of metabolites and impurities, and other adverse effects. Data on human toxicology, the no observable effect level, acceptable daily intake, and proposed and safety directions
- Results of metabolic and toxicokinetic studies in laboratory and target animals
- Complete, detailed proposed use patterns for the product, including dose rate, regimen, and proposed withholding period; data showing the nature, level and safety of residues and metabolites in livestock and poultry

tissues, eggs, and milk and the effect of any major variables; included should also be the fate of residues during storage, processing and cooking; and finally a proposed MRL and data on MRL status in Australia, other countries, and Codex.
- Information about the overseas registration status of the product/active constituent, use patterns and MRLs overseas, export intervals, labeling, and compliance with overseas MRLs.
- Data on potential occupational exposure of workers to the active constituent, end-use product, and residues; health conditions contraindicating use of the product; occupational health monitoring including atmospheric and biological monitoring.

The NRA gives full consideration to all data presented for the registration of a product to ensure that the product meets accepted standards for safety and efficacy. Within the first month of receiving an application, the NRA Registration Processing Section screens each application for completeness, and advises applicants if they must submit further information, including the number of copies of data it requires. It has the right to refuse registration if insufficient data are presented or it the data presented demonstrate that the product is either not effective or not safe for humans, animals, the environment, and trade. Applicants have the right to obtain a formal written statement from the NRA setting out the findings of an evaluation, with references to the materials on which those finding were based, and reasons for the NRA decision. Applications must be in writing and should be lodged with the NRA Corporate Secretary within 28 days of a decision.

Maximum residue limits are set for all types of raw food commodities in which the use of veterinary drugs is required for efficient practice. When the use of the drug is likely to leave residues in foods, the NRA makes a determination as to the likely maximum level of residue that could occur in the product when the compound is used as approved. This is given to another Commonwealth authority, the Australia New Zealand Food Authority (ANZFA), which assesses the impact of dietary intake and, if acceptable, promulgates relevant MRLs that are legal limits governing the allowable levels of the defined residue in foods. These MRLs are adopted into State food laws where they take legal force as benchmark against which residues in products can be measured to ascertain whether the drug has been used in the approved manner (Table 11.8).

Registration of veterinary products is not indefinite. In addition to registering new drugs, the NRA is required under legislation to conduct regular reviews of registered veterinary drugs to ensure that they meet contemporary regulatory standards for safety and efficacy. As more scientific data about the possible harmful effects or the longer-term impacts of drugs become available, the NRA reassesses older registered chemicals for their possible harmful effects on human

TABLE 11.8 Maximum Residue Limits (MRLs) for Veterinary Medicinal Products in Foodstuffs of Animal Origin According to Australian Regulation

Compound(s)	Residue definition	Animal species	Tissue	MRLs (μg/kg)	Other provisions
ANTIBACTERIAL DRUGS					
Amoxycillin	Amoxycillin	Mammalian, poultry	Meat	10	MRL for salmonids is temporary
			offal	10	
		Cattle, sheep	Milk	10	
		Salmonids	Not specified	10	
Ampicillin	Ampicillin	Horse	Meat	10	
			offal	10	
Apramycin	Apramycin	Mammalian	Meat	50	
			offal	2000	
		Poultry	Meat	50	
			offal	1000	
Benzyl G penicillin	Benzyl G penicillin	Mammalian	Meat	60	
			offal	60	
		Not specified	Milk	1.5	
		Not specified	Eggs	18	
Ceftiofur	Desfuroylceftiofur	Cattle	Meat	100	
			offal	2000	
			fat	500	
			milk	100	
Cefuroxime	Cefuroxime	Cattle	Meat	100	
			offal	100	
			milk	100	
Cephalonium	Cephalonium	Cattle	Meat	100	
			offal	100	
			milk	20	
Chlortetracycline	Chlortetracycline	Cattle, pig, sheep, poultry	Meat	100	MRLs for cattle and sheep tissues and milk are temporary
			offal	600	
		Not specified	Milk	20	
		Not specified	Eggs	200	

(continued)

TABLE 11.8 Continued

Compound(s)	Residue definition	Animal species	Tissue	MRLs (μg/kg)	Other provisions
Clavulanic acid	Clavulanic acid	Cattle	Meat	10	
			offal	10	
			milk	10	
Cloxacillin	Cloxacillin	Cattle	Milk	10	
Erythromycin	Erythromycin	Mammalian	Meat	300	
			offal	300	
		Not specified	Milk	40	
		Not specified	Eggs	300	
Flavophospholipol (bambermycin)	Flavophospholipol (bambermycin)	Not specified	Eggs	20	
Kitasamycin	Kitasamycin	Pig, poultry	Meat	200	
			offal	200	
		Not specified	Eggs	200	
Lincomycin	Lincomycin	Mammalian (except sheep)	Meat	200	
			offal	200	
		Poultry	Meat	100	
			offal	100	
		Goat	Milk	100	
		Not specified	Eggs	200	
Neomycin	Neomycin	Mammalian	Meat	500	
			offal	500	
			fat	20	
		Not specified	Milk	20	
Novobiocin	Novobiocin	Cattle	Meat	100	Refers to milk fat content
			offal	100	
			milk	100	
Oleandomycin	Oleandomycin	Mammalian	Meat	100	
			offal	100	

Drug		Species	Tissue	MRL	Notes
Oxolinic acid	Oxolinic acid	Salmon	Not specified	10	MRL for salmonids is temporary
Oxytetracycline	Oxytetracycline	Mammalian, poultry	Meat	250	
			offal	250	
		Not specified	Milk	100	
		Not specified	Eggs	300	
		Salmonids	Not specified	200	
Procaine penicillin	Procaine penicillin	Mammalian	Meat	100	
			offal	100	
		Not specified	Milk	2.5	
		Not specified	Eggs	30	
Spectinomycin	Spectinomycin	Mammalian (except sheep), poultry	Meat	1000	
			offal	1000	
		Goat	Milk	2000	
			Eggs	2000	
Spiramycin	Spiramycin	Not specified	Meat	100	
		Pig, poultry	offal	1000	
Streptomycin, dihydrostreptomycin	Streptomycin or dihydrostreptomycin	Mammalian	Meat	300	
			offal	300	
		Not specified	Milk	200	
		Not specified	Eggs	200	
Sulfadiazine	Sulfadiazine	Mammalian, poultry	Meat	100	
			offal	100	
		Cattle	Milk	100	
Sulfadimidine	Sulfadimidine	Mammalian	Meat	100	
			offal	100	
		Poultry	Meat	100	Except turkey
			offal	100	
Sulfadoxine	Sulfadoxine	Mammalian	Meat	100	
			offal	100	
		Cattle	Milk	100	

(continued)

TABLE 11.8 Continued

Compound(s)	Residue definition	Animal species	Tissue	MRLs (µg/kg)	Other provisions
Sulfaquinoxaline	Sulfaquinoxaline	Poultry	Meat	100	Temporary MRLs
			offal	100	
Sulfatroxazole	Sulfatroxazole	Mammalian	Meat	100	
			offal	100	
		Cattle	Milk	100	
Tetracycline	Tetracycline	Not specified	Milk	100	
Tiamulin	Tiamulin	Pig, poultry	Meat	100	
			offal	100	
Tilmicosin	Tilmicosin	Cattle, pig	Meat	50	
			offal	1000	
Trimethoprim	Trimethoprim	Mammalian, poultry	Meat	50	
			offal	50	
		Cattle	Milk	50	
Tylosin	Tylosin	Cattle	Meat	100	
			offal	100	
		Pig, poultry	Meat	200	
			offal	200	
			fat	100	
		Not specified	Milk	50	
		Not specified	Eggs	200	
ANTHELMINTHIC DRUGS					
Abamectin, avermectin B₁	Sum of avermectin B₁ₐ, avermectin B₁ᵦ and Δ-8,9 isomer of avermectin B₁ₐ	Cattle	Meat	5	
			offal	100	
			fat	100	
			milk	5	
		Sheep	Meat	50	Refers to meat fat content
			offal	50	

Albendazole, albendazole sulfoxide, netobimin	Sum of albendazole, its sulfoxide, sulfone and 2-aminosulfone metabolites, expressed as albendazole	Cattle, goat	Meat	100	
			offal	100	
		Sheep	Meat	200	
			offal	3000	
Clorsulon	Clorsulon	Cattle	Meat	100	
			offal	100	
Closantel	Closantel	Sheep	Meat	2000	
			offal	5000	
Coumaphos	Sum of coumaphos and its oxygen analogue, expressed as coumaphos	Cattle, poultry	Meat	1000	The two meat and the milk value refers to meat and milk fat content
			offal	1000	
		Pig, sheep, goat	Meat	500	
			offal	500	
		Not specified	Milk	100	
		Not specified	Eggs	50	
Dichlorvos	Dichlorvos	Mammalian, poultry	Meat	50	
			offal	50	
		Not specified	Milk	20	
		Not specified	Eggs	50	
Doramectin	Doramectin	Cattle	Meat	10	MRLs for sheep tissues are temporary
			offal	100	
			fat	100	
		Sheep	Meat	2.5	Refers to meat fat content
			offal	2.5	
Eprinomectin	Eprinomectin B_{1a}	Cattle	Meat	100	
			offal	2000	
			fat	500	
			milk	30	
		Deer	Meat	100	
			offal	2000	

(continued)

TABLE 11.8 Continued

Compound(s)	Residue definition	Animal species	Tissue	MRLs (μg/kg)	Other provisions
Febantel	Febantel	Cattle, sheep, goat	Meat	100	
			offal	500	
		Not specified	Milk	500	
			milk fat	4000	
Fenbendazole	Fenbendazole	Cattle, pig	Meat	100	MRLs for pig tissues are temporary
			offal	100	
		Sheep, goat	Meat	500	
			offal	500	
		Not specified	Milk	100	
Ivermectin	Sum of ivermectin isomers	Mammalian	Meat	10	
			offal	10	
		Pig	Fat	20	
		Sheep	Fat	50	
Levamisole	Levamisole	Mammalian	Meat	100	
			offal	1000	
		Poultry	Meat	100	
			offal	100	
		Goat	Milk	100	
		Not specified (except goat)	Milk	300	
Mebendazole	Mebendazole	Mammalian	Meat	20	
			offal	20	
		Not specified	Milk	20	
Morantel	Morantel	Mammalian	Meat	300	
		Cattle, sheep, goat	Offal	2000	
		Pig	Offal	5000	
		Not specified	Milk	100	

The three meat and the milk value refers to meat and milk fat content

Substance	Animal	Tissue	Value
Moxidectin	Cattle	Meat	1000
		offal	500
		milk	2000
	Sheep	Meat	500
		offal	50
	Deer	Meat	1000
		offal	200
Nitroxynil	Cattle, sheep, goat	Meat	1000
		offal	1000
Oxfendazole	Mammalian	Meat	100
		offal	3000
Oxyclozanide	Not specified	Milk	100
	Cattle, sheep, goat	Meat	500
		offal	2000
Parbendazole	Not specified	Milk	50
	Mammalian	Meat	100
		offal	100
Praziquantel	Not specified	Milk	100
	Sheep	Meat	50
		offal	50
Rafoxanide	Cattle, sheep, goat	Meat	100
		offal	200
		fat	200
Thiabendazole	Sum of thiabendazole and 5-hydroxythiabendazole, expressed as thiabendazole	Mammalian	Meat	200
		offal	200
	Not specified	Milk	50
Triclabendazole	Cattle, sheep, goat, deer, horse	Meat	200
		offal	500

(continued)

TABLE 11.8 Continued

Compound(s)	Residue definition	Animal species	Tissue	MRLs (μg/kg)	Other provisions
ANTICOCCIDIAL AND OTHER ANTIPROTOZOAL DRUGS					
Amprolium	Amprolium	Poultry	Meat	500	
			offal	1000	
			eggs	4000	
Diclazuril	Diclazuril	Chicken	Meat	200	
			offal	1000	
Dimetridazole	Dimetridazole	Pig, poultry	Meat	5	
			offal	5	
Dinitolmide (zoalene)	Dinitolmide	Poultry	Meat	3000	
			offal	6000	
			fat	2000	
Ethopabate	Ethopabate	Poultry	Meat	5000	
			offal	15000	
Halofuginone	Halofuginone	Poultry	Meat	50	
			offal	1000	
Imidocarb	Imidocarb	Cattle	Meat	1000	
			offal	5000	
			milk	200	
Lasalocid	Lasalocid	Mammalian, poultry Not specified	Meat	50	
			offal	50	
			Eggs	50	
Maduramicin	Maduramicin	Poultry	Meat	100	
			offal	1000	
Monensin	Monensin	Cattle	Meat	50	
			offal	50	
			milk	10	
		Goat	Meat	50	
			offal	50	
		Poultry	Fat	500	

Compound	Substance	Animal	Tissue	Value	Note
Narasin	Narasin	Cattle	Meat	50	
			offal	50	
		Poultry	Meat	100	
			offal	100	
Nicarbazin	Nicarbazin	Poultry	Meat	5000	Refers to meat fat content
			offal	20000	
Salinomycin	Salinomycin	Cattle	Meat	50	
			offal	500	
		Pig	Meat	100	
			offal	100	
		Poultry	Meat	100	
			offal	500	
Toltrazuril	Sum of toltrazuril, its sulfoxide and sulfone metabolites, expressed as toltrazuril	Not specified	Eggs	20	
		Pig	Meat	1000	
			offal	2000	
		Chicken	Meat	2000	
			offal	5000	
ANTIMICROBIAL GROWTH PROMOTERS					
Avoparcin	Avoparcin	Mammalian, poultry	Meat	100	
			offal	100	
		Not specified	Milk	10	
Bacitracin	Bacitracin	Chicken	Meat	500	
			offal	500	
			fat	500	
		Not specified	Milk	500	
		Not specified	Eggs	500	
Olaquindox	Sum of olaquindox and all metabolites that reduce to 2-(N-2-hydroxyethylcarbamoyl)-3-methyl quinoxalone, expressed as olaquindox	Pig, poultry	Meat	300	
			offal	300	

(continued)

TABLE 11.8 Continued

Compound(s)	Residue definition	Animal species	Tissue	MRLs (μg/kg)	Other provisions
Virginiamycin	Virginiamycin	Cattle, pig, poultry	Meat	100	
			offal	200	
			fat	200	
		Sheep	Meat	100	
			offal	200	
		Cattle	Milk	100	
		Not specified	Eggs	100	
ANABOLIC HORMONAL-TYPE GROWTH PROMOTERS					
Norgestomet	Norgestomet	Mammalian	Meat	0.1	
			offal	0.1	
Trenbolone acetate	Sum of trenbolone acetate and 17 alpha-, and 17 beta-trenbolone, both free and conjugated, expressed as trenbolone	Cattle, pig	Meat	2	MRLs for pig tissues are temporary
			offal	10	
Zeranol	Zeranol	Cattle	Meat	5	
			offal	20	
SEDATIVES AND β-BLOCKERS					
Azaperone	Azaperone	Pig	Meat	200	
			offal	200	
CORTICOSTEROIDS					
Dexamethasone	Dexamethasone	Cattle, pig, horse	Meat	100	
			offal	100	
		Cattle	Milk	50	

health, occupational health and safety, the environment, efficacy, and implications for trade. This authority can further grant permits to provide for off-label use, and conduct programs allowing minor uses of drugs.

11.5.2 Residue Control

Apart from MRL setting, NRA and ANZFA authorities are also responsible for inspection of the primarily exported animal products, while State and Territory authorities are responsible for inspection of products destined for domestic markets.

In Australia, extensive monitoring of edible animal products for residues is carried out at both National and State levels to ensure that residues are within established standards and do not pose risks to consumers. Residues monitoring is further a trade requirement, either mandatory or as an expectation, of importing countries allowing market access to Australian food products. Some major importing countries of Australian products require a Government residue monitoring program in the country of origin, as a condition of entry for certain products. These include the United States and European Union, both of which formally audit the operations and results of National Residue Survey programs. In addition, Canada, Mexico, Japan, and Korea have conditions of entry similar to the United States. Most countries require that imported food commodities be certified as complying with agreed chemical residues limits.

Since 1961, the main Commonwealth government agency involved in residue monitoring has been the National Residue Survey (NRS), in the National Office of Food Safety of the Department of Agriculture, Fisheries and Forestry, Australia (AFFA). Through its residue monitoring programs, this agency how covers a wide range of food commodities including fisheries and aquaculture products, eggs, and honey, as well as meat destined for the domestic and export markets. NRS is also delivering residue monitoring services to industry clients on a full cost recovery basis. As such it must meet all government requirements, operate essentially on a commercial fee-for-service basis with client industries, and work cooperatively with state and government agencies with complementary responsibilities. In addition, NRS also provides technical support to the Australian Quarantine and Inspection Service (AQIS) in AFFA, which also carries out extensive monitoring and investigations as part of the export inspection and certification process.

Another Commonwealth government agency also involved in residue monitoring is the Market Basket Survey within ANZFA. This agency is responsible for the Australian Total Dietary Survey that estimates the total dietary burden of pesticides and contaminants. This agency examines levels in food purchased from retail outlets in all capital cities throughout a calendar year. In this way, ANZFA is able to estimate the residues contained in the average Australian diet.

Besides the above-mentioned Commonwealth agencies, state and territory authorities are also responsible for the regulation and control of the use of veterinary drugs. The Departments of Primary Industries or Agriculture in each state and territory are also involved in monitoring drug residues in food destined for human consumption within Australia. Moreover, many industry groups, such as the state dairy marketing bodies, conduct residue testing programs in Australia. They do this mainly to monitor their own practices as part of their overall quality assurance programs. Meat processors at abattoirs test livestock for veterinary chemicals, whereas some of the large food wholesalers and retailers also monitor the products they buy. They do this to check on suppliers and to provide assurance to themselves on behalf of their customers.

NRS conducts residue programs that involve monitoring, surveillance, and compliance programs. Monitoring programs aim to obtain a statistically valid profile of the occurrence of a residue in a commodity by a randomized sampling process. Surveillance programs are used to obtain information about a known or potential residue problem by a targeted sampling process. Compliance programs control procedures to prevent the normal marketing from specific sources of products known to be contaminated. By now, NRS surveillance and compliance programs have related only to cattle, while monitoring programs cover a wide range of animal, fish, and plant commodities.

Monitoring programs are used to check randomly selected samples for residues of a range of agricultural chemicals, veterinary drugs, stock-feed additives, environmental contaminants, and some metals. Drug residue data on edible animal products are obtained through a national monitoring survey based on commodity-drug combinations derived from Australian veterinary practice, and the requirements of export and domestic markets. The data collected facilitate certification of commodities for export and domestic consumption. Monitoring programs ensure industries maintain access to, and a competitive advantage in, important and potential markets NRS residue monitoring data are increasingly being used to audit the effectiveness of industry-operated quality assurance programs.

In 1997–1998, NRS monitoring programs involved management of about 26,000 samples. A key component of the operation of these programs was a unique sample identification number with which outgoing and incoming information were linked. Sample requests were generated and sent to sample collection points; they specified the commodity-tissue to be collected and the time period for that collection. Once collected, samples were transferred in containers provided by NRS either to specified laboratories or the NRS Central Receival and Dispatch (CRAD) facility in Canberra. At CRAD, samples were aggregated, repacked, and forwarded to laboratories. Laboratories reported analytical results to NRS, which were then verified and entered into the NRS database. State agencies were immediately notified of any results over permitted limits.

NRS contracts public and private sector laboratories to analyze samples for chemical residues. Laboratories are selected on the basis of a proficiency testing program, accreditation by the National Association of Testing Authorities for the particular residue test when feasible, and a competitive tendering process. NRS conducts a proficiency testing program, including interlaboratory checks in which identical material is supplied for analysis to a number of laboratories, and blind checks in which samples of known residue content are mixed with normal samples to permit a comparison of results and laboratory performance. New Zealand laboratories participate in the program as well. The system developed by NRS is now achieving international recognition.

NRS works closely with client industries and those considering involvement in NRS monitoring programs to develop cost-effective programs and implement appropriate funding mechanisms. The preferred and usual method of funding residue monitoring programs is by levy, usually imposed at the request of an industry. Statistical validity is an essential component of a monitoring program, but decisions on sample size must reflect the capacity of an industry to meet costs. A sampling strategy was developed to achieve viable compromises between requirements of statistical validity and costs.

NRS monitoring programs and the operational and administrative arrangements that support them are driven primarily by the needs of participating industries to maintain access to key markets. In addition these programs establish a bank of objective and scientifically valid data to underpin quality assurance programs and assist in resolving residue-related incidents. The data gathered by NRS monitoring programs also contribute to the establishment of scientifically based national and international standards for residues in food and thus, indirectly, to the improved functioning of the international agricultural trading system. In meeting the objectives of industry, NRS monitoring programs also contribute to the achievement of government goals of enhancing the value of Australian products and improving market access.

In addition to monitoring programs, NRS is involved in programs designed specifically to assess the residue status of some commodities in specific circumstances. These surveillance programs focus on commodities from specific areas or farms with a higher risk of residues, to help identify, investigate, or delineate the extent of a residue problem. NRS also assists with the management of data for surveillance programs conducted by other agencies. To date all surveillance programs have been concerned with cattle.

The samples in surveillance programs are not taken at random and the results do not reflect the overall residue status of a commodity. Consequently they are reported separately from other NRS results. Surveillance programs are generally developed under the auspices of the Residue Management Group (RMG, now SAFEMEAT), which was formed in 1994 to provide industry leadership in the development of a strategic approach to residue management in the cattle industry. NRS is involved in coordinating such programs; receiving and collating the results; making payments to state governments, laboratories, and abattoirs; and auditing the operational and financial aspects of the programs.

During 1997–1998, NRS implemented and managed a surveillance testing programs called National Antibacterial Residue Minimization Program on veterinary drug residues. This was a joint program between industry, state and Commonwealth governments combining extension, analytical, and regulatory aspects that focused on the minimization of antibacterial residues in cattle.

Residue monitoring is technically demanding and expensive, and is generally used as a check rather than a control. Monitoring involves a time-lag of several weeks between the collection of a sample and receipt of the analytical results. Recall and destruction of produce contravening the MRL are often not possible. If routine monitoring reveals a residue problem, the source of supply is traced as far as possible and action is taken to avoid future occurrences. This has occasionally meant the quarantining of properties, preventing them from selling products until problems have been rectified. If problems are persisting and the source is difficult to control, programs of quality control will be implemented by processors to prevent product contravening an MRL from reaching the market or consumer.

In 1997, the NRA introduced a compliance program known as the Hormonal Growth Promoters Audit program. The objective was to monitor compliance with controls on hormonal growth promoters usage in the cattle industry in order to maintain access to the EU cattle market. This program was introduced following concerns voiced by the EU about Australian meat and meat products containing hormonal growth promoters. The control system, of which importers, wholesalers, and retailers are part, ensures continued trade in these products with the European Union.

Control of supply and use of hormonal growth promoters has been the responsibility of state and territory governments, which have enacted appropriate legislation to implement the control system. The supply of these drugs is controlled by requiring that all suppliers be registered; that all importers, manufacturers, and suppliers keep records; and by regular audits of these records. These audits are conducted by the NRA. Control of use is achieved through the auditing of supply records; identification of treated livestock; keeping of records related to the treatment, keeping, and sale of livestock; and auditing of these controls. These audits are conducted by the states and territories.

The system is also liable to audit by EU auditors at any time. Should the auditors find systematic deficiencies in the procedures or in the enforcement of the procedures, Australian trade with the European Union could be jeopardized. Adhering to the requirements of the control system, maintaining good records, and accounting for every dose of hormonal growth promoters will ensure that suppliers do not jeopardize Australias trading reputation with the European Union.

Currently there are 277 suppliers of hormonal growth promoters in Australia. The majority of these are in Queensland, where most hormonal growth promoters are used. Over the past year, the NRA has audited 80 premises, with a yearly target of 102. This means that every premises is likely to be audited every 3 years. During an audit, the auditor checks the suppliers records to ensure that each entry is complete and that a purchases declaration has been received for each supply of hormonal growth promoters. Stock on hand at last audit and subsequent acquisitions are also calculated, to ensure that all units of hormonal growth promoters are accounted for.

In the past year, the NRA found 20 minor breaches of the regulations, such as stock on hand not being consistent with records, monthly returns not being provided to the state or territory department, or records not being kept for 2 years. In these instances, the audit issued a report on the deficiencies with either suggestions for rectifying them or a letter advising that the permission to supply hormonal growth promoters had been withdrawn. Auditors also detected 26 major breaches, including failure to obtain a purchaser declaration before supply, incomplete declarations, and failure to keep proper records. Critical breaches of audit requirements lead to prosecution, whereas failure to comply may result in prosecution, with penalties of up to $1000.

11.6 REGULATORY OUTLINE IN CANADA

Canadian regulatory requirements closely parallel those used by the United States as provided for under the terms of the United States–Canada Free Trade Agreement. Nevertheless, both countries retain their individual processes, responsibilities, and terminology. Thus, both countries require the same toxicological data and use identical methods for calculating safe concentrations. Specifically, the countries use the same safety and consumption factors, and a human body weight of 60 kg when calculating safe concentrations. Identical methods are also used for estimating tolerances or MRLs. Tolerance is the term used in the United States, while MRL is the term favored in Canada. In Canada, however, the analytical method proposed by the drug sponsor is usually reviewed by a desk audit, not through actual testing in a regulatory laboratory as in the United States. The MRLs for veterinary medicinal products in foodstuffs of animal origin according to Canadian Regulations are presented in Table 11.9.

11.6.1 Safety Assessment

In Canada, the registration of veterinary drugs is the responsibility of the Bureau of Veterinary Drugs, Health Protection Branch, Federal Department of Health, acting under the Food and Drugs Act and Regulations. The registration of a veterinary drug in Canada starts with an application in which the sponsor includes

TABLE 11.9 Maximum Residue Limits (MRLs) for Veterinary Medicinal Products in Foodstuffs of Animal Origin According to Canadian Regulation

Compound(s)	Residue definition	Animal species	Tissue	MRLs (μg/kg)	Other provisions
ANTIBACTERIAL DRUGS					
Ampicillin	Ampicillin	Cattle, swine	Edible tissue	10	
		Not specified	Milk	10	
Apramycin	Apramycin	Swine	Kidney	100	
Cephapirin	Cephapirin	Cattle	Edible tissue	100	
		Not specified	Milk	20	
Chlortetracycline	Chlortetracycline	Cattle	Muscle	100	
			liver	100	
			kidney	100	
		Calves	Muscle	1000	
			fat	1000	
			liver	4000	
			kidney	4000	
		Swine	Muscle	1000	
			fat	200	
			liver	2000	
			kidney	4000	
		Sheep	Muscle	100	
			liver	500	
			kidney	1000	
		Chicken, turkey	Muscle	1000	
			fat	1000	
			skin	1000	
			liver	1000	
			kidney	4000	
Dihydrostreptomycin	Dihydrostreptomycin	Not specified	Milk	125	

Erythromycin	Erythromycin	Swine	Edible tissue	100
		Chicken, turkey	Edible tissue	125
		Not specified	Milk	50
Gentamicin	Gentamicin	Swine	Kidney	400
		Turkey	Edible tissue	100
Neomycin	Neomycin	Calves	Edible tissue	250
Novobiocin	Novobiocin	Cattle, chicken, turkey	Edible tissue	1000
Penicillin G	Penicillin G	Cattle	Edible tissue	50 IU/ml
		Turkey	Edible tissue	10
		Not specified	Milk	0.01 IU/ml
Polymyxin B	Polymyxin B	Not specified	Milk	4 IU/ml
Spectinomycin	Spectinomycin	Chicken	Edible tissue	100
Streptomycin	Streptomycin	Not specified	Milk	125
Sulfachlorpyridazine	Sulfachlorpyridazine	Cattle, swine	Edible tissue	100
Sulfadimethoxine	Sulfadimethoxine	Cattle	Edible tissue	100
		Not specified	Milk	10
Sulfaethoxypyridazine	Sulfaethoxypyridazine	Cattle	Edible tissue	100
sulfamethazine	Sulfamethazine	Cattle, swine, chicken, turkey	Edible tissue	100
Sulfathiazole	Sulfathiazole	Swine	Edible tissue	100
Tetracycline	Tetracycline	Calves, swine, sheep, chicken, turkey	Edible tissue	250
Tiamulin	8-alpha-hydroxymutilin	Swine	Liver	400

(continued)

TABLE 11.9 Continued

Compound(s)	Residue definition	Animal species	Tissue	MRLs (μg/kg)	Other provisions
Tylosin	Tylosin	Cattle, swine, chicken, turkey	Muscle fat liver kidney	200 200 200 200	
Anthelminthic drugs					
Ivermectin	22,23-dihydro-avermectin B_{1a}	Cattle Sheep	Liver Liver	15 30	
Levamisole hydrochloride	Levamisole	Cattle, swine, sheep	Edible tissue	100	Calculated as levamisole hydrochloride
Pyrantel tartrate	N-methyl-1,3-propanediamine	Swine	Muscle liver kidney	1000 10000 10000	Calculated as pyrantel tartrate
Thiabendazole	Sum of thiabendazole and total 5-hydroxythiabendazole metabolites (free form, glucuronide and sulfate conjugates)	Cattle, goat, sheep	Edible tissue	100	
		Not specified	Milk	50	
ANTICOCCIDIAL AND OTHER ANTIPROTOZOAL DRUGS					
Amprolium	Amprolium	Chicken, turkey	Muscle liver kidney eggs	500 1000 1000 7000	

Buquinolate	Buquinolate	Chicken	Muscle	100
			fat	400
			skin	400
			liver	400
			kidney	400
Clopidol	Clopidol	Chicken, turkey	Muscle	5000
			liver	15000
			kidney	15000
Decoquinate	Decoquinate	Cattle, goat, chicken	Muscle	1000
			fat	2000
			chicken skin	2000
			liver	2000
			kidney	2000
Dinitolmide (zoalene)	Dinitolmide, including the metabolite 3-amino-5-nitro-o-toluamide	Chicken	Muscle	3000
			fat	2000
			liver	6000
			kidney	6000
		Turkey	Muscle	3000
			fat	3000
			liver	3000
Monensin	Monensin	Cattle	Edible tissue	50
Nicarbazin	N,N¹-bis(4-nitrophenyl) urea	Chicken	Muscle	4000
			skin	4000
			liver	4000
			kidney	4000
Robenidine hydrochloride	Robenidine	Chicken	Muscle	100
			fat	200
			skin	200
			liver	100
			kidney	100

Calculated as robenidine hydrochloride

(continued)

TABLE 11.9 Continued

Compound(s)	Residue definition	Animal species	Tissue	MRLs (μg/kg)	Other provisions
ANTIMICROBIAL GROWTH PROMOTERS					
Arsanilic acid	Arsenic	Swine, chicken, turkey	Muscle	500	
			liver	2000	
			eggs	500	
Nitarsone	Arsenic	Turkey	Muscle	500	
			liver	2000	
Roxarsone	Arsenic	Swine, chicken, turkey	Muscle	500	
			liver	2000	
			eggs	500	
CORTICOSTEROIDS					
Hydrocortisone	Hydrocortisone	Not specified	Milk	10	

all data required by the Bureau of Veterinary Drugs for a six-step evaluation process. Evaluation is based on metabolism and depletion studies to acquire information on the depletion of total residues following treatment and to identify residues of toxicological concern, on comparative metabolism studies to ascertain suitability of laboratory test species for toxicity studies; on toxicity and carcinogenicity tests to determine toxic effects, a NOEL, an ADI, and to establish safe concentrations of total residues; on metabolism studies in the target species to identify a target tissue, a marker residue and an MRL; on development of a regulatory analytical method for the marker residue sensitive enough to detect residues quantitatively at the MRL level; and on establishment of a withdrawal period to ensure safe use of approved drug.

In Canada, the federal mandate for food control rests with four departments: Health Canada, Agriculture and Agri-Food Canada, Department of Fisheries and Oceans, and Industry Canada. A cooperative relationship exists among departments with the ultimate goal of creating a harmonized and streamlined national food control system. All four departments ensure the application of food safety standards in their areas of responsibility to prevent or eliminate human health and safety threats created through chemical, biological, physical, or other hazards.

The safety of food from the view of veterinary drug residues is ensured by a number of activities including establishment of MRLs for animal drugs in foods (Health Canada [HC]), designing and implementing inspection and laboratory testing programs to ensure compliance of products with safety standards (Health Canada, Department of Fisheries and Oceans, Agriculture and Agri-Food Canada), registering processing plants and slaughter plants to ensure that facilities meet standards (Agriculture and Agri-Food Canada, Department of Fisheries and Oceans), inspecting processing and slaughter plants (Agriculture and Agri-Food Canada, and Department of Fisheries and Oceans in registered plants and HC in nonregistered plants), inspecting meat animals and poultry ante- and postmortem (Agriculture and Agri-Food Canada), inspecting retail food (Industry Canada), and certifying products for import and export trade (Agriculture and Agri-Food Canada, Department of Fisheries and Oceans).

The provincial governments also have food regulatory programs covering their jurisdictions and these programs are being integrated into the Canadian Food Inspection System. Provincial responsibilities in food control are shared between provincial agriculture and health ministries. For most food inspection programs, provinces are involved only with clients producing and marketing a product within that province. The federal government is involved with products shipped interprovincially or internationally. Federal provincial committees in Agriculture and Health coordinate existing programs and are working toward a fully coordinated Canadian food inspection system.

Provincial legislation provides inspection standards for agrifood products, including dairy, meat, and honey. These responsibilities include provision of regulatory and advisory services regarding farm facility standards, recommended production practices, and dairy inspection. Municipal governments are responsible for enforcing provincially mandated legislation on food control. Food inspections are carried out by public health inspectors hired either by the local health unit or provincial government.

11.6.2 Residue Control

In Canada, routine monitoring of drug residues in edible animal tissues is an integral part of the Canadian federal meat inspection system of the Food Production and Inspection Branch, Federal Department of Agriculture and AgriFood. Monitoring for antibiotic residues in cultured fish is the responsibility of the Inspection Service Branch, Federal Department of Fisheries and Oceans.

Unlike the meat and fish industry, the Canadian dairy industry has developed a system in collaboration with regulatory authorities by which the lead role in product testing is taken by the industry itself, with regulatory monitoring conducted primarily by provincial authorities. Testing is usually conducted on bulk tank milk received at the dairy prior to processing for human consumption. Dairy products intended for export, however, are subject to federal inspection, and additional testing of retail meat and dairy products for drug residues may be conducted by the Canadian Federal Department of Health.

The Canadian veterinary drug residue control program operates in the monitoring, surveillance, and compliance modes. Monitoring is designed to provide profile information on the occurrence of drug residues in predefined animal populations. Monitoring information is normally obtained through a statistically based selection of random samples from healthy-appearing animals. The sampled lots are not held and are usually passed into consumer channels before the results are known. No direct enforcement action is taken on the basis of monitoring alone. The monitoring subprogram is conducted in support of setting MRLs, to discern residue trends, to respond to international commitments, to identify potential problem areas for surveillance activities, and to access the effectiveness of control programs.

Surveillance is designed to verify suspected problems of potential health risk suggested in the monitoring subprogram, and is directed at targeted populations. The program identifies samples in violation of Canadian Acts and Regulations, and triggers further investigation as part of compliance action. If warranted, product is detained until test results indicate the appropriate course of action. The sampling approach to surveillance is referred to as biased or directed sampling. Violative results must be verified by prescribed laboratory techniques before any follow-up control action is taken. Education is an important element in correcting problems once they are identified.

Compliance action is taken as a regulatory control measure to prevent the marketing or to remove from the market a product known to be contaminated or adulterated. It presupposes that enforcement regulations or guidelines relevant to the situation are in existence. The compliance action is always directed at the party considered to be legally responsible. The product is detained until test results indicate the appropriate disposition. The sampling approach for compliance testing is referred to as in-depth sampling. The establishment of a chain of custody of the sample is essential if legal proceedings are expected to occur.

Drug monitoring is conducted at the slaughter plants by veterinary meat inspectors who test both a random selection of slaughter animals, according to a national survey plan, and also any suspect animals. When results from inplant screening tests are positive, or when an inspector has reason to suspect the presence of antibiotic residues even if the test kit result is negative, the carcass is retained pending laboratory testing of kidney and muscle tissues. A maximum turnaround time of 4 days from receipt to reports has been established for these held carcass samples. Testing to confirm positive inplant test results from slaughter plant meat samples is conducted within laboratories of the Food Production and Inspection Branch, Agriculture and Agri-Food Canada. Shipment of sample to the laboratory can add another 1–3 days to this time. The average laboratory turnaround time for these samples, using the current testing scheme, is under 2 working days.

11.7 REGULATORY OUTLINE IN JAPAN

Established in 1947, the Japanese Food Sanitation Law, which describes standards and criteria of foods, was the first essential law in Japan on food safety. According to this law, meat, eggs, milk, dairy products, fish, and shellfish should not contain any antibiotic or synthetic antibacterial substances.

In Japan, the principal legal regulations dealing with feed additives and veterinary drugs is the Pharmaceutical Affairs Law established in 1960. Table 11.10 summarizes the compounds currently regulated as medicinal or feed additives by the Pharmaceutical Affairs Law and the Law Concerning Safety Assurance and Quality Improvement of Feed in Japan (74).

On the basis of these legal regulations, foods are analyzed for residues of synthetic antibacterials and antibiotics used as feed additives or veterinary drugs. The analytical methods approved by the Japanese Government are published as two volumes. Volume I contains microbial inhibition tests organized by the Veterinary Sanitation Division, the Ministry of Health and Welfare, using antibiotic-sensitive strains of bacteria as test organisms. Volume II contains approved chemical methods for synthetic antibacterials. National surveys are conducted by the Veterinary Sanitation Division, Environmental Health Bureau, Ministry of Health and Welfare. Samples are collected from both urban and rural prefectures

TABLE 11.10 Veterinary Drugs Regulated as Medicinal or Feed Additive Agents in Japan

Class	Medicinal	Feed additive	Class	Medicinal	Feed additive
Aminoglycosides	Apramycin	Destomycin A	Macrolides	Erythromycin	Kitasamycin
	Destomycin A			Josamycin	
	Dihydrostreptomycin			Kitasamycin	
	Fradiomycin			Mirosamycin	
	Gentamicin			Oleandomycin	
	Hygromycin B	Hygromycin B		Sedecamycin	
	Kanamycin			Spiramycin	
	Spectinomycin			Terdecamycin	
	Streptomycin			Tylosin	Tylosin
β-Lactams	Amoxycillin		Tetracyclines	Chlortetracycline	Chlortetracycline
	Ampicillin			Doxycycline	
	Cloxacillin			Oxytetracycline	Oxytetracycline
	Dicloxacillin			Tetracycline	
	Mecillinam		Polyethers	Monensin	Lasalocid
	Nafcillin			Salinomycin	Monensin
	Penicillin G				Salinomycin
	Cephalonium				Avilamycin
	Cephazolin		Polysaccharides	Flavophospholipol	Flavophospholipol
Polypeptides	Bacitracin	Avoparcin		Bicozamycin	Bicozamycin
	Colistin	Bacitracin	Others	Chloramphenicol	
	Enramycin	Colistin		Fosfomycin	
		Enramycin		Lincomycin	
		Noshiheptide		Novobiocin	
	Thiopeptin	Thiopeptin			Polynactin
	Virginiamycin	Virginiamycin		Tiamulin	

and are sent for analysis to Government laboratories, including those of the Meat Inspection Offices, the Market Food Inspection Offices, and the Institutes of Public Health.

In recent years, public concern over the presence of drug residues in meat products has grown rapidly. To prevent the occurrence of drug residues, the law prescribes that animals are not to be slaughtered shortly after the drugs are administered or while the concentration of the drugs remains at therapeutically effective levels. However, instances of illegal or extralabel usage of drugs are occasionally found.

Since legal regulation for drug residues in foods at a level that would not produce any hazard to the health of the consumer was not available, in January, 1994, the Japanese Health and Welfare Ministry requested the Food Hygiene Investigative Committee to determine MRLs for those antibiotics, antibacterial agents, and hormones that have not been banned. Based on a November, 1995, report from the Food Sanitation Investigation Council, ministerial ordinances and notifications have been amended for six types of veterinary drug residues, including oxytetracycline. Standards for other veterinary drugs will gradually be set after deliberation by the Food Sanitation Investigation Council, once there are sufficient data to make a safety evaluation. In addition to antibacterial agents and hormones, tolerances are to be set for residual anthelminthics. Tolerances established for these compounds will be based on a consideration of the toxicological data and the establishment of a NOEL in experimental animals.

REFERENCES

1. K.N. Woodward, in Xenobiotics and Food-Producing Animals (D.H. Hutson, D.R. Hawkins, G.D. Paulson, and C.B. Struble, Eds.), American Chemical Society, Washington, DC (1992).
2. World Health Organization, in Evaluation of Certain Veterinary Drug Residues in Food, Thirty-sixth Report of the Joint FAO/WHO Expert Committee on Food Additives, Technical Report Series 799, World Health Organization, Geneva (1990).
3. World Health Organization, in Principles for the Safety Assessment of Food Additives and Contaminants in Food, Environmental Health Criteria 70, World Health Organization, Geneva, p. 75 (1987).
4. World Health Organization, in Principles for the Safety Assessment of Pesticide Residues in Food, Environmental Health Criteria 104, World Health Organization, Geneva, p. 76 (1990).
5. E.J. Bigwood, CRC Crit. Rev. Toxicol., 2:41 (1973).
6. M.K.J. Perez, Toxicol. Environ. Health, 3:837 (1977).
7. World Health Organization, in Evaluation of Certain Veterinary Drug Residues in Food, Thirty-second Report of the Joint FAO/WHO Expert Committee on Food Additives, Technical Report Series 763, World Health Organization, Geneva (1988).

8.   World Health Organization, in Evaluation of Certain Veterinary Drug Residues in Food, Thirty-fourth Report of the Joint FAO/WHO Expert Committee on Food Additives, Technical Report Series 788, World Health Organization, Geneva (1989).

9.   K.N. Woodward, in Food Contaminants: Sources and Surveillance (C. Creaser and R. Purchase, Eds.), Royal Society of Chemistry, London, p. 99 (1991).

10. C.L. Barry, and G.M. Mac Eachern, J. Assoc. Off. Anal. Chem., 66:4 (1983).

11. M. Gilliam, and R. Argauer, J. Environ. Entom., 10:479 (1981).

12. M. Gilliam, and S. Taber, J. Invert. Pathol., 31:128 (1978).

13. M. Gilliam, S. Taber, and R. Argauer, J. Apic. Res., 18:208 (1979).

14. K.N. Woodward, in Xenobiotics and Food-Producing Animals (D.H. Hutson, D.R. Hawkins, G.D. Paulson, and C.B. Struble, Eds.), American Chemical Society, Washington, DC (1992).

15. V. Burgat-Sacaze, A. Rico, and J.-C. Panisset, in Drug Residues in Animals (A.G. Rico, Ed.), Academic Press, Inc., Orlando, FL, p. 1 (1986).

16. A.Y.H. Lu, G.T. Miwa, and P.G. Wislocki, Rev. Biochem. Toxicol., 9:1 (1988).

17. L.H.M. Vroomen, M.C.J. Berghmans, P.J. van Bladeren, J.P. Groten, A.C.J. Wissink, and H.A. Kuiper, Drug Metab. Rev., 22:663 (1990).

18. P.G. Wislocki, and A.Y.H. Lu, Drug Metab. Rev., 22:649 (1990).

19. S. Sved, and B. Foster, Drug Metab. Rev., 22:849 (1990).

20. P. Evrard, and G. Maghuin-Rogister, Food Addit. Contam., 5:59 (1987).

21. J.E. Baer, T.A. Jacob, and F.J. Wolf, J. Toxicol. Environ. Health, 2:895 (1977).

22. Food and Drug Administration, in General Principles for Evaluating the Safety of Compounds in Food-Producing Animals, Food and Drug Administration, Rockville, MD (1986).

23. R.C. Livingston, in Agricultural Uses of Antibiotics (W.A. Moats, Ed.), American Chemical Society, Washington, DC, p. 129 (1986).

24. Federal Food, Drug, and Cosmetic Act, As Amended, the Food Additives Amendments of 1958, 72 Stat. 1784, 85th Cong., 2nd session, p. 331 (1958).

25. Food and Drug Administration, Fed. Reg., 52:49572 (1987).

26. J.H. Farmer, R.L. Kodell, and D.W. Gaylor, Soc. Risk Anal., 2:27 (1982).

27. Food and Drug Administration, in Proposed Guideline. Microbiological Testing of Antimicrobial Drug Residues in Food, Food and Drug Administration, Rockville, MD (1993).

28. J.D. MacNeil, and R.L. Ellis, in Chemical Analysis of Antibiotics Used in Agriculture (H Oka, H. Nakazawa, K.-I. Harada, and J.D. MacNeil, Eds.), AOAC International, Arlington, VA, p. 2 (1995).

29. B. Schwab, and J. Brown, in Agricultural Uses of Antibiotics (W.A. Moats, Ed.), American Chemical Society, Washington, DC, p. 137 (1986).

30. Food Safety and Inspection Service (FSIS), in Compound Evaluation and Analytical Capability National Residue Program Plan, US Department of Agriculture, Washington, DC, (1993).

31. Food Safety and Inspection Service (FSIS), in Compound Evaluation and Residue Information, US Department of Agriculture, Washington, DC, (1994).

32. Official Journal of the European Communities, No. L317, Brussels, p. 1 (1981).

33. Official Journal of the European Communities, No. L317, Brussels, p. 16 (1981).

34. Official Journal of the European Communities, No. L373, Brussels, p. 15 (1990).
35. Official Journal of the European Communities, No. L214, Brussels, p. 31 (1993).
36. Official Journal of the European Communities, No. L15, Brussels, p. 17 (1987).
37. Official Journal of the European Communities, No. L97, Brussels, p. 1 (1992).
38. Official Journal of the European Communities, No. L214, Brussels, p. 1 (1993).
39. Official Journal of the European Communities, No. L224, Brussels, p. 1 (1990).
40. Official Journal of the European Communities, No. L83, Brussels, p. 14 (1992).
41. Official Journal of the European Communities, No. L73, Brussels, p. 8 (1993).
42. Official Journal of the European Communities, No. L311, Brussels, p. 18 (1992).
43. Official Journal of the European Communities, No. L93, Brussels, p. 10 (1993).
44. Official Journal of the European Communities, No. L264, Brussels, p. 1 (1993).
45. Official Journal of the European Communities, No. L270, Brussels, p. 1 (1970).
46. Official Journal of the European Communities, No. L319, Brussels, p. 13 (1984).
47. Official Journal of the European Communities, No. L235, Brussels, p. 39 (1996).
48. K.N. Woodward, in General and Applied Toxicology (B. Ballantyne, T. Mars, and P. Turner, Eds.), MacMillan, Basingstoke, UK, p. 1105 (1993).
49. Official Journal of the European Communities, No. L275, Brussels, p. 36 (1986).
50. J.F. Kay, and C.E. Penny, in Residues of Veterinary Drugs in Food, Proc. Euroresidue III Conf., Veldhoven, 1996 (N. Haagsma and A. Ruiter, Eds.), Fac. Vet. Med., Univ. Utrecht, The Netherlands, p. 596 (1996).
51. Official Journal of the European Communities, No. L351, Brussels, p. 39 (1989).
52. Official Journal of the European Communities, No. L118, Brussels, p. 75 (1993).
53. Council of the European Communities, in The BCR Programme on Applied Metrology and Chemical Analysis. Projects and Results 1988–92, Report EUR 14800 (1992).
54. Official Journal of the European Communities, No. L223, Brussels, p. 18 (1987).
55. Official Journal of the European Communities, No. L286, Brussels, p. 33 (1990).
56. Official Journal of the European Communities, No. L118, Brussels, p. 64 (1993).
57. Official Journal of the European Communities, No. L118, Brussels, p. 75 (1993).
58. Council of the European Communities, in Veterinary Drug Residues. Residues in Food-Producing Animals and Their Products: Reference Materials and Methods (RJ Heitzman, Ed.), Luxembourg, Report EUR 14126 (1992).
59. Council of the European Communities, in Veterinary Drug Residues. Residues in Food-Producing Animals and their Products: Reference Materials and Methods (RJ Heitzman, Ed.), Blackwell Scientific Publications, Report EUR 15127-EN, Oxford, UK (1994).
60. R.W. Stefany, and L.A. van Ginkel, in Veterinary Drug Residues (W.A. Moats and M.B. Medina, Eds.), American Chemical Society, Washington, DC, p. 23 (1995).
61. Official Journal of the European Communities, No. L368, Brussels, p. 17 (1991).
62. Official Journal of the European Communities, No. L66, Brussels, p. 37 (1989).
63. Official Journal of the European Communities, No. L15, Brussels, p. 29 (1987).
64. Official Journal of the European Communities, No. L145, Brussels, p. 35 (1988).
65. R.J. Maxwell, A.A.M. Stolker, and A.R. Lightfield, J. High Resol. Chromatogr., 18: 231 (1995).
66. A. Preiss, G. Balizs, L. Benesch-Girke, T. Gude, A. Boenke, and R. Kroker, in Residues of Veterinary Drugs in Food, Proc. Euroresidue II Conf., Veldhoven, May

3–5, 1993 (N. Haagsma, A. Ruiter, and P.B. Czedik-Eysenberg, Eds.), Fac. Vet. Med., Univ. Utrecht, The Netherlands, p. 558 (1993).

67.　A. Boenke, Anal. Chim. Acta, 275:3 (1993).

68.　L.A. van Ginkel, R.W. Stephany, H.J. van Rossum, and M. Bos, in Residues of Veterinary Drugs in Food, Proc. Euroresidue II Conf., Veldhoven, May 3–5, 1993 (N. Haagsma, A. Ruiter and P.B. Czedik-Eysenberg, Eds.), Fac. Vet. Med., Univ. Utrecht, The Netherlands, p. 308 (1993).

69.　L.A. van Ginkel, R.W. Stephany, A. Spaan, and S.S. Sterk, Anal. Chim. Acta, 275: 75 (1993).

70.　L.A. van Ginkel, R.W. Stephany, and H.J. van Rossum, J. AOAC Int., 75:554 (1992).

71.　Official Journal of the European Communities, No. L15, Brussels, p. 29 (1987).

72.　Official Journal of the European Communities, No. L145, Brussels, p. 35 (1988).

73.　R.W. Stephany, and L.A. van Ginkel, Fresenius J. Anal. Chem., 338:370 (1990).

74.　H. Nicosia, in Chemical Analysis of Antibiotics Used in Agriculture (H. Oka, H. Nakazawa, K.-I. Harada, and J.D. MacNeil, Eds.), AOAC International, Arlington, VA, p. 31 (1995).

75.　World Health Organization, in Evaluation of Certain Veterinary Drug Residues in Food, Thirty-eighth Report of the Joint FAO/WHO Expert Committee on Food Additives, Technical Report Series 815, World Health Organization, Geneva (1991).

76.　World Health Organization, in Evaluation of Certain Veterinary Drug Residues in Food, Fortieth Report of the Joint FAO/WHO Expert Committee on Food Additives, Technical Report Series 832, World Health Organization, Geneva (1993).

77.　World Health Organization, in Toxicological Evaluation of Certain Veterinary Drug Residues in Food WHO Food Additives Series, No. 33 (1994).

78.　World Health Organization, in Evaluation of Certain Veterinary Drug Residues in Food, Forty-seventh Meeting of the Joint FAO/WHO Expert Committee on Food Additives, WHO Food Additive Series 38, World Health Organization, Rome, (1996).

79.　World Health Organization, in Evaluation of Certain Veterinary Drug Residues in Food, Forty-eighth Report of the Joint FAO/WHO Expert Committee on Food Additives, Technical Report Series 879, World Health Organization, Geneva (1997).

80.　World Health Organization, in Evaluation of Certain Veterinary Drug Residues in Food, Fiftieth Meeting of the Joint FAO/WHO Expert Committee on Food Additives, WHO Food Additive Series 41, World Health Organization, Rome, (1998).

81.　Joint FAO/WHO food standards programme codex alimentarius commission, report of the 11th session of the codex committee on residues of veterinary drugs in foods, Alinorm 99/31, Washington, DC, 15–18 September 1998.

82.　World Health Organization, in Evaluation of Certain Veterinary Drug Residues in Food, Fifty-second Meeting of the Joint FAO/WHO Expert Committee on Food Additives, WHO Food Additive Series 43, World Health Organization, Rome, (1999).

83.　Official Journal of the European Communities, No. L224, Brussels, p. 1 (1990).

84.　Official Journal of the European Communities, No. L205, Brussels, p. 1 (1998).

85.　Official Journal of the European Communities, No. L205, Brussels, p. 7 (1998).

86.　Official Journal of the European Communities, No. L205, Brussels, p. 10 (1998).

87. Official Journal of the European Communities, No. L343, Brussels, p. 8 (1998).
88. Official Journal of the European Communities, No. L102, Brussels, p. 58 (1999).
89. Official Journal of the European Communities, No. L118, Brussels, p. 23 (1999).
90. Official Journal of the European Communities, No. L118, Brussels, p. 28 (1999).
91. Official Journal of the European Communities, No. L122, Brussels, p. 24 (1999).
92. Official Journal of the European Communities, No. L122, Brussels, p. 30 (1999).

12

Global Harmonization of Regulatory Requirements

The legislation on the use of veterinary drugs in food-producing animals is regulated by many authorities throughout the world, all concerning the quality, efficacy, and safety of the use of these agents. However, considerable variation in the regulatory process is recognized to occur within different countries; licensing requirements may range from highly controlled to minimal inspection.

In some developing countries, there is no legal framework for prescription of veterinary drugs and, in some cases, they can be marketed without any type of review process by a regulatory authority. As food laws in many developing countries reflect their primary need to ensure an adequate supply of safe and wholesome food for the rapidly expanding population, drugs are usually more widely used in food-producing animals and under less rigorous systems of control than in the developed world. However, this can cause problems to the developed world, particularly with exports of animal products from developing countries.

Harmonized legislation relating to food safety does not exist even among countries of the developed world, and, therefore, a barrier to international food trade is often produced due to distortion of the conditions of competition in the market. Usage of veterinary drugs in any country usually complies with domestic MRLs in the edible animal products. Problems emerge, however, when these products are exported to markets where MRLs for a particular drug have not been established and default tolerances apply. In these cases, noncompliance of the imported product is the direct result of a drug not being needed or registered in the importing country and the procedural default tolerance being applied. All food importing or exporting countries run the risk of encountering such situations, which may have a significant impact on trading relationships; weaken consumer confidence; and impose considerable dislocation, uncertainty and, costs on exporting countries. Nevertheless, such situations, even when differences in dietary habits and agricultural practices are taken into account, rarely place consumer health and safety at risk.

Some critical differences in risk assessment procedure lead to confusing situations on a worldwide basis. These differences are due to some very controversial areas of safety issues including the calculation of the acceptable daily intake (ADI), the assignment of the ADI to maximum residue limit (MRL)/tolerance, the validation of the analytical methods needed to regulate drug residues, and the fitness of legislation to toxicology.

12.1   ACCEPTABLE DAILY INTAKE

A comparison of the worldwide risk assessment procedures for animal drug residues in food reveals different approaches in the establishment of the ADIs (Table 12.1). Major differences among regulatory agencies concern the number and type of genotoxicity studies required, the number of teratology studies required, the route of administration, the length of time for which the toxicology studies are conducted, the need for chronic versus subchronic or carcinogenic studies, the number of species in which reproductive toxicity studies are required, and the number of generations required per species (1). Differences in establishing an ADI continue with the safety factor applied to extrapolate from short-term animal studies to life time exposure in humans. Different safety factors can be applied for the same set of data and the resulting ADI can differ by as much as 10-fold.

Other particularly controversial issues of hazard and risk assessment that urgently need harmonization refer to the potential impact of residues of antimicrobial drugs on the human gut flora, the impact of bound residues, and the impact of residues at injection site on the calculation of ADIs.

Emergence of resistance among zoonotic pathogens has become an issue of increasing worldwide concern. While the phenomenon of induction of resistance is well known, there is no evidence for the supposed effects in humans in vivo as a result of ingestion of food contaminated with drug residues. At present, no standardized procedure exists to assess such effects, nor, indeed, are the effects themselves described adequately.

Despite the lack of agreed guidelines for the tests involved, tests do exist and they comprise studies in human volunteers, studies in germ-free rats the intestines of which harbor human gut bacteria, and in vitro studies with bacterial populations. However, the selection of the most appropriate test system remains an open question. All tests investigate minimum inhibitory concentrations (MICs) that can be used in ADI calculations; however, such ADI calculations tend to

TABLE 12.1   Approaches of Major Regulatory Authorities in Setting ADIs and MRLs

Features	FAO/WHO	European Union	United States
Genotoxicity	Required	Required	Required
Acute toxicity	Required	Required	Required
Short-term toxicity	Required	Required	Required
Reproduction	Required	Required	Required
Teratogenicity	Required	Two studies	One study
Oncogenicity	Required	Required	Required; threshold higher than European Union
Human microflora	Required	Required	Not required
Expert report	Required	Required	Not required
Safety factor	200–2000	100–1000; 1000 for studies shorter than 90 days	100–1000; 1000 for studies shorter than 90 days
Depletion of residues	Total/marker residue in two studies	Total/marker residue in four studies	Total/marker residue in target tissues only
MRL setting	MRL for each tissue	MRL for each tissue	MRL for target tissue only

be very conservative and may lead to long withdrawal periods for antibacterial substances.

Most recently, the entire area of antimicrobial resistance has raised its European head again. While the avoparcin story is well known, the Food and Agriculture Organization/World Health Organization (FAO/WHO) and the European Union (EU) are now embarking on a new program of resistance monitoring and surveillance. This is of particular importance in the veterinary domain. The future of feed additives, fluoroquinolones and macrolides, and questions relating to overuse of veterinary antibiotics are now being closely scrutinized, and monitoring programs upon which to make future decisions are now being initiated. It remains to be seen what lies ahead for feed additives and some of the therapeutic antibiotics widely used in veterinary medicine. In the meantime, many scientists face the calculation of ADIs based upon microbiological data as an interim and added safety measure, while others regard it as dubious science.

As a result of these considerations, a fundamental addition to the registration process in some countries is currently the evaluation of resistance concerns preapproval and the monitoring of susceptibility of zoonotic and/or target animal pathogens postapproval, as a critical part of the registration process. In some jurisdictions, issues arising for a particular product have to be addressed before renewal of a marketing authorization.

Another subject of scientific debate is still the bioavailability and toxicity of bound residues (2). Data on this particular topic are sparse but tend to suggest the absence of hazardous effects of bound residues rather than the contrary. Answers that remain to be provided on this subject concern the relevance of these toxicological effects and, if the effects are viable, the best and most reliable method by which they can be measured and evaluated for a specific compound. As long as these questions are not answered satisfactorily, any attempt to address them can only be considered as a shot in the dark and a potential waste of finance and time. The industry is prepared to perform any additional safety evaluation as long as the answers are reasonable and can result in a greater guarantee of protection for the consumer.

JECFA has addressed this issue and has recommended a systematic approach to the problem (3, 4). It suggests use of a mild extraction procedure to determine residues that are clearly bioavailable. This is followed by a more vigorous extraction using acids or enzymatic techniques to assess whether potentially biologically active compounds may be released in vivo. These studies can be backed up by relay methodologies by which tissues from treated animals are fed to laboratory species and the release of drug-related moieties measured. The Committee stressed the need to treat each drug on a case-by-case basis rather than laying down strict protocols to deal with bound residues as a common issue.

In addition, current Food and Drug Administration (FDA) guidelines outline a series of short-term and in vitro tests for the safety assessment of bound residues together with their chemical characterization (5). A study of reversibility of adduct formation is also included and as with the Joint FAO/WHO Expert Committee on Food Additives (JECFA) recommendation, drugs are investigated in an individual manner. It seems likely that the JECFA and FDA approaches, at least in general terms, will become widely adopted in this particular area of hazard and risk assessment.

Likewise, differences in the risk assessment procedures among different regulatory authorities might assume even more significance if the potential for violative residues at injection site were to be taken into consideration (6). This might become the case if certain countries decide to use this issue as a trade barrier. To make things worse, most countries do not have a formal surveillance program for monitoring residues at injection sites. Routine residue monitoring programs that use liver or kidney as the preferred sampling tissues cannot detect such residues. Even with port-of-entry programs that use meat as the sample tissue for analytical testing, the chances of detecting injection site residues are actually very low.

Recent Australian and Canadian studies (7–10) on residues at injection sites indicate that injection site residues of certain drugs are at levels high enough to cause public health and trade concerns. Major concerns raised by these studies are that in a significant number of cattle severe tissue reactions occur at the injection site, which adversely affect the quality of the carcass and also create an animal welfare issue. These tissue reactions lead to residues at the injection sites that persist beyond the withdrawal period whereas, in some cases, they can cause such an extremely variable residues depletion so that withdrawal periods cannot be readily established. Lesions at the injection sites are not always obvious on visual inspection and cannot be identified and discarded during trimming and processing of the carcass. Moreover, the presence or absence of violative residues in samples of kidney, liver, and muscle cannot be used as a reliable indicator of the fate of residues at an injection site.

Until recently, regulatory authorities have not insisted on information about residues that persist at or near the injection site when establishing ADIs or MRLs. Even though some countries currently require injection-site residue depletion studies, there are no so far clear guidelines, with the exception of the EU-issued ones, on how this information can be used or on the value of this information in determining the contribution of drug residues in edible tissues to the total daily intake. Hence, there exists a need for a harmonized approach to all aspects of residues at injection sites, including the elaboration of MRLs and withdrawal periods if they are to be considered important in terms of consumer safety and trade. A summary of the current position of major regulatory authorities toward the issue of residues at injection site and its contribution in establishing ADIs, MRLs and withdrawal periods is presented in Table 12.2.

In the absence of adequate information on the potential hazard of residues at injection site to the consumer, it is also difficult for most national authorities to develop a practical policy when evaluating injectable veterinary drugs to compensate for any potential risk posed by residues at injection sites. Because of this difficulty, greatly varying regulatory options are followed worldwide (11). According to one option, evaluation of injection site residues may not be necessary in view of the perceived extremely low incidence of these residues. According to another option, depletion studies of residues at injection site should be taken into account when establishing withdrawal periods to ensure that theses residues are not higher than the MRLs.

The latter option has been opposed, however, by sections of the veterinary drug and meat industry for several reasons. One reason is that the probability of meat consumption from an injection site is estimated to occur only once in the

TABLE 12.2   Position of Major Regulatory Authorities on Residues at Injection Site

Country/organization	Regulatory approach
FAO/WHO	Residues at injection site are assessed and comments made where appropriate, but results are not used in setting ADI and MRL.
EU	Specific guidelines have been prepared and depletion studies of residues at injection site are required, but results are not factored into the MRL; the withdrawal period is set at the point where residues are depleted below muscle MRL.
US, Canada	Tolerance/MRL is based on ordinary tissue. When residues are 10-fold higher at the injection site, the withdrawal period is adjusted relative to the difference.
Australia	Residues at injection site are not taken into account when establishing MRL and withdrawal period (currently under review).
Japan	Depletion studies of residues at injection site are required; the withdrawal period is established on the basis of ordinary tissue.

lifetime of only 1 : 20 consumers. Another reason is that for drugs with a good safety profile, establishment of withdrawal periods on the basis of depletion studies at injection site would be not necessary and would be prohibitively expensive. In addition, the hazard for contamination of meat with zoonotic or other microbes is far greater than the hazard posed by residues at injection site. Accidental and unintended ingestion of injection site residues by consumers is also recognized as not adding any toxicological concern to lifetime exposure of the drug involved. Furthermore, this option could lead to long withdrawal periods that could jeopardize a number of injectable drugs that are important for the food animal industry.

According to a third option, evaluation of injection site residues on ad hoc basis should be carried out depending on the pharmacological and toxicological profile of the drug, its potential to initiative hypersensitivity, and its persistence and irritability. Even though most authorities favor the third option, none so far has vocalized its policy on the matter, except the European Union.

12.2   ASSIGNMENT OF THE ADI TO MRL/TOLERANCE

MRL/tolerance is the highest concentration of the marker residue allowed in milk, eggs, and edible tissues. Observed values below the MRL/tolerance in marketed commodities are deemed safe for human consumption even if residues are present in measurable concentrations. Observed values that exceed MRL/tolerances in marketed commodities are violative but not necessarily a food safety concern because human safety is based on chronic exposure.

Differences in MRL/tolerances more often reflect differences in the use of that compound in a particular country, or in the choice of safety factors, food consumption values, or the analyte used in monitoring programs. The United States will, but does not always, assign tolerances when preslaughter drug withdrawal period is zero, Generally, the European Union assigns an MRL even when withdrawal periods are not required.

The MRL/tolerances for a certain drug are normally calculated from the ADI determined for that compound. However, the amount of the ADI assigned to the MRL is not consistent among regulatory agencies. Generally, the European Union does not assign all of the ADI, even when seemingly justified; it includes all of the four edible tissues plus milk and eggs in calculating residue daily consumption that must be equal or less than one ADI.

In contrast, the United States frequently assigns 100% of the ADI to each of the edible tissues (12). For those drugs, however, used in dairy cattle or laying hens, it reserves 50% of the ADI for milk or 20% for eggs, and the remainder for each of the four edible tissues: muscle, liver, kidney and fat.

The United States uses food consumption data and food factors in conjunction with the ADI to calculate the tolerance of residues in edible tissues. The calculation starts with an estimate of the safe concentration of the total drug residues by dividing the ADI by food factors that reflect the contribution of the edible tissues to the daily diet. Following analysis of the depletion of the total residues from the edible tissues, a target tissue is selected for residue monitoring. The residue whose concentration is in known relationship to the total residues in the target tissue is selected as the marker residue. The tolerance is the concentration of the marker residue in the target tissue, which ensures that the total residues in each edible tissue are below their safe concentration.

The MRL is the EU equivalent of the US tolerance. Since in addition to consumption figures the relative distribution of residues between edible tissues is considered in the calculation of the MRL, practical withdrawal periods can be set for products containing the active substances concerned. This is an important point that differentiates the approach used to set MRLs in the Europe from the approach used by the United States to set residue tolerances. At least two tissues, one on the carcass and one organ meat, have to be designated as target tissues.

The daily consumption figures used by the European Union, although similar to those proposed by JECFA, differ from the food factors employed in the United States. There is currently much debate over whether these daily consumption values represent a realistic food intake for the commodities involved. One could say that they neither take into account the so-called extreme consumer who might at an instance eat large daily quantities of liver nor do they represent international food consumption. It cannot be accepted, for example, that 300 g muscle can cover both the US and developing world consumption of beef. Nevertheless JECFA, through the Codex Alimentarius system attempts to recommend MRL values that will be universally applicable. For these reasons, some might say limitations, what might be seen as average values for food consumption must be adopted if a practical solution is to be found.

Table 12.3 shows the impact of the different evaluation procedures on the MRL/tolerance of a model drug. The same set of safety and residue data would

TABLE 12.3   Calculation of the US Tolerance and the EU MRL for a Model Drug

Experimental data on a model drug
    NOEL   0.3 mg/kg × day
    Total residues   liver > kidney > muscle > milk > fat
    Marker residue   constitutes 50% of the total residues
USA
    Safety factor: 1000
    ADI = NOEL × 60 kg (hypothetical human body weight)/Safety factor
    ADI = 0.3 mg/kg × day × 60 kg/1000 = 0.018 mg per person per day
    Safe concn = ADI/Food factor × 0.5 kg/day

Food commodity	Food factor	Safe concentration (ppb)
Muscle	1	9
Liver	0.5	72
Kidney	0.33	109
Fat	0.25	144

Tolerance of the marker residue in the target tissue liver: 36 ppb
EU
    Safety factor: 100
    ADI = NOEL × 60 kg (hypothetical human body weight)/Safety factor
    ADI = 0.3 mg/kg × day × 60 kg/100 = 0.18 mg per person per day

Food commodity	Total residues (ppb)	Daily food intake (kg)	Total residue intake (μg)	Relative distribution	Acceptable residue intake (μg)	Acceptable residue concn (ppb)
Muscle	200	0.3	60	0.067	12	40
Liver	4800	0.1	480	0.536	96.5	965
Kidney	1600	0.05	80	0.089	16	320
Fat	120	0.05	6	0.007	1.3	26
Milk	180	1.5	270	0.301	54.2	36
Total			896		180 (ADI)	

MRL of the marker residue in the target tissue liver : 482 ppb
MRL of the marker residue in the target tissue muscle : 20 ppb

result in a tolerance of 36 ppb for the marker residue in the target tissue liver in the United States while in the European Union the equivalent MRL value would be 482 ppb. Consequently, the calculated withdrawal periods will differ considerably as well.

Apart from differences in the establishment of the MRL/tolerance values, different procedures are also used for the calculation of the withdrawal period. Even in countries where similar MRLs have been established, similar drugs may differ greatly with respect to the withdrawal periods established by the national authorities. A greater degree of harmonization would be possible if a standard approach for calculating the withdrawal period was adopted throughout the world.

Presently, some countries including the United States and a few Member States of the European Union use statistical methods to establish withdrawal periods. However, most countries employ a simple method: the withdrawal period is set at the time point when residues in all tissues in all the animals have depleted to below the respective MRL values. When one has determined that time point, the estimation of a safety span also has to be considered in order to compensate for uncertainties of the biological variability. The dimensions of a safety span depend on various, not easy to specify, factors determined by the study design, the quality of the data, and the pharmacokinetic properties of the drug. Hence, an overall recommendation on the estimation of the safety span cannot be provided. An approximate guide for the safety span is likely to be a value of 10–30% of the time period when all observations are below the MRL. As an alternative, the safety span might be calculated from the tissue depletion curve as a value of possibly one to three times the half-life.

When considering the establishment of withdrawal periods for parenterally administered drugs, it is important to take into account the residues at the injection site. For drugs for which the target tissue or one of the target tissues is muscle, national authorities set withdrawal periods on the basis of the MRL for muscle. The injection site and its residues should be treated as normal muscle and the withdrawal period should be based on residue depletion to below the MRL at the injection site as well. Where muscle is not a target tissue and hence there is no MRL for muscle, national authorities should ensure that the withdrawal period is established to ensure that the ADI is not exceeded when the usual food package is consumed. Here, the usual food package of 300 g of muscle should be considered to include the injection site.

12.3 ANALYTICAL METHODS FOR RESIDUES DETERMINATION

Differences exist among regulatory agencies in establishing the relationship of the marker residue to total residues, and standardizing the conditions under which analytical methods will be required. Some countries require microbiological methods for antibiotics for which there is no known relationship to total residues of toxicological concern. Other countries such as the United States require an analytical method only for the marker residue in the target tissues. The European Union normally requires an analytical method for several tissues even when incurred residues are not present. It has not been generally specified whether analytical methods are needed always or only when withdrawal periods are indicated. Moreover, there are no standardized procedures for accounting for analytical method validation needs. This results in a continuing need for reliable analytical methods for use in determining whether or not the marker residue exceeds the MRL at the time a commodity is marketed, and in thus ensuring, compliance with national regulations as well as international requirements in the area of drug residues in food. Understanding the importance of mentioned differences might substantially improve harmonization efforts.

The reliability of a method can be determined by assessing certain method performance criteria including, specificity, accuracy, precision, limit of detection and quantitation, sensitivity, applicability, and practicability as appropriate (13). This very often requires that an extensive collaborative study be undertaken to obtain the necessary data. Methods that have successfully undergone this performance review testing have been considered to be validated for the purpose of the analysis (14).

The ideal validated method would be the one that has progressed fully through a collaborative study in accordance with international protocols for the design, conduct, and interpretation of method performance studies. A typical study of a determinative method conducted in accordance with the internationally harmonized International Organization for Standardization (ISO)/International Union for Pure and Applied Chemistry (IUPAC)/AOAC International (AOAC) protocol would require a minimum of up to five test materials including blind replicates or split-level samples to assess within-laboratory repeatability parameters, and eight participating laboratories (15). Included with the intended use should be recommended performance criteria for accuracy, precision and recovery.

Validation attempts in the field of drug residue analysis have demonstrated that the requirement for a full collaborative trial at the ideal level, while desirable, is sometimes impractical. Limiting factors for completing ideal multilaboratory validation studies are usually the high cost, lack of sufficient expert laboratories willing to participate in such studies, and overall time constraints. Hence, a three-laboratory validation study is often applied (16).

In cases in which this less stringent model cannot be used, alternative validation schemes may be used (17). These include a two-laboratory validation protocol similar to the AOAC International Peer Verified Method Protocol, or a single-laboratory validation approach. With any of the alternative validation schemes, the Joint FAO/IAEA Expert Consultation on Validation of Analytical Methods for Food Control strongly encourages that the validation work be conducted according to the principles outlined below:

- Laboratories carrying out the validation studies should operate under a suitable quality system based upon internationally recognized principles.
- Laboratories should have in operation a periodic, independent, third-party assessment mechanism of their whole validation process carried out by an accreditation agency, a Good Laboratory Practice authority, or one or more collaborating laboratories. As an alternative, the laboratory carrying out the validation may submit the validation work for peer review to be assessed by an appropriate organization. Such an independent assessment and review helps to ensure the transferability of the validated method from the originating laboratory to other laboratories.
- Analytical methods are assessed in respect to internationally accepted general analytical performance criteria for selection of methods of analysis, with emphasis on the assessment of the limit of quantitation rather than the limit of detection (18).
- The validation work should be carefully documented in an expert validation report in which it is unambiguously stated for which matrices and analyte levels the method has been found to perform in a satisfactory manner.

While the provision of suitably validated analytical methods is a necessary requirement for ensuring compliance with MRLs, the method alone is not sufficient to ensure creditable analytical measurements. In addition to selecting suitable methods, the analyst must demonstrate that the method is operating under statistical control in the laboratory and is performed to meet performance specifications as required by the analytical problem. This means that all methods should be applied in an environment with appropriate quality assurance procedures and performance evaluation checks.

Performance characteristics of residue methods are often only determined for major food animal species. The Joint FAO/IAEA Expert Consultation on Validation of Analytical Methods for Food Control (17) has discussed the issue of the availability of suitable analytical methods for determining compliance of residues in tissues of the so-called minor species with established MRLs. The Consultation has concluded that if metabolism and related pharmacokinetic data are similar in minor species to those in major species, only the recovery of the analytes in the minor species needs to be determined. If the recovery remains stable, there is no need to study the method performance any further. If the recovery is not stable the full set of performance data should be determined.

Chemical analytical methods used in veterinary drug residue depletion studies in target animals constitute a potential source of suitable methods for determining compliance of tissue residues with established MRLs. In some situations, these methods may have been used in several laboratories conducting depletion studies in the same analyte/tissue combination. Often, however, the information on these analytical methods may not have been studied or processed any further for their suitability as regulatory methods. At the national level many methods are available that are used for routine, but in many cases these methods have not been subjected to interlaboratory validation trials.

An analytical method must be properly validated if it is to be used at the national level for enforcement purposes. Validated methods stand on their own merits in contested legal actions in national courts. This situation has been recognized by all nations and international organizations. Initiatives to harmonize method validation criteria and approaches are currently being considered.

12.4   COMPLIANCE OF LEGISLATION WITH TOXICOLOGY

Although toxicology, through its risk assessment procedures and the establishment of the ADI, gives a base to legislation for prevention of public health risks from drug residues in food, some exceptions show that toxicology and legislation do not always fit together.

Toxicology and legislation in the field of health protection are related subjects but they do not use identical procedures. Toxicology follows scientific methods in the assessment of risks using results of experiments or epidemiological analyses. The final result will be a figure of a dose that is probably harmless for humans. Legislation, on the other hand, has to consider these scientific recommendations but has not always to follow them. The decision sometimes or mostly has to consider many other aspects, such as public opinion, right or wrong risk acceptance, political reliability, and social consequences.

Drug examples for which toxicology and legislation do not always fit together are the nitroimidazoles, the growth-promoting sex hormones, and the recombinantly produced somatotropins.

Nitroimidazoles are regulated within the European Union as both veterinary medicinal drugs and feed additives. As veterinary medicinal drugs, they are regulated under the Veterinary Medicines Directives 81/851/EEC and 81/852/EEC, which are dealt with by one Directorate General (19, 20), while as feed additives they are regulated under Directive 70/524/EEC, which is handled by a different Directorate General (21). Due to safety risk concerns, use of nitroimidazoles including ronidazole, ipronidazole, and dimetridazole as veterinary medicinal drugs has been prohibited in the European Union for administration to food-producing animals. Nevertheless, ipronidazole and dimetridazole, paradoxically, are still approved for use as feed additives in feedstuffs. For the latter use, formal MRLs and, consequently, residue monitoring are not required.

In order to avoid contradictory drug regulations and to ensure consumer safety, the European Union has recently initiated elaboration of an amendment of Council Directive No 87/153/EEC. The draft of this amended Commission Directive specifies for the first time a procedure for the establishment of MRLs for feed additives in animal-derived food. It is based on the ADI concept and on standard food packages similar to those used for the safety assessment of veterinary medicinal drugs.

The growth-promoting sex hormones have been used for many years in both the European Union and the United States to increase body weight gain in immature calves. Three naturally occurring sex steroids, (estradiol, progesterone, and testosterone), and two synthetic compounds, (zeranol and trenbolone acetate) are still used legally in US cattle and sheep (22). All growth-promoting hormone products used in the United States are manufactured in the form of ear implants. Approximately 63% of all cattle and about 90% of the fed cattle in the United States are implanted. In large commercial feedlots, the rate approaches 100%.

As fattening agents, these hormones have several economic, health, and environmental benefits. The resulting beef is leaner, less feed is needed to produce the same amount of meat, and animals produce less waste. When steers and heifers are implanted with growth promoters, they grow significantly faster than nonimplanted animals. Using implants allows the cattle grower to realize an 8–12% increase in carcass weight per unit of feed. Growth implants can reduce the total cost of beef production by $50–80 per steer. If implants were banned, the average retail price of all cuts of beef would increase by 10–15%, or about 20- to 30 cents per pound (23).

Despite those advantages, use of these growth-promoting agents has been prohibited in the European Union since 1989. As a consequence, a ban has been implemented on imports of red meat from animals treated with growth-promoting hormones, cutting off US beef exports to the European Union valued at about $100 million annually.

The issue over the use of hormones as growth promoters in cattle goes back to the 1980s. In 1980, a health scandal in Italy raised suspicions about school lunches containing veal that may have contained hormone residues. Diethylstilbestrol (DES), a synthetic drug that can promote weight gain and muscle development in animals, was detected in veal samples (24). The scandal sparked a consumer boycott of veal, and Italy adopted measures to restrict imports of veal from EC Member States, particularly France, where hormones were authorized. In July 1981, the EU Council adopted Directive 81/602 to prohibit the use of hormones, except for therapeutic purposes. The Council postponed action for five hormones (estradiol, progesterone, testosterone, trenbolone acetate, and zeranol), calling for a Commission report no later than July 1, 1984. Member state regulations were to apply until the Council made a decision on these substances.

The Commission set up a Scientific Working Group on Anabolic Agents in Animal Production, which was composed of 22 notable European scientists, to determine whether use of these five hormones as growth promoters posed any health risk (25). In 1982, an interim report by this Working Group concluded that the three natural hormones (estradiol, progesterone, and testosterone), would not present any harmful effects to the health of the consumer when used under appropriate conditions as growth promoters in farm animals. The Group also reported that further research was necessary on the two synthetic hormones. The report was approved by the EU Veterinary Committee in November, 1982, and the Working Group continued to collect and evaluate information on trenbolone and zeranol during 1983 and 1984.

In June, 1984, the EU Commission proposed amending Directive 81/602 to allow the use of natural hormones, and in July the EU Council president requested the European Parliament for an opinion on this proposal. In October, 1985, the European Parliament adopted a resolution on the Commission's proposal. The resolution claimed that scientific information about the five hormonal substances was far from complete and that considerable doubt therefore exists about the desirability of their use and of their effect on human health. It endorsed a ban on zeranol and trenbolone on the grounds that their safety has not been conclusively proven, and rejected the proposed authorization of the three natural hormones except for therapeutic purposes.

In November, 1985, the Commission submitted to the Council a draft regulation that would ban natural hormones, except for therapeutic purposes, and banned synthetic hormones altogether. In December, 1985, the Commission's proposal to amend Directive 81/602 to prohibit use of anabolics was adopted by the Council and became Council directive EC 85/649. The directive banned the use of natural hormones except for therapeutic purposes and absolutely banned the use of synthetic hormones. The directive also imposed a trade clause that required Member States to prohibit importation from third countries of live animals and of meat from animals to which have been administered in any way whatever substances with a thyreostatic, estrogenic, androgenic, or gestagenic action. Member States were required to bring this directive into force no later than January 1, 1988.

In September, 1986, the United States raised the EU hormone ban in the Committee on Technical Barriers to Trade of the General Agreement on Tariffs and Trade (GATT). In 1987, after a series of informal bilateral discussions, the United States invoked dispute settlement under the Tokyo Round Agreement on Technical Barriers to Trade. Formal bilateral consultations were held on two occasions without a satisfactory resolution. The United States then requested that the matter be referred to a group of technical experts. The European Union blocked the formation of the technical expert group, and the dispute went unresolved.

In June 1987, the JECFA established acceptable daily intake levels and acceptable residue limits for zeranol and trenbolone acetate and decided that these levels were not needed for the naturally occurring hormones. With respect to the natural hormones, the JECFA explained that residues resulting from use of these compounds as growth promoters in accordance with good veterinary and and animal husbandry practice are unlikely to pose a hazard to human health (26).

In November, 1987, largely in response to complaints from exporting countries, the European Union delayed application of the hormone ban to imports for 1 year until January 1, 1989. In December, 1987, the CVDCAC agreed on safe limits for trenbolone and zeranol, and agreed that limits were unnecessary for the three natural hormones. In December, 1987, President Ronald Reagan announced, and suspended, retaliatory tariff increases on certain EU imports. Throughout 1988, the United States and the European Union negotiated but were unable to resolve the dispute.

In November, 1988, the EU Commission notified the United States that the hormone directive would apply to all meat, including pork and horse-meat. The US Department of Agriculture (USDA) informed the European Union that the United States has no hormonal substances approved for use in pork or horse-meat. The Commission indicated that the United States needed a residue testing program for these meats to be in compliance with the directive. In December, 1988, the European Union approved a counterretaliation list, but implementation was postponed until January, 1989. On January 1, 1989, the European Union hormone ban and the US retaliation measures took effect.

In June, 1991, the full Codex Commission met. The three natural hormones were on the agenda for a final decision, after a lengthy eight-stage approval process. The European Union arranged for an unprecedented vote on the hormones. Due to the EU focus on nonscientific criteria and to many delegations being unprepared for a vote, the Commission decided to postpone a final decision until its next meeting in the summer of 1993.

In 1993, the issue of the role of science in the Codex decisionmaking process was delegated to the Committee on General Principles. With participation by both the United States and the European Union, the Committee developed four principles that reenforced the preeminent role of science. In January, 1995, the GATT Uruguay Round Agreement and the Sanitary and Phytosanitary text were implemented. In July, 1995, the four principles developed by the Codex committee were presented to the full Codex Commission. During a lengthy debate, a diverse set of countries gave strong support to the preeminent role of science in the Codex decision-making process, and the principles were adopted despite EU opposition. In addition, the Codex Commission decided that MRLs were not necessary for the three natural hormones and adopted MRLs for trenbolone and zeranol.

From November 29 to December 3, 1995, the European Union held its Scientific Conference on Growth Promotion in Meat Production. The conference concluded that there was no evidence of health risk from the five hormones approved for use in the United States. On January 18, 1996, the European Parliament voted 366 to 0 out of 626 total Parliamentarians for a resolution to maintain the ban. On January 22, the Agriculture Council discussed the final report of the Hormone Conference and also reaffirmed its commitment to maintaining the ban.

In 1996, the United States and Canada launched separate World Trade Organization (WTO) dispute settlement panel cases against the European Union hormone ban. The WTO Agreement on Sanitary and Phytosanitary Measures, an important part of the Uruguay Round, protects exporters against the use of health-related measures as disguised barriers to trade. It has several provisions that relate directly to the EU hormone ban. Under the SPS Agreement, all health or safety measures must be based on sound scientific principles, whereas these measures must be based on the concepts of risk assessment. The WTO dispute settlement panel issued its final ruling on June 30, 1997. It found that the EU ban on imports of beef violated several of the provisions of the WTO Agreement on Sanitary and Phytosanitary Measures. The European Union, however, has appealed the ruling.

The issue of hormones have received widespread publicity in recent years. Belief that residues of hormones represent a real hazard is a misconception not supported by experience or by the results of government monitoring of the beef supply. Overwhelming scientific evidence has shown that beef from cows treated with US-approved compounds is completely safe (27).

Despite the small increase in estradiol, progesterone, and testosterone in meat from treated animals, the levels of these hormones are far less than those naturally found in meat from sexually mature animals. Estradiol levels in muscle from cattle in late pregnancy are 3–80 times greater than those found in the muscle of estradiol-treated heifers. The concentration of progesterone in muscle from pregnant cattle is likewise more than 20 times higher than that occurring in progesterone-treated steers. Muscle from mature bulls contains approximately eight times the level of testosterone found in testosterone-treated heifers. Consequently, there is no such thing as hormone-free beef (28, 24). All beef, and all other meats, naturally contain hormones at extremely low levels. Moreover, a number of other foods including milk and milk products, eggs, cabbage, and soybean oil contain naturally occurring hormonally active substances at levels far exceeding those found in meat from treated cattle.

Because these compound are naturally occurring in humans and in food-producing animals, the consumer is exposed throughout his or her lifetime to large quantities of these hormones through daily production and to much lesser quantities from food from unmedicated animals. For estradiol and progesterone, prepubertal boys synthesize the least whereas prepubertal girls synthesize the least amount of testosterone per day (29). Prepubertal boys produce per day 100–3000 times the amount of estradiol and more than 500 times the amount of progesterone that would be expected to occur in 500 g meat from treated animals. Similarly, prepubertal girls produce 600–900 times the amount of testosterone that would be expected to be present in 500 g meat from treated animals.

On the other hand, as a result of hormone implants the average amount of estrogen can be increased in a 3 oz serving of beef from 1.3 ng in a sample from a nonimplanted steer to 1.9 ng in a sample from a steer implanted 100 or so days prior to slaughter. If it is realized, however, that the average nonpregnant human female produces 480,000 ng estrogen/day by normal physiological body processes, the increased body load of estrogen occasioned by eating 3 oz beef from an implanted steer (total of 480,001.9 versus eating 3 oz beef from a nonimplanted steer, total 480,001.2) is of no physiological or medical consequence to the consumer (30). Therefore, consumers will not be at risk by eating meat from animals treated with estradiol: the amount of added hormone is negligible compared to the consumer's own daily production rate.

The same situation applies to testosterone and progesterone. Unlike the naturally occurring hormones, there is no daily production rate for the synthetic compounds trenbolone acetate and zeranol. Therefore, the FDA requires toxicological testing in animals to determine a safe level in meat for these compounds. When FDA approved zeranol and trenbolone, it determined that residues were well below a safe concentration and therefore no residue tolerance was required (25). Due to consumer concerns, testing procedures for zeranol were put into place in the early 1980s but were discontinued in the late 1980s because no residue violations were found.

It is obvious, therefore, that the EU decision to ban the growth-promoting hormones, both natural and synthetic, in beef production has no scientific basis. There is little doubt that the ban was initially developed, in large part, in response to consumer pressure by the widely publicized illegal use of DES in veal calves in Italy several years ago. This publicity caused some antitechnology activists to seek a ban on all hormone products.

Of course, consumers have the right to be able to buy safe food. If consumers want to buy beef from untreated cattle, and producers are able to market it as such in a way consistent with truth-in-labeling principles, there may be no objection. However, the evidence indicates that the EU ban is not ensuring a safe beef supply. There are widespread reports of use of illegal and often dangerous hormones, and low consumer confidence is contributing to a declining beef consumption.

The exact cause of the profound antihormone sentiment among the European public is unclear, but seems to be related to the European farm price support systems, which were resulting in costly excess production of beef. Political figures who wanted to reduce the mountain of surplus beef utilized government action on hormones as one way to reduce beef production. By making growth hormones illegal, they were able to remove competing US imports and those from other nations that utilized growth hormones to a large extent. The EU hormone ban in 1989 was in response to beef supplies, not to health risks. It appears that the

European Union used the hormone issue to create a nontariff trade barrier to preclude importation of US beef into EU Member States (29–31).

Recombinant bovine somatotropin (rBST) is another example of a drug that complicates the trade of dairy products between the United States and the European Union. This substance has been one of the most extensively studied animal drug products. In the mid-1980s, the FDA Center for Veterinary Medicine first determined that food products from rBST-treated cows are safe for human consumption. Since that time, the agency has authorized rBST testing on more than 20,000 cows in the United States. In 1990, FDA scientists summarized more than 120 studies all concerning the safety of milk and meat from dairy cows treated with rBST (32). This review allowed FDA to conclude that milk and meat from cows treated with rBST, under conditions authorized by FDA, are safe within the meaning of the Federal Food, Drug and Cosmetic Act.

The FDA conclusion that rBST poses no risk to human health has been affirmed by a variety of scientific reviews conducted by the National Institutes of Health, the Congressional Office of Technology Assessment, Canadian and EU regulatory agencies, and by the Health and Human Services Office of Inspector General. Apart from the FDA, the Joint FAO/WHO Expert Committee on Food Additives also stated in 1993 that edible products from rBST-treated animals do not pose any risks to humans (33). In 1998, the Committee reconfirmed, after examining new evidence, that there are no food safety or health concerns related to bovine somatotropin residues in products such as milk and meat from treated animals (14). In arriving at its conclusion, the Committee considered several concerns including the likelihood of mastitis increase in rBST-treated cows and the risk of insulin-dependent diabetes mellitus. The Committee concluded that rBST neither increases the incidence of mastitis above that expected from the greater milk yield nor represents an additional risk for the development of diabetes mellitus.

In view of these findings, FDA has placed no restriction on the commercial use of milk and meat from cows treated with rBST. In contrast, the European Union has opposed the use of this hormone, thus complicating the trade of dairy products with the United States. Council Decision 94/936/EC states that rBST is an issue that gives rise to considerable interest among consumers, agricultural, and industry interests. In this context, concerns have been expressed about the safety to humans, animals, and the environment; the quality of milk; the economic and social consequences in agriculture; the climate for research and development, industrial competitiveness, and trade implications.

A major food safety issue addressed by the European Union concerns the increase in the level of circulating insulin-like growth factor (IGF-I) in the target animal and its increased excretion in the milk as a consequence of the administration of rBST. There has been epidemiological evidence for an association between circulating IGF-I levels and the relative risk of breast and prostate cancer (34–36).

It is worthwhile to emphasize that these retrospective studies refer to a time interval in which exposure to dairy products originated exclusively from non-rBST-treated animals.

IGF-I, a single chain polypeptide, is a physiological constituent of bovine milk. During lactation, a typical IGF-I profile in cow's milk varies from 150 ng/ml after parturition, to 25 ng/ml at the end of the first week of lactation, to 1–5 ng/ml at day 200 of lactation (37, 38). However, data on the actual amount of IGF-I in milk are inconsistent since the physiological levels show a considerable variation depending on the age of animals, state of lactation, and nutritional status (39, 40). On the other hand, the IGF-I concentration in human breast milk at weeks 6–8 is 22 ng/ml.

As a consequence of rBST treatment, a two- to fivefold increase of IGF-I has been reported in several studies (32). JECFA cited average control values for IGF-I in milk of 3.7 ng/ml for untreated cows, and a significant increase to an average of 5.9 ng/ml as a consequence of rBST treatment (41). These levels correspond to amounts several times lower than the total amount of IGF-I secreted daily in the gastrointestinal tract of humans. These findings justify the argument that the additional amounts of IGF-I ingested with milk from treated animals will not result in any adverse effects. Nevertheless, further concerns have been expressed by the EU about the role of milk casein, which may hypothetically increase the resistance of exogenous and possibly endogenous IGF-I towards proteolytic cleavage and inactivation, thus constituting a potential health hazard (42).

12.5 HARMONIZATION INITIATIVES

Registration of veterinary drugs has become an industry in its own right. The requirements for registering and marketing veterinary pharmaceutical products have expanded enormously over the past 30 years so that a separate industry has grown up to cater to a massive volume of data and a plethora of regulation. However, the pharmaceutical industry is becoming increasingly unwilling to invest in the research and development of newly synthesized veterinary products. There is a considerable danger that increasing the complexity and nature of the data required of pharmaceutical companies will inevitably result in reduction in the range and number of new products available to the veterinary profession for treatment and prevention of animal disease.

A major factor jeopardizing the maintenance of some of the existing drugs that have been in common use for decades is the need to generate data for calculating MRLs. This factor may lead to a reduction in licensed proven products and create the potential for a rise in unlicensed or illegal products, leading in turn to a genuine hazard to human health. Therefore, a revisionary approach in which genuine international dialogue will take place leading to significant international harmonization seems to be indispensable.

The initiative to begin the harmonization process came in 1983 when the first International Technical Consultation on Veterinary Drug Registration (ITCVDR) was held. As global harmonization of the MRLs was becoming increasingly essential for unconstrained world trade of animal-derived food products, international initiatives to harmonize the regulatory requirements and evaluation procedures for animal drug residues in milk, eggs, and edible tissues of food-producing animals began to develop as a lofty but necessary goal. Since then a series of government and industry initiatives has been developed as follows:

- The Codex Alimentarius Committee on Residues of Veterinary Drugs in Foods in 1985.
- The US FDA and the European Union have held regular bilateral meetings for the last decade to discuss common areas of interest. This has involved mutual exchange of guidelines for consultation.
- Meetings on harmonization of veterinary biologicals were held in 1992 in Ploufragan, France; in 1994 in Arlington, Virginia, US; and in 1995 in Singapore.
- In 1993, the Global Harmonization of Standards (GHOST) discussion document was published by FEDESA. This sets out a program for the international harmonization of registration requirements for veterinary pharmaceuticals and biologicals.
- Following discussions at ITCVDR and Office International des Epizooties (OIE) conferences, the OIE set up an ad hoc group on the harmonization of veterinary medicinal products in 1994.
- Preparatory work carried out by this OIE ad hoc group led to establishment of an International Cooperation on Harmonization of Technical Requirements for Registration of Veterinary Medicinal Products (VICH).

The need for international harmonization of standards and approach to residue issues has gained new urgency as a result of provisions in the General Agreement on Tariffs and Trade (GATT). The GATT provisions on sanitary and phytosanitary measures call for the use of Codex Alimentarius standards as reference points in resolving international trade disputes with regards to food standards including MRLs. This is currently the subject of discussion by many worldwide regulatory agencies and other parties including consumers, food producers, and drug manufacturers.

Harmonization of standards and evaluation procedures in the area of consumer safety will strengthen public confidence in the safety of food stuffs of animal origin, decrease trade barriers for food commodities and veterinary medicinal products, and help to reduce the amount of animal experimentation. In any proposals to overcome these problems, protecting consumer health and safety is paramount. The simplest solution would be for all countries to harmonize their MRLs. This has been attempted several times without success, possibly due to the fact that differing regional dietary habits and agricultural practices have not been taken into account, but more likely due to differing trade interests among food-importing countries.

Notwithstanding these differences, the United Nations (UN), in a continuing effort to protect the world population against harm from every sector while facilitating world trade, instituted the Codex Alimentarius Commission through which controls may be established over virtually every category of food entering the human body. The Codex Alimentarius Commission, according to official UN documents, is an intergovernmental body that currently has 157 member governments, representing over 98% of the world consumers. One of the main tasks of the Committee is to establish worldwide harmonized MRLs. The standards, guidelines, and recommendations of the Commission are used by the World Trade Organization as reference points. While noncompulsory, the UN claims that the work of Codex has been widely accepted because it is based on sound scientific risk assessment.

Despite being an extensive listing, the Codex MRLs do not cover all the drugs used in modern agriculture. Some notable omissions include a number of new-generation drugs that have come onto the market in the last 5–10 years. Moreover, Codex processes are slow, and despite efforts to accelerate them, they have generally failed to keep pace with demand. However, provisions of the Sanitary and Phytosanitary Measures Agreement (SPS Agreement) concluded under the Uruguay Round of Trade Negotiations, will place far greater importance on Codex Standards, including MRLs.

Under the SPS agreement, if an importing country's MRL is more stringent than the Codex MRL for the same drug/commodity combination, the importing country may be required to justify scientifically why it cannot accept the Codex MRL. These provisions will improve the flow of international trade and help reduce the number of different national MRLs. Default tolerances will be subject to the same treatment as MRLs established after full scientific evaluation of the chemicals concerned.

Because it will take time for the SPS Agreement to have a significant impact, alternative ways of managing most of the residue problems currently present in international food trade are also being examined. They are based on different concepts including that of the temporary tolerance, the adoption of MRLs by reference, the categorization of residue incidents, and the response and pipeline clearance strategies.

The concept of temporary tolerance applies in situations where importing countries have not established MRLs for particular commodity/drug combinations, and therefore default tolerances apply. It aims to establish a temporary procedure under which international food trade can be kept unrestricted while more permanent solutions can be negotiated.

In practice, an exporting country would identify those commodity/drug combinations most likely to generate residue incidents in key export markets and, through agreed channels, would provide the regulatory authorities of importing countries with the chemical evaluation data it normally uses in its registration processes. The objective is that a review of the supplied evaluation data would lead to a temporary tolerance for the particular drug/commodity combination being established at, or about, the level applicable in the exporting country. Assuming that the exporting country employs acceptable scientifically based evaluation procedures to establish its MRL, there should be no threat to consumer health and safety. Moreover, it would be consistent with the SPS Agreement procedures.

The concept of adoption of MRLs by reference aims to establish a permanent mechanism under which an importing country with no established MRLs for particular commodity/residue combinations will automatically apply the Codex MRL to relevant imported products. For those situations in which the Codex has not yet established MRLs, the MRL of the exporting country, or that of an agreed third country, would automatically be applied, provided that the MRLs have been determined by scientifically based chemical evaluation procedures. This mechanism already applies in a number of EU countries and is consistent with EU directives.

Bilateral arrangements between national drug registration authorities to recognize mutually the evaluation and registration procedures would be a logical follow on to this process. These agreements, as well as the regular exchange of information and possibly personnel exchanges, would lead to greater confidence in the registration processes of each country. In turn, this would lead to greater and speedier acceptance of the overall integrity of national drug registration processes.

The concept of the categorization of residue incidents is based on development of a system to categorize residue incidents according to response actions needed to deal with them, while at the same time enhancing consumer confidence in food safety. A scientifically sound classification of residue incidents together with regulatory strategies that reassure consumers and inform import control agencies of the appropriate ways to handle residue issues are likely to go a long way towards defusing sensitivities associated with minor incursions above MRLs. This is especially true in cases where import tolerances are set at zero, or near zero, because the chemicals concerned have not been evaluated by the importing country.

This can be effected through scientifically sound and transparent assessment of the risks presented to consumers by drug residues in foods. It also seeks to minimize the impact on the trade of residue incidents by establishing the basis for a predictable and stable regulatory response to specific detection cases. By this system, ad hoc and unscientific decisions would be avoided, consumer concerns would be addressed, and the uncertainties, delays, costs, and disruptions to trade would be avoided.

Under the proposal, residue incidents would be categorized into risk groups, which in turn would be used to determine the nature and severity of any response actions needed. Criteria for such categorizations would be determined by the impact consumption of a particular food would have on the dietary intake of consumers, measured as a proportion of the Acceptable Daily Intake. This approach recognizes that chemical residues occasionally consumed at concentrations marginally above MRL rarely present a risk to public health, whereas they may do so at higher concentrations.

The concept of the response and pipeline clearance strategies aims to making the control strategy more effective. Controls designed specifically for raw material inputs would be implemented in the country of origin to screen out contaminated material from the food chain. In the case of slaughter animals, these controls might be exercised on the farm, at the abattoir, or at a later stage during the processing line.

Apart from the Codex Alimentarius Commission, the EU is also concerned with the harmonization of pertinent regulations that differ among the Member States, thus permitting free circulation in the market of food of animal origin (43). Up to now considerable progress in establishing EU-harmonized MRLs has been made for many drugs, whereas a number of other old and new drugs are under investigation.

Even when Community MRLs have been established, similar products in various member states may differ greatly with respect to the withdrawal times established by national authorities. Most member states employ a simple method by which the withdrawal time is set at the time when residues in all tissues in all the animals have depleted to below the respective MRL values. In addition, some member states then add an additional safety period if, for example, there are large variations in the depletion data set or other shortcomings are found in the studies. On the other hand, some other member states use statistical methods to establish withdrawal times. A greater degree of harmonization would be possible if a standard approach for calculating the withdrawal time was adopted throughout the European Union. Moreover, this would aid both the centralized and the decentralized procedures.

It becomes evident that the best approach to ensuring that food commodities do not exceed their MRLs is to have in place comprehensive management systems and, where necessary, regulatory controls covering all aspects of the registration and use of veterinary drugs. Drug registration procedures must not only focus on matters such as toxicology, chemistry, environmental, and consumer protection, but also on the potential impact chemical residues can have on international trade.

As a result of a Free Trade Agreement (FTA), the United States and Canada have also made substantial harmonization efforts (44). One intention of the FTA was to remove tariff and nontariff barriers to trade in agricultural and nonagricultural products. In this area, the major goals included halting the growth in new barriers to agricultural trade and phasing out the barriers that existed; freezing the present level of trade-distorting agricultural subsidies and phasing out the use of subsidies over time; and harmonizing, among others, food regulations to ease trade. To implement certain provisions of the agreement on technical regulations and standards, the US Center for Veterinary Medicine, the Canadian Bureau of Veterinary Drugs, and Agriculture Canada established several working groups including a group on Veterinary Drug Tolerances.

The primary charges to the Working Group on Veterinary Drug Tolerances were to harmonize the procedures used for evaluating new animal drugs, performing risk assessments and calculating MRL/tolerances, and harmonizing the MRL/tolerances for approved drugs with the goal of having the same figures in each country. The first of these charges was met early in the negotiations. Both countries agreed to require the same toxicological data and to use identical procedures for calculating safe concentrations and tolerances. Specifically, the countries agreed to use the same safety and food factors and human body weight (60 kg) when calculating safe concentrations (45, 46). The procedures adopted by the US and Canada were consistent with those used by the European Union and JECFA.

As a result of these harmonization efforts, Canada published an index of 38 drugs for which MRL/tolerances have been harmonized through the FTA (47). The United States and Canada prepared also a second index of drugs for which there are different MRL/tolerances between the two countries. An amalgamation of both of these indexes is presented in Table 12.4.

The working group concluded that there appeared to be little or no human food safety significance to the MRL/tolerance figures that differed. In some instances, the differences were attributed to the use of different average human body weights (50 versus 60 kg) in calculating the safe concentration. In other cases, the difference reflected each country coming to its own conclusion on the detection limit of a particular analytical method. The working group determined that an effort to make MRL/tolerance figures identical for every drug would be resource-demanding and might not prove fruitful. Accordingly, the working group recommended that the two countries find an appropriate procedure for recognizing and accepting the MRL/tolerances of each country when it is concluded that there is no human food safety concern.

Such a procedure that is based on use of the ADI as the safety standard for reaching conclusions on the acceptability of residues in food has been recently reported in the literature (48). By this procedure, the equivalence of different MRLs for the same veterinary drug can be determined by predicting, with varying

TABLE 12.4 Harmonization of Tolerances (MRLs) Between the United States and Canada

Drug (marker)	Matrix	MRL (ppb)
Ampicillin	Swine and bovine tissues; milk	10
Amprolium	Chicken and turkey muscle	500
	Chicken and turkey liver and kidney	1000
	Eggs	7000
Apramycin	Swine kidney	100
Arsanilic acid (arsenic)	Swine, chicken, and turkey muscle; eggs	500
	Swine, chicken, and turkey liver	2000
Bacitracin	Milk	0.02 IU/ml for US 0.05 IU/ml for Canada
Buquinolate	Chicken muscle	100
	Chicken liver, kidney, skin and fat	400
Ceftiofur	Bovine kidney	None for US 6800 for Canada
Cephapirin	Milk	20
	Bovine tissues	100
Chlortetracycline	Bovine liver, kidney, and muscle; sheep muscle	100
	Swine fat	200
	Sheep liver	500
	Chicken and turkey muscle, liver, skin, and fat; swine muscle; calf fat and muscle; sheep kidney	1000
	Swine liver	2000
	Swine, chicken, and turkey kidney; calf liver and kidney	4000
Clopidol	Chicken and turkey muscle	5000
	Chicken and turkey liver and kidney	15,000
Cloxacillin	Milk	10 for US 30 for Canada
Decoquinate	Bovine, goat, and chicken muscle	1000
	Bovine and goat kidney, liver and fat; chicken kidney, liver, skin and fat	2000
Dihydrostreptomycin	Milk	125
Erythromycin	Milk	50
	Swine tissues	100
	Chicken and turkey tissues	125

(continued)

TABLE 12.4   Continued

Drug (marker)	Matrix	MRL (ppb)
Fenbendazole	Bovine liver	800 for US
		450 for Canada
	Swine liver	None for US
		4500 for Canada
Gentamicin	Turkey tissues	100
	Swine kidney	400
Halofuginone HBr	Chicken liver	160 for US
		100 for Canada
Hydrocortisone	Milk	10
Ivermectin (22,23-dihydroavermectin B_{1a})	Bovine liver	15
	Sheep liver	30
	Swine liver	20 for US
		15 for Canada
Lasalocid	Bovine liver	700 for US
		650 for Canada
	Chicken skin and fat	300 for US
		350 for Canada
Levamisole HCl	Bovine, sheep, and swine tissues	100
Maduramicin	Chicken skin and fat	380 for US
		400 for Canada
Monensin	Bovine tissues	50
Morantel tartrate (N-methyl-1,3-propane diamine)	Bovine liver	700 for US
		500 for Canada
Narasin	Chicken fat	None for US
		500 for Canada
Neomycin	Bovine tissues	250
	Milk	150 for US
		250 for Canada
Nicarbazin (N,N^1-bis(4-nitrophenyl)urea)	Chicken muscle, liver, kidney, and skin	4000
Nitarsone (arsenic)	Turkey muscle	500
	Turkey liver	2000
Novobiocin	Bovine, chicken, and turkey tissues	1000
	Milk	100 for US
		125 for Canada
Penicillin G	Milk	0.01 IU/ml
	Turkey tissues	10
	Bovine tissues	50

TABLE 12.4 Continued

Drug (marker)	Matrix	MRL (ppb)
Polymyxin B	Milk	4.0 IU/ml
Pyrantel tartrate (N-methyl-1,3-propane diamine)	Swine muscle	1000
	Swine liver and kidney	10000
Robenidine HCl	Chicken muscle, liver, and kidney	100
	Chicken skin and fat	200
Ronnel (sum of parent and 2,4,5-trichlorophenol-containing metabolites)	Bovine, sheep and goat fat	10,000 for US 7500 for Canada
Roxarsone (arsenic)	Swine, chicken, and turkey muscle; eggs	500
	Swine, chicken, and turkey liver	2000
Salinomycin	Chicken skin and fat	None for US 350 for Canada
Spectinomycin	Chicken tissues	100
Streptomycin	Milk	125
Sulfachlorpyridazine	Bovine and swine tissues	100
Sulfadimethoxine	Milk	10
	Bovine tissues	100
Sulfaethoxypyridazine	Bovine tissues	100
Sulfamethazine	Bovine, swine, chicken, and turkey tissues	100
Sulfathiazole	Swine tissues	100
Tetracycline	Bovine, swine, sheep, chicken, and turkey tissues	250
Thiabendazole (sum of parent and 5-hydroxy-thiabendazole metabolites	Milk	50
Tiamulin (8-alpha-hydroxymutilin)	Swine liver	400
Tylosin	Bovine, swine, chicken and turkey muscle, liver, kidney and fat	200
Zoalene (sum of parent and 3-amino-5-nitro-o-toluamide)	Chicken fat	2000
	Chicken and turkey muscle; turkey liver and fat	3000
	Chicken liver and kidney	6000

Source: From Ref. 47.

degrees of conservatism, whether there is a realistic possibility that use of a particular MRL will result in a dietary intake of residues that exceeds another country's ADI for the drug. The prediction is made using the so-called estimated maximum residue intake, (EMDI) model (49). The EMDI is an estimate of drug residue intake that is calculated using the equation, EMDI = MRL × 90th percentile food consumption data for approved species/60 kg human body weight.

Since this model assumes that in those species in which a drug is approved, 100% of the animals are treated with the drug, the EMDI is actually an overestimation of the real veterinary drug residue intake. It also uses exaggerated values for food consumption of edible animal products: the 90th percentile consumer represents the heavy eater of meat who usually consumes two or three times more than the average, or the 50th percentile, consumer. It finally assumes that all edible animal products contain residues at the MRL level, although very few animal products actually contain residues at that very high level. Because it is unlikely that, on the same day, the 90th percentile consumer of beef, for example, will also be the 90th percentile consumer of chicken, it is not valid to add together the estimated residue intake from beef and chicken by the 90th percentile consumer of each since unrealistic estimates of the exposure of consumers to residues would result. In order to add together exposure from different sources, the WHO prescribes that the 50th percentile consumer data be used (50).

An example of the application of this procedure for testing the equivalence of the albendazole or ivermectin MRLs for which differences exist between the United States and JECFA is presented in Table 12.5. Differences between US and JECFA MRLs for albendazole are due to use of different safety factors and to the JECFA consideration of good veterinary practice. That is, JECFA considered practical conditions of use of the drug and set MRLs consistent with that use; accordingly, the entire ADI is likely not to be consumed. On the other hand, the United States always uses the entire ADI in setting MRLs for edible tissues.

The intake estimates for albendazole and ivermectin predict that use of the US MRLs will not result in residues above the ADI established by JECFA, and, conversely, that use of the JECFA MRLs will not result in dietary exposure to residues above the US ADI (51). In most cases, only small amounts of the ADI would be consumed. Based on these estimates, the US and JECFA MRLs for each drug would be considered equivalent for trade purposes.

In a similar fashion, dietary intake estimates can be made for lasalocid and halofuginone, two drugs that have disparate MRLs in the United States and Canada (51). The data presented in Table 12.6 predict that use of the US MRLs will not result in residues above the ADI established by Canada, and, conversely that use of the Canadian MRLs will not result in dietary exposure to residues above the US ADI. Although some of the percentages in Table 12.6 appear substantial, it should be taken into account that the estimates would have been much smaller had less conservative factors been included in the calculations. Based on these

TABLE 12.5 Testing of Equivalence of US and JECFA MRLs for Albendazole and Ivermectin

	Albendazole		Ivermectin	
	US	JECFA	US	JECFA
NOEL (mg/kg)	5	5	0.2	0.1
Safety factor	1000	100	1000	100
ADI (mg/kg)	0.005	0.05	0.0002	0.001
MRL bovine muscle (mg/kg)	0.6	0.1	0.025	Not established
MRL bovine liver (mg/kg)	1.2	5	0.1	0.1 (0.35 on a total residue basis)
90% intake bovine muscle (kg)[a]	0.155	0.155	0.155	0.155
Estimated maximum daily intake for imported bovine muscle (mg/kg)	0.000026 (5.2% of US ADI)	0.00155 (3.1% of JECFA ADI)	Not established	0.000065 (6.5% of JECFA ADI)
90% intake bovine liver (kg)[a]	0.02	0.02	0.02	0.02
Estimated maximum daily intake for imported bovine liver (mg/kg)	0.0017 (33% of US ADI)	0.0004 (0.8% of JECFA ADI)	0.000117 (58% of US ADI)	0.0000333 (3.3% of JECFA ADI)

[a] The intake values cited for muscle and liver come from a National Food Consumption Survey conducted by the Market Research Corporation of America (MRCA) in 1977–1978.
Source: From Ref. 51.

TABLE 12.6   Testing of Equivalence of US and Canada MRLs for Halofuginone and Lasalocid

	Halofuginone		Lasalocid	
	US	Canada	US	Canada
NOEL (mg/kg)	0.07	0.0625	1	1
Safety factor	100	100	100	100
ADI (mg/kg)	0.0007	0.000625	0.01	0.01
MRL chicken muscle (mg/kg)	0.1	0.06	1.2 (MRL applies to beef also)	1 (MRL applies to beef also)
90% intake chicken muscle (kg)[a]	0.054	0.084	0.054	0.084
Estimated maximum daily intake for imported chicken muscle (mg/kg)	0.000054 (8% of US ADI)	0.00014 (27% of Canada ADI)	0.0009 (9% of US ADI)	0.0017 (17% of Canada ADI)
90% intake beef muscle (kg)[a]	Not applicable	Not applicable	0.155	0.206
Estimated maximum daily intake for imported beef muscle (mg/kg)	Not applicable	Not applicable	0.0026 (26% of US ADI)	0.0041 (41% of Canada ADI)

[a] The US intake values come from a National Food Consumption Survey conducted by the Market Research Corporation of America (MRCA) in 1977–1978.
Source: From Ref. 51.

estimates, the US and Canada MRLs for each drug would be considered equivalent for trade purposes.

In 1996, the VICH program was officially launched among the European Union, Japan, and the United States (52). Among the objectives of the VICH is to provide a forum for a constructive dialogue between regulatory authorities and the veterinary medicinal products industry on the real and perceived differences in the technical requirements for product registration in the three jurisdictions, with the expectation that such a process may serve as a catalyst for a wider international harmonization. VICH should identify areas in which modifications in technical requirements or greater mutual acceptance of research and development procedures could lead to a more economical use of human, animal, and material resources, without compromising safety. It has also to make recommendations on practical ways to achieve harmonization on technical requirements affecting registration of veterinary products and to implement these recommendations in these regions. Once adopted, the VICH recommendations should replace corresponding regional requirements. These recommendations should focus on the essential scientific requirements needed to address a topic and should eliminate unnecessary or redundant requirements. The VICH has been conducted in a transparent and cost-effective manner and provides the opportunity for public comment on recommendations at the draft stage.

Labeling, better education in the use of farm chemicals, on-farm management, regular monitoring of known residue problems, and selected testing of the raw materials presented for processing are some of the considerations needed to ensure the compliance of food products with public health concerns and residue regulations. Other considerations include maintaining an appropriate analytical capability, conducting regular residue surveys, and collecting and exchanging data on residue status and trends. It is essential, however, that residue incidents are not created through the bureaucratic practice of ascribing default tolerances to residues of drugs for which registration has not been sought in importing countries.

In achieving this target, all countries should seek common, science-based, international standards. FSIS should continue to ensure that equivalent inspection systems and standards for meat and poultry products exist in all countries exporting such products to the United States, especially in light of the better US safety standards expected under Hazard Analysis Critical Control Points (HACCP). FDA also should evaluate the food safety systems of other countries, with the purpose of entering into agreements with those countries having food safety systems that offer equivalent levels of public health protection to those of the United States or that can provide assurance that their products will be in compliance with FDA requirements.

It is clear that the fundamental tenets of safety, quality, and efficacy should remain but considerable scope exists to produce a more easily understood core of requirements among which the subject of risk analysis should also be included. International harmonization cannot be mandatory either for government or for industry. Nevertheless, a commitment can and should be entered into both by individual governments and by pharmaceutical associations to accept specific guidelines that have drawn up and agreed. Such a commitment would preempt the demands to provide additional data requirements unless the scientific validity of such requirements were proven (53).

A radical revision of veterinary registration by an internationally accepted group of specialists would result in advantages to government, industry, and consumers. Governments would be assured that all essential parameters are covered, industry that unnecessary bureaucratic and unscientific demands are not being made, and consumers that standards are laid down by independent experts without political interference and without the fear that industrial influence is exerting pressure. Fundamentally, the timber for harmonization already exists in sets of standards drawn up by the FDA, European Union and many countries individually. It only remains to suggest one way in which these multidisciplinary and multinational facets may be drawn together into a single potentially acceptable entity.

Increased harmonization offers clear benefits for public health. It can increase the safety and quality of food produced and sold in foreign countries or food imported from other countries, as more countries participate in the international standard setting process. Harmonization benefits industry by replacing many different standards with one international standard that must be met. In the long run, harmonization will bring cost savings to industry, open markets, enhance opportunities for export, and, in some cases, lessen the time needed to bring new products to market.

REFERENCES

1. M. Miller, and C.C. Miller, J. Vet. Pharmacol. Ther., 20:299 (1997).
2. L. Desplenter, J. Frens, B. Schmit, and C. Verschueren, in Residues of Veterinary Drugs in Food, Proc. Euroresidue Conf., Noordwijkerhout, May 21–23, 1990 (N. Haagsma, A. Ruiter, and P.B. Czedik-Eysenberg, Eds.), Fac. Vet. Med., Univ. Utrecht, The Netherlands, p. 154 (1990).
3. World Health Organization, in Evaluation of Certain Veterinary Drug Residues in Food, Thirty-sixth Report of the Joint FAO/WHO Expert Committee on Food Additives, Technical Report Series 799, World Health Organization, Geneva (1990).
4. World Health Organization, in Evaluation of Certain Veterinary Drug Residues in Food, Thirty-fourth Report of the Joint FAO/WHO Expert Committee on Food Additives, Technical Report Series 788, World Health Organization, Geneva (1989).
5. N.E. Weber, and S.D. Brynes, in Residues of Veterinary Drugs in Food, Proc. Euroresidue Conf., Noordwijkerhout, May 21–23, 1990 (N. Haagsma, A. Ruiter, and P.B. Czedik-Eysenberg, Eds.), Fac. Vet. Med., Univ. Utrecht, The Netherlands, p. 404 (1990).
6. P. Bette, Assessment of the Safety for the Consumer of Residues of Veterinary Medicinal Products in Intramuscular Injection Sites, Draft Paper, 31 May, Boehringer Ingelheim Vetmedica GmBH, Germany (1994).
7. Anonymous, Antibacterial Residues at Injection Sites in Food-producing Animals, Report of the Animal Research Institute, QDPI, Brisbane, Australia (1992).
8. Anonymous, Report of the Working Party on Residues of Long Acting Antibiotics at Injection Sites, National Registration Authority, Camberra, Australia (1995).

9. G.O. Korsrud, J.O. Boison, M.G. Papich, W.D. Yates, J.D. MacNeil, E.D. Janzen, R.D. Cohen, D.A. Landry, G. Lambert, M.S. Yong, and J.R. Messeir, Can, J. Vet. Res., 57:223 (1993).

10. T.J. Nicholls, G.D. McLean, N.L. Blackman, and I.B. Stephens, Austr. Vet. J., 71: 393 (1994).

11. World Health Organization, in Injection Site Residues of Veterinary Drugs, Codex Committee on Residues of Veterinary Drugs in Foods, Ninth Session, Joint FAO/WHO Food Standards Programme, Washington, DC (1995).

12. P. Bette, Proc. of the 6th EAVPT Inter. Congress (P. Lees, Ed.), European Association for Veterinary Pharmacology and Therapeutics, Blackwell Scientific Publications, Edinburgh, UK, p. 70 (1994).

13. Veterinary International Cooperation on Harmonization (VICH), in Guideline on Validation of Analytical Procedures: Methodology, EMEA/CVMP/590/98-Final, London, UK (1998).

14. M. Thompson, and R. Wood, Pure Appl. Chem., 67:649 (1995).

15. W. Horwitz, Pure Appl. Chem., 67:331 (1995).

16. International Organization for Standardization (ISO/IEC), in General Requirements for the Competence of Calibration and Testing Laboratories, International Organization for Standardization, ISO Guide 25, Geneva (1990).

17. World Health Organization, in Validation of Analytical Methods for Food Control, Joint FAO/IAEA Expert Consultation 2–4 December 1997, Vienna, Austria, Food and Agriculture Organization of the United Nations, FAO Food and Nutrition Paper No 68, Rome (1998).

18. World Health Organization, in Methods of Analysis and Sampling, FAO/WHO, ALINORM 97/23A, Report of the 21st Session of the Codex Committee, paras 20–23, FAO, Rome (1997).

19. Official Journal of the European Communities, No. L317, Brussels, p. 1 (1981).

20. Official Journal of the European Communities, No. L317, Brussels, p. 16 (1981).

21. Official Journal of the European Communities, No. L270, Brussels, p. 1 (1970).

22. Food and Drug Administration, in The Use of Hormones for Growth Promotion in Food-Producing Animals, Food and Drug Administration, Center for Veterinary Medicine, Rockville, MD, August (1988).

23. H. Ritchie, in Animal Agriculture on the Stand: Are Modern Production Practices Safe?, Michigan State University, April 20 (1991).

24. B. Hoffman, Proc. of the Health Aspects of Residues of Anabolics in Meat, Vol. 59, p. 16 (1982).

25. G.E. Lamming, Vet. Rec., 121:389 (1987).

26. World Health Organization, in Residues of Some Veterinary Drugs in Animals and Foods, Thirty-second Report of the Joint FAO/WHO Expert Committee on Food Additives, Food and Nutrition paper, No 41, World Health Organization, Geneva (1988).

27. J.A. Smith, in Science-Driven Solutions to Food Safety Dilemmas-A Progress Report, US Department of Agriculture, November 29 (1991).

28. G.R. Foxcroft, in Drug Residues in Animals (A. Rico, Ed.), Academic Press, Orlando, FL, p. 147 (1986).

29.   S.F. Sundlof, and J. Cooper, in Veterinary Drug Residues, Food Safety (W.A. Moats and M.B. Medina, Eds.), American Chemical Society, Washington, DC, p. 5 (1996).

30.   G.C. Smith, in The Safety of Beef, Colorado State University, September (1991).

31.   H.J. Hapke, in Residues of Veterinary Drugs in Food, Proc. Euroresidue II Conf., Veldhoven, May 3–5, 1993 (N. Haagsma, A. Ruiter and P.B. Czedik-Eysenberg, Eds.), Fac. Vet. Med., Univ. Utrecht, The Netherlands, p. 51 (1993).

32.   J.C. Juskevich, and C.G. Guyer, Science, 249:875 (1990).

33.   World Health Organization, in Evaluation of Certain Veterinary Drug Residues in Food, Fortieth Meeting of the Joint FAO/WHO Expert Committee on Food Additives, WHO Food Additive Series 31, World Health Organization, Rockville, US, p. 149 (1993).

34.   V. Brower, Nature Biotechnology, 16:223 (1998).

35.   J.M. Chan, M.J. Stampfer, E. Giovannucci, P.H. Gann, J. Na, P. Wilkinson, C.H. Hennekens, and N. Pollack, Science, 279:563 (1998).

36.   J.L. Resnik, D.B. Reichart, K. Huey, N.J. Webster, and B.L. Seely, Cancer Res., 58:1159 (1998).

37.   J.L.C.G. Prosser, Lancet, 2:8621 (1988).

38.   R.-J. Xu, Food Rev. Int., 14:1 (1998).

39.   P.G. Campbell, and C.R. Baumrucker, J. Endocrinol., 120:21 (1989).

40.   P.V. Malven, H.H. Head, R.J. Collier, and F.C. Buonoma, J. Dairy Sci., 70:2254 (1987).

41.   World Health Organization, in Evaluation of Certain Veterinary Drug Residues in Food, Fifth Meeting of the Joint FAO/WHO Expert Committee on Food Additives, WHO Food Additive Series 41, World Health Organization, Rome, p. 125 (1998).

42.   T. Kimura, Y. Murakawa, M. Ohno, S. Ohtani, and K. Higaki, J. Pharmacol. Exp. Ther., 283:611 (1997).

43.   C. Verschueren, in GHOST-Global Harmonization of Standards, FEDESA, Brussels, Belgium (1993).

44.   S.D. Brynes, and M.S. Yong, in Residues of Veterinary Drugs in Food, Proc. Euroresidue II Conf., Veldhoven, May 3–5, 1993 (N. Haagsma, A. Ruiter and P.B. Czedik-Eysenberg, Eds.), Fac. Vet. Med., Univ. Utrecht, The Netherlands, p. 226 (1993).

45.   Food and Drug Administration, in General Principles for Evaluating the Safety of Compounds Used in Food-Producing Animals, Food and Drug Administration, Center for Veterinary Medicine, Rockville, MD (1986).

46.   Anonymous, in Preparation of Veterinary New Drug Submissions, Drugs Directorate Guideline, Bureau of Veterinary Drugs, Health Protection Branch, Health and Welfare, Canada (1991).

47.   Canada Gazette, Part I, p. 3539 (1990).

48.   S.C. Fitzpatrick, S.D. Brynes, and G.B. Guest, J. Vet. Pharmacol. Ther., 18:325 (1995).

49.   G.B. Guest, and S.C. Fitzpatrick, in Predicting the Dietary Intake of Veterinary Drugs, ILSI Monographs (I. MacDonald, Ed.), Springer-Verlag, p. 205 (1991).

50.   World Health Organization, in Guidelines for Predicting Dietary Intake of Pesticide Residues, World Health Organization, Geneva, p. 8 (1989).

51.   S.D. Brynes, S.F. Sundlof, A. Vilim, G. Lambert, M.S. Yong, and S.C. Fitzpatrick, in Residues of Veterinary Drugs in Food, Proc. Euroresidue III Conf., Veldhoven,

1996 (N. Haagsma and A. Ruiter, Eds.), Fac. Vet. Med., Univ. Utrecht, The Netherlands, p. 296 (1996).

52. Veterinary International Cooperation on Harmonization (VICH), in Guideline on Validation of Analytical Procedures: Methodology, EMEA/CVMP/591/98-Final, London, UK (1998).

53. A.R.M. Kidd, Proc. of the 6th EAVPT Inter. Congress (P. Lees, Ed.), European Association for Veterinary Pharmacology and Therapeutics, Blackwell Scientific Publications, Edinburgh, UK, p. 67 (1994).

13

Incidence of Violative Residues in Foods

The use of drugs in food-producing animals inevitably results in the appearance of drug-related residues in milk, meat, and eggs. Antimicrobial residues occur more frequently than desired; violative residues occur much less frequently, but in definitely significant numbers.

Calves have the highest potential for violative antibiotic residues. Bob veal calves under 150 pounds have the greatest potential residue problem since these animals can be slaughtered before administered drugs can deplete to acceptable levels. Cows can also represent a significant source of residues because animals performing poorly or with chronic health problems may be slaughtered before drug depletion occurs. Generally, all animals that are culled from herds, regardless of species, pose residue problems.

13.1 RESIDUES IN THE UNITED STATES

Three decades ago, a survey of animals slaughtered in four US states indicated that 27% of the swine sampled were treated with antimicrobial drugs before slaughter. Some 10% of those cases resulted from lack of adherence to withdrawal periods or from exceeding the levels cleared for feeding of the antimicrobial substances. Among beef cattle, a total of 9% were found positive to antimicrobials with 2% attributed to penicillin residues. In veal calves, 17% contained antibiotic residues with 7% ascribed to penicillin. Twenty-one percent of the market lambs contained antimicrobial residues, 4% with penicillin residues. Chickens exhibited a 26% contamination by antimicrobials, 6% containing penicillin residues (1).

446

Chapter 13

In 1975, a United States Department of Agriculture (USDA) survey showed that 5.3% of the 529 carcasses sampled were positive for antibiotic residues (2). Only 17 of the 5301 samples (0.3%) were positive for penicillin, whereas 12 of 728 samples (1.6%) were positive for sulfonamides. Nonspecific antimicrobial activity was found in 154 of the 5301 samples (2.9%) analyzed.

In the period 1976–1978, violative residues were found in all animal species marketed (3). Although the USDA data (Table 13.1) contain listings of several species and the frequency with which violative residues were found, nonviolative residues occurred in many more animals. Species with the lowest frequency were poultry and cattle, whereas swine and veal calves exhibited the highest frequency

TABLE 13.1 Samples Exceeding Tolerances for Antibiotics and Sulfonamides over the Period 1976–1978 in the United States

Species	Antibiotic samples	Violations (%)	Sulfonamide samples	Violations (%)
1976				
Cattle	545	1.3	476	0.9
Calves	1378	8.6	327	3.7
Sheep, goats	70	7.1	100	1.0
Swine	247	1.6	1493	9.4
Chickens	155	0.6	331	0.3
Turkeys	258	0.0	648	2.5
Geese, ducks	160	0.6	265	0.0
1977				
Cattle	1739	1.3	175	2.3
Calves	1120	4.1	166	3.0
Sheep goats	176	1.1	12	0.0
Swine	449	1.3	9461	13.1
Chickens	366	0.0	1	0.0
Turkeys	450	0.7	445	0.9
Geese, ducks	161	0.6	206	0.5
1978				
Cattle	1769	2.6	243	0.8
Calves	1409	6.7	216	2.8
Sheep, goats	210	2.4	40	15.0
Swine	1399	5.4	6687	9.7
Chickens	470	1.7	119	0.8
Turkeys	447	3.3	443	4.4
Geese, ducks	175	1.1	148	0.0

Source: From Ref. 3.

TABLE 13.2 Violative Residue Rates (%) for Antibacterials in Several Animal Species During 1979–1983 in the United States

Species	1979	1980	1981	1982	1983
Mature cattle	2.2	—	—	—	0.2
Chickens	0.0	—	—	—	0.0
Turkeys	2.4	—	—	—	0.01
Bob veal	7.8	3.9	7.3	6.1	7.7
Swine	10.0	6.8	8.7	7.0	9.2

figures. The high frequency of violative residues in veal calves was attributed to the high levels of antibiotics and sulfonamides incorporated in the diets of those animals for prophylactic purposes. The high incidence of violative residues in swine was reflective of the recycling problem with sulfonamides. Although the medicated feeds were usually withdrawn 7–10 days before animals were marketed, many of the replacement feeds were contaminated with sulfonamides, causing a cycling of sulfonamides and the appearance of unwanted residues in the tissues.

The residue profile seen over the years 1976–1978 is similar to that seen in the following years. Table 13.2 lists the violative residue rates for antibacterials in several animal species for the years 1979–1983. The residue violation rate in mature cattle and poultry was very low. Chickens, in particular, had almost a zero violation rate due possibly to highly integrated US chicken-producing operations. In addition, the violation rate for turkeys was still very low although turkeys were mostly raised by independent producers.

The violation rate, however, was not low for all species. Bob veal calves exhibited a very high violation rate relative to the other species. This was attributed to the fact that bob veals were given drugs to keep them alive until they could be marketed and, thus, the likelihood of withdrawal periods being followed was not high. The violation rate in swine was also relatively high due primarily to residues of sulfamethazine. The high violation rate for sulfamethazine in swine was attributed to several factors including the tendency of this substance to adhere to feed-mixing equipment and to contaminate the nonmedicated feeds, the tendency of pigs to be coprophagic, and the refusal of some producers to follow the recommended withdrawal period.

In the period 1988–1989, the drug residue profile in edible animal products does not change. Data complied by the FSIS National Residue Program during 1988 showed that chlortetracycline, erythromycin, gentamicin, neomycin, oxytetracycline, penicillins, streptomycin, tetracycline, and tylosin were the antibiotics most often present in the samples analyzed (Table 13.3). During the same period,

TABLE 13.3   Samples Exceeding Tolerances for Antibiotics and Sulfonamides during 1988–1989 in the United States

Species	Monitoring sample units			Surveillance sample units		
	Tested/ violative	Violations (%)	Types of antibacterials[a]	Tested/ violative	Violations (%)	Types of antibacterials[a]
1988						
Antibiotics						
Horses	305/3	0.98	g	32/0	0.00	—
Cattle	1228/4	0.33	c,e,g	339/41	12.09	b,c,d,e,f,g,h,i
Calves	—	—	—	3394/88	2.59	a,c,d,e,f,g,h
Chickens	409/0	0.00	—	533/1	0.19	a
Turkeys	541/1	0.18	g	451/1	0.22	g
Ducks	319/0	0.00	—	2/0	0.00	—
Geese	75/0	0.00	—	—	—	—
Swine	1381/10	0.72	a,b,d,f,g	756/11	1.45	a,e,g,h
Sheep	337/2	0.59	h	497/9	1.81	d,f,g,h
Goats	280/1	0.36	g	1/0	0.00	—
Total samples	4875/21	0.43	—	6005/151	2.51	
Sulfonamides						
Horses	306/2	0.65	r	2/0	0.00	—
Cattle	944/1	0.10	r	107/7	6.54	n,r
Calves	—	—	—	1186/18	1.52	q,r,t
Chickens	944/1	0.10	n	15/0	0.00	—
Turkeys	883/4	0.45	n	59/6	10.16	r
Swine	1936/35	1.81	n,r	3015/171	5.67	n,r
Sheep	344/3	0.87	n,r	2/0	0.00	—
Goats	103/0	0.00	—	—	—	—
Total samples	5460/46	0.82		4386/202	4.60	
1989						
Antibiotics						
Horses	306/3	0.98	a,e,f	2/0	0.00	—
Cattle	627/6	0.96	d,e,f	584/47	8.05	c,d,e,f,g
Calves	3106/33	1.06	c,d,e,f,g	591/13	2.20	c,d,e,f
Chickens	597/0	0.00	—	12/0	0.00	—
Turkeys	488/0	0.00	—	24/0	0.00	—
Ducks	325/0	0.00	—	—	—	—
Geese	69/1	1.45	f	—	—	—
Swine	1913/6	0.31	f,g,h	505/13	2.57	c,d,g
Sheep	320/0	0.00	—	6/0	0.00	—
Goats	287/3	1.04	f,g	9/0	0.00	—
Total samples	8038/52	0.65		1733/74	4.27	

(continued)

TABLE 13.3 Continued

Species	Monitoring sample units			Surveillance sample units		
	Tested/ violative	Violations (%)	Types of antibacterials[a]	Tested/ violative	Violations (%)	Types of antibacterials[a]
Sulfonamides						
Horses	302/1	0.33	n	2/0	0.00	—
Cattle	632/1	0.16	r,t	186/7	3.76	n,r,t
Calves	1221/5	0.41	n,r,t	198/7	3.53	r,t
Chickens	922/0	0.00	—	9/0	0.00	—
Turkeys	819/5	0.61	n	108/4	3.71	n,s
Ducks	332/0	0.00	—	—	—	—
Geese	68/0	0.00	—	—	—	—
Swine	3883/43	1.11	r	1060/111	10.47	l,n,r,q
Sheep	342/7	2.05	n,r	1/0	0.00	—
Goats	108/0	0.00	—	1/0	0.00	—
Total samples	8629/62	0.72		1569/129	8.22	

[a] Antibiotics: a, chlortetracycline; b, erythromycin; c, gentamicin; d, neomycin; e, oxytetracycline; f, penicillins; g, streptomycin; h, tetracycline; i, tylosin; j, chloramphenicol. Sulfonamides: k, sulfabromomethazine; l, sulfachlorpyridazine; m, sulfadiazine; n, sulfadimethoxine; o, sulfaethoxypyridazine; p, sulfamethoxypyridazine; q, sulfapyridine; r, sulfamethazine; s, sulfaquinoxaline; t, sulfathiazole
Source: From Refs. 47 and 48.

the particular sulfonamides found were sulfamethazine, sulfadimethoxine, sulfapyridine, and sulfathiazole. The antibiotics found in the 1989 survey were the same as in 1988, but the sulfonamides included sulfamethazine, sulfadimethoxine, sulfathiazole, sulfaquinoxaline, sulfapyridine, and sulfachlorpyridazine.

Overall, the incidence of violative residues of antibiotics was less than 1% in 1988. Beef cattle, calves, and swine all exhibited a relatively high frequency of violative residue levels. Because of the drug usage patterns, this was not unexpected. Chickens, turkeys, and ducks had a low incidence of violative residues, probably reflecting subtherapeutic use rather than disease prevention and treatment use. Violative sulfonamide residues were generally at a low incidence in the monitoring samples. However, surveillance samples taken when there was a prior history of violative residues or suspicion that residues were present presented a somewhat different profile. In the surveillance samples, cattle, calves, and swine showed a greater percentages of violative samples. No chloramphenicol was found in either the monitoring or surveillance samples for 1988 and 1989.

In the period 1992–1994, the drugs and groups of drugs screened by the National Residue Program included antibiotics, sulfonamides, ivermectin, halofuginone, levamisole, and morantel tartrate. The microbial assays applied by FSIS for monitoring antibiotics could detect chlortetracycline, oxytetracycline, tetracy-

cline, penicillins, erythromycin, gentamicin, neomycin, streptomycins, and tylosin. Penicillins could be detected but not identified: the FSIS laboratory methodology could not differentiate among penicillin G, amoxycillin, ampicillin,
cloxacillin and other members of the β-lactam group of antibiotics. Likewise,
streptomycin could not be differentiated from dihydrostreptomycin residues. The
sulfonamides that could be detected by FSIS laboratories included sulfachlorpyridazine, sulfamethazine, sulfadimethoxine, and sulfathiazole.

The kidney was the target tissue analyzed for antibiotics. When violative
residues were found in the kidney, the liver of that animal was subsequently
analyzed. When violative residues were also found in the liver, muscle tissue
was then analyzed. For sulfonamides, the target tissue was liver. When the liver
contained violative levels, muscle tissue was also analyzed.

Tables 13.4, 13.5, and 13.6 present the results of the monitoring program
testing for antibiotics and ivermectin, sulfonamides and halofuginone, and levamisole and morantel tartrate, respectively, over the period 1992–1994. In these
tables, calves are not presented as a single class but divided into four categories,
because calves, historically, have been identified as a problem population for
antibiotic violations. These categories included bob calves up to 3 weeks of
age or 150 pounds in weight, formula-fed calves 150–250 pounds in weight,
nonformula calves that are 250–400 pounds in weight, and heavy calves over
400 pounds in weight.

Table 13.7 provides information on the antibiotic and sulfonamide violations detected during 1992–1994. Sample sizes differed in the various animal
slaughter classes in different years. Thus, it would not be appropriate to attribute
undue significance to the number of violations detected of an individual compound. Table 13.7 does provide relevant information about the specific compounds that produced violative residue concentrations in food animals during that
period. Residue violations for more than one compound might occasionally occur
in the same animal.

Analysis of the 1993 tissue residue data revealed that FSIS reported 3809
animals containing violative residues. The Food and Drug Administration (FDA),
in cooperation with participating states, conducted follow-up investigation on
1207 (32%) of the reported violations to determine the responsible individuals,
prevent future occurrence of residues by that person, provide official warning of
the violation, and take necessary enforcement actions. The drugs most frequently
identified as causing antibiotic residues included penicillin (20%), streptomycin
(10%), oxytetracycline (10%), sulfamethazine (9%), tetracycline (4%), gentamicin (4%), and neomycin (3%). Sulfamethazine was the most frequently cited
sulfonamide. A total of 35% of the reported violative residues were samples
positive to the calf antibiotic and sulfonamide test (CAST).

The animal slaughter classes most often associated with residues in 1993
were culled dairy cows, veal calves, and market hogs. Residues associated with

TABLE 13.4   National Residue Monitoring Program Results for Antibiotics and Ivermectin over the Period 1992–1994 in the United States

	1992		1993		1994	
Slaughter class	Tested/ violative	Violations (%)	Tested/ violative	Violations (%)	Tested/ violative	Violations (%)
Antibiotics						
Horses	101/0	0.0	309/12	3.9	NT	—
Bulls	7/0	0.0	350/0	0.0	406/0	0.0
Beef cows	90/0	0.0	671/1	0.1	527/1	0.2
Dairy cows	NT	—	260/4	1.5	424/0	0.0
Heifers	129/0	0.0	344/0	0.0	341/0	0.0
Steers	194/0	0.0	333/0	0.0	339/0	0.0
Bob calves	294/4	1.4	489/9	1.8	455/3	0.7
Formula-fed calves	325/1	0.3	537/1	0.2	547/0	0.0
Non-formula-fed calves	287/1	0.3	303/3	1.0	409/1	0.2
Heavy calves	295/1	0.3	308/1	0.3	493/1	0.2
Sheep	24/0	0.0	291/1	0.3	302/0	0.0
Lambs	317/2	0.6	351/2	0.6	364/2	0.5
Goats	88/0	0.0	318/0	0.0	431/0	0.0
Market hogs	327/6	1.8	322/1	0.3	326/4	1.2
Boars/stags	55/0	0.0	444/0	0.0	455/2	0.4
Sows	256/0	0.0	532/1	0.2	540/3	0.6
Young chickens	297/0	0.0	489/0	0.0	499/0	0.0
Mature chickens	330/0	0.0	498/0	0.0	525/0	0.0
Young turkeys	308/2	0.6	520/3	0.6	530/1	0.2
Mature turkeys	186/0	0.0	246/2	0.8	258/0	0.0
Ducks	108/0	0.0	356/1	0.3	139/1	0.7
Geese	26/0	0.0	3/0	0.0	44/0	0.0
Ivermectin						
Horses	94/2	2.0	NT	—	NT	—
Bulls	22/0	0.0	NT	—	NT	—
Beef cows	285/3	1.0	405/0	0.0	317/2	0.6
Dairy cows	238/0	0.0	161/0	0.0	256/0	0.0
Heifers	131/0	0.0	339/0	0.0	351/0	0.0
Steers	275/0	0.0	332/1	0.3	332/0	0.0
Formula-fed calves	323/0	0.0	338/1	0.3	319/1	0.3
Non-formula-fed calves	303/0	0.0	289/4	1.4	233/1	0.4
Heavy calves	290/0	0.0	312/3	1.0	291/1	0.3
Sheep	23/0	0.0	NT	—	296/0	0.0
Lambs	329/0	0.0	282/1	0.3	357/0	0.0
Goats	285/1	0.4	312/2	0.6	254/2	0.8
Market hogs	328/0	0.0	318/0	0.0	309/0	0.0
Boards/stags	65/0	0.0	267/0	0.0	282/0	0.0
Sows	262/0	0.0	324/0	0.0	329/0	0.0

NT, not tested.
Source: From Ref. 49.

TABLE 13.5 National Residue Monitoring Program Results for Sulfonamides and Halofuginone over the Period 1992–1994 in the United States

Slaughter class	1992		1993		1994	
	Tested/ violative	Violations (%)	Tested/ violative	Violations (%)	Tested/ violative	Violations (%)
Sulfonamides						
Horses	103/0	0.0	306/2	0.6	NT	—
Bulls	7/0	0.0	350/0	0.0	366/0	0.0
Beef cows	97/1	1.0	672/1	0.1	513/1	0.2
Dairy cows	NT	—	261/3	1.1	401/2	0.5
Heifers	131/0	0.0	348/0	0.0	343/0	0.0
Steers	195/0	0.0	338/0	0.0	340/0	0.0
Bob calves	290/2	0.7	489/7	1.4	515/1	0.2
Formula-fed calves	329/2	0.6	537/1	0.2	520/0	0.0
Non-formula-fed calves	306/3	1.0	300/2	0.7	397/0	0.0
Heavy calves	291/0	0.0	309/2	0.6	463/1	0.2
Sheep	24/0	0.0	292/0	0.0	299/0	0.0
Lambs	336/0	0.0	351/0	0.0	363/0	0.0
Goats	100/0	0.0	317/1	0.3	268/0	0.0
Market hogs	3969/37	0.9	322/0	0.0	325/1	0.3
Boars/stags	141/1	0.7	442/7	1.6	455/3	0.7
Sows	529/2	0.4	532/3	0.6	542/7	1.3
Young chickens	312/0	0.0	487/0	0.0	506/1	0.2
Mature chickens	315/0	0.0	491/0	0.0	524/0	0.0
Young turkeys	312/0	0.0	524/1	0.2	521/3	0.6
Mature turkeys	195/2	1.0	243/2	0.8	259/3	1.2
Ducks	100/0	0.0	353/0	0.0	137/0	0.0
Geese	27/0	0.0	3/0	0.0	41/0	0.0
Halofuginone						
Young chickens	301/1	0.3	311/1	0.3	309/0	0.0
Young turkeys	311/0	0.0	321/0	0.0	320/0	0.0

NT, not tested.
Source: From Ref. 49.

injectable drugs accounted for approximately 46% of the violations. This was followed by the oral route and the intramammary route. Most of the drugs that caused the residues were purchased from a feed/farm supply store or veterinarian. The primary cause of residue violations was failure to adhere to the approved withdrawal periods. Other causes included failure to keep proper animal identification and treatment records and extralabel use exceeding recommended dosage. The feeding of colostrum containing drug residues to bob veal was also viewed as a possible risk factor in causing residue violations. Veterinarians contributed

TABLE 13.6 National Residue Monitoring Program Results for Levamisole and Morantel Tartrate over the Period 1993–1994 in the United States

Slaughter class	1993		1994	
	Tested/ violative	Violations (%)	Tested/ violative	Violations (%)
Levamisole				
Bulls	354/0	0.0	375/0	0.0
Beef cows	406/0	0.0	329/1	0.3
Dairy cows	177/0	0.0	229/0	0.0
Heifers	335/0	0.0	345/0	0.0
Steers	340/0	0.0	340/0	0.0
Formula-fed calves	343/0	0.0	325/0	0.0
Heavy calves	305/0	0.0	294/0	0.0
Sheep	304/2	0.7	294/2	0.7
Lambs	361/0	0.0	358/1	0.3
Goats	308/0	0.0	266/0	0.0
Market hogs	328/1	0.3	314/1	0.3
Boars/stags	268/0	0.0	279/1	0.4
Sows	339/0	0.0	329/0	0.0
Morantel tartrate				
Bulls	362/0	0.0	360/0	0.0
Beef cows	106/0	0.0	405/1	0.2
Dairy cows	163/0	0.0	251/0	0.0
Heifers	340/0	0.0	351/0	0.0
Steers	331/0	0.0	249/0	0.0
Formula-fed calves	343/0	0.0	326/0	0.0
Non-formula-fed calves	290/0	0.0	242/0	0.0
Heavy calves	312/0	0.0	294/0	0.0

Source: From Ref. 49.

to 3% of the violative residues via extralabel use compared with 9% by the producer. The failure of producers to adhere to the withdrawal period recommended by the veterinarian accounted for 2% of the primary causes of residue violations.

Analysis of the 1994 tissue residue data revealed that FSIS reported 2514 animals containing violative residues. FDA, in cooperation with participating states, conducted follow-up investigation on 1076 (45%) of the reported violations. The drugs most frequently identified as causing antibiotic residues included penicillin (21%), oxytetracycline (10%), sulfamethazine (10%), streptomycin (6%), tetracycline (5.2%), neomycin (4.1%), gentamicin (3.7%), and sulfadimeth-

TABLE 13.7 Antibiotics and Sulfonamides Responsible for Violative
Residues in Food Animals from 1992 to 1994 in the United States

Slaughter class	Antibiotic violations	Sulfonamide violations
Horses	10 streptomycin, 2 penicillin	2 sulfamethazine, 1 sulfadimethoxine
Beef cows	1 neomycin, 1 erythromycin	1 sulfamethazine, 1 sulfadimethoxine, 1 sulfadoxine
Dairy cows	3 gentamicin, 1 penicillin, 1 neomycin, 1 tetracycline	3 sulfadimethoxine, 2 sulfamethazine
Bob calves	6 neomycin, 6 gentamicin, 1 erythromycin, 4 penicillin, 1 tetracycline	8 sulfamethazine, 2 sulfadimethoxine
Formula-fed calves	1 tetracycline, 1 oxytetracycline	3 sulfamethazine
Non-formula-fed calves	2 penicillin, 2 streptomycin, 1 neomycin, 1 oxytetracycline, 1 erythromycin	4 sulfamethazine, 1 sulfadimethoxine
Heavy calves	1 penicillin, 1 erythromycin, 1 tetracycline, 1 oxytetracycline	3 sulfamethazine
Sheep	1 penicillin, 1 streptomycin	—
Lambs	4 tetracycline, 2 streptomycin, 1 penicillin	—
Goats	—	1 sulfamethazine
Market hogs	1 penicillin, 1 neomycin, 1 oxytetracycline, 6 tetracycline, 2 chlortetracycline	36 sulfamethazine, 2 sulfadimethoxine, 1 sulfathiazole
Boars/stags	1 penicillin, 1 gentamicin	10 sulfamethazine, 1 sulfathiazole
Sows	4 penicillin	8 sulfamethazine, 2 sulfadimethoxine, 1 sulfathiazole, 1 sulfachlorpyridazine
Young chickens	—	1 sulfaquinoxaline
Young turkeys	1 pencillin, 1 streptomycin, 4 tetracycline, 1 chlortetracycline	2 sulfadimethoxine, 2 sulfaquinoxaline
Mature turkeys	2 tetracycline	5 sulfadimethoxine
Ducks	2 chlortetracycline	

Source: From Ref. 49.

oxine (3.4%). Sulfamethazine was again the most frequently cited sulfonamide. A total of 30% of the reported violative residues were samples that gave positive results with the CAST test.

In 1994, the animal slaughter class most often associated with residues were bob veal calves, culled dairy cows, both beef and cull cows, and market hogs. Residues associated with injectable drugs accounted for approximately 42% of the violations. This was followed by the oral route and the intramammary route. Most of the drugs that caused the residues were purchased from a feed/farm supply store or veterinarian. The primary cause of residue violations was failure to adhere to the approved withdrawal periods. Other causes included failure to keep proper animal identification and treatment records and extralabel use exceeding recommended dosage.

Table 13.8 presents total violative animals and residues for the years 1991–1994 in the United States. It becomes evident that violations were steadily decreased each year since 1991. No major changes in the drug groups, slaughter classes, and drug use patterns have contributed to violative residues. Ignoring labeled withdrawal periods continued to be a major source of drug residue violations.

Lower levels of violative samples were detected in the US monitoring program of 1996 (Table 13.9). FSIS data indicated that the great majority of the 134.3 million head of livestock and 8.1 billion birds were free of violative residues when they were slaughtered in federally inspected plants (4). Only 50 of 31,748 monitoring samples showed violative concentrations of residues. The percentage of violations for all samples and all residues shown in Table 13.9 is not necessarily representative of the percentage that were violative in the livestock population as a whole. The percentage occurrence of violations or positive findings can be considered representative only within a slaughter class/compound pair.

In the 1996 monitoring program, 14 antibiotic violations were found in 7375 samples from all slaughter classes monitored for antibiotics. Multiple antibiotic violations were found in at least one bob veal calf sample.

TABLE 13.8 Total Violative Animals and Residues for the Years 1991–1994 in the United States

Year	Violative animals	Violative residues
1991	4339	5072
1992	4325	4960
1993	3809	4283
1994	2514	2937

TABLE 13.9   Monitoring Program Results of the 1996 National Residue Program in the United States

| | Antibiotic violations | | | | Sulfonamide violations | | | |
| | Monitoring | | | Enforcement testing | Monitoring | | | Enforcement testing |
Slaughter class	Analyses/ violations	Violative (%)	Types of drugs[a]	Analyses/ violations	Analyses/ violations	Violative (%)	Types of drugs[a]	Analyses/ violations
Bulls	118/0	0.0	—		119/0	0.0	—	
Beef cows	521/0	0.0	—		522.0	0.0	—	
Dairy cows	540/0	0.0	—		543/0	0.0	—	
Heifers	111/0	0.0	—		114/0	0.0	—	
Steers	112/0	0.0	—		109/0	0.0	—	
Bob calves	531/7	1.3	a,b,c,d		526/4	0.8	k	
Formula-fed calves	524/1	0.2	e		525/0	0.0	—	
Non-formula calves	351/0	0.0	—		355/1	0.3	k	
Heavy calves	460/3	0.7	b,d		465/0	0.0	—	
Cattle			b,d,e,f,g,h	65/8			k,l,n	18/12
Sheep	309/0	0.0	—		303/0	0.0	—	
Lambs	586/0	0.0	—		363/2	0.6	k	
Sheep/Lambs			—	8/0			e,k	4/1
Goats	300/0	0.0	—		298/1	0.3	k,l	3/1
Market hogs	319/0	0.0	—		320/2	0.6	k,l	
Boars/Stags	539/0	0.0	—		540/3	0.6	k	
Sows	518/1	0.2	d		528/3	0.6	k	
Swine			—	22/0			k,l	12/4
Young chickens	299/0	0.0	—		468/0	0.0	—	
Mature chickens	119/0	0.0	—		119/0	0.0	—	
Chickens			—	1/0			—	1/0
Young turkeys	399/0	0.0	—		391/0	0.0	—	
Mature turkeys	145/0	0.0	—		223/0	0.0	—	
Turkeys			—	4/0		—	—	—
Ducks	545/0	0.0	—		413/0	0.0	—	
Geese	29/0	0.0	—		40/1	2.5	k	
Rabbits			c	17/2	—	—	—	—

[a] Antibiotics: a = neomycin; b = tetracycline; c = streptomycin; d = penicillin; e = chlortetracycline; f = oxytetracycline; g = gentamicin; h = erythromycin. Sulfonamides: j = sulfachlorpyridazine; k = sulfamethazine; l = sulfadimethoxine; m = sulfathiazole; n = sulfadiazine
Source: From Ref. 4.

In addition, a total of 14 sulfamethazine and 3 sulfadimethoxine violations occurred among 7824 samples from all slaughter classes monitored for sulfonamides. Bob calves exhibited four sulfonamides violations, sows and boar/stags three, and lambs and market hogs two. One sulfonamide violation was observed in each of non-formula-fed veal, goats, and geese. Swine exhibited 24 violative samples of 15,600 analyses in swine in 1996; violative levels of sulfadimethoxine were reported in the muscle of one animal. Violative levels of sulfamethazine were reported in the muscle of 15 animals, in the muscle and liver of 7 animals, and in the liver of 1 animal.

Residues of arsenical compounds were tested in 1056 monitoring samples of poultry. Three violations were detected in each of young chicken and turkey samples. Testing for ivermectin residues showed that 6 of 3327 samples taken from 10 production classes contained violative residues; two violations occurred in dairy cows, two in goats, and one in each of bulls and heavy calves. In contrast, no violations from halofuginone were found among the 1196 monitoring samples taken from 472 young chickens, 213 mature chickens, 400 young turkeys, and 111 mature turkeys. Violations from levamisole were also not found in 4101 samples from 14 animal production classes.

Apart from monitoring testing, FSIS conducted numerous in-plant tests during 1996 to detect the presence of antibiotic and sulfonamide residues in meat and poultry. A total of 41,995 analyses were carried out on samples from horses, cattle, sheep/lambs, goats, and ostriches using the swab tests on premises (STOP) step. A figure of 266 of the 292 violations found concerned cattle. In cattle, the STOP specific violative residue cases reported were 105 for penicillin, 71 for oxytetracycline, 34 for tetracycline, 18 for gentamicin, 16 for sulfadimethoxine, 24 for streptomycin, 24 for sulfamethazine, 9 for chlortetracycline, 2 for erythromycin, and 9 for neomycin. The specific violative residue cases reported for horses were eight for penicillin, two for streptomycin, and one for oxytetracycline. In sheep/lambs the violative cases were limited to one for tetracyline and one for penicillin, whereas in swine they were limited to four for penicillin, five for tetracycline, one for chlortetracycline, three for oxytetracycline, and one for sulfamethazine. In goat, only one sample was found violative and concerned tetracycline; in unnamed species the violative sample found concerned oxytetracycline. These results compare well with the results of the fiscal year 1995: FSIS tested 83,524 samples using the STOP test and found 888 violations.

In addition, a total of 21,045 analyses were carried out on samples of bob veal calves using the Calf Antibiotic and Sulfa Test. There were 169 violations including 20 for penicillin, 11 for streptomycin, 29 for tetracycline, 1 for erythromycin, 29 for neomycin, 14 for oxytetracycline, 4 for chlortetracycline, 36 for gentamicin, 14 for sulfamethazine, 6 for sulfamethoxazole, 3 for sulfadimethoxine, and 2 for sulfathiazole. Analogous surveys conducted in 1995 showed 848 violative specimens of the 58,197 samples tested.

Furthermore, 156,078 samples from cattle, sheep/lambs, goats, swine, and other animals were screened for antibiotics and sulfonamide drug residues using the fast antimicrobial screen test (FAST) developed in 1991 to replace CAST and STOP. There were 1022 violations for cattle and 2 for swine samples. In cattle, violative cases included 335 for penicillin, 142 for streptomycin, 128 for tetracycline, 28 for erythromycin, 48 for neomycin, 174 for oxytetracycline, 17 for chlortetracycline, 109 for gentamicin, 87 for sulfamethazine, 22 for sulfamethoxazole, 141 for sulfadimethoxine, 7 for sulfachlorpyridazine, 2 for tylosin, and 19 for sulfathiazole. In swine, violative samples were limited to one for oxytetracycline and one for penicillin. Analogous surveys conducted in 1995 showed 804 violative specimens of the 68,139 samples tested.

In the fiscal year 1996, FSIS and FDA also began a joint survey of formula-fed veal at slaughter for the presence of clenbuterol residues. Since clenbuterol persists far longer in retinal tissue than in other tissues, eyeballs except liver and muscle tissue samples were also used in this survey. FDA first analyzed the eyeballs with an enzyme-linked immunosorbent assay (ELISA) screening assay. When eyeballs were found to contain clenbuterol, the liver of that animal was subsequently analyzed. When violative residues were also found in the liver, muscle tissue was also analyzed.

The FDA/FSIS survey lasted to 1997. Only 1 of the 499 eyeball samples gave a positive result with the ELISA screen, but the presence of clenbuterol could not be confirmed in this sample. Confirmatory analysis showed that this animal contained residues of the β-agonist fenoterol.

13.2   RESIDUES IN THE EUROPEAN UNION

Within the European Union, each member state is obliged to monitor food-producing animals and their products for residues of legally and illegally used veterinary drugs and to present a National Residue Monitoring Plan that takes into account the specific situation in its country. Aspects that must be covered in the National Plan are a description of the authorities and laboratories involved in the implementation and execution of the National Plan, drugs to be analyzed, methods for screening and confirmation, action levels, animal species, and number of samples to be taken in relation to the number of slaughtered animals in the previous years. The frequency of sampling is dependent on the group of drugs and animal species; when positive samples are identified, sampling intensity has to be increased. Differences exist between member states in terms of the species sampled, number of samples taken, sampling methods, matrices for analysis, methods of analysis, range of screened drugs, and detection levels used in determining positive results.

During the last decade, antibiotic use in food-producing animals was increasingly directed against specific conditions and less toward general therapy or disease prevention. Nevertheless, some antibiotics with specific withdrawal periods continue to be fed at subtherapeutic levels, creating the potential for residues in the animals at the time of slaughter. As a result, antibiotics currently account for many of the residue violations within the European Union.

Another issue of high public concern within the European Union is the illegal use of hormones and hormone-like growth-promoting substances in food-producing animals. Since the European ban on anabolic steroids in 1986, alternative chemicals, particularly β-agonists, have been introduced and are used in the black market as growth-promoting agents. Most of the black-market designer agents have not been given names suggested by their chemical structures. Instead, their names have been assigned so as to provide a practical taxonomy in maintaining a catalog of this rapidly growing list of relatively simple to synthesize growth promoters. A typical list of the β-agonists used illegally within the European Union for fattening purposes includes clenbuterol, clenproperol, clenpenterol, clencyclohexerol, brombuterol, salbutamol, mabuterol, mapenterol, pirbuterol, terbutaline, fenoterol, cimaterol, and cimbuterol (5).

Since 1987, the European Commission has received the monitoring plans of EU member states concerning anabolic steroids and thyreostats, and since 1988 concerning other drugs. The use of stilbenes, stilbene derivatives, their salts and esters, and thyreostatic drugs in all animal species has been prohibited in the European Union since 1981, as well as the use of natural or synthetic hormones for fattening purposes. Administration of drugs with estrogenic, androgenic, or gestagenic action is only allowed for therapeutic reasons under specified conditions, such as fertility disorders, in those member states where these substances are authorized. The only β-agonist registered for veterinary use in cattle, horses, and pets in almost all European countries is clenbuterol. None of the member states has authorized the use of clenbuterol or any other β-agonist for repartitioning purposes, and national action levels used in determining positive results have been adopted by each EU country (Table 13.10).

TABLE **13.10** Action Levels for β-Adrenergic Agonists Within EU Member States

Country	Matrix	Level of action in matrices (1993)
Belgium	Liver	1 μg/kg
Denmark	Liver	250/100 ppt clenbuterol, 5/1 μg/kg salbutamol,
	Urine	3/1 μg/kg other β-agonists
France	Urine	1 μg/kg
Germany	Urine	1 μg/kg
Greece	Liver	1 μg/kg
	Urine	
Ireland	Urine	1 μg/kg
Italy	Urine	0.2–5 μg/kg
Luxembourg	Urine	2 μg/kg
Netherlands	Liver	1 μg/kg clenbuterol, salbutamol, mabuterol,
	Urine	mapenterol
		2 μg/kg cimaterol, terbutaline, broombuterol
Portugal	Urine	1 μg/kg
Spain	Liver	1–2 μg/kg
	Urine	
	Feed	
United Kingdom	Liver	Detection limit: 0.5–1 μg/kg
	Urine	

Source: From Ref. 5.

At present, approximately 30,000 animals in EU Member States are examined each year for the presence of residues of β-agonists. For residue surveillance of β-agonists, it is essential to identify the proper matrices for detection of residues with respect to potential accumulation of the drug, ease of sampling, and extractability of residues. Species examined for β-agonist residues are cattle, sheep, goats, swine, horses, poultry, and rabbits. Results of the monitoring vary substantially between member states; positive samples taken at the farm or in the slaughterhouse vary in the range of 0–7%.

An extensive EU survey on growth promoters was carried out in 1994 by the Belgian Consumers Organization in 12 member states in cooperation with the National Consumers Organizations (6). A total of 1183 beefsteaks samples and 936 liver samples purchased in retail stores across Europe were analyzed for the presence of anabolic hormones and β-agonists. The number of samples per country was determined on the basis of the size of each country, but a minimum of 60 samples was considered necessary to provide a representative picture of the use of growth promoters in each country. In beefsteaks, 19 positive samples were identified (1.6%); 1 sample contained acetoxyprogesterone, 2 boldenone, 1 megestrol acetate, 2 methylboldenone, 8 methyltestosterone, and 5 nortestosterone. Synthetic estrogens were not detected in any sample. In liver, 92 samples (10%) were found positive to β-agonists. In each case, clenbuterol was identified as the only β-agonist residue. Examination of the relative incidence of the positive samples within the tested 12 EU member states revealed that contamination was higher in Spain and Belgium, and absent in Denmark.

13.2.1   Austria

A survey carried out in Austria between 1991 and 1993 demonstrated that the incidence of residues of veterinary drugs and hormones in edible tissues of slaughtered animals was almost negligible (7). In particular, urine samples obtained from calves, cows, and swine were tested for the presence of residues of stilbenes, zeranol, trenbolone and 19-nortestosterone. Blood samples were examined for 17-β-estradiol and 17-β-testosterone. Furthermore, urine samples from calves, beef cattle, and thyroid gland specimens were tested for the presence of β-agonists and thyreostatic substances. None of the samples gave evidence of illegal use of these substances in Austria.

In addition, kidney fat from calves, beef cattle, dairy cows, and swine was tested for the presence of gestagens; muscle tissues from calves, beef cattle, and swine for nitrofuran residues; and swine muscle for tranquilizer residues. None of these samples was found to contain residues of the investigated analytes. In contrast, a considerable number of swine samples taken from one slaughterhouse were found to be contaminated with chloramphenicol at levels exceeding 5 ppb during 1991 and 1992 but not during 1993.

13.2.2 Belgium

In Belgium, monitoring of drug residues is carried out at both the slaughterhouses by the Institute for Veterinary Inspection of the Belgian Ministry of Public Health and at farms by the Veterinary Inspection Service of the Ministry of Agriculture. Under both monitoring programs, sampling may be either random or directed. In the random sampling, carcasses are chosen at random according to EU Directive 96/23/EC and not confiscated. In the directed sampling suspected carcasses are analyzed and confiscated awaiting the result of the analysis.

In 1997, the random sampling at farm for hormonal residues revealed 68 positive results of 5142 samples examined (1.3%). The levels from directed sampling were 195 of 3540 samples (5.5%). These figures are much higher than those obtained at the slaughterhouse level, where only 6 of 692 samples (0.9%) were found positive for hormonal residues during random sampling, and 35 of 4092 samples (0.9%) during directed sampling. All positive samples were from cattle and included injection sites, fat, skin, feces, and urine. Most of the positive samples contained testosterone, progesterone, estradiol, methylboldenone, and stanozolol. Some samples were contaminated with trenbolone acetate, ethylestrenol, norethandrolone, chlortestosterone acetate and its metabolite, nortestosterone, acetoxyprogesterone, methyltestosterone, medroxyprogesterone, and fluoxymestrone. These results are very encouraging if one considers the evolution of hormonal residues in edible animal products in Belgium over the period 1988–1997 (Table 13.11).

Apart from hormonal residues, samples randomly sampled at slaughterhouses in 1997 were also examined for potential presence of corticosteroids and

TABLE 13.11 Results of Directed Sampling at Belgian Slaughterhouses for Hormonal Residues over the Period 1988–1997

Year	Amount	Positives	Positives (%)
1988	4164	484	12
1989	2874	469	16
1990	3120	934	30
1991	5719	686	12
1992	4497	490	11
1993	3065	230	7.5
1994	3003	309	10.3
1995	5196	161	3.1
1996	5574	208	3.7
1997	4092	35	0.9

Source: From Ref. 50.

β-agonists. The corticosteroid dexamethasone, in particular, has been frequently encountered in feeds, urine, and feces of cattle. Given the possibility that residues of this drug might be present in animal products such as liver, 435 liver samples from 155 pigs and 280 beef cattle, originating from slaughterhouses in the Flemish region of Belgium over a 9 month period starting January, 1995, were screened for dexamethasone (8).

Results showed that only one pig liver sample (0.65%) and five beef liver samples (1.79%) contained dexamethasone residues exceeding the MRL of 2.5 ppb set by the Commission Regulation 1441/95 (9). It is of interest, however, to note that the concentrations found in 3 of the 5 beef livers examined were more than 10 times the MRL. The results drawn for beef livers were found to be in remarkably good agreement with the results of feces analysis carried out in the same period at the State Laboratory in 2000 cattle feces. Approximately 1.55% of these samples were also found positive for dexamethasone. Dexamethasone residues were found in 15 of 515 samples taken from cattle at the slaughterhouse level, no information is available as to whether the level of these residues exceeded the official MRL. No positive samples of β-agonists were found in a total of 1886 samples collected from cattle, calf, pigs, and sheep during 1997.

In 1997, the percentage of slaughterhouse samples found positive for antibiotics differed based on the method of sampling, being higher in the case of directed sampling (Table 13.12). An analogous trend has appeared in the evolution of antibiotic residues over the period 1992–1997 (Table 13.13).

In 1997, no samples were found positive for sulfonamides, chloramphenicol, phenylbutazone, nitrofurans, oxfendazole/fenbendazole, or acetylsalicylac-

TABLE 13.12   Results of Random versus Directed Sampling at Belgian Slaughterhouses for Antibiotic Residues in 1997

Species	Samples	Sample type	Positives	Positives (%)
Random sampling				
Cattle	400	Kidney	7	2.4
Calf	1227	Kidney	10	1.1
Swine	2604	Kidney	66	2.5
Sheep	30	Kidney	0	0.0
Directed sampling				
Cattle	8992	Kidney	788	8.8
Calf	1375	Kidney	169	12.3
Swine	7038	Kidney	196	2.8
Sheep	27	Kidney	0	0.0
Horses	299	Kidney	33	11.0

Source: From Ref. 50.

TABLE 13.13 Results of Random versus Directed
Sampling at Belgian Slaughterhouses for Antibiotic
Residues (%) over the Period 1992–1997

Year	Random sampling	Directed sampling
1992	7.3	4.7
1993	15.3	4.2
1994	15.3	4.2
1995	2.0	5.1
1996	2.4	6.2
1997	1.9	6.7

Source: From Ref. 50.

ides from a total of 102, 235, 52, 234, 242, and 111 samples, respectively. In
swine, 1 of 103 samples was found positive for dimetridazole/ronidazole, whereas
6 of 192 samples were positive for carazolol, and 25 of 341 samples were positive
for tranquillizers. The evolution of chloramphenicol, sulfonamides, and tranquil-
lizer residues over the period 1992–1997 is presented for comparison purposes
in Table 13.14.

13.2.3 Denmark

In the period 1984–1994, 1076 samples of various animal products including
broilers, bovine liver, and swine liver and muscle, and 323 samples of fish including trout from sea and pond farming and salmon were analyzed for veterinary
drug residues by the National Food Agency of Denmark (10). The animal products
were monitored for residues of carbadox, olaquindox, benzimidazoles, levami-

TABLE 13.14 Evolution of Chloramphenicol, Sulfonamides, and
Tranquilizers Residues Over the Period 1992–1997 in Belgium

	Number of positive results as a fraction of total samples					
Type of drugs	1992	1993	1994	1995	1996	1997
Chloramphenicol	12/4782	0/2351	1/302	11/279	1/303	0/235
Sulfonamides	4/302	5/301	7/301	9/288	1/299	0/102
Tranquilizers	2/100	6/100	6/300	17/288	9/301	25/341

Source: From Ref. 50.

TABLE 13.15 Veterinary Drug Residues in Pond-Farmed Trout in Denmark

Veterinary drug	Year	Number of samples	Number of findings	Limit of determination (μg/kg)	Findings (μg/kg) min–max
Furazolidone	1991	49	0	4	—
Malachite green/ leucomalachite green	1991	49	2	4	4–5
Malachite green	1998	49	13	2	15–214
	1989	20	6	5	5–17
Oxolinic acid	1991	49	0	50	—
Oxytetracycline	1990	25	0	20	—
	1991	49	1	13	13
Sulfadiazine	1991	49	0	20	—
Sulfamerazine	1984	52	2	20	40–90
	1988	49	6	10	13–76
	1991	49	1	20	230
Trimethoprim	1991	49	0	50	—

Source: From Ref. 10.

sole, dimetridazole and ronidazole; the fish products were examined for residues of furazolidone, malachite/leucomalachite green, oxolinic acid, oxytetracycline, sulfadiazine, sulfamerazine, and trimethoprim.

Residues were only detected in 1 sample of swine liver that contained 80 ppb carbadox, and in 31 fish samples all coming from pond farming (Table 13.15). The most frequent residue found in fish was malachite green. During 1988–1989, residues of malachite green were also detected in 19 fish samples, and in two fish samples in 1991. During the period 1984–1988, low levels of sulfamerazine were detected in eight samples; in 1991 an atypical high level of sulfamerazine (230 ppb) was detected in one sample. During 1992 and 1993, monitoring of 215 liver and urine samples collected at the farm level and 601 samples collected at the slaughter level gave no evidence for illegal use of β-agonists in food-producing animals (11).

13.2.4 Germany

In 1991 and 1992, muscle, kidney, and liver samples that gave positive results in a *Bacillus subtilis* inhibitor test were further analyzed to identify and quantify the drug residues responsible for the inhibition (12). Antimicrobial substances were identified in 45% of the samples analyzed. In most cases, the found residues

TABLE 13.16 Drug Residues and their Concentration Range in Kidney, Muscle, and Liver Samples from a Total of 529 Animals in Germany

Type of drugs	Number of samples	Concentration range (μg/kg)
Tetracyclines	151	10–13,500
Sulfonamides	82	14–33,600
N^4-acetylsulfonamides	59	6–36,000
Chloramphenicol	60	0.5–100,000
Penicillins	5	5–65
Dapsone	2	20–450
Quinolones	2	12–250
Nitroimidazoles	1	300

Source: From Ref. 12.

originated from tetracyclines, sulfonamides, and chloramphenicol, and occurred at concentrations far above the MRL values defined by the European Union (Table 13.16). Higher residue concentrations of several drugs were present in tissues of animals that had been subjected to emergency slaughter. Presumably, these drugs had been administered shortly before slaughtering so that the withdrawal periods could no longer be followed. In addition to the analysis of inhibitor-positive samples, a number of inhibitor-negative muscle samples from animals exhibiting inhibitor-positive kidneys were also examined in the same study. Most of these samples (53%) were found to contain residues, partially in concentrations exceeding the EU MRLs to a percentage of 69%.

The incidence of tetracycline residues in turkeys has been also studied recently (13). During meat inspection, suspicious flocks were identified by fluorescence detection in bones. A total of 85 flocks showed significant fluorescence in bones. When bones, liver, kidney, and muscle of these animals were analyzed for tetracyclines, residues of tetracycline, chlortetracycline, oxytetracycline, or doxycycline were found in 83 flocks. These results suggest that the detection of fluorescence in bones might be a useful screening method for tetracycline residues in poultry carcasses.

In 1993, the incidence of antimicrobials in car tanker milk and the suitability of different tests for the detection of antimicrobials on the MRL level has been examined in Northern Germany using an integrated detection system (14). This system comprised microbial inhibitor tests for screening, immunochemical tests for preliminary confirmation, and high-performance liquid chromatography (HPLC) for final confirmation either in a parallel or a subsequent fashion in case of positive or questionable screening results.

Results showed a total of 2.8% of the samples (n = 2972) to be inhibitor positive by the Delvotest SP test; further examination identified 1.7% as β-lactam antibiotics, and 1.1% as sulfonamides and dapsone. The percentage of chloramphenicol suspicious samples determined by the Charm II test was amazingly high; however, tests for confirmation were not available and contamination of the samples by residues of the chloramphenicol-based preservative azidiol could not be excluded with certainty. Low concentrations of streptomycins were also detected in 5.7% of the samples (n = 1221), but the MRL was not exceeded. Macrolide and tetracycline residues were not found in significant levels. Model trials with commercially applied yoghurt cultures confirmed how important the compliance to MRLs can be to dairy industry; compared to antibiotic-free milk, a pH of 5.0 was reached with a delay of 15 min in the case of contamination with cloxacillin; 30 min in the case of penicillin, spiramycin, and tylosin; and 45 min in the case of oxytetracycline contamination.

Antimicrobial residues in natural honey may result from direct contamination after antibiotic treatment of bacterial honey-bee diseases, and from carryover if antibiotics are used for plant protection in fruit farming during blossom. Use of antimicrobials is not approved for treatment of bees colonies in many countries, but unauthorized drug use cannot be excluded. Nevertheless, MRLs have not been set so far for honey. Substances of concern are tetracycline, oxytetracycline, streptomycin, and sulfathiazole (15). Given the possibility that residues may occur, 10 commercial honey samples in Germany were tested for tetracycline, chlortetracycline, and oxytetracycline residues. The survey revealed only one positive sample containing 15.7 ppb of the drugs (16). These results are encouraging since in an earlier study (17) conducted also in Germany, tetracycline was found at levels as high as 1.5–5.1 ppm in 3 of 54 samples.

In the same survey, honey from producers in Southwest Germany (Oberschwaben) and commercial honey from the area of Munich were also screened for potential presence of streptomycin residues. Results showed that more than 50% of the commercial honey samples contained detectable concentrations of streptomycin residues at a maximum level of 100 ppb. These findings demonstrate the need for further and more intense control measures for drug residues in honey.

Another major issue of concern for the regulatory authorities in Germany is the illegal use of β-agonists in food-producing animals. Both random monitoring and targeted surveillance are carried out for the potential presence of residues of β-agonists in veal calves, young bovine, cows, poultry, swine, and lambs (11). At the farm level, only urine and blood samples were collected before 1995, but thereafter feed, milk, and feces were also taken. At the slaughterhouse level, a great variety of samples including urine, blood, liver, kidney, bile, muscle, and retina/choroid were collected. The incidence of positive samples was found to be highest in veal calves followed by young cattle. Clenbuterol was the only β-agonist detected in all surveys. Samples from cows and swine were negative.

TABLE 13.17 Random Monitoring of Clenbuterol Concentrations in Veal Calves in 1994 and 1995 in Germany[a]

	Number of positive samples (total number of samples)			
	1994	%	1995	%
Farm phase				
Urine	7 (449)	15.5	37 (379)	9.8
Blood	39 (270)	14.4	9 (534)	1.7
Slaughter phase				
Urine	59 (393)	12.8	17 (324)	5.2
Liver	15 (159)	9.4	2 (211)	0.9
Retina/choroid	0 (23)	0.0	0 (36)	0.0
Eye (other parts)	7 (46)	15.2	13 (53)	24.5

[a] Method of detection: ELISA/GC-MS (sensitivity < 0.5 μg/kg).
Source: From Ref. 11.

The number of samples positive to clenbuterol from veal calves at farms and slaughterhouses during the period 1994–1995 is presented in Table 13.17. A decrease in the percentage of positive samples of urine and blood taken at both farms and slaughterhouses from 1994 through 1995 was observed.

13.2.5 Ireland

Several sampling programs were developed during the period 1989–1994 in Northern Ireland to monitor veterinary drug abuse in the local meat industry (18). Random survey of residues in swine, sheep and cattle was performed by the National Monitoring Program, whereas targeted survey of cattle suspected of being treated with growth promoters were carried out by the Meat Inspection Scheme. Between 1989 and 1994, increasing numbers of urine, bile, liver, retina, and hair samples were collected to implement these programs. Specific on farm surveys were further conducted and samples of suspected animals, medicinal products, and feedstuffs were also collected.

Results indicated a low incidence of clenbuterol contamination in cattle liver during 1992–1994, with 3 positive of 151 liver samples in 1992 and 1 positive of 219 samples in 1994. Results of targeted sampling from cattle indicated high percentages of clenbuterol positive carcasses during 1990 and 1991, with 43 of 121 samples and 139 of 286 samples showing detectable residues, respectively. Despite the substantial increase in the number of samples analyzed over succeeding years, the number of positive results steadily declined, thus giving strong

TABLE 13.18 Results of Targeted Testing Programs for β-Adrenergic Agonists Abuse in Cattle in Northern Ireland's National Surveillance Scheme (Meat Inspection Scheme [MIS] and On-Farm Follow-up Sampling [OFFUS])

Location and year	Matrices	No. of carcasses	Positive findings (%)
Slaughterhouse (MIS)			
1990	Urine, bile, liver	121	35.5
1991	Bile, liver	286	48.6
1992	Liver, retina	1831	6.2
1993	Retina, liver	1861	5.6
1994	Retina, liver	973	1.5
		No. of samples	
On farm (OFFUS)			
1991	Urine	276	19.2
1992	Urine	853	3.8
1993	Urine	237	8.4
1994	Urine	51	0.0
	Hair	61	27.9

Source: From Ref. 11.

evidence that abuse was also on the decline (Table 13.18). Specific onfarm surveys have indicated that in 1994 all tested urine samples were negative for clenbuterol, but 17 of 61 hair samples were positive (27.9%), indicating that clenbuterol abuse still has not been abandoned (11).

Monitoring for ionophore residues in eggs produced in North Ireland was also carried out in 1994 (19). Narasin, monensin, and salinomycin were detected in 1, 6, and 2 eggs, respectively, of the 161 eggs totally surveyed. In all cases, the concentrations detected were less than 2.5 ppb.

In contrast, lasalocid residues were present at concentrations ranging from 0.3 to 129 ppb in 107 eggs (66.6%). This difference in the incidence of ionophore residues in eggs was explained on the basis of the relative ability of the tested ionophores to accumulate in eggs. Since the abilities of monensin, salinomycin, and lasalocid are in the ratio 0.12, 3.3, and 63 ng/g egg per mg/kg feed, respectively, the potential for monensin and salinomycin to cause residues in eggs is very low as compared with lasalocid. In 1995, a granular formulation of lasalocid premix was introduced into United Kingdom that decreased the carryover of this drug from medicated to unmedicated feeds. Six months after the introduction of this formulation, the incidence of lasalocid residues in eggs decreased to 21%.

A study was also undertaken to investigate the presence of antibiotics in a total of 397 feedstuffs and 11 premixes, 161 of which were declared free of medication and 247 were medicated (20). Among the 247 medicated samples, 83 (35.2%) contained undeclared antimicrobials, of which 59 (23.9%) were at a level sufficient to allow quantification by HPLC. Among the 161 unmedicated samples, 71 (44.1%) were found to contain detectable antimicrobials, of which 42 (26.1%) contained concentrations that could be quantified by HPLC. The most frequently identified contaminants were chlortetracycline (15.2%), sulfonamides (6.9%), penicillin (3.4%), and ionophores (3.4%). Three samples contained ionophores, one sample sulfamethazine, and one sample monensin at therapeutic or supratherapeutic levels; the remainder were at subtherapeutic levels. However, all feeds contaminated with sulfamethazine were sufficient to cause violative tissue residues if fed to animals immediately prior to slaughter.

13.2.6 Italy

In 1991, a survey of the swine sector in Italy noted a relatively high contamination of feedstuffs with veterinary drugs. The contamination concerned more than two-thirds of the controlled industrial animal feed producers (21). Not declared drugs, principally carbadox, olaquindox, and sulfamethazine, were found in 29 of 193 feed samples (15%) collected from 10 different feed producers. For some of these feeds, the relatively high drug levels could caused appearance of residues in the urine of the live swine and further in the offal taken from slaughterhouses. Positive findings in both urine and offal accounted for 10 of the 520 samples analyzed.

In 1992, the situation improved markedly owing to the activity of involvement, information, and pressure made on farmers and feed producers on the residue problem. In spite of the higher number of analyzed samples both at the farm and slaughterhouse levels, feed contamination showed a value of only 4.4%. The contaminated feeds contained carbadox and sulfamethazine and originated from four different feedstuffs industries out of 9 totally examined. The concentrations recorded on positive samples were in the range 0.5–28 ppm, while in 1991 the levels ranged from 0.05 to 88 ppm.

During the period June, 1994, to June, 1996, a monitoring program for analyzing nicarbazin residues in several animal matrices was also carried out (22). The results of this program showed that nicarbazin residues occurred only in some egg samples.

In the period 1992–1993, extensive surveillance for the potential presence of β-agonists in veal calves, young cattle, and cows was carried out (11). A total of 7121 and 5883 urine samples collected at the slaughter phase in 1992 and 1993, respectively, were tested. Analysis results revealed 264 positive samples (3.7%) in 1992 and 397 positive samples (6.7%) in 1993.

Monitoring results of anabolic drug residues in animals from the Campania and Calabria regions of Italy during the period 1994–1995 have been also reported (23). Tested substances included 17-β-estradiol, 17-β-testosterone, progesterone, boldenone, trenbolone, nandrolone, diethylstilbestrol, zeranol, dienestrol, hexestrol, corticosteroids, and β-agonists. The results suggested illegal use of β-agonists in bovine breeding. They further indicated that eyeball could be used as a more appropriate matrix than urine for the detection of such residues.

13.2.7 The Netherlands

Since 1989, control of the illegal use of hormonal growth promoters in the Netherlands has intensified. Random sampling as well as targeted sampling on suspect farms is performed by the National Inspection Service for Livestock and Meat within the framework of the Annual National Program. The number of samples collected for examination represents 1% of the slaughtered cattle younger than 1 year, 100 slaughtered cattle older than 1 year, and 100 pigs. Samples are assayed for a variety of hormone-like substances including clenbuterol, salbutamol, mabuterol, mapenterol, cimaterol, terbutalin, and 17-β-estradiol. Since 1993, samples have also been screened for the presence of bromobuterol and since 1995 for clenproperol.

Monitoring results of random sampling during the period 1989–1995 showed the presence of β-agonists in veal calves, young cattle, and cows, but not in samples from pigs, sheep, and horses at a level ≥1 ppb (11). Most of the positive samples contained clenbuterol, with other β-agonists occurring only marginally. However, since 1990 the presence of clenbuterol in the urine of young cattle was clearly decreased, from about 11% to almost 0.4% in 1995. A similar decrease in the number of positive liver samples was observed since the time systematic monitoring started in 1992.

Between 1993 and 1995, more than 250 farms were also inspected, and more than 4000 urine samples and 400 feeds were also examined for potential presence of β-agonists (24). During that period, the percentage of positive urine samples from suspected animals decreased from 30% to less than 5%, and the percentage of positive feed samples was in the range 11–15%. Most positive samples contained clenbuterol and some mabuterol, bromobuterol, and salbutamol in addition to clenbuterol. In a few cases, more than one β-agonist was detected in urine whereas various synthetic anabolic hormones were also found in feeds.

Next to the Annual National Program, the control on the illegal use of growth promoters in veal calves and beef cattle is also conducted by the Foundation for Quality Guarantee and the Cattle Quality Inspection, respectively. Every year, about 40,000 samples, mainly urine samples from groups of calves and cattle at the farm level, are randomly collected. The inspectors take $\sqrt{n}$ samples from each group at random. For example, if 144 calves are present in a group, 12 calves are sampled. Samples are analyzed for the presence of β-agonists, estrogenic and androgenic steroids, and corticosteroids.

TABLE 13.19 Number of Groups of Calves with Urine Positive for Growth Promoters over the Period 1991–1995 in the Netherlands

Compound	1991	1992	1993	1994	1995
Clenbuterol	4	4	6	7	6
Mabuterol	1	0	0	0	0
Mapenterol	10	2	0	0	0
Salbutamol	0	2	3	0	0
Estradiol-17β	5	2	0	0	1

Source: From Ref. 51.

The combined result of these activities is shown in Table 13.19. In 1991, the year of the establishment of the Foundation for Quality Guarantee of the Veal Calf Sector, mapenterol, clenbuterol, and 17-β-estradiol were detected; in 1994 and 1995 samples contained only clenbuterol.

13.2.8 Portugal

The potential use of β-agonists in bovine for growth-promoting purposes has been investigated in Portugal during 1991–1993 (25). A total of 1031 urine samples were screened for potential presence of clenbuterol, clenpenterol, clenproperol, mabuterol, mapenterol, bromobuterol, tulobuterol, and salbutamol residues. Results showed that 24 samples were contaminated with clenbuterol and one sample with salbutamol residues.

Apart from β-agonists, bovine products in Portugal have been found contaminated with antibiotic residues. Presence of violative penicillin residues in commercialized milk in Portugal has been recently confirmed (26).

13.2.9 Spain

In fulfillment of the EU and Spanish legislation, the Basque areas started monitoring clenbuterol residues in food-producing animals in 1990 (27). Between 1990 and 1994, a total of 3559 samples of urine and liver were collected at slaughterhouses, farms, refrigerated storehouses, and retailers, and analyzed to determine clenbuterol residues. At slaughterhouses, only urine was collected in 1990, only liver in 1991, and both liver and urine in 1992–1994. At farms, only urine was collected, whereas at refrigerated storehouses and retailers only liver was collected. The total number of samples according to the type of outlet was 2482 at slaughterhouses, 336 at farms, and 741 at refrigerated storehouses and retailers. In 1991 and 1992, control of clenbuterol residues was fully random but only 29

TABLE 13.20 Number of Samples Positive for Clenbuterol Residues over the Period 1990–1994 in the Basque Country of Spain

		Positive results		
Year	Number of samples	Slaughterhouses	Farms	Refrigerated storehouses/retailers
1990	29	—	—	—
1991	21	1	—	—
1992	1068	21	1	14
1993	957	21	1	48
1994	1484	37	0	10

Source: From Ref. 27.

and 21 samples were collected, respectively. Since 1992, the number of samples increased, reaching 1484 in 1994.

Clenbuterol residues were detected in a total of 154 samples. Yearly results according to the kind of outlet are summarized in Table 13.20. As shown by these data, the number of positive samples increases with the number of the samples analyzed. This fact proves an extended illegal use of this substance in the Basque areas of Spain that is higher than that of other drugs illegally used in cattle feeding.

Illegal use of clenbuterol in bovine animals has been detected in other regions of Spain as well (11). In 1992 and 1993, a total of 5294 and 3988 samples, respectively, of urine, liver, and feeds collected at the farm level were analyzed. Analysis results showed 59 positive samples (1.1%) in 1992 and 36 positive samples (0.9%) in 1993. In the same period, a total of 6515 and 7040 samples collected at the slaughter level in 1992 and 1993, respectively, were also tested. Analysis results revealed 268 positive samples (4.4%) in 1992 and 343 positive samples (3.4%) in 1993. Analysis results from veal liver samples collected from a slaughterhouse in Catalonia, Spain, showed that in 9 of 16 samples of contaminated veal liver the concentrations of clenbuterol were in the range 19–5395 ppb.

In Spain, screening of antibacterial residues in meat and kidney samples is also performed using the four-plate test. Inhibitor-positive samples are sent to the Spanish National Reference Laboratory for antimicrobial residues, and a seven-plate postscreening test is applied to all samples to identify, prior to final confirmation, antibiotics or antibiotic groups including tetracyclines, β-lactams, aminoglycosides, and macrolides. When 634 inhibitor-positive muscle and kidney samples originated from the Spanish National Residue Program during 1994 and 1995 were postscreened, 83% of the positive results in the postscreening test were tetracycline residues, 7.5% β-lactams, 5% neomycin and gentamicin, 1.7% erythromycin and related macrolides, 1.7% streptomycin, and less than 0.5% tylosin and quinolones (28). Only 1% of the samples contained unidentified microbial inhibitors caused by antibiotics or complex antibiotic mixtures that did not correspond to the standard antibiotic used.

13.2.10 United Kingdom

Between May, 1986, and December, 1990, over 35,000 analyses were conducted in the United Kingdom for surveillance for veterinary drug residues in food. The results drawn from these analyses allow the incidence and concentrations of drug residues in the national food supply to be assessed (29). Although a very large number of samples were analyzed, a rather small number of samples were found to contain violative residues that mainly concerned sulfonamides in swine, and oxolinic acid and oxytetracycline in farmed fish. However, the incidence of sulfonamide residues in a range of swine tissues from home-produced and imported sources showed a significant decline over the period 1986–1990 (Table 13.21).

Both farmed salmon and trout were not found to contain residues of malachite green or dichlorvos. However, a total of 20 of 92 salmon samples contained residues of oxytetracycline at a maximum level of 0.22 ppm, whereas a total of 15 of 92 salmon samples contained residues of oxolinic acid at a maximum level of 0.03 ppm. In addition, a total of 5 of 128 trout samples contained residues of oxytetracycline at a maximum level of 0.18 ppm, whereas a total of 34 out of 128 trout samples contained residues of oxolinic acid at a maximum level of 0.36 ppm. A seasonal pattern of residues was not apparent for salmon, but for trout a higher incidence of oxolinic acid residues was observed in spring and summer months.

Over the period 1991–1992, a total of 173 sheep liver samples and 204 cattle liver samples were collected in the United Kingdom to be screened for the

TABLE 13.21 Swine Tissue Samples Analyzed for Sulfonamides Between 1986 and 1990 in the United Kingdom

Year	Samples examined	Positive samples	Violative samples	Violative samples (%)
1986	513	124	58	11.3
1987	422	100	73	17.3
1988	1309	208	111	8.5
1989	1380	139	75	5.4
1990	1318	134	69	5.2

Source: From Ref. 29.

presence of levamisole residues (30). Results showed that five sheep and four cattle liver samples contained levamisole at concentrations above 10 ppb.

A total of 140 archived imported liver samples collected in 1991 were also analyzed. It was found that 16 samples, all imported from New Zealand, contained levamisole residues at concentrations in the range 15–53 ppb. The archived samples were from consignments exported from New Zealand before the introduction of the EU MRL of 10 ppb.

A further 62 samples of imported sheep liver were collected in 1992 and analyzed. These samples included 56 samples from New Zealand, 9 of which contained levamisole at concentrations in the range 15–254 ppb. Surveillance of sheep liver for residues of levamisole continued in 1993. A total of 66 samples of sheep liver were purchased from retail outlets throughout the United Kingdom and analyzed; 24 of the samples were home-produced and the remaining 42 samples were imported from New Zealand. Home-produced samples were found not to contain residues of levamisole. In contrast, four of the samples from New Zealand contained residues of levamisole at concentrations in the range 16–174 ppb.

More recent surveillance indicates that the incidence of veterinary drug residues above MRLs is falling. Results from the 1994 UK surveillance programs showed that a total of approximately 0.2% of all samples analyzed contained violative residues (31). By way of comparison, the total in excess of MRLs in 1993 was also 0.2%, whereas in 1992 the figure was 0.48%. A total of 5 of 86 samples of imported swine kidney contained residues of tetracyclines in excess of the MRL. Apart from tetracyclines, 1.7% of the swine kidney samples were found to contain residues of sulfonamides above the MRL, compared with 1.5% in 1993. This is likely to have resulted from the increased use of sulfonamides to treat respiratory disease. Residues of nicarbazin were determined in 8 samples, residues of sulfonamides in 11 samples, and residues of lasalocid in 46 of the 429 egg samples analyzed. One sample contained residues of sulfadiazine at a level of 924 ppb.

The reasons for both the nicarbazin and sulfonamide contamination were not established but might result from feed contamination or on-farm management practices. The lasalocid contamination has been shown to be due to trace level carryover during feed production. As a result, the formulation of the lasalocid was changed from a powder to a granular form to reduce the carryover.

In addition, a total of 36 of 220 samples (16%) of trout contained residues of malachite green in the range 2–33 ppb; a total of 41 of 409 salmon samples contained residues of ivermectin in the range 2–30 ppb. Although the MRL of 100 ppb set for bovine liver cannot be directly extrapolated to salmon, it is considered unlikely that, at the concentrations of ivermectin being determined in salmon, the ADI for this substance is being exceeded. There is therefore unlikely to be a consumer hazard arising from these residues.

TABLE 13.22 Incidence of Nicarbazin in Eggs in the United Kingdom during 1995–1997

Report	Date published	Date of analysis	Free range analyzed	Free range detected	Other analyzed	Other detected	Range (ppb)	Mean (ppb)
MAVIS 18	April 1996	Jan–Dec 1995	214	21	213	16	10–900	–
MAVIS 21	Jan 1997	Feb–Nov 1996	108	14	108	13	8–270	48
MAVIS 23	July 1997	Jan–Jun 1997	26	1	29	2	46–83	61

MAVIS, Medicines Act Veterinary Information Service.
Source: From Ref. 32.

Despite increased sampling, no evidence has been found for the use of stilbene, β-agonists, or thyreostatic substances. A total of 13 cattle had elevated concentrations of natural hormones, but the subsequent onfarm visits established that no illegal use had taken place. Random sampling during the period 1994–1995 of liver and urine samples of young cattle, and liver samples of cows, sheep, and swine did not reveal samples with concentrations of clenbuterol or salbutamol above action levels (32). Nonstatutory surveillance of β-agonists in cattle and calf liver also showed no samples exceeding the action levels.

In the United Kingdom one of the chemicals monitored regularly is the coccidiostat nicarbazin, which is not licensed for use in laying hens and, therefore, any positive samples create cause for concern. The results of surveillance of the incidence of nicarbazin in eggs during the period 1996–1997 are presented in Table 13.22.

13.3 RESIDUES IN AUSTRALIA

In Australia, drug residue data on animal products are obtained through a national monitoring survey based on commodity–drug combinations derived from Australian agricultural and veterinary practice, and the requirements of export and domestic markets. The data collected facilitate certification of commodities for export and domestic consumption. The monitoring programs ensure that industries maintain access to, and a competitive advantage in, important markets. They also support agricultural and food promotions in new and potential markets. Drug residue monitoring data are increasingly being used to audit the effectiveness of industry-operated Quality Assurance programs.

During 1997–1998 beef, sheep, and pork were the main commodities monitored, but horse, deer, emu, ostrich, poultry, and eggs were also covered. Over 20,000 samples were collected on which about 29,000 chemical analyses were conducted during 1997. Drug residues were not detected in any of the horse,

TABLE 13.23   National Residue Survey Results during 1997–1998 in Australia

Drug(s)	Tissue	Samples	Residues < MRL	Residues > MRL	% Compliance
CATTLE					
Hormones					
Stilbenes	Feces	114	0	No MRL	—
Stilbenes	Feces[a]	202	0	No MRL	—
Stilbenes	Urine	125	0	No MRL	—
Stilbenes	Liver	286	0	0	100.0
Zeranol	Feces	114	9	No MRL	—
Zeranol	Feces[a]	202	5	No MRL	—
Zeranol	Urine	125	0	No MRL	—
Zeranol	Liver	286	0	0	100.0
Trenbolone	Feces[a]	202	0	No MRL	—
Trenbolone	Urine	122	0	No MRL	—
Trenbolone	Liver	120	0	0	100.0
19-nortestosterone	Urine	281	0	No MRL	—
Melengestrol acetate	Fat	304	0	0	100.0
β-Agonists					
Screen	Urine	284	0	No MRL	—
Antimicrobials					
Sulfonamides	Liver	613	0	0	100.0
Antibiotics	Kidney	617	1	2	99.7
Chloramphenicol	Muscle	296	0	0	100.0
Nitrofurans	Muscle	157	0	0	100.0
Nitrofurans	Serum	93	0	No MRL	—
Anthelminthics					
Macrocyclic lactones	Liver	293	0	0	100.0
Benzimidazoles	Liver	283	1	1	99.6
Levamizole	Liver	287	0	0	100.0
Triclabendazole	Liver	291	0	0	100.0
SHEEP					
Hormones					
Stilbenes	Liver	296	0	0	100.0
Zeranol	Liver	296	0	0	100.0
Trenbolone	Liver	297	0	0	100.0
19-nortestosterone	Urine	272	0	No MRL	—
β-Agonists					
Screen	Urine	290	0	No MRL	—
Antimicrobials					
Antibiotics	Kidney	297	0	0	100.0
Chloramphenicol	Muscle	296	0	0	100.0

(continued)

TABLE 13.23 Continued

Drug(s)	Tissue	Samples	Residues < MRL	Residues > MRL	% Compliance
Anthelminthics					
Macrocyclic lactones	Liver	288	6	1	99.6
Benzimidazoles	Liver	298	5	0	100.0
Closantel	Liver	289	4	0	100.0
Levamizole	Liver	284	1	0	100.0
SWINE					
Hormones					
Stilbenes	Liver	97	0	0	100.0
Antimicrobials					
Antibiotics	Kidney	721	95	34	95.3
Dimetridazole	Muscle	154	0	0	100.0
Sulfonamides	Liver	594	5	4	99.3
Anthelminthics					
Macrocyclic lactones	Liver	149	0	0	100.0
Levamizole	Liver	149	0	0	100.0

[a] Collected on farm.
Source: From Ref. 52.

deer, emu, ostrich, poultry, and egg commodities. The National Residue Survey results for beef, sheep, and pork are summarized in Table 13.23.

During 1997–1998, no evidence of the illegal use of hormones for growth-promoting purposes was detected in any of the samples tested from cattle, sheep, and pigs, although trenbolone and zeranol are registered for use as growth pro-moters in cattle. No residues of trenbolone were detected, but zeranol and zeara-lenone residues were detected in 2 and 14 samples from cattle, respectively. The source of this contamination was presumably attributed to *Fusarium* spp. known to infest improved rye grass pastures, producing the mycotoxin zearalenone, which can then be ingested by cattle and detected in urine, feces, and liver. The zearalenone toxin can be metabolized in the ruminant to zeranol, which is indistinguishable from zeranol administered as a growth promoter.

Samples from cattle, sheep, horse, poultry, and ratite were tested for the β-agonists clenbuterol, salbutamol, and cimaterol. Clenbuterol has restricted use and is registered as a tocolytic agent for the facilitation and postponement of parturition in cattle and sheep and as a bronchodilator and expectorant in horses. No residues were detected in any of the samples tested.

Three classes of anthelminthics were also monitored: macrocyclic lactones, benzimidazoles, and levamisole. Samples were taken from cattle, sheep, pigs, and ostriches. Only 2 of 2613 samples contained residues above the MRL. These were for fenbendazole in a cattle sample and avermectin in a sheep sample.

In Australia, the general antimicrobial screen is performed on kidney and is able to detect β-lactam, aminoglycoside, tetracycline, and macrolide antimicrobials and to identify the class of antimicrobial compound present. Where the screen test identifies a class of compounds, confirmation and quantitation are done by the specific HPLC or gas chromatographic (GC) method appropriate for the class of antimicrobial.

In the general screen for antimicrobials, 36 of 2112 samples from cattle, sheep, pigs, horses, deer, poultry, and ratites had residues above the MRL. Two of these samples were from cattle and the residues found were oxytetracycline and dihydrostreptomycin. The remaining 34 noncompliant samples were from 721 pig samples tested in the general screen. From these samples 19 were due to chlortetracycline, 14 due to oxytetracycline, and 1 to neomycin.

An additional factor in the high level of noncompliance is that the Australian MRLs in offal (0.05 mg/kg for chlortetracycline and 0.25 mg/kg for oxytetracycline) are significantly lower than those now recommended by Codex Alimentarius (0.60 mg/kg for both compounds). Thus, the registration data, withdrawal periods, and MRLs for these compounds are currently being reviewed by the responsible bodies in Australia, namely the National Registration Authority and the Australia New Zealand Food Authority.

In addition, specific testing was performed for chloramphenicol in muscle, nitrofurans in muscle and serum, dimetridazole in muscle of pigs and poultry, and sulfonamides in liver. In Australia, chloramphenicol is not registered for use in food animals and nitrofurans are only available as a topical preparation for use in companion animals. No residues of either of these compounds were detected. No residues of dimetridazole were detected in pig and poultry samples. Sulfonamide residues were monitored in cattle and pigs. No residues were detected in 613 cattle samples. In 594 pig liver samples analyzed, 9 residues of sulfamethazine (sulfamethazine) were detected, 4 of which were above the MRL.

13.4   RESIDUES IN OTHER COUNTRIES

13.4.1   Canada

An overview of the results of the Canadian Veterinary Drug residue control program during the fiscal years 1990/1991–1994/1995 shows that all meat and poultry commodities produced or imported during that period in Canada were totally free of violative residues of many veterinary drugs including chloramphenicol, benzimidazoles, nitrofurans, coccidiostats, zeranol, diethylstilbestrol and stilbenes, trenbolone acetate, melengestrol acetate and other hormonal anabolics, clenbuterol and other β-agonists, tranquillizers and β-blockers, and thyreostats (33). A few violations that occurred in the fiscal years 1993/1994 and 1994/1995 for home-produced commodities concerned residues of antibiotics, sulfonamides, carbadox, nitroimidazoles, and ivermectin (Table 13.24).

TABLE 13.24 Five-Year Compliance Summary for Meat and Poultry Commodities in Canada

	1990/91		1991/92		1992/93		1993/94		1994/95	
Drugs	n	Violation (%)	n	Violation (%)	n	Violation (%)	n	Violation (%)	n	Violation (%)
Antibiotics										
Beef	14,767	0.0	17,018	0.1	17,276	0.1	14,472	0.1	12,798	0.1
Veal	3001	0.0	3782	0.1	4382	0.0	4898	0.5	5068	0.6
Mutton	261	0.0	306	0.0	492	0.0	690	0.3	601	0.4
Pork	19,916	0.0	21,310	0.2	22,536	0.2	21,662	0.5	25,001	1.0
Horse	1258	0.0	884	0.0	1176	0.0	718	0.4	681	0.0
Chicken	671	0.0	961	0.4	747	0.0	1288	0.0	1265	0.0
Other	803	0.0	674	0.0	534	0.0	951	0.1	1303	0.0
Subtotal	40,677		44,935		47,143		44,679		46,717	
Sulfonamides										
Beef	390	0.0	434	0.0	373	0.0	385	0.0	1294	0.0
Veal	527	1.1	346	1.3	411	1.1	936	1.3	1923	0.3
Mutton	78	0.0	82	0.0	64	0.0	50	0.0	122	0.0
Pork	66,519	0.4	71,093	0.3	50,707	0.3	74,195	0.3	81,309	0.2
Chicken	177	0.0	216	0.0	170	0.0	114	0.0	148	0.0
Turkey	59	0.0	79	0.0	83	0.0	72	0.0	92	0.0
Other	—	—	18	0.0	1	0.0	29	0.0	111	0.0
Subtotal	67,750		73,068		51,809		75,781		84,999	
Carbadox										
Pork	539	1.1	608	0.7	772	0.3	879	0.1	412	0.5
Other	—	—	—	—	83	0.0	114	0.0	42	0.0
Subtotal	539		608		855		993		454	
Nitroimidazoles										
Pork	304	0.0	293	0.0	299	0.0	486	0.4	385	0.3
Turkey	72	0.0	70	0.0	58	0.0	107	1.9	60	0.0
Other	—	—	—	—	56	0.0	18	0.0	—	—
Subtotal	376		363		413		611		445	
Ivermectin										
Beef	209	0.0	192	0.0	202	0.0	427	0.2	397	0.5
Mutton	49	0.0	63	0.0	151	0.0	138	0.0	106	0.0
Pork	151	0.0	147	0.0	196	0.0	46	0.0	220	0.0
Other	—	—	—	—	2	0.0	67	0.0	66	0.0
Subtotal	409		402		551		678		789	
Hormonal substances: clenbuterol and other agonists										
Veal	374	0.0	422	0.0	576	0.3	234	0.8	281	0.7
Pork	—	—	—	—	—	—	23	0.0	24	0.0
Other	—	—	—	—	—	—	48	0.0	25	0.0
Subtotal	374		422		576		305		330	
Imported meat & poultry products										
Antibiotics	1156	0.5	2150	0.5	2316	0.0	4841	0.0	3590	0.1
Sulfa drugs	1789	0.5	2007	0.0	2010	0.0	3618	0.1	3091	0.0
Hormones	1197	0.0	1890	0.1	2802	0.1	2518	0.0	1546	0.0
Imported total	4142		6047		7128		10977		8227	

Source: From Ref. 53.

TABLE 13.25   Antibiotics Residues in Edible Animal Products in Japan

Sample		Number of samples	1990 Penicillin positives	Tetracycline positives
Meat	Bovine	594	1	—
	Swine	910	3	13
	Chicken	301	—	—
Fish	Yellowtail	40	—	—
	Bream	72	—	—
	Salmon	1	—	—
	Carp	53	—	—
	Trout	38	—	—
	Sweetfish	12	—	—
	Eel	67	—	—
	Mackerel	—	—	—
	Tilapia	—	—	—
	Flatfish	—	—	—
Eggs		—	—	—
Honey		137	2	13
Total		2224	6	26

Source: From Ref. 54.

13.4.2   India

A survey of veterinary drug use and residues in milk has been carried out in Hyderabad, India (34). The results of this survey showed that oxytocin and oxytetracycline were frequently used in veterinary formulations. As a result, a total of 9% of the marketed milk samples and 73% of the individual animal milk samples of the 205 milk samples analyzed in this survey contained oxytetracycline residues. Residual concentrations ranged from 0.2 to 1.4 ppm in marketed milk and from 0.2 to 6.7 ppm in samples obtained from individual buffaloes. In contrast, none of the government dairy samples analyzed was found to contain oxytetracycline residues. Maximum oxytetracycline intake by humans through consumption of such contaminated milk was calculated at the level of 0.045 mg/kg body weight (bw)/day.

13.4.3   Japan

Results of a national survey conducted by the Ministry of Health and Welfare on residual antibiotics in domestic meat and fish in Japan for the fiscal years 1990–1992 are presented in Table 13.25. Samples were collected at the urban

	1991				1992	
Number of samples	Penicillin positives	Tetracycline positives	Aminoglycoside positives	Number of samples	Penicillin positives	Tetracycline positives
1866	5	—	—	1939	1	—
4974	7	5	1	3063	1	9
612	—	1	—	3116	—	1
88	—	—	—	103	—	—
83	—	—	—	134	—	—
10	—	—	—	20	—	—
61	—	—	—	57	—	—
73	—	—	—	86	—	—
51	—	—	—	118	—	—
93	—	—	—	128	—	—
1	—	—	—	4	—	—
13	—	—	—	14	—	—
10	—	—	—	20	—	—
341	—	1	—	608	—	—
210	—	8	—	354	—	7
8486	12	15	1	9764	2	17

and rural prefectures, and were analyzed by approved biological assays in the laboratories of Meat Inspection Offices, Market Food Inspection Offices, and Institutes of Public Health. Results showed that the livestock products available to consumers contained a relatively low incidence of antibiotic residues.

Since over 60% of all antibiotics used in Japan for veterinary purposes are tetracyclines (35), targeted surveys of tetracycline residues in animal tissues have become of particular importance for public health agencies in Japan (36, 37). In 1991, a limited survey in the Aichi prefecture of residual tetracyclines in tissues collected from 64 cattle and 68 hogs of 1358 slaughtered animals that did not pass inspection at slaughterhouses due to presence of disease symptoms was conducted (38). Among 271 kidney, liver, and other organ samples, 49 (18.1%) were positive to oxytetracycline, 5 (1.8%) to chlortetracycline, and 5 (1.8%) to doxycycline, respectively. One cattle kidney sample was positive to both oxytetracycline and doxycycline, whereas tetracycline was not detected in any of the samples.

Among the 128 kidney samples (62 cattle and 66 hogs), 22.6% (19 cattle and 10 hogs) were positive to tetracyclines (cattle, 30.6%; hogs, 15.1%). Among the 100 liver samples (45 cattle and 55 hogs), 15% were positive to tetracyclines (cattle, 22.2%; hogs, 9.0%). The highest residue level was found in a hog kidney and amounted to 33.6 ppm oxytetracycline, while the lowest was 0.05 ppm oxytetracycline in a cattle kidney. Average concentrations of residual oxytetracycline in kidney, liver, and other organs were 1.62, 0.67, and 0.29 ppm for cattle; and 12.37, 3.41, and 3.56 ppm for hogs, respectively. Chlortetracycline and doxycycline concentrations were in the range of 0.15–4.80 ppm and 0.53–4.18 ppm, respectively.

A similar survey was also conducted from January, 1992, to December, 1994 (39). Among a total of 39 animals (9 cattle and 30 hogs), 11 animals (28.5%) were positive to oxytetracycline, and 7 animals (17.9%) to chlortetracycline. Percentage frequencies of tetracycline residues were 22.2% (2 of 9) and 30.0% (9 of 30) in cattle and hogs, respectively. However, tetracycline and doxycycline residues were not detected in any sample. Kidney showed higher incidence of tetracycline residues and 1.6–6.9 times higher residual concentrations than liver or other matrices, indicating that inspection of this tissue is the most effective means of ensuring food safety.

13.4.4   Kuwait

In Kuwait, a total of 350 samples including 230 sheep urine, 30 beef meat, and 90 chickens were screened for the presence of residues of trenbolone acetate (40). The results obtained showed that the trenbolone acetate levels in the urine ranged from 0.1 to 0.9 ppb and in the muscle tissue from 0.02 to 0.05 ppb, none of the figures exceeding the MRL of 2 ppb set by the Food and Agriculture Organization/World Health Organization (FAO/WHO).

In addition, a total of 146 sheep urine and 87 chicken muscle samples from birds sold in local markets and originating from Brazil, Denmark, France, and Turkey were tested for residues of diethylstilbestrol and ethinylestradiol (41). Although some of the samples were positive to both analytes by an immunochemical screening assay, confirmatory analysis by GC–mass spectroscopy (MS) showed that none of the samples contained residues of the examined steroids.

13.4.5   Malaysia

In Malaysia there are over 10,000 poultry breeders and 2500 pig farms. Since use of antibiotics is unavoidable for preventing animal diseases, livestock breeders have been told to conform to Good Farming Practices to minimize or eliminate drug residues. As a result, in 1996 only 1.1% of 300 samples taken from 7 poultry processing plants tested positive to antibacterials. Similarly, only 5.7% of 300 samples taken from cattle abattoirs and 17.5% of 300 samples taken from pig abattoirs were tested positive for antibacterial residues.

13.4.6 Poland

In Poland, samples of muscle, kidneys, and liver from cattle, swine, horses, and poultry are taken four times per year by veterinary inspectors at slaughterhouses to be analyzed for drug residues. Between 1992 and 1996, 5733 samples of cattle, swine, horse, and chickens muscle were analyzed to determine residues of sulfonamides, nitrofurans, and nitroimidazoles; 2613 samples of cattle and swine liver to determine β-agonists; and 1661 samples of cattle and swine kidney to determine violative levels of tranquilizers and β-blockers. No residues of the mentioned groups of drugs above MRL were detected in the examined samples (42). However, nonviolative residues of sulfamethazine, sulfadimethoxine, sulfathiazole, furazolidone, nitrofurazone, nitrofurantoin, metronidazole, dimetridazole, azaperone, chlorpromazine, propiopromazine, carazolol, clenbuterol, and salbutamol could be detected in the corresponding target samples.

13.4.7 Slovenia

In 1986, a monitoring program for potential presence of sulfonamide residues in food of animal origin was introduced in Slovenia (43). A total of 225 samples including muscle, liver, kidney, canned ham, egg, and milk were collected and analyzed. Results showed that only one canned ham sample was contaminated with sulfamethazine at a level of less than 50 ppb.

In 1987, a total of 342 samples including muscle, liver, canned ham, and eggs were also surveyed. Results showed that four samples of swine muscle were contaminated with each of sulfamethazine, sulfadimethazine, or sulfadimethoxine at levels of less than 50 ppb to 170 ppb, whereas six canned ham samples contained sulfamethazine at levels of less than 50 ppb to 50 ppb.

In 1988, a total of 477 samples including muscle, liver, kidney, canned ham, and milk were collected and analyzed. Results showed only one canned ham sample contained sulfadimethazine at a level of 100 ppb.

Apart from edible animal products, urine samples from slaughtered animals were also screened for sulfonamide residues over the period 1986–1988. In 1986 and 1987, only 2 urine samples from swine of the examined 280 urine samples of slaughtered cattle and swine were found positive for sulfonamides. Thus, the 1988 survey was directed only to slaughtered swine. Results showed that only 8 of 278 urine samples were positive for sulfonamides.

13.4.8 Switzerland

During the period 1981–1990, the Federation of Migros Cooperatives, which is the central organization of a Swiss retail company, has made a survey on the potential presence of antibiotic residues in marketed meat using the EU official

TABLE 13.26   Results of Antibacterial Residue Surveys over the Period 1981–1990 in Switzerland

	Veal		Beef		Swine		Total	
Year	Meat samples	Positive (%)	Meat samples	Positive (%)	Meat samples	Positive (%)	Meat samples	Positive (%)
1981	609	7.06	619	0.16	713	2.10	1941	3.04
1982	540	1.67	105	0.00	628	0.48	1273	0.94
1983	582	3.61	0	0.00	689	1.60	1271	2.52
1984	8	0.00	0	0.00	8	0.00	16	0.00
1985	390	3.59	0	0.00	545	0.18	935	1.60
1986	166	1.20	0	0.00	258	0.00	424	0.47
1987	269	0.74	0	0.00	307	0.33	576	0.52
1988	59	3.39	12	0.00	209	0.96	280	1.43
1989	80	0.00	30	0.00	51	3.92	161	1.24
1990	53	1.89	36	0.00	52	0.00	141	0.71

Source: From Ref. 44.

Four-Plate microbiological test. The results of the survey (Table 13.26) showed that the percentage of positive results declined over the tested period, falling down to less than 1% in the final year of the survey (44).

In the following years, the survey for drug residues continued but focused on veterinary drugs commonly used in animal husbandry such as sulfonamides and tetracyclines, and on chloramphenicol. Screening was carried out using the Charm II test, while confirmation of positive results involved HPLC or GC-MS. The results obtained are summarized in Table 13.27.

During 1992, the number of positive samples for sulfonamide residues was relatively high and the concentration of the substances, particularly sulfametha-

TABLE 13.27   Results of Sulfonamides, Chloramphenicol, and Tetracyclines Residues Surveys from 1992 to 1995 in Switzerland

		Sulfonamides			Chloramphenicol			Tetracyclines		
Year	Samples	Positives	%	Violations (>100 ppb)	Positives	%	>1 ppb	Positives	%	Violations (>100 ppb)
1992	300	43	14.3	11	6	2.0	2	15	5.0	1
1993	678	89	13.1	37	66	9.7	5	9	1.3	4
1994	703	57	8.1	18	40	5.7	0	61	8.7	36
1995	667	40	6.0	15	18	2.7	3	18	2.7	3

Source: From Ref. 44.

zine, was sometimes in the ppm level. The amount of sulfonamides residues decreased over the period 1992–1995, dropping to less than 500 ppb in the last year. Many samples considered positive for chloramphenicol by the Charm II test during 1993 and 1994 were confirmed as negative by GC-MS analysis. In 1995, two of the three positive samples for chloramphenicol were from injection sites from swine.

13.4.9 Taiwan

From January to June, 1985, a total of 1080 samples from fresh milk, swine liver and muscle, chicken liver and muscle, and hen eggs marketed at three cities located at the middle area of Taiwan were collected and analyzed for antibiotic residues (45). The positive rates found in the screen tests were 22.2% for milk, 21.1% for swine liver, 12.7% for swine muscle, 49.4% for chicken liver, 19.4% for chicken muscle, and 1.1% for hen eggs.

Further qualitative and quantitative analysis showed that penicillin, tetracycline, neomycin, streptomycin, erythromycin, and unidentified microbial inhibitors were responsible for 57.5%, 22.5%, 2.5%, 0%, 6.8%, and 17.5%, respectively, of the positive fresh milk samples; 20.7%, 22.5%, 6.8%, 0%, 6.8%, and 37.9%, respectively, of the positive swine liver; 14.3%, 21.4%, 7.1%, 0%, 0%, and 57.2%, respectively, of the positive swine muscle; 0%, 8.5%, 0%, 0%, 0%, and 91.5%, respectively, of the positive chicken liver; and 0%, 6.3%, 0%, 0%, 0%, and 93.7%, respectively, of the positive chicken muscle. The quantities of penicillin, tetracycline, and neomycin residues found in the positive samples were mostly below 0.03 IU/ml (91.3%), 0.31 ppm (66.6%) and 0.5 ppm (100%), respectively, in fresh milk; although they all were higher than 0.03 IU/ml (100%), 0.32 ppm (100%), and 1 ppm (100%), respectively, in all other samples. Erythromycin was detectable in only two samples of swine liver: 0.075 and 0.1 ppm.

13.4.10 Yugoslavia

Programs for monitoring drug residues have been established in Yugoslavia with the task of maintaining the safety of meat and meat products. Within the framework of these programs, samples of fat, muscle, kidney, and liver tissues are collected regularly by veterinary inspectors at random at the slaughterhouses. At least 0.01% of the overall number of slaughtered animals that originate from the same region are examined yearly.

During the period 1972–1989, the potential presence of antibiotics in a total of 17,200 liver, kidney and muscle tissue samples was examined (46). Rela-

TABLE 13.28   Residues of Antibiotics in Swine and Cattle Tissues over the
Period 1972–1989 in Yugoslavia

Tissue	Swine		Cattle	
	Samples examined	Positive samples (%)	Samples examined	Positive samples (%)
Muscle	1324	3.68	375	1.90
Liver	1311	4.04	376	2.17
Kidney	1320	4.26	378	2.71

Source: From Ref. 46.

tively small numbers of samples were found positive for antibiotics (Table 13.28).
The number of positive cattle tissues was 50% lower than the number of positive
swine samples. Differences in antibiotic occurrence among the tissues of the same
animal were also significant.

Since 1975, the potential presence of diethylstilbestrol residues has been
also examined. By 1989, 4 cattle liver samples of a total of 4864 liver samples
were found positive for diethylstilbestrol.

During 1985–1989, a total of 2374 kidney samples were analyzed for chloramphenicol. A total of 11 of 1477 pig kidneys tested positive, whereas all of the
897 cattle kidney samples were negative. In 1989, testing for dimetridazole was
also introduced in the monitoring program. A total of 520 muscle tissue samples
were tested, but none gave a positive result.

REFERENCES

1. W. Huber, Adv. Vet. Sci. Comp. Med., 15:101 (1971).
2. H.C. Mussman, Fed. Proc., 34:197 (1975).
3. US Department of Agriculture, in Objective Phase Biological Residue Reports, US
   Department of Agriculture, January 1976-December 1978 (1979).
4. Food Safety and Inspection Service (FSIS), in 1996 Residue Program Species-Specific Results, US Department of Agriculture, Office of Public Health and Science,
   Chemistry and Toxicology Division, Washington, DC (1998).
5. R.W. Stephany, and L.A. van Ginkel, in Veterinary Drug Residues, Food Safety
   (W.A. Moats, and M.B. Medina, Eds.), American Chemical Society, Washington,
   DC (1996).
6. R. Remy, and W. de Debeuckelaere, in Residues of Growth Promoting Substances
   in Meat (R. Remy, and W. de Debeuckelaere, Eds.), Verbruikers Unie-Test-Aankoop
   S.V., Brussels, Belgium (1994).

7. J. Kofer, and K. Fuchs, Wiener Tieraztliche Monartsschrift., 82:3 (1995).

8. K. Vanoosthuyze, E. Daeseleire, D. Courtheyn, J. Vergammen, and C. van Peteghem, in Residues of Veterinary Drugs in Food, Proc. Euroresidue III Conf., Veldhoven, 1996 (N. Haagsma and A. Ruiter, Eds.), Fac. Vet. Med., Univ. Utrecht, The Netherlands, p. 953 (1996).

9. Official Journal of the European Communities, No. L143, Brussels, p. 22 (1995).

10. A.M. Sorensen, M. Green, A. Buchert, and M. Vahl, in Residues of Veterinary Drugs in Food, Proc. Euroresidue III Conf., Veldhoven, 1996 (N. Haagsma, and A. Ruiter, Eds.), Fac. Vet. Med., Univ. Utrecht, The Netherlands, p. 872 (1996).

11. H.A. Kuiper, M.Y. Noordam, M.M.H. van Dooren-Flipsen, R. Schilt, and A.H. Roos, J. Anim. Sci., 76:195 (1998).

12. B. Bergner, B. Bourgeois, M. Edelhauser, F. Klein, R. Lippold, M. Mollers, and D. Pletscher, in Residues of Veterinary Drugs in Food, Proc. Euroresidue II Conf., Veldhoven, May 3–5, 1993 (N. Haagsma, A. Ruiter and P.B. Czedik-Eysenberg, Eds.), Fac. Vet. Med., Univ. Utrecht, The Netherlands, p. 186 (1993).

13. M. Kuhne, Fleischwirtschaft, 78:369 (1998).

14. G. Suhren, P. Hammer, and W. Heeschen, Kiel. Milchwirts. Forschung., 46:237 (1994).

15. K. Weiss, in Biennen-Pathologie (K. Weiss, Ed.), Ehrenwirth Verlag, Munchen, Germany (1990).

16. E. Usleber, R. Dietrich, E. Martlbauer, and W. Unglaub, in Residues of Veterinary Drugs in Food, Proc. Euroresidue III Conf., Veldhoven, 1996 (N. Haagsma and A. Ruiter, Eds.), Fac. Vet. Med., Univ. Utrecht, The Netherlands, p. 948 (1996).

17. U. Jurgens, Z. Lebensm. Unters. Forsch., 173:356 (1981).

18. C.T. Elliott, H.D. Shortt, D.G. Kennedy, and W.J. Mccaughey, Vet. Q., 18:41 (1996).

19. D.G. Kennedy, P.J. Hughes, and W.J. Blanchflower, Food Addit. Contam., 15:535 (1998).

20. L. Lynas, D. Currie, W.J. Mccaughey, J.D.G. Mcevoy, and D.G. Kennedy, Food Addit. Contam., 15:162 (1998).

21. M. Marchetti, R. Laffi, M. Zucchi, and V. Ramazza, in Residues of Veterinary Drugs in Food, Proc. Euroresidue II Conf., Veldhoven, May 3–5, 1993 (N. Haagsma, A. Ruiter, and P.B. Czedik-Eysenberg, Eds.), Fac. Vet. Med., Univ. Utrecht, The Netherlands, p. 479 (1993).

22. P. Gallo, and L. Serpe, Ind. Aliment. 36:618 (1997).

23. P. Gallo, and L. Serpe, Ind. Aliment. 35:1302 (1996).

24. C.J.M. Arts, M.J. van Baak, C.P.V. van der Weg, A.C. Tas, and J. van der Greef, in Residues of Veterinary Drugs in Food, Proc. Euroresidue III Conf., Veldhoven, 1996 (N. Haagsma, and A. Ruiter, Eds.), Fac. Vet. Med., Univ. Utrecht, The Netherlands, p. 207 (1996).

25. F. Ramos, M.C. Castilho, and M.I.N. Dasilveira, J. AOAC Int., 81:544 (1998).

26. E. Marques-Fontes, S. Martins, and B. Carrapico, Toxicol. Letters, 1:85 (1996).

27. E. Hidalgo, G. Herrero, M. Azpiri, M.L. Macho, J.M. Escudero, and J. Carcia, in Residues of Veterinary Drugs in Food, Proc. Euroresidue III Conf., Veldhoven, 1996 (N. Haagsma, and A. Ruiter, Eds.), Fac. Vet. Med., Univ. Utrecht, The Netherlands, p. 501 (1996).

28. V. Calderon, J.A. Berenguer, J. Gonzalez, and P. Diez, in Residues of Veterinary
     Drugs in Food, Proc. Euroresidue III Conf., Veldhoven, 1996 (N. Haagsma and A.
     Ruiter, Eds.), Fac. Vet. Med., Univ. Utrecht, The Netherlands, p. 305 (1996).
29. J.F. Kay, in Residues of Veterinary Drugs in Food, Proc. Euroresidue II Conf.,
     Veldhoven, May 3–5, 1993 (N. Haagsma, A. Ruiter, and P.B. Czedik-Eysenberg,
     Eds.), Fac. Vet. Med., Univ. Utrecht, The Netherlands, p. 404 (1993).
30. Ministry of Agriculture, Fisheries and Food (MAFF), in Surveillance for Clenbuterol
     and Levamisole, Food Surveillance Information Sheet, Joint Food Safety and Stan-
     dards Group, UK (1993).
31. J.F. Kay, and C.E. Penny, in Residues of Veterinary Drugs in Food, Proc. Euroresidue
     III Conf., Veldhoven, 1996 (N. Haagsma, and A. Ruiter, Eds.), Fac. Vet. Med., Univ.
     Utrecht, The Netherlands, p. 596 (1996).
32. Ministry of Agriculture, Fisheries and Food (MAFF), Medicines Act Veterinary
     Information Service (MAVIS), Veterinary Medicines Directory, UK (1996).
33. E. Neidert, and P.W. Saschenbrecker, in Residues of Veterinary Drugs in Food, Proc.
     Euroresidue III Conf., Veldhoven, 1996 (N. Haagsma and A. Ruiter, Eds.), Fac. Vet.
     Med., Univ. Utrecht, The Netherlands, p. 185 (1996).
34. R.V. Sudershan, and R.V. Bhat, Food Addit. Contam., 12:645 (1995).
35. Japan Ministry of Agriculture, Forestry and Fisheries, Ann. Rep. Nat. Vet. Assay
     Lab., 20:50 (1983).
36. T. Fujimoto, and T. Oka, Ann. Rep. Fukuoka Inst. Public Health, 8:50 (1983).
37. H. Terada, M. Asanoma, and Y. Sakabe, Eisei Kagaku, 30:138 (1984).
38. H. Oka, Y. Ikai, N. Kawamura, and J. Hayakawa, J. Assoc. Off. Anal. Chem., 74:
     894 (1991).
39. H. Oka, Y. Ikai, J. Hayakawa, N. Ishikawa, S. Shibata, F. Saito, S. Ohmi, K. Ando,
     M. Kawada, and K. Nakahishi, J. Food Hyg. Soc. Japan, 36:759 (1995).
40. W.N. Sawaya, K. Lone, T. Saeed, A. Husain, and S. Khalafawi, Food Addit. Contam.,
     15:151 (1998).
41. W.N. Sawaya, K. Lone, A. Husain, B. Dashti, and S. Alzenki, Food Chem., 63:563
     (1998).
42. A. Posyniak, J. Zmudzki, J. Niedzielska, and S. Semeniuk, J. Vet. Pharmacol. Ther.,
     20:306 (1997).
43. M. Komar, J. Marinsek, K. Sinigoj-Gacnik, S. Ivanc, and M. Milohnoja, in Residues
     of Veterinary Drugs in Food, Proc. Euroresidue Conf., Noordwijkerhout, May 21–23,
     1990 (N Haagsma, A Ruiter, and PB Czedik-Eysenberg, Eds.), Fac. Vet. Med., Univ.
     Utrecht, The Netherlands, p. 246 (1990).
44. C. Roland, L. William, and D. Roland, in Residues of Veterinary Drugs in Food,
     Proc. Euroresidue III Conf., Veldhoven, 1996 (N. Haagsma and A. Ruiter, Eds.),
     Fac. Vet. Med., Univ. Utrecht, The Netherlands, p. 320 (1996).
45. T.-C. Chung, in An examination of Antibiotic Residues in Animal Products Marketed
     at the Middle Area of Taiwan, Department of Veterinary Medicine, National Chung
     Hsing University, Taiwan (1986).
46. V. Visacki, A. Spiric, G. Vojinovic, and N. Radovic, in Residues of Veterinary Drugs
     in Food, Proc. Euroresidue Conf., Noordwijkerhout, May 21–23, 1990 (N. Haagsma,
     A. Ruiter, and P.B. Czedik-Eysenberg, Eds.), Fac. Vet. Med., Univ. Utrecht, The
     Netherlands, p. 376 (1990).

47. National Residue Program, 1988, Domestic Residue Data Book, Washington, DC, 1988.
48. National Residue Program, 1989, Domestic Residue Data Book, Washington, DC, 1989.
49. T. Kindred, B. Patel, and J. Walcott, in Residues of Veterinary Drugs in Food, Proc. Euroresidue III Conf., Veldhoven, 1996 (N. Haagsma, and A. Ruiter, Eds.), Fac. Vet. Med., Univ. Utrecht, The Netherlands, p. 175 (1996).
50. Veterinary Inspection Service, Monitoring Programs 1997, Ministry of Agriculture, Belgium (1998).
51. C.J.M. Arts, M.J. van Baak, C.P.V. van der Weg, A.C. Tas, and J. van der Greef, in Residues of Veterinary Drugs in Food, Proc. Euroresidue III Conf., Veldhoven, 1996 (N. Haagsma and A. Ruiter, Eds.), Fac. Vet. Med., Univ. Utrecht, The Netherlands, p. 207 (1996).
52. Bureau of Rural Sciences, National Residue Survey 1997 Results, Australia (1998).
53. E. Neidert, and P.W. Saschenbrecker, in Residues of Veterinary Drugs in Food, Proc. Euroresidue III Conf., Veldhoven, 1996 (N. Haagsma and A. Ruiter, Eds.), Fac. Vet. Med., Univ. Utrecht, The Netherlands, p. 185 (1996).
54. H. Nakazawa, in Chemical Analysis for Antibiotics Used in Agriculture (II. Oka, H. Nakazawa, K.-I. Harada, and J.D. MacNeil, Eds.), AOAC International, Arlington, VA, p. 43 (1995).

14

Factors Influencing the Occurrence of Residues in Foods

In modern agricultural practice, where herd and flock health is controlled and adequate records are maintained, detection of violative drug residues in the edible animal products is unlikely (1). Whenever they appear, violative residues are the result of inadvertent contamination due to management mistakes or to individual variations in animals' ability to eliminate drugs. Therefore, factors of management and/or biological origin should always be considered by farmers, veterinarians, and regulatory agencies for a safe and wholesome food supply.

14.1 MANAGEMENT

Failure to abide by the approved label instructions is by far the leading cause of illegal residues detected in edible animal products. Noncompliance with proper withdrawal periods was responsible for 46% and 54% of the cases of violative residues monitored in the fiscal years 1990 and 1991, respectively, in the United States. Failure to comply with approved withdrawal periods was also identified as the most common cause of the drug violations monitored in the fiscal year 1993 by the Food Safety and Inspection Service of the Food and Drug Administration (FDA). Livestock species producing most violations were the bob veals, with approximately 40%, followed by cull cows with 30%.

Inadequate recordkeeping and inadequate cow identification are among the common causes of failure to observe withdrawal periods. It specifically applies to milk after lactational or dry-cow intramammary infusions for therapy of mastitis, injection of antibiotics for therapy of foot rot, or treatment of teats with udder creams and ointments.

Occasionally, the withdrawal period is not known to the farmer because of an incorrectly labeled formulation. In a few cases, it is deliberately not obeyed or only partly, for instance by milking out of only the treated udder quarters instead of all quarters. Numerous situations have also occurred in which the farmer used a few different medications on a cow and followed the withdrawal period on just one, and thought the milk was safe.

Sometimes farmers may be victims of sabotage by a disgruntled employee who adds drugs to the milk. In the case of coccidiostats, the relatively short withdrawal periods may tempt the farmer to leave out the required switch to a coccidiostat-free final feed. There have been also cases in which farmers have bought cows that supposedly had not been treated, but were. Dairy farmers should always test milk from newly purchased animals before adding it to the tank. An additional problem is that the withdrawal period will probably never be obeyed in case of emergency-slaughtered animals.

Violative residues can also occur when drugs are used by nonapproved routes of administration, or given to nonapproved species (2). In the fiscal year 1993, the Food Safety and Inspection Service reported 3809 cases of violative residues for all species of livestock; based on gathered information on 1,015 violative animals, the FDA reported that approximately 46% of the violations were caused by drugs administered parenterally while 20% were caused by drugs administered orally through boluses (10%), feed additives (9%), and drinking water (1%).

Extralabel use is another source of food contamination. The application of a drug in a dosage exceeding the labeled dosage can result in an increase in elimination half-life, or in the dose-dependent pharmacokinetics. This is usually the result of some rate-limiting process in drug metabolism. These errors may result not only in very high residues but also in adverse toxicological effects on the treated animals, as in the case of swine given elevated dosages of carbadox (3, 4).

Apart from noncompliance with approved label instructions, a high percentage of residue violations has also been connected with errors from improperly trained personnel and family members. Residues are not, however, always the personnel's fault. Farmers are also negligent. They rely on memory when it comes to which cows they have treated, or they forget to notify members or other milkers who then milk a treated cow into the tank. Perhaps they mark cows in one manner only: the leg band falls off or the chalk wears off. Some producers paint the hind quarters but fail to take the mark off once the cow's milk is clear. An extensive onfarm review based on investigations of 20 cases of antibiotic adulteration in milk representing 797,436 pounds of dumped milk by a major US milk cooperative demonstrated that management mistakes were to blame in all cases. All antibiotic adulterations were confirmed on the farm and attributed to an act under the control of the producer, such as the milker milked the hospital pen into tank, moved 18 of 19 dried cows to dry pen, milker milked treated cow, and cow lost leg band.

Even when proper management procedures are followed, various feeding errors such as failure to clean feed mixing and delivery equipment properly, delivery of the wrong feed by the feed mill, or improper feed storage at the farm can cause residue violations (5, 6). Large variations in drug content of medicated feeds may occur as a result of improperly formulated premixes or inefficient mixing. The actual content may differ considerably from what is declared by the manufacturers (7). Even disorders in animals, as a result of drug intoxication associated with erroneous inclusion of drugs in feed, were reported (8, 9). Pharmaceutical premixes should be formulated such so homogenous mixing is ensured and dusting and segregation are prevented.

Low-level inadvertent contamination of animal feeds with drugs both on the farm and in commercial feed production unit is a well-known phenomenon (7, 10). This can take place at different levels of the animal feed production chain. Animal feeds or drinking water may be contaminated by carryover of drugs from former batches of medicated feed or water. It is generally recognized within the feed milling industry that even with an adequate manufacturing process in plants producing medicated feeds, an approximately 5% carryover from one feed batch to the next batch is technically unavoidable.

Because of that carryover, drug-free final feeds for species for which use of a certain drug is approved provided a withdrawal period is followed may get contaminated with the drug, whereas feeds intended for animal species for which the drug is not approved at all may be contaminated. Although the carryover of a few percent of a feed medicated at a low level with a drug is not generally expected to produce a serious problem, the wide extent of use of feed additives enlarges the risk of a continuous feed contamination. It is therefore necessary that feeds and therapeutic drugs be processed in a manner that prevents feed contamination.

A sound example of accidental feed contamination with drugs has been provided by a report on an incidence of violative residues of sulfamethazine in swine (11). The electrostatic attraction of powdered sulfamethazine to the metallic milling or storage equipment was implicated as the source of feed contamination in that case. The problem was reduced by using granular forms of the drug, which lessened the production of drug dust during feed preparation (12).

In an investigation on the potential contamination of swine, broiler, and layers feeds by veterinary drugs, more than 50% of the studied feeds were found contaminated with medicinal feed additives or therapeutic drugs at levels generally less than 5 ppm (13). However, the question as to whether these relatively low drug concentrations in the feeds would cause violative residues in swine and poultry meat and in eggs could not be absolutely answered.

Microbiologically active residue levels equivalent to 30–50 ppb narasin or salinomycin have been detected in eggs from hens given feeds containing 5 ppm of these drugs (13), but no residues could be detected when the feeds contained the same level of monensin (14). On the other hand, the unintended presence of 1 ppm sulfamethazine in swine feeds has been reported responsible for residues concentrations above 0.1 ppm in the liver when the feed was used during the withdrawal period (10).

Processing of dead 19-nortestosterone-injected animals in rendering plants and the commercial use of the fat thus produced in some milk replacers can also provoke positive results (15) when fed to veal calves due to presence of 19-nortestosterone in the bovine fat (16). It is possible, therefore, for a farmer who has not used illegal hormone cocktails or indeed any form of hormone treatment on his animals to be caught out because positive levels of banned hormonal substances are detected in urine samples from his livestock, due to presence of these substances in the feed they have been given. Farmers who have not indulged in illegal practices are consequently unfairly suspected, whereas farmers who have adopted such practices, producing animals with high levels of additional hormones, are difficult to trace.

Noncompliance with good animal husbandry can also produce residue violations. Drugs excreted in the urine and feces may be recycled to tissues, after ingestion by the animals, causing accidental residue levels (10). Recirculation of drug residues through litter (17) or processed streams in slaughterhouses can be other sources of contamination (18). In this context, administration of nicarbazin to free-range hens has given rise to much longer-lasting residues in their eggs compared with those laid by hens held in cases (19). Residue contamination of litter and drinking water has been also considered responsible for the appearance of residues in swine meat at the low ppb level (20); pigs are coprophagic and as little as 23 ppm sulfamethazine in their feces can cause recycling of violative residues to their tissues.

Pig kidneys in several countries including the United Kingdom and the United States have been found to contain residues of sulfamethazine at levels above the maximum residue limit (MRL) of 100 ppb (21, 22). The level of violations in the United Kingdom during 1980–1983 reached around 20% of all pig kidneys tested, but it declined steadily thereafter to reach the figure of 6% in 1989 (23). It might have been tempting at one stage to suggest that the withdrawal periods were of insufficient duration and that pharmacokinetic studies could be useful to throw some light on the problem. However, the real reasons are complex and involve carryover of the drug in the feces and urine of treated pigs, contamination of nonmedicated feed with medicated feed, contamination of drinking water at slaughterhouses with feces from treated animals, and failure to observe withdrawal periods (24–26).

Direct contamination may sometimes also occur in the animal product itself. Inadequate flushing of antibiotic-contaminated discarded milk from milking equipment has resulted in violative residues in the entire bulk tank (27–29). It has been estimated that contaminated milk from a single cow treated with 200 mg penicillin has the potential to contaminate the combined milk of up to 8000 cows if mixed in bulk tanks (30).

In aquaculture, an unpredictable sudden lowering of water temperature during fish medication can also result in very high residues in fish tissue unless the withdrawal period is increased and observed accordingly. As an example, the predicted withdrawal period for oxolinic acid in muscle tissue of rainbow trout ranges from 28 days at 16 °C to 60 days at 10 °C and to 140 days at 5 °C (31, 32). Both the salinity and the pH of the surrounding water can also affect drug pharmacokinetics in fish. It has been reported, for example, that tissue concentrations of drug residues in tissues of sea-water trout decreased to undetectable levels by 72 h, whereas in the freshwater trout levels peaked at 48 h and were detectable for at least 224 h (33). In fish, many pharmacokinetic parameters including the total intake of the medicated feed; the gastric emptying time; the intestinal motility; and the absorption, biotransformation, and excretion rate of drugs depend on the temperature, pH, and salinity of the water.

14.2 BIOLOGICAL PROCESSES

These are factors governed by biological processes taking place in the animal itself. They will influence the levels of drug residues in animal tissues as well as the time course of drug elimination, which, in turn, depends on the pharmacokinetic profile of the drug.

Several drugs in several species are known to exhibit different pharmacokinetic profiles when the animals are sick. Many of the disease conditions for which drugs are utilized exert an effect upon drug elimination, and therefore may have a bearing on drug residues present in slaughtered animals. Fever, for example, has been shown almost to double the elimination half-life of gentamicin given to febrile rabbits, and to induce change in the distribution volumes of gentamicin in horses and sheep (34–36). Several drugs including trimethoprim in the calf, sulfamethazine and oxytetracycline in the goat, and oxytetracycline in the pig have also shown prolonged plasma elimination half-lives in feverish or infected animals (37).

On the other hand, the volume of distribution is significantly increased for orally administered trimethoprim in feverish rabbits compared with their healthy counterparts and absorption is reduced (38). The significance of these changes can be appreciated if one considers that the total body clearance of a drug is directly related to the distribution volume, and inversely related to half-life. In addition, feverish pigs show reduced elimination half-lives when oxytetracycline is given orally (39). It appears that disease-induced variations in the oral drug intake may also influence the drug absorption and elimination profile. It has been shown that absorption of drugs following oral administration can be altered by fever in young goats, possibly due to inhibition of reticule–rumen motility (40).

In some cases, the same disease states exert no effect on drug pharmacokinetics as with amoxycillin and chloramphenicol in calves, and ampicillin and sulfamethazole in goats. Although feverish pigs show reduced elimination half-lives when oxytetracycline is given orally, there is no apparent effect after intravenous administration, which suggests an effect on gastrointestinal absorption (39).

In other cases, the same disease states exert a different effect on drug pharmacokinetics depending on the drug and the animal species (41). Elimination of sulfadimethoxine or amoxycillin from pigeons was distinctly accelerated in case of Coccidia (42) or *Salmonella* infection (43). However, significant differences in the residue profile, compared to healthy chickens, were observed neither in that of sulfamethazine nor in that of its acetyl metabolite after oral administration to chickens infected with Coccidia (44).

Renal failure will result in a diminished elimination of drugs that are primarily secreted, such as penicillins and aminoglycosides, and therefore in a longer half-life of the drug (45). Likewise, liver disease may result in a capacity-limited biotransformation, and consequently in a slower elimination of the drug. Bacterial pneumonia in calves may also result in increased serum oxytetracycline concentrations, a condition that can cause prolonged elimination (46).

The serum-protein binding ability, which varies between animals and is also influenced by the disease state of the animal, will also determine the free diffusible concentration. This, in turn, will have an effect on the elimination of drug residues as well as on their penetration in eggs or milk. This effect will be more pronounced for drugs with a higher tendency for protein binding such as sulfonamides, doxycycline, and cloxacillin (47).

Apart from the pathophysiological condition of the animal, the mode of drug application may also significantly influence the pharmacokinetic profile of a drug (48, 49). For example, drug residues may persist at the injection site for prolonged periods of time (2). In a study in which various sulfonamides and trimethoprim were injected intramuscularly into swine, detectable residues were found at most sites 6 days after the injection, and with the sulfonamides at 30 days in almost half of the animals (50). Other drugs such as dihydrostreptomycin persist for up to 60 days, while positive residues of chloramphenicol are found at 7 days postinjection. Sodium and procaine penicillin, neomycin, tylosin, and oxytetracycline residues have also been determined at 24 h or more postinjection (51).

The persistence of residues at intramuscular injection sites may be due in part to the irritant response produced in the muscle (52). Chloramphenicol, tylosin, penicillins, dihydrostreptomycin, and oxytetracycline have been shown to produce local irritation at the site of injection, leading to residue persistence; this may be exacerbated by the solvent used. However, residues do not persist with proper injection of drugs and use of formulations that do not cause severe irritation (52), as has been demonstrated with one oxytetracycline product that produced little irritation (53–55).

Next to the health state, other physiological states of the animal, such as age, gender, or anatomy, can significantly influence the rate of drug elimination. Most important age-related factors are those related to renal function, drug distribution volume, degree of protein binding, drug metabolism, and biliary excretion (56).

The rate of renal function development is species dependent. Several studies have indicated that while the calf may have nearly adult renal function by the second day of its life (57, 58), it will take up to a week in the lamb to reach adult function (59). As an example, the elimination half-life of sulfamethazone is 13.5 h in a 1-day-old bovine, and only 6 h in an adult (51). However, except for bob veal, renal function may not play a significant role in residue violations.

Unlike renal function, hepatic maturation is generally believed to be a two-stage process with the major development completed at 4 weeks postpartum and the second stage completed by about 10 weeks of age. In sheep, for example, the activity of a number of hepatic drug-metabolizing enzymes was found to be relatively low in animals aged up to 6 months compared with adult individuals (60). This finding helps to account for the relatively long half-lives of sulfadoxine and trimethoprim in neonatal calves and lambs, and for the significant half-lives, which shorten with increasing age.

Drugs that are primarily eliminated by hepatic mechanisms often demonstrate age-dependent pharmacokinetics. Chloramphenicol, a drug primarily eliminated by hepatic processes, has a half-life of 11.7 and 6.1 h in day-old calves and pigs, and 4.4 and 0.8 hours at 8 weeks or older, respectively (61, 62). Thus, the use of drugs in young animals presents a greater potential for residue problems. Similar pharmacokinetic variation and problems could no doubt be observed as a process of aging, although most animals raised for food are slaughtered before this process has any influence on the elimination of antibiotics (63).

Similar considerations can also be made for animals of different gender. Antipyrine plasma elimination, for example, in rats and cattle show gender differences that, to some extent, cannot be mediated by sex hormones. In contrast, clearance of antipyrine and sulfamethazine in female dwarf goats markedly decreases following implantation of the anabolic steroid trenbolone (64).

Abnormal drug elimination or metabolism occurs when a combination of drugs is used. Induction or inhibition of hepatic enzymes, as with an androgen hormone, can result in a decreased or increased persistence of drug residues (65). These observations may have implications for withdrawal periods since residue depletion studies are often conducted with animals of similar gender.

Differences in the physiology and anatomy of the udder, the level of milk production, and the stage of lactation may sometimes be the cause of residue violations in milk. Failure to observe the proper withdrawal period after prophylactic and therapeutic use for mastitis might be simply due to some variation from the established milk-out rates (66).

These and other factors of biological origin are no doubt involved in the persistence of violative residues following (especially) emergency slaughter, and are the reasons for the selective sampling of those animals showing signs of drug injection, mastitis, or any condition that may have required drug therapy. Mentioned examples lead one to wonder whether residues studies ought to be conducted in sick animals rather than in healthy ones or to question whether pharmacokinetic studies should be conducted in both sick and healthy animals so that withdrawal periods might be adjusted when disease states are shown to affect drug clearance.

REFERENCES

1. D. Meisinger, and C.D. van Houweling, J. Am. Vet. Med. Assoc., 188:134 (1986).
2. H.C. Mussman, Fed. Proc., 34:197 (1975).
3. E. Goren, Tijdschr. Diergeneeskd., 108:350 (1983).
4. M.J.A. Nabuurs and E.J. van der Molen, J. Vet. Med., 36:209 (1989).
5. R.F. Bevill, J. Am. Vet. Med. Assoc., 185:1124 (1984).
6. R.F. Hall, Compend. Contin. Ed., 8:200 (1986).
7. G.H.M. Counotte, T. Eefting, and A. Bosch, Tijdschr. Diergeneesk., 109:339 (1984).
8. F.W. van Schie, Tijdschr. Diergeneesk., 107:428 (1982).
9. D.A. Rice and C.H. McMurray, Vet. Rec., 113:495 (1983).
10. R.F. Bevill, J. Am. Vet. Med. Assoc., 185:1124 (1984).
11. M.K. Cordle, J. Anim. Sci., 66:413 (1988).
12. M.C. Rosenberg, J. Am. Vet. Med. Assoc., 187:704 (1985).
13. M.M.L. Aerts, in Residues of Veterinary Drugs in Edible Products. An Analytucal Approach, Thesis, University of Amsterdam (1990).
14. E. Kolsters, C.A. Kan, M.M.L. Aerts, in Determination of Ionophoric Antibiotics in Eggs, Depletion Studies with Laying Hens, RIKILT Report, Wageningen, The Netherlands (1989).
15. E. Rattenberger, and P. Matzke, Arch. Lebensmittelhyg., 39:21 (1988).
16. M. Rapp, and H.H.D. Meyer, J. Chromatogr., 489:181 (1989).
17. K.E. Webb, and J.P. Fontenot, J. Anim. Sci., 41:1212 (1975).
18. P. Dorn, C. Schwarzer, and E. Rattenberger, Dtsch. Tierartzl. Wschr., 93:70 (1986).
19. A. Friedrich, H.M. Hafez, and H. Woernle, Tierartzl. Umsch., 39:769 (1984).
20. P. Dorn, C. Schwarzer, and E. Rattenberger, Dtsch. Tierärztl. Wochenschr., 93:70 (1986).

21. K. Lawrence, Pig. Vet., 24:88 (1990).
22. J.D. McKean, Agripractice, 9:15 (1988).
23. Ministry of Agriculture, Fisheries and Food (MAFF), in Annual Report 1989–90, Veterinary Medicines Directorate, London, UK (1990).
24. W.J. McCaughey, J.N. Campbell, and C.T. Elliott, Vet. Rec., 126:113 (1990).
25. W.J. McCaughey, C.T. Elliott, and S.R.H. Crooks, Vet. Rec., 128:125 (1990).
26. W.J. McCaughey, C.T. Elliott, and S.R.H. Crooks, Vet. Rec., 126:351 (1990).
27. A.G. Rauws, Tijdschr. Diergeneeskd., 110:932 (1985).
28. K.E. Pugh, P.G. Henry, and J.M. Evans, Vet. Rec., 101:313 (1977).
29. J. Egan and F. O'Connor, Farm Food Res., 14:26 (1983).
30. D.F. Wishart, Vet. Annual, 23:71 (1983).
31. H.V. Bjorklund, A. Eriksson, and G. Bylund, Aquaculture, 102:17 (1992).
32. S.O. Hustvedt, T. Storebakken, and R. Salte, Aquaculture, 92:109 (1991).
33. N. Ishida, Aquaculture, 102:9 (1992).
34. H. Halkin, M. Lidji, and E. Rubinstein, J. Pharm. Exp. Ther., 216:415 (1981).
35. R.C. Wilson, J.N. Moore, and N. Eakle, Am. J. Vet. Res., 44:1746 (1983).
36. R.C. Wilson, D.D. Goetsch, and T.L. Huber, Am. J. Vet. Res., 45:2495 (1984).
37. S.M. Anika, J.F.M. Nouws, H. van Gough, J. Nieuwenhuis, T.B. Vree, and A.S.J.-P.A.M. van Miert, Res. Vet. Sci., 46:386 (1986).
38. O. Ladefoged, Zbl. Vet. Mcd., 26:580 (1979).
39. A. Pijpers, E.J. Schoevers, H. van Gough, L.A.M.G. van Leengoed, I.J.R. Visser, A.S.J.P.A.M. van Miert, and J.H.M. Versheijden, J. Vet. Pharmacol. Ther., 13:320 (1990).
40. A.S.J.P.A.M. van Miert, H. van Gogh, and J.G. Wit, Vet. Rec., 99:480 (1976).
41. J.F.M. Nouws, T.B. Vree, M.M.L. Aerts, and J. Grondel, Arch. Lebensmittelhyg., 37:69 (1986).
42. J. vom Bruch, in Untersuchungen zur Pharmakokinetic und Wirkung von Intramuskular, Oral und Uber das Trinkwasser Appliziertem Sulfadimethoxin an Kokzidieninfizierten Adulten Tauben, Thesis, University of Munchen, Germany (1986).
43. J. Krieg, in Pharmakokinetische Untersuchungen von Amoxicllin bei der Gesunden und Specifisch Geschadigten Adulten Taube, Thesis, University of Munchen, Germany (1986).
44. N. Haagsma, in Control of Veterinary Drug Residues in Meat, Thesis, University of Utrecht, The Netherlands (1988).
45. T.E. Powers, J.D. Powers, and K.J. Varma, J. Am. Vet. Med. Assoc., 192:250 (1988).
46. J.G. Clark, C. Adams, D.G. Addis, J.R. Dunbar, D.D. Hinman, and G.P. Lofgreen, Vet. Med./Small Anim. Clinician, 69:1542 (1974).
47. G. Ziv, and F.G. Sulman, Antimicrob. Agents Chemother., 2:206 (1977).
48. J.F.M. Nouws, Vet. Q., 6:80 (1984).
49. E.C. Firth, J.F.M. Nouws, F. Driessen, P. Schmaetz, K. Peperkamp, and W.R. Klein, Am. J. Vet. Res., 47:2380 (1986).
50. F. Rasmussen, and O. Svendsen, Res. Vet. Sci., 20:55 (1976).
51. J.F.M. Nouws, T.B. Vree, J. Holtkamp, M. Baakman, F. Driessen, and P.J.M. Guelen, Vet. Q., 8:224 (1986).
52. A.G. Rauws, Tijdschr. Diergeneeskd., 110:932 (1985).

53. M. Dagorn, P. Guillot, and P. Sanders, Vet. Q., 12:166 (1990).
54. J.F.M. Nouws, Ann. Rec. Vet., 21:145s (1990).
55. J.F.M. Nouws, A. Smulders, and M. Rappalini, Vet. Q., 12:129 (1990).
56. C.R. Short and C.R. Clarke, J. Am. Vet. Med. Assoc., 185:1088 (1984).
57. R.G. Dalton, Br. Vet. J., 124:371 (1968).
58. R.G. Dalton, Br. Vet. J., 124:451 (1968).
59. D.P. Alexander and D.A. Nixon, Nature, 194:483 (1962).
60. J.C. Kawalek, and K.R. El Said, Am. J. Vet. Res., 51:1736 (1990).
61. R. Reiche, M. Mulling, and H.H. Frey, J. Vet. Pharmacol. Ther., 3:95 (1980).
62. O. Svendsen, Acta Vet. Cand., 176:1 (1976).
63. J. Koch-Weser, D.J. Greenblatt, E.M. Sellers, and R.I. Shader, N. Eng. J. Med., 306: 1081 (1982).
64. R.F. Witkamp, G.A.E. van Klooster, and A.S.J.P.A.M. van Miert, in Residues of Veterinary Drugs in Food, Proc. Euroresidue Conf., Noordwijkerhout, May 21–23, 1990 (N. Haagsma, A. Ruiter, and P.B. Czedik-Eysenberg, Eds.), Fac. Vet. Med., Univ. Utrecht, The Netherlands, p. 415 (1990).
65. A.J. Glazko, Therap. Drug Monit., 9:320 (1987).
66. J. Egan, F. O'Connor, and J. Connolly, Irish J. Food Sci. Tech., 5:129 (1981).

15

Costs of Residues in the Livestock Industry

Food safety starts with the producer. Livestock producers recognize and support consumer demand for high quality, safe, and wholesome meat, milk, and eggs. The rewards for higher quality will be new and larger markets for the product. Profit is the primary goal of any livestock producer and is a prerequisite to a successful industry.

Accomplishing these goals depends, in part, upon the production of residue-free edible animal products. Producers can prevent violative residue levels by following withdrawal periods, incorporating residue preventive procedures designed to avoid contamination of equipment or storage areas into routine management practices, and identifying treated animals with individual markings or group records. Through a well-planned and executed residue avoidance program at the farm level, livestock producers can reduce the economic risks of residues in their individual operations and their collective marketplace.

Buyers, both overseas and domestic, have become more discerning in selecting their suppliers. Buyers do not limit their inspections of operations to the manufacturing plant. Buyers can be seen combing through producer records and operations as they reach a decision on suppliers. If producers cannot document through recordkeeping, management practices, and analytical testing that they produce what the buyer of the manufactured end product wants, the processor loses the sale and in turn reduces the amount of products he or she can receive.

Recordkeeping and quality management will become as much a part of producing raw commodities as they now are in processing foods. That reality motivated leaders in the industry to construct programs such as the California

Dairy Quality Assurance Program. This program attempts to learn exactly what the producer needs in terms of technology, management practices, training, recordkeeping, equipment, veterinary care, and any other parts of the production business that contribute to the ability to market the product from the perspective of food quality and safety.

Residues have the potential to cause significant monetary losses to livestock industry. The livestock producer can have direct financial losses from violative drug residues through condemnations of carcasses at slaughter, rejection of milk, increased production costs, test costs, and regulatory action.

For meat two types of tissue sampling are carried out in all federally inspected slaughterhouses through the US Department of Agriculture (USDA) meat and poultry inspection program. In targeted sampling, tissue samples are obtained before and after slaughter from animals of producers who have had previous violations or from animals that show evidence of recent medication to be submitted to targeted testing. Evidence of recent medication is provided by swellings around injection sites, discoloration of muscles or locations under the skin, discoloration of bowel or internal organs, and unusual odors. The samples are sent to USDA laboratories for testing and the carcasses are retained until the test results are available. The carcasses are condemned if the tissue tests confirm the presence of violative residues. Even when the tests reveal the carcasses are residue-free, carcass value is nevertheless reduced because of the time it takes to get the test results back.

In residue surveys, tissue samples are also collected at random to be submitted to routine testing. If a violative residue is found, the producer is notified and the animals are held in the farm, and tested until they are proven to be residue-free. To provide this proof, producers are allowed to submit a small number of animals for residue evaluation. The marketing status of the producer is reevaluated based on the tissue test results. The carcasses are retained usually for 14–30 days until the test results are available and will be condemned if the results indicate the presence of violative residues. In many cases, producers incur additional expenses for the packer to debone, freeze, and store the retained carcasses.

Even when no violative residues are found, the carcasses usually depreciate in value a great deal while awaiting the test results. To reduce testing time, the producers may apply to an approved laboratory to have the samples analyzed at their own expense. In the event a violative residue is found, the producer has to submit another group of animals for residue evaluation. This procedure may be repeated until analysis data of tissue samples indicate a residue-free status. In the meantime, the livestock producer is often confronted with increased production costs due to overcrowding caused by inability to market the animals on a timely basis. In addition, weight gains are slowed, feed efficiency becomes poorer, and the value of the product is lowered because of accumulation of excessive finish.

Residues can also lead to regulatory action under the US federal food and drug laws. Producers whose animals are found to contain illegal drug residues may be held legally responsible for the shipment of adulterated food in interstate commerce. In some cases, prosecution of offenders under these rules will result in monetary fines and possible jail sentences. These potential penalties are in addition to the economic difficulties encountered because of the market restrictions.

On July 24, 1996, a US livestock dealer was sentenced to 6 months in jail followed by 12 months of supervised release, a $2500 fine, and the Court's special assessment fee, because he offered at least 150 animals for slaughter for human consumption that contained illegal levels of a variety of new animal drugs (1). New animal drugs are approved by the Food and Drug Administration (FDA) with strict use requirements, including a specified time period to withdraw an animal from treatment prior to marketing, to ensure that the drug has depleted from edible tissue to a level that will not present harm to the consuming public. Many of the detected illegal residues were thousands of times higher than the permitted levels or they were residues of drugs not approved for use in those animals. This was the first prosecution of a livestock dealer in the United States for illegal residues, and should send a strong message to others in the livestock dealing industry to take seriously their responsibility to ensure that they do not pass on adulterated food to the consumer.

Producers can suffer economic losses from residues in a number of indirect ways. Many of these losses are unobserved but are encountered as a part of the cost of being in livestock production. Such losses may occur from reduced performance and effectiveness, reduced new product development, regulatory costs, condemnations, and loss of consumer confidence and market share.

Frequently, the source of the contamination can be traced to small quantities of medicated feed remaining in the feed mixing and handling equipment. These small quantities get mixed into the next batch of feed and may become a potential source of residues. Thorough cleaning of the equipment and proper ration sequencing during feed processing can help avoid such contamination. Properly identifying feeders or pens can also be very helpful in identifying and monitoring animals on medicated feeds. Producers who wish to determine the residue status of their animals before slaughter should test feed, urine, saliva, or serum in several representative animals for the presence of drug or chemical residues. Such test procedures can help producers to certify the residue-free status of their animals prior to shipment for slaughter, but are costly.

Improper drug usage that results in violative residues can cause the FDA to revoke or restrict a marketing license. Fear of this has resulted in drug companies that develop fewer new products. New product development is an expensive and time-consuming process, since it often takes several years of successful marketing for a new product to recover research and development expenses. Costs of testing, ingredients, potentially useful drugs, and monitoring programs to help producers verify residue-free status are additional costs indirectly shared by the entire industry.

For milk, the US Pasteurized Milk Ordinance requires that all bulk milk tankers be sampled and analyzed for animal drug residues. Information released from the National Milk Drug Residue Data Base showed that a total of 4,179,108 tested samples from October 1, 1993 to September 30, 1994 were reported by states participating in the data base program. Of these samples, 3693 were positive, resulting in the disposal of slightly more than 68 million pounds of milk. From October 1, 1994, to September 30, 1995, nearly 4000 tankers tested violative out of the 4 million samples taken from all 50 states and Puerto Rico. As hundreds of producers are painfully aware, this milk was rejected for human consumption. This is good news for the consumer since none of this milk reached the grocery store.

One could say that good news for the consumer is also good news for a dairy producer. This is correct for the entire milk industry because the disposition of these 4000 loads of milk may not mean anything, but for the individual dairy producer this is a disaster. For example, how could the milk producer explain this to his banker, tell his insurance company he contaminated a load of milk, discuss the matter with his wife, inform his veterinarian, share this information with his employees, or inform his milk buyer? The list could go on.

Detection of a violative drug residue is always a disaster that threatens the smaller milk producer much more than the large producer. Recently a veterinarian that consulted with 130 herds with 150,000 cows indicated to the US Dairy Quality Assurance center that none of the herds had a violative load of milk in over 6 months. In contrast, an insurance company that insures smaller dairies reported that 10% of their 9000 clients had a claim in over 12 months.

Compounding the size-of-farm issue is that discarding your own milk is costly, but the loss is your production costs and large dairies own the majority of the milk in the tanker. Compare this with the small producer: most of the milk in the tank belongs to the neighbors and the producer or perhaps his or her insurance company must pay the market value for the loss. It is questionable how much longer dairy farmers will be able to buy farm liability insurance that covers truckloads of milk they might contaminate with drug residues. Dairy farmers may very well have to pay higher premiums and higher deductibles and face limits on the number of incidents their policies will cover, or the industry may determine that residue milk is uninsurable.

Producers are not the only ones who suffer economic losses from residues. Consumers also share in some of these losses through higher prices and reduced consumption of livestock products. Some consumers lose confidence in the wholesomeness of their food supply. Although the residues found in meat, milk, and eggs are generally at extremely small levels and the number of residue-containing samples is quite low, consumers can be frightened by the ghost of contamination on the grocery counters. The significance of this perception in reducing animal products' consumption cannot be measured, but should not be ignored. Removal of this fear should be the goal of everyone involved with animal agriculture.

REFERENCES

1. Food and Drug Administration, in Sentencing in Residue Case, Food and Drug Administration, Center for Veterinary Medicine, Rockville, MD (1997).

16

Residue Avoidance Management

Collaboration between national authorities, producers, and the food industry in sharing the responsibility and burden of assuring consumers that their food is safe and wholesome appears most promising to meeting the challenge of residue avoidance. Residue avoidance is based on the notion that enforcement of legislation may be more effective when combined with cooperative educational programs and communication with all involved groups. Within this framework, the Food and Drug Administration (FDA) has set up an educational and cooperative residue prevention plan called the Residue Avoidance Program.

The Residue Avoidance Program stresses education rather than regulation. Within this program, the FDA began in 1978 to educate swine farmers about the use of sulfonamides in pigs (1). As a result, the sulfa residue violations in pigs had declined from 10 to 4.4% by 1980 (2). The success of this initial program led to increased funding for developing educational programs on residue avoidance in other food animal species as well. For all classes of livestock and poultry, the average violation rate detected by residue monitoring decreased from 2.58% in 1978 to 0.52% in 1982. However, the effect of the Residue Avoidance Program was not consistent, because residue violations increased again in 1983 (3, 4).

The Residue Avoidance Program is based on a voluntary residue control agreement signed between Food Safety and Inspection Services (FSIS) and the federal slaughtering establishment that has official responsibility for the animal or poultry production. The first agreement called "Memorandum of Understanding" was signed with a turkey establishment in 1976. Since then, FSIS has received many requests for participation as the Residue Avoidance Program renewed interest in the poultry industry and stimulated new interest in the red-meat industry.

507

The agreement requires producers for the establishment to control all elements of production to prevent drug residues. In implementing this strategy, FSIS has worked with constituent groups to encourage adoption of producer-driven voluntary food safety initiatives and to coordinate efforts to identify animal production practices that have the potential to eliminate drug residues in edible animal products.

The Milk and Dairy Beef Quality Assurance Program can be considered a result of such initiatives and efforts. It is a voluntary program designed to reduce the incidence of violative drug residues in milk and dairy beef by educating producers on proper management and drug usage procedures. The goal is to help producers evaluate their operations in conjunction with their veterinarian, thus creating a valid working relationship between the veterinarian and the dairy producer. The dairy operator or employee and the veterinarian follow a Producer Manual that combines information and questions to complete the evaluation process. The program is based on the Hazard Analysis Critical Control Point (HACCP) concept, and suggests that adapting certain principles and taking into account some hints can significantly reduce drug residue violations in beef or milk (Tables 16.1, 16.2).

The Milk and Dairy Beef Quality Assurance Program is referenced under the grade "A" Pasteurized Milk Ordinance (PMO) and under the US Department of Agriculture (USDA) Manufacturing Grade Milk Standards. It is often used by the FDA in their follow-up activities after meat residue infractions in veal and dairy beef. Under the PMO, producers whose grade "A" permit has been suspended due to violative drug residues in the milk, cannot be reinstated until the producer and a licensed veterinarian have completed the Milk and Dairy Beef Drug Residue prevention Protocol and have signed a certificate for display in the milk-house. Many endorsements for the program have been received from veterinarians, extension dairy agents, extension veterinarians, state agriculture

TABLE 16.1   Principles for Reducing Drug Residue Violations in Beef According to the US Milk and Dairy Beef Quality Assurance Program

Principle 1	Identify and track all treated animals.
Principle 2	Maintain a system of records that permits a paper trail of drugs used in each animal.
Principle 3	Properly label, store, and account for all drug products and medicated feeds used in the operation.
Principle 4	Purchase prescription drugs only through veterinarians who have a valid client/patient relationship on the farm.
Principle 5	Educate all employees and family members on proper drug use.

TABLE 16.2 Hints for Preventing Antibacterial Residues in Milk and Dairy Products According to the US Milk and Dairy Beef Quality Assurance Program

Identification hints	Treatment hints	Check hints
Treated cows marked	Recommended dosage	Factory check suspect cows
Blackboard/whiteboard to denote treated cows	Registered brand	Recently purchased cows
Communication to all milkers	Segregation of treated cows	
Cows treated by veterinarian	Treated cows milked last	
	Correct withholding period	
	Inclusion of milk from partially treated udders	
	Inclusion of milk following other treatments, such as footrot, Injections, etc.	
	Short rest period of cows treated with dry cow therapy	
	Use dry cow therapy to reduce lactation treatment and endure colostrum is withheld for eight milkings after calving	

officials, producer organizations, veterinary associations, and regulatory agencies including the FDA, FSIS, and the Animal and Plant Health Inspection Service.

Within the framework of the Residue Avoidance Program, producers have also had much success in implementing preventive measures to address the problem of drug residues at the animal production level. As a result of these efforts, animals such as bob veal calves, cull dairy cows, and market hogs, which were singled out by the FDA to be a major problem just a few years ago, are not of concern regarding drug residues any more.

Someone once said that a bob veal calf is a calf ready to die on the way to market. Even in these times of low calf prices, it does not make sense to calve weak animals. It also does not make sense not to care for the calf after birth. The problem of antibiotics in bob veal calves is a dairy producer's problem. It is not a special-fed veal producer's problem. If the calf is not raised with pride and no effort is made to capture a quality premium, the calf is destined to be bob veal and probably given antibiotics. The quality premium comes if the calf can be a special-fed veal calf, or a replacement heifer, or an animal that will be fed out in the feedlot. To capture the quality premium, many family farmers turn the calves over to the farm wife for care. The principle here is that it takes tender loving care to produce a quality calf. Other suggested principles include calving in clean, sanitized, dry, and well-ventilated maternity areas; feeding high-quality colostrum within 2h of birth; dipping the navel in 7% tincture of iodine soon after birth; feeding high-quality milk replacer without antibiotics; and not marketing calf until 3 days old.

FSIS monitors the agricultural practices, and verifies that the production controls are being applied as agreed. The producers utilize USDA-accredited laboratories, at their expense, to analyze feed and other products for contamination before using them on the farm. The producer also has a representative number of animals or birds sampled prior to presenting the entire flock or herd for slaughter. In the case of large food animals, urine or blood may be used in lieu of tissue samples. The establishments perform 10–30 times the number of tests normally conducted by FSIS. The program has been very successful: violative residues in food-producing animals have declined dramatically. Residue violations are now rarely found in an industry that once had repeated residue problems.

In addition, FSIS has implemented a nationwide interagency computerized information database known as the Residue Violation Information System (RVIS), to review, sort, cross-reference, and manage all residue data obtained by FSIS, FDA, or other agencies from residue violation cases. This includes names and addresses of sellers and producers, dealers, and the results of investigations.

In the fiscal year 1996, FSIS laboratories began using RVIS to coordinate the supplying of FDA districts with portions of known violative samples to support FDA field investigations of preharvest drug misuse. RVIS is also being used, with controlled industry access, in a pilot project with the National Milk Producers Federation to encourage quality assurance programs on dairy farms with residue violations in dairy beef and newborn veal calves sent to slaughter.

In the fiscal year 1995, when FSIS assumed responsibility for egg product inspection, FSIS started residue testing of processed eggs and incorporated all processed egg sample residue data into RVIS. USDA has also implemented a swine identification program to trace hogs back to their farm of origin. A number of industry and consumer groups have urged the department to broaden the program to include other species, to control not only residues but also animal disease.

Another information database that originated with the Residue Avoidance Program in 1982 is the Food Animal Residue Avoidance Databank (FARAD).

This is a multistate collaborative effort funded by the US Department of Agriculture Extension Service as a repository of residue avoidance information and educational materials. FARAD has evolved into an expert-mediated residue avoidance decision support system, and its focus is the production of safe food of animal origin (5).

Over the years, the database files of which FARAD is composed have been refined, expanded, and linked into an integrated program for widespread distribution to producers, veterinarians, and others who have responsibility for ensuring the safety of foods derived from animals. The FARAD Professional Guide to Residue Avoidance Management (FARAD Program) is a Windows-based program developed in two versions: one for producers and one for veterinarians. The veterinary version differs from the producer version in that it includes a subroutine to assist the veterinarian in deciding on preslaughter intervals and milk discard times when drugs are used in an extralabel manner. Extralabel drug use is not permitted by producers. The program allows producers to choose over-the-counter products that satisfy their needs, or alerts them to the need for veterinary assistance with prescription drugs. When this information is not sufficient, direct access to FARAD experts is available through the FARAD Regional Access Centers at the Universities of California and Illinois and at North Carolina State University.

A significant improvement in the FARAD is the recent inclusion of detailed indications for use in the approved drug file. This allows the user of the FARAD program quickly to search the entire list of approved products for a particular disease. Thus, approved treatments can be alternatively examined in the light of economic factors and withdrawal periods (6). Work is currently underway to extrapolate pharmacokinetic data across species by using the extensive pharmacokinetic data in FARAD to develop allometric algorithms. This will be especially useful in those cases in which minimal data are available in the species of interest and yet a decision is still needed. The goal is to establish robust algorithms and to identify those compounds for which extrapolation is not possible.

The challenge of food safety requires careful preventive measures throughout the chain of production, processing, transportation, and handling at the retail level. End-product testing has been for many decades the most widely used tool to ensure the safety of food. However, there is a growing awareness that end-product testing cannot by itself ensure food safety. The current tool in wide use in the food industry is the Hazard Analysis Critical Control Points (HACCP) program. End-product testing is a very useful supplement to HACCP to ensure that effective systems are in place.

The HACCP program is a quality assurance system used all around the world to ensure the quality and safety of food. The system works on the concept that prevention is better than cure. The original HACCP concept for food safety was developed at Pillsbury in the 1960s. HACCP was first conceived when Pillsbury was asked to design and manufacture the first space foods for Mercury flights. As they moved onto Gemini with its more complex foods and longer flights, the problems were magnified. By the time the Apollo program landed on the moon, HACCP was developed in the United States.

The European Union is being guided with regards to the HACCP approach by the deliberations taking place at the Food and Agriculture Organization and the World Health Organization of the United Nations and the pertinent Codex Alimentarius Committees. Codex has initiated a working group to formalize a worldwide approach and application of HACCP principles. The concepts incorporated in the Canadian model, the Food Safety Enhancement Program (FSEP), are consistent with the Codex approach to HACCP.

For the implementation of the HACCP system, clear guidance is needed. This is of special importance concerning the role of regulatory agencies, the responsibilities of the food industries, and the training needs of people, who will be involved in using the system. Consideration needs to be given to the specific problems that the developing world will face in its implementation. HACCP is a tool using seven principles to access hazards and to establish control systems that focus on prevention rather than relying mainly on end-product testing (Table 16.3). Its application can aid inspection by regulatory authorities and promote international trade by increasing confidence in food safety.

In the years immediately ahead, maximum use will be made of residue avoidance and cooperative residue programs directed toward generic prevention of problems through appropriate controls at all critical stages of production. Such programs are expected to address the public health problem with the best weapons

TABLE 16.3   HACCP Principles

Principle 1	List potential hazards, assess the likelihood of occurrence, and identify the preventive measures for their control
Principle 2	Determine the critical control points
Principle 3	Establish the critical limits
Principle 4	Establish monitoring procedures to control the critical control points
Principle 5	Establish the corrective actions to be taken when monitoring indicates that a particular critical control point is out of control
Principle 6	Establish verification procedures to confirm that the HACCP system is working effectively
Principle 7	Establish documentation concerning all procedures and records appropriate to HACCP principles and their application

available, that is, solid scientific understanding and systematic prevention, giving thus rise to the challenge for a common goal, which is the production of abundant, healthy, and safe products.

REFERENCES

1. Food and Drug Administration, FDA Consumer, 13:14 (1979).
2. G.W. Meyerholz, in Agriculture Programs, Livestock and Veterinary Sciences, Residue Avoidance Program Summary, US Department of Agriculture Extension Service, Office of the Administrator, Washington, DC (1983).
3. D. Meisinger and C.D. van Houweling, J. Am. Vet. Med. Assoc., 188:134 (1986).
4. P.C. Bartlett, J.H. Kirk, and E.C. Mather, Compend. Cont. Ed. Pract. Vet., 7:S124 (1985).
5. S.F. Sundlof, A.L. Craigmill, and J.E. Riviere, J. Am. Vet. Med. Assoc., 198:816 (1991).
6. A Craigmill, J. Riviere, and S. Sundlof, Proc. of the 6th EAVPT Inter. Congress (P. Lees, Ed.), European Association for Veterinary Pharmacology and Therapeutics, Blackwell Scientific Publications, Edinburgh, UK, p. 72 (1994).

17

Stability of Residues During Food Processing

Inspection of carcasses with regard to drug residues is not always carried out immediately after slaughter. Tissue samples collected at slaughterhouses for residue testing are usually packed with freezer bags in insulated containers and shipped to regulatory laboratories, where they may be stored for various periods of time in a cooled state pending analysis.

The choice of storage temperature, which has traditionally been $-20\,°C$, necessitates some knowledge of the effect of temperature on the stability of the analyte in question. Such information is also of value to residue-testing laboratories in establishing the validity of laboratory sample-handling for routine sample analysis; in setting up appropriate handling, storage, and turnaround times for interlaboratory residue programs, and in selecting suitable residue–matrix combinations for the preparation of reference materials.

Information about the effect of temperature on the stability of drug residues in foods is also important from a toxicological point of view. Many edible animal products do not directly enter the human food chain but are frequently frozen or submitted to some kind of cure and processing waiting marketing. Almost all edible animal products and byproducts are not consumed raw but require some kind of heat processing or cooking, such as frying, boiling, or roasting, before consumption. These handlings can cause denaturation of proteins, elevation of temperature, loss of water and fat, and pH variations that can eventually result in change of concentration, chemical nature, chemical reactions, or altered solubility of the drug residues originally present in a particular food commodity. Many

515

drugs are chemically unstable to some extent, and therefore may undergo degradation during storage and/or cooking or processing to consumable foods.

The assumption that postprocessing loss of drug activity reflects reduced levels of the drug in the food commodity is not well founded and indeed may raise more questions than answers, particularly when information regarding the types of chemical alterations that drug residues undergo during food processing is unavailable. It is always important to consider the possibility that new chemical compounds with greater toxicity than the parent drug may be formed during food processing.

In this respect, it is not only of interest to know whether the parent drug is simply degraded or not but, as for the metabolites produced by the living animal, it is of importance what degradation products are formed in the ready-to-eat foods. Questions must be also raised in regard to health effects due to ingestion of cooking degradation products of metabolites of the drug, since as they may possess potentially harmful biological activity similar to or different from that exhibited by the initial metabolites.

Although most edible animal products are consumed after cooking or some type of processing, none of the required studies for veterinary drug licensing includes the effect of such treatments on the amount and nature of the potentially present residues. Most information about drug residues in edible animal products and government regulatory considerations are directed toward raw products. Only relatively few studies have been reported concerning the effect these treatments may have on residues, and therefore on the dietary exposure of these chemicals and any breakdown products to the consumer. However, in most of these studies only the decrease of antimicrobial activity or of the amount of the parent drug is measured, the cause of this decrease rarely being described or suggested. A discussion of the stability characteristics of groups of drugs potentially present as residues in foods is provided below.

17.1 RESIDUES OF ANTIBACTERIAL DRUGS

17.1.1 Aminoglycosides

Published studies on the effect of storage and cooking on aminoglycoside residues are limited to streptomycin and neomycin. In most studies, streptomycin was shown to be fairly resistant to storage. No measurable loss of the antimicrobial activity of streptomycin residues in meat was observed after storage at either 4 °C or −18 °C for 14 days (1, 2).

Cooking can cause some loss of the antimicrobial activity of streptomycin and neomycin, the loss being dependent on both the temperature and the matrix. When milk and water matrices were heated at 100 °C for 30 min, the microbiological inactivation of neomycin was determined at 25% and 35%, respectively, whereas that of streptomycin was at 33% and 41.7%, respectively (3). When muscle and kidney tissue matrices containing both drugs were heated at 100 °C for 2 h, no loss of antimicrobial activity was observed in muscle, but a 50% loss was determined in kidney (1). However, complete loss of activity could be observed when muscle tissue samples were cooked for 20 min at 120 °C.

In eggs, little or no activity loss was determined after various cooking procedures including frying, poaching, scrambling, or hard boiling (4, 5). In milk, both drugs were also relatively stable; a total of 1320 min heating at 71 °C was found necessary for complete loss of the antimicrobial activity of the streptomycin added in milk.

Little or no loss of antimicrobial activity was further observed after fermentation of raw sausages containing streptomycin (6). However, smoking/scalding processes could cause a 32–45% reduction of the streptomycin activity (7). When semi- or fully preserved sausages were heated at 90–95 °C for 1 h, the microbiological activity of the contained streptomycin exhibited a 50% reduction of the initial dose (8); however, some of the initial activity could be demonstrated in the juices exuded from the heated sausages even when the temperature was raised to 120–125 °C.

Neomycin residues were also found to be quite stable in chicken muscle extracts heated at 100 °C for 5 h (9, 10). Unlike chicken muscle extracts, milk favored the loss of the contained neomycin when heated under similar conditions; no more than 0–25% of the original activity could be determined after heating at 100 °C for 5 h (9, 10).

17.1.2 Amphenicols

Investigation on the stability of chloramphenicol during storage showed that the drug was rapidly degraded in spiked bovine liver tissue (11). Extensive postmortem degradation of chloramphenicol in liver tissue has been reported by other workers as well (12, 13) and attributed to cytochrome P-450-mediated metabolism *in vitro* that led to oxidation and glucuronic acid conjugation of the compound.

Use of piperonyl butoxide, a potent cytochrome P-450 inhibitor, has been recommended as an effective means for preventing the degradation of chloramphenicol. Since addition of this substance to liver homogenates could result in a recovery enhancement from about 30% to 60%, it was suggested that incurred tissue samples taken for analysis should be frozen immediately after excision and homogenized in water containing 2.5% piperonyl butoxide (11).

Recently, the stability of chloramphenicol in both spiked and incurred calf tissues has been further investigated (14). The same favorable effect of piperonyl butoxide on the stability of chloramphenicol has been observed in both liver and kidney tissues. Moreover, the stability of chloramphenicol in these organs was found to be a function of the storage time, temperature, and the presence of piperonyl butoxide.

Without addition of piperonyl butoxide to the analyzed samples, recovery from liver was determined at 63% after a 5 min storage and at 9% after a 30 min storage at room temperature. At 1 °C and 4 °C, the recovery figures for liver after 1 h of storage were 44% and 40%, respectively. The same results were obtained when kidney tissue samples were stored under similar conditions.

Addition of piperonyl butoxide allowed a high enough recovery value to be maintained for longer times. After 30 min storage at room temperature in presence of piperonyl butoxide, recovery was found to be as high as 71% for both liver and kidney tissue samples. Nevertheless, lower concentrations than those initially determined were found when the same samples were reanalyzed after long-term storage at −20 °C. This difference was not established when tissues were not ground before freezing but immediately cut into cubes and frozen at −20 °C, even in the absence of piperonyl butoxide. By this treatment, the stability of chloramphenicol was quite good and no degradation was observed during an 85-day storage at −20 °C. Results of other pertinent stability studies by high-performance liquid chromatography (HPLC) lent support to this finding (15). When muscle tissue from chloramphenicol-treated rabbits was immediately frozen at −20 °C, there was no significant loss or degradation of the analyte during a 30 day storage. Thus, it was eventually concluded that piperonyl butoxide was not sufficient to prevent a decrease in the chloramphenicol content of samples stored for a long time (14).

Several investigations on the stability of chloramphenicol during thermal treatment have been also carried out. Chloramphenicol has been found quite stable to heating when added to water or milk. Even after 2 hours of boiling, no more than 8% loss of its amount could be observed by physicochemical methods of analysis (16). Application of microbiological methods has shown, however, a 33.3–35% reduction in the activity of chloramphenicol after heating the milk or water samples at 100 °C for 30 min (3).

The stability of chloramphenicol is also markedly affected by emulsifying, curing, and cooking processes (17). Successive losses of about 50% for each of these processing steps have been recorded. When incurred pork or beef muscle tissue was minced at 2–3 °C to form an emulsion product, chloramphenicol concentration was reduced from about 48 ppb to 11 ppb (17). Processing the emulsion product in casings at 68 °C without added cure resulted in a 25% additional reduction of chloramphenicol, while the combined effect of curing and heating accelerated the loss of chloramphenicol. Chloramphenicol could not survive the 122 °C canning process, in both the cured and uncured products. On the other hand, when beef steaks with incurred chloramphenicol residues were grilled or roasted for 120 min, the microbiological inactivation of the contained residues was not found to be extensive (2).

17.1.3 β-Lactams

The stability of several β-lactam antibiotic in aqueous solutions is pH dependent. Optimum stability for monobasic penicillins in general is exhibited at pH 6–7, while for the amphoteric penicillins this coincides with the isoelectric point (18). A fast degradation occurs at both acidic and basic conditions. At pH 2.6, acid-labile β-lactams such as penicillin G, methicillin, and nafcillin disappear almost completely while acid-resistant compounds like penicillin V and isoxazolyl penicillins survive (19).

Most studies on the effect of storage on β-lactam residues have been directed toward penicillin G. Kidney tissue samples containing penicillin G showed some loss of microbiological activity when stored at 4 °C (1), whereas incurred tissues held in a walk-in cooler at 4 °C for about 2 weeks or stored in freezer at −20 °C over the same period were also found to contain lower penicillin G levels than were present initially (20). The lactate ester of penicilloic acid has been identified as the major decomposition product of penicillin G formed during the storage of incurred beef and chicken samples at −2 °C or room temperature (21).

A study on the storage stability of penicillin G in milk showed that about 60% could be destroyed within 48 h at 2 °C, while 75% could be destroyed at 22 °C (22). The loss of penicillin G was attributed to the hydrolytic activity of the enzyme β-lactamase produced by both gram-negative and gram-positive bacteria of the raw milk. This was confirmed by analogous experimentation with UHT milk, in which penicillin G did not show any decrease under mentioned storage conditions.

The stability of penicillin G has been further investigated in spiked bovine plasma samples that were stored at either room temperature or at −20 °C and −70 °C (23). Results showed that the half-life of penicillin G at −20 °C was 75 days. The degradation of the spiked penicillin G was so rapid that even plasma samples stored at −70 °C should be analyzed within a month of storage to ascertain no more than a small percentage loss of the analyte.

Unlike spiked penicillin G, incurred residues in bovine plasma showed a slower rate of degradation. The half-life was estimated at 276 days for storage at −20 °C (24). Further experimentation showed that incurred residues in tissues stored at −20 °C decreased more rapidly than in plasma. Losses of up to 20% were observed in kidney and liver samples stored at −20 °C after as little as 10 days of storage. On the other hand, gluteal muscle samples stored at the same temperature showed within 10 days of storage losses of nearly 50% of the initial residue present. However, penicillin G residues in tissue samples stored at −76 °C remained stable.

Analogous findings were reported by other workers who studied the stability of both spiked and incurred residues of penicillin G in ovine liver during storage at −20 °C for 3 months (25). If we assume that the rate of loss followed a first-order kinetic decay, the mean half-life of penicillin G was estimated at 62 days for the spiked tissues and 71 days for the tissues with incurred residues. This is not in direct agreement with the results of a previous pertinent study in which a longer half-life of 114 days for incurred residues in bovine liver stored at -20 °C was predicted (24). The difference between these studies could be due to the way the tissues were prepared; in the former study tissues were blended prior to storage, while in the latter tissues were stored without blending.

The above findings suggest that if testing laboratories do not adjust their analytical and sample storage protocols according to the extent to which penicillin G decreases in tissues and biological fluids stored in conventional freezers, quantitative analyses conducted on such samples may not reflect concentrations at time of sample submission.

Apart from storage stability studies, numerous investigations have been also carried out on the effect of various heat treatments such as those applied in pasteurization, evaporation, and drying processes on the stability of penicillin G residues. Early published work was based on measurement of the reduction of microbiological activity, whereas more recent work was based on results of physicochemical analytical techniques.

Microbiological tests have indicated that penicillin G is stable to heat. Pasteurization temperatures and times commonly applied to milk and milk products are inadequate for inactivation of the antibiotic if it is present (26–29). At 71 °C, a total of 1705 min was required to inactivate completely penicillin G in milk, whereas at boiling temperatures or above, all data indicated that a portion of the penicillin activity in milk survived boiling for 60 min or autoclaving at 15 psi steam pressure for 15–30 min (26, 29). Milk from treated cows retained some of its antimicrobial activity even after conversion to dried skim milk powder (30).

Cooking procedures exert similar effects. Penicillin G was not consistently inactivated by 90 min heating at 100 °C in water, milk, and beef extracts, except in extracts of chicken muscle, in which it was less stable (10). In another study, the microbiological activity of penicillin G in buffer and buffered meat homogenates at pH 5.0 and 7.0 was studied (31). Penicillin G was found less stable at pH 5.0 than at 7.0. It was not totally inactivated by 60 min at 100 °C in any of the media, but it could be inactivated within 60 min at 117 °C or 121 °C.

More recent physicochemical assays have also confirmed that the thermal stability of penicillin G is pH-dependent (32). At 100 °C, the half-life of penicillin G was given a value of 45 min in pure aqueous solutions, a value of 25 min at pH 5.5, and a value of 8 min at pH 8.2. In cooking oil heated at 180 °C and 140 °C, the half-life of penicillin G was estimated at 18 min and 45 min, respectively (32).

In general, penicillin G in meat is not stable to cooking. Following treatment at 100 °C for 10 min or longer, a marked decrease in microbiological activity in pork or rabbit meat has been observed although residues in rabbit kidney were more stable (9, 33). The loss is usually proportional to the harshness of the cooking regimen; where fluids are released during the cooking process, over half of the residue sometimes passes from the solid tissue into the cooking medium (34).

Various degradation products of penicillin G have been demonstrated in the cooked meat (21). The major product formed after cooking was identified as the lactate ester of penicilloic acid. Moreover, formation of bound residues was also suggested.

The stability of penicillin G in various types of sausages has been studied as well. In smoked/scalded products, the antimicrobial activity was found to be reduced to about 45% (7). However, complete inactivation was observed in semi- and fully preserved sausages and during the preparation of raw fermented sausages (6, 8). It was suggested that the latter inactivation might be due to the action of penicillinase-producing organisms.

Procaine penicillin and ampicillin are other β-lactams for which the stability of residues in meat has been investigated. Significant levels of the original activity of procaine penicillin remained following rare and medium cooking of spiked hamburgers, steaks, and pork chops (35); after well-done cooking conditions, however, only a small percentage of the initial activity could be seen in the cooked products. Ampicillin concentrations in meat, on the other hand, decrease with both storage at − 20 °C and cooking (2). When beef steaks with incurred ampicillin residues were grilled or roasted for 120 min, microbiological inactivation of the contained residues occurred to some extent (2).

17.1.4 Macrolides

The stability of oleandomycin has been found to be highly dependent on the type of the food matrix in which it is contained; a milk matrix, for example, considerably increases the loss of the antimicrobial activity of oleandomycin upon heating (9). Nevertheless, both oleandomycin and spiramycin have generally shown considerable thermostability when heated in water, milk, and meat extracts (9).

17.1.5 Nitrofurans

The instability of nitrofurans in meat or liver has been well documented (36–38). Hence, a major concern from a regulatory point of view has arisen regarding the stability of nitrofuran residues during transport of the samples from the collection place to the testing facility.

With muscle tissue that has been stored frozen and then thawed and kept at room temperature, furazolidone has been shown to disappear within a few hours after spiking (37). The drop in concentration was much more rapid in incurred than in spiked muscle. A rapid decrease of parent furazolidone in swine muscle tissue from 61 to 2 ppb was also observed even when samples were stored at − 30 °C for 4 weeks.

Additional studies have demonstrated that incurred residues of furaltadone and furazolidone in tissues of veal calves are rapidly decreased postmortem. Two h after slaughtering, only traces of the parent drugs could be determined in muscle and kidney tissues, whereas residues of the parent drugs could no longer be detected in the liver (39). In chicken liver, furazolidone is also rapidly degraded postmortem; more than 95% of a furazolidone dose spiked to a liver tissue sample kept at 32 °C could be degraded in 15 min (40).

The cause of the postmortem decrease of furazolidone residues has not yet been elucidated. There have been indications that it might be due to some tissue enzymes remaining active for long periods after animal death, but it cannot be excluded that bound residues are formed as well since in vivo and in vitro studies have shown formation of such residues (41, 42). Heat denaturation of the enzymes involved by microwaving treatment improved the stability during storage, but there was still a decrease of about 50% that could be due to either accelerated breakdown during heating or occlusion of the drug in the denatured protein matrix.

Due to the rapid and extensive metabolism of nitrofurans in animals, thermostability studies on residues of the parent compounds are not relevant and not published. Instead, the effect of cooking on the concentrations of both the bound and extractable 3-amino-2-oxazolidinone, the main furazolidone metabolite, in incurred swine tissues has been investigated (43). Total 3-amino-2-oxazolidinone concentrations were not found to be significantly reduced in liver, kidney, or muscle following frying, grilling, or microwaving.

Unlike in meat and liver, no further metabolism of nitrofurans occurs in egg during its long development time. As a result, considerable concentrations of the parent drugs may be encountered in eggs from treated birds (44, 45). Stability studies on incurred residues of furazolidone, furaltadone, nitrofurazone, and nitrofurantoin in eggs stored for 65 weeks under different storage temperatures and packaging materials have been reported (45). Storage at − 20 °C or − 80 °C for 65 weeks of lyophilized or original egg samples had no effect on the concentrations of furazolidone initially present in the egg samples.

On the other hand, the type of the packaging material did not exert any effect on the residue levels at a storage temperature of − 20 °C. At 4 °C, nitrofuran residues remained stable when the egg samples were stored in glass or polypropylene tubes, but a loss of 60–70% was observed when a laminated foil was used. At 20 °C, all four nitrofurans exhibited marked residue reduction, the losses being 30–50% for glass tubes, 40–60% for polypropylene tubes, and 100% for laminated foil.

17.1.6 Quinolones

The influence of baking on enrofloxacin and ciprofloxacin residues in flatfish has been investigated (46). Both drugs showed excellent thermal stability.

Studies on the fate of residues of oxolinic acid and flumequine in salmon after cooking have shown that residues of the former drug could be detected in both boiled and baked muscle of treated fish even though no residues were present before cooking (47). In contrast, muscle samples of fish treated with flumequine were consistently negative after cooking provided they were also negative before cooking. It appears that cooking allowed some of the reservoir residues of oxolinic acid to be released into the muscle.

Further investigation showed that some amounts of both the quinolones investigated could also leak out into the boiling water or the juice exuded from the baked fish. Therefore, cooking may reveal residues of quinolones that could not be detected in the raw fish muscle before preparation. It is of value to note that none of the quinolones used in this study showed any degradation at the temperatures reached when the fish were cooked.

These findings lend support to the notion that residues of quinolones can be withheld in certain tissues of fish for prolonged periods after the end of treatment (48). Residues of oxolinic acid seem to be especially trapped in fish backbone and skin, whereas residues of flumequine predominate in fish backbone. These reservoirs appear to act as depots from which the drugs are slowly released into other tissues.

17.1.7 Sulfonamides

The stability of sulfonamide residues in animal tissues during frozen storage has been investigated in several studies, most of which dealt with sulfamethazine (2, 49–54). Early studies suggested a 10% decrease in sulfamethazine levels in frozen calf liver samples stored for 40 days (49), and a 12.6% or 13.9% decrease in spiked sulfamethazine residues in swine liver or muscle tissues, respectively, after 15 days of storage at -20 °C (2).

Results of more recent studies have confirmed previous findings also providing evidence that the drug was transformed during storage to the N_4-glucopyranosyl derivative that is the reaction product of sulfamethazine with glucose (53, 54). A decrease of about 50% in the sulfamethazine content of incurred and spiked pig muscle samples was found after 15 months of frozen storage (55). No loss of the amount of sulfamethazine in ground swine muscle was observed by other workers after storage at -20 °C for either 3 months (56) or 21 days (52); in the latter case, extension of the storage time from 21 to 43 days was found, nevertheless, to cause a loss of about 15%. Although there is some discrepancy between those results, the trend of decreasing sulfamethazine levels during prolonged storage at -20 °C is clear in most studies.

Apart from sulfamethazine, the stability of several other sulfonamides including sulfathiazole, sulfachlorpyridazine, sulfaquinoxaline, and sulfadimethoxine in spiked pig liver frozen at -20 °C have been investigated over a period of 6 months (57). In this study, storage stability values expressed as decay half-lives were found to be 567 days for sulfadimethoxine, 457 days for sulfamethazine, 312 days for sulfachlorpyridazine, 291 days for sulfathiazole, and 271 days for sulfaquinoxaline. To gain information on the effect of alternative storage conditions, the stability of the least stable sulfonamide, sulfaquinoxaline, was further investigated under accelerated decay conditions (57). When swine liver tissue spiked with sulfaquinoxaline was stored in a refrigerator at 4 °C to accelerate degradation, a decay half-life of 11 days was observed. Although these results suggested sulfaquinoxaline to be an unstable sulfonamide, another study on frozen spiked swine liver showed that sulfamerazine degraded with the much lower half-life of 14 days and that sulfadiazine was even less stable (58).

It is of interest to note that in the above-mentioned studies all examined compounds exhibited a rapid initial decrease during tissue homogenization, the decrease being as high as 65% for sulfaquinoxaline but only 10–25% for the rest of the sulfonamides (57). Such a decrease has been also exhibited in model systems containing sulfamethazine and riboflavin and was attributed to photodegradation of the sulfonamide (59). A similar behavior was obtained when crude polar liver extracts spiked with sulfamethazine were exposed to fluorescent light for 1 h; the same photodegradation product as observed in model systems of sulfamethazine and riboflavin, was formed (60). Therefore, procedures for determining sulfonamides in liver, an organ containing relatively large amounts of riboflavin, must be carried out in subdued light to prevent possible loss due to photochemical reactions.

Another storage stability study in which metabolites of sulfaquinoxaline and sulfadimethoxine were also involved was recently reported (61). The results of this study demonstrated that, unlike the parent drugs, the N_4-acetyl derivatives of sulfaquinoxaline and sulfadimethoxine did not depleted in spiked chicken liver and tissues during frozen storage for 1 year at -20 and -70 °C. The transformation of the parent compounds, which depleted approximately 35% in liver tissue at -20 °C, to their N_4-glucopyranosyl derivatives was negligible, suggesting that products other than glucosides resulted during the storage period. These results demonstrate the need for both regulatory agencies and testing laboratories to be aware of potential errors associated with improper transport, storage, and handling of tissue samples submitted for residue testing.

The stability of sulfonamide residues during preparation, cooking, and processing of foods has also been examined. Sulfonamides are examples of heat-stable compounds. Sulfamethazine was shown (56) to be stable in boiling water at 100 °C, but in cooking oil at 180 °C or 260 °C losses were observed, indicating half-lives of about 2 h or 5 min, respectively. Little or no effect on the antimicrobial activity was observed in meat from sulfamethazine-treated bovine animals under normal household preparation methods, such as roasting or grilling steaks (2). Tissues containing sulfamethazine that were minced and chilled or canned at 122 °C showed no apparent loss of the drug (13). Sulfamethazine was found to be stable in milk after boiling for 15 min as well (62).

When a dose of radiolabeled sulfamethazine was administered singly to a pig, no loss of sulfamethazine could be detected in the obtained pig loin, liver, and cured ham after application of various cooking procedures (63). Levels of the N_4-acetyl metabolite of sulfamethazine were not altered by cooking, but the N_4-glucoside metabolite exhibited cooking-related declines of up to 70%. Liver, which contained high concentrations of the glucoside metabolite, exhibited an increase in sulfamethazine as a result of cooking, and this could be only explained by heat-related hydrolysis of the sulfamethazine–glucoside complex. These results indicate that cooking does not destroy but may increase sulfamethazine in pork products.

Boiling, roasting, grilling, frying, pressure cooking, and microwaving cooking processes had no significant effect on the concentration of sulfamethazine residues in incurred animal tissue once allowance was made for weight loss during cooking (56). Migration from the tissue into the surrounding liquid or meat juices was observed during the cooking processes. It is of interest to note that the analytical method used in this investigation included an acid-extraction step that back-converted the N_4-metabolites to the parent compound. The findings of this investigation show that surveillance data obtained from measurements on raw tissue are applicable for use in consumer exposure estimates and dietary intake calculations.

Unlike with sulfamethazine, cooking processes such as baking, frying, and smoking could cause an average 46.1% reduction of sulfadimethoxine and 54% reduction of ormetoprim from raw fillets of channel catfish (64). In this study, however, allowance for weight loss during cooking was not made.

Sulfonamides, although stable compounds, can show chemical reactivity towards endogenous tissue components or to additives. Thus, during raw fermented sausage preparation, apart from a 25% leaching out of sulfamethazine in the brine, bound residues at a percentage of about 20% along with several reaction products with endogenous components were formed (65, 66). In addition, various compounds, such as the hydroxydesamino sulfamethazine and desamino sulfamethazine, which are both products of the reaction of sulfamethazine with nitrite, the sausage additive, were found to be present.

Addition of cure to spiked pork muscle tissue resulted in loss of sulfamethazine at approximately 48%, 20%, and 40% for chilling at 2–3 °C, heating at 68 °C, and canning at 122 °C treatments, respectively (17). The effect of sterilization and fermentation on the amount of sulfamethazine residues in the final product has been also established (67). No decrease of sulfamethazine was observed during the preparation of luncheon meat, while in the raw fermented product, after a ripening period of 1 month, only 20% of the original amount was still present. These results are in line with pertinent investigations conducted with sulfachlorpyridazine (68).

The stability of sulfadimethoxine during raw fermented sausage preparation was also investigated in a model study (69). Sulfadimethoxine content decreased by about 30% during brining but remained constant during further ripening in the climate room. In this study, both N^4-glucopyranosyl- and desaminosulfadimethoxine, and bound residues, were formed in the sausages as well.

17.1.8   Tetracyclines

Tetracycline antibiotics are generally considered relatively unstable compounds. Oxytetracycline posseses limited stability in aqueous solutions and shows specific and base catalysis, with overall hydrolysis observed to follow pseudo-first-order kinetics. The maximum stability of this drug is exhibited at pH 2, whereas the optimum stability ranges from pH 1 to 3, which accounts for the recent finding (70) that oxytetracycline has greater heat stability at pH 3 than at pH 6.9.

During storage, minimal, if any, reducing effects have been observed on the oxytetracycline microbiological activity in muscle, liver, and kidney tissue kept at 4 °C and at −20 °C for 6 months (2).

The thermal stability of oxytetracycline in liquid media, as indexed by the antimicrobial activity retained following heating at 71 °C, has been shown to be much less than that of other antibiotics such as aminoglycosides and β-lactams (71, 72). Recent investigation on the thermostability of oxytetracycline in water and vegetable oil showed that the drug is unstable in water at 100 °C with a half-life of 2 min, but more stable in oil at 180 °C with a half-life of 8 min.

The results of the oxytetracycline thermostability experiments in liquid media are not totally representative of the actual cooking and processing conditions, since the length of time at a particular temperature to which antibiotic residues may be subjected during cooking, is relatively more difficult to determine (73). Characteristically different thermostability values of oxytetracycline activity have been shown in various food matrices (9). Thus, oxytetracycline was more stable in salmon tissue than in simple buffer systems of the same pH (70), and also more stable in milk than in chicken or beef muscle samples that heated at 100 °C (9). Using microbiological methods, a heat treatment at 100 °C for 10–15 min has been found in many instances sufficient to inactivate oxytetracycline and chlortetracycline to nondetectable residues (9). However, prolonged heat treatment at 100 °C for 40 min has been also used to inactivate tetracycline residues totally in poultry meat and eggs (33, 74).

The effect of a range of cooking processes including microwaving, boiling, roasting, grilling, braising, and frying, on oxytetracycline residues in incurred animal tissues has been thoroughly investigated (75). Substantial net reductions in oxytetracycline residues of 35–94% were observed, with temperature during cooking having the largest impact on the loss. Other workers also found that the reduction in antimicrobial activity of oxytetracycline during grilling or roasting of beef steaks was temperature dependent but never exceeded a 50% reduction (2, 4). Migration from the tissue into the surrounding liquid or meat juices was also observed during the cooking processes. In addition, some workers showed complete inactivation of oxytetracycline with canning in glass and tin containers but very little loss of oxytetracycline activity with smoke or scalding processing (6–8).

These findings on meat cooking agree well with recent pertinent studies on fish cooking. It was observed that frying, baking, and smoking could not completely eliminate high levels of oxytetracycline residues from fillets of channel catfish (76, 77). The oxytetracycline content of incurred salmon tissue was reduced by about 60% when fish patties were cooked at 100 °C for 15 min (70). The residual amounts of oxytetracycline in the patties corresponded to the levels of chlortetracycline detected when ground beef patties and frankfurters from incurred animals were cooked at 136 °C for 10 min (78), but they were far greater than those reported for oxytetracycline in breaded oysters and crab cakes, in which 3.6% and 7.5%, respectively, of the antimicrobial activity was retained (79). The obvious inconsistency of these studies should be due to their different detection principle since physicochemical assays in general offer greater specificity than the microbiological assays.

Tetracyclines have the tendency to form chelates with bivalent metal ions. As a consequence of their affinity to calcium, tetracyclines tend to accumulate in the bones of treated animals. Although their chelates with calcium show considerable stability, tetracyclines can be extracted from bones containing these drugs and, therefore, may be present in soups and meals when bones from treated animals are cooked (80, 81). The extractability of chlortetracycline from bone tissue is strongly pH-dependent, being higher at low pH values. This can be easily explained by the dependence of the dissociation constant of the chelate from the pH value.

Early microbiological investigations (80, 81) on the effect of processing on the tetracycline content in bones showed that the thermal stability of chlortetracycline was higher in ground bones than in meat; at a cooking temperature of 110 °C for 1 h, 50% of the drug present in ground bones could be inactivated (81).

Recent studies, in which raw chicken muscle tissues and wet-milled bones incurred with oxytetracycline were used to manufacture meat patties, cans, and hamburgers that were cooked by boiling, frying, microwaving, and autoclaving, showed that oxytetracycline was completely degraded only when cans with chicken bones and muscle tissues were autoclaved at 120 °C for 60 min; other cooking processes exerted only a partial effect (82, 83). Thus, boiling and stir-frying degraded 39–49% of the residues in chicken muscle and 8–34% in the hamburgers, whereas microwaving and deep-frying degraded 53–75% of the residues in muscle and 42–61% in the hamburgers. Residues in chicken muscle tissues were, generally, more labile to heat degradation than those in the bones.

When the effect of cooking procedures on oxytetracycline incurred tissues of cultured eel and ayu was also investigated (83), it was observed that residues in edible tissues of fish were more labile to degradation than those in bones. Although residual oxytetracycline in fish muscle and liver could be reduced to about 70–80% with boiling, baking, or frying, the reduction in bones never exceeded the range of 30–50%.

The stability of oxytetracycline in sausages can also depend on the particular procedure applied for their preparation. Thus, no loss of antimicrobial activity was observed during raw fermented sausage preparation (6), but oxytetracycline was completely inactivated in semi- and fully preserved sausages (7, 8).

These early results are in direct agreement with recent findings on the stability of oxytetracycline residues in sausages (84). When ground meat from lambs treated with oxytetracycline was packed in a sausage casing and cooked in boiling water, the level of oxytetracycline residues was reduced to 95% within 30 min. Microwave cooking for 8 min to a final temperature of 98–102 °C reduced the concentration of oxytetracycline about 60%, whereas frying for 8 min to a final internal temperature of 81 °C reduced oxytetracycline residues about 17%. In all cases, the extent of the degradation was related to the final temperature reached, which was higher for microwave and boiling than for frying cooking.

Certain food additives can also influence significantly the rate of oxytetracycline degradation in both aqueous and tissue media. Pertinent studies (85) in aqueous media showed that orthophosphates increase the rate of oxytetracycline degradation, but pyrophosphates, tripolyphosphates, hexametaphosphates, and nitrites decrease this rate. The degradation of oxytetracycline was found to occur at a slower rate in porcine tissue than in aqueous media. Addition of orthophosphates to tissue had no effect on the rate of oxytetracycline degradation, but addition of polyphosphates increased this rate. On the other hand, nitrites in tissue increased the degradation at 60 °C but decreased it at 80 °C. Inclusion of calcium chloride significantly decreased the rate of oxytetracycline degradation in both aqueous and tissue matrices.

17.2   RESIDUES OF ANTHELMINTHIC DRUGS

17.2.1   Albendazole

To determine the stability of albendazole residues in milk upon storage at − 18 °C from 3 to 8 months, both incurred and spiked milk samples containing all three albendazole metabolites, namely albendazole sulfoxide, albendazole sulfone, and albendazole 2-aminosulphone, were used. Results showed that the 3 month storage did not produce any change in the concentration of the analytes in both spiked and incurred samples (86). A similar concentration profile was also observed after the 8 month storage for the spiked but not for the incurred milk samples. For the latter samples, the concentration of all analytes was found to be higher, the increase being higher in the case of the 2-aminosulphone metabolite. This increase suggested some release of albendazole residues that were bound to milk constituents in the incurred samples during the 8 month storage. The intense precipitation of milk constituents observed in all samples stored for 8 months lends support to this explanation.

Since not all milk enters the human food chain directly, but most of the milk produced is normally subjected to some kind of processing for preparation of various dairy products, the fate of incurred albendazole residues during cheese-making, ripening, and storage has been also investigated (87). Albendazole residues in dairy products would be of major concern if the transfer and accumulation were significant.

Results showed that about 70% from each major albendazole metabolite initially present in milk could be distributed in the whey. The remaining 30% appeared in the produced cheese at residue levels higher than those initially present in milk (688 ppb versus 445 ppb, or 450 ppb versus 230 ppb for albendazole sulfoxide; 890 ppb versus 608 ppb, or 1502 ppb versus 783 ppb for albendazole sulfone; 19 ppb versus 15 ppb, or 161 ppb versus 105 ppb for albendazole-2-aminosulfone). Ripening and storage of the prepared cheeses resulted in decrease of the sulfoxide metabolite to 225 ppb or 206 ppb, increase of the sulfone metabolite to 1181 ppb or 1893 ppb, whereas it had no effect on the 2-aminosulfone metabolite.

17.2.2 Oxfendazole

The thermal stability of oxfendazole has been examined in both water and cooking oil (88). Some evidence of instability was observed in boiling water after 3 h. This instability was associated with hydrolysis of the carbamate group of the oxfendazole molecule and formation of an amine byproduct. In hot cooking oil at 150 °C or 180 °C, the half-life of oxfendazole was 15 min or 6 min, respectively. The instability was also associated with the formation of the amine byproduct, which increased as the concentration of the parent drug decreased.

The effect of cooking on incurred residues of oxfendazole in cattle liver has been also investigated (88). However, the results drawn from this study are inconclusive due to several variable factors. One such factor is the unstable equilibrium between oxfendazole, oxfendazole sulfone, and fenbendazole in the incurred tissue. Other factor is the overall instability of oxfendazole and its metabolites in tissue during frozen storage. Another factor is the variable distribution of the residues within the tissue used for the study and the effect of protein binding on the extractability of the residues from the tissue. It was nevertheless observed that cooking did not destroy oxfendazole residues, although it affected the point of equilibrium between oxfendazole, oxfendazole sulfone, fenbendazole, and some other metabolites in the incurred tissue. It was further suggested that storage time decreases the residue concentrations in liver.

17.2.3   Levamisole

Storage stability studies (89) in muscle tissue from treated swine showed that freezing at -20 °C for 1 month could result in a 29% decrease of levamisole residues, while chilling at 5 °C for 5 days did not show any decreasing effect. The high decrease noted in the frozen muscle was reported to be due to the high dripping losses of levamisole with tissue water owing to the significant temperature fluctuations that occurred during the frozen storage.

Heat stability studies (90) with standard levamisole have indicated that the substance is stable in boiling water at 100 °C, but unstable in cooking oil at 260 °C, with a half-life of about 5 min. Cooking stability studies with animal tissues showed that boiling, roasting, frying, stir-frying, smoking, stewing, pressure-cooking, grilling, and microwaving cooking processes did not exert any significant decreasing effect on the stability of levamisole residues in a range of fortified and incurred samples (90). A net loss of levamisole was observed in these cooking processes, but the lost levamisole was present either in the cooking liquid or in the exuded juices. Most observed changes in swine and beef muscle containing incurred residues were well within the precision limits of the analytical method, once allowance for weight loss during cooking was made to counter the apparent concentration increase.

Processing procedures such as canning of swine muscle tissue at 121 °C for 60 min resulted in a 62% decrease of levamisole residues, whereas curing in a 33% decrease of the drug concentration. These results lend support to previous pertinent findings also reporting a substantial decrease of levamisole residues during curing and canning (89). The high loss of levamisole during canning was attributed to the extreme cooking conditions applied, while the loss after curing was attributable to leakage of the water-soluble drug from muscle into the aqueous curing solution.

17.2.4   Ivermectin

The effect of heating on aqueous solutions of ivermectin is difficult to study due to the very low solubility of the compound in water. Thus, the stability of ivermectin has been only investigated on incurred tissue samples. When a series of incurred pig and cattle muscle and liver samples and salmon muscle samples were subjected to various cooking processes, some loss of ivermectin was observed but the loss was associated with the leakage of the fat from the tissue samples during the cooking process and not to degradation of the drug itself. In one case, this leakage amounted to about 50% of the total residues (91).

If allowance for weight loss during cooking is not made, stability studies will definitely show that the drug is unstable to typical cooking conditions, although this is certainly an illusion. In such a study, the decrease of the ivermectin residues was found to reach to 45% or 50% when an ordinary culinary preparation of minced beef muscle from a bull treated with ivermectin was submitted to boiling or frying, respectively (92, 93).

17.3 RESIDUES OF ANTICOCCIDIAL DRUGS

17.3.1 Dinitolmide

Following administration to chickens, dinitolmide, also known as zoalene, is primarily metabolized to the 3-amino-5-nitro-o-toluamide and 5-amino-3-nitro-o-toluamide metabolites, which exhibit a high tendency to bind to tissues. It has been shown that these dinitolmide metabolites deplete from frozen liver tissues stored up to 1 year at − 20 °C, but not at − 70 °C (94). A slight loss of the 5-amino-3-nitro-o-toluamide also occurs in thigh muscle stored at − 20 °C. It has been suggested that the depletion of the dinitolmide metabolites should be partially the result of their transformation to glucopyranosyl derivatives as both the α- and β-anomers of the 5-amino-3-nitro-o-toluamide conjugate have been observed in tissue extracts.

17.4 RESIDUES OF ANTIMICROBIAL GROWTH PROMOTERS

17.4.1 Lasalocid

As has been demonstrated by stability experiments at 100 °C in aqueous buffer solutions, lasalocid is relatively stable to heat in neutral and acidic conditions, but unstable in alkaline conditions (95). Thus, the drug exhibits stability at pH 5.5 and 7.0, but instability at pH 10.0 with a half-life of 30 min. Lasalocid is also not stable in sunflower cooking oil heated at 180 °C, with a half-life of 15 min.

In incurred chicken muscle, lasalocid residues were found to be stable to cooking. Residues in raw tissue from the treated chickens were found to be evenly distributed in edible muscle. Chicken was cooked by microwaving, boiling, roasting, frying, and grilling. Less than 5% of the residue was found in juices that came out of the meat when it was cooked by microwave and roasting.

Unlike with muscle, cooking decreased the amount of residues measured in eggs. Frying decreased residues by 59%, whereas scrambling reduced it by 27%.

These results are consistent with the mentioned pH-dependence of lasalocid stability: chicken muscle is known to be at about pH 5.7, egg yolk at about pH 6.0–6.8, whereas egg white pH can be as high as 9.0–10.0. The loss of lasalocid in egg should therefore be due to the base-catalyzed hydrolysis of lasalocid.

17.4.2 Salinomycin

Although use of salinomycin in laying hens is not approved, residue levels of salinomycin in eggs, due to cross-contamination of the laying hens' feeds between different batches, have been reported (96). The amounts of salinomycin residues in eggs from hens accidentally given medicated feed for broilers may reach to the level of about 400 ppb, whereas the presence of residues may persist for 8 days after withdrawal because salinomycin has the tendency to accumulate in the egg yolk (97, 98).

The stability of salinomycin during egg cooking has been investigated by exposing incurred eggs to thermal treatment at 80–90 °C for 5 min, with no fat or water added (98). Results of HPLC analyses showed that the exposure of eggs to temperature had no effect on the level of residues present before treatment.

17.4.3 Carbadox

In the presence of light, carbadox undergoes complete degradation within 6 h. Because of its known instability to light, carbadox stability in aqueous solutions has been extensively studied (16). Stored at room temperature in the dark, carbadox remains stable in solution for at least 1 week. Even when carbadox solutions were heated to 100 °C in the dark, a loss of only 20% occurred.

In view of these observations, uncooked samples of spiked kidney samples were stored under laboratory lighting for various periods corresponding to the cooking periods normally applied, to be examined for possible carbadox loss. Results showed that samples experienced only marginal loss over the cooking periods subsequently used. All samples were then subjected to boiling, baking, and frying and the water and oil from the first and last processes were checked for residues of carbadox. The drug completely disappeared within 15 min after boiling at 100 °C, within 20 min after baking at 100 °C, and within 8 min after frying at 120 °C.

17.4.4 Olaquindox

Since olaquindox is structurally similar to carbadox, stability studies have been conducted in a manner similar to carbadox (16). The results obtained paralleled the carbadox findings. In the presence of light, olaquindox completely disappeared from its aqueous solutions within 80 min. When samples of kidney tissue spiked with the drug were subjected to various cooking processes including boiling at

100 °C, baking at 110 °C, and frying at 160 °C, olaquindox completely disappeared within 15 min, 40 min, and 8 min, respectively.

17.5 RESIDUES OF ANABOLIC HORMONAL-TYPE GROWTH PROMOTERS: SOMIDOBONE

This polypeptide hormone constitutes one form of the recombinant bovine somatotropins used to increase milk production in dairy cows. Several studies have been performed in the United States, United Kingdom, and Germany to determine the concentrations of this drug in milk (99, 100).

Since the highest detectable level of somidobone found in milk from treated animals is 4.2 ppb, the effect of heat treatment on residues of this drug has been investigated in fresh, nonpasteurized milk spiked with somidobone in the range 0–20 ppb (101). It was found that pasteurization with the high-temperature–short-time technique at 72–78 °C for 15 s reduced the concentration of the drug by 70–79% of the initial dose. Batch pasteurization at 63–65.5 °C for 30 min reduced drug concentration by 94–95%, whereas no drug could be detected when milk was subjected to either direct or indirect UHT treatment at 133–142 °C for 2–4 s. These results agree well with other findings also demonstrating an 85–90% reduction upon pasteurization (102).

17.6 RESIDUES OF β-ADRENERGIC AGONISTS: CLENBUTEROL

Literature stability studies on residues of β-agonists in food are limited to clenbuterol. This is possibly due to the fact that many farmers throughout Europe continue to use this drug in cattle for increasing carcass weight, despite the European Community's ban on growth-promoting agents since 1985 (103). Because clenbuterol residues concentrate mainly in the liver of treated animals, stability studies have primarily targeted liver, but urine and muscle tissue have also been examined.

Clenbuterol has been found stable in lyophilized urine of veal calves kept at a temperature range of 4–37 °C for 1 year (104). In addition, boiling, braising, grilling, roasting, and microwaving have no net effect on clenbuterol residues in fortified and incurred tissues (105, 106). There is, however, some observed migration of residues from the tissue into the surrounding medium or meat juices during cooking.

In contrast to other cooking processes, frying has been found to exert a vanishing effect on clenbuterol residues, which is temperature dependent (106). The deeper the frying, the higher the vanishing effect (105). This is in agreement with other thermostability studies indicating that clenbuterol is stable in boiling

water at 100 °C, but unstable in cooking oil at 260 °C with a half-life of about
5 min (105).

17.7 RESIDUES OF SEDATIVE DRUGS

17.7.1 Azaperone

Stability studies have shown azaperone to be quite stable upon heating. When
samples of kidney, liver, bacon, and injection sites from pigs treated with azaperone were heat-pasteurized, no losses of the concentrations of the parent drug and
its main metabolite, azaperol, occurred (107).

17.7.2 Diazepam

The stability of diazepam and its metabolites (oxazepam, temazepam, and demeth-
yldiazepam) when present in liver of treated bulls has been studied (108). Following boiling in water for 1 h, the oxazepam metabolite was the most unstable of
the compounds studied, being degraded to an extent of approximately 50%. The
parent drug and the other metabolites were more stable: they were all present,
after treatment, at levels corresponding to 79–89% of the initial concentrations.

17.8 CONCLUSION

Drug stability studies show that regulatory authorities with responsibility for
residue monitoring programs might need to review the adequacy of arrangements
for sampling, dispatch, and transport of field samples to testing laboratories. The
rapid degradation, for example, of sulfaquinoxaline at refrigerator temperatures
suggests that refrigeration of samples may not be sufficient to maintain sample
integrity. It appears, nevertheless, that the minimum requirement is for samples
to be received at the laboratory frozen and then stored in the frozen condition
prior to analysis.

Residue-testing laboratories might also need to review their sample preparation processes and consider modifying or eliminating tissue homogenization prior
to residue extraction. Suppliers of proficiency-testing services should also question whether certain drugs are appropriate to include in such studies. For example,
liver spiked with sulfaquinoxaline, sulfadiazine, or sulfamerazine is not suitable
for preparation of spiked interlaboratory check samples or reference materials.

The information provided by the drug stability studies during food cooking
and processing demonstrate how subtle the prediction of consumer exposure to
drug residues may be. Some drugs, such as chloramphenicol and sulfamethazine,
are stable to cooking and, therefore, data obtained from surveillance of raw samples for residues of those drugs can be assumed to be directly applicable in
calculating dietary exposure and consumer intake.

Other drugs are unstable to cooking and, therefore, residues may be transformed to various derivatives or to a mixture of fragments of the initial compounds. When new products are formed, their identity should be established and their toxicity assessed. When an increase in the residues level is observed, it is possible that metabolites have been converted back into the parent compound after exposure to heat, or the cooking may have reversed an effect of drug binding. This is the case with meat from fish treated with oxolinic acid. Sometimes cooking may also affect the equilibrium between the parent drug and its metabolites, as found in the raw tissue, and sometimes new products may be formed, or a combination of these processes may occur, as is observed with residues of oxfendazole.

Even if drug stability during cooking is established in some tissue types, this data cannot be extrapolated for all tissue types, as demonstrated in the case of lasalocid, which was shown to be stable to cooking in chicken muscle, but not in egg where the pH is higher. Also, if a drug is stable, it may or may not exude from the tissue with juices into the surrounding medium during the cooking process.

Unfortunately, all cooking studies to date are not sufficiently comprehensive. To conduct a study for a single analyte and include all the possible food and tissue types, cooking or processing methods and times, pH values likely to be encountered such as cooking with vinegar or baking with sodium bicarbonate, solvent effects, such as cooking in wine, would be a very time-consuming and expensive task. Only a small selection of foods and recipes may be used for each analyte to indicate what may happen during cooking and processing.

REFERENCES

1. M. van Schothorst, in Antibiotic Residues in Slaughter Animals, Thesis, University of Utrecht, The Netherlands (1969).
2. J.J. O'Brien, N. Campbell, and T. Conaghan, J. Hyg. Camb., 87:511 (1981).
3. S. Konecny, Veternarstvi, 28:409 (1978).
4. J.M. Inglis and S.E. Katz, J. Assoc. Off. Anal. Chem., 61:1098 (1978).
5. S.E. Katz and P.R. Levine, J. Assoc. Off. Anal. Chem., 61:1103 (1978).
6. G. Scheibner, Monatsch. Veterinaermed., 27:941 (1972).
7. G. Scheibner, Monatsch. Veterinaermed., 27:161 (1972).
8. G. Scheibner, Monatsch. Veterinaermed., 27:745 (1972).
9. C. Pilet, and B. Toma, Rec. Med. Vet., 145:897 (1969).
10. C. Pilet, B. Toma, J. Muzet, and F. Renard, Cahier. Med. Vet., 6:227 (1969).
11. R.M. Parker and I.C. Shaw, Analyst, 113:1875 (1988).
12. J.F.M. Nouws and G. Ziv, Tijdschr. Diergeneeskd., 103:725 (1978).
13. T.J. Haley, Ecotoxicol. Environ. Safety, 2:9 (1978).
14. P. Sanders, P. Guillot, M. Dagorn, and J.M. Delmas, J. Assoc. Off. Anal. Chem., 74:483 (1991).

15. M.H. Costa, M.E. Soares, J.O. Fernandes, M.L. Bastos, and M. Ferreira, in Residues of Veterinary Drugs in Food, Proc. Euroresidue II Conf., Veldhoven, May 3–5, 1993 (N. Haagsma, A. Ruiter, and P.B. Czedik-Eysenberg, Eds.), Fac. Vet. Med., Univ. Utrecht, The Netherlands, p. 246 (1993).

16. T. Hassett, A.L. Patey, and G. Shearer, in Residues of Veterinary Drugs in Food, Proc. Euroresidue Conf., Noordwijkerhout, May 21–23, 1990 (N. Haagsma, A. Ruiter, and P.B. Czedik-Eysenberg, Eds.), Fac. Vet. Med., Univ. Utrecht, The Netherlands, p. 211 (1990).

17. R.L. Epstein, V. Randecker, P. Corrao, J.T. Keeton, and H. Russell Cross, J. Agric. Food Chem., 36:1009 (1988).

18. J.O. Miners, J. Liq. Chromatogr., 8:2827 (1985).

19. M. Petz, in Analysis of Antibiotic Drug Residues in Food Products of Animal Origin (V.P. Agarwal, Ed.), Plenum Press, New York, p. 147 (1992).

20. J.O. Boison, C.D.C. Salisbury, W. Chan, and J.D. MacNeil, J. Assoc. Off. Anal. Chem., 74:497 (1991).

21. A.M. DePaolis, S.E. Katz, and J.D. Rosen, J. Agric. Food Chem., 25:1112 (1991).

22. R. Guay, P. Cardinal, C. Bourassa, and N. Brassard, Int. J. Food Microb., 4:187 (1987).

23. B. Wiese, and K. Martin, J. Pharm. Biomed. Anal., 7:107 (1989).

24. J.O. Boison, G.O. Korsrud, J.D. MacNeil, W.D.G. Yates, and M.G. Papich, J. AOAC Int., 75:974 (1992).

25. H.-E. Gee, K.-B. Ho, and J. Toothhill, J. AOAC Int., 79:640 (1996).

26. H. Katznelson, and E.G. Hood, J. Dairy Sci., 32:961 (1949).

27. W.A. Krienke, Am. Milk Rev., 11:24 (1950).

28. F.C. Storrs and W. Hiett Brown, J. Dairy Res., 21:337 (1954).

29. F. Vigue, J. Am. Vet. Med. Assoc., 124:377 (1954).

30. H.C. Hansen, G.E. Wiggins, and J.C. Boyd, J. Milk Food Technol., 13:359 (1950).

31. J. Tropilo, Med. Weter., 41:276 (1985).

32. M.D. Rose, G. Shearer, and W.H.H. Farrington, in Residues of Veterinary Drugs in Food, Proc. Euroresidue III Conf., Veldhoven, 1996 (N. Haagsma and A. Ruiter, Eds.), Fac. Vet. Med., Univ. Utrecht, The Netherlands, p. 829 (1996).

33. S. Buncic and M. Dakic, Technol. Miesa, 22:66 (1981).

34. M.D. Rose, J. Bygrave, W.H.H. Farrington, and G. Shearer, Analyst, 122:1095 (1997).

35. S.E. Katz, C.A. Fassbender, A.M. dePaolis, and J.D. Rosen, J. Assoc. Off. Anal. Chem., 61:564 (1978).

36. J.J. Laurensen and J.F.M. Nouws, J. Chromatogr., 472:321 (1989).

37. G. Carignan, A.I. MacIntosh, and S. Sved, J. Agric. Food Chem., 38:716 (1990).

38. R.J. McCracken, W.J. Blanchflower, C. Rowan, M.A. McCoy, and D.G. Kennedy, Analyst, 120:2347 (1995).

39. J.F.M. Nouws and J.J. Laurensen, Vet. Q., 12:56 (1990).

40. O.W. Parks and L.F. Kubena, J. Assoc. Off. Anal. Chem., 73:526 (1990).

41. L.H.M. Vroomen, M.C.J. Berghmans, P. van Leeuwen, T.D.B. van der Struijs, P.T.H. de Vries, and H.A. Kuiper, Food Addit. Contam., 3:331 (1986).

42. L.A.P. Hoogenboom, M. van Kammen, M.C.J. Berghmans, J.H. Koeman, and H.A. Kuiper, Food Chem. Toxicol., 29:321 (1991).

43. R.J. McCracken and D.G. Kennedy, Food Addit. Contam., 14:507 (1997).
44. N.A. Botsoglou, D. Kufidis, A.B. Spais, and V.N. Vassilopoulos, Arch. Geflugelkd., 53:163 (1989).
45. A. Oeser and M. Petz, in Residues of Veterinary Drugs in Food, Proc. Euroresidue III Conf., Veldhoven, 1996 (N. Haagsma, and A. Ruiter, Eds.), Fac. Vet. Med., Univ. Utrecht, The Netherlands, p. 765 (1996).
46. M. Horie, K. Saito, Y. Hoshino, H. Terada, and H. Nakazawa, J. Food Hyg. Soc. Jpn. 38:329 (1997).
47. I. Steffenak, V. Hormazabal, and M. Yndestad, Acta Vet. Scand. 35:299 (1994).
48. I. Steffenak, V. Hormazabal, and M. Yndestad, Food Addit. Contam., 8:777 (1991).
49. S.C. Murtha, T.L. Brown, B. Chamberlain, and C.E. Lee, J. Agric. Food Chem., 25:556 (1977).
50. P.W. Saschenbrecker, and N.A. Fish, Can. J. Comp. Med., 44:338 (1980).
51. B.L. Cox, and L.F. Krzeminski, J. Assoc. Off. Anal. Chem., 65:1311 (1982).
52. N. Haagsma, R.J. Nooteboom, B.G.M. Gortemaker, and M.J. Maas, Z. Lebensm. Unters. Forsch., 181:194 (1985).
53. D.D. Giera, R.F. Abdulla, J.L. Occolowitz, D.E. Dorman, J.L. Mertz, and R.F. Sieck, J. Agric. Food Chem., 30:260 (1982).
54. O.W. Parks, J. Assoc. Off. Anal. Chem., 67:566 (1984).
55. G. Alfredsson and A. Ohlsson, Food Addit. Contam., 15:302 (1998).
56. M.D. Rose, W.H.H. Farrington, and G. Shearer, Food Addit. Contam., 12:739 (1995).
57. G.K. Thomas, R.G. Millar, and P.W. Anstis, J. AOAC Int., 80:988 (1997).
58. R.G. Millar, P. Armishaw, M.G. Wilson, and J.M. Majewski, Fresenius I Anal. Chem., 352:28 (1995).
59. O.W. Parks, J. Assoc. Off. Anal. Chem., 68:1232 (1985).
60. M. Sher Ali, J.D. White, R.S. Bakowski, and E.T. Phillippo, J. AOAC Int., 76: 1309 (1993).
61. O.W. Parks, J. AOAC Int., 77:486 (1994).
62. T. Hassett, A.L. Patey, and G. Shearer, in Residues of Veterinary Drugs in Food, Proc. Euroresidue II Conf., Veldhoven, May 3–5, 1993 (N. Haagsma, A. Ruiter, and P.B. Czedik-Eysenberg, Eds.), Fac. Vet. Med., Univ. Utrecht, The Netherlands, p. 415 (1993).
63. L.J. Fischer, A.J. Thulin, M.E. Zabic, A.M. Booren, R.H. Poppenga, and K.J. Chapman, J. Agric. Food Chem., 40:1677 (1992).
64. D.H. Xu, J.M. Grizzle, W.A. Rogers, and C.R. Santerre, Food Addit. Contam. Food Res. Int., 29:339 (1996).
65. L.A. Smit, L.A.P. Hoogenboom, M.C.J. Berghmans, and N. Haagsma, Z. Lebensm.-Unters. Und-Forsch., 198:480 (1994).
66. L.A. Smit, N. Haagsma, and A. Ruiter, Z. Lebensm.-Unters. Und-Forsch., 206:94 (1998).
67. N. Haagsma and J.T. van Elteren, Proc. 32nd Eur. Meeting of Meat Research Workers, Ghent, Belgium, p. 481 (1986).
68. L.I. Ellerbroek and G. Steffen, Int. J. Food Sci. Technol., 26:479 (1991).
69. A. Koole, L.A. Smit, and N. Haagsma, in Residues of Veterinary Drugs in Food, Proc. Euroresidue Conf., Noordwijkerhout, May 21–23, 1990 (N. Haagsma, A.

Ruiter, and P.B. Czedik-Eysenberg, Eds.), Fac. Vet. Med., Univ. Utrecht, The Netherlands, p. 829 (1990).

70. D.D. Kitts, C.W.Y. Yu, R.G. Aoyama, H.M. Burt, and K. McErlane, J. Agric. Food Chem., 40:1977 (1992).

71. K.M. Shahani, J. Dairy Sci., 40:289 (1957).

72. K.M. Shahani, J. Dairy Sci., 41:382 (1958).

73. W.A. Moats, J. Food Prot., 51:491 (1988).

74. I. Yonova, Vet.-Med. Nauki, 8:75 (1971).

75. M.D. Rose, J. Bygrave, W.H.H. Farrington, and G. Shearer, Food Addit. Contam., 13:275 (1996).

76. T.S. Huang, W.X. Du, M.R. Marshall, and C.I. Wei, J. Agric. Food Chem., 45:2602 (1997).

77. W.X. Du, M.R. Marshall, D.H. Xu, and C.R. Santerre, J. Food Sci., 62:119 (1997).

78. O.I. Escanilla, A.F. Carlin, and J.C. Ayres, Food Technol., 13:520 (1959).

79. M.E. Bernarde, J. Am. Diet. Assoc., 33:1145 (1957).

80. K.O. Honikel, Fleischwirtschaft, 56:722 (1976).

81. K.O. Honikel, U. Schmidt, W. Woltersdorf, and L. Leistner, J. Assoc. Off. Anal. Chem., 61:1222 (1978).

82. S.Y. Hsu, J. Chin. Agric. Chem. Soc., 35:573 (1997).

83. R. Maruyama, and K. Uno, J. Food Hyg. Soc. Jpn., 38:425 (1997).

84. A. Ibrahim, and W.A. Moats, J. Agric. Food Chem., 42:2561 (1994).

85. R.W. Fedeniuk, P.J. Shand, and A.R. Mccurdy, J. Agric. Food Chem., 45:2252 (1997).

86. D.J. Fletouris, N.A. Botsoglou, I.E. Psomas, and A.I. Mantis, Anal. Chim. Acta, 345:111 (1997).

87. D.J. Fletouris, N.A. Botsoglou, I.E. Psomas, and A.I. Mantis, J. Food Prot., 61:1484 (1998).

88. M.D. Rose, G. Shearer, and W.H.H. Farrington, Food Addit. Contam., 14:15 (1997).

89. S.Y. Hsu, and R.L. Epstein, in Residues of Veterinary Drugs in Food, Proc. Euroresidue II Conf., Veldhoven, May 3–5, 1993 (N. Haagsma, A. Ruiter and P.B. Czedik-Eysenberg, Eds.), Fac. Vet. Med., Univ. Utrecht, The Netherlands, p. 387 (1993).

90. M.D. Rose, L.C. Argent, G. Shearer, and W.H.H. Farrington, Food Addit. Contam., 12:185 (1995).

91. M.D. Rose, W.H.H. Farrington, and G. Shearer, Food Addit. Contam., 15:157 (1998).

92. P. Slanina, J. Kuivinen, C. Ohlsen, and L.G. Ekstrom, Food Addit. Contam., 6:475 (1989).

93. J. Kuivinen and P. Slanina, Vaar Foeda, 38:280 (1986).

94. O.W. Parks, J. AOAC Int., 76:698 (1993).

95. M.D. Rose, L. Rowley, G. Shearer, and W.H.H. Farrington, J. Agric. Food Chem., 45:927 (1997).

96. C.A. Kan, H.W. van Gend, and M.M.L. Aerts, in Residues of Veterinary Drugs in Food, Proc. Euroresidue Conf., Noordwijkerhout, May 21–23, 1990 (N. Haagsma, A. Ruiter, and P.B. Czedik-Eysenberg, Eds.), Fac. Vet. Med., Univ. Utrecht, The Netherlands, p. 231 (1990).

97. K. Sinigoj-Gacnik, in Residues of Veterinary Drugs in Food, Proc. Euroresidue Conf., Noordwijkerhout, May 21–23, 1990 (N. Haagsma, A. Ruiter, and P.B. Czedik-Eysenberg, Eds.), Fac. Vet. Med., Univ. Utrecht, The Netherlands, p. 859 (1990).
98. M.M.L. Aerts, in Residues of Veterinary Drugs in Edible Products, An Analytical Approach, Thesis, Free University, Amsterdam (1990).
99. C.M. Zwickl, H.W. Smith, and P.H. Bick, J. Agric. Food Chem., 38:1358 (1990).
100. D. Schams, in Use of Somatotropin in Livestock Production (K. Sejzsen, M. Vestergaard, and A. Neimann-Sorensen, Eds.), Elsevier Applied Science, Amsterdam, The Netherlands, p. 192 (1989).
101. M.R. Coleman, H.W. Smith, C.M. Zwickl, C.H. Marsden, P.H. Bick, M.L. Heiman, F.C. Tinsley, J. Saunders, and J. Wilkinson, in Residues of Veterinary Drugs in Food, Proc. Euroresidue Conf., Noordwijkerhout, May 21–23, 1990 (N. Haagsma, A. Ruiter, and P.B. Czedik-Eysenberg, Eds.), Fac. Vet. Med., Univ. Utrecht, The Netherlands, p. 134 (1990).
102. P.P. Groenewegan, B.W. McBride, and J.H. Burton, J. Dairy Sci., 72:6 (1989).
103. J.F. Martinez-Navarro, Lancet, 336:1311 (1990).
104. L.A. van Ginkel, R.W. Stephany, H.J. van Rossum, and M. Bos, in Residues of Veterinary Drugs in Food, Proc. Euroresidue II Conf., Veldhoven, May 3–5, 1993 (N. Haagsma, A. Ruiter and P.B. Czedik-Eysenberg, Eds.), Fac. Vet. Med., Univ. Utrecht, The Netherlands, p. 308 (1993).
105. M.D. Rose, G. Shearer, and W.H.H. Farrington, Food Addit. Contam., 12:67 (1995).
106. F. Ramos, M.C. Castilho, and M.I.N. Silveira, in Residues of Veterinary Drugs in Food, Proc. Euroresidue II Conf., Veldhoven, May 3–5, 1993 (N. Haagsma, A. Ruiter, and P.B. Czedik-Eysenberg, Eds.), Fac. Vet. Med., Univ. Utrecht, The Netherlands, p. 563 (1993).
107. A.G. Rauws and M. Olling, J. Vet. Pharmacol. Ther., 1:57 (1978).
108. M.-de-L. Bastos and M.E. Soares, J. Agric. Food Chem., 41:965 (1993).

18

Consumer Perceptions and Concerns

Years ago, food was produced and processed in the proximity of our home, cooked in our kitchen, and consumed in the same place of preparation. Today, food can be produced in Australia, processed and packed in the United Kingdom, and distributed in various countries on the same or different continents. In addition, the number of foodstuffs offered to the consumer is a hundred to a thousand times greater than in the beginning of this century.

Production methods, particularly in the field of edible animal products, are currently at the leading edge of technology and it may be that, temporarily at least, production technology is surpassing control technology. This causes a series of problems, and a number of serious incidents of food poisoning in various countries have focused public attention on the object as never before. The fortunate assumption that the food we eat today is totally safe has been rudely disturbed by these events, which have led to healthy food of good quality becoming a political issue. The press, the public, and politicians have doubts concerning the efficacy of food inspection services, their resources and competence, the adequacy of food hygiene standards and regulations, the rigor of epidemiological surveys, and the health of the food systems as a whole.

In Western countries, governments have been put under pressure through campaigns to create and strengthen food laws to give protection to consumers and to ensure an adequate and safe food supply. Food has been a main item on the consumer agenda for as long as consumer organizations have been active. Pertinent studies and tests have been carried out, and as a result numerous articles have been published in consumer magazines informing and educating consumers

542 Chapter 18

about the food they eat. As a result, concerns about an adequate food supply and the discussion of food security have been replaced by increasing concerns about food safety and the adequacy of controls. This is demonstrated by the numerous public debates about food issues and the growing market for products with a healthy image.

Attitude studies show that food scares have undermined consumer confidence in both products and control systems. A survey conducted in 1994 by the Food Marketing Institute indicated that 72% of the respondents believed that residues were something of a hazard, 3% thought that residues were not a hazard, and 1% were not sure (1). Consumer reliance on food safety almost doubled in 1996–1997; surveys conducted in the United States on the level of confidence among consumers in the safety of their food showed that residues of antibiotics and hormones in poultry and livestock were seen as serious hazards by 43% of the shoppers queried about specific health hazards in their food supply (2). Consumers believed that their food was safe enough to eat but some underlying concerns prevented them from expressing complete confidence in the food supply. Consumers had generally very limited knowledge of the government's role in regulating the safety of food supply, and, therefore, not as much trust. It is evident that food safety is one of the most visible and emotional issues confronting affluent societies (3).

Concerns with antibiotic use have centered on the potential development of antibiotic-resistant strains of bacteria, and allergic or physiological responses. Customer perceptions about food safety differed by gender, age, and education level. Women were more concerned about quality control and pesticides than men, whereas consumers with at least some college education were more concerned with spoilage and bacteria/germs contamination than those with only a high school education.

In contrast to Western countries, concerns of consumer organizations in developing countries about food supply and consumers' access to food are still high. This is due to the fact that for many third world consumers access to food is a matter of life and death. Food standards and regulations are minimal and in some cases even nonexistent in these countries, since the technological means to control food quality is often missing due to lack of funds. Food adulteration is therefore a common annoyance and danger to consumers' health.

In view of the present situation where the role of governments as regulators becomes less important, consumer organizations in both developed and developing countries face a shift from national regulatory approaches to agreements that will be settled at the regional and international level. Producers, industry, and retailers are very well organized at the regional and international level. They have good access to the new food bureaucracy and are involved in the decisionmaking process at a very early stage. Consumer organizations also have to become professional negotiating partners and become recognized as such. The European Community and at the international level, the Codex Alimentarius Commission are more and more becoming the bodies that develop the guidelines for food standards.

Rules for setting international food standards must respect consumer demands and consumer protection should be their first aim. It is consumers who eat food, who pay for it, and who face the consequences of the risks inherent in evaluation procedures. Consumer concern about whether selected food attributes constitute some health hazard presents a complex picture, frequently giving a different view from that of the scientist. Where concern exists, it relates to lack of awareness or trust in regulatory procedures. A recent study (4) shows that part of this distrust is due to the human tendency to remember and focus on those areas where recommended practices change. Some consumers see it as a weakness of the regulatory decisions when dietary or safety recommendations change. It is said, for example, that if you trace back far enough, people were once advised to have a breakfast of bacon and eggs; then egg consumption was discouraged because of cholesterol, and bacon because of high fat. Now, recommendations appear to change again as some scientists report that eggs are not so bad after all.

Food means more to consumers than a simple set of formulas. The way people look upon their food is based on certain norms, values, and traditions. The preparation of food, food habits, and food consumption are all part of a culture. These cultures are decisive in laying down rules on which occasions what kind of food is eaten. Food consumption patterns are imbedded in social and cultural life. This is reflected by the fact that consumption patterns are different in different countries.

Consumers want to keep control over what they eat and what is in their food. Cholesterol and saturated fat content have been perceived by the public as less serious than microbial pathogens or chemical residues (1) because consumers can count fat intakes by reading the labels and many have been diligent in this respect. In doing so, consumers can avoid fat. However, it is impossible to avoid drug residues. Too many questions are being asked on the use of and need for drugs in food-producing animals, the findings of antibiotic residues in food, and the illegal (in several countries) use of hormones. In developing countries, consumers also ask questions about contaminated food, lack of controls, and low safety standards. Food hygiene, in general, is becoming a major issue in both developed and developing countries.

Consumers are not willing to accept foreign and unknown substances in their food except if they are useful, they are savory, and will increase the nutritional value or taste of food. For instance, the presence of antibiotic residues in milk reduces the desire to drink it, although these agents are harmless in the levels detected. Public opinion sometimes is not correct. It is not necessary to explain the reason: it may depend on public information disseminated by some reporters in the newspapers or on television. Nevertheless, public opinion is the base for political decisions, if there is a majority for this opinion.

Consumers want to exercise their right to choose. Consumer choice is a leading consumer principle. It is viewed by consumer organizations as a prime condition to establish consumer sovereignty in the marketplace. Sometimes, however, consumers cannot be provided with a choice; for example, because of the high costs involved in separating bovine somatotropin-treated milk from untreated milk, it is unlikely that treated and untreated milk will be sold separately. Consumers are denied a choice between alternatives and thus the introduction of bovine somatotropin should not be allowed. To exercise consumer choice, it is necessary to know from what to choose and about what to choose. Consumers find it increasingly difficult to access food products in terms of quality, health, price, and nutrients. This puts heavy requirements on the labeling of foodstuffs.

However, consumer choice has its limitations. It does not automatically follow that more choice is always desirable or necessary. Linked to the satisfaction of consumer choice is the availability of information.

The introduction of new technologies, for example, genetic modification, raises questions on the ethical, cultural, and religious level. Our world is in a stage of rapid change in which people are exposed to an increasing number of new drugs, technical products, and waste materials. The introduction of new products and technologies to the market should take place with careful consideration. Public opinion is increasingly concerned about the harmful effects they might have, not only obvious toxicity, but also long-term effects that are hard to detect or affect only few people exposed separately, or genetic damage, among others. Public opinion does not differentiate between the possibility of a harmful effect and the reality of this effect (i.e., between hazard and risk). This may lead to a growing conflict between consumer interest and producer interest. Consumers become more interested in food items that have changed little from their original state and/or that are made in an animal-friendly and environmentally sound way. Producers are interested in gaining more consumers and creating new markets. They try to bring many new products on the market, which does not always reflect consumer demands.

The developments through which governments want to arrive at internationally accepted food standards should be a careful balancing of criteria and include consumer interests. Safety assessments as such, without looking at other consumer interests, is a far too narrow approach. At the moment, safety is used as the only criterion to assess products. Even in the few cases in which other criteria have been added, safety has been looked upon as the most relevant. For consumer organizations, this approach is no longer sufficient. Safety assessments are based on scientific evidence, which clearly has its limitations. Science is not free of values and expert statements address values as well as facts. Experts can change their minds and scientific evidence therefore is often uncertain. Sometimes scientists reach different conclusions although they assess the same evidence.

In the debates on food, scientific questions have played a prominent role. However, food problems are about public choices and thus involve more than scientific assessments. Good science is absolutely essential for sound policy choices, but it cannot make the value judgments to decide which choice is best for consumers. It is consumers who take the risk when buying and eating the new products. They should therefore be involved in the assessment procedures. Government bodies should work together with consumer groups to adapt assessment techniques and further develop procedures and a consumer checklist of issues that should be considered when judging food substances or processes.

In the area of risk communication, the regulatory agencies should continue to be flexible in the way information is presented to the public regarding drug residues. Continuing efforts are needed to combat false and misleading consumer perceptions of the hazards of drug residues in the tissues of food animals.

The public is repeatedly presented with information that is conflicting, often times misleading, and usually critical of food regulatory agencies. For example, food scientists can tell consumers that today's milk is the best it's ever been and they know it is. Most dairy farmers and most dairy practitioners are currently diligent in ensuring that illegal drugs are not allowed to contaminate our milk supply. However, this is not enough when consumers hear that drug residues are present in milk. They do not know whom to believe. Rarely are they told that there is great difference between residues and violative residues from a toxicological point of view. However, such concerns, whether warranted or not, can do serious damage to milk's good image and affect consumer behavior. If the milk cannot be sold, there is no need for it to be produced. In this case, industry's best defense and the approach that promises the greatest public health advantage for the consumer is information. Perception becomes more important than reality.

The extent to which perception can become reality has been demonstrated over time; for example, consumer activism in the 1960s led to the enactment of the Wholesome Meat Act of 1967 and the Wholesome Poultry Products Act of 1968. Food safety became again a sensitive political topic during the early 1990s. Widely publicized cases of food contamination, foodborne illness and death became front page headlines in newspapers and in *Time* and *Newsweek* magazines. This awakening of the American public was particularly marked by concern over drugs, pesticides, and other chemical residues in foods. Then in 1993, with the foodborne outbreak of *Escherichia coli* O157:N7, consumers were further riveted as national attention was focused on the vulnerability of our food chain to disease-causing pathogens and possible drug and chemical residues. This outbreak caused many Washington DC-based consumer advocacy groups to exert pressure, via lobbying Congress and demanding that policymakers do something to ensure a safe food supply.

It is currently very easy to get time in the press by claiming knowledge of some danger in the food supply. Several groups have seized this opportunity with the issue of drug residues and antimicrobial resistance. For example, *Escherichia coli* O157:H7 is now recognized as an important human pathogen (5). The mode of transmission is primarily through the food; however, person-to-person transmission also has been identified in some day care center and nursing home outbreaks (6). Illness and death due to this pathogen have placed cattle under increased scrutiny. Special interest groups are ready to make accusations and establish blame wherever they can. Once again, industry's best defense is information. Recordkeeping as to antibiotic use and factors correlated with the presence of *Escherichia coli* O157:H7 are essential to create an informed public. Should a crisis arise in this area, producers, veterinarians, and regulators need data to quantify drug use and industry practices.

Concern about drug residues may sometimes be fueled by marketing practices and promotional material, produced by some industry and special interest groups. Some stores advertise that their products are free of such agents as hormones, steroids, and antibiotics. This advertisement creates an impression of difference when none exists. This could be considered deceptive advertising, and it contributes to consumer anxiety about the safety of animal production practices. A widespread consumer perception is that poultry is loaded with growth hormones, although these are never in fact used in poultry industry. In a consumer survey conducted in California, 10% of persons surveyed said they were eating less poultry because of concern about hormone residues (7).

In addition, faulty food testing procedures may create an impression that residues are more prevalent than is actually the case. It has been suggested, without supporting evidence, that cases of premature menarche observed in Puerto Rico were a result of growth hormone residues in chickens (8).

Concern may also arise from information dissemination by special interest groups that use the potential of health concerns to promote their organization. The example of bovine somatotropin illustrates this practice. The US Foundation on Economic Trends initiated a vigorous campaign questioning milk's safety from cows receiving supplemental bovine somatotropin. Other, more moderate, groups have echoed this concern. The health and environmental benefits of use of bovine somatotropin in cattle were not told. Consumers never heard that bovine somatotropin allows the animals to use feed more efficiently which is an environmental benefit since fewer resources will be used and less manure produced. Neither were they told that use of growth hormones in beef cattle has an insignificant effect on muscle estrogen level but increases the ratio of lean muscle to fat (2). Research indicated that consumer concerns stopped increasing by the time leading medical and health groups affirmed the safety of milk produced from cows receiving bovine somatotropin (9). With the exception of Wisconsin, where the bovine somatotropin debate became highly politicized, the effectiveness of this fear campaign was limited (10), and milk sales across the United States were again increased.

Inappropriate animal care and management can also contribute to a declining confidence in the production and regulation systems (7). Consumers in Western countries are becoming more critical of the way cattle is raised in intensive production. Most countries in the world have become more urbanized and people have less knowledge of farm practices and challenges. As a result, people are very sensitive to pictures of animals that are ill or injured. Animal welfare has become a consumer issue: consumers have expressed an interest in buying free-range eggs and hormone-free beef. Also consumers are looking at safety in relation to animal welfare from an ethical point of view. This aspect is even outlined in the Dutch food legislation. A product advertised in a trade publication as being capable to turn a cow "into a factory" is not well received by the public and may tarnish the reputation of integrity and responsibility of the whole food industry.

Because consumers get most of their information from the media (11, 12), responsible presentation of food safety issues is needed. When US newspaper editors, who cover food safety issues, were asked about where they receive the information they write about, government agencies and consumer groups received the highest scores as communicators with the media on food safety issues with 60% and 54%, respectively; food manufacturers and processors received the lowest. When the editors were asked about who provides the best source of information, government agencies and universities both received scores of 77% in the credibility of information on food safety, whereas food manufacturers and processors were described as the least useful sources.

Recent surveys have shown that more than one-fourth (29%) of United States consumers rely primarily on themselves to ensure the food they eat is safe (1). Surprisingly, consumers' reliance was higher on manufacturers than government, with scores of 23% and 20%, respectively; this is a dramatic change compared to 1988, when three times as many consumers relied on the government as on industry. Therefore, continuous information to consumers, particularly by health authorities, on the purpose of various food animal production practices and each person's responsibility in ensuring food safety is essential to create an informed public and to contribute further to public confidence.

A total of 88% of the US newspaper editors believed that the public would put the heaviest responsibility for food safety on the government. According to editors, consumers see food producers as the next most responsible for food safety, while seeing themselves as the least responsible. Consumers believe food safety could be improved by the government developing and enforcing strict regulations, producers and processors following strict standards, and consumers adopting safe handling practices (13). Consumers know that regulators cannot be everywhere, but they expect high compliance from a regulatory and checking system with enforcement that is rigorous and poses significant fines.

Producers might rethink standards based on voluntary compliance. If standards are not followed universally, the entire industry may suffer from lost public confidence and lost sales. Given today's sensitivities and the huge selection of options in the supermarket, consumers will readily abandon entire food categories on the slightest suspicion. Therefore, continued alertness and sensitivity to the concerns of an urban public are necessary. Consumer concerns should be addressed by vigorous safety testing, monitoring, enforcement, responsible advertising, and information dissemination.

REFERENCES

1. J.E. Riviere, Agri-practice, 13:11 (1992).
2. Food Marketing Institute, Trends in the United States, Consumer Attitudes and the Supermarket, 1998, Food Marketing Institute, Washington, DC (1998).
3. Food Marketing Institute, Trends in the United States, Consumer Attitudes and the Supermarket, 1988, Food Marketing Institute, Washington, DC (1988).
4. C.M. Bruhn, S. Peterson, P. Phillips, and N. Sakovich, J. Food Safety, 12:315 (1992).
5. L.W. Riley, R.S. Remis, S.D. Helgerson, H.B. McGee, J.G. Wells, B.R. Davis, R.J. Herbert, E.S. Olcott, L.M. Johnson, N.T. Hargrett, P.A. Blake, and M.L. Cohen, N. Engl. J. Med., 308:681 (1983).
6. N.V. Padhye and M.P. Doyle, J. Food Prot., 55:555 (1992).
7. C.M. Bruhn, in Veterinary Drug Residues, Food Safety (W.A. Moat and M.B. Medina, Eds.), American Chemical Society, Washington, DC, p. 18 (1996).
8. W.A. Moats, and M.B. Medina, Veterinary Drug Residues, Food Safety (W.A. Moats and M.B. Medina, Eds.), American Chemical Society, Washington, D.C., p. vii (1996).
9. T.J. Hoban, in Consumer Awareness and Acceptance of Bovine Somatotropin (BST), North Carolina State University (1994).
10. L.B. Bradford, F.H. Buttel, and D.B. Jackson-Smith, American Association for the Advancement of Science, Annual Meeting, Atlanta, GA, (1995).
11. Center for Produce Quality, in Fading Scares—Future Concerns: Trends in Consumer Attitudes Toward Food Safety, Produce Marketing Association, Alexandria, VA (1992).
12. T.J. Hoban, and P.A. Kendall, in Consumer Attitudes about the Use of Biotechnology in Agriculture and Food Production, North Carolina State University, Raleigh, NC (1992).
13. Food Marketing Institute, Trends in the United States, Consumer Attitudes and the Supermarket, 1994, Food Marketing Institute, Washington, DC (1994).

19

The Analytical Challenge

Since the main objectives of the regulatory control of residues of veterinary drugs are to ensure a safe and wholesome food supply and to take regulatory action after identification of adulterated products, analysts are usually challenged to analyze, often on a routine basis, for a wide range of physicochemically and structurally highly different compounds, some of which may be used illegally or entered unexpectedly the food chain via contamination of animal feeds. This challenge may be better comprehended considering the number of the veterinary drugs currently available in the market. Several hundred active veterinary drugs are commercially available, and at least 75 of them are being used more or less extensively in food-producing animals.

The extremely low concentrations at which drug residues occur often in meat, milk, or eggs represent by themselves a major analytical challenge. The concentration of drugs and metabolites in foods of animal origin is in many cases at the part per billion or even in the part per trillion level, thus necessitating use of selective separation and sensitive detection procedures. The analytical challenge in detecting 1 part per billion may be better described by considering the difficulty in identifying five named individuals in the whole world population. Even with the great variety of the currently available separation/detection systems, it is not always possible to achieve the desired detection limit at an acceptable precision without prior application of some form of special sample preparation procedure, such as derivatization of the analyte (1–5). Factors responsible for analyte losses during sample preparation are becoming most critical at low concentrations and can adversely affect the reliability of analytical results.

Moreover, most of the drug administered to food-producing animals is enzymatically oxidized, reduced, or hydrolyzed, in phase I of the metabolic process, to give more polar forms that can be readily excreted from the animal organism. The number of these metabolites in the edible animal products may range from 0, as in the case of aminoglycosides (6), to more than 20 as, for example, with chlorpromazine (7). Many of such metabolites must be identified and quantitatively determined, particularly in cases in which the metabolites are more toxic than the parent drug, as has been clearly demonstrated in the case of the desoxy metabolite of carbadox in swine (8).

The parent drug or metabolites produced in phase I can also be biotransformed, during phase II of the metabolic process, to water-soluble conjugates, primarily by glucuronidation, sulfatation, acetylation, or conjugation with glycine. Direct determination of these conjugates is often very difficult because they are very polar and often poorly extractable compounds. Furthermore, the possibility of formation of several different conjugates from the same parent compound or from a primary metabolite makes analytical results difficult to interpret as pertinent synthesized standards are usually not available in the market. In this case, cleavage of these conjugates by hydrolysis with hydrochloric acid or by enzymatic incubation with β-glucuronidase or arylsulfatase may be a necessary sample preparation step. In many instances, however, the enzyme itself and decomposition products formed during the deconjugation step may give rise to chromatographic interferences as it has been noted in the analysis of chloramphenicol residues in milk (8).

Besides, for those drugs where information is available with regard to relevant metabolites such as for sulfonamides, chloramphenicol, or carbadox, the analytical methods should be capable of detecting both the parent compound and metabolites. For drugs such as nitrofurans, for which the metabolic profile has not been fully elucidated, the analysis has to be necessarily focused solely on the parent compound. In the latter case, however, the presence of structurally related but unknown metabolites may interfere with the analysis and further confirmation is normally required. Furthermore, serious analytical difficulties may sometimes come out even when the drug is not significantly metabolized, as in the case of the aminoglycosides class of drugs for which specific reference standards corresponding to the individual components of each drug, which are needed for quantification, are not commercially available.

The analytical challenge becomes greater when one considers the multitude of endogenous compounds are normally present in such complex biological matrices, often at concentrations much higher than the analytes themselves. Many of these endogenous compounds have reactive functional groups that can interfere with the detection of the compounds of interest, if they are not sufficiently separated by some type of sample cleanup prior to analysis. Although analyte isolation from the matrix may be superfluous in the case of a very selective detection technique, procedures for selective extraction of the analyte, removal of coextractants, and sensitive and specific detection should be equal to this challenge. Hence, in developing a suitable analytical method for drug residues in foods, the chemical composition of the sample should always be taken into account by the analyst is faced with this challenge. Although the regulatory control of residues of veterinary drugs in meat, milk, or eggs is generally performed by analyzing the particular edible animal product, it is sometimes equally attractive for screening purposes to perform the analysis on body fluids such as urine, plasma, or saliva. These matrices are generally easier to collect and analyze and they usually contain elevated levels of drug residues.

Urine is a biological matrix easily amenable to extraction with organic solvents since it does not readily produce emulsions or foams due to the absence of proteins or lipids. The most serious disadvantage of urine analysis is the great number of endogenous components with molecular weights ranging from about 17 up to 70,000, which may interfere with the analysis of drug residues.

Its composition varies with the animal species and particularly the animal diet. As a result, its color may vary from dark amber to pale, while its pH can vary from 4 to 9. Upon standing, urine gradually throws out CO_2 and becomes more alkaline, favoring the precipitation of the dissolved phosphates and organic salts. It is therefore essential that urine samples be buffered to a certain pH prior to analysis, and that the analytical method be validated for a variety of urine samples obtained at different time points from different animals and species.

Many drugs are excreted in the urine as conjugates. Since the free nonconjugated drug fraction shows usually a large intra- and interanimal variation, it is customary to treat urine samples with an enzymatic combination of β-glucuronidase/arylsulfatase in order to release the conjugated fraction. However, the added enzyme itself and decomposition products formed during the deconjugation process may give rise to an increase in chromatographic interference.

Unlike urine, plasma contains about 7% proteins and a substantial amount of lipids, salts, and enzymes, especially esterases. The pH of plasma is approximately 7.4. Despite its complex nature, plasma exhibits a composition that hardly varies within the animal species and the diet, except for the lipid content, which is diet-dependent.

Because of the high affinity between some drugs and plasma proteins, one can differentiate between the free or unbound and total concentration of the drug. Binding proteins in plasma include albumin, α-acid glycoprotein, lipoproteins, and γ-globulins (9). Although the free fraction of a drug can be considered the physiologically active portion that governs the residue level in tissues, for screening purposes the total drug content will be measured in most cases because the free drug concentration may be extremely low when the drug is highly protein-bound. After establishment of the percentage protein binding, the result of the free fraction assay is then supposed to correlate with the tissue residue level. In practice, however, the free fraction is to some extent concentration-dependent, decreasing at lower drug levels (10), whereas it is greatly influenced by the pathological state of the animal (9).

Analysis of saliva can sometimes replace the analysis of plasma samples since a constant ratio between plasma and saliva concentrations can exist for a number of drugs. The amount of the analyte excreted in saliva depends on both the degree of protonation and the extent of protein binding, implying that neutral analytes that do not tend to bind to proteins can be found in relatively high concentrations in this matrix.

A much more frequently analyzed matrix in the field of drug residues in foods is milk. Cow milk has a pH value of 6.7, and contains 3.3% proteins, mainly casein (78%); 3.7% lipids, mainly triglycerides; and 4.7% carbohydrates, mainly lactose. The composition of milk is influenced by genetic factors, the physiological condition of the animal, climate, and the diet (11). Apart from that, the composition may change upon storage as a result of oxidation, enzymatic conversions, and growth of microorganisms. Milk contains a number of naturally occurring microorganism-inhibiting substances that can be inactivated by heating (12). These include the enzymes peroxidase and lysozyme, a number of immuno-globulins that may agglutinate gram-positive bacteria, and lactoferrin, which inhib-its the analytically important bacteria *B. stearothermophilus* and *B. subtilis.*

As a matrix, milk can be considered an emulsion of fat particles in an aqueous milk plasma. However, the membrane of these fat particles is much more complex than an ordinary emulsion globule membrane, and consists of a mixture of water, proteins, lipids, enzymes, minerals, phosphatides, and other compounds. Moreover, milk plasma is not homogenous, being a colloidal solution of globular proteins and a dispersion of lipoproteins and casein micelles. Globular proteins and lipoproteins constitute the proteins of serum, whereas the casein micelles consist of casein proteins, inorganic salts, water, and enzymes. Casein micelles can be precipitated by acidification to pH 4.6 or by heating above 120°C. Serum proteins are not precipitated at this pH but become insoluble upon heating above 80°C.

Because of the physicochemically different phases in milk, drugs will some-times be distributed unevenly and may remain predominantly in one phase after, for example, acidification or decreaming. Table 19.1 gives some examples of the distribution of a number of antibacterial drugs over cream, casein, and whole goat milk, as established by radiolabeled studies (13). The distribution depends both on the residue concentration range and the route of administration. The latter can be explained by the trapping of the more lipophilic compounds by the fat globules during their formation in the milk-secreting cells in the udder cavity. Since drug residues are transported from the bloodstream to the milk within the udder by passive diffusion, nondissociated apolar compounds are most easily transported, and it is therefore unlikely that polar drug conjugates such as glucu-ronides will be found in milk (13). When a drug is added after the fat globule is

TABLE **19.1**   Distribution of Radiolabeled Antibacterials over Cream, Casein, and Whole Goat Milk

Antibacterial	Administration route	Distribution of the drug in cream/whole milk	Distribution of the drug in casein/whole milk
Benzylpenicillin	Intramammary infusion	0.3–0.5	1.0–1.1
	Intramuscular injection	1.0–2.1	0.8–3.2
Chloramphenicol	Intramammary infusion	1.1–2.3	2.2–24.8
	Intramuscular injection	7.4–8.1	22.4–24.5
DH-Streptomycin	Intramammary infusion	0.3–0.6	1.3–400
	Intramuscular injection	1.0	260
Spiramycin	Intramammary infusion	0.4–0.9	1.5–22.8
	Intramuscular injection	0.9	22.6
Tetracycline	Intramammary infusion	0.4–0.7	2.0–22.4
	Intramuscular injection	1.1–3.2	25.6–726

Source: From Ref. 13.

formed, as in the case of intramammary injection or even when spiking a sample, the enrichment in the fat globules apparently does not take place to the same extent. As in plasma, drugs can also be protein-bound in milk. Therefore, the distribution of a drug residue over the various milk phases should be established for each individual drug.

In contrast to milk, where samples are primarily derived from cows, meat analysis has to be performed in samples of a widely different animal origin including cattle, lamb, swine, poultry, and fish. Muscle is a complex matrix with a pH of 5.7, composed of muscle fibers, various types of connective tissue, adipose tissue, cartilage, and bones. Sarcoplasmic proteins such as myoglobin, and glycolytic enzymes are soluble in water while the myofibrillar proteins such as myosin and actin are soluble in concentrated salt solutions (14). The connective tissue proteins, collagen and elastin, are insoluble in both solvents.

Fish muscle tissue, in particular, is a very peculiar matrix because of its high content of nonprotein nitrogen. Nonprotein nitrogen content in fish is much higher than that in terrestrial animals, amounting to 9–18% of the total nitrogen content (15). This implies that the nonprotein nitrogen amounts to 1.5–4% of the total fish weight but only 1% of the total weight of a terrestrial animal. Nonprotein nitrogen represents a class of ionogenic matrix components that, in most fish species, is mainly composed of amino acids, creatine and creatinine, trimethylamine oxide, nucleotides, amides, and ammonia. These fish components have the potential to create extractability problems to drugs or metabolites that occur in a charged form.

Apart from differences between muscle tissues from various parts of an animal, there are qualitative and quantitative differences in composition between animal species. Therefore, analytical methods will always have to be tested on material from each individual species, since differences in fat composition, in the presence of species-specific proteins, and in colored components such as in the case of myoglobin in poultry and beef may influence both the extraction and the separation of the analytes. As an example, a recovery higher than 70% was obtained for furazolidone after spiking chicken and veal calf muscle tissue but only 10% after spiking pork tissue (16). In this study, the recovery from pork meat could markedly be improved by addition to the aqueous extraction solvent of about 25% acetonitrile, an observation indicating binding of furazolidone to pork-specific proteins.

Apart from muscle, other tissues such as liver and kidney are frequently used as target matrices in residues monitoring due to their relatively higher residue content. However, liver in particular contains highly active enzyme systems such as the cytochrome P450 complex, which can lead to postmortem metabolism of the contained drugs (17, 18). To inhibit the cytochrome P450 activity in liver samples, piperonyl butoxide may be used as a very effective inactivation agent. When piperonyl butoxide was added to chloramphenicol-incurred bovine liver homogenates prior to analysis, the recovery of chloramphenicol increased to 60% compared with the 30% recovery without addition of piperonyl butoxide (17).

Special handling is also required when eggs are to be analyzed. Eggs consist of two distinct compartments, egg white and egg yolk, with a very different composition. Egg white constitutes about 60% of the total egg weight and is essentially a colloidal aqueous dispersion of 10.5% globular glycoproteins including ovalbumin, ovotransferin, ovomucoid, lysozyme, and ovomucin. Egg yolk constitutes a more complex matrix that contains particulate granules consisting of a mixture of high-density lipoproteins, phosvitin, and low-density proteins suspended in a micellar protein solution (19). Egg yolk lipids are mainly composed of triglycerides (64%), phospholipids (28%), and cholesterol (5%). The fatty acid composition of the yolk lipids depends to some extent on the composition of the diet of the hens. The content of yolk pigments and, therefore, the color of the egg likewise depend on the specific feeds given to the hens. Therefore, the diet of the laying hens can largely determine interferences potentially present in the analyzed eggs.

The high lipid content of the yolk makes it an apolar medium, while egg white is relatively polar. One can thus expect differences in the concentrations of polar and apolar drugs in the two egg compartments. Table 19.2 gives a few examples of this (8).

TABLE 19.2 Distribution of Ionophoric Coccidiostats and Flumequine in Egg Yolk and Egg White after Oral Medication to Laying Hens

Drug	Medication period (days)	Medication level (ppm)	Mean level (ppb)		Ratio, yolk/egg white
			Yolk	Egg white	
Flumequine	10[a]	90	400	2000	0.2
Monensin	7[b]	110	100	150	0.7
Narasin	7[b]	70	1000	250	4.0
Salinomycin	7[b]	60	1500	50	30.0

[a] Water medication
[b] Feed medication
Source: From Ref. 20.

When one wishes to determine drug residues separately in yolk and egg white, it is also advisable to separate these compartments immediately after laying because of reported diffusion from yolk to egg white (20). As with urine samples, it is also necessary to buffer egg samples prior to analysis, because the pH of the egg white may vary between 7.6 and 9.4 depending on the storage time, although while yolk pH is always in the narrower range of 6.0–6.8 (19).

Due to the wide range of matrices encountered in drug residues analyses and, also, the wide range of different classes of drugs, it is not possible to consider a typical analytical methodology. In developing a suitable analytical scheme, a number of certain physicochemical properties of the analyte(s) should also be taken into account by the analyst faced with this challenge.

Normally, most physicochemical properties including the solubility index and absorptivity data of the analytes are readily accessible in literature. Some particular properties, however, such as the pK values, are often not readily approachable or partially only known although they can be of great importance when estimating the liquid–liquid partitioning behavior of drugs and their metabolites. Primary physicochemical properties of drugs commonly used in animal farming are listed in Table 19.3.

It is well known, for example, that compounds with functional groups possessing free electrons behave as acids if they are proton-donors or as bases if they are proton-acceptors. Thus, the carboxylic acid function is moderately weakly acidic, with a pK in water of about 4.5–5.0. Its acidic function, however, is much stronger than that of the corresponding alcohol and phenol due to the high stabilization energy of the carboxylate ion. On the other hand, the amine group function is moderately weakly alkaline, with pK values in the range 8–10. As a consequence, the pK values of the primary amine function of amphetamine and dopamine are 9.9 and 8.8, respectively; the pK values of the secondary amine

TABLE 19.3   Primary Physicochemical Properties of Drugs Commonly Used in Animal Farming

Drug	Source	Classification	Formula	Mol. weight	UV max (nm)	pK values	Soluble	Slightly soluble	Almost insoluble
Albendazole	Synthetic	Benzimidazole	$C_{12}H_{15}N_3O_2S$	265			DMSO, DMF, HOAc, acids, bases	EtOAc	H_2O, hexane, toluene, petroleum ether
Amoxicillin	Semisynthetic	β-Lactam	$C_{16}H_{19}N_3O_5S$	365	230, 248, 291	2.8, 7.2	H_2O, MeOH, DMF, EtOH, DMSO		Hexane, EtOAc, ACN
Amphotericin B	S. nodosus	Antifungal	$C_{47}H_{73}NO_{17}$	924	345, 363, 382, 406		DMSO, DMF	Alkalies, acids	H_2O (pH 6–7)
Ampicillin	Semisynthetic	β-Lactam	$C_{16}H_{19}N_3O_4S$	349		2.7, 7.3	H_2O, MeOH, EtOH, acetone, DMF, DMSO	$CHCl_3$	Hexane, petroleum ether, ether, EtOAc.
Apramycin	S. tenebrarius	Aminoglycoside	$C_{21}H_{41}N_5O_{11}$	540		8. 5, 7.8, 7.2, 6.2, 5.4	H_2O	Lower alcohols	
Arsanilic acid	Synthetic	Organic arsenical	$C_6H_8AsNO_3$	217			Amyl alcohol	H_2O, EtOH, HOAc	Acetone, ether, benzene, $CHCl_3$
Avermectin B_{1a} B_{1b}	Synthetic	Macrocyclic lactone	$C_{48}H_{72}O_{14}$ $C_{47}H_{70}O_{14}$	872 858	237, 245, 253		MeOH, EtOH, $CHCl_3$, acetone, isopropanol, toluene	H_2O, BuOH, cyclohexane	
Avilamycin A C	S. viridochromogenes	Polyether	$C_{61}H_{88}Cl_2O_{32}$ $C_{61}H_{90}Cl_2O_{32}$	1403 1405	227,286 228,284			MeOH	
Avoparcin A B	S. candidus	Peptide	$C_{89}H_{101}ClN_9O_{36}$ $C_{89}H_{100}Cl_2N_9O_{36}$	1900	280, 300		H_2O, DMF, DMSO	MeOH	
Bacitracin A	B. subtilis and B. licheniformis	Peptide	$C_{66}H_{103}N_{17}O_{16}S$	1421	251, 287	8.8	H_2O, MeOH, EtOH, DMF	Acetone, dioxane	Hexane, toluene, petroleum ether, ether, $CHCl_3$
Bambermycin A B_1, B_2 and C	S. bambergiensis	Aminoglycoside	Complex		258		H_2O, MeOH, DMF	Ether, EtOAc	Benzene, $CHCl_3$

Name	Source	Class	Formula	MW	UV λ_{max}	pKa	Soluble	Slightly soluble	Insoluble
Bithionol	Synthetic	Substituted phenol	$C_{12}H_6Cl_4O_2S$	356			Alkali, acetone	EtOH	H_2O
Cambendazole	Synthetic	Benzimidazole	$C_{14}H_{14}N_4O_2S$	302	252, 319	4.8, 10.5	EtOH, DMSO, DMF	Acetone, benzene	H_2O, isooctane
Carbadox	Synthetic	Quinoxaline dioxide	$C_{11}H_{10}N_4O_4$	262	3C3, 366, 373		DMF, MeOH, EtOH, DCM, CHCl$_3$		H_2O
Cephalosporin C	Cephalosporium	β-Lactam	$C_{16}H_{21}N_3O_8S$	415	260	2.6, 3.1, 9.8	H_2O	Ether, EtOH	
Cephapirin	Cephalosporium	β-Lactam	$C_{17}H_{16}N_3NaO_5S_2$	445			H_2O		
Chloramphenicol	Synthetic	Amphenicol	$C_{11}H_{12}Cl_2N_2O_5$	323	278	5.5	H_2O, MeOH, EtOH, EtOAc, ether, acetone, DMF	Toluene, CHCl$_3$	Hexane, petroleum ether, isooctane
Chlorothiazide	Synthetic	Diuretic	$C_7H_6ClN_3O_4S_2$	296	225, 280	8–10	H_2O, EtOH,	MeOH	Hexane, petroleum ether, isooctane
Chlortetracycline	S. aureofaciens	Tetracycline	$C_{22}H_{23}ClN_2O_8$	479	230, 263, 368	3.3, 7.4, 9.3	H_2O, MeOH, DMF	EtOH, EtOAc, dioxane, acetone	Hexane, toluene, ether, petroleum ether, CHCl$_3$
Clenbuterol	Synthetic	β-Agonist	$C_{12}H_{18}Cl_2N_2O$	277			H_2O, MeOH, DMF	CHCl$_3$	Benzene
Clindamycin	Semisynthetic	Lincosamide	$C_{18}H_{33}ClN_2O_5S$	425		7.6	H_2O, EtOH		
Clopidol	Synthetic	Anticoccidial	$C_7H_7Cl_2NO$	192	227, 267, 325		DMF, MeOH	ACN	H_2O
Clorsulon	Synthetic	Anthelminthic	$C_8H_8Cl_3N_3O_4S_2$	381					
Closantel	Synthetic	Salicylanilide	$C_{22}H_{14}Cl_2I_2N_2O_2$	663	230, 261	2.7	H_2O, MeOH, EtOH, dioxane, DMF, DMSO	EtOAc, CHCl$_3$, acetone	Hexane, petroleum ether, ether, isooctane
Cloxacillin	Semisynthetic	β-Lactam	$C_{19}H_{18}ClN_3O_5S$	436					
Colistin	B. colistinus	Peptide	$C_{53}H_{100}N_{16}O_{13}$	1168			H_2O, MeOH, DMF, DMSO	Dioxane	EtOH, ether, EtOAc, CHCl$_3$, acetone, hexane
Coumaphos	Synthetic	Organophosphate	$C_{14}H_{16}ClO_5PS$	363			DMSO	CHCl$_3$, acetone	H_2O

(continued)

TABLE 19.3 Continued

Drug	Source	Classification	Formula	Mol. weight	UV max (nm)	pK values	Soluble	Slightly soluble	Almost insoluble
Dexamethasone	Synthetic	Corticosteroid	$C_{22}H_{29}FO_5$	392	239		EtOH, acetone, CHCl$_3$	H$_2$O	
Diazepam	Synthetic	Sedative	$C_{16}H_{13}ClN_2O$	285		3.4	EtOH, DMF, CHCl$_3$, acetone, benzene	H$_2$O	
Dichlorophen	Synthetic	Substituted phenol	$C_{13}H_{10}Cl_2O_2$	269			EtOH, MeOH, ether, isopropyl ether, petroleum ether	Toluene	H$_2$O
Dichlorvos	Synthetic	Organophosphate	$C_4H_7Cl_2O_4P$	221		2.7	EtOH	H$_2$O, EtOAc, CHCl$_3$	Hexane, petroleum ether, isooctane, benzene
Dicloxacillin	Semisynthetic	β-Lactam	$C_{19}H_{17}Cl_2N_3O_5S$	470			H$_2$O, MeOH, EtOH, acetone, DMF, DMSO		
Dienestrol	Synthetic	Anabolic	$C_{18}H_{18}O_2$	266		MeOH, EtOH, ether, acetone, CHCl$_3$		H$_2$O, dil acids	
Diethylstilbestrol	Synthetic	Anabolic	$C_{18}H_{20}O_2$	268			MeOH, EtOH, ether, CHCl$_3$		H$_2$O
Dihydrostreptomycin	Semisynthetic	Aminoglycoside	$C_{21}H_{41}N_7O_{12}$	584		8.8	H$_2$O, MeOH, DMF	EtOH	Hexane, petroleum ether, isooctane
Dimetridazole	Synthetic	Nitroimidazole	$C_5H_7N_3O_2$	141			EtOH, acids	H$_2$O, ether, CHCl$_3$, benzene	
Doxycycline		Tetracycline	$C_{22}H_{24}N_2O_8$	462	267, 351		H$_2$O, MeOH, dioxane, DMF		Hexane, pet ether, isooctane
Efrotomycin	S. lactamdurans	Peptide	$C_{59}H_{88}N_2O_{20}$	1145	232, 327				

Name	Source	Class	Formula	MW	λ	pH	Soluble	Slightly soluble	Insoluble
Enrofloxacin	Synthetic	Quinolone	$C_{19}H_{22}FN_3O_3$	359			ACN, MeOH	H_2O	Hexane, petroleum ether, isooctane, toluene
Erythromycin	S. erythreus	Macrolide	$C_{37}H_{67}NO_{13}$	734	280	8.8	H_2O, MeOH, EtOH, acetone, ACN, EtOAc, CHCl$_3$, ether, DMF	Hexane, toluene, isooctane	Petroleum ether,
Estradiol-17β	Ovaries	Sex hormone	$C_{18}H_{24}O_2$	272	225, 280		EtOH, acetone, dioxane		H_2O
Ethopabate	Synthetic	Anticoccidial	$C_{12}H_{15}NO_4$	237	267, 298		ACN, MeOH, EtOH, acetone	EtOAc, DCM, isopropanol	H_2O, isooctane
Fenbendazole	Synthetic	Benzimidazole	$C_{15}H_{13}N_3O_2S$	299			DMSO	EtOAc	H_2O, hexane, petroleum ether, isooctane
Florfenicol	Synthetic	Amphenicol	$C_{12}H_{14}Cl_2FNO_4S$	358			H_2O, MeOH, EtOH, DMF		Hexane, petroleum ether, isooctane
Flubendazole	Synthetic	Benzimidazole	$C_{16}H_{12}FN_3O_3$	313			DMSO		H_2O, hexane, isooctane
Flumequine	Synthetic	Quinolone	$C_{14}H_{12}FNO_3$	261			Alkali, EtOH, DMF		H_2O
Furaltadone	Synthetic	Nitrofuran	$C_{13}H_{16}N_4O_6$	324			EtOH, DMSO, DMF	H_2O	Hexane, isooctane
Furazolidone	Synthetic	Nitrofuran	$C_8H_7N_3O_5$	225	265, 352		DMSO, DMF	DCM	Hexane, H_2O
Furosemide	Synthetic	Diuretic	$C_{12}H_{11}ClN_2O_5S$	331		4–5	Alkali, MeOH, EtOH, acetone, DMF	H_2O, CHCl$_3$	Hexane, petroleum ether, isooctane
Gentamicin C$_1$ C$_2$ C$_{1a}$	M. purpurea	Aminoglycoside	$C_{21}H_{43}N_5O_7$ $C_{20}H_{41}N_5O_7$ $C_{19}H_{39}N_5O_7$	477 453 449		8.2	H_2O, DMF, DMSO	MeOH, ether, CHCl$_3$, acetone	Hexane, EtOH, petroleum ether, ether, EtOAc
Gentian violet	Synthetic	Dye	$C_{25}H_{30}ClN_3$	408			H_2O, EtOH, CHCl$_3$	Ether	

(continued)

TABLE 19.3 Continued

Drug	Source	Classification	Formula	Mol. weight	UV max (nm)	pK values	Soluble	Slightly soluble	Almost insoluble
Halofuginone	Synthetic	Anticoccidial	$C_{16}H_{17}BrClN_3O_3$	415			MeOH, DMF		$CHCl_3$, DCM, acetone
Hexestrol	Synthetic	Anabolic	$C_{18}H_{22}O_2$	270			MeOH, EtOH, ether, acetone,	$CHCl_3$, benzene	H_2O, dil acids
Hydrochlorothiazide	Synthetic	Diuretic	$C_7H_8ClN_3O_4S_2$	298	226, 271, 317	7.9, 9.2	Alkalies, MeOH, EtOH, acetone		H_2O, hexane, petroleum ether, isooctane
Hygromycin B	Synthetic	Anthelminthic	$C_{20}H_{37}N_3O_{13}$	527		7.1, 8.8	H_2O, MeOH, EtOH, DMF		Hexane, petroleum ether, isooctane, cyclohexane
Indomethacin	Synthetic	Anti-inflammatory	$C_{19}H_{16}ClNO_4$	358	230, 260, 319	4.5	EtOH, acetone, ether		H_2O
Ivermectin B_{1a} B_{1b}	Synthetic	Macrocyclic lactone	$C_{48}H_{74}O_{14}$ $C_{47}H_{72}O_{14}$	874 860	238, 245		Methyl ethyl ketone, propylene glycol	H_2O	Hexane, petroleum ether, isooctane, cyclohexane
Kanamycin A, C B	S. kanamyceticus	Aminoglycoside	$C_{18}H_{36}N_4O_{11}$ $C_{18}H_{37}N_5O_{10}$				H_2O	DMF, ether, dioxane	MeOH, EtOH, hexane, EtOAc, acetone, $CHCl_3$
Ketoprofen	Synthetic	Anti-inflammatory	$C_{16}H_{14}O_3$	254	255		EtOH, DMF, $CHCl_3$, EtOAc, acetone, ether		H_2O
Lasalocid	Streptomyces?	Polyether	$C_{34}H_{54}O_8$	591	248, 318		MeOH, EtOH, DMF, $CHCl_3$, ACN, DCM, EtOAc	H_2O	
Levamisole	Synthetic	Imidazothiazole	$C_{11}H_{12}N_2S$	204					Hexane, petroleum ether, isooctane

Name	Source	Class	Formula	MW	UV (nm)	pKa	Solubility		
Lincomycin	*S. lincolnensis*	Lincosamide	$C_{18}H_{34}N_2O_6S$	406		7.6	H_2O, MeOH, EtOH, DMF	Acetone, $CHCl_3$	Hexane, ether, petroleum ether
Malachite green	Synthetic	Dye	$C_{23}H_{25}ClN_2$	365	616.9		H_2O, MeOH, EtOH, amyl alcohol		Ether
Mebendazole	Synthetic	Benzimidazole	$C_{16}H_{13}N_3O_3$	295			Formic acid, DMSO	EtOAc	H_2O, EtOH, $CHCl_3$, ether, hexane, isooctane
Methylene blue	Synthetic	Dye	$C_{16}H_{18}ClN_3S$	320	609, 668		H_2O, EtOH, $CHCl_3$		Ether
Methylthiouracil	Synthetic	Thyreostatic	$C_5H_6N_2OS$	142			Alkalies	H_2O, EtOH, ether, acetone	$CHCl_3$, benzene
Metronidazole	Synthetic	Nitroimidazole	$C_6H_9N_3O_3$	171			H_2O, EtOH	DMF, $CHCl_3$, ether	
Monensin	*S. cinnamonensis*	Polyether	$C_{36}H_{62}O_{11}$	671		6.6	MeOH, EtOH, DMF, $CHCl_3$, ACN, DCM, EtOAc	H_2O	
Nalidixic acid	Synthetic	Quinolone	$C_{12}H_{12}N_2O_2$	232	256, 318, 328	8.6	$CHCl_3$, ACN, DCM, EtOAc, toluene	MeOH, EtOH	H_2O, ether
Narasin	*S. aureofaciens*	Polyether	$C_{43}H_{72}O_{11}$	755	285	7.9	MeOH, $CHCl_3$, DMF, ACN, DCM, DMSO, EtOAc, acetone, benzene	H_2O	H_2O
Natamycin	*S. natalensis*	Antifungal	$C_{33}H_{47}NO_{13}$	666	220, 280, 290, 303, 318		DMSO, DMF	Acids	Ether, higher alcohols, esters, dioxane, ketones

(continued)

Table 19.3 Continued

Drug	Source	Classification	Formula	Mol. weight	UV max (nm)	pK values	Soluble	Slightly soluble	Almost insoluble
Neomycin A B, C	S. fradiae	Aminoglycoside	$C_{12}H_{26}N_4O_6$ $C_{23}H_{46}N_6O_{13}$	322 454		8.3	H_2O	MeOH, ether, EtOH, acetone	Hexane, toluene, petroleum ether, CHCl$_3$, EtOAc
Nicarbazin	Synthetic	Carbanilide	$C_{19}H_{18}N_6O_6$	426	298				H_2O
Niclosamide	Synthetic	Salicylanilide	$C_{13}H_8Cl_2N_2O_4$	327				EtOH, ether, CHCl$_3$	H_2O
Nithiazide	Synthetic	Antiprotozoal	$C_6H_8N_4O_3S$	216		7.3			
Nitrofurantoin	Synthetic	Nitrofuran	$C_8H_6N_4O_5$	238	266, 370	7.2	Acetone, DMF, DMSO	H_2O, EtOH	Hexane, petroleum ether, isooctane
Nitrofurazone	Synthetic	Nitrofuran	$C_6H_6N_4O_4$	198	260 , 375		Alkalies, DMF, DMSO		Ether, H_2O, EtOH
Nitroxynil	Synthetic	Substituted phenol	$C_7H_3IN_2O_3$	290			EtOH, acetone CHCl$_3$, DMF, DMSO,	H_2O, MeOH	
Nosiheptide	S. actuosus	Macrolide	$C_{51}H_{43}N_{13}O_{12}S_6$	1222	242, 322		CHCl$_3$, DMF, DMSO	MeOH, EtOH, EtOAc, benzene	H_2O, petroleum ether
Novobiocin	S. spheroides	Antibacterial	$C_{31}H_{36}N_2O_{11}$	613	248, 307, 324, 350	4.3, 9.1	H_2O, MeOH, EtOH, acetone, DMF	EtOAc, ether, CHCl$_3$	Hexane, toluene, isooctane
Nystatin A$_1$	S. noursei, S. aureus	Antifungal	$C_{47}H_{75}NO_{17}$	925	290, 307, 322		MeOH, ethylene glycol, DMSO, DMF	H_2O, EtOH, CHCl$_3$, benzene	Hexane, isooctane, petroleum ether
Olaquindox	Synthetic	Quinoxaline dioxide	$C_{12}H_{13}N_3O_4$	263			H_2O	MeOH, acetone, EtOH	
Oleandomycin	S. antibioticus	Macrolide	$C_{35}H_{61}NO_{12}$	688	286–289		H_2O, MeOH, EtOH, BuOH, acetone, CHCl$_3$, EtOAc, DMF	Ether, toluene	Hexane, petroleum ether, isooctane
Oxacillin	Semisynthetic	β-Lactam	$C_{19}H_{19}N_3O_5S$	40 1	232, 259	2.7	H_2O, MeOH, EtOH, DMSO, DMF	Hexane, acetone	Petroleum ether, EtOAc, ether, CHCl$_3$

Oxfendazole	Synthetic	Benzimidazole	$C_{15}H_{13}N_3O_3S$	315			DMSO, DMF	EtOAc	Hexane, petroleum ether, isooctane
Oxibendazole	Synthetic	Benzimidazole	$C_{12}H_{15}N_3O_3$	249			DMSO, DMF	EtOAc	Hexane, petroleum ether, isooctane
Oxolinic acid	Synthetic	Quinolone	$C_{13}H_{11}NO_5$	261			MeOH, ACN, DCM, EtOAc, CHCl$_3$	H$_2$O	Hexane, benzene
Oxytetracycline	S. rimosus	Tetracycline	$C_{22}H_{24}N_2O_9$	460	249, 276, 353	3.3, 7.3, 9.1	H$_2$O, MeOH, EtOH, EtOAc, acetone, DMF	Ether, CHCl$_3$	Hexane, toluene, petroleum ether
Penicillin G	Penicillium culture	β-Lactam	$C_{16}H_{18}N_2O_4S$	333	257, 263, 277	2.8	H$_2$O, MeOH, EtOH, dioxane, DMF, DMSO	Hexane, EtOAc, acetone	Toluene, petroleum ether, ether, CHCl$_3$
Penicillin V	Penicillium culture	β-Lactam	$C_{16}H_{18}N_2O_5S$	350	263, 268, 274	2.7	H$_2$O, MeOH, DMF, DMSO	EtOH, acetone, ether, EtOAc, CHCl$_3$	Hexane, toluene, petroleum ether
Phenylbutazone	Synthetic	Anti-inflammatory	$C_{19}H_{20}N_2O_2$	308	239.5	4.5		H$_2$O	
Polymyxin B$_1$, B$_2$	B. polymyxa	Peptide	$C_{56}H_{98}N_{16}O_{13}$, $C_{55}H_{96}N_{16}O_{13}$			8–9	H$_2$O	MeOH, EtOH, acetone	Hexane, toluene, EtOAc, CHCl$_3$
Progesterone	Corpus luteum	Sex hormone	$C_{21}H_{30}O_2$	314	240		EtOH, acetone, dioxane		H$_2$O
Pyrantel tartrate	Synthetic	Tetrahydropyrimidines	$C_{15}H_{20}N_2O_6S$	356	312				
Rafoxanide	Synthetic	Salicylanilide	$C_{19}H_{11}Cl_2I_2NO_3$	626			MeOH, EtOH, CHCl$_3$, EtOAc, acetone	ACN, acetone	H$_2$O
Ronidazole	Synthetic	Nitroimidazole	$C_6H_8N_4O_4$	200		1.2		H$_2$O	Hexane, benzene
Roxarsone	Synthetic	Organic arsenical	$C_6H_6AsNO_6$	233			MeOH, EtOH, HOAc, acetone, alkalies	H$_2$O	EtOAc, ether

(continued)

TABLE 19.3 Continued

Drug	Source	Classification	Formula	Mol. weight	UV max (nm)	pK values	Soluble	Slightly soluble	Almost insoluble
Salinomycin	S. albus	Polyether	$C_{42}H_{70}O_{11}$	751	284	6.4	MeOH, EtOH, DMF, CHCl₃, ACN, DMSO, acetone		H_2O
Sedecamycin	S. griseofuscus	Macrolide	$C_{27}H_{35}N\ O_8$	501.6	228		MeOH, EtOAc, CHCl₃		Hexane, petroleum ether
Spectinomycin	S. spectabilis	Aminoglycoside	$C_{14}H_{24}N_2O_7$	332		6.9, 8.7	H_2O, MeOH, DMF, DMSO	Dioxane	EtOH, hexane, ether, EtOAc, acetone
Spiramycin I	S. ambofaciens	Macrolide	$C_{43}H_{74}N_2O_{14}$		231		H_2O, MeOH, EtOH, EtOAc, DMF acetone, ether, CHCl₃	Hexane, petroleum ether, isooctane	
II			$C_{45}H_{76}N_2O_{15}$						
III			$C_{46}H_{78}N_2O_{15}$						
Stanozolol	Synthetic	Anabolic steroid	$C_{21}H_{32}N_2O$	328	223			MeOH, EtOH, EtOAc, ether	Hexane, toluene, petroleum ether, acetone, CHCl₃
Streptomycin A	S. griseus	Aminoglycoside	$C_{21}H_{39}N_7O_{12}$	582	280, 318		H_2O		
B			$C_{27}H_{49}N_7O_{17}$	743					
Sulfadiazine	Synthetic	Sulfonamide	$C_{10}H_{10}N_4O_2S$	250	242, 254	6.4	Acids and alkalies	EtOH, CHCl₃, ether, acetone	H_2O, hexane
Sulfadimethoxine	Synthetic	Sulfonamide	$C_{12}H_{14}N_4O_4S$	310	268	6.2		EtOH, CHCl₃, ether, acetone	H_2O, hexane, isooctane
Sulfamethazine	Synthetic	Sulfonamide	$C_{12}H_{14}N_4O_2S$	278	243, 258, 301	2.6, 7.4	H_2O, acids and alkalies, ether	EtOH, CHCl₃	Hexane, petroleum ether, isooctane
Sulfanilamide	Synthetic	Sulfonamide	$C_6H_8N_2O_2S$	172	250, 262, 269	10.4, 11.6	Acids and alkalies	H_2O, EtOH	Ether, petroleum ether, CHCl₃, hexane
Sulfaquinoxaline	Synthetic	Sulfonamide	$C_{14}H_{12}N_4O_2S$	300	252, 360	5.5	EtOH, acetone, alkalies		H_2O, ether

Name	Source	Class	Molecular Formula	MW	λmax	pKa	Solubility		
Sulfathiazole	Synthetic	Sulfonamide	$C_9H_9N_3O_2S_2$	255	257, 283	7.2	Acetone, H_2O	EtOH	Ether, petroleum ether, CHCl$_3$, hexane
Sulfisoxazole	Synthetic	Sulfonamide	$C_{11}H_{13}N_3O_3S$	267	263, 264	4.7	H_2O	EtOH, ether	CHCl$_3$, hexane, petroleum ether
Testosterone	Testes	Sex hormone	$C_{19}H_{28}O_2$	288	238		EtOH, acetone, ether, dioxane		H_2O
Tetracycline	S. viridifaciens	Tetracycline	$C_{22}H_{24}N_2O_6$	444	220, 268, 355	3.3, 7.7, 7.7	H_2O, MeOH, EtOH, CHCl$_3$, DMF, dioxane	Toluene, ether, EtOAc, acetone	Hexane, petroleum ether, isooctane
Thiabendazole	Synthetic	Benzimidazole	$C_{10}H_7N_3S$	201	298		DMSO, DMF	EtOH, MeOH, EtOAc	
Thiamphenicol	Synthetic	Amphenicol	$C_{12}H_{15}Cl_2NO_5S$	356	224		H_2O, EtOH, MeOH, EtOAc, DMSO, DMF		Hexane, petroleum ether, isooctane
Thiopeptin	S. tateyamensis	Peptide			230–250, 295, 305		DMSO, DMF, CHCl$_3$, dioxane, pyridine	MeOH, EtOAc, acetone	H_2O, hexane, petroleum ether, ether, benzene
Thiouracil	Synthetic	Thyreostatic	$C_4H_4N_2OS$	128			Alkalies	H_2O	EtOH, ether, acids
Tiamulin	Semisynthetic	Antibacterial	$C_{28}H_{47}NO_4S$	494				Acetone	
Tobramycin	S. tenebrarius	Aminoglycoside	$C_{18}H_{37}N_5O_9$	467			H_2O		
Trenbolone	Synthetic	Anabolic steroid	$C_{18}H_{22}O_2$	270	239, 340.5		MeOH, EtOH DMF, hot acetone		
Tribromsalan	Synthetic	Salicylanilide	$C_{13}H_8Br_3NO_2$	450				H_2O	H_2O
Trichlormethiazide	Synthetic	Diuretic	$C_8H_8Cl_3N_3O_4S_2$	381	225, 270	8.6	H_2O, MeOH, EtOH,		Hexane, petroleum ether, isooctane

(continued)

TABLE 19.3 Continued

Drug	Source	Classification	Formula	Mol. weight	UV max (nm)	pK values	Soluble	Slightly soluble	Almost insoluble
Triclabendazole	Synthetic	Benzimidazole	$C_{14}H_9Cl_3N_2OS$	360			DMSO		H_2O, hexane, petroleum ether, isooctane
Trimethoprim	Synthetic	Diamainopyrimidine	$C_{14}H_{18}N_4O_3$	290		6.6	$CHCl_3$, MeOH	H_2O	Hexane, ether, benzene
Tylosin	S. fradiae	Macrolide	$C_{46}H_{77}NO_{17}$	916	282	7.1	H_2O, MeOH, EtOH, acetone, EtOAc, ether, $CHCl_3$, DMF, DMSO	Hexane	Petroleum ether, isooctane
Virginiamycin M_1, S_1	S. virginiae	Peptide	$C_{28}H_{35}N_3O_7$ $C_{43}H_{49}N_7O_{10}$	525 795	216 305		$CHCl_3$, DMF	MeOH, EtOH, EtOAc	H_2O, petroleum ether
Xylazine	Synthetic	Sedative	$C_{12}H_{16}N_2S$	220			Dil acids, $CHCl_3$, benzene, acetone	Petroleum ether	H_2O, alkalies
Zeranol	Synthetic	Anabolic	$C_{18}H_{26}O_5$	322	218, 265, 304		MeOH, EtOH		

ACN, acetonitrile; MeOH, methanol; EtOH, ethanol; BuOH, butanol; EtOAc, ethyl acetate; ether, diethyl ether; HOAc, acetic acid; DCM, dichloromethane; DMF, dimethylformamide; DMSO, dimethylsulfoxide.

function of ketamine and phenylefrine are 7.5 and 10.1, respectively; whereas the pK of the tertiary amine function of cocaine is 8.4. However, these pK values can be shifted dramatically if aromatic functions are introduced adjacent to the amine function. For example, the pK of the primary amine function in aniline is shifted to about 4.6, whereas in benzocaine it is about 2.5. Electron-withdrawing functions neighboring an amine function can change the basic character of the group into a neutral function, as in primary and secondary amides, or even into an acidic function, as in sulfonamides and barbiturates (5).

Established physicochemical properties are sometimes strongly influenced by the intrinsic possibility of the analytes to form hydrogen bonds with other potential hydrogen-bonding compounds. However, the carboxylic acid hydrogen bond is much stronger than the corresponding hydrogen bond in the analogous alcohols and amines, because of the high degree of polarization of the former. Furthermore, carboxylic acids, and to some extent alcohols and phenols, are able to form additional hydrogen bonds by the negative oxygen of the carbonyl dipole resulting in cyclic dimers in the solid as well as in the liquid phases of the carboxylic acid. Hydrogen-bonding effects are primarily responsible for the high solubility of carboxylic acids and lower alcohols in polar, proton-donated solvents; except for the carboxylic acids with long saturated or unsaturated chains or large aromatic systems, the solubility in very aprotic solvents will be limited.

The intrinsic possibility of an analyte to form hydrogen bonds is another important factor in liquid chromatographic separations, because the majority of the stationary phases are still based on polar materials such as silica, which have a strong tendency to form hydrogen bonds. In a number of chromatographic processes, this hydrogen-bonding tendency is, however, an undesirable retention-influencing parameter. Except for the possibility of hydrogen-bonding formation of the analyte during the chromatographic process, the hydrogen-bonding capability of matrix polar compounds including amino acids, peptides, or vitamins may also induce their bonding to the analyte during the sample preparation process, converting a simple analysis to a difficult task.

Apart from hydrogen-bonding forces, a number of other interactions of varying importance may also occur between the analyte and matrix components. Including in this category are covalent, ionic, dipole–dipole, induced dipole–dipole, and dispersion interactions that have a force of 100–300 kcal/mol, 50–200 kcal/mol, 3–10 kcal/mol, 2–6 kcal/mol, and 1–5 kcal/mol, respectively (5). Covalent binding, for example, of nitroimidazole, nitrofuran, and benzimidazole residues to macromolecular matrix components is the cause of the more or less persistent nonextractable residues appearing in foods (11, 21, 22).

REFERENCES

1. J.F. Lawrence and R.W. Frei, in Chemical Derivatization in Liquid Chromatography (J.F. Lawrence and R.W. Frei, Eds.), J. Chromatogr. Libr. Vol. 7, Elsevier, Amsterdam (1976).

2. K. Blau and G.S. King, in Handbook of Derivatives for Chromatography (K. Blau and G.S. King, Eds.), Heyden & Son, London (1978).

3. D.R. Knapp, in Handbook of Analytical Derivatization Reactions (D.R. Knapp, Ed.), Wiley-Interscience, New York (1979).

4. R.W. Frei and J.F. Lawrence, in Chemical Derivatization in Analytical Chemistry (R.W. Frei and J.F. Lawrence, Eds.), Vol. 2, Plenum Press, London (1982).

5. H. Lingeman and W.J.M. Underberg, in Detection-Oriented Derivatization Techniques in Liquid Chromatography (H. Lingeman and W.J.M. Underberg, Eds.), Marcel Dekker, Inc., New York, pp. 1–50 (1990).

6. M. Wenk, S. Vozeh, and F. Follath, Clin. Pharmacokin., 9:475 (1984).

7. J. Chamberlain, in Analysis of Drugs in Biological Fluids (J. Chamberlain, Ed.), CRC Press, Inc., Boca Raton, FL, USA (1985).

8. M.M.L. Aerts, in Residues of Veterinary Drugs in Edible Products, Thesis, Free University of Amsterdam, The Netherlands (1990).

9. J.J.H.M. Lohman, in Plasma Protein Binding of Drugs, Implications for Therapeutic Drug Monitoring, Thesis, Leiden, The Nerherlands (1986).

10. G. Ziv, and F.G. Sulman, Antimicrob. Agent Chemother., 2:206 (1977).

11. V. Burgat-Sacaze, A. Rico, and J.-C. Panisset, in Drug Residues in Animals (A.G. Rico, Ed.), Academic Press, Inc., Orlando, FL, p. 1 (1986).

12. P. Walstra and M.C. van der Haven, in Course on Dairy Technology (P. Walstra and M.C. van der Haven, Eds), Agricultural University of Wageningen, Wageningen, The Netherlands (1977).

13. G. Ziv and F. Rasmussen, J. Dairy Sci., 58:938 (1975).

14. R.A. Lawrie, in Meat Science (R.A. Lawrie, Ed.), Pergamon Press, Oxford, U.K. (1979).

15. N.F. Haard, in Fish and Fishery Products (A. Ruiter, Ed.), CAB International, Wallingford, Oxon, UK, pp. 77–115 (1995).

16. M.M.L. Aerts, W.M.J. Beek, and U.A. Th. Brinkman, J. Chromatogr., 500:453 (1990).

17. R.M. Parker and I. Shaw, Analyst, 113:1875 (1988).

18. J.F.M. Nouws, Arch. Lebensmittelhyg., 32:103 (1981).

19. M. Bennion, in The Science of Food (M. Bennion, Ed.), Harper & Row, San Francisco, CA, USA, pp. 383–406 (1980).

20. M.F. Geertsma, J.F.M. Nouws, J.L. Grondel, M.M.L. Aerts, T.B. Vree, and C.A. Kan, Vet. Q., 9:67 (1987).

21. M.M.L. Aerts, A.C. Hogenboom, and U.A.Th. Brinkman, J. Chromatogr. B, 667:1 (1995).

22. A.Y.H. Lu, G.T. Miwa, and P.G. Wislocki, Rev. Biochem. Toxicol., 9:1 (1988).

20

Sample Preparation

The success of an analytical method for determining drug residues in edible animal products is determined by a number of independent factors. However, the sample preparation procedure can most directly influence the overall analytical result.

Sample preparation includes all techniques that involve handling the sample before detection begins. The intent of sample preparation is to extract efficiently the analytes and isolate them relatively free of interfering matrix components that could obscure the final detection, identification, and quantification process.

In many cases, the sample preparation procedure makes up the weakest link in the whole analytical procedure. Owing to the wide range of matrices encountered in food of animal origin and, also, the wide range of different groups of drug residues, a typical sample preparation scheme cannot be established. Instead, the extent of sample preparation depends strongly on the concentration of the analyte, the composition of the matrix, and the detection system chosen.

If analysis is to be attempted with a detection system of only moderate selectivity, a substantial cleanup procedure may be required in order to enhance the concentration of the extracted trace residue while decreasing the concentration of possible interfering substances in the sample matrix. This is the case with most of the relatively nonspecific physicochemical detection systems used in residue analysis. Occasionally a sample may be suitable for direct physicochemical analysis after an extraction and concentration step. However, the majority of edible animal products need extensive cleanup to separate the compounds of interest from animal lipids and other natural organic substances prior to detection. For such detection systems, there has been a general rule dictating that the cleaner sample, the better the result obtained.

When a more specific detection system is used instead, a rigorous sample cleanup may not be necessary. This is actually the case with most of the microbiological and immunochemical detection systems applied in residue analysis. Owing to the selectivity and sensitivity of their detection principle, homogenization with an aqueous buffer is often the only treatment required prior to analysis. Moreover, these detection systems are usually independent of the sample size as, in many cases, a single drop of milk or tissue fluid is sufficient to carry out a successful analysis.

Sample preparation procedures commonly used in the field of drug residues analysis are briefly described below. Since some of these overlap and cannot be strictly separated, the intent of the authors is to attempt to outline the complexity of the sample preparation issue rather than to give a comprehensive listing of the relevant literature.

20.1 SELECTION OF BASIC ANALYTICAL EQUIPMENT

In starting a residue analysis in foods, the choice of proper vials for sample preparation is very important. Available vials are made of either glass or polymeric materials such as polyethylene, polypropylene, or polytetrafluoroethylene. The choice of the proper material depends strongly on the physicochemical properties of the analyte. For a number of compounds that have the tendency to irreversible adsorption onto glass surfaces, the polymer-based vials are obviously the best choice. However, the surface of the polymer-based vials may contain phthalates or plasticizers that can dissolve in certain solvents and may interfere with the identification of analytes. When using dichloromethane, for example, phthalates may be the reason for the appearance of a series of unexpected peaks in the mass spectra of the samples. Plasticizers, on the other hand, fluoresce and may interfere with the detection of fluorescence analytes. Thus, for handling of troublesome analytes, use of vials made of polytetrafluoroethylene is recommended. This material does not contain any plasticizers or organic acids, can withstand temperatures up to 500 K, and lacks active sites that could adsorb polar compounds on its surface.

The color of the vial wall may also be of importance when photolabile compounds are analyzed. In these circumstances, brown vials are generally used, although in some special cases, green, blue, or red vials may be more appropriate. However, the dyes in the colored vials may sometimes interfere with the analysis. In such cases, transparent vials should be used: photodegradation of the samples can also be avoided by wrapping the vials in aluminum foil.

The type of pipette used for addition or transferring of solvents is another issue of importance. Automated micro- or macropipettes in the volume range of 5–10,000 μl with disposable wetting polypropylene tips are commonly used for this purpose. These pipettes have some advantages over the classic glass pipettes, including ease of operation and elimination of cross-contamination. The mean accuracy of this type of pipettes is 1% in volume of the sample size. However, their accuracy may be unfavorably influenced when solvents with relatively high vapor pressure are processed.

Mixing of solutions and dissolution of standards are usually carried out by means of vigorous mixing devices (vortex-mixer). Sometimes, dissolution is also performed by using microwave irradiation for a few seconds up to 1 min, or by ultrasonic vibration for 5–15 min. On the other hand, homogenization of solid samples is usually carried out by high-speed blending mixing devices, particularly the so-called ultraturrax.

Evaporation and heating are two different procedures that can nevertheless be performed concurrently in an evaporation/heating device. This device consists of an aluminum thermostatted block with holes to allow insertion of vials. On top of the block, a plate is fixed containing an evaporator tip above each hole. These evaporator tips can be used to blow nitrogen or helium over the samples for evaporating the contents of the vials to dryness at ambient or higher temperatures. Nitrogen or helium should be used instead of air to prevent degradation of the analytes by oxidation. When only evaporation of the samples at ambient tempera-ture is needed, simple homemade evaporation systems can be used instead.

20.2 SAMPLING/STORAGE

Proper sampling requires knowledge of the purpose for which sampling is re-quired. The precise method of sampling depends heavily on the particular food commodity and the nature of the tested analyte. For example, fresh meat should be separated as completely as possible from any bone to be further passed three times through food chopper, and mixed thoroughly after each grinding (1).

Following sampling, proper storage of biological specimens is absolutely essential in maintaining sample integrity. If the sample cannot be analyzed imme-diately, it must be stored under conditions that minimize microbial degradation, chemical or photochemical decomposition, metabolism of the analyte in enzyme-containing matrices, or loss of volatile components prior to analysis. Normally, the specimens are rapidly cooled in liquid nitrogen and kept frozen in the absence of light for transport and storage. For most drugs, storage at $-18°C$ is adequate for long-term storage, whereas lower temperatures ranging from -40 to $-70°C$ are normally recommended for very long storage times.

Freezing of samples should be executed carefully. If the freezing of samples is not rapid enough, part of the water may freeze out and the analyte concentration of the remaining solution can rise until crystallization occurs. This can lead to analyte losses, because the crystallized particles in such samples cannot readily redissolve during the thawing process, as has been observed with residues of the drug mitomycin C even with microwave-assisted heating (2).

Freeze-drying is another technique that may be applied for preparing biological samples for long-term storage. Samples are frozen in a dry ice–acetone bath or in liquid nitrogen to be subsequently placed in a freeze-dryer where water is removed by vacuum sublimation (3). However, derivatization of the analytes prior to the freeze-drying process is sometimes necessary to eliminate losses during the last stages of the sublimation procedure.

Following storage, frozen samples have to be submitted to thawing prior to analysis. Thawing is usually performed in the unopened containers or plastic bags at ambient temperature. To hasten thawing, however, samples may be warmed in a water bath held at a temperature of approximately 40°C. Another choice is to use microwave irradiation, which is an excellent technique for rapid thawing of samples frozen at 253 K (4). However, thawing is not always the recommended procedure for frozen meat samples, since such solidified samples may be cut into chunks and then submitted to the pulverizing action of a kitchen blender (5). Other common methods used for reducing sample particle size include chopping, cutting, blending, grinding, macerating, and mincing.

20.3   PROTEIN DENATURATION

Before applying a sample preparation procedure, the degree of drug–protein binding should be known since it can never be assumed that the selected procedure will destroy this binding (6). This step is most critical when there is a hint of binding of the drug to proteins. Determination of the degree of drug–protein binding can be carried out using dialysis or ultrafiltration techniques (7, 8).

Sometimes the easiest way to destroy drug–protein binding is to dilute the sample with a physiological saline solution. For instance, for isoxazolyl penicillins with a binding percentage of over 95%, dilution with 9 volumes of 0.9% sodium chloride solution can be sufficient (9). Alternative widely used techniques are based on either protein denaturation or enzymatic/chemical hydrolysis of the drug–protein complexes (10–12).

Protein denaturation in a food sample can be effected by a variety of means including addition of various protein-precipitating reagents, sample boiling, or use of microwave irradiation. Precipitation of sample proteins can be performed with a great number of reagents including hydrochloric acid (13), perchloric acid (14), tungstic acid (15), trichloroacetic acid (16, 17), acetonitrile (18–21), ethanol (22), acetone (23), methanol (24, 25), ammonium sulfate (26), or ammonium chloride (27).

With the use of the inorganic sulfates or chlorides, protein precipitation does occur but the process is reversible. This does not occur when acids or organic solvents are used for protein precipitation, since the biological activity of the proteins in this case is irreversibly destroyed. On the other hand, use of mineral or organic acids, although valuable for deproteinization purposes, has raised problems with regard to precision and accuracy of the analysis due to occasional adsorption and/or occlusion of the analytes in the precipitate. Unlike acids, use of water-miscible organic solvents has consistently offered, with proper pH adjustment, almost quantitative recoveries for a large number of drugs in a simple and rapid way (18–25, 28).

Methanol and acetonitrile are the most frequently used water-miscible organic solvents for protein denaturation. The main advantage of using methanol for protein precipitation is that a clear supernatant is obtained and a flocculent precipitate is formed. Acetonitrile, on the other hand, gives a hazy supernatant with a fine precipitate. The compatibility of these solvents with the reversed-phase liquid chromatographic eluents commonly used for separation purposes is an added advantage.

As an example, the denaturating procedure using acetonitrile requires mixing of 1 volume of sample homogenate with 1–4 volumes of the solvent, the ratio depending on the composition of the sample itself. Residues are uniformly distributed in the melange formed by the addition of the organic solvent and, therefore, lengthy multiple extractions of the precipitate are not required. However, this procedure may lead to coextraction of water-insoluble compounds and considerable dilution of the sample. One way to overcome this problem is to add dichloromethane that removes acetonitrile and water-insoluble interferences, leading to an increased concentration of the analyte in the aqueous supernatant.

Microwave irradiation is a particularly attractive technique because it can denature both quaternary and tertiary structures of proteins within 1 s (10). Dissociation of drug–protein complexes can also be achieved by heating the samples in hydrochloric acid or by incubation with subtilisin-A or proteinase-K, which are nonspecific proteolytic enzymes that hydrolyze peptide bonds (29–32). Overnight incubation at 60°C in enzyme suspensions of pH 9 containing, for example, subtilisin-A constitutes a well-established procedure for solubilizing tissue proteins and releasing drug residues that are covalently bound to the proteins. Compared with other pertinent methods, digestion with subtilisin-A is less elaborate and yields higher recoveries of the residues for a number of toxicologically important compounds. However, extensive grinding and homogenization of the tissues prior to digestion are necessary, whereas the maximal action of subtilisin-A is achieved at a pH range 8–10, which excludes its use to compounds that are not stable under these conditions. It is also not yet clear to what extent the covalently bound residues are liberated under these enzymic digestion conditions.

Enzyme systems such glucuronidase or sulfatase can further be used for hydrolyzing the conjugates formed during drug metabolism with glucuronic and sulfuric acid, respectively. This treatment is very important because direct isolation of these conjugates is laborious and time-consuming due to their highly hydrophilic nature and their ionization at physiological pH values. Moreover, their detection by application of microbiological methods is not possible, while their detection by physicochemical methods, although feasible, is generally difficult. Such drug conjugates can only be detected in their intact form by immunochemical methods and, therefore, in that case deconjugation procedures are not needed.

Protein denaturation is most important for another reason as well. The presence of proteins in the extracts of the samples favors the formation of persistent emulsions during subsequent liquid–liquid extractions. This makes for further handling problematic and can cause rapid deterioration or even clog the analytical liquid chromatographic colum. It also stops unwanted metabolism of the analytes, thus eliminating artifact formation during analysis. Alternative procedures usually applied to stop enzyme activity in enzyme-containing matrices include rapid cooling in liquid nitrogen and addition of enzyme inhibitors such as piperonyl butoxide (10, 11).

20.4   EXTRACTION/CLEANUP

Extraction/cleanup have been recognized as the most critical steps in any analytical process. Traditional solvent extraction techniques such as solid–liquid and liquid–liquid extractions are still very popular. These techniques are time tested, and analysts are familiar with the processes and procedures. However, they are often time-consuming and labor-intensive, and usually require large volumes of organic solvents.

During the last two decades, regulatory pressure towards increased productivity and reduction of the organic solvents used for extraction has created an increasing demand for alternative faster and more automated sample preparation procedures. The research in this challenging topic has been stimulated and there has been more activity in the area of sample preparation in the past 10 years than at any time in history. New sample preparation technology that holds promise for increasing accuracy and throughput in sample preparation has been introduced. We have seen considerable advances in this area, in particular with the introduction of sorbents with high affinity and/or selectivity for solid-phase extraction of an ever-expanding list of analytes from various matrices. Nevertheless, the demand for quicker, more generic extraction procedures is still on the rise. This is mainly because the time available to develop new assay extraction methods, as well as the time to process a batch of samples once the method has been validated, has been significantly compressed.

Some of the newer procedures use the same basic principles as the older extraction methods but provide fast and easy-to-use options and generally consume less organic solvent. For the most part, they have higher initial purchase price than the traditional methods. Examples include supercritical fluid extraction, accelerated solvent extraction, and automated solid-phase extraction and microextraction. Modular systems are now readily available that automate these procedures and bridge them to analytical instruments, such as gas chromatography (GC), mass spectrometry (MS), or high-performance liquid chromatography (LC). These techniques are environmentally sound since they incorporate low-volume or solvent-free extractions, and, in most cases, they can also increase the efficiency of the extraction.

The new procedures, in general, have a small but growing number of advocates, but they are not still widely applied in the analytical laboratory. As a whole, advanced sample preparation technology has been comparatively slow in gaining widespread acceptance in drug residues analysis in foods. People are reluctant to change the way they do things. Therefore, a lot of new technology has been neglected although government regulatory agencies are becoming more flexible in accepting new methods. Supercritical fluids, for example, have many advantages and supercritical fluid extraction may become the most fruitful area for foods and pharmaceuticals in the near future, but the inertia to change has been great.

20.4.1 Solid–Liquid Extraction

Solid–liquid extraction can take many forms: shake-filter, homogenization, sonication, and microwave-assisted solvent extraction. The shake-filter procedure merely involves adding a solvent to the sample and agitating it to allow the analytes to dissolve into the surrounding liquid until they are completely isolated. This technique works well when the analyte is very soluble in the extracting solvent and the physical state of the sample provides the extracting medium with a great surface area per unit mass. Samples that are in a finely divided form can be extracted more rapidly than samples in the formds of lumps or chunks. Using hot extraction solvents may speed up the extraction process. Following shaking, the dispersion is filtered, decanted, or centrifuged to separate the solution from insoluble solids. The shake-filter technique can be performed in batches, which helps in increasing the overall sample throughput.

To get faster and more complete extractions, analysts can use homogenization or sonication procedures. In the homogenization procedure, organic or aqueous solvent is added to the sample, and the sample is homogenized in a blender to a finely divided state. Small, well-dispersed sample specimen promotes the efficiency of the extraction. Following homogenization, either filtration or centrifugation techniques may be used for separating liquid and solids. The latter is the preferable technique in the field of drug residue analysis, because filter papers may turn out to be good adsorbers for analytes usually present in trace concentrations, and/or they may be significant sources of interfering compounds, has been demonstrated (33) in the analysis of furazolidone residues in eggs.

Sonication in the presence of solvent is also an alternative, very effective procedure to maximize extraction yield. Ultrasonic agitation allows more intimate solid–liquid contact, whereas the gentle heating generated during sonication can further aid the extraction process. In this technique, sample in a finely divided state is placed in a vial, solvent is added, and the vial is immersed in an ultrasonic bath to be submitted to ultrasonic radiation. An ultrasonic probe or cell disrupter can also be used instead. Ultrasonic agitation is a safe and rapid procedure that allows for multiple samples to be extracted simultaneously.

Another solid–liquid extraction procedure that has been evolved from a little known, scarcely used technique to a crucial step in many current sample preparation methods is microwave-assisted solvent extraction. Although microwave sample digestion techniques have been used widely in analytical laboratories, microwave-assisted extraction is a relatively new technique still being explored as an alternative to conventional solvent extraction (34–37). In microwave-assisted extraction, the sample can be placed in either a pressure vessel or a vessel heated at atmospheric pressure. The latter appoach is commonly known as Soxwave extraction. The solvent usually contains a component with a high-dielectric constant, so that it can be heated by microwaves. Chemical substances absorb microwave energy roughly in proportion to their dielectric constants: the higher the value of the dielectric constant, the higher the level of microwave-energy absorption.

Analysts have a choice when using microwave-assisted solvent extraction. They can use either a microwave-absorbing extraction solvent with a high dielectric constant or a non-microwave-absorbing extraction solvent with a low dielectric constant. In the former approach, both sample and solvent are placed in a closed vessel, microwave radiation heats the solvent to a temperature higher than its boiling point, and the hot solvent extracts rapidly the analytes under moderate pressure. In the latter approach, either an open or a closed vessel may be used (38–40). In this procedure, the solvent does not become hot because it absorbs very low levels of microwave radiation. The sample that usually contains water or other compounds possessing a high dielectric constant absorbs, in contrast, high microwave radiation and releases the heated analytes into the surrounding cool liquid, which is selected according to its solubility characteristics. Since it is performed under atmospheric or low pressure conditions, the second approach is more gentle and is particularly recommended for use with heat-sensitive or thermally labile analytes.

Microwave-assisted solvent extraction offers many advantages. It uses less solvent than conventional liquid–liquid extraction. Users can control the heat exchange between the sample and the solvent by selecting extraction solvents based on their microwave-absorbing abilities. Many other experimental parameters including the heating time, pulsed versus continous heating, stirring versus nonstirring, closed versus open containers, and outside cooling versus noncooling of vessels are also available. Multiple samples can be extracted simultaneously, resulting in increased throughput. The technique is safe because laboratory workers are not exposed to the extraction solvents in most cases.

20.4.2 Membrane Extraction

Membrane extraction offers attractive alternatives to conventional solvent extraction through the use of dialysis or ultrafiltration procedures (41). The choice of the right membrane depends on a number of parameters such as the degree of retention of the analyte, flow rate, some environmental characteristics, and the analyte recovery. Many early methods used flat, supported membranes, but recent membrane technology has focused on the use of hollow fibers (42–45). Although most membranes are made of inert polymers, undesired adsorption of analytes onto the membrane surface may be observed, especially in dilute solutions and when certain buffer systems are applied.

Dialysis procedures are relatively slow when mass transfer is based only on diffusion. These procedures do not offer particular selectivity when they are concurrently used for extraction and cleanup purposes, because many low-molecular-weight sample components along with the analyte can pass through the membrane. Dialysis systems must be renewed frequently, automation is difficult except for the continous-flow systems, and there is a significant temperature dependence.

To increase selectivity, a diphasic dialysis membrane approach has been recently introduced in the determination of chloramphenicol in milk (46). In this procedure, dialysis tubing filled with ethyl acetate is introduced into a flask containing the sample, and the extraction is performed by shaking for 5 h. This type of dialysis may overcome some of the classic dialysis problems, since only low-molecular-weight compounds that are more lipid-soluble will pass into the organic phase, while other compounds of higher molecular weight will remain in the aqueous phase. This procedure is promising but does not provide any advantages over liquid extraction methods in terms of reduction in sample preparation time or in improvement in analytical capability.

Ultrafiltration is an alternative procedure somewhat similar to dialysis: it involves use of molecular mass cut-off filters to remove proteinaceous material. It is based on the selective retainment of analytes by convective solvent flow through an anisotropic membrane. Compounds with dimensions larger than the specified membrane cut-off will nearly quantitatively be retained, whereas compounds with smaller dimensions will pass the membrane together with the solvent. To achieve the desired ultrafiltration, the equipment must be designed to obtain a high transport flow over the membrane and to diminish the effect of increasing macromolecular concentration just above the membrane, which is the major problem in ultrafiltration (47). Nowadays, ultrafiltration membranes with cut-off values ranging from a molecular weight of 500 to 300,000 are commercially available.

As with dialysis, a limitation with ultrafiltration procedures is that any low-molecular-weight proteinaceous material will pass through the filter. However, ultrafiltration offers some distinct advantages over classic dialysis because temperature effects are less pronounced, a minimum of exchange solvent is required, and automation is simple. One of the major advantages of the ultrafiltration procedure is its speed; by applying a hollow fiber ultrafiltration system a flow rate of 100 L/h can be obtained. Furthermore, the combination of several ultrafiltration membranes can allow isolation of a group of analytes with a very narrow molecular weight range. In addition, protein removal by ultrafiltration eliminates interferences and low-recovery problems inherent to most of the conventionally protein-precipitation methods (48, 49). Ultrafiltration procedures have been widely applied in the analysis of tetracycline (50, 51) and penicillin (52, 53) residues in milk.

20.4.3   Liquid–Liquid Extraction

Liquid–liquid partitioning constitutes the most common form of solvent extraction. It is a relatively simple, rapid, and flexible procedure that is readily applicable to all types of matrices and a wide range of analytes ranging from fairly polar to nonpolar compounds (54). Despite the fact that they are simple and rapid, liquid–liquid extractions may result in highly selective isolation (55, 56). However, they also necessitate use of toxic and inflammable solvents, favor formation of emulsions, may cause sample losses by occlusions or adsorption onto glass surfaces, and are often laborious and costly.

Liquid–liquid extractions involve the separation of analytes from interferences by partitioning the sample between two immiscible solvents. In most cases, one of the liquids is an aqueous solvent and the other is an organic solvent. The selectivity and efficiency of the extraction process are governed by the choice of the solvent pair. In aqueous and organic solvent pairs, the more hydrophilic compounds prefer the aqueous phase and the more hydrophobic compounds will be found in the organic phase.

It is often, preferable to isolate the analytes of interest in the organic solvent, because the analyte can be generally concentrated by evaporation of the solvent. However, care should be exercised during evaporation, since traces of acids or alkalis present in the extract may degrade acid- or base-labile drug residues when solvent volume approaches dryness (33, 57), unless a small quantity of a "keeper" solvent such as ethylene glycol has been introduced. If reversed-phase chromatography is going to be employed for final analysis, the analytes can be also isolated in the aqueous phase, because this phase can be injected directly into the reversed-phase column.

Organic solvents that are miscible with water such as low-molecular-weight alcohols, ketones, aldehydes, and acetonitrile are unsuitable for liquid–liquid extractions. On the other hand, organic solvents immiscible with water are suitable if they are volatile enough, show compatibility with the detection system, and possess polarity and hydrogen-bonding properties that enhance partitioning of the analytes in the organic phase. Among these provisions, polarity is usually the most important factor in choosing the extraction solvent. The closer the solvent polarity is to the analyte polarity, the higher the extraction efficiency may be. The best solvent for a selective extraction procedure is the most apolar solvent with which the drug can be extracted with sufficient efficiency. An increase in selectivity can also be attained by the addition of inorganic salts that favor the trasfer of the analyte from the aqueous to the organic phase through a salting-out effect.

Apart from polarity, extraction efficiency is also determined by the sample/solvent volume ratio, and the intensity and duration of mixing. A thorough mixing may generate an cnormous interfacial area that ensures intimate contact between the two phases, which aids mass transfer. Due to this vigorous mixing, emulsion formation is always a possibility in liquid–liquid extraction, particularly for samples containing surfactants or fatty matrices. Emulsification can be avoided by using larger volumes of the extracting solvent or by less vigorous mixing of the samples. Methods that may be used for breaking up emulsions include centrifugation, addition of salts to the aqueous phase, addition of a small amount of a different organic solvent, and filtration of the emulsion through glass-wool or phase-separation filter paper.

The pH of the sample/solvent system is also most important in the development of an efficient extraction scheme. The undissociated molecule of the analyte is soluble in a nonpolar organic solvent. Therefore, alkalinization of samples prior to extraction favors the partition of a basic drug into water-immiscible organic solvents, due to suppression of its ionization. For an efficient liquid–liquid partition cleanup, the extracted basic analyte can be back-extracted into an acidic aqueous solution that can in turn be basified to favor reextraction of the analyte into the organic solvent. Acidic analytes can likewise be extracted by taking advantage of their pK value and partitioning characteristics. However, the analyte may occasionally be chemically unstable in the pH range necessary for an efficient liquid–liquid extraction. To overcome this problem, the analyte can be derivatized in the biological sample with an appropriate reagent to form a suitable derivative that can be subsequently quantitatively extracted. Amphoteric analytes show an optimum extraction pH that in any case should be accurately determined (58), but the extraction of neutral analytes is independent of the pH value.

Nevertheless, it may sometimes be proven extremely difficult to extract highly polar drug residues from edible animal products at any pH value. In that case, a possible solution is salting out by addition of sodium sulfate until the aqueous phase of the sample disappears (59) or use of a freeze-drying technique. After freeze-drying, the resulting solid residue can be dry-extracted with a suitable organic solvent and in this way freeze-drying can be of great help. An alternative solution may be sample deproteinization with acetonitrile followed by addition of ammonium sulfate until the acetonitrile phase separates. When this procedure was applied to the analysis of tetracycline residues in milk (60), salting out was not considered the predominant extraction mechanism since addition of sodium sulfate was found to be unable to promote extraction.

The efficiency of an extraction process can be greatly improved by applying ion-pairing techniques. In these techniques, specific ions are directly added to the sample in order to enable ionic analytes of opposite charge to be transferred from the aqueous homogenates into the organic solvents as neutral, well-extractable complexes (60–65). However, many similarly charged endogenous compounds can be coextracted as well. The extent of extraction is predominantly controlled by the nature and concentration of the ion-pairing reagent. The polarity of the solvent influences also the ion-pair extraction ability and, in many instances, hydrogen-accepting or hydrogen-donating properties are of importance (66). An example of effective ion-pairing extraction is the treatment of some corticosteroid glucuronic acid conjugates with tetrapentylammonium cations; the resulting ion-pairs become fairly lipophilic and readily extractable with chloroform (67).

Apart from improving extractions, ion-pairing techniques can also improve liquid–liquid partition cleanup. Examples of effective ion-pairing cleanup procedures have been described in the analysis of tetracycline (60) and penicillin (68) residues in milk; using tetrabutylammonium reagent, the resulting ion pairs turned out to be fairly lipophilic and readily extractable with organic solvents.

For difficult separations, multiple extractions are frequently carried out, although in many cases the background is also coextracted. Using multiple extractions, polar interferences may sometimes be transferred from the aqueous into organic solvents that can dissolve minute amounts of water. This problem cannot be eliminated by simple presaturation of the extraction solvent but only by washing the extract with small amounts of water (58). Another relevant issue to be considered in trace residue analysis concerns the purity of the organic solvents, since they can introduce solvent impurities into the sample extract. Therefore, the need for high solvent purification should not be overlooked in some applications.

Classic liquid–liquid extraction generally requires a great deal of handling and, thus, analysts frequently turn to automation (69–73). A number of autosamplers and workstations have been developed for LC and GC that can perform all or a portion of the extraction and concentration process. Most of these systems use their liquid dispensing and mixing capabilities to perform liquid–liquid extraction in sample vials. Some systems mix the layers by alternately sipping the solvents into the autosampler needle and dispelling the contents back into the sample vial (69). In other cases, the units use vortex mixing to spin the vial at a high rate of speed (70, 71). After the mixing is complete, the autosampler waits for a specified period of time until the phases separate. By controlling the depth of the needle, either the top layer or the bottom layer can be removed for injection or further sample preparation.

Most of autosamplers use volumes of sample in the milliliter range. Larger volumes can be better handled with robotic systems, which, however, are of limited speed. In contrast to autosamplers, which are cartesian three-dimension programmable systems, robotic systems are anthropomorphic devices working with a programmable arm. Sample processors have a high rate of accuracy and precision, allow a high throughput of samples, posses sufficient flexibility, and are far less expensive than robotic systems. However, the use of autosamplers for the analysis of drug residues in foods can be a source of major analytical problems associated with the stability of the analytes. Decomposition of the analytes may occur during extended stay of samples at laboratory temperature and light in the autosampler pending analysis. Therefore, cooling of the autosampler vial holder and/or exclusion of daylight may be a necessity in some applications (74).

A specific form of liquid–liquid extraction is the use of the time- and solvent-saving diatomaceous earth columns (75, 76). Although they contain solid diatomaceous earth, these columns are not considered to constitute solid-phase extraction systems, because the transfer of the analytes from the aqueous to the organic phase obeys all the laws of classic liquid–liquid extraction. The sorbent in the column is a special grade of flux-calcined, high-purity diatomaceous earth (77). An aqueous sample is applied to the sorbent and the sample is partitioned over the porous matrix as a stationary phase. The analytes are eluted with a water-immiscible organic solvent. The high surface area of the packing aids efficient, emulsion-free interactions between the aqueous sample, which is absorbed by the diatomaceous earth, and the organic extraction solvent. This technique is especially applicable to the isolation of lipophilic compounds from liquid aqueous samples or homogenates, because the material can hold four times its weight in water. In principle, every classic liquid–liquid extraction can be transferred to a diatomaceous earth procedure. In comparison with the classic liquid–liquid extraction, the application of prefabricated or manually packed diatomaceous earth columns offers distinct advantages including the substantial reduction of emulsification during the extraction process and a high recovery increase (78, 79). A major disadvantage is that relatively large volumes of the organic solvent are needed.

20.4.4 Solid-Phase Extraction

Liquid–liquid extractions, although valuable in sample preparation procedures, are often time-consuming, laborious, and costly, necessitating multiple partitioning in order to achieve adequate isolation of the analytes. Thus, whenever distribution problems exist or the partition coefficients of the analytes do not favor their extraction from the aqueous biological sample into a water-immiscible organic solvent, solid-phase extraction (SPE) techniques are preferably used to effect extraction and get reasonably clear extracts.

SPEs offer distinctive advantages over conventional liquid–liquid extractions. They are relatively fast, require small sample size, eliminate emulsification problems, provide the possibility of performing both cleanup and preconcentration of the extract in one analytical step, and offer high precision. Another great advantage of SPEs over liquid–liquid extractions is solvent savings. Unlike liquid–liquid extractions that often require hundreds of milliliters for single or multiple extractions, SPEs require only a few milliliters of solvents for analyte extraction and cleanup.

SPEs can afford a high degree of selectivity through use of either a selective sorbent or an appropriate combination of several different sorbents. Their contribution toward improving extraction selectivity can further be increased by applying, prior to the SPE, a liquid–liquid extraction in order to remove highly lipophilic endogenous components from the matrix (80). These advantages have made SPE sample preparation techniques very popular over the last decade (54, 81).

Most current SPE sample preparations are performed using SPE cartridges. Most often, the cartridge is made by polypropylene or polyethylene to eliminate irreversible adsorption of the analytes onto its inner surface. The cartridges usually comprise a disposable medical-grade plastic syringe barrel manually packed or prefabricated with porous particles with an average diameter of 40 μm. The packing is contained with bottom and top frits usually constructed of porous PTFE or metal. SPE cartridges are available in a wide variety of sizes, with packing capacities normally in the range of 100–500 mg suitable sorbents. Many automated SPE devices and robotics adaptations are also available (82).

In general, SPE procedures are relatively simple to perform; the cartridge is solvated and then conditioned with appropriate solvents. Sorbent solvation is a very important step, particularly in the case of chemically bonded hydrophobic sorbents, because it can open the hydrocarbon chains and increase the surface area of the sorbent (83). The sample homogenate is subsequently applied on the cartridge and forced to pass through by hydrostatic pressure, or pressure obtained by means of a syringe, or by suction using a special vacuum device. After a washing-up step with an eluent that does not elute the analytes but removes unretained matrix components (cleanup step), the analytes are eluted selectively from the cartridge with a solvent of sufficient eluotropic strength that enrichment of the extract can be effected concurrently. Elution of the analytes can be executed with reduced pressure or pressurized force by means of a syringe, followed by centrifugation. The elution rate is very important in obtaining accurate and precise results.

Extensive information about the type of solvents and their volumes needed for solvation and conditioning of any sorbent, and for washing and elution of any type of analyte by means of SPE, is available in the literature (83, 84). In many methods, a C_{18} sorbent cartridge is selected, activation is made with 2–3 ml methanol, conditioning with 2–3 ml water, washing with 2–3 ml water, and elution with 2–3 ml acidified or basified aqueous methanol. Hence, when reviewing the literature on SPE applications, one can be forgiven for thinking that there is a universal SPE technique for extracting any analyte. The universal application of this approach merely shows that there is a general lack of knowledge of the sorption chemistry taking place during analyte isolation by SPE.

According to some general principles, for chemically bonded silica sorbent cartridges, analytes corresponding to about 1–5% of the sorbent weight can be retained, 20-bed volumes of washing solvent can be applied, and elution should be executed with less than 5-bed volumes. Since the bed volume of a 100 mg cartridge is only about 150 µl, use of a large volume of washing water will remove much of the solvating methanol and affect the orientation of the hydrocarbon chains and, hence, the precision of the method.

In general, SPE isolates sample components on the basis of the principles of liquid chromatography. The sample passes over the stationary phase, and the analytes are separated according to the degree to which each component is partitioned or adsorbed by the stationary phase. The objective of an SPE scheme based on chromatographic principles is either to retain the analyte on the stationary phase thus allowing isolation of the analyte and cleanup, or to elute it rapidly in the smallest possible volume prior to analysis. This differs substantially from liquid chromatography, which requires good peak shape and relatively short retention times. As a result, the breakthrough volume, which is determined by the capacity factor of the analyte on the sorbent, is very important in SPEs in controlling the amount of sample and the solvent volume that can be applied to the column before the analyte is washed off (85). While the capacity factors should be in the range of 1–10 in liquid chromatography, they should ideally be higher than 1000 for retention and less than 0.001 for elution when using SPEs for analyte isolation (86).

Nowadays, a plethora of polar, nonpolar, or ion-exchange sorbents, originally designed for normal-phase, reversed-phase, and ion-exchange liquid chromatography, respectively, is marketed for SPE applications. Similarly to liquid chromatography, the sorbent is chosen in such a way that the interactions between the stationary phase and the analyte will be stronger than the interactions between the analyte and the mobile phase. For selective isolation of the analytes, solvents must have the weakest solvent strength possible in combination with the chosen sorbent. For instance, if a choice must be made between a C_8 or a C_{18} stationary phase, the former must be selected because it can be used in combination with a lower-strength solvent that contains less organic modifier and more water. Moreover, the extraction will work provided that the interactions between the stationary phase and the analyte are greater than those between the analyte and the matrix.

Hydrophobic sorbents including octadecyl, octyl, diphenyl, cyclohexyl, phenyl, butyl, ethyl, methyl, and copolymers of styrene and divinylbenzene can be applied for retaining nonpolar to medium polar analytes. In this list, the styrene–divinylbenzene copolymer phases such as PRP-1 and XAD-2 are the most nonpolar phases, while the methyl phase is the least nonpolar one. The analytes are adsorbed onto the hydrophobic materials by means of van der Waals interactions and, to some extent, by hydrophobic bonding or dipole–dipole interactions.

PRP-1 is a highly cross-linked material with outstanding chemical resistance. The major disadvantage of this material is its limited efficiency. However, the efficiency can be increased significantly by the addition of 1% dichloromethane to the eluting solvent (87). Addition of dichloromethane causes some swelling of the material and, thus, an increase of pressure resistance.

Amberlite XAD-2 hardly swells or shrinks upon hydration of its structure, and because of its macroreticular structure it can be used for cleanup of urine and plasma samples. Since analytes are adsorbed onto the column by means of the same interactions as in chemically bonded stationary phases, XAD-2 can be used for the simultaneous isolation of acidic, basic, and neutral analytes. An interesting application of the XAD-2 resin is the isolation of sulfate and glucuronic acid conjugates from biological samples, which is troublesome with conventional liquid–liquid extraction methods (88). One of the disadvantages of XAD-2 is that the pretreatment, cleaning, wetting, and equilibration of the column itself are rather time-consuming. However, in comparison with the chemically bonded phases, XAD-2 can be used in the entire pH range 1–14.

For extraction of polar to medium polar analytes, polar sorbents including silica, alumina, magnesium silicate, diol, aminopropyl, and cyanopropyl materials are used. The cyanopropyl phase is a sorbent of medium polarity and can be applied in the normal as well as in the reversed-phase mode. The aminopropyl phase can be used in both the normal or reversed-phase mode, and as a weak anion exchanger, but it should not be used in combination with aldehydes and ketones. Because of its mixed retention mechanism, isolations that are not possible with the usual hydrophobic or ion exchange materials can be executed on this material. It is important to realize that with these polar sorbents in adsorption chromatography, the pure adsorption mechanisms including dipole–dipole and dipole-induced dipole interactions are replaced by a liquid–liquid partition equilibrium with increasing solvent strength of the eluent.

Ion-exchange sorbents allow extraction of ionic hydrophilic analytes that are difficult or impossible to isolate with liquid–liquid extraction. The applied sorbents are permeable hydrophilic polymers or hydrophilic polymers bound to silica containing a fixed concentration of acidic and/or basic functions on the surface. In the anion exchange mode, the sorbent surface is covered with positively charged groups, such as aminopropyl, primary/secondary amine, and quaternary ammonium, which bind reversibly to anionic solutes, whereas in the cation-exchange mode the surface contains negatively charged groups, such as carboxylic and sulfonic, which bind reversibly to cationic solutes. A severe drawback of the use of ion exchange sorbents is that, because of the limited capacity of the resin-based materials, a precipitation step should be introduced in the procedure when the matrix under investigation contains a relatively high concentration of ionic components (89).

The choice of the washing and eluting solvents for a particular sorbent is most critical when SPE procedures are applied. Since SPE procedures aim to isolate analytes within a narrow polarity range while keeping all other sample components totally unretained or completely retained, a number of physicochemical and other parameters should always be taken into consideration (5, 6). The physicochemical properties of the analyte including its molecular weight, solubility, polarity and acidity, the composition and sorption behavior of the sorbent including its polarity and stability, the nature of the matrix, and the forces of the different interactions between the analyte and the sorbent, the analyte and the matrix, and the sorbent and the matrix are all parameters that can greatly help in optimizing an SPE procedure.

The correlation between solvent strength and solvent polarity depends on the polarity of the applied sorbent. For polar sorbents, solvent strength increases by increasing the solvent polarity. However, for nonpolar sorbents, the solvent strength is increased by decreasing the solvent polarity (83, 84). A general outline for selecting proper solvent strength and polarity in certain SPE applications is presented in Table 20.1. By proper selection of the type of sorbent and the elution solvents, a great variety of antibacterials, anthelminthics, anticoccidials and other antiprotozoals, anabolic hormonal-type growth promoters, and miscellaneous drugs of a wide range of physicochemical properties can be isolated from complex biological samples (Table 20.2).

The key to employing SPE procedures successfully is to understand the nature of the bonded silica surface. On a typical C_{18} surface, the siloxane structure of the silica binds a permanent layer of water molecules, which is removed only by heating. Protruding from the water layer are the bonded silica chains, whereas dispersed between them are molecules of water and the conditioning solvent. This configuration is controlled by solvation, because the higher the organic content the more extended the chains. Thus, swelling or shrinking is expected to occur during the application and elution stages of the extraction. Residual silanols are also present on this surface and can play an additional role in the extraction process because the analytes can bind to the solid phase by hydrogen bonding, dipole–dipole interactions, hydrophobic dispersion forces, and electrostatic interactions. Any or all of these forces can be involved during an extraction, and the mastery of these forces will determine the specificity of the extraction.

TABLE 20.1   General Recommendations for Using Solid-Phase Extraction
(SPE) for Sample Preparation

| Handling sequence | Type of SPE | | | |
| | Reversed-phase | Normal-phase | Ion exchange | |
			Cationic	Anionic
Sorbent polarity	Low	High	High	High
Analyte polarity	Low	High	Acidic	Basic
Conditioning solvent polarity	High (methanol)	Low (chloroform)	Water	Water
Washing solvent polarity	High (water)	Low (hexane)	Basic	Acidic
Eluting solvent polarity	Decreased (methanol)	Increased (methanol)		
Elution order	Decreasing polarity	Increasing polarity	Decreasing ionization	Decreasing ionization

The energies involved in the various bonding forces vary considerably. Hydrophobic bonding energies from dipole–dipole, dipole-induced dipole, and dispersive interactions range from 1 to 10 Kcal/mol. Hydrogen bonding between suitable polar groups has an energy of 5–10 Kcal/mol, whereas electrostatic or ionic interactions between oppositely charged species involve energies of 50–200 Kcal/mol. Many analytes are amines, which, if positively charged, will interact with the silanol groups on the surface of the solid phase. These interactions are very strong and will only be broken by a pH shift to ensure that either the amine or the silanol is unionized.

The pK of a silanol group is not easy to determine because it is influenced by the surrounding environment; however, at a pH of 2, the silanol is uncharged. Above this pH value it becomes increasingly dissociated and able to influence an extraction by virtue of its negative charge. Therefore, if a mixed-retention mechanism is present, the influence of residual silanols should be either reduced or enhanced, depending on the extraction mechanism desired.

To reduce the influence of silanol groups during an isolation, the residual silanols must be masked by using a competing base such as triethylamine or

TABLE 20.2 Applications of SPE Cleanup in the Analysis of Drug Residues in Edible Animal Products

Drug	Matrix	Type of SPE	Washing solvent	Eluting solvent	Ref.
ANTIBACTERIALS					
Aminoglycosides	Animal tissues	Sep-Pak Silica	H_2O, EtOH, H_2O	EtOH	181
Amphenicols	Animal tissues	Sep-Pak Silica	DCM	ACN/H_2O	182, 183
	Animal tissues	Extract-Clear C_{18}	ACN/acetate buffer	ACN	184
	Animal tissues	Sep-Pak C_{18}	H_2O, pet. ether	Ether	185
	Animal tissues	Baker Silica	Hexane	MeOH	186
	Animal tissues	Baker-10 C_{18}	H_2O, MeOH/H_2O	ACN	187
	Animal tissues	Sep-Pak C_{18}	—	MeOH/HCl	188
	Animal tissues	Sep-Pak Florisil	Hexane, ether	Ether/MeOH	189
	Animal tissues	Extrelut	—	DCM	190–192
	Animal tissues	Sep-Pak Silica	Pet. ether, EtOAc/ hexane	EtOAc/hexane	192
	Animal tissues	Sep-Pak C_{18}	ACN	ACN	193
	Animal tissues	Sep-Pak Silica	ACN	EtOAc	
	Eggs	Sep-Pak Silica	DCM	ACN/H_2O	183
	Eggs	Sep-Pak Silica	Hexane	Acetone	194
	Fish	Sep-Pak Florisil	Hexane, ether	Ether/MeOH	189
	Liver	Bond Elut Silica	EtOAc/hexane, hexane	Phosp. buffer	195
	Meat	Sep-Pak Silica	EtOAc/hexane, ether/hexane	Ether	196
	Meat	Chem Elut CE 1020	—	EtOAc	197
	Milk	Extrelut QE,	—	EtOAc	198
		Bakerbond C_{18}	H_2O	MeOH	
	Milk, serum	Extrelut-3	—	EtOAc	199
	Urine	Bakerbond C_{18},	H_2O, H_2O/MeOH	H_2O/MeOH	200
		Bakerbond C_{18}	H_2O	MeOH	

(continued)

TABLE 20.2 Continued

Drug	Matrix	Type of SPE	Washing solvent	Eluting solvent	Ref.
Cephalosporins	Milk	Sep-Pak C$_{18}$	H$_2$O, DCM	MeOH/ACN	201
	Milk	Sep-Pak C$_{18}$	Phosp. buffer, ACN/H$_2$O	ACN/H$_2$O	202
	Milk	Sep-Pak C$_{18}$	H$_2$O	ACN	203
	Milk	Bond-Elut C$_{18}$	Amm. acetate soln	MeOH	204
	Animal tissues	Bond-Elut C$_{18}$,	Phosp buffer, NaOH soln	ACN/H$_2$O	205
		Bond-Elut LRC SAX,	H$_2$O	ACN/HOAc	
		Bond-Elut LRC SCX		ACN/NaCl soln	
Macrolides	Animal tissues	Baker Silica	DCM	MeOH	206
	Animal tissues	Bond-Elut C$_{18}$	H$_2$O	MeOH/acetate buffer	207
	Animal tissues	Bond-Elut diol	CHCl$_3$, H$_2$O	MeOH/amm. acetate soln	208
	Animal tissues	Bond-Elut SCX	H$_2$O, 0.1M K$_2$HPO$_4$	MeOH	209
	Fish	Bond-Elut-NH$_2$	DCM, DCM/MeOH	DCM/MeOH	210
	Fish	Sep-Pak C$_{18}$	H$_2$O/MeOH, H$_2$O	H$_2$O/ACN	211
	Milk	Sep-Pak C$_{18}$	H$_2$O, NH$_4$OH/H$_2$O, H$_2$O	MeOH/HOAc	212
Nitrofurans	Animal tissues	Extract-Clean C$_{18}$	ACN/acetate buffer	ACN	184
	Animal tissues	Bond-Elut NH$_2$	DCM/hexane, CHCl$_3$/ hexane	CHCl$_3$/MeOH	213
	Animal tissues	Extrelut 1	—	EtOAc	214
	Animal tissues	Sep-Pak Silica	DCM/pet. ether, pet. ether	MeOH, EtOAc/MeOH	215
	Animal tissues	Bakerbond C$_{18}$	H$_2$O	ACN contg NH$_3$	216

Nitrofurans	Eggs	Sep-Pak Silica	DCM/pet. ether, pet. ether	MeOH, EtOAc/MeOH	215
	Fish	Bond-Elut C$_{18}$	H$_2$O	MeOH	217
	Fish	Bond-Elut NH$_2$	DCM/hexane, CHCl$_3$/hexane	CHCl$_3$MeOH	218
	Milk	Sep-Pak C$_{18}$	—	0.1M sodium perchlorate/ACN contg 0.5% HOAc	219
Penicillins	Shrimp	Bond-Elut C$_{18}$	H$_2$O	H$_2$O	220
	Animal tissues	Sep-Pak C$_{18}$	NaCl soln, MeOH/H$_2$O/ NaCl soln	H$_2$O	15
	Animal tissues	Bond-Elut C$_{18}$	NaCl soln, H$_2$O	Phosp. buffer/ACN	221
	Animal tissues	Bond-Elut C$_{18}$	Phosp. buffer	MeOH/H$_2$O	222
	Animal tissues	Bond-Elut C$_{18}$	NaCl soln	ACN	223
	Animal tissues	Isolute C$_{18}$	NaCl scln/H$_2$O	Phosp. buffer/ACN	224
	Eggs	Bond-Elut C$_{18}$	NaCl scln/H$_2$O	Phosp. buffer/ACN	225
	Fish	Sep-Pak Florisil		ACN/H$_2$O	226
	Fish	Sep-Pak C$_{18}$	TCA soln/H$_2$O	ACN	227
	Milk	Sep-Pak C$_{18}$	H$_2$O, MeOH/H$_2$O contg NaCl/18-crown-6 ether	MeOH/H$_2$O	228
	Milk	Sep-Pak C$_{18}$	Phosp. buffer, ACN/H$_2$O	ACN/H$_2$O	202
	Milk	tC$_{18}$ Sep-Pak	H$_2$O	ACN	229
	Milk	Bond-Elut C$_2$	H$_2$O/ACN	H$_2$O/ACN	230
	Milk	Baker-10 C$_{18}$	—	MeOH	231
	Milk	Bond-Elut C$_{18}$	NaCl soln H$_2$O	Phosp. buffer/ACN	232
	Milk, meat, cheese	tC$_{18}$ Sep-Pak	NaCl soln H$_2$O	Phosp. buffer/ACN	233
	Muscle	tC$_{18}$ Sep-Pak	Phosp. buffer	ACN	234, 235

(continued)

TABLE 20.2 Continued

Drug	Matrix	Type of SPE	Washing solvent	Eluting solvent	Ref.
Quinolones	Fish	Sep-Pak C_{18}	H_2O, MeOH/H_2O	MeOH	236
	Fish	Baker-10 NH_2	Hexane/EtOAc	Oxalic acid/ACN/ MeOH	237
	Fish	Baker-10 C_{18}	Buffer/MeOH	MeOH/ammoniac soln	238
	Fish	Bond-Elut C_{18}	MeOH/H_2O	MeOH	239
	Fish	Baker-10 NH_2	Hexane/EtOAc	Oxalic acid/ACN	240
	Milk	Bond-Elut PRS	MeOH, H_2O, MeOH	MeOH/NH_4OH	241
Streptomycin, dihydrostreptomycin	Animal tissues	IEC Bakerbond	H_2O	Phosp. buffer	242
Sulfonamides	Milk	Bakerbond C_{18}	H_2O, hexane	MeOH	243
	Milk	Cyclobond-I	Phosp. buffer	ACN/H_2O	244
	Milk	Bond-Elut C_8	H_2O	MeOH	245
	Honey	Sep-Pak Florisil	ACN/DCM	MeOH/DCM	246
	Animal tissues	Sep-Pak Silica	Hexane	DCM/acetone	247
	Animal tissues	Bond-Elut C_{18}	H_2O	ACN contg TEA	248
	Animal tissues	Bond-Elut C_{18}	H_2O	MeOH	249
	Animal tissues	Bakerbond C_{18}	H_2O, hexane	MeOH	250
	Animal tissues	Tandem Sep-Pak Silica and Sep-Pak C_{18}	DCM	Phosp. Buffer	251
	Animal tissues	Sep-Pak C_{18}	H_2O	MeOH	252
	Animal tissues	Sep-Pak C_{18}	H_2O	ACN	253
	Animal tissues	Baker-10 NH_2	Hexane	ACN/H_3PO_4	254
	Animal tissues	Sep-Pak Silica	—	ACN	255
	Fish	Bond-Elut C_{18}	H_2O	MeOH	217
	Fish	Baker-10 NH_2	Hexane	ACN/H_3PO_4	254
	Eggs	Bond-Elut C_{18}	H_2O	ACN contg TEA	248
	Eggs	Baker-10 NH_2	Hexane	ACN/H_3PO_4	254
	Eggs	Sep-Pak Silica	—	ACN	255

	Sample	SPE	EDTA/McIlvaine buffer	ACN/EDTA/McIlvaine buffer	
Tetracyclines	Animal tissues	Sep-Pak C_{18}		ACN/EDTA/McIlvaine buffer	256
	Animal tissues	Bond-Elut CH	H_2O	MeOH	257
	Animal tissues	Baker-10 C_{18}	H_2O	EtOAc, MeOH/EtOAc	258
	Animal tissues	Baker-10 C_{18}	H_2O	Oxalic acid/MeOH	259
	Animal tissues	Baker-10 COOH	EtOAc	Oxalic acid/ACN	260
	Animal tissues	Bond-Elut C_{18}	H_2O	MeOH/ACN	261
	Animal tissues	Bond-Elut C_{18}	H_2O	EtOAc, MeOH/EtOAc	262
	Animal tissues	Sep-Pak C_{18}, Bond-Elut SCX	H_2O	MeOH	263
	Animal tissues	SDB-RPS cation-exchange extraction membrane	0.1M HCl	MeOH/HCl, MeOH contg NH_4	264, 265
	Animal tissues	Isolute Cyclohexyl	H_2O	MeOH	266
	Fish	Bond-Elut C_{18}	H_2O	Oxalic acid/MeOH	267, 268
	Fish	Baker-10 COOH	EtOAc	Oxalic acid/ACN	260
	Fish	Bakerbond C_{18}	—	MeOH	269
	Milk	ENVI-Chrom P	H_2O	MeOH	270
	Milk, meat, cheese	Sep-Pak C_{18}	H_2O	Oxalic acid/MeOH	271
	Eggs	Bond-Elut C_{18}	H_2O	Oxalic acid/MeOH	272
	Eggs	Baker-10 COOH	EtOAc	Oxalic acid/ACN	260
	Honey	Baker-10 C_{18}, Baker-10 COOH	MeOH	EtOAc, Oxalic Acid/MeOH/ACN	273
	Honey	Baker-10 C_{18}, Baker-10 COOH	H_2O, EtOAc, —	EtOAc/MeOH, Oxalic acid/MeOH/ACN	274

(continued)

TABLE 20.2 Continued

Drug	Matrix	Type of SPE	Washing solvent	Eluting solvent	Ref.
Trimethoprim	Meat	Sep-Pak C_{18}	0.05M, pH 3, phosp. buffer contg 5 mM pentanesulfonic acid	ACN/phosp. buffer	275
ANTHELMINTHICS					
Albendazole	Bovine liver	Sep-Pak C_{18}	H_2O, toluene	EtOAc	276, 277
Albendazole-2-aminosulfone	Milk	Bond-Elut SCX	Phosp. buffer, ACN, EtOAc, MeOH	H_2O/NH_3	278
Avermectin B_1	Meat, plasma	PT C_{18}	—	MeOH	279
Closantel	Animal tissues, plasma	Bond-Elut C_{18}	—	ACN	280
Clorsulon	Bovine kidney	Bond-Elut CH	H_2O	ACN	281, 282
	Milk	Bond-Elut CH	H_2O	ACN	283
Coumaphos	Honey	Tandem Sep-Pak C_{18}	H_2O	DCM/hexane	284
Eprinomectin	Bovine tissues	Bond-Elut NH_2	DCM, toluene	EtOH/EtOAc	285, 286
Fenbendazole	Bovine liver	Bond-Elut Silica	DCM	MeOH/DCM	287
Ivermectin	Animal tissues	Sep-Pak Silica	—	$CHCl_3$	288
	Animal tissues	Bakerbond C_{18},	H_2O/ACN	Methyl *tert.* butyl ether	289
		Sep-Pak Silica	—	$CHCl_3$	
	Animal tissues	Bond-Elut C_{18},	—	ACN	290
		Bond-Elut Silica	—	$CHCl_3$	
	Bovine liver	Sep-Pak Alumina-B,	DCM/EtOAc, acetone	MeOH	291
		Supelclean LC-Silica	—	$CHCl_3$	

Drug	Matrix	SPE column	Solvent	Eluent	Ref.
Ivermectin	Bovine serum	Sep-Pak C₁₈	H₂O/ACN	ACN/DCM	292
	Bovine tissues	Sep-Pak Silica	—	ACN	293
	Meat, liver	Sep-Pak C₁₈	—	ACN	294
	Milk	Bond-Elut C₁₃	—	ACN	295
		Supelclean LC-Silica	—	CHCl₃	
	Milk	Bond-Elut Silica	EtOAc/hexane	EtOAc/MeOH	296
		Bond-Elut Silica	—	CHCl₃	
	Muscle, serum	Bond-Elut C₁₈	H₂O/ACN	Methyl *tert.* butyl ether	297
Levamisole	Milk	Sep-Pak C₁₈	—	EtOAc	298
Luxabendazole	Serum, urine	Sep-Pak C₁₈	—	H₂O/DMF	299
Mebendazole	Fish	Bakerbond Silica	EtOAc/hexane	MeOH/HOAc	300
Moxidectin	Bovine tissues	Sep-Pak Florisil	—	Hexane	301
Thiabendazole	Plasma	Supelclean LC18	H₂O, H₂O/MeOH	MeOH	302
Thiabendazole, 5-hydroxythiabendazole	Meat	Extrelut-20	Hexane	DCM	303
	Milk	Bond-Elut PRS	EtOAc	ACN/phosp. buffer	304
Fenbendazole and metabolites	Liver, urine, plasma	Chem-Elut	—	DCM	305
Mebendazole and two metabolites	Fish	Bakerbond NH₂	EtOAc/hexane, isooctane	MeOH	306
Four benzimidazoles	Milk	Bond-Elut Silica	DCM	MeOH/DCM	307
Five anthelminthics	Milk	Bond-Elut C₁₈	ACN/H₃PO₄	ACN	308
Five benzimidazoles	Bovine tissues	Bond-Elut Silica	DCM	MeOH/DCM	309
Eight benzimidazoles	Animal tissues	Prep-Elute C₂	H₂O	EtOAc	310

(continued)

TABLE 20.2 Continued

Drug	Matrix	Type of SPE	Washing solvent	Eluting solvent	Ref.
Eight benzimidazoles	Meat	Sep-Pak C_{18}, Sep-Pak Florisil	— —	ACN CHCl$_3$/MeOH contg TEA	311
ANTICOCCIDIALS AND OTHER ANTIPROTOZOALS					
Dimetridazole	Bovine muscle	Sep-Pak Silica	DCM	Amm. acetate soln	312
	Swine tissues	Bond-Elut Silica	DCM	EtOAc	313
	Poultry tissues and eggs	Bakerbond Silica	DCM or toluene, hexane	Acetone	314
Halofuginone	Chicken serum	Bond-Elut C_8	H$_2$O/HOAc, MeOH-HOAc, H$_2$O/HOAc	H$_2$O/ACN/HOAc contg decylamine	315
Imidocarb	Bovine kidney	Bond-Elut CBA	MeOH	MeOH contg TFA	316
Lasalocid	Chicken tissues and eggs	Bond-Elut Silica	CHCl$_3$	CHCl$_3$/MeOH	317
Monensin	Bovine tissues and milk	Sep-Pak Silica	DCM	DCM/MeOH	318
	Chicken tissues	Sep-Pak Silica	DCM	CHCl$_3$/MeOH	319
	Chicken tissues	Sep-Pak Silica	CHCl$_3$, CHCl$_3$/ hexane	CHCl$_3$/MeOH	320
Nicarbazin	Chicken tissues	Sep-Pak Alumina-B	DMF, hexane	MeOH	321
	Chicken tissues	Tandem Sep-Pak Alumina-B	DMF	MeOH	322, 323
	Eggs	Bond-Elut Silica	CHCl$_3$/hexane	CHCl$_3$/ACN	324
Salinomycin	Chicken skin and fat	Bond-Elut Silica, Bond-Elut C_{18}	DCM	DCM/MeOH	325
	Chicken tissues	Sep-Pak Silica	H$_2$O, MeOH/H$_2$O DCM/MeOH	MeOH DCM/MeOH	326

Semduramicin	Chicken liver	Bond-Elut C$_8$, Bond-Elut Silica	H$_2$O, MeOH/H$_2$O DCM/isooctane, EOAc	EtOAc DCM/MeOH	327
Nitroimidazoles	Animal muscle	Baker-10 C$_{18}$	—	MeOH	328
ANABOLIC HORMONAL-TYPE GROWTH PROMOTERS					
Diethylstilbestrol	Bovine muscle	Sep-Pak C$_{18}$	H$_2$O, MeOH/H$_2$O	MeOH/H$_2$O	329
Nortestosterone, methyltestosterone	Bovine muscle	Baker Florisil	EtOH/pet. ether	EtOH/pet. ether	330
Stanozolol and two hydroxy metabolites	Urine	Clean Screen DAU	HOAc, MeOH	EtOAc/NH$_4$OH	331
Zearalenone, α-zearalenol	Urine	Bond-Elut C$_{18}$, Sep-Pak Silica	H$_2$O/MeOH	Acetone CHCl$_3$/MeOH	332
Zearalenone, α-zearalenol, β-zearalenol	Milk	Bond-Elut NH$_2$	— DCM/hexane	MeOH	333
Trenbolone, epitrenbolone	Bovine tissues	Bakerbond C$_{18}$, Baker Silica	H$_2$O/MeOH Acetone/benzene	H$_2$O/MeOH Acetone/benzene	334
Thirteen steroid hormones	Meat	Bond-Elut C$_8$, Bond-Elut Silica, Bond-Elut NH$_2$	H$_2$O, H$_2$O/MeOH EtOAc/hexane	MeOH EtOAc/hexane EtOAc/MeOH	335
Thirty steroid hormones	Fatty tissues	Bond-Elut C$_{18}$	H$_2$O, H$_2$O/MeOH, hexane	MeOH	336
OTHER DRUGS					
Acriflavine, proflavine	Fish	Bakerbond C$_{18}$	—	—	337

(continued)

TABLE 20.2 Continued

Drug	Matrix	Type of SPE	Washing solvent	Eluting solvent	Ref.
β-Adrenergic agonists	Hair, urine	Isolute C_{18}	H_2O, H_2O/MeOH	MeOH	338
	Liver, muscle	Baker-WCX	H_2O, EtOH	EtOH contg NH_4OH	339
	Liver, urine	Bakerbond Alumina, Bond-Elut Certify	ACN, HOAc, MeOH	H_2O, DCM/PrOH contg NH_3	340
	Urine	Baker-10 C_{18}	NaOH soln, MeOH	MeOH	341
	Urine	Bond-Elut Certify, Bakerbond C_{18}	HOAc, MeOH	EtOAc contg NH_4Cl, MeOH	342
	Urine	Clean Screen DAU	—	EtOAc contg NH_3	343
Anti-inflammatory drugs	Plasma	Bakerbond C_{18}	Ascorbic acid soln, H_2O	Ether/hexane	344
Corticosteroids	Meat	Bond-Elut C_8, Bond-Elut Silica	H_2O, H_2O/MeOH	H_2O/MeOH, EtOAc	335
	Milk, liver	Bakerbond C_{18}	H_2O, H_2O/acetone, H_2O/MeOH, DCM/hexane, EtOAc/hexane	EtOAc	345
Dexamethasone	Bovine tissues	Bond-Elut C_{18}	H_2O, H_2O/MeOH, hexane	H_2O/MeOH	346
Flunixin	Milk	Bakerbond C_{18}	—	EtOAc	347
	Urine	Bond-Elut Certify II	H_2O, MeOH, hexane	HOAc/hexane	348
Gentian violet, leukogentian violet	Fish	Tandem Bakerbond Alumina and Bond-Elut PRS	ACN; H_2O, ACN, amm. acetate buffer	ACN; ACN/amm. acetate buffer	5

Analyte	Tissue	Column	Wash/Load	Elution	Ref.
Malachite green and metabolites	Fish	Tandem Bakerbond Alumina and Bond-Elut PFS	ACN	ACN / ACN/acetate buffer, MeOH contg hydroxylamine	349–351
	Fish	Bakerbond C_{18}	—	ACN/H_2PO_4 soln contg pentane sulfonic acid	352
	Fish	Bakerbond sulphonic acid	MeOH/citric acid contg ascorbic acid, H_2O, MeOH	NH_3, MeOH	353
Malachite green, gentian violet and metabolites	Fish	Tandem Bakerbond Alumina and Bond-Elut PRS	ACN / H_2O, ACN/amm. acetate buffer	ACN / ACN/amm. acetate buffer	354,355
Phenylbutazone, oxyphenbutazone	Plasma	Isolute C_{18}	Phosp. buffer, hexane	Hexane/EtOAc	356
Sedatives and β-blockers	Kidney	Baker diol	Ether, EtOH, ACN/H_2O	ACN/H_2O contg amm. acetate	357
	Kidney	Sep-Pak C_{18}	H_2SO_4 soln	ACN/H_2SO_4 soln	358
	Liver, kidney	Bond-Elut C_{18}	H_2SO_4 soln	ACN/H_2SO_4 soln	359
Thyreostatics	Thyroid gland	Sep-Pak Silica	Pet. ether, hexane	Hexane/EtOAc	360
Thyreostatics	Thyroid gland	Sep-Pak Silica	Pet. ether, hexane	Hexane/EtOAc	360
	Thyroid gland, urine	Sep-Pak Silica	$CHCl_3$	$CHCl_3$/MeOH	361

ACN, acetonitrile; MeOH, methanol; EtOH, ethanol; PrOH, propanol; BuOH, butanol; EtOAc, ethyl acetate; ether, diethyl ether; pet. ether, petroleum ether; HOAc, acetic acid; DCM, dichloromethane; THF, tetrahydrofuran; TEA, triethylamine; DMF, dimethylformamide; TFA, trifluoroacetic acid; TCA, trichloroacetic acid; EDTA, ethylenediaminetetraacetic acid; contg, containing; soln, solution; phosph., phosphate; amm., ammonium.

ammonium acetate. As an alternative, ion suppression can be employed by choosing a pH value at which either the silanol (pH < 4) or the ionizable groups on the analyte molecule are uncharged. If silanol activity cannot be reduced using the above suggestions, increasing the ionic strength of the conditioning solvent, sample, and washing solvent may be tried as a means to compete with the silanols and prevent analyte bonding.

To enhance the influence of silanol groups during an isolation, a conditioning buffer with a pH value higher than 4 should be used to ensure that the residual silanol groups are ionized. A buffer is recommended as the second conditioning solvent because water can have a variable pH value and has little buffering capacity. An application of this approach has been described in the determination of salbutamol in plasma using a silica sorbent activated by successive aliquots of methanol and water. Plasma was passed through the cartridge and the positively charged salbutamol was extracted by ionic interaction with the silanol groups. The stationary phase was washed with water and then acetonitrile. Because the retention mechanism was essentially ionic, acetonitrile was used as a washing solvent to remove material bound by nonpolar bonding because it did not have the capacity to interfere with the binding. Elution of the analyte was effected by methanol containing 0.5% ammonium acetate.

The following points outline the stages of an optimized SPE procedure:

- Wet the sorbent with methanol to open up the hydrocarbon chains and thus to increase the surface area available for interaction with the analyte, and to remove residues from the packing material that might interfere with the analysis. Failure to carry out this stage effectively will result in poor recoveries of analytes due to reduced retention on the column and interference peaks.
- Wash the sorbent bed with LC-grade water or a suitable buffer. This will remove excess methanol and prepare the surface for the sample. This conditioning step should be as similar as possible in polarity, ionic strength, and pH value to the sample being extracted. It is not necessary to use a large volume of solvent since three to four times the bed volume of the cartridge is usually sufficient.
- Apply the sample, allow it to flow through the sorbent bed, and discard the waste. Biological samples are generally viscous and, whenever possible, must be diluted to speed passage through the sorbent bed. All samples must be centrifuged prior to extraction to remove particulate matter that could block the column. If a large volume of sample is used, the column may no longer be wetted and a reduction in recovery will be observed. To overcome this problem, 3–5% methanol should be added to a large volume sample prior to processing. This will help in maintaining the equilibrium between the stationary and mobile phases. Flow

rates through the sorbent bed should be controlled and, if an analyte is strongly protein bound, slower flow rates may be used to achieve good analyte recovery.

- Wash the column with water or a suitable solvent to remove endogenous compounds selectively from the sample matrix, which might interfere with the subsequent chromatography.

- Elute the sample with a suitable solvent and collect the eluent for immediate analysis or further sample preparation. The volume of the eluting solvent should be as small as possible to avoid dilution of the extract and destroy of sensitivity.

SPE procedures can be performed either off-line or on-line with the chromatographic separation. The main advantage of the application of on-line SPE is the ease of automation. In general, off-line procedures can be easily transformed to online procedures, although some problems may arise in the compatibility of the solvents used for SPE and the analytical column.

Major advantages of SPE are the possibilities of performing cleanup and preconcentration of the sample in one step, and using several precolumns in series to achieve the desired degree of purification for complicated samples. One of the drawbacks of the system is the fact that frozen and thawed plasma sometimes contains solid particles (fibrins) that can block the SPE cartridges, but the application of specially constructed frits can solve this problem. Major limitations of packed-bed SPE cartridges can be considered the restricted flow rate and channeling. Restricted flow rates are due to the low ratio of cross-sectional area to bed mass, which hampers the ability to decrease processing time. Channeling is caused by the inherent difficulty of packing loose particles, thus requiring the use of excess bed mass to retain the desired analyte quantitatively. Channeling in packed beds causes nonuniform flow, reducing reproducibility and sorption capacity.

SPE disc technology through rigid disc and membrane disc formats provides a way around the above-listed limitations of packed-bed SPE columns. SPE discs closely resemble membrane filters; they are flat, usually 1 mm or less in thickness, with diameters varying in size. Some disks are sold loose, and users must install them in a filter holder. Others are sold preloaded in disposable holders with Luer fittings (82).

Rigid disc microcolumns contain an extraction disc made of rigid glass fiber material with a silica-bonded phase. Several sizes of rigid extraction discs are available, and each addresses different processing requirements. Varying the diameter, thickness, and porosity of the extraction discs produces various bed masses that have measured void volumes in the range 10–50 μl. Rigid extraction discs can also contain any of the bonded-phases used in conventional packed-bed SPEs. In practice, however, discs are available in only a limited number of phases.

In some designs, a glass fiber filter is supported above the extraction disc to prefilter samples containing particulates without clogging the extraction disc. Because of the rigid disc design, frits to support the extraction disc are not necessary. The polyethylene frits used in conventional SPE columns may be a source of contamination (90) and have a large surface area and void volume.

Rigid disc microcolumns require special handling procedures that differ significantly from conventional packed-bed SPEs. The small bed mass requires reduced volumes during processing. Column conditioning, selective washes, and elution require only 3–5 void volumes each (91). Another characteristic of the small bed mass is a reduction in the amount of the weakly retained compounds, which provides a cleaner extract (92). The rigid disc microcolumns retain the analytes at the top surface of the disc, the capacity of the extraction efficiency not being a problem in most cases. Because of the high ratio of flow area to bed volume, a moderate pressure differential yields high flow rates. With the rigid disc microcolumn configuration, the channeling observed with packed columns is eliminated.

In addition, analysts can create a multimodal SPE column by stacking several discs with differing bonded phase in the disc holder. With the proper chemical design, such multimodal systems can provide customized separation protocols. The stacking order of the discs depends on the particular physicochemical characteristics of the analysis under way. The general rule is to place the disc with the more selective extraction mechanism on top of the less selective adsorbent.

As far as the membrane disc microcolumns is concerned, they contain an extraction disc made of packing-impregnated polytetrafluoroethylene or polyvinyl chloride materials. Membrane discs address the channeling that occurs with packed columns, but they can become clogged like membrane filters when processing samples containing particulates. Among the various approaches used to overcome the flow limitations of the membrane discs, creation of a depth filter above the membrane is the most effective way of preventing clogging, although it increases the column void volume (93). Membrane disc microcolumns with strong cation-exchange properties were recently successfully used to extract a number of β-agonists including clenbuterol, bromobuterol, mabuterol, clenproperol, and mapenterol residues from urine (94).

In general, both configurations of modern SPE disc technology offer distinct advantages over conventional SPE packed columns due primarily to combination of reduced bed mass, large flow area, and rigid structure. With proper selection of extraction conditions and bonded phases, SPE discs require significantly less sample, solvent, and processing time than packed SPE columns.

Another relatively new SPE approach originally developed for the analysis of volatile organic compounds in environmental samples is solid-phase microextraction (SPME). This technique has gained acceptance for a wide variety of additional applications for the isolation of organic compounds from aqueous solutions at sub-ppb levels (95, 96). SPME offers several advantages for sample preparation, including reduced time per sample, lower cost, less sample manipulation, elimination of organic solvents, and reduced analyte losses.

SPME uses a polymer-coated fused-silica fiber, typically 1 cm $\times$ 100 μm, that is fastened into the end of a fine stainless steel tube contained in a syringelike device and protected by an outer stainless steel needle. In use, the plunger of the device is depressed to expose the fiber to the sample matrix so that the organic compounds to be sorbed onto the fiber. The plunger is retracted at the end of the sampling time, and then it is depressed again to expose the fiber to a desorption interface for analysis typically by GC or LC. In a recent variation of this technique, the so-called in-tube SPME, the polymer is not coated on a fiber but on the inside of a fused-silica capillary before analysis by LC.

In SPME, the process is controlled by diffusion of analytes from the surrounding solution through a thin, static, aqueous layer located around fiber. An equilibrium is established, and because nonpolar organic compounds have a high distribution ratio in the nonpolar fiber, excellent quantification and recovery of analytes are possible. Although the most common polymeric material used for coating is polydimethylsiloxane, a polyacrylate-film fiber provides more efficient extractions for polar semivolatile analytes such as phenols (97). The SPME process has recently been automated using an autosampler in which the standard autosampler needle has been replaced by a fused-silica fiber (98). With the continued introduction of new SPME fibers, and the possible application of micro-LC columns to in-tube SPME, the future is promising for application of these technologies to drug residue analysis.

20.4.5 Matrix Solid-Phase Dispersion

Application of SPE technology requires samples to be in a liquid, relatively nonviscous, particulate-free and homogenous state. Many edible animal products, however, start out in forms that are not directly applicable to SPE. This fact presents problems for analysts trying to find the best process for obtaining analytes that are in solution and free from tissue debris and for reducing the semisolid sample to a liquid extract. Semisolid samples such as animal tissues constitute some of the most difficult samples to disrupt and homogenize. On the other hand, readily homogenized liquid samples such as milk present fewer complications in terms of disruption and homogeneity, but they may be too viscous or they may contain particulates that hinder rapid SPE analysis. Analysts often encounter emulsions and may need to perform several centrifugations, reextractions, and complex sample manipulations to render samples into suitable forms. To remedy many of these complications a new technique was introduced in 1989 (99). Called matrix solid-phase dispersion (MSPD), this technique allows analysts to prepare, extract, and purify any sample in a simultaneous process.

The MSPD technique involves the mixing of a bonded phase-solid support and a tissue matrix in a glass mortar, and the blending with a glass pestle to produce a nearly homogenous dispersion of tissue cell membranes and matrix components. The blending of tissue with C_{18}-coated silica proceeds rapidly and smoothly, producing a semidry material. This has been observed to be the case with fat, liver, or muscle tissues. Tissue dissolution onto a solid support can also be conducted with C_3, C_8, as well as polymeric phases. The semidry material can be packed into a column from which different drug residues can be eluted based on their solubilities in the polymer/tissue matrix. In this approach, drugs can be rapidly isolated based on their distribution in the polymer/tissue matrix and polarity of the solvents used. The extracts so obtain often require no further processing prior to instrumental analysis.

The sample is disrupted completely and distributed over the surface as a function of interactions with the support, the bonded phase, and the tissue matrix components themselves. The solid support acts as an abrasive that promotes sample disruption, whereas the bonded phase acts as a lipophilic, bound solvent that assists in sample disruption and lysis of cell membranes. The MSPD process disrupts cell membranes through solubilization of the component phospholipids and cholesterol into the C_{18} polymer matrix, with more polar substituents directed outward, perhaps forming a hydrophilic outer surface on the bead. Thus, the process could be viewed as essentially turning the cells inside out and forming an inverted membrane with the polymer bound to the solid support. This process would create a pseudo-ion exchange-reversed-phase for the separation of added components. Therefore, the C_{18} polymer would be modified by cell membrane phospholipids, interstitial fluid components, intracellular components and cholesterol, and would possess elution properties that would be dependent on the tissue used, the ratio of C_{18} to tissue employed and the elution profile performed (99–104).

The interactions observed between the individual components and the target analytes in MSPD are greater and different, in part, from SPE. They appear between the analyte and the solid support, the analyte and the bonded phase, the analyte and the dispersed matrix, the matrix and the solid support, and the matrix and the bonded phase; all of the above components interact with the elution solvents, and the dynamic interactions of all of the above occur simultaneously. As a result, both the bonded phase and the solid support are expected to affect the results (99–104).

For applications that require a lipophilic bonded phase, C_8 and C_{18} phases may be used interchangeably. The best ratio of sample to solid support-bonded phase is 1 : 4. However, this ratio is dependent on the application. Lower ratios have been used successfully, and samples have been scaled up to 2 g from the typical 0.5 g used in most MSPD procedures. The isolation of more polar analytes from biological samples is assisted by the use of polar solid supports-phases and less polar analytes by less polar phases.

Studies on solid supports have shown that the pore size of the silica-based sorbents is of little importance in MSPD, but it should be considered as could vary with the sample. Particle size is of greater importance since particles as small as 3–20 μm can lead to extended solvent elution times and plugged MSPD columns. However, 40 μm particles with 60 Angstrom pores have been used extensively and successfully. Sorbents that have a blended range of particle size such as 40–100 μm work equally well and can be used in most applications (101, 103). These materials also tend to be less expensive. Depending on the application, analysts can also use non-end-capped materials and materials with a range of carbon loading. Different applications may benefit, suffer, or be unaffected by these parameters, but workers should consider them to obtain the best extraction efficiency and the cleanest sample.

Conditioning the sorbent to be used for MSPD can greatly enhance analyte recovery and, also, speed up the process of blending and dispersion. It is essential to condition the column sorbent with a solvent that breaks the surface tension differences that may exist between the sample and solid support-bonded phase. The MSPD performance can also be affected by addition of acids, bases, or ion-pairing reagents to the matrix at the time of blending or to the solvents used for washing or analyte elution. The ionization or suppression of ionization of analytes and sample components can greatly affect the nature of interactions of specific analytes with the blend and the eluting solvents. MSPD is characterized by elution and retention properties that appear to be a mix of partition, adsorption, and paired-ion paired-component chromatography that is unique.

The washing and eluting solvents and their usage sequence are of utmost importance to the success of MSPD. Analysts can vary elution profiles to obtain ideal analytical results by isolating the analyte or cleaning the column with each solvent step. The nature of the MSPD column and the range of interactions permit isolation of a range of different polarity analytes or an entire class of compounds in a single solvent or in different solvents passed through the column. The analytes in MSPD tend to be eluted in fractions that are somewhat inconsistent with expected solubility behavior. This inconsistency may be due to the fact that the elution of a sample removes analytes but simultaneously fractionates the sample components. These characteristics make MSPD readily amenable to multiresidue isolation and analysis. Table 20.3 provides a list of recent MSPD applications for the extraction and analysis of various matrices and drug residues.

In some cases, the eluate from a MSPD column is adequately clean. However, additional steps are often required to remove coeluted matrix components either by using other solid-phase materials packed at the bottom of the MSPD column or by eluting analytes from the MSPD column directly onto a second SPE

TABLE 20.3 Examples of Matrix Solid-Phase Dispersion (MSPD) for the Analysis of Drug Residues in Edible Animal Products

Drug	Matrix	MSPD material	Washing solvent	Eluting solvent	Ref.
Aminoglycosides	Bovine tissues	Bondesil Cyanopropyl	Hexane, EtOAc, H$_2$O, MeOH/H$_2$O	H$_2$O, 0.05 M H$_2$SO$_4$	362
	Bovine kidney	Bondesil Cyanopropyl	Hexane, EtOAc, MeOH, H$_2$O	0.1 M HCl	363
Cephapirin	Bovine muscle	C$_{18}$	Hexane, benzene, EtOAc	MeOH	100
Chloramphenicol	Meat	C$_{18}$	Hexane, DCM	EtOAc	364
	Milk	C$_{18}$	Hexane, benzene	EtOAc	365
Flunixin	Milk	Silica gel	DCM-hexane	EtOAc	347
Furazolidone	Chicken muscle	C$_{18}$	Hexane	DCM	366
	Meat	C$_{18}$	Hexane, DCM	EtOAc	364
	Milk	C$_{18}$	Hexane	DCM	367
	Swine muscle	C$_{18}$	Hexane	EtOAc	368
Ivermectin	Bovine liver	C$_{18}$	Hexane	DCM/EtOAc	291
	Milk	C$_{18}$	H$_2$O	EtOAc	296
Moxidectin	Bovine tissues	C$_{18}$	Hexane	DCM/EtOAc	369
Nicarbazin	Chicken tissues	C$_{18}$	Hexane	ACN	321
	Meat	C$_{18}$	Hexane, DCM	EtOAc	364
Oxolinic acid	Catfish muscle	C$_{18}$	Hexane	ACN, MeOH	370
Penicillins	Bovine muscle	C$_{18}$	Hexane, benzene, EtOAc	MeOH	100

Sulfonamides	Bovine and swine muscle	C_{18}	Hexane	DCM	371
	Catfish muscle	C_{18}	Hexane	DCM	372
	Catfish muscle	C_{18}	Hexane	DCM	373
	Meat	C_{18}	Hexane	DCM	364
	Milk	C_{18}	Hexane	DCM	374, 375
	Salmon muscle	C_{18}	Toluene/hexane	DCM	376
	Swine muscle	C_{18}	Hexane	DCM	377
Tetracyclines	Milk	C_{18} + EDTA – oxalic acid	Hexane	ACN/EtOAc	271, 378
	Fish	C_{18} + EDTA – oxalic acid	Hexane	ACN/MeOH	379
Thiabendazole, mebendazole	Meat	C_{18}	Hexane, DCM	EtOAc	364
Virginiamycin	Meat	C_{18}	Hexane, DCM	EtOAc	364
Five benzimidazoles	Bovine liver	C_{18}	Hexane	ACN	380
Seven benzimidazoles	Milk	C_{18}	Hexane	DCM/EtOAc	381
Eight benzimidazoles	Animal tissues	Diatomaceous earth	–	EtOAc	382

Abbreviations as in Table 20.2.

column for sample cleanup and analyte enrichment. Other alternatives include the use of classic liquid–liquid extraction for final sample cleanup prior to analysis.

MSPD can greatly reduce sample manipulation, solvent usage and disposal, and working time. In most cases, MSPD generally requires 95% less solvent and 90% less time than classic sample preparation procedures. It can also eliminate emulsification problems, but the number and amounts of coextracted components also greater adversely affect the detection limit of the final analysis.

20.4.6 Restricted-Access Media

Although not a real sample preparation procedure, direct injection of the sample into the LC can save hours of sample-preparation time. Packing materials for this technique have been available in many versions for nearly a decade, but the technique is still relatively unknown to many analysts, even those involved in food analysis.

The packing material first described for direct injection of biological samples was prepared by simply saturating the accessible adsorption sites of a C_{18} reversed-phase silica with human plasma proteins (105). After saturation, the human plasma proteins were denatured at the external surface, and their native conformation was destroyed. With this treatment, the proteins formed a hydrophilic layer with weak ion-exchange properties, which provided protection from contact with the sample proteins, whereas the alkyl ligands inside the pores remained unchanged and thus served for analyte retention. The retention behavior of the saturated phase did not alter with this treatment, but the efficiency was reduced dramatically. Such protein-coated columns have shown a lifetime of several months (106).

Many variations on this theme that allow repetitive, direct injection and chromatographic analysis of untreated sample matrices including tissue homogenates, milk, plasma, and saliva (107–112) have appeared since the original publication. These packings have been described generically as restricted-access media because they are generally characterized by a limited accessibility of macromolecular compounds to the adsorption sites of the porous supports.

On the basis of the separation mechanism, restricted-access media can be classified into physical or chemical diffusion barrier types. The limited accessibility of the former type is due to the pore structure of the support that represents physical diffusion barriers for macromolecular compounds. The restricted access of the latter type is due to covalently or adsorptively bonded synthetic or natural polymers that cover the support surface, preventing macromolecules from being adsorbed on or denatured by the column packing material.

The usual base materials for LC restricted-access media are porous silica supports, which limit the pH range of the mobile phases to 2–8. Polymer-based stationary phases have also been used as restricted-access media and are characterized by a high chemical stability throughout the entire pH range but, depending on the polymer type and the mobile phase, their mechanical stability is lower and their hydrophobicity is higher than that of the silica-based supports. In addition, polymer supports show much lower separation efficiency than the silica supports. When using 10 μm particles, the efficiency rarely exceeds 30,000 theoretical plates/m, while conventional silica supports of the same particle size can provide an efficiency of 50,000 theoretical plates/m (113). Some specifications of commercially available restricted-access media are presented in Table 20.4.

Besides the above differentiation, restricted-access media can be further subdivided on the basis of the topochemistry of the bonded phase. Packings with a uniform surface topochemistry show a homogenous ligand coverage, whereas packings with a dual topochemistry show a different chemical modification of the pore internal surface and the particle external surface (114). Restricted-access media of the former type are divided into mixed-mode and mixed-function phases, bonded-micellar phases, biomatrix, binary-layered phases, shielded hydrophobic phases, and polymer-coated mixed-function phases. Restricted-access media of the latter type include the Pinkerton's internal surface reversed-phase, Haginaka's internal surface reversed-phase diol, alkyl-diol silica, Kimata's restricted-access media, dual-zone phase, tris-modified Styrosorb, Svec's restricted-access media, diphil sorbents, Ultrabiosep phases, Bio Trap phases, and semipermeable surface phases.

Mixed-mode and mixed-function phases combine different chromatographic modes, such as size exclusion and affinity chromatography, or different functionalities, such as hydrophilic and hydrophobic ligands. Well-known phases of this type are those based on hydrophilic materials that are nonadsorptive for proteins, that is, porous glass materials modified by diol ligands or porous polymeric supports (115). Subsequent modification of these materials with affinity ligands provided adsorbents that were highly specific for particular groups of analytes.

Mixed-function phases synthesized by a reaction of porous base silica gels with a hydrophilic and a hydrophobic trifunctional silane followed by hydrolysis of the oxirane ring have been also developed (116, 117). Since both diol and alkyl or aryl ligands are randomly distributed on the inner and outer support surface, these mixed-function phases are suitable for analysis of hydrophilic and hydrophobic substances in samples of biological origin. Column efficiency is not significantly influenced after 500 injections of 20 μl serum (116). However, two repetitive injections are usually needed to saturate the hydrophobic ligands of the support surface with proteins prior to the final analysis of a protein-containing sample (118).

Bonded-micellar phases are porous unmodified silica supports with an adsorptively bonded detergent layer (119). In these phases, the hydrophilic sites of the detergent molecules are directed to the outside, which prevents the adsorption

TABLE 20.4 Specifications of Typical Commercially Available Restricted-Access Media

Name	Type	Surface chemistry	Column dimensions	Lifetime
Bio Trap 500	Protein-coated external phase	Internal: C_{18} External: α-1-acid glycoprotein	Precolumn: 10 × 3.0 mm	500 injections of 10 μl plasma
Capcell Pak MF	Polymer-coated mixed function phase	Mixed function C_1, phenyl, or C_8 and polyoxyethylene	Analytical: 50, 100 and 150 × 4.6 mm	>500 injections of 20 μl serum
ChromSpher 5 Biomatrix	Mixed-function phase	Ligand with phenyl, alkyl and hydroxyl groups	Precolumn: 50 × 4.6 mm Analytical: 150 × 4.6 mm	>500 injections of 20 μl plasma
Hisep	Shielded hydrophobic phase	Polyoxyethylene-polymer with disubstituted aromates	Precolumn: 20 × 4.6 mm Analytical: 150 and 250 × 4.6 mm	>1000 injections of 10 μl serum
ISRP GFF II	Internal surface reversed-phase	Internal: glycyl-L-phenylalanyl-L-phenylalanine External: glycine	Analytical: 50, 150 and 250 × 4.6 mm	>500 injections of 10–20 μl serum
LiChrospher ADS	Alkyl-diol silica internal phase	Internal: C_{18}, C_8 or C_4 External: diol	Precolumn: 25 × 4.0 mm	>200 injections of 500 μl plasma
Semipermeable surface	Polymer-coated external phase	Internal: C_8 External: polyoxyethylene-polymer	Analytical: 150 × 4.6 mm	>500 injections of 20 μl serum
Ultrabiosep	Protein-coated external phase	Internal: C_8 External: protein	Analytical: 150 and 250 × 4.6 mm	>250 injections of 20 μl plasma

of protein while low-molecular-weight analytes can reach the hydrophobic C_{10}-alkyl chains of the detergent and are retained. Size exclusion is not due to the pores in the base silica but to the density of the adsorbed detergent molecules. Major disadvantage of these phases is the gradual loss of their restricted-access properties as the detergent molecules, which are not covalently fixed to the surface, may be washed out from the column after their association with samples' proteins.

Comparable to the bonded-micellar phases are the binary-layered phases. These phases are also covered by a ligand that possesses both hydrophilic and hydrophobic functions. Diol groups at the outside prevent adsorption of matrix proteins, and methoxypropyl chains shielded by the diol functionalities serve as adsorption sites for very hydrophobic analytes (120).

Also based on porous silica support, the so-called Biomatrix phases contain a ligand that combines both hydrophilic and hydrophobic properties in the same molecule. Nonpolar analytes interact with the hydrophobic phenyl and alkyl moieties of the ligand, while the hydrophobic outer part of the ligand is supposed to be the result of hydroxyl groups that prevent the adsorption of proteins.

Pinkerton's internal surface reversed-phase supports are designed to enable large biomolecules to be eluted quickly at or near the void volume of the column and to retain small molecules such as drugs and drug metabolites beyond the void volume. Early packings consisted of porous particles that had glycyl-L-phenylalanyl-L-phenylalanine bonded to silica (121). By exposing the bonded particles to carboxypeptidase, the phenylalanine was removed from the outer surface, creating a diol–glycine hydrophilic phase outside the pores. Because the enzyme could not penetrate inside the pores, the packing retained its inner hydrophobic surface characteristics. The negative charge of the carboxyl group of the amino acids both at the external and internal surface provided also weak cation-exchange properties and delayed elution of positively charged analytes and matrix compounds (122). When a serum sample was injected, proteins and other large biomolecules were excluded from the packing by repulsion from the hydrophilic surface group, whereas small molecules diffused into the pores interacting with the hydrophobic surfaces by a reversed-phase mechanism. This packing material can be used for acidic as well as basic compounds. When the packing material was used in a guard column of 10×3.0 mm (internal diameter) I.D. packed with 5 μm spherical particles, about 1000 serum injections could be made before the column should be replaced (121).

For synthesis of the commercially available GFF-II version of the Pinkerton's internal surface reversed-phase, monofunctional instead of trifunctional silane has been used in order to prepare more homogenous surfaces (123). Compared with the first version, GFF-II shows significantly improved selectivity, retention capacity, and separation efficiency as demonstrated in the analysis of trimethoprim (124).

Compared with the Pinkerton's internal surface reversed-phase packing, alkyl-diol silica phases provide significantly increased retention capacity. These phases are based on silica supports that react with 3-glycidoxypropyl-methyldimethoxysilane. Acidic hydrolysis of the epoxy groups leads to a diol-modified silica. In the next synthesis step, this silica is esterified with fatty acids of different chain length and is covered with alkanoyl ligands on both external and internal surfaces. Similarly to the synthesis of the Pinkerton's internal surface reversed-phase packing, enzymes are used to differentiate both surfaces (125). These diol-modified supports with the hydrophobic pore surface display several distinct properties. Their size exclusion limit is a molecular weight of about 15,000, whereas their retention capacity remains the same even when injecting a total serum volume of 100 ml in 500 μl injections (126).

In contrast to the internal surface reversed-phases described above, Kimata's internal surface reversed-phases are synthesized without use of enzymes. These C_1, C_8, C_{18}, and phenylethyl-modified porous silica supports are treated with HCl at 100°C for 5 h to cleave preferentially the ester bonds at the external surface (127). Hydrolysis inside the pores is extremely slow because of hydrolysis products that are enriched in the pores, low wettability, and the presence of air bubbles. The generated silanol groups are reacted with 3-glycidoxypropyl-trimethoxysilane, which is then hydrolyzed to hydrophilic diol groups. Several variations of Kimata's supports with different hydrophobicity exist, so these phases can be used for analyzing a broad spectrum of analytes.

A completely different way of surface differentiation, specifically pore-size-specific functionalization of special supports, has been recently described with Svec's restricted-access media that are characterized by easy synthesis, quantitative protein recovery, and high column stability (128, 129). The shielded hydrophobic phases comprise porous silica with a layer of a polyoxyethylene polymer as a hydrophilic network, which includes hydrophobic regions that have substituted aromatics serving as hydrophobic adsorption sites for small analytes (130). The hydrophilic polymer layer is impermeable to macromolecules to prevent the retention of matrix proteins from biological samples. These phases have been used for the determination of many drugs in serum and plasma including diuretic and inflammatory agents (131, 132). Users can solve problems with the retention of hydrophilic analytes by adding ion-pairing reagents to the mobile phase.

The polymer-coated mixed-function phases are also porous silica modified by a multistep process (133). In the first step, the silica particles are covered with a layer of a silicone polymer that diminishes the negative effects of the silica surface. Following coverage, hydrophobic styrene groups representing the analyte adsorption sites are introduced. In the next step, hydrophilic properties are given to the material by coverage with biocompatible non-protein-adsorbing ligands, such as polyoxyethylene and oligoglyceryl groups. These phases are generally characterized by higher retention capacities, better protein exclusion, and faster mass transfer of small molecules.

The so-called diphil sorbents fit into the class of protein-coated supports. In these phases, silica-modified particles are saturated with albumin, and the adsorbed and denatured protein layer is stabilized with glutaric dialdehyde (134). Due to their structure, these sorbents exhibit both hydrophilic and organophil (diphil) properties that give them their name.

Comparable to the other protein-coated supports are the Ultrabiosep and the BioTrap phases. The former are composed of C_4, C_8, or C_{18} reversed-phase silica supports covered with a biological polymer which is not described in the literature (135). The latter are commercially available as Bio Trap Acid or Bio-trap Amine precolumns (136). They are C_{18}-modified silica supports covered with α-1-acid glycoprotein as a biocompatible layer. Due to the immobilized protein, this type of reversed-phase material also possesses weak ion-exchange properties.

The semipermeable surface phases constitute restricted-access media in which the hydrophilic properties are provided by a semipermeable layer of poly-oxyethylene that covers reversed-phase silica supports (137). In the first generation semipermeable surface phases, the polymer layer was adsorbed by means of nonionic detergents of either the Tween (polyoxyethylene sorbitane fatty acid ester, branched structure) or the Brij (polyoxyethylene fatty acid ether, linear structure) type. In these phases, the hydrophobic part of the detergent molecules is adsorbed on the alkyl chains of the support so that the detergent sites can form a hydrophilic layer on which the polyoxyethylene can anchor. A major disadvantage of the first-generation phases was the gradual washing out of the detergent and the polymer over the time. As a result, a second generation of semipermeable surface phases was developed, where the polyoxyethylene layer was covalently bonded to the silica matrix so that detergents were no longer required. Comprised of polyoxyethylene-covered C_8, C_{18}, cyano, and phenyl-modified base silica supports, these second-generation semipermeable surface phases are characterized by their high stability with organic solvents, quantitative protein recovery, and high separation efficiency.

The major application of the restricted-access media is in the LC analysis of drugs and metabolites in body fluids. Samples may be run in single-column, coupled-column, or column-switching mode. In the single-column mode, the sample is injected directly into the restricted-access media column under conditions in which the undesired matrix, mainly proteins, will pass through the column unretained. The drugs and metabolites are then eluted from the column by gradient elution. In the coupled-column mode, a short restricted-access media column serves as the precolumn or initial column, and the drugs and metabolites are transferred to a secondary column after matrix elution through a column-switching valve. The drugs are then separated using a reversed-phase column that provides a better separation and a cleaner chromatogram than that formed with the single-column mode.

20.4.7 Supercritical Fluid Extraction

Supercritical fluids have been used for many years by the food industry as solvents for extracting caffeine from coffee and tea, and for isolating aromas and flavors from spices and herbs. However, their application in sample preparation procedures was delayed until the late 1980s, when pumping systems for supercritical fluids became available through the rise of interest in supercritical fluid chromatography. Since then, increasing concerns over environmental pollution, disposal costs, and exposure of analysts to harmful organic solvents have placed supercritical fluid extraction (SFE), a sample preparation procedure that is still in an evolutionary state, in an outstanding position (138).

Supercritical fluids are substances that are above their critical temperature and pressure. Every substance has a point in its gaseous phase where, if the pressure is raised while the temperature is held constant above its critical temperature, it will exhibit properties of both a gas and a liquid. This means that it is dense like a liquid but, like a gas, has no surface tension.

Density is a factor in the solvating power of a supercritical fluid; the more dense the fluid, the more powerful its solvent strength. Since changing the temperature and pressure within the supercritical phase changes the density, a supercritical fluid can be made to possess a wide range of solvent power. This property together with its increased diffusion and lower viscosity makes supercritical fluid an attractive extraction medium.

Carbon dioxide has been by far the supercritical fluid of choice for analytical SFE (139). The selection of CO_2 was initially based on its widespread use in supercritical fluid chromatography, its low critical temperature, and the high degree of nonideality that the gas exhibits even at relatively low levels of compression (140, 141). In general, CO_2 mimics the solubilizing behavior of nonpolar to moderately polar solvents. At low densities (0.2–0.45 g/ml), the solubilizing power of CO_2 is similar to that of hexane, as the density increases the polarity gradually changes, so that at about 0.6 g/ml CO_2 behaves more like the moderately polar solvent methylene chloride.

However, CO_2 does not always work the best for all analytes. It is not very polar, so in cases where the extracted analyte is polar, small amounts of organic modifiers such as methanol, ethanol, or isopropyl alcohol must be added to increase the polarity of the solvent (142). Methanol is the most commonly used modifier because it is the least toxic of the polar solvents that can be used. Other modifiers are water, acetonitrile, tetrahydrofuran, and methylene chloride. The addition of a small percentage of modifier to the solvent can increase the efficiency of the extraction by 100%. Changes in polarity with small additions of modifiers can be dramatic; a solubilizing power equivalent to that of a 50% acetonitrile in water has been achieved with less than 5% organic modifier added to CO_2 (143).

Apart from CO_2, several alternative supercritical fluids as far as the polarity index is concerned have been described (144). Nitrous oxide, with a small permanent dipole moment of 0.17 D, was one of the first tested alternatives. It is now avoided due to the risk of oxidation and explosion particularly when the matrix organic content is high (145–151). Other alternatives such as freons or water/ methanol are also limited because of environmental hazards or critical temperatures and pressures too high for convenient use, respectively. Chlorodifluoromethane or freon-22 is nonflammable, has a large dipole moment of 1.29 D, and is believed to be less ozone-depleting than older freon-11 and freon-12. However, it is very expensive, has a relatively high critical temperature of 96°C, and is still damaging since it contains chlorine. Trifluoromethane, also known as fluoroform or freon-23, has a large dipole moment of 1.65 D, critical temperature and pressure lower than those of CO_2, and is believed to be less hazardous to the atmosphere than freon-22 because it does not contain chlorine. Critical properties and dipole moments of several supercritical fluids are presented in Table 20.5.

In combination with temperature, the SFE pressure control, through density variation, the solvating power of CO_2. For CO_2, low pressures such as 75 bar (1090 psi, 80°C, d = 0.15 g/ml) correlate to a solvent power analogous to pentane. For higher pressures such as 380 bar (5550 psi, 40°C, d = 0.95 g/ml), the solvent power is more similar to liquid solvents such as methylene chloride, carbon

TABLE 20.5 Critical Properties and Dipole Moments of some Typical Supercritical Fluids

Extraction fluid	Critical temperature (°C)	Critical pressure (atm)	Dipole moment (debye)
CO_2	31.3	72.9	0.96
N_2O	36.5	72.5	0.94
C_2H_4	9.9	50.5	–
NH_3	132.5	112.5	0.40
$n\text{-}C_5$	196.6	33.3	0.51
$n\text{-}C_4$	152.0	37.5	0.50
CCl_2F_2	111.8	40.7	1.12
CHF_3	25.9	46.9	1.65
CH_3OH	240	78.5	1.70
H_2O	374.1	218.3	1.85

tetrachloride, toluene, and benzene. Thus, a chemical change or benefit can occur from adjusting physical parameters such as pressure and temperature.

When selecting the pressure for an extraction, a good rule of thumb is that the lower the analyte molecular weight, the less pressure density is required for compound solubilization. A second consideration for selecting a pressure level relates to polarity and polar interactions; the more polar an analyte is or the more tightly it is bound to the matrix, the greater the pressure-density required for the dissolution and removal of the analyte from the matrix.

Temperature is an important but complex parameter for controlling the extraction. At a particular density, an infinite number of combinations of temperature and pressure yield the same value of density. For example, with temperature-setting precision of 1°C from 40°C to 120°C, 80 combinations of temperature and pressure yield a density of 0.050 g/ml. Temperature and density vary inversely and nonlinearly. Choosing a low-temperature–high-density (relatively low pressure) combination often yields fast, efficient extractions. Although analysts can obtain fast, efficient results when working with high pressures (high densities) and temperatures, the extraction may contain other solutes that can interfere with the analysis.

Supercritical CO_2 should not be perceived as capable of extracting only the desired target analyte since coextractives are frequently dissolved in as well, just as in liquid extractions. Since the dissolution power of a supercritical fluid is exponentially proportional to its fluid density, rapid and exhaustive extractions can be best handled by conducting the extractions at high pressures. Extraction selectivity for a particular species in SFE can be achieved at low temperatures (32–60°C) and low densities, but usually at the expense of solute solubility. A low temperature–density procedure is useful for thermally sensitive compounds. In some cases, good reasons exist for using higher temperatures, including thermal contribution in terms of enthalpy and phase transfer kinetics. On the one hand, the extraction of nonpolar analytes at the extraction temperature of 80°C is better than at 40°C. On the other hand, this advantage can also reach a point of diminishing returns; 80°C also proves to be a more advantageous temperature than 120°C at constant pressure. This phenomenon is probably very complicated, so users should exercise caution in extrapolating these results to general cases as the role of increasing temperature at constant density has not been yet elucidated.

To ensure overall extraction of a polar solute, the pressure or density must be increased or a modifier must be added to the extraction fluid after an initial low-pressure extraction. In this way, the analyte of interest can be collected separately from the oily interference. Polar solutes may be removed more easily from matrices with higher moisture content. It is believed that the analyte is solubilized in the entrained water and removed from the matrix with physical removal of water. Since polar analytes benefit from the presence of water in samples, water has been added as a mobile phase modifier to enhance extraction recoveries (152).

For extraction of nonpolar analytes, drying agents are mixed with the matrix to adsorb moisture before extraction. Hydromatrix (Celite 566) has been used frequently. Sodium sulfate, and calcium sulfate (Drierite) are also used to dehydrate the matrix. Ratios of sample to drying agent of 1 : 1 up to 1 : 5 have been reported, but no rules of thumb exist for determining this ratio.

Application of SFE necessitates a CO_2 source, a pump to pressurize the fluid, an oven containing the extraction vessel, a restrictor to maintain a high pressure in the extraction line, an analyte collection vessel, and an overall system controller. CO_2 is drawn from the bottom of the tank with a dip tube because the liquid is the more dense of the two phases. The substantial vapor pressure of the CO_2 at ambient temperature helps to displace the liquid into the pump. CO_2 remains a liquid throughout the pumping or compression zones and passes through small-diameter metal tubing as it approaches the extraction vessel. A preheating zone in front of the extraction vessel allows supercritical temperature, pressure, and density conditions to be applied immediately to the analyte matrix in the vessel.

The fluid enters the extraction vessel containing the sample matrix that is mixed with a drying agent such as sodium sulfate. With this process, analytes are rapidly dissolved in the supercritical fluid, while water is retained by the sodium sulfate. Following extraction, the supercritical fluid exits the extraction vessel and passes through the restrictor. At the restrictor zone, the temperature is usually raised significantly because, as the fluid passes through the restrictor, the fluid cools and expands to a gas at atmospheric pressure. Heating the restrictor zone can help avoid plugging and too rapid precipitation of the analytes in the collection vessel that contains a small amount of organic solvent (2–30 ml). As an alternative to trapping in an organic solvent, some commercial systems allow collection of the analytes on sorbent traps containing 20–40 μm LC, GC, or SPE solid packing materials that may be cryogenically cooled.

Extractions can be carried out in dynamic, static, or combination modes. In the dynamic mode, the supercritical fluid continuously flows through the sample in the extraction vessel and out the restrictor to the trapping vessel. In the static mode, the supercritical fluid circulates in a loop containing the extraction vessel for some period of time before being released through the restrictor to the trapping vessel. In the combination mode, a static extraction is performed for some period of time, followed by a dynamic extraction.

Current practices in analytical SFE are organized into off-line and on-line procedures, despite their common physicochemical basis. Off-line SFE, the current method in fashion, offers more flexibility with respect to extracting different sample sizes and types, as well as in the choice of the final analytical method. On-line procedures are usually combinations of SFE with ancillary techniques such as GC, LC, supercritical fluid, or gel permeation chromatography.

SFE manifests its best advantages when extracting analytes from solid and semisolid rather than liquid samples. A primary limitation in extracting analytes from liquid sample matrices is the mechanical difficulty of retaining the liquid matrix in the extraction vessel. To extract a liquid sample by SFE successfully, analysts must first mix it with a solid material, such as diatomaceous earth or alumina, so that the sample is no longer free-flowing. Control of sample matrix effects is critical in SFE to limit coextractives, moderate the influence of moisture, and improve the efficiency of the extraction. Recent studies have shown that the addition of both inert and active sorbents to the sample matrix can improve the efficiency of SFE (153).

SFE has been efficiently applied to extract specific drug residues such as sulfonamides and melengestrol from edible animal products (154–157). Polar analytes, in general, remain an analytical challenge because of their lower solubility in supercritical CO_2 and their partitioning equilibria, which favor an aqueous medium. The optimal SFE system for drug residues has yet to be further explored by investigating the possibility of altering the solubility characteristics of the supercritical fluid through addition of low levels of organic cosolvents or special additives. Analysts would have an easy time if they could simply take a reference book from the bookshelf, look up the appropriate analyte–matrix pair, and use the appropriately stated instructions for application of SFE. However, because analytical SFE is relatively immature, this approach is the exception rather than the rule. The degree of SFE maturity is currently analogous to the technology of LC in the 1970s.

Supercritical fluids, in general, are inexpensive, contaminant-free, and less costly to dispose of safely than conventional organic solvents. Extracts are obtained under mild conditions that minimize thermal degradation, they are usually solvent-free or in a concentrated form, and no evaporation steps are needed prior to the final assay. However, the disadvantages of SFE should not be also ignored. As with all extraction methods, there are analytes and matrices for which SFE is not suitable. Some compounds are insoluble and may need solvent extraction. Aqueous matrices can cause problems and samples may need to be freeze-dried. Like all single-step extractions, SFE has only limited selectivity, but some distinction can be made between analytes by careful selection of temperature and pressure.

Commercial SFE systems have been on the market for only the past 5 years. Currently available systems are not perceived as being ready to perform routine extraction work. It is believed, however, that although no single analytical technique can hope to solve the diversity of sample preparation problems confronting analysts, analytical SFE will eventually take its rightful place among other sample preparation methods.

20.4.8 Immunoaffinity Chromatography

Immunoaffinity chromatography (IAC) is an elegant sample preparation procedure that is at least equivalent to but in most cases superior to other analytical sample preparation procedures. IAC is based on the selective and reversible interaction between the analyte molecule and an antibody raised against it. Generally, the antibody, immobilized on a support, is transferred to a small column. The sample solution is drawn through the column by gravity flow or by means of a peristaltic pump. Use of a pump is a preferred procedure because ensures a constant flow through the column during loading and offers the possibility to process more columns simultaneously.

As a result of the immunochemical interaction, the analyte molecules are retained by the immobilized antibodies, while matrix components fail to interact and pass through the column. Remaining unretained components can be fully removed from the column by a phosphate buffer saline washing-up step. Following washing, adsorbed analytes are desorbed from the column by means of a buffer of greater ionic strength or lower pH than the adsorption buffer; the partition equilibrium for the analyte molecules shifts from the ligand to the buffer, thus eluting the analytes (158–161).

The first requirement for preparing IAC matrices is an antiserum. Synthesis of immunogens and the processes of immunization and purification of the antibodies are not exclusively related to IAC but are essential parts of all immunochemical procedures and are discussed in Chapter 28. Following its production, the antibody has to be bound to a solid support in such a manner that it does not lose appreciable activity. In most cases, the antibodies are covalently bound to supports such as polyacrylamide, trisacryl, agarose, dextran, and cellulose. Prior to coupling, the supports must be activated using reagents such as cyanogen bromide, periodate, triazine, carbonyldiimidazole, or N-hydroxysuccinimide. Activated supports such as cyanogen bromide-activated Sepharose, and carbonyldiimidazole-activated Trisacryl are available. The cyanogen bromide coupling procedure has some disadvantages; the isourea link introduced is quite unstable, and charged isourea groups are formed that are responsible for undesirable nonspecific binding due to ion-exchange effects (162).

In coupling procedures, the covalent binding of the immunoglobulin to the carrier proceeds usually through interaction of its amino groups. Such immunoaffinity sorbents generally exhibit lower analyte capacity than that theoretically calculated, due mainly to partial inactivation of the antibodies during immobilization and to shielding of the analyte-binding sites resulting from random immobilization of the immunoglobulin molecules on the support (163).

It is also possible to immobilize antibodies by physicochemical interactions. Group-specific adsorbents including immobilized protein-A, which is a cell wall component produced by several strains of *Staphylococcus aureus;* immobilized protein-G, which is a recombinant form of a bacterial cell wall protein isolated from group G *Streptococcus;* and immobilized (strept)avidin immunosorbent can be used for this purpose. Protein-A and protein-G are able to bind specifically to the crystallizable fragment (Fc) of immunoglobulin G (164), whereas (strept)avidin has an extraordinary high affinity to biotin. The binding of antibodies via the Fc portions to protein-A leaves the analyte-combining site in the corrected orientation for the binding of the analyte (159–161). Antibodies coupled to the matrix by their analyte-binding area are immunochemically inactive and are therefore responsible for a limited column capacity.

For high-performance IAC, the preferred solid support is a glass bead solid support coated with either protein-A or protein-A covalently linked with the antibody through a carbodiimide bond (165, 166). In either case, protein-A binds to the Fc portion of the antibody so that the combining sites are oriented to the mobile phase. Once the protein is attached, the IAC matrix is packed into the column either as a slurry or dry. Pump-slurry techniques use buffers with a low salt content, such as Tris or 0.01 M phosphate buffer to minimize friction and denaturation of the immobilized antibody (16). If the solid support consists of glass beads, the packing can be freeze-dried after antibody attachment and packed dry.

The maximum amount of analyte that can be bound to an immunoaffinity column depends on both the number and the orientation of the antibody molecules on the sorbent. However, the binding efficiency of an immunoaffinity column may vary with the flow rate, the concentration of the analyte, and the nature of the sample solution. The amount of analyte practically retained is usually always smaller than that theoretically calculated. It may approximate the theoretically calculated amount only when low flow rates combined with low analyte concentrations pass through the column, and the medium of the sample solution is close to the physiological conditions. The former condition favors a strong binding reaction, because the number of analyte molecules passing through the column per time unit greatly influences this retention. As a result, retention in IAC can be improved with sample dilution, but the time of analysis inevitably also increases. Optimal flow rates are functions of the solvent systems used during isolation of the analytes and the gradient system used for the elution. Flow rates between 0.4 and 4.0 ml/min are common.

A continuing source of concern is the operating pressure of an immunoaffinity column. Excessively pressures will generate shear-type forces that could cause destruction of the antibody-support bond and lower the efficiency of the column. In general, pressures should not exceed the value of $0.34 \cdot 10^6$ Pa to prevent loss of immobilized antibody (167). This condition meets the major restriction of all immunoaffinity cleanup procedures, which is the need to use aqueous extracts. Analytes extracted from the original sample with organic solvents cannot be submitted to antibody-mediated cleanup unless they are transferred into an aqueous solution. If water-miscible organic solvents are used for extraction, dilution of the extract with water or an aqueous buffer is often an attractive alternative.

To elute the analytes from an IAC matrix, specific conditions within the column have to be applied. The elution procedure depends on the nature of the antibody–analyte bond, which is generally of weak physical nature. Since the types of physical bonds involved in immunochemical interactions vary considerably among the different anibody–analyte systems, each antibody-mediated cleanup procedure has its own optimal conditions for elution (168).

In general, elution can be made by either specific or nonspecific desorption. Specific desorption can be achieved, for example, by ligand competition and cosubstrate elution. Nonspecific desorption can be accomplished by a variety of different procedures, all aiming at dissociation of the antibody–analyte complex. It has been estimated that, without prior breaking of the antibody–analyte bond, an elution volume of approximately 25 L would be needed to elute 10 ng from a 1 ml column with a capacity of 20 ng. In order to decrease this elution volume to 5 ml, the conditions within the column must be altered to such a degree that the affinity constant is reduced from 5.10^{11} L/mol to about 10^8 L/mol. However, the elution conditions must be chosen in such a way that the reduction of the affinity constant is a reversible process. Otherwise the antibody will be damaged and the repeated use of the immunoaffinity column will be strongly restricted. This is of major importance from an economic point of view, because several milligrams of antibodies are required for the preparation of only one immunoaffinity column.

Reduction of the affinity constant can be achieved by means of a variety of different procedures including a linear pH gradient or a linear chaotropic-ion gradient elution using ions such as chlorides, perchlorates, thiocyanides, or trichloroacetates, changing the polarity by using solvents such as methanol or ethanol, changing the temperature, altering the ionic strength, or adding in the eluent denaturing agents such as urea, guanidine, and detergents (162). Best results are obtained using pH gradients but chaotropic gradients may be also necessary when the affinity of the antibody–analyte complex is high.

The conditions that can improve the elution of the analyte are not always compatible with the IAC matrix. It has long been established that changing the polarity of the aqueous eluent by adding methanol or ethanol, or using denaturing agents, antibodies may be inactivated to some extent. Also, chaotropic ions have the tendency to reduce hydrophobic interactions and can cause some antibody denaturation. In addition, as the column temperature rises, antibodies have a tendency to denature slowly; the lower the temperature, the longer the life of the column and the better the peak resolution (167). Therefore, the less vigorous elution solvent has to be chosen in practice. It is common experience that IAC matrices are generally very stable as long as the elution conditions are not too extreme.

The extent to which the immunoaffinity column can be reused depends mainly on the nature of the analyzed samples as well as the stability of the antibody and the support. The most important step is to remove any of the material physically adsorbed to the antibody so that the column may be reused with reproducibility. All that it is required for a column to be reequilibrated is the passage of several volumes of the starting buffer. Table 20.6 presents an outline of commercial column protocols used during analysis of steroid and β-agonist residues in urine. Most columns have been shown to last at least 100 runs, provided that the sample is properly defatted and does not contain solid particles (169).

Selectivity in IAC depends on the specificity of the immobilized antibody and, thus, monoclonal antibodies are preferentially used. In that case, a large amount of sample can be subjected to immunoaffinity cleanup without any retention of matrix components. This opens the possibility to determine very low concentrations of drug residues in edible animal products. For example, 20 ng chloramphenicol in 1 L milk can be determined with a recovery of 99% when 1 L of defatted milk is submitted to immunoaffinity cleanup. The chromatograms obtained after LC analysis were as clean as those obtained when 10 ml milk containing the same amount of chloramphenicol was also submitted to immunoaffinity cleanup (170).

Polyclonal antibodies that will recognize the basic molecular structure for all the members of a drug group may also be used whenever the analytical problem requires analysis of several members within the same group. In that case, the multispecific antibody should have sufficient affinity for all analytes while allowing retained drugs to be eluted from the column as discrete peaks.

Immunoaffinity cleanup was first applied in drug residue analysis for the determination of chloramphenicol in swine muscle tissue by LC (113). The IAC column was prepared using monoclonal antibodies originally developed for an enzyme-linked immunosorbent assay (ELISA) method (171) specific for chloramphenicol. Meat samples were extracted with water, and a concentrated phosphate buffer was added to the filtered extracts before immunoaffinity cleanup. A phosphate buffer was used in the washing process, whereas chloramphenicol was eluted from the column with a glycine/sodium chloride solution of pH 2.8. For subsequent LC analysis, this eluate was extracted with ethyl acetate, evaporated, and reconstituted in the mobile phase. The same analytical scheme was later successfully applied for the determination of chloramphenicol in eggs and milk as well (170, 172).

Use of polyclonal antibodies in immunoaffinity cleanup of drug residues was first made in the determination of trenbolone in bovine urine by thin layer chromatography–liquid chromatography (TLC-LC) (173). The polyclonal antibody used was capable to bind both the active form 17-β-trenbolone and its

TABLE 20.6   Immunoaffinity-Column Protocols Recommended for Steroid and β-Adrenergic Agonist Residue Analysis in Urine by Column Manufacturers

| Steroids immunoaffinity columns | | β-Agonists immunoaffinity columns | | |
Protocol I	Protocol II	Protocol I	Protocol II	Protocol III
Nortestosterone, diethylstilbestrol, zeranol	Nortestosterone, diethylstilbestrol, trenbolone, zeranol	β-Agonists	β-Agonists	β-Agonists
Urine deconjugation	Urine deconjugation	Urine deconjugation		
Column equilibration	Column equilibration	Column equilibration	Column equilibration	Column equilibration
Urine loading (0.25 ml). Leave 5 min	Urine loading (3 ml)	Urine loading (0.25 ml). Leave 5 min	Urine loading (3 ml)	Urine loading (4 ml)
Washing with 4 ml extraction buffer 1:10	Washing with 5 ml EtOH/H_2O (10:90)	Washing with 8 ml extraction buffer 1:10	Washing with 5 ml H_2O	Washing with 2 × 4 ml wash buffer
Washing with 5 ml H_2O		Washing with 2 ml extraction buffer 1:100		Washing with 5 ml H_2O
Repetition of both washes				
Gentle aspiration		Gentle aspiration		
Addition of acetone/H_2O (95:5). Leave 5 min. Elution	Elution with 3 ml EtOH/H_2O (70:30)	Addition of EtOH/HOAc (96:4), pH 3.5–4.0. Leave 5 min. Elution	Elution with 3 ml EtOH (0.5M NaCl: 0.58%) HOAc (50:50), pH 3.5	Elution with 4 ml EtOH/H_2O (70:30), pH 5.0
Washing with acetone/H_2O (95:5)	Washing with 3 ml EtOH/H_2O (80:20)	Washing with 10 ml EtOH/HOAc (96:4), pH 3.5–4.0	Washing with 3 ml EtOH/H_2O (80:20)	Addition of 15 ml elution buffer
Washing with 10 ml H_2O	Washing with 10 ml PBS	Washing with 10 ml H_2O	Washing with 10 ml PBS	Equilibration with 20 ml wash buffer

Abbreviations as in Table 20.2.

major metabolite 17-α-trenbolone. A similar procedure has been described for the determination of 17-β-nortestosterone and one of its major metabolites, 17-α-nortestosterone in bovine urine and bile by LC and/or GC-MS (174). In both procedures, the compounds eluted from the IAC column with aqueous ethanol without any adverse effect on the binding capacity of the sorbent. Immunoaffinity cleanup using polyclonal antibodies has further been used in the determination of diethylstilbestrol, dienestrol, and hexestrol in urine and plasma by GC-MS (175), and zeranol in milk using IAC with subsequent measurement by ELISA (176).

Multi-immunoaffinity cleanup (MIAC), in which different polyclonal antibodies were combined in one column, has also been described (169, 177). A mixture of two different polyclonal antibodies was coupled to one support for the determination of nortestosterone and methyltestosterone in bovine muscle tissue by GC-MS (174), whereas seven individual IAC matrices were combined in a single column for the analysis of seven anabolics including nortestosterone, methyltestosterone, trenbolone, zeranol, diethylstilbestrol, testosterone, and estradiol, in muscle tissue by LC (169). The latter procedure has been also applied in an online automated sample preparation method for the determination of the same analytes in urine at the low ppb level (169). In this method, enzymatically hydrolyzed urine samples were directly injected by means of an automated injector onto the immunoaffinity column. Following elution, the analytes were trapped in a preconcentration column to be directed by column-switching to the analytical column. Methods based on the same analytical strategy have also been developed for the determination of clenbuterol in urine by LC (177), and for the analysis of both 17-β-nortestosterone and 17-α-nortestosterone in urine (178) and muscle tissue (179) of calves. Recently, immunoaffinity cleanup has been described in the multiresidue determination of several anabolic steroids and β-agonists in urine, including zeranol, diethylstilbestrol, nortestosterone, trenbolone, clenbuterol, and cimaterol (180).

However, to become a truly popular technique, more is required for IAC. The availability of IAC materials is the major factor that will determine its success. With rare exceptions, most analytical laboratories are not equipped to produce antibodies. On the other hand, custom preparation of antibodies is subject to uncertainty about the quality of the final product and to a waiting period typically of 6–24 months before the serum becomes available.

IAC, in its various forms, is therefore dependent upon the commercial availability of such reagents. All too often, antibodies are proprietary products used for some other analytical purpose and are unavailable to the analytical scientist. By now, commercially available immunoaffinity columns and sorbents are limited to applications regarding hormones, β-agonists, and corticosteroids. When commercialization of antibody production for analytical purposes becomes commonplace, IAC will then realize its potential.

REFERENCES

1. K. Helrich, AOAC, Official Methods of Analysis (K. Helrich, Ed.), 15th Edition, Association of Official Analytical Chemists, Arlington, VA, Sec. 970.84 (1990).
2. L.M.L. Stolk, A. Fruijtier, and R. Umans, Pharm. Weekbl., Sci. Ed., 8:286 (1986).
3. R.A. Chalmers, in Methodological Developments in Biochemistry, Vol. 5 (E. Reid, Ed.), Elsevier, Amsterdam, p. 121 (1976).
4. L. Keusters, L.M.L. Stolk, H. Umans, and P. van Asten, Pharm. Weekbl., Sci. Ed., 8:194 (1986).
5. L.G. Rushing, S.F. Webb, H.C. Thompson, Jr., J. Chromatogr. B, 674:125 (1995).
6. J.J.H.M. Lohman, Pharm. Weekbl., Sci. Ed., 8:302 (1986).
7. P.J. Green and M.J. Yucis, Clin. Chem., 28:1237 (1982).
8. J.A. Sophianopoulos, S.J. Durham, A.J. Sophianopoulos, H.J. Ragsdale, and W.O. Cropper, Arch. Biochem. Biophys., 187:132 (1978).
9. U.R. Tjaden, R.A.M. van der Hoeven, J.A.C. Bierman, H.J.E.M. Reeuwijk, H. Lingeman, and J. van der Greef, Chromatographia, 24:597 (1987).
10. M. Rubenstein, S. Stein, and S. Udenfriend, in Hormonal Proteins and Peptides, Vol. 9 (M. Rubenstein, S. Stein, and S. Udenfriend, Eds.), Academic Press, New York, (1985).
11. Z. Deyl, J. Hyanek, and M. Horakova, J. Chromatogr., 379:177 (1986).
12. B. Shaikh, E.H. Allen, and J.C. Gridley, J. Assoc. Off. Anal. Chem., 68:29 (1985).
13. Y. Onji, M. Uno, and K. Tanigawa, J. Assoc. Off. Anal. Chem., 67:1135 (1984).
14. R. Bocker and C.J. Estler, Arzneim. Forsch., 29:1690 (1979).
15. H. Terada, M. Asanoma, and Y. Sakabe, J. Chromatogr., 318:299 (1985).
16. I. Nordlander, H. Johnsson, and B. Osterdahl, Food. Addit. Contam., 4:291 (1987).
17. D.N. Gilbert and S.J. Kohlhepp, Antimicrob. Agents Chemother., 30:361 (1986).
18. W.A. Moats, J. Agric. Food Chem., 31:880 (1983).
19. W.A. Moats, J. Chromatogr., 317:311 (1984).
20. W.A. Moats, E.W. Harris, and N.C. Steele, J. Assoc. Off. Anal. Chem., 68:413 (1986).
21. W.A. Moats, J. Chromatogr., 358:253 (1986).
22. A.I. MacIntosh and G.A. Neville, J. Assoc. Off. Anal. Chem., 67:958 (1984).
23. A.E. Mooser and M. Rychener, in Residues of Veterinary Drugs in Food, Proc. Euroresidue Conf., Noordwijkerhout, May 21–23, 1990 (N. Haagsma, A. Ruiter, and P.B. Czedik-Eysenberg, Eds.), Fac. Vet. Med., Univ. Utrecht, The Netherlands, p. 284 (1990).
24. W.A. Moats and L. Leskinen, J. Assoc. Off. Anal. Chem., 71:776 (1988).
25. W.A. Moats and L. Leskinen, J. Agric. Food Chem., 36:1297 (1988).
26. L.C. Nicholls, in Toxicology in the Scientific Investigation of Crime (L.C. Nicholls, Ed.), Butterworth, London, (1956).
27. H.M. Stevens, J. Forens. Sci. Soc., 7:184 (1967).
28. B. Wiese and K. Martin, J. Pharm. Biomed. Anal., 7:95 (1989).
29. E. Daeseleire, A. De Guesquiere, and C. Van Peteghem, Z. Lebensm. Unters. Forsch., 192:105 (1991).
30. M.D. Osselton, M.D. Hammond, and P.J. Twitchett, J. Pharm. Pharmacol., 29:460 (1977).

31. M.D. Osselton, J. Forensic Sci. Soc., 17:189 (1977).
32. E. Horne, A. Cadogan, M. OKeeffe, and L.A.P. Hoogenboom, Analyst, 121:1463 (1996).
33. N.A. Botsoglou, J. Agric. Food Chem., 36:1224 (1988).
34. J.R.J. Pare, U.S. patent 5002784 (1991).
35. J.R.J. Pare, Eur. Pat. Appl. EP 485668 A1 (1992).
36. F.I. Onuska and K.A. Terry, Chromatographia, 36:191 (1993).
37. V. Lopez-Avila, R. Young, and W.F. Beckert, Anal. Chem., 66:1097 (1994).
38. J.R.J. Pare, U.S. patent 5338557 (1994).
39. B.W. Renoe, Am. Lab., 26:34 (1994).
40. J.R.J. Pare, J.M.R. Belanger, and S.S. Stafford, Trends Anal. Chem., 13:176 (1994).
41. D. Warren, Anal. Chem., 56:1529A (1984).
42. M.E. Bier and R.G. Cooks, Anal. Chem., 59:597 (1987).
43. J.C. Tou, D.C. Ruff, and P.T. DeLassus, Anal. Chem., 62:593 (1990).
44. M.A. Lapack, J.C. Tou, and C.G. Enke, Anal. Chem., 62:1265 (1990).
45. S.J. Bauer and R.G. Cooks, Am. Lab., 25:36 (1993).
46. J. Bayo, M.A. Moreno, J. Prieta, S. Diaz, G. Suarez, and L. Dominguez, J. AOAC Int., 77:854 (1994).
47. M.C. Porter, in Handbook of Separation Techniques for Chemical Engineers (P.A. Schweitzer, Ed.), McGraw-Hill, New York (1979).
48. R. Achari, J. Chromatogr. Sci., 21:278 (1983).
49. J. Blanchard, J. Chromatogr., 226:455 (1981).
50. M.H. Thomas, J. Assoc. Off. Anal. Chem., 72:564 (1989).
51. B. Roudaut and M. Garnier, in Residues of Veterinary Drugs in Food, Proc. Euroresidue II Conf., Veldhoven, May 3–5, 1993 (N. Haagsma, A. Ruiter and P.B. Czedik-Eysenberg, Eds.), Fac. Vet. Med., Univ. Utrecht, The Netherlands, p. 596 (1993).
52. K. Tyczkowska, R.D. Voyksner, and A.L. Aronson, J. Chromatogr., 490:101 (1989).
53. R.F. Straub and R.D. Voyksner, J. Chromatogr., 647:167 (1993).
54. R.D. McDowall, J.C. Pearce, and G.S. Murkitt, J. Pharm. Biomed. Anal., 4:3 (1986).
55. J.-M. Wal, J.-C. Peleran, and G.F. Bories, J. Assoc. Off. Anal. Chem., 63:1044 (1980).
56. G.S.F. Bories, J.-C. Peleran, and J.-M. Wal, J. Assoc. Off. Anal. Chem., 66:1521 (1983).
57. N.A. Botsoglou, D.C. Kufidis, A.B. Spais, and B.N. Vassilopoulos, Archiv. Geflugelk., 53:163 (1989).
58. M. Uihlein, in Practice of High Performance Liquid Chromatography (H, Engelhardt, Ed.), Springer-Verlag, Berlin, Germany, p. 160 (1986).
59. A. Haussler and P. Hajdu, Arznei.-Forsch./Drug Res., 14:710 (1964).
60. D.J. Fletouris, J.E. Psomas, and N.A. Botsoglou, J. Agric. Food Chem., 38:1913 (1990).
61. N.A. Botsoglou, B.N. Vassilopoulos, and D.C. Kufidis, Chimica Chronika, New Series, 13:37 (1984).
62. M. Patthy, J. Chromatogr., 275:115 (1983).
63. W.A. Moats, J. AOAC Int., 76:535 (1993).
64. W.A. Moats, J. AOAC Int., 77:41 (1994).

65. G. Weiss, P.D. Duke, and L. Gonzales, J. Agric. Food Chem., 35:905 (1987).
66. D.J. Fletouris, J.E. Psomas, and A.J. Mantis, Chromatographia, 32:436 (1991).
67. D.J. Fletouris, J.E. Psomas, and A.J. Mantis, J. Agric. Food Chem., 40:617 (1992).
68. B. Fransson, and G. Schill, Acta Pharm. Suec., 12:107 (1975).
69. J.P. Bell, R.A. Simpson, and R.L. Cunico, Am. Lab., 18:94 (1986).
70. V.A. Nau and L.B. White, Am. Lab., 24:64 (1992).
71. R.E. Majors and K.D. Fogelmann, Am. Lab., 25:40W (1993).
72. G.L. Hawk, and P.F. Hensley, Am. Lab., 27:35 (1995).
73. J.X. Duggan, Am. Lab. News, 28:50F (1996).
74. R.C. Simpson and P.R. Brown, LC, 3:537 (1985).
75. J. Breiter, Clin. Chem. Biochem., 14:46 (1976).
76. J. Breiter and R. Helger, Z. Klin. Chem. Biochem., 13:254 (1975).
77. J. Breiter, Kontakte, 3:9 (1977).
78. S.J. Dickson, W.T. Cleary, A.W. Missen, E.A. Queree, and S.M. Shaw, J. Anal. Toxicol., 4:74 (1980).
79. J. Breiter, R. Helgar, and H. Lang, Forensic Sci., 7:131 (1976).
80. H. Lingeman, G.W.M. Meussen, C. van der Zouwen, W.J.M. Underberg, and A. Hulshoff, in Bioactive Analytes: Including CNS Drugs, Peptides, and Enantiomers (E. Reid, B. Scales, and I.D. Vdilson, Eds.), Plenum Press, New York, p. 343 (1986).
81. B. Tippins, Int. Lab., 17:28 (1987).
82. R.E. Majors, LC-GC Int., 6:336 (1993).
83. J.T. Baker, Application Guide, Vols. 1 and 2, Philipsburg, NJ, USA (1984).
84. Sorbent Extraction Technology Handbook, Analytichem International Inc., Harbor City, CA, USA (1985).
85. T. Kawasaki, M. Maeda, and A. Tsuji, J. Chromatogr., 233:61 (1982).
86. R.E. Shoup and G.S. Mayer, Anal. Chem., 54:1164 (1982).
87. H.J.E.M. Reeuwijk and U.R. Tjaden, J. Chromatogr., 353:339 (1986).
88. M.P. Kullberg and C.W. Gorodetzky, Clin. Chem., 20:177 (1974).
89. M.W.F. Nielen, R.W. Frei, and U.A.Th. Brinkman, J. Chromatogr., 317:557 (1984).
90. G.A. Junk, M.J. Avery, and J.J. Richard, Anal. Chem., 60:1347 (1988).
91. D.D. Blevins and S.K. Schultheis, LC-GC Int., 7:70 (1994).
92. G.M. Hearna and D.O. Hall, Am. Lab., 25:28H (1993).
93. C. Markell, D.F. Hagen, V.A. Bunnelle, LC-GC Int., 4:10 (1991).
94. K. Vanoosthuyze and C. van Peteghem, in Residues of Veterinary Drugs in Food, Proc. Euroresidue III Conf., Veldhoven, 1996 (N. Haagsma and A. Ruiter, Eds.), Fac. Vet. Med., Univ. Utrecht, The Netherlands, p. 958 (1996).
95. D. Louch, S. Motlagh, and J. Pawliszyn, Anal. Chem., 64:1187 (1992).
96. C.L. Arthur, D.W. Potter, K.D. Buchholz, S. Motlagh, and J. Pawliszyn, LC-GC Int., 5:656 (1992).
97. R.E. Shirey, in The Supelco Reporter, Supelco Corporation, Bellefonte, PA, USA, p. 8 (1994).
98. J.R. Berg, Am. Lab., 25:18 (1993).
99. S.A. Barker, A.R. Long, and C.R. Short, J. Chromatogr., 475:353 (1989).
100. S.A. Barker and R. Haley, Int. Lab., 46:16 (1992).

101. S.A. Barker and A.R. Long, J. Liq. Chromatogr., 15:2071 (1992).
102. S.A. Barker, Chemtech, 23:42 (1993).
103. S.A. Barker, A.R. Long, and M.E. Hines, J. Chromatogr., 629:23 (1993).
104. S.A. Barker, LC-GC Int., 11:719 (1998).
105. H. Yoshida, I. Morita, T. Masujima, and H. Imai, Chem. Pharm. Bull., 30:2287 (1982).
106. H. Yoshida, I. Morita, T. Masujima, and H. Imai, Chromatographia, 19:466 (1984).
107. D. Westerlund, Chromatographia, 24:155 (1987).
108. Z.K. Shibabi, J. Liq. Chromatogr., 11:1579 (1988).
109. K. Kimata, R. Tsuboi, K. Hosoya, N. Tanaka, and T. Araki, J. Chromatogr., 515: 1361 (1990).
110. K.K. Unger, Chromatographia, 31:507 (1991).
111. T.C. Pinkerton, J. Chromatogr., 544:19 (1991).
112. D.J. Anderson, Anal. Chem., 65:434R (1993).
113. J. Haginaka, TrAC, 10:17 (1991).
114. K.-S. Boos and A. Rudolphi, LC-GC Int., 11:84 (1998).
115. K.-S. Boos, J. Lintelmann, and A. Kettrup, J. Chromatogr., 600:189 (1992).
116. J. Haginaka, J. Wakai, and H. Yasuda, J. Chromatogr., 535:163 (1990).
117. J. Haginaka and J. Wakai, J. Chromatogr., 596:151 (1992).
118. J. Haginaka and J. Wakai, Chromatographia, 29:223 (1990).
119. B. Feibush and C.T. Santasania, J. Chromatogr., 544:41 (1991).
120. N. Nimura, H. Itoh, and T. Kinoshita, J. Chromatogr., 689:203 (1995).
121. I.H. Hagestam, and T.C. Pinkerton, Anal. Chem., 57:1757 (1985).
122. S.E. Cook, and T.C. Pinkerton, J. Chromatogr., 368:233 (1985).
123. I.H. Hagestam and T.C. Pinkerton, J. Chromatogr., 351:239 (1986).
124. I.H. Hagestam and T.C. Pinkerton, J. Chromatogr., 368:77 (1986).
125. K.-S. Boos, A. Walfort, and F. Eisenbeiss, German Patent DE 4130475 (1991).
126. S. Vielhauer, A. Rudolphi, K.-S. Boos, D. Seidel, B. Meiser, and B. Reichart, J. Chromatogr., 666:315 (1995).
127. K. Kimata, R. Tsuboi, K. Hosoya, N. Tanaka, and T. Araki, J. Chromatogr., 515: 73 (1990).
128. V. Smigol, F. Svec, and J.M.J. Frechet, J. Liq. Chromatogr., 17:891 (1994).
129. V. Smigol, F. Svec, and J.M.J. Frechet, Anal. Chem., 66:2129 (1994).
130. D.J. Gisch, B.T. Hunter, and B. Feibush, J. Chromatogr., 433:264 (1988).
131. S.H.Y. Wong, L.A. Butts, and A.C. Larsen, J. Liq. Chromatogr., 11:2039 (1988).
132. C.T. Santasania, J. Liq. Chromatogr., 13:2605 (1990).
133. T. Kanda, H. Kutsuno, Y. Ohtsu, and M. Yamaguchi, J. Chromatogr., 672:51 (1994).
134. S.J. Bogoslovski, K.A. Sakodynskii, and A.A. Serdan, in Diphil Sorbents for Direct Sample Injection of Drugs in Biological Matrices, 19th Int. Symp. Chromatogr., Aix-en-Provence, France (1992).
135. M.J. Gonzalez, High Resol. Chromatogr., 16:129 (1993).
136. J. Hermansson and A. Grahn, J. Chromatogr., 660:119 (1994).
137. L.J. Gluntz, J.A. Perry, B. Invego, H. Wagner, T.J. Szezerba, J.D. Rateike, and P.W. Gluntz, J. Liq. Chromatogr., 15:1361 (1992).
138. Milton Roy, in Sample Preparation Accessory (SPA), Milton Roy, LDC Division, Riviera Beach, FL, USA.

139. S.B. Hawthorne, Anal. Chem., 62:633A (1990).
140. J.F. Deye, T.A. Berger, and A.G. Anderson, Anal. Chem., 62:615 (1990).
141. S. Bowadt and S.B. Hawthorne, J. Chromatogr., 703:549 (1995).
142. T.S. Reighard and S.V. Olesik, Crit. Rev. Anal. Chem., 26:1 (1996).
143. M.E.P. McNally, J. AOAC Int., 79:380 (1996).
144. R.C. Weast, in CRC Press Handbook of Chemistry and Physics, 68th Edition CRC Press, Boca Raton, FL (1987).
145. F.I. Onuska and K.A. Terry, J. High Resol. Chromatogr., 12:3 (1989).
146. S.B. Hawthorne, D.J. Miller, and J.J. Langenfeld, J. Chromatogr. Sci., 28:2 (1990).
147. S.B. Hawthorne, D.J. Miller, J.J. Langenfeld, and M.D. Burford, Anal. Chem., 64: 1614 (1992).
148. N. Alexandrou, M.J. Lawrence, and J. Pawliszyn, Anal. Chem., 64:301 (1992).
149. F.I. Onuska and K.A. Terry, J. High Resol. Chromatogr., 14:829 (1991).
150. N. Alexandrou, Z. Miao, M. Colquhoun, J. Pawliszyn, and C. Jennison, J. Chromatogr. Sci., 30:351 (1992).
151. E. Sauvage, J.-L. Rocca, and G.J. Toussaint, J. High Resol. Chromatogr., 16:234 (1993).
152. M.E.P. McNally, Anal. Chem., 67:302A (1995).
153. J.W. King and M.L. Hopper, J. AOAC Int., 77:375 (1992).
154. K. Bartle, N. Din, A.A. Clifford, A. McCormack, and L. Castle, J. Chromatogr. Sci., 35:31 (1997).
155. O.W. Parks, R.J. Shadwell, A.R. Lightfield, and R.J. Maxwell, J. Chromatogr. Sci., 34:353 (1996).
156. J.W. Pensabene, W. Fiddler, and O.W. Parks, J. Chromatogr. Sci., 35:270 (1997).
157. M.T. Combs, M. Ashraf-Khorassani, and L.T. Taylor, J. Chromatogr. Sci., 35:176 (1997).
158. N. Cook, LC-GC Int., 5:869 (1987).
159. T.M. Phillips, J. Liq. Chromatogr., 3:962 (1985).
160. T.M. Phillips, N.S. More, W.D. Queen, and A.M. Thompson, J. Chromatogr., 327: 205 (1985).
161. T.M. Phillips, N.S. More, W.D. Queen, and A.M. Thompson, J. Chromatogr., 327: 213 (1985).
162. P.D.G. Dean, W.S. Johnson, and F.A. Middle, in Affinity Chromatography, a Practical Approach (P.D.G. Dean, W.S. Johnson, and F.A. Middle, Eds.), IRL Press, Oxford, UK (1985).
163. V.S. Prisyaznoy, M. Fusek, and Y.B. Alakhov, J. Chromatogr., 424:243 (1988).
164. G. Rule and J.D. Henion, J. Chromatogr., 582:103 (1992).
165. J.W. Coding, in Monoclonal Antibodies: Principles and Practice (J.W. Coding, Ed.), 2nd Edition, Academic Press, Orlando, FL (1986).
166. E.S. Golub and D.R. Green, in Immunology: A Synthesis (E.S. Golub and D.R. Green, Eds.), 2nd Edition, Sinauer Associates, Sunderland, MA (1991).
167. S.E. Katz and M. Siewierski, J. Chromatogr., 624:403 (1992).
168. C.J. van Oss, R.J. Good, and M.K. Chaudhury, J. Chromatogr., 376:111 (1986).
169. L.A. Van Ginkel, J. Chromatogr., 564:363 (1991).
170. C. Van de Water, D. Tebbal, and N. Haagsma, J. Chromatogr., 478:205 (1989).

171. C. Van de Water and N. Haagsma, J. Assoc. Off. Anal. Chem., 73:534 (1990).
172. C. Van de Water and N. Haagsma, J. Chromatogr., 566:173 (1991).
173. L.A. Van Ginkel, H. Van Blitterswijk, P.W. Zoontjes, D. Van den Bosch, and R.W. Stephany, J. Chromatogr., 445:385 (1988).
174. L.A. Van Ginkel, R.W. Stephany, H.J. Van Rossum, H. Van Blitterswijk, P.W. Zoontjes, R.C.M. Hooijschuur, and J. Zuydendorp, J. Chromatogr., 489:95 (1989).
175. R. Bagnati, M.G. Castelli, L. Airoldi, M.P. Oriundi, A. Ubaldi, and R. Fanelli, J. Chromatogr., 527:267 (1990).
176. J.I. Azcona, M.M. Abouzied, and J.J. Pestka, J. Food Prot., 53:577 (1990).
177. W. Haasnoot, M.E. Ploum, R.J.A. Paulussen, R. Schilt, and F. Huf, J. Chromatogr., 519:323 (1990).
178. A. Farjam, G.L. de Jong, R.W. Frei, U.A.Th. Brinkman, W. Haasnoot, W. Hammers, A.R.M. Schilt, and F.A. Huf, J. Chromatogr., 452:419 (1988).
179. W. Haasnoot, R. Schilt, A.R.M. Hamers, A. Huf, A. Farjam, R.W. Frei, and U.A.Th. Brinkman, J. Chromatogr., 489:157 (1989).
180. S.R.H. Crooks, C.T. Elliott, C.S. Thompson, and W.J. McCaughey, J. Chromatogr., 690:161 (1997).
181. V.P. Agarwal, J. Liq. Chromatogr., 12:613 (1989).
182. M. Ramos, Th. Reuvers, A. Aranda, and J. Gomez, J. Liq. Chromatogr., 17:385 (1994).
183. L.A. van Ginkel, H.J. van Rossum, P.W. Zoontjes, H. van Blitterswijk, G. Ellen, E. van der Heeft, A.P.J.M. de Jong, and G. Zomer, Anal. Chim. Acta, 237:61 (1990).
184. M. Gips, M. Bridzy, S. Barel, and S. Soback, in Residues of Veterinary Drugs in Food, Proc. Euroresidue II Conf., Veldhoven, May 3–5, 1993 (N. Haagsma, A. Ruiter and P.B. Czedik-Eysenberg, Eds.), Fac. Vet. Med., Univ. Utrecht, The Netherlands, p. 313 (1993).
185. A. Simonella, L. Torreti, and C. Filipponi, J. High Res. Chromatogr., 555:555 (1989).
186. N. Haagsma, C. Schreuder, and E.R.A. Rensen, J. Chromatogr., 363:353 (1986).
187. R.L. Epstein, C. Henry, K.P. Holland, and J. Dreas, J. AOAC Int., 77:570 (1994).
188. J.R. Nelson, K.F.T. Copeland, R.J. Forster, D.J. Campbell, and W.D. Black, J. Chromatogr., 276:438 (1983).
189. T. Nagata and M. Saeki, J. Liq. Chromatogr., 15:2045 (1992).
190. M.M.L. Aerts, H.J. Keukens, and G.A. Werdmuller, J. Assoc. Off. Anal. Chem., 72:570 (1989).
191. R.M. Parker and I.C. Shaw, Analyst, 113:1875 (1988).
192. H.J. Keukens, W.M.J. Beek, and M.M.L. Aerts, J. Chromatogr., 352:445 (1986).
193. C. Hummert, B. Luckas, and H. Siebenlist, J. Chromatogr., 668:53 (1995).
194. J.F.M. Nouws, J. Laurensen, and M.M.L. Aerts, Arch. Lebensmittelhyg., 38:7 (1987).
195. B. Roudaut, J. Liq. Chromatogr. Rel. Technol., 19:1097 (1996).
196. J.P. Abjean, J. AOAC Int., 77:1101 (1994).
197. A.M. Di Pietra, V. Piazza, V. Andrisano, and V. Cavrini, J. Liq. Chromatogr., 18: 3529 (1995).

198. P.J. Kijak, J. AOAC Int., 77:34 (1994).
199. K. Yoshida and F. Kondo, J. Liq. Chromatogr., 17:2625 (1994).
200. K.P. Holland, A.C. Henry, R.T. Wilson, J.S. Dreas, and R.B. Ashworth, J. AOAC Int., 78:483 (1995).
201. A.I. MacIntosh, J. Assoc. Off. Anal. Chem., 73:880 (1990).
202. K.O. Dasenbrock and W.R. LaCourse, Anal. Chem., 70:2415 (1998).
203. P.G. Schermerhorn, P.-S. Chu, and M.A. Ngoh, J. AOAC Int., 81:973 (1998).
204. P.J. McNeilly, V.B. Reeves, and E.J.I. Deveau, J. AOAC Int., 79:844 (1996).
205. M.G. Beconi-Barker, R.D. Roof, L. Millerioux, F.M. Kausche, T.J. Vidmar, E.B. Smith, J.K. Callahan, V.L. Hubbard, G.A. Smith, and T.J. Gilbertson, J. Chromatogr., 729:229 (1996).
206. L.J.-Y Keng and J.O.K. Boison, J. Liq. Chromatogr., 15:2025 (1992).
207. W. Chan, G.C. Gerhardt, and C.D.C. Salisbury, J. AOAC Int., 77:331 (1994).
208. B. Delepine, D. Hurtaud-Pessel, and P. Sanders, J. AOAC Int., 79:397 (1996).
209. M. Horie, K. Saito, R. Ishii, T. Yoshida, Y. Haramaki, and H. Nakazawa, J. Chromatogr., 812:295 (1998).
210. M. Janecek, M.A. Quilliam, M.R. Bailey, and D.H. North, J. Chromatogr., 619:63 (1993).
211. W. Luo, E.B. Hansen, C.Y.W. Ang, and H.C. Thompson, J. AOAC Int., 79:839 (1996).
212. M.A. Ngoh, J. AOAC Int., 79:652 (1996).
213. W.J. Blanchflower, R.J. McCracken, and D.G. Kennedy, in Residues of Veterinary Drugs in Food, Proc. Euroresidue II Conf., Veldhoven, May 3–5, 1993 (N. Haagsma, A. Ruiter and P.B. Czedik-Eysenberg, Eds.), Fac. Vet. Med., Univ. Utrecht, The Netherlands, p. 201 (1993).
214. L.H.M. Vroomen, M.C.J. Berghmans, and T.D.B. Van Der Struijs, J. Chromatogr., 362:141 (1986).
215. L. Kumar, J.R. Toothill, and K-B Ho, J. AOAC Int., 77:591 (1994).
216. T. Juszkiewicz, A. Posyniak, S. Semeniuk, and J. Niedzielska, in Residues of Veterinary Drugs in Food, Proc. Euroresidue II Conf., Veldhoven, May 3–5, 1993 (N. Haagsma, A. Ruiter and P.B. Czedik-Eysenberg, Eds.), Fac. Vet. Med., Univ. Utrecht, The Netherlands, p. 401 (1993).
217. M. Horie, K. Saito, Y. Hoshino, N. Nose, H. Nakazawa, and Y. Yamane, J. Chromatogr., 538:484 (1991).
218. O.B. Samuelsen, J. Chromatogr., 528:495 (1990).
219. T. Galeano Diaz, A. Guiberteau Cabanillas, M.I. Acedo Valenzuela, C.A. Correa, and F. Salinas, J. Chromatogr., 764:243 (1997).
220. H.S. Rupp, R.K. Munns, and A.R. Long, J. AOAC Int., 76:1235 (1993).
221. J.O.K. Boison, C.D.C. Salisbury, W. Chan, and J.D. MacNeil, J. Assoc. Off. Anal. Chem., 74:497 (1991).
222. V. Hormazabal and M. Yndestad, J. Liq. Chromatogr. & Rel. Technol., 21:3099 (1998).
223. H.-E. Gee, K.-B. Ho, and J. Toothill, J. AOAC Int., 79:640 (1996).
224. J.A. Tarbin, W.H.H. Farrington, and G. Shearer, Anal. Chim. Acta, 318:95 (1995).
225. W. Chan and C.D.C. Salisbury, in Residues of Veterinary Drugs in Food, Proc. Euroresidue II Conf., Veldhoven, May 3–5, 1993 (N. Haagsma, A. Ruiter, and P.B.

Czedik-Eysenberg, Eds.), Fac. Vet. Med., Univ. Utrecht, The Netherlands, p. 236 (1993).

226. T. Nagata and M. Saeki, J. Assoc. Off. Anal. Chem., 69:448 (1986).

227. C.Y.W. Ang, W. Luo, E.B. Hansen, J.P. Freeman, and H.C. Thompson, J. AOAC Int., 79:389 (1996).

228. H. Terada and Y. Sakabe, J. Chromatogr., 348:379 (1985).

229. L.K. Sorensen, B.M. Rasmussen, J.O. Boison, and L. Keng, J. Chromatogr., 694: 383 (1997).

230. V. Hormazabal, and M. Yndestad, J. Liq. Chromatogr., 18:2467 (1995).

231. K. Takeba, K. Fujinuma, T. Miyazaki, and H. Nakazawa, J. Chromatogr., 812:205 (1998).

232. J.O.K. Boison, L.J.-Y Keng, and J.D. MacNeil, J. AOAC Int., 77:565 (1994).

233. P. Kubalec, E. Brandsteterova, and A. Bednarikova, Z. Lebensm. Unters Forsch., 205:85 (1997).

234. J.O. Boison and L.J.-Y. Keng, J. AOAC Int., 81:1113 (1998).

235. J.O. Boison and L.J.-Y. Keng, J. AOAC Int., 81:1267 (1998).

236. M. Horie, K. Saito, Y. Hoshino, N. Nose, E. Mochizuki, and H. Nakazawa, J. Chromatogr., 402:301 (1987).

237. Y. Ikai, H. Oka, N. Kawamura, M. Yamada, K.-I. Harada, M. Suzuki, and H. Nakazawa, J. Chromatogr., 477:397 (1989).

238. B. Brinkmann, N. Haagsma, and H. Buning-Pfaue, in Residues of Veterinary Drugs in Food, Proc. Euroresidue Conf., Noordwijkerhout, May 21–23, 1990 (N. Haagsma, A. Ruiter, and P.B. Czedik-Eysenberg, Eds.), Fac. Vet. Med., Univ. Utrecht, The Netherlands, p. 123 (1990).

239. M. Horie, and H. Nakazawa, J. Liq. Chromatogr., 15:2057 (1992).

240. N. Haagsma, M. van Roy, and B. G. M. Gortemaker, in Residues of Veterinary Drugs in Food, Proc. Euroresidue II Conf., Veldhoven, May 3–5, 1993 (N. Haagsma, A. Ruiter, and P.B. Czedik-Eysenberg, Eds.), Fac. Vet. Med., Univ. Utrecht, The Netherlands, p. 337 (1993).

241. J.E. Roybal, A.P. Pfenning, S.B. Turnipseed, C.C. Walker, and J.A. Hurlbut, J. AOAC Int., 80:982 (1997).

242. G.C. Gerhardt, C.D.C. Salisbury, and J.D. MacNeil, J. AOAC Int., 77:334 (1994).

243. J. Unruh, E. Piotrowski, D.P. Schwartz, and R.A. Barford, J. Chromatogr., 519: 179 (1990).

244. V.K. Agarwal, in Analysis of Antibiotic/Drug Residues in Food Products of Animal Origin (V.K. Agarwal, Ed.), Plenum Press, New York (1992).

245. E. Zomer, S. Saul, and S.E. Charm, J. AOAC Int., 75:987 (1992).

246. M. Horie, K. Saito, N. Nose, and H. Nakazawa, J. AOAC Int., 75:786 (1992).

247. G. Balizs, L. Benesch-Girke, and S.A. Hewitt, in Residues of Veterinary Drugs in Food, Proc. Euroresidue II Conf., Veldhoven, May 3–5, 1993 (N. Haagsma, A. Ruiter, and P.B. Czedik-Eysenberg, Eds.), Fac. Vet. Med., Univ. Utrecht, The Netherlands, p. 155 (1993).

248. S. Horii, C. Momma, K. Miyahara, T. Maruyama, and M. Matsumoto, J. Assoc. Off. Anal. Chem., 73:990 (1990).

249. M. Horie, K. Saito, Y. Hoshino, N. Nose, N. Hamada, and H. Nakazawa, J. Chromatogr., 502:371 (1987).

250. J. Unruh, D.P. Schwartz, and R.A. Barford, J. AOAC Int., 76:335 (1993).

251. N. Haagsma, R.J. Nooteboom, B.G.M. Gortemaker, and M.J. Maas, Z. Lebensm. Unters. Forsch., 181:194 (1985).

252. J.O.K. Boison and L.J.-Y. Keng, J. AOAC Int., 77:558 (1994).

253. J.O. Boison and L.J.-Y. Keng, J. AOAC Int., 78:651 (1995).

254. Y. Ikai, H. Oka, N. Kawamura, J. Hayakawa, M. Yamada, K.-I. Harada, M. Suzuki, and H. Nakazawa, J. Chromatogr., 541:393 (1991).

255. K. Takatsuki and T. Kikuchi, J. Assoc. Off. Anal. Chem., 73:886 (1990).

256. J.R. Walsh, L.V. Walker, and J.J. Webber, J. Chromatogr., 596:211 (1992).

257. W.J. Blanchflower, R.J. McCracken, and D.A. Rice, Analyst, 114:421 (1989).

258. Y. Ikai, H. Oka, N. Kawamura, M. Yamada, K.-I. Harada, and M. Suzuki, J. Chromatogr., 411:313 (1987).

259. H. Oka, H. Matsumoto, K. Uno, K.-I. Harada, S. Kadowaki, and M. Suzuki, J. Chromatogr., 325:265 (1985).

260. N. Haagsma and P. Scherpenisse, in Residues of Veterinary Drugs in Food, Proc. Euroresidue II Conf., Veldhoven, May 3–5, 1993 (N. Haagsma, A. Ruiter, and P.B. Czedik-Eysenberg, Eds.), Fac. Vet. Med., Univ. Utrecht, The Netherlands, p. 342 (1993).

261. J.M. Degroodt, B.W. de Bukanski, and S. Srebrnik, J. Liq. Chromatogr., 16:3515 (1993).

262. H. Oka, Y. Ikai, Y. Ito, J. Hayakawa, K. Harada, M. Suzuki, H. Odani, and K. Maeda, J. Chromatogr., 693:337 (1997).

263. S. Horii, J. Liq. Chromatogr., 17:213 (1994).

264. S.M. Croubels, K.E.I. Vanoosthuyze, and C.H. Van Peteghem, J. Chromatogr., 690: 173 (1997).

265. S.M. Croubels, H. Vermeersch, P. De Backer, M.D.F. Santos, J.P. Remon, and C.H. Van Peteghem, J. Chromatogr., 708:145 (1998).

266. W.J. Blanchflower, R.J. McCracken, A.S. Haggan, and D.G. Kennedy, J. Chromatogr., 692:351 (1997).

267. H. Bjorklund, J. Chromatogr., 432:381 (1988).

268. G.J. Reimer and L.M. Young, J. Assoc. Off. Anal. Chem., 73:813 (1990).

269. R.G. Aoyama, K.M. McErlane, H. Erber, D.D. Kitts, and H.M. Burt, J. Chromatogr., 588:181 (1991).

270. M.C. Carson, M.A. Ngoh, and S.W. Hadley, J. Chromatogr., 712:113 (1998).

271. E. Brandsteterova, P. Kubalec, L. Bovanova, P. Simko, A. Bednarikova, and L. Machackova, Z. Lebensm. Unters Forsch., 205:311 (1997).

272. W. Chan and C.D.C. Salisbury, in Residues of Veterinary Drugs in Food, Proc. Euroresidue II Conf., Veldhoven, May 3–5, 1993 (N. Haagsma, A. Ruiter and P.B. Czedik-Eysenberg, Eds.), Fac. Vet. Med., Univ. Utrecht, The Netherlands, p. 238 (1993).

273. H. Oka, Y. Ikai, N. Kawamura, K. Uno, M. Yamada, K.-I. Harada, M. Uchiyama, H. Asukabe, Y. Mori, and M. Suzuki, J. Chromatogr., 389:417 (1987).

274. H. Oka, Y. Ikai, N. Kawamura, K. Uno, M. Yamada, K.-I. Harada, and M. Suzuki, J. Chromatogr., 400:253 (1987).

275. E. Brandsteterova, P. Kubalec, and L. Machackova, Z. Lebensm. Unters Forsch., 204:341 (1997).

276. J. Markus and J. Sherma, J. AOAC Int., 75:1129 (1992).
277. J. Markus and J. Sherma, J. AOAC Int., 75:1135 (1992).
278. P.S. Chu, R.Y. Wang, T.A. Brandt, and C.A. Weerasinghe, J. Chromatogr., 620: 129 (1993).
279. J. Li and C. Qian, J. AOAC Int., 79:1062 (1996).
280. G. Stoev, J. Chromatogr., 710:234 (1998).
281. J. Markus and J. Sherma, J. AOAC Int., 75:937 (1992).
282. J. Markus and J. Sherma, J. AOAC Int., 75:942 (1992).
283. F.J. Schenck, R. Wagner, and W. Bargo, J. Liq. Chromatogr., 16:513 (1993).
284. M.A.F. Muino and J.S. Lozano, Analyst, 118:1519 (1993).
285. L.D. Payne, V.R. Mayo, L.A. Morneweck, M.B. Hicks, and T.A. Wehner, J. Agric. Food Chem., 45:3501 (1997).
286. J.M. Ballard, L.D. Payne, R.S. Egan, T.A. Wehner, G.S. Rahn, and S. Tom, J. Agric. Food Chem., 45:3507 (1997).
287. K. Helrich, AOAC, Official Methods of Analysis (K. Helrich, Ed.), 15th Edition, 2nd Supplement (1991), Association of Official Analytical Chemists, Arlington, VA, Sec. 991.17 (1991).
288. K.P. Reising, J. AOAC Int., 75:751 (1992).
289. G. Dusi, M. Curatolo, A. Fierro, and E. Faggionato, J. Liq. Chromatogr. Rel. Technol., 19:1607 (1996).
290. C.D.C. Salisbury, J. AOAC Int., 76:1149 (1993).
291. F.J. Schenck, S.A. Barker, and A.R. Long, J. AOAC Int., 75:655 (1992).
292. D.D. Oehler and J.A. Miller, J. Assoc. Off. Anal. Chem., 72:59 (1989).
293. Th. Reuvers, R. Diaz, M. Martin de Pozuelo, and M. Ramos, Anal. Chim. Acta, 275:353 (1993).
294. J.M. Degroodt, B.W. de Bukanski, and S. Srebrnik, J. Liq. Chromatogr., 17:1419 (1994).
295. P.J. Kijak, J. AOAC Int., 75:747 (1992).
296. F.J. Schenck, J. Liq. Chromatogr., 18:349 (1995).
297. C.M. Dickinson, J. Chromatogr., 528:250 (1990).
298. C.G. Chappell, C.S. Creaser, and M.J. Shepherd, J. Chromatogr., 626:223 (1992).
299. M.L. Alvarez-Bujidos, A. Ortiz, R. Balana, J.C. Cubria, D. Ordonez, and A. Negro, J. Chromatogr., 578:321 (1992).
300. J.G. Steenbaar, C.A.J. Hajee, and N. Haagsma, J. Chromatogr., 615:186 (1993).
301. A. Khunachak, A.R. Dacunha, and S.J. Stout, J. AOAC Int., 76:1230 (1993).
302. M. Alvinerie, J.F. Sutra, M. Badri, and P. Galtier, J. Chromatogr., 674:119 (1995).
303. B.W. de Bukanski, J.M. Degroodt, and H. Beernaert, Z. Lebensm. Unters Forsch., 193:130 (1991).
304. R.V. Arenas and N.A. Johnson, J. AOAC Int., 78:642 (1995).
305. S.A. Barker, L.C. Hsieh, and C.R. Short, Anal. Biochem., 155:112 (1986).
306. C.A.J. Hajee and N. Haagsma, J. AOAC Int., 79:645 (1996).
307. S.S.C. Tai, N. Cargile, and C.J. Barnes, J. Assoc. Off. Anal. Chem., 73:368 (1990).
308. K. Takeda, T. Itoh, M. Matsumoto, H. Nakazawa, and S. Tanabe, J. AOAC Int., 79:848 (1996).
309. L.W. LeVan and C.J. Barnes, J. Assoc. Off. Anal. Chem., 74:487 (1991).

310. R.T. Wilson, J.M. Groneck, A.C. Henry, and L.D. Rowe, J. Assoc. Off. Anal. Chem., 74:56 (1991).
311. A.M. Marti, A.E. Mooser, and H. Koch, J. Chromatogr., 498:145 (1990).
312. M. Ramos, A. Aranda, Th. Reuvers, and R. Jimenez, Anal. Chim. Acta, 275:317 (1993).
313. D.R. Newkirk, H.F. Righter, F.J. Schenck, J.L. Okrasinski, and C.J. Barnes, J. Assoc. Off. Anal. Chem., 73:702 (1990).
314. A. Cannavan, and G. Kennedy, Analyst, 122:963 (1997).
315. R.C. Beier, L.D. Rowe, M.I. Abd El-Aziz Nasr, M.H. Elissalde, and L.H. Stanker, J. Liq. Chromatogr., 17:2961 (1994).
316. J.A. Tarbin and G. Shearer, J. Chromatogr., 577:376 (1992).
317. J.A. Tarbin and G. Shearer, J. Chromatogr., 579:177 (1992).
318. J.W. Moran, J.M. Turner, and M.R. Coleman, J. AOAC Int., 78:668 (1995).
319. K. Takatsuki, S. Suzuki, and I. Ushizawa, J. Assoc. Off. Anal. Chem., 69:443 (1986).
320. J.W. Moran, J.M. Rodewald, A.L. Donoho, and M.R. Coleman, J. AOAC Int., 77: 885 (1994).
321. F.J. Schenck, S.A. Barker, and A.R. Long, J. AOAC Int., 75:659 (1992).
322. M.G. Leadbetter and J.E. Matusik, J. AOAC Int., 76:420 (1993).
323. J.L. Lewis, T.D. Macy, and D.A. Garteiz, J. Assoc. Off. Anal. Chem., 72:577 (1989).
324. M.H. Vertommen, A. Van Der Laan, and H.M. Veenendaal-Hesselman, J. Chromatogr., 481:452 (1989).
325. G.P. Dimenna, J.A. Creegan, T.B. Turnbull, and G.J. Wright, J. Agric. Food Chem., 34:805 (1986).
326. G.P. Dimenna, F.S. Lyon, F.M. Thompson, J.A. Creegan, and G.J. Wright, J. Agric. Food Chem., 37:668 (1989).
327. J.F. Ericson, A. Calcagni, and M.J. Lynch, J. AOAC Int., 77:577 (1994).
328. E.T. Mallinson, A.C. Henry, and L. Rowe, J. AOAC Int., 75:790 (1992).
329. Th. Reuvers, E. Perogordo, and R. Jimenez, J. Chromatogr., 564:477 (1991).
330. L.A. Van Ginkel, R.W. Stephany, H.J. Van Rossum, H.M. Steinbuch, G. Zomer, E. Van De Heeft, and A.P.J.M. De Jong, J. Chromatogr., 489:111 (1989).
331. V. Ferchaud, B. Le Bizec, M.-P. Montrade, D. Maume, F. Monteau, and F. Andre, J. Chromatogr., 695:269 (1997).
332. J. Plasencia, C.J. Mirocha, R.J. Pawlosky, and J.F. Smith, J. Assoc. Off. Anal. Chem., 73:973 (1990).
333. P.M. Scott and G.A. Lawrence, J. Assoc. Off. Anal. Chem., 71:1176 (1988).
334. S.H. Hsu, R.H. Eckerlin, and J.D. Henion, J. Chromatogr., 424:219 (1988).
335. S. Hartmann and H. Steinhart, J. Chromatogr., 704:105 (1997).
336. L. Van Look, Ph. Deschuytere, and C. Van Peteghem, J. Chromatogr., 489:213 (1989).
337. S.M. Plakas, K.R. El Said, E.L.E. Jester, F.A. Bencsath, and W.L. Hayton, J. AOAC Int., 80:486 (1997).
338. Y. Gaillard, A. Balland, F. Doucet, and G. Pepin, J. Chromatogr., 703:85 (1997).
339. J.F. Lawrence and C. Menard, J. Chromatogr., 696:291 (1997).

340. L. Leyssens, C. Driessen, A. Jacobs, J. Czech, and J. Raus, J. Chromatogr., 564: 515 (1991).
341. H.H.D. Meyer, L. Rinke, and I. Dursch, J. Chromatogr., 564:551 (1991).
342. C.T. Elliott, C.S. Thompson, C.J.M. Arts, S.R.H. Crooks, M.J. van Baak, E.R. Verheij, and G.A. Baxter, Analyst, 123:1103 (1998).
343. F. Ramos, C. Santos, A. Silva, and M.I.N. da Silveira, J. Chromatogr., 716:366 (1998).
344. P. Gowik, B. Julicher, and S. Uhlig, J. Chromatogr., 716:221 (1998).
345. Ph. Delahaut, P. Jacquemin, Y. Colemonts, M. Dubois, J. De Graeve, and H. Deluyker, J. Chromatogr., 696:203 (1997).
346. P. Shearan, M. O'Keeffe, and M.R. Smyth, Analyst, 116:1365 (1991).
347. H.S. Rupp, D.C. Holland, R.K. Munns, S.B. Turnipseed, and A.R. Long, J. AOAC Int., 78:959 (1995).
348. S.M.R. Stanley, N.A. Owens, and J.P. Rodgers, J. Chromatogr., 667:95 (1995).
349. S.M. Plakas, K.R. El Said, G.R. Stehly, and J.E. Roybal, J. AOAC Int., 78:1388 (1995).
350. J.E. Roybal, A.P. Pfenning, R.K. Munns, D.C. Holland, J.A. Hurlbut, and A.R. Long, J. AOAC Int., 78:453 (1995).
351. S.B. Turnipseed, J.E. Roybal, H.S. Rupp, J.A. Hurlbut, and A.R. Long, J. Chromatogr., 670:55 (1995).
352. A. Swarbrick, E.J. Murby, and P. Hume, J. Liq. Chrom. & Rel. Technol., 20:2269 (1997).
353. C.A.J. Hajee and N. Haagsma, J. Chromatogr., 669:219 (1995).
354. L.G. Rushing and H.C. Thompson, J. Chromatogr., 688:325 (1997).
355. L.G. Rushing and E.B. Hansen, J. Chromatogr., 700:223 (1997).
356. M.R. Taylor and S.A. Westwood, J. Chromatogr., 697:389 (1995).
357. L.A. Van Ginkel, P.L.W.J. Schwillens, and M. Olling, Anal. Chim. Acta, 225:137 (1989).
358. M.D. Rose and G. Shearer, J. Chromatogr., 624:471 (1992).
359. H.J. Keukens and M.M.L. Aerts, J. Chromatogr., 464:149 (1989).
360. B. Le Bizec, F. Monteau, D. Maume, M.P. Montrade, C. Gade, and F. Andre, Anal. Chim Acta, 340:201 (1997).
361. W.J. Blanchflower, P.J. Hughes, A. Cannavan, M.A. McCoy, and D.G. Kennedy, Analyst, 122:967 (1997).
362. L.G. McLaughlin and J.D. Henion, J. Chromatogr., 591:195 (1992).
363. F.J. Schenck, Lab. Inf. Bull., 7:3559 (1991).
364. S. Le Boulaire, J.-C. Bauduret, and F. Andre, J. Agric Food Chem., 45:2134 (1997).
365. A.R. Long, L.C. Hsieh, A.C. Bello, M.S. Malbrough, C.R. Short, and S.A. Barker, J. Agric. Food Chem., 38:427 (1990).
366. M.M. Soliman, A.R. Long, and S.A. Barker, J. Liq. Chromatogr., 13:3327 (1990).
367. A.R. Long, L.C. Hsieh, M.S. Malbrough, C.R. Short, and S.A. Barker, J. Agric. Food Chem., 38:430 (1990).
368. A.R. Long, L.C. Hsieh, M.S. Malbrough, C.R. Short, and S.A. Barker, J. Assoc. Off. Anal. Chem., 74:292 (1991).
369. M. Alvinerie, J.F. Sutra, D. Capela, P. Galtier, A. Fernandez-Suarez, E. Horne, and M. O'Keeffe, Analyst, 121:1469 (1996).

370. H.H. Jarboe and K.M. Kleinow, J. AOAC Int., 75:428 (1992).

371. L.V. Walker, J.R. Walsh, and J.J. Webber, J. Chromatogr., 595:179 (1992).

372. C.C. Walker and S.A. Barker, J. AOAC Int., 77:1460 (1994).

373. A.R. Long, L.C. Hsieh, M.S. Malbrough, C.R. Short, and S.A. Barker, J. Assoc. Off. Anal. Chem., 73:868 (1990).

374. A.R. Long, C.R. Short, and S.A. Barker, J. Chromatogr., 502:87 (1990).

375. A.R. Long, M.D. Crouch, and S.A. Barker, J. Assoc. Off. Anal. Chem., 74:667 (1991).

376. G.J. Reimers and A. Suarez, J. AOAC Int., 75:979 (1992).

377. A.R. Long, L.C. Hsieh, M.S. Malbrough, C.R. Short, and S.A. Barker, J. Agric. Food Chem., 38:423 (1990).

378. A.R. Long, L.C. Hsieh, M.S. Malbrough, C.R. Short, and S.A. Barker, J. Assoc. Off. Anal. Chem., 73:379 (1990).

379. A.R. Long, L.C. Hsieh, M.S. Malbrough, C.R. Short, and S.A. Barker, J. Assoc. Off. Anal. Chem., 73:864 (1990).

380. A.R. Long, M.S. Malbrough, L.C. Hsieh, C.R. Short, and S.A. Barker, J. Assoc. Off. Anal. Chem., 73:860 (1990).

381. A.R. Long, L.C. Hsieh, M.S. Malbrough, C.R. Short, and S.A. Barker, J. Assoc. Off. Anal. Chem., 72:739 (1989).

382. S.A. Barker, T. McDowell, B. Charkhian, L.C. Hsieh, and C.R. Short, J. Assoc. Off. Anal. Chem., 73:22 (1990).

21

Derivatization

Drug residues that do not sufficiently absorb or fluoresce are usually submitted, prior to their analysis by physicochemical techniques, to some type of derivatization aimed primarily at enhancing analyte detectability. Furthermore, formation of relatively nonpolar derivatives offers advantages for a successful extraction and cleanup.

In choosing a derivatization procedure for a certain analyte, a number of provisions must be taken into account. The derivatizing reagent should be selective for a single functional group, nontoxic, able to introduce a high degree of sensitivity, stable over prolonged period of time, and capable to react rapidly and quantitatively with the analyte under mild conditions yielding a single derivative with a minimum of manipulation. The derivative should exhibit stability over time and possess favorable chromatographic properties. Fluorescence, ultraviolet-visible, enzymatic, and photochemical derivatization procedures have all been used with varying success within the field of drug residues analysis. Examples of derivatizing reagents commonly used in food analysis for drug residues are presented in Table 21.1.

21.1 FLUORESCENCE DERIVATIZATION

Although various fluorescence-labeling derivatization reagents have been used in drug residues analysis, those replacing active hydrogens of hydroxyl, sulfydryl, or amino groups account for most applications.

21.1.1 Amino Group

One of the most widely used reagents for introduction of a fluorophor into primary and secondary amines is 5-dimethylaminonaphthalene-1-sulfonyl chloride, com-

TABLE 21.1 Commonly Used Derivatizing Agents in the Analysis of Drug Residues in Edible Animal Products

Drug	Matrix	Derivatizing agent	Detection mode	Ref.
β-Adrenergic agonists	Animal tissues	Phosgene	GC-EI-MS	1
	Bovine hair and urine	Trimethylboroxine	GC-EI-MS	2
	Bovine liver	N,O-Bis(trimethylsilyl)-trifluoroacetamide (BSTFA)	GC-CI-MS	3
	Bovine liver and urine	N-Methyl-N-(trimethylsilyl)-trifluoroacetamide (MSTFA)	GC-PICI-MS-MS	4
	Bovine liver and urine	N,O-Bis(trimethylsilyl)-trifluoroacetamide (BSTFA)	GC-FT-IR	5, 6
	Bovine urine	Methyl- and butylboronic acid	GC-EI-MS	7
	Bovine urine	N,O-Bis(trimethylsilyl)-trifluoroacetamide (BSTFA), N-Methyl-N-(tetr-butyldimethylsilyl)-trifluoroacetamide (MTBSTFA)	GC-CI-MS	8
	Bovine tissues and plasma	Pentafluoropropionic anhydride	GC-NICI-MS	9
Albendazole	Bovine liver	N-Methyl-N-(tetr-butyldimethylsilyl)-trifluoroaceta mide (MTBSTFA)	GC-EI-MS and GC-MID-MS	10
Anticoccidials	Bovine liver	9-Anthryldiazomethane	LC-Fluorometric	11, 12
	Bovine tissues and milk	Vanillin	LC-UV	13
	Chicken tissues	9-Anthryldiazomethane	LC-Fluorometric	14
	Chicken tissues	Vanillin	LC-UV	15, 16
	Chicken tissues	Potassium ferricyanide	LC-Fluorometric	17
Anti-inflammatory drugs	Plasma, urine	N,O-Bis(trimethylsilyl)-trifluoroacetamide (BSTFA)	GC-EI-MS	18
	Plasma, urine	Methyl iodide	GC-EI-MS	19

Analyte	Matrix	Derivatization reagent	Detection	References
3-Amino-2-oxazolidinone (furazolidone metabolite)	Swine tissues	2-Nitrobenzaldehyde	MS-TSP	20
Carbadox and metabolites	Animal tissues	NaOH	LC-Vis	21, 22
Chloramphenicol	Egg powder	Trimethylsilyl-N,N-dimethylcarbamate	GC-ECD	23
	Animal tissues, milk, eggs, shrimp	Chlorotrimethylsilane, pyridine, hexamethyldisilazane	GC-ECD	24–30
	Meat, milk	Chlorotrimethylsilane, pyridine, hexamethyldisilazene	GC-NICI-MS	31, 32
	Milk	Heptafluorobutyric anhydride	GC-NICI-MS	33
	Meat, eggs	N,O-Bis(trifluoromethylsilyl)-acetamide	GC-NICI-MS	34
	Meat, milk, eggs	Diazomethane, heptafluorobutyric anhydride	GC-NSTD	35
	Urine	Chlorotrimethylsilane, pyridine, hexamethyldisilazane	GC-ECD	36
Chloramphenicol, florfenicol, thiamphenicol	Milk	N,O-Bis(trimethylsilyl)-trifluoroacetamide (BSTFA)	G C-ECD	37
Clorsulon	Kidney	Methyl iodide	GC-EI-MS and GC-MID-MS	38
Diethylstilbestrol	Meat	Heptafluorobutyric acid anhydride	GC-EI-MS	39
Diethylstilbestrol, dienestrol, hexestrol	Plasma, urine	Pentafluorobenzyl bromide	GC-NICI-MS	40
Corticosteroids	Milk, liver	Pyridinium chlorochromate	GC-NICI-MS	41
Eprinomectin	Bovine tissues	Trifluoroacetic anhydride	LC-Fluorometric	42
Erythromycin	Animal tissues	Acetic anhydride, pyridine	GC-SIM-MS	43

(continued)

TABLE 21.1 Continued

Drug	Matrix	Derivatizing agent	Detection mode	Ref.
Flumequine	Fish	H_2SO_4	LC-Fluorometric	44
Gentamicin	Bovine tissues	o-Phthalaldehyde	LC-Fluorometric	45
Indomethacin	Plasma, urine	N-Methyl-N-(tert.-butyldimethylsilyl)-trifluoroaceta mide (MTBSTFA)	GC-ECD	46
Ivermectin	Animal tissues	Methylimidazole, acetic anhydride	LC-Fluorometric	47–49
	Meat, liver	Methylimidazole, trifluoroacetic anhydride	LC-Fluorometric	50
	Milk	Methylimidazole, acetic anhydride	LC-Fluorometric	51, 52
Malachite green, gentian violet and metabolites	Fish	PbO_2	LC-UV	53–57
17α-methyltestosterone and two metabolites	Fish	3α-Hydroxysteroid dehydrogenase,	LC-Fluorometric	58
Moxidectin	Bovine tissues	Methylimidazole, acetic anhydride	LC-Fluorometric	59
	Bovine tissues	Methylimidazole, trifluoroacetic anhydride	LC-Fluorometric	60
	Plasma	Methylimidazole, trifluoroacetic anhydride	LC-Fluorometric	61
Neomycin	Animal tissues, milk	o-Phthalaldehyde	LC-Fluorometric	62–65
Nortestosterone, methyltestosterone	Bovine muscle	Heptafluorobutyric acid anhydride	GC-NICI-MS	66
19-Nortestosterone, testosterone, trenbolone	Urine	Carboxymethoxylamine, pentafluorobenzyl bromide, N,O-Bis(trimethylsilyl)-trifluoroacetamide (BSTFA)	GC-NICI-MS	67

Analyte	Matrix	Reagent	Detection	Reference
Oleandomycin	Animal tissues	Acetic anhydride, pyridine	GC-SIM-MS	43
Penicillins	Fish	Formaldehyde	LC-Fluorometric	68
	Meat, milk	Diazomethane	GC-NSTD	69–71
	Meat, milk, eggs	1,2,4-Triazole-mercuric chloride	LC-UV	72–74
	Meat, milk, cheese	1,2,4-Triazole-mercuric chloride	LC-UV	75
	Milk	4-Bromomethyl-7-methoxycoumarin	LC-Fluorometric	76
	Milk	Dansylhydrazine	LC-Fluorometric	77
	Milk	Salicylaldehyde	LC-Fluorometric	78
	Milk	Formaldehyde	LC-Fluorometric	79
	Milk	1,2,4-Triazole-mercuric chloride	LC-UV	80, 81
	Muscle	Formaldehyde	LC-Fluorometric	82
	Tissues	Imidazole-mercuric chloride	LC-UV	83
	Tissues	1,2,4-Triazole-mercuric chloride	LC-UV	84–86
Pirlimycin	Tissues	Iodoacetamide	LC-UV	87
	Milk	9-Fluorenylmethyl chloroformate	LC-UV	88
Quinolones	Fish	Sodium tetrahydroborate	GC-SIM-MS	89
Quinoxaline-2-carboxylic acid (carbadox metabolite)	Swine tissues	Methanolic sulfuric acid	GC-SIM-MS	90–92
	Swine tissues	Methanolic sulfuric acid	GC-ECD	93
Roxarsone	Swine tissues	NaOH	LC-Vis	94
Spiramycin	Animal tissues	Acetic anhydride, pyridine	GC-SIM-MS	43
Stanozolol and two hydroxy metabolites	Urine	Heptafluorobutyric acid anhydride	GC-EI-MS	95

(continued)

TABLE 21.1 Continued

Drug	Matrix	Derivatizing agent	Detection mode	Ref.
Steroid hormones	Meat	N,O-Bis(trimethylsilyl)acetamide	GC-EI-MS	96
Steroid hormones	Meat	Heptafluorobutyric acid anhydride, N-Methyl-N-(trimethylsilyl)-trifluoroacetamide (MSTFA)	GC-EI-MS	97
Steroid hormones and corticosteroids	Meat	N-Methyl-N-(trimethylsilyl)-trifluoroacetamide (MSTFA)	GC-EI-MS	98
Streptomycin, dihydrostreptomycin	Animal tissues, milk	1,2-Naphthoquinone-4-sulfonic acid	LC-Fluorometric	99, 100
Sulfonamides	Animal liver	Diazomethane	GC-ECD tandem PICI-MS	101
	Animal tissues	p-Dimethylaminobenzaldehyde (DMBA)	LC-Vis	102
	Animal tissues	Diazomethane, pentafluoropropionic anhydride, diethylamine	GC-SIM-MS	103
	Animal tissues	Diazomethane	GC-ECD	104
	Animal tissues, eggs	Diazomethane	GC-SIM-MS	105
	Chicken muscle	Fluorescamine	LC-Fluorometric	106
	Fish	Fluorescamine	LC-Fluorometric	107
	Meat	Fluorescamine	LC-Fluorometric	108
	Milk	Fluorescamine	LC-Fluorometric	109, 110
	Milk, eggs, fish	o-Phthalaldehyde	LC-Fluorometric	111

Analyte	Matrix	Reagent	Detection	Reference
Milk, eggs, meat		p-Dimethylaminobenzaldehyde (DMBA)	LC-Vis	112
	Swine tissues	Diazomethane	GC-PICI-MS	113, 114
	Swine tissues	N-Methyl-bis(trifluoroacetamide), diazomethane	GC-PPINICI-MS	115
Tetracyclines	Swine tissues	Diazomethane	GC-SIM-MS	116
	Animal tissues, eggs	Zirconyl chloride	LC-Fluorometric	117, 118
	Animal and fish tissues	$Mg(OAc)_2$	LC-Fluorometric	119
Thiabendazole, 5-hydroxythiabendazole	Bovine tissues	Trimethylanilinium	GC-SIM-MS	120
Thyreostatics	Bovine muscle	Methyl iodide	GC-SIM-MS	121
	Thyroid gland	7-Chloro-4-nitrobenzo-2-oxa-1,3-diazole	TLC-MS	122
	Thyroid gland	Pentafluorobenzyl bromide, N-methyl-N-(trimethylsilyl)-trifluoroacetamide (MSTFA)	GC-NICI-MS or GC-PICI-MS	123
Tiamulin	Urine	Methyl iodide	GC-NPD	124
Trenbolone, epitrenbolone	Swine liver	Pentafluoropropionic anhydride	GC-ECD	125
	Bovine tissues	N,O-Bis(trimethylsilyl)-trifluoroacetamide (BSTFA)	GC-EI-MS	126
Zearalenone, α-zearalenol	Urine	Tri-Sil BT	GC-MS-MS	

MS, Mass spectrometry; EI, electron impact; CI, chemical ionization; MID, multiple ion detection; PICI, positive-ion chemical ionization; NICI, negative-ion chemical ionization; SIM, selected ion monitoring; TSP, thermospray; PPINICI, pulsed positive ion–negative ion chemical ionization; ECD, electron-capture detector; NPD, nitrogen/phosphorous detector; NSTD, nitrogen-selective thermionic detector; FT-IR, Fourier transform infrared spectrometry.

monly called dansyl chloride (128–134). This reagent is capable of reacting with alcohol, phenol, and thiol groups as well (135, 136). Alternative dansylation reagents include 5-dibutylaminonaphthalene-1-sulfonyl chloride and 5-methyl-phenylaminonaphthalene-1-sulfonyl chloride (137, 138).

Derivatization is performed in either aqueous or nonaqueous solvents under alkaline conditions. Most widely used compound for rendering the reaction mixture alkaline is triethylamine since this base does not lead to undesirable byproducts and can be completed in a short time. The dansylated products are relatively stable, exhibit high sensitivity, and offer a detection limit is often at the picogram level.

Whenever only primary amines need to be derivatized, fluorescamine often constitutes the reagent of choice. Fluorescamine, although nonfluorescent itself, can react with primary amines forming highly fluorescent pyrrolinones (139–144). Aliphatic primary amines favor derivatization reaction at pH 8–9, whereas primary aromatic amines exhibit optimal reactivity at pH 3–4. Secondary amines are also fully reactive with fluorescamine but their products do not fluoresce. However, secondary amines can be detected with fluorescamine if they are converted to primary amines by oxidation with N-chlorosuccinimide prior to their fluorescamine derivatization (145, 146). Alcohols can also interact with fluorescamine but this reaction is reversible; as a result, alcohols just slow down the reaction rate of fluorescamine with primary amines. On the other hand, tertiary amines and guanidines are not reactive at all with fluorescamine.

The derivatization reaction is performed at ambient temperature by simply mixing the aqueous sample extract with a phosphate buffer of appropriate pH and then adding the fluorescamine solution in acetonitrile under vigorous stirring. Acetonitrile is the solvent of choice for preparing fluorescamine solutions, because the net fluorescence decreases with a decrease in polarity of the organic solvent in the order acetonitrile, acetone, dioxane, and tetrahydrofuran.

Besides fluorescamine, several other reagents can react with primary amines yielding fluorescent products. A reagent whose structure is closely related to that of fluorescamine is 2-methoxy-2,4-diphenyl-(2H)-furanone (147). Another widely used reagent that reacts with primary amines yielding fluorescent isoindole derivatives in presence of thiols such as ethanethiol, 3-mercapto-1-propanol or 2-mercaptoethanol is o-phthalaldehyde (OPA) (148–159). The fluorescence of the OPA derivatives is somewhat higher than those of fluorescamine, but their stability is lower because the formed fluorescent iso-indole derivatives undergo spontaneous rearrangement with time. Secondary amines cannot be detected with OPA unless they are previously oxidized with chloramine T, N-chlorosuccinimide, or sodium hypochlorite (160–162).

Other reagents used for fluorescence derivatization are the so-called Edman-type isothiocyanate compounds, namely fluoresceinisothiocyanate (163), 9-isothiocyanatoacridine (164), 4-dimethylamino-1-naphthylisothiocyanate (165), or

BOC-aminophenyl- and BOC-aminoethylphenyl-isothiocyanate (166). These reagents can also react with primary amines to give fluorescent thioureido derivatives.

A number of other reagents are also available for derivatizing both primary and secondary amines. The chloroformate-type reagents such as 9-fluorenylmethylchloroformate (167) and 2-naphthylchloroformate (168) allow the prechromatographic derivatization of primary and secondary amines, whereas 1,2-naththoylenebenzimidazole-6-sulfonyl chloride has been specifically designed for prechromatographic derivatization of aliphatic primary and secondary amines. Pre- and postchromatographic derivatization of primary and secondary amines can also be carried out with nonfluorescent reagents including 4-fluoro-7-nitrobenzo-2-oxa-1,3-diazole, and 4-chloro-7-nitrobenzo-2-oxa-1,3-diazole (169–173). Although these reagent are also capable of reacting with phenolic hydroxyl and sulfydryl groups, their higher reactivity toward amino groups makes them attractive for selective derivatization. Guanidino compounds can also be readily derivatized using 9,10-phenanthrenequinone, a reagent that yields fluorescent 2-aminophenanthrimidazoles (174, 175).

21.1.2 Hydroxyl and Sulfydryl Group

For derivatization of hydroxyl groups, several fluorescent reagents containing carbonyl nitrile as the reacting group have been developed. Pyrene-1-carbonylnitrile (176), 1-anthroylnitrile (177–179), and 4-dimethylamino-1-naphthoylnitrile (180) are all derivatizing agents capable of reacting with both primary and secondary hydroxyl groups under mild conditions yielding highly fluorescent esters. In contrast, 9-anthroylnitrile reacts only with primary hydroxyl groups (177).

Carbonylazides can also be used for fluorescent labeling of both primary and secondary hydroxyl groups. Including in this class of reagents are 7-methoxycoumarin-3-carbonylazide and 7-methoxycoumarin-4-carbonylazide (181).

For prechromatographic fluorescence labeling of sulfydryl groups, a number of dansyl derivatives have been also proposed. Dansylaziridine reacts selectively with sulfydryl groups (182), whereas N-chlorodansylamide, a nonfluorescent derivatizing agent, yields the highly fluorescent dansylamide (183, 184). Prechromatographic labeling of sulfydryl groups can also be performed with several maleimide derivatives containing potential fluorophores, such 1-anilinonaphthyl- (185), 9-acridinyl- (186, 187), p-(2-benzimidazoyl)phenyl- (188), p-(2-benzoxazoyl)-phenyl- (189), 7-dimethylamino-4-methylcoumarin (190, 191), or 1-pyrenyl- groups (192, 193). These reagents, most of which do not show any significant fluorescence, can react selectively with sulfydryl groups under mild conditions yielding highly fluorescent derivatives. Apart from the above, certain diazole derivatives including 4-fluorobenzo-2-oxa-1,3-diazole-7-sulfonate, and 4-fluoro-7-sulfamoylbenzo-2-oxa-1,3-diazole can also serve for prechromatographic labeling of sulfydryl groups (194, 195). Fluorescent derivatives can further be produced when OPA reacts from sulfydryl groups in presence of a primary amine.

21.1.3   Carboxylic and Carbonyl Groups

Several alkylating agents have been developed for the fluorescent labeling of the carboxylic group. The first developed 4-bromomethyl-7-methoxycoumarin and 4-hydroxy-7-methoxycoumarin derivatization reagents provided esters with lower quantum yields than those produced from the later-developed 4-bromomethyl-6,7-dimethoxycoumarin (196–202). The esters formed from 4-bromomethyl-7-acetoxycoumarin underwent facile hydrolysis with alkalis to yield highly fluorescent 7-hydroxycoumarin. Accordingly, the procedure involving chromatographic separation of the methoxycoumarin esters followed by alkaline hydrolysis of the eluate was recommended (203). Similar alkylating reagents including 1-bromoacetylpyrene (204), 9-(chloromethyl)-anthracene (205), naphthacyl bromide (206), and panacyl bromide (207) are also available.

Other well-known labeling reagents for the carboxylic group are certain diazoalkane derivatives, such as 4-diazomethyl-7-methoxycoumarin and 9-anthryldiazomethane, which are highly reactive but generally lack stability (208–210). Some *O*-alkyl isourea derivatives including N,N′-dicyclohexyl-methylisourea and N,N′-diisopropyl-O-(7-methoxycoumarin-4-yl)-methylisourea have been also used for derivatization of the carboxylic group; these reagents can be readily prepared from equimolar amounts of carbodiimide and alcohol (211, 212).

Fluorescent amines can also be employed for labeling the carboxylic group, provided it will be activated prior to its coupling with the amines. For this purpose, carbodiimide derivatives such as the N,N′-dicyclohexylcarbodiimide or N-ethyl-N′-(3-dimethylaminopropyl)carbodiimide have been widely used (213, 214). Addition of 1-hydroxybenzotriazole is often effective for suppressing the formation of N-acylisourea derivatives. Activation of carboxylic acids can be also attained through use of 2-bromo-1-methylpyridinium and N,N′-carbonyldiimidazole, although oxalyl or thionyl chloride can be used for preparing acid chlorides (215). 9,10-Diaminophenanthrene condenses with carboxylic acids, resulting in fluorescent phenanthroimidazole derivatives (216). In this condensation reaction, methyl polyphosphate is used as solvent. Derivatization of α-keto acids with o-phenylenediamine produces 2-quinoxalinol (217–219).

Several reagents for derivatization of carbonyl groups are also available. Dansylhydrazine reacts with carbonyl groups in the presence of trichloroacetic acid, yielding highly fluorescent dansylhydrazones that exhibit, however, limited stability. In addition, fluorescent hydrazones can be produced from carbonyl-containing compounds after their reaction with 4-hydrazino-2-oxa-1,3-diazole or

4'-hydrazino-2-stilbazole. Whenever selective fluorescent labeling of the oxo-methylene group is required, as in the case, for example, of acetophenone, N'-methylnicotinamide chloride may be considered the best choice.

21.2 ULTRAVIOLET-VISIBLE DERIVATIZATION

Ultraviolet-visible (UV-Vis) detection in liquid chromatography is often hampered by the poor spectral properties of the analytes at the applied analytical wavelengths. In this respect, a variety of pre- and postchromatographic derivatization reactions have been proposed for improving UV-Vis detectability.

21.2.1 Amino Group

Primary and secondary amino groups are most commonly labeled by nucleophilic substitution reactions. Widely used labels, introducing nitrophenyl chromophores, include 1-fluoro-2,4-dinitrobenzene, 2,4,6-trinitrobenzenesulfonic acid, and 4-fluoro-3-nitrotrifluoromethylbenzene. The former reagent reacts with amino groups to form substituted aromatic amines. It is commonly used prechromato-graphically as a label for aminoglycosides including neomycin (220, 221), tobra-mycin (222–225), amikacin (226, 227), gentamicin, and sisomicin (223–225). The kinetics of these labeling reactions are complicated (222). To label all amino groups present in the aminoglycosides while preventing both hydrolytic degrada-tion of the derivatives and hydroxyl derivatization, accurately standardized reac-tion conditions must be followed since this derivatization process requires a fairly long reaction time (20–30 min) at high temperature (333–373 K) in alkaline solution (pH 9). However, some workers (227) succeeded in derivatizing amikacin in serum within 5 min using 0.05 M sodium hydroxide–methanol as a reaction medium.

2,4,6-Trinitrobenzenesulfonic acid has been also used for the prechromato-graphic derivatization of aminoglycosides in alkaline media (228, 229). A major advantage of this label is the fact that hydroxyl groups cannot be concurrently derivatized, thus increasing, the selectivity. Unlike prementioned labels, 4-fluoro-3-nitrotrifluoromethylbenzene does not react with compounds such as amino acids that contain additional polar groups (230). This reagent does not react with sec-ondary amines either.

Amino groups can also be derivatized using acyl chlorides that form amides. A number of suitable acyl chlorides including p-chloro-, p-methoxy-, p-nitroben-zoyl-, p-tolyl-, and p-nitro-benzenesulfonyl chloride have been successfully used for sensitive UV-Vis derivatization of nonabsorbing amine compounds (231). Among all those amide derivatives, p-methoxybenzamides appear more attractive because they exhibit high molar absorptivity at the convenient analytical wave-length of 254 nm. After derivatization in tetrahydrofuran–sodium hydroxide solution, the derivatives are extracted with chloroform and analyzed by LC. Polyfunctional amines, in general, can be derivatized as well within 5 min at room temperature using p-tolylbenzenesulfonyl chloride (232).

In addition, primary amino groups are sometimes derivatized using isothiocyanates as labels (233). These labels have replaced earlier used isocyanate reagents that also reacted with hydroxyl groups, carboxylic groups, and water, and hence lacked sensitivity and selectivity (234). Although isothiocyanates react with secondary amines, alcohols, and phenols (235), they exhibit an amino-group affinity higher than that for the other functional groups. Moreover, the isothiocyanate derivatization reaction is pH-independent. Phenylisothiocyanate is the reagent most widely employed for prechromatographic derivatization of aliphatic and aromatic amines (234). The selectivity of this reaction, however, is limited by the presence of alcohols and water, although it appears that the amino function is most reactive. p-Phenylbenzoylisothiocyanate, another often used label, has the added advantage of a high wavelength of absorption that limits interferences from nonspecific absorbance originating from the matrix (236).

Tertiary amines can also be selectively derivatized with citric acid on acetic acid anhydride, a mixture that is mixed with the eluent after chromatography and then heated to 393 K to develop a violet–red color (237). Absorbance is measure at 550 nm but some compounds can show strongly tailing peaks.

21.2.2   Carboxylic Group

Most popular for derivatization of the carboxylic group are certain phenacyl and naphthacyl bromide reagents that react to form the corresponding phenacyl- and naphthacyl-carboxylates (238, 239). These halides readily alkylate carboxylic acids but the reaction yield is far from complete. The reaction is nonselective because many other compounds can undergo alkylation with these reagents, but selectivity can be increased through use of crown ethers that activate the carboxylic function. Crown ethers complex the cation of the neutralized acid, thus activating the anion to react in a nucleophilic substitution reaction with the halide. In general, neutralization of the solutions prior to derivatization is carried out with potassium hydroxide or carbonates (240–242). Activation of carboxylic acids can be also achieved with some tertiary amines that act as hydrobromide scavengers. Triethylamine (243, 244) and N,N′-diisopropylethylamine (245–249) are tertiary amines frequently used for this purpose.

These alkylating derivatization reactions can be accomplished within 15 min at a temperature of 353 K using acetonitrile (250, 251) or dimethylformamide (245–248) as derivatization solvents. The average yield under such conditions is often higher than 97%. Although the presence of small amounts of water does not influence the reaction yield significantly (238), removal of excess water can be achieved by extraction of the acids from the biological samples using water-immiscible organic solvents or by applying a solvent-demixing technique (241).

This technique can be also applied when the water-miscible acetonitrile is added to the serum sample for extracting the analytes. Following the addition of acetonitrile, the solution is saturated with potassium chloride so that the water and acetonitrile phases separate and derivatization is performed in the acetonitrile layer. Such alkylating procedures have been applied for prechromatographic derivatization of various drug residues with carboxylic groups, including penicillins (252) and barbiturates (253).

In contrast to prechromatographic derivatization, postchromatographic derivatization of carboxylic acids is generally very limited. A literature survey shows a few applications only in the case of penicillins. In the most prominent of these methods (254, 255), penicillins are extracted from serum or urine to be separated by reversed-phase liquid chromatography and subsequently derivatized with a reagent containing imidazole and mercuric chloride. In this reaction, opening of the beta-lactam ring initially occurs and the resulting intermediate rearrangement reacts with mercuric chloride to form a mercuric mercaptide that can be detected at 310 nm (254, 255).

Several other reagents for derivatization of carboxylic acids and related compounds have been described in the literature. Most reports concern derivatization with 2-nirophenylhydrazine after activation of the carboxylic group with N,N'-dicyclohexylcarbodiimide (256) or 1-ethyl-3-(dimethylaminopropyl)carbodiimide (257), but the performance of this derivatization has not been yet thoroughly tested. Prostaglandins can be derivatized by alkylating the carboxyl group with diazomethane (258). Subsequently, the keto function of the methylated compounds is derivatized with p-nitrobenzylhydroxylamine in pyridine to form the corresponding p-nitrobenzyloxime derivative. The advantage of this reaction is that high background absorbance raised after labeling of the carboxylic group can be avoided.

21.2.3   Hydroxyl and Sulfydryl Groups

Hydroxyl-containing compounds are very suitable for transformation into esters, enabling detection improvement when proper labels are introduced. Most commonly, benzoyl chlorides with various spectroscopic properties are used, but phenyldimethylsilylchloride or phenylisocyanates are also applied.

Benzoyl chlorides, like other acyl chlorides, react readily with alcohols to form the corresponding esters (259). The reaction requires 19 h to be completed, and it has been studied in the analysis of carbohydrates, aminosugars, and glycosides (260). Because the preparation of acyl derivatives of monosaccharides is difficult, phenyldimethylsilyl chloride has been also investigated as an alternative label (261). After dissolving the analytes in dimethylformamide and addition of imidazole, the solution was heated at 373 K for 1 h, the label was added, and the reaction was allowed to proceed for more than 6 h. However, the molar absorptivities of the derivatives obtained were generally very low. Phenylisocyanate reagents have been also applied for derivatization of aliphatic alcohols prior to liquid chromatographic (LC) analysis (262). Most suitable solvents for this reaction were found to be dimethylformamide, acetonitrile, and dioxane.

As far as derivatization of the sulfydryl group is concerned, this is complicated and lacks sensitivity. It is usually performed, after separation of the analytes on a C_{18} column, using 6,6'-dithiodinicotinic acid or 5,5'-dithio-2-nitrobenzoic acid at pH values over 6 or 7.5, respectively, whereas the formed derivatives are detected at 344 or 412 nm, respectively (263). The selectivity of the latter reaction is higher due to the higher analytical wavelength but the alkaline medium is disadvantageous in view of the risk of oxidation of the thiol compounds. Using the above reagents for derivatization of disulfides, a reduction step to form the corresponding thiols is necessary prior to derivatization.

21.3 ENZYMATIC DERIVATIZATION

Enzymatic derivatization offers major advantages over alternative procedures. The selectivity of an enzyme for its substrate along with the sensitivity offered by modern analytical instrumentation makes enzymatic derivatization a powerful tool in the field of drug residue analysis.

Enzymes can be used in several ways in chromatographic applications to improve selectivity or to enhance the detector response. Applications may involve enzymes with either a broad specificity toward a group of related compounds or a high specificity toward a particular compound. In the field of drug residue analysis, most current applications concern enzymatic reactions taking place in separate reactors incorporated in LC systems before or after the analytical column. Reactors with immobilized enzymes have proven to be suitable in such continuous flow systems.

The enzyme catalyzes the conversion of the analyte to a corresponding product. Determination of the amount of this product or of a specific coformed byproduct or, alternatively, measurement of the concentration decrease of a coreactant agent by means of a suitable LC detector can allow estimation of the analyte level in the injected sample.

The specific effect of the inclusion of an enzyme in a chromatographic system is difficult to predict. Although there is no general description of the effects of organic mobile phases on the enzyme activity, changes in the structure of the enzyme, in its specific binding, solvation, competition at the active site, and shifting equilibria are obvious. Increased bleeding of the enzyme from the matrix may occur due to reaction of the organic solvent with the enzyme–matrix bonds, whereas enzymes can be denatured whenever large concentrations of organic solvents are used. Nevertheless, the presence of small amounts of organic solvents may sometimes increase the activity, as has been observed in the case of immobilized β-glucuronidase and a mobile phase containing up to 10% methanol (264–266). Other constituents of the mobile phase, such as buffers and metal ions, may also act as inhibitors or activators of the enzyme activity.

Changes in the activity of enzymes may also occur by a variety of other parameters including temperature, pH, and ionic strength. Temperature can affect both the activity and the stability of the enzymes. For most enzymes, the reaction velocity doubles with a temperature increase of 10°C but potential enzyme denaturation may also occur (265).

Another important parameter is the acidity of the system. Since the relation between enzyme activity and pH often shows an optimum, buffers are regularly used in enzymatic derivatization to control the pH. Use of buffers, however, can cause increase of the ionic strength of the system, thus changing the tertiary structure of the enzyme and either making it more accessible for the substrate or blocking its active sites. Therefore, optimization of the chromatographic system is recommended for each specific system.

Enzymes can be immobilized on several support materials using several procedures. Most common is the direct linking of the enzyme to the matrix. The popularity of this procedure can be explained by the simplicity and the efficiency of the coupling procedure and the increased stability of the enzyme. After activation of the matrix, the enzyme solution is brought into contact with the matrix and the unbound enzyme is washed out. The yield of immobilization and the activity of the bonded enzyme are governed by the activation step, as the binding of the enzyme should take place at amino acid residues that are not essential for its activity.

The number of relevant applications, especially those dealing with immobilized enzyme reactors, increases steadily (267, 268). Immobilization of enzymes on suitable matrices permits their reuse, thus creating the possibility to perform more experiments with the same batch of enzymes, which cuts down the cost of the analysis.

An enzyme reactor with immobilized 3α-hydroxysteroid dehydrogenase has been successfully used for the analysis of residues of 17α-methyltestosterone in trout by high-performance liquid chromatography (HPLC) (269). Following their separation by reversed-phase chromatography, the major tissue metabolites of 17α-methyltestosterone, namely 5α-androstane-17α-methyl-3α,17β-diol, and 5β-androstane-17α-methyl-3α,17β-diol, were enzymatically modified in the presence of a coreactant, nicotinamide-adenine dinucleotide (NAD), to the corresponding ketone. The position at 3α was enzymatically oxidized, and NADH, the reduced form of NAD, was produced as a coproduct and subjected to fluorescence detection. Reoxidation of NADH to NAD provides the possibility for electrochemical detection.

Enzyme reactors with immobilized β-glucuronidase have been also applied for the determination of glucuronide conjugates in urine. The glucuronides either prior (270–273) or after (274, 275) their separation by LC were enzymatically hydrolyzed to glucuronic acid and the aglycon. After the enzymatic hydrolysis, either a specific detection of the parent aglycon was applied or the produced glucuronic acid was determined. The latter approach, based on reduction of the glucuronic acid in presence of lucigenin, resulted in a more generic method for the detection of glucuronides leading to a chemiluminescent product. Most frequently the enzyme was immobilized by the glutaraldehyde crosslinking procedure on aminopropyl beads.

Using immobilized β-glucuronidase reactors, estriol and estradiol glucuronides have been determined in urine by a column-switching technique (270, 271). Both glucuronides were hydrolyzed by the immobilized enzyme at pH 7. The steroid mixture was subsequently separated by gradient elution on a reversed-phase column, to be finally detected by UV absorbance at 280 nm. In this procedure, the activity of enzyme did not alter even after 150 h continuous run and exposure to a mobile phase containing 10% methanol. When a separate reversed-phase precolumn was inserted in the LC system, additional sample purification and shorter analysis time could be attained (272).

A postchromatographic β-glucuronidase procedure has been also used for the analysis of phenolic glucuronides, such as those produced from trimethoprim (274). The enzymatic analysis of these glucuronides provided the production of the corresponding phenolic compounds, which were measured by both UV and electrochemical detection.

The wide variety of enzymes available gives for promise enzymatic derivatization to become a potent analytical tool in the future. Better understanding and theoretical formulations will lead to commercial availability of immobilized enzymes and consequently to more ready use of them. Since in such systems a low content of organic cosolvent in the mobile phase can only be tolerated (whereas a compromise has to be made as far as the optimum mobile phase pH is concerned), artificial enzymes, which are synthetic polymer chains having functional groups that mimic the biocatalytic activity of natural enzymes, are currently being synthesized and investigated as a means to overcome such limitations (276).

21.4 PHOTOCHEMICAL DERIVATIZATION

An elegant approach to increase the selectivity and specificity of the analyte after its elution from a chromatographic column is to apply an online photochemical reaction for which suitable reactors are now commercially available. Photochemical reactions can be applied for various purposes, as, for example, to increase the detectability by converting weakly or nonfluorescing analytes into highly fluorescent products or to create electroactive products that can be detected with photoconductivity, photoionization, or photoelectrochemical detectors. Photoconductivity reactions use UV irradiation to generate new products that have different conductivity properties, whereas photoionization reactions form ions and electrons that are collected and detected. In photoelectrochemical reactions, light encroaches upon the working electrode of the detector in order to convert a nonelectroactive product to an electrophore.

Photochemical reactions are dependent on the composition of the mobile phase, the reaction time, and the wavelength and intensity of the irradiation. All these parameters should be considered for optimization of the sensitivity and specificity of a photochemical reaction. The advantage of using a postchromatographic photoreaction over more conventional reactions is the absence of additional pumps and mixing devices for reagent addition, since photons are the only reagent actually needed. This is very promising because analytical procedures do not have to be changed except to add the reactor between column exit and the detector, and to use it in an on/off mode.

When using photochemical reactions, a gain in fluorescence output or electroactivity not only lowers detection limits but also contributes to confirm an analytical result. Examples are the conversion of diethylstilbestrol to a fluorescent hexahydrophenanthrene (277), and the conversion of fenbendazole to fluorescent species (278). The fluorescence of photoconverted diethylstilbestrol can further be enhanced by a subsequent online postchromatographic derivatization with bisulfite to the highly fluorescent phenanthrenediol (279). Another example of photolytic derivatization is the postchromatographic conversion of penicillins and cephalosporins into electroactive species that can be detected by an amperometric detector (280).

This type of derivatization seems promising for the detection of drugs and metabolites with phenolic groups. A recent application on the determination of chlorophenols in surface water showed that the dansyl derivatives of phenols are readily convertible to the highly fluorescent dansyl-OH and dansyl-OCH$_3$ products after postchromatographic irradiation (281). Fluorescence gain factors of up to 8000-fold were obtained for chlorophenol derivatives with a low native fluorescence.

REFERENCES

1. R.T. Wilson, J.M. Groneck, K.P. Holland, and A.C. Henry, J. AOAC Int., 77:917 (1994).
2. Y. Gaillard, A. Balland, F. Doucet, and G. Pepin, J. Chromatogr., 703:85 (1997).
3. P. Gonzalez, C.A. Fente, C. Franco, B. Vazquez, E. Quinto, and A. Cepeda, J. Chromatogr., 693:321 (1997).
4. L. Leyssens, C. Driessen, A. Jacobs, J. Czech, and J. Raus, J. Chromatogr., 564: 515 (1991).

5. L.A. van Ginkel, R.W. Stephany, and H.J. van Rossum, J. AOAC Int., 75:554 (1992).

6. T. Visser, M.J. Vredenbregt, A.P.J.M. de Jong, L.A. van Ginkel, H.J. van Rossum, and R.W. Stephany, Anal. Chim. Acta, 275:205 (1993).

7. F. Ramos, C. Santos, A. Silva, and M.I.N. da Silveira, J. Chromatogr., 716:366 (1998).

8. J.A. van Rhijn, H.H. Heskamp, M.L. Essers, H.J. van de Wetering, H.C.H. Kleijnen, and A.H. Roos, J. Chromatogr., 665:395 (1995).

9. J. Girault and J.B. Fourtillan, J. Chromatogr., 518:41 (1990).

10. J. Markus and J. Sherma, J. AOAC Int., 75:1135 (1992).

11. E.E. Mertinez and W. Shimoda, J. Assoc. Off. Anal. Chem., 68:1149 (1985).

12. E.E. Mertinez and W. Shimoda, J. Assoc. Off. Anal. Chem., 69:637 (1986).

13. J.W. Moran, J.M. Turner, and M.R. Coleman, J. AOAC Int., 78:668 (1995).

14. K. Takatsuki, S. Suzuki, and I. Ushizawa, J. Assoc. Off. Anal. Chem., 69:443 (1986).

15. J.F. Ericson, A. Calcagni, and M.J. Lynch, J. AOAC Int., 77:577 (1994).

16. J.W. Moran, J.M. Rodewald, A.L. Donoho, and M.R. Coleman, J. AOAC Int., 77: 885 (1994).

17. H. Takahashi, T. Sekiya, M. Nishikawa, and Y.S. Endoh, J. Liq. Chromatogr., 17: 4489 (1994).

18. A.K. Singh, Y. Jang, U. Mishra, and K. Granley, J. Chromatogr., 568:351 (1991).

19. G. Gonzales, R. Ventura, A.K. Smith, R. de la Torre, and J. Segura, J. Chromatogr., 719:251 (1996).

20. R.J. McCracken and D.G. Kennedy, J. Chromatogr., 691:87 (1997).

21. M.M.L. Aerts, W.M.J. Beek, H.J. Keukens, and U.A.Th. Brinkman, J. Chromatogr., 456:105 (1988).

22. G.M. Binnendijk, M.M.L. Aerts, H.J. Keukens, and U.A.Th. Brinkman, J. Chromatogr., 541:401 (1991).

23. L. Weber, in Residues of Veterinary Drugs in Food, Proc. Euroresidue Conf., Noordwijkerhout, May 21–23, 1990 (N. Haagsma, A. Ruiter, and P.B. Czedik-Eysenberg, Eds.), Fac. Vet. Med., Univ. Utrecht, The Netherlands, p. 394 (1990).

24. S. Fabiansson, T. Nilsson, and J. Backstrom, J. Sci. Fd Agric., 27:1156 (1976).

25. R. Malisch, U. Sandmeyer, and K. Kypke-Hutter, Lebensmittelchem. Gerichl. Chem., 38:11 (1984).

26. J.R. Nelson, K.F.T. Copeland, R.J. Forster, D.J. Campbell, and W.D. Black, J. Chromatogr., 276:438 (1983).

27. D. Arnold and A. Somogyi, J. Assoc. Off. Anal. Chem., 68:984 (1985).

28. R.K. Munns, D.C. Holland, J.E. Roybal, J.M. Storey, A.R. Long, G.R. Stehly, and S.M. Plakas, J. AOAC Int., 77:596 (1994).

29. Th. Gude, A. Preiss, and K. Rubach, J. Chromatogr., 673:197 (1995).

30. M.H. Akhtar, C. Danis, A. Sauve, and C. Barry, J. Chromatogr., 696:123 (1995).

31. P.J. Kijak, J. AOAC Int., 77:34 (1994).

32. R.L. Epstein, C. Henry, K.P. Holland, and J. Dreas, J. AOAC Int., 77:570 (1994).

33. J.M. Wal, J.C. Peleran, and G. Bories, J. Chromatogr., 168:179 (1979).

34. L.A. van Ginkel, H.J. van Rossum, P.W. Zoontjes, H. van Blitterswijk, G. Ellen, E. van der Heeft, A.P.J.M. de Jong, and G. Zomer, Anal. Chim. Acta, 237:61 (1990).

35. H. Holtmannspotter and H.P. Thier, Dtsch. Lebensm. Rundsch., 78:347 (1982).
36. K.P. Holland, A.C. Henry, R.T. Wilson, J.S. Dreas, and R.B. Ashworth, J. AOAC Int., 78:483 (1995).
37. A.P. Pfenning, M.R. Madson, J.E. Roybal, S.B. Turnipseed, S.A. Gonzales, J.A. Hurlbut, and G.D. Salmon, J. AOAC Int., 81:714 (1998).
38. J. Markus and J. Sherma, J. AOAC Int., 75:942 (1992).
39. C.H. Van Peteghem, M.F. Lefevere, G.M. Van Haver, and A.P. De Leenheer, J. Agric. Food Chem., 35:228 (1987).
40. R. Bagnati, M.G. Castelli, L. Airoldi, M.P. Oriundi, A. Ubaldi, and R. Fanelli, J. Chromatogr., 527:267 (1990).
41. Ph. Delahaut, P. Jacquemin, Y. Colemonts, M. Dubois, J. De Graeve, and H. De-luyker, J. Chromatogr., 696:203 (1997).
42. L.D. Payne, V.R. Mayo, L.A. Morneweck, M.B. Hicks, and T.A. Wehner, J. Agric. Food Chem., 45:3501 (1997).
43. K. Takatsuki, S. Suzuki, N. Sato, I. Ushizawa, and T. Shoji, J. Assoc. Off. Anal. Chem., 70:708 (1987).
44. N. Haagsma, L.M.J. Mains, W. van Leeuwen, and H.W. van Gend, in Residues of Veterinary Drugs in Food, Proc. Euroresidue Conf., Noordwijkerhout, May 21–23, 1990 (N. Haagsma, A. Ruiter, and P.B. Czedik-Eysenberg, Eds.), Fac. Vet. Med., Univ. Utrecht, The Netherlands, p. 206 (1990).
45. V.P. Agarwal, J. Liq. Chromatogr., 12:613 (1989).
46. R. Krishna, K.W. Riggs, M.P.R. Walker, E. Kwan, and D.W. Rurak, J. Chromatogr., 674:65 (1995).
47. F.J. Schenck, S.A. Barker, and A.R. Long, J. AOAC Int., 75:655 (1992).
48. K.P. Reising, J. AOAC Int., 75:751 (1992).
49. G. Dusi, M. Curatolo, A. Fierro, and E. Faggionato, J. Liq. Chrom. & Rel. Technol., 19:1607 (1996).
50. J.M. Degroodt, B.W. De Bukanski, and S. Srebrnik, J. Liq. Chromatogr., 17:1419 (1994).
51. P.J. Kijak, J. AOAC Int., 75:747 (1992).
52. F.J. Schenck, J. Liq. Chromatogr., 18:349 (1995).
53. S.M. Plakas, K.R. El Said, G.R. Stehly, and J.E. Roybal, J. AOAC Int., 78:1388 (1995).
54. L.G. Rushing and H.C. Thompson, J. Chromatogr., 688:325 (1997).
55. J.E. Roybal, A.P. Pfenning, R.K. Munns, D.C. Holland, J.A. Hurlbut, and A.R. Long, J. AOAC Int., 78:453 (1995).
56. L.G. Rushing, S.F. Webb, and H.C. Thompson, J. Chromatogr., 674:125 (1995).
57. C.A.J. Hajee and N. Haagsma, J. Chromatogr., 669:219 (1995).
58. J.P. Cravedi and G. Delous, J. Chromatogr., 564:461 (1991).
59. A. Khunachak, A.R. Dacunha, and S.J. Stout, J. AOAC Int., 76:1230 (1993).
60. M. Alvinerie, J.F. Sutra, D. Capela, P. Galtier, A. Fernandez-Suarez, E. Horne, and M. O'Keeffe, Analyst, 121:1469 (1996).
61. M. Alvinerie, J.F. Sutra, M. Badri, and P. Galtier, J. Chromatogr., 674:119 (1995).
62. B. Shaikh, E.H. Allen, and J.C. Gridley, J. Assoc. Off. Anal. Chem., 68:29 (1985).
63. V.P. Agarwal, J. Liq. Chromatogr., 13:2475 (1990).

64. B. Shaikh and J. Jackson, J. Liq. Chromatogr., 12:1497 (1989).

65. B. Shaikh and J. Jackson, J. AOAC Int., 76:543 (1993).

66. L.A. Van Ginkel, R.W. Stephany, H.J. Van Rossum, H.M. Steinbuch, G. Zomer, E. Van De Heeft, and A.P.J.M. De Jong, J. Chromatogr., 489:111 (1989).

67. R. Bagnati and R. Fanelli, J. Chromatogr., 547:325 (1991).

68. C.Y.W. Ang, W. Luo, E.B. Hansen, J.P. Freeman, and H.C. Thompson, J. AOAC Int., 79:389 (1996).

69. U. Meetschen and M. Petz, in Residues of Veterinary Drugs in Food, Proc. Euroresidue Conf., Noordwijkerhout, May 21–23, 1990 (N. Haagsma, A. Ruiter, and P.B. Czedik-Eysenberg, Eds.), Fac. Vet. Med., Univ. Utrecht, The Netherlands, p. 267 (1990).

70. U. Meetschen and M. Petz, Z. Lebensm. Unters. Forsch., 193:337 (1991).

71. U. Meetschen and M. Petz, J. Assoc. Off. Anal. Chem., 73:373 (1990).

72. J.O.K. Boison, C.D.C. Salisbury, W. Chan, and J.D. MacNeil, J. Assoc. Off. Anal. Chem., 74:497 (1991).

73. J.O.K. Boison, L.J.-Y Keng, and J.D. MacNeil, J. AOAC Int., 77:565 (1994).

74. J. Haginaka, J. Wakai, H. Yasuda, and T. Uno, Anal. Sci., 1:73 (1985).

75. P. Kubalec, E. Brandsteterova, and A. Bednarikova, Z. Lebensm. Unters Forsch., 205:85 (1997).

76. K. Berger and M. Petz, in Residues of Veterinary Drugs in Food, Proc. Euroresidue Conf., Noordwijkerhout, May 21–23, 1990 (N. Haagsma, A. Ruiter, and P.B. Czedik-Eysenberg, Eds.), Fac. Vet. Med., Univ. Utrecht, The Netherlands, p. 119 (1990).

77. R.K. Munns, W. Shimoda, J.E. Roybal, and C. Vieira, J. Assoc. Off. Anal. Chem., 68:968 (1985).

78. W. Luo, E.B. Hansen, C.Y.W. Ang, J. Deck, J.P. Freeman, and H.C. Thompson, J. Agric. Food Chem., 45:1264 (1997).

79. C.Y.W. Ang and W. Luo, J. AOAC Int., 80:25 (1997).

80. E. Verdon and P. Couedor, J. Chromatogr., 705:71 (1998).

81. L.K. Sorensen, B.M. Rasmussen, J.O. Boison, and L. Keng, J. Chromatogr., 694:383 (1997).

82. W. Luo, C.Y.W. Ang, and H.C. Thompson, J. Chromatogr., 694:401 (1997).

83. J.A. Tarbin, W.H.H. Farrington, and G. Shearer, Anal. Chim. Acta, 318:95 (1995).

84. H.-E. Gee, K.-B. Ho, and J. Toothill, J. AOAC Int., 79:640 (1996).

85. J.O. Boison and L.J.-Y. Keng, J. AOAC Int., 81:1113 (1998).

86. J.O. Boison and L.J.-Y. Keng, J. AOAC Int., 81:1267 (1998).

87. M.G. Beconi-Barker, R.D. Roof, L. Millerioux, F.M. Kausche, T.J. Vidmar, E.B. Smith, J.K. Callahan, V.L. Hubbard, G.A. Smith, and T.J. Gilbertson, J. Chromatogr., 729:229 (1996).

88. D.N. Heller, J. AOAC Int., 80:975 (1997).

89. K. Takatsuki, J. AOAC Int., 75:982 (1992).

90. M.J. Lynch and S.R. Bartolucci, J. Assoc. Off. Anal. Chem., 65:66 (1982).

91. M.J. Lynch, F.R. Mosher, R.P. Schneider, H.G. Fouda, and J.E. Risk, J. Assoc. Off. Anal. Chem., 74:611 (1991).

92. G.J. de Graaf, Th.J. Spierenburg, and A.J. Baars, in Residues of Veterinary Drugs in Food, Proc. Euroresidue Conf., Noordwijkerhout, May 21–23, 1990 (N. Haag-

sma, A. Ruiter, and P.B. Czedik-Eysenberg, Eds.), Fac. Vet. Med., Univ. Utrecht, The Netherlands, p. 203 (1990).
93. M.G. Lauridsen, C. Lund, and M. Jacobsen, J. Assoc. Off. Anal. Chem., 71:921 (1988).
94. L.G. Croteau, M.H. Akhtar, J.M.R. Belanger, and J.R.J. Pare, J. Liq. Chromatogr., 17:2971 (1994).
95. V. Ferchaud, B. Le Bizec, M.-P. Montrade, D. Maume, F. Monteau, and F. Andre, J. Chromatogr., 695:269 (1997).
96. H.-J. Stan and B. Abraham, J. Chromatogr., 195:231 (1980).
97. E. Daeseleire, A. De Guesquiere, and C. Van Peteghem, J. Chromatogr., 562:673 (1991).
98. S. Hartmann and H. Steinhart, J. Chromatogr., 704:105 (1997).
99. G.C. Gerhardt, C.D.C. Salisbury, and J.D. MacNeil, J. AOAC Int., 77:334 (1994).
100. G.C. Gerhardt, C.D.C. Salisbury, and J.D. MacNeil, J. AOAC Int., 77:765 (1994).
101. J.E. Matusik, R.S. Sternal, C.J. Barnes, and J.A. Sphon, J. Assoc. Off. Anal. Chem., 73:529 (1990).
102. L.V. Bui, J. AOAC Int., 76:966 (1993).
103. R.M. Simpson, F.B. Suhre, and J.W. Shafer, J. Assoc. Off. Anal. Chem., 68:23 (1985).
104. K. Helrich, AOAC, Official Methods of Analysis (K. Helrich, Ed.), 15th Edition, Association of Official Analytical Chemists, Arlington, VA, Sec. 982.41 (1990).
105. K. Takatsuki and T. Kikuchi, J. Assoc. Off. Anal. Chem., 73:886 (1990).
106. E.J. Simeonidou, N.A. Botsoglou, I.E. Psomas, and D.J. Fletouris, J. Liq. Chromatogr., 19:2349 (1996).
107. T.A. Gehring, L.G. Rushing, and H.C. Thompson, J. AOAC Int., 80:751 (1997).
108. N. Takada and Y. Akiyama, J. Chromatogr., 558:175 (1991).
109. N. Takeda and Y. Akiyama, J. Chromatogr., 607:31 (1992).
110. C.-E. Tsai and F. Kondo, J. AOAC Int., 78:674 (1995).
111. P. Vinas, C.L. Erroz, N. Campillo, and M. Hernandez-Cordoba, J. Chromatogr., 726:125 (1996).
112. M.M.L. Aerts, W.M.J. Beek, and U.A.Th. Brinkman, J. Chromatogr., 435:97 (1988).
113. J.E. Matusik, C.G. Guyer, J.N. Geleta, and C.J. Barnes, J. Assoc. Off. Anal. Chem., 70:546 (1987).
114. K. Helrich, AOAC, Official Methods of Analysis (K. Helrich, Ed.), 15th Edition, Association of Official Analytical Chemists, Arlington, VA, Sec. 982.40 (1990).
115. A.E. Mooser and H. Koch, J. AOAC Int., 76:976 (1993).
116. G. Carignan and K. Carrier, J. Assoc. Off. Anal. Chem., 74:479 (1991).
117. S.M. Croubels, K.E.I. Vanoosthuyze, and C.H. Van Peteghem, J. Chromatogr., 690: 173 (1997).
118. S.M. Croubels, H. Vermeersch, P. De Backer, M.D.F. Santos, J.P. Remon, and C.H. Van Peteghem, J. Chromatogr., 708:145 (1998).
119. N. Haagsma and P. Scherpenisse, in Residues of Veterinary Drugs in Food, Proc. Euroresidue II Conf., Veldhoven, May 3–5, 1993 (N. Haagsma, A. Ruiter, and P.B. Czedik-Eysenberg, Eds.), Fac. Vet. Med., Univ. Utrecht, The Netherlands, p. 342 (1993).

120. W.J.A. VandenHeuvel, J.S. Wood, M. DiGiovanni, and R.W. Walker, J. Agric. Food Chem., 25:386 (1977).

121. G.Y.F. Yu, E.J. Murby, and R.J. Wells, J. Chromatogr., 703:159 (1997).

122. K. De Wasch, H.F. De Brabander, L.A. van Ginkel, A. Spaan, S.S. Sterk, and H.D. Meiring, J. Chromatogr., 819:99 (1998).

123. B. Le Bizec, F. Monteau, D. Maume, M.P. Montrade, C. Gade, and F. Andre, Anal. Chim Acta, 340:201 (1997).

124. R. Schilt, J.M. Weseman, H. Hooijerink, H.J. Korbee, W.A. Traag, M.J. van Steenbergen, and W. Haasnoot, J. Chromatogr., 489:127 (1989).

125. J.R. Markus and J. Sherma, J. AOAC Int., 76:451 (1993).

126. S.H. Hsu, R.H. Eckerlin, and J.D. Henion, J. Chromatogr., 424:219 (1988).

127. J. Plasencia, C.J. Mirocha, R.J. Pawlosky, and J.F. Smith, J. Assoc. Off. Anal. Chem., 73:973 (1990).

128. R.W. Frei, W. Santi, and M. Thomas, J. Chromatogr., 116:365 (1976).

129. P.J. Meffin, S.R. Harapat, and D.C. Harrison, J. Pharm. Sci., 66:583 (1977).

130. N.D. Brown, R.B. Sweett, J.A. Kintzios, H.D. Cox, and P.B. Doctor, J. Chromatogr., 164:35 (1979).

131. C.E. Werkhoven-Goewie, U.A. Th. Brinkman, and R.W. Frei, Anal. Chim. Acta, 114:147 (1980).

132. S. Courte and N. Bromet, J. Chromatogr., 224:162 (1981).

133. J.P. Sommadossi, M. Lemar, J. Necciari, Y. Sumirtapura, J.P. Cano, and J. Gaillot, J. Chromatogr., 228:205 (1982).

134. N.A. Farid and S.M. White, J. Chromatogr., 275:458 (1983).

135. G.J. Schmidt, F.L. Vandemark, and W. Slavin, Anal. Biochem., 91:636 (1978).

136. K. Yamada, E. Kayama, Y. Aizawa, and K. Oka, J. Chromatogr., 223:176 (1981).

137. H. Kamimura, H. Sasaki, and S. Kawamura, J. Chromatogr., 225:115 (1981).

138. R.D. Cory, R.R. Becker, R. Rosenbluth, and I. Isenberg, J. Am. Chem. Soc., 90: 1643 (1968).

139. S. Udenfriend, S. Stein, P. Boehlen, W. Dairman, W. Leimgruber, and M. Weigele, Science, 178:871 (1972).

140. S.E. Walker and P.E.J. Coates, J. Chromatogr., 223:131 (1981).

141. A.J. Sedman and J. Gal, J. Chromatogr., 232:315 (1982).

142. R.W. Frei, L. Michel, and W. Santi, J. Chromatogr., 126:665 (1976).

143. A. Licht, R.L. Bowman, and S. Stein, J. Liq. Chromatogr., 4:825 (1981).

144. K. Imai, J. Chromatogr., 105:135 (1975).

145. M. Weigele, S. de Bernardo, and W. Leimgruber, Biochem. Biophys. Res. Commun., 50:352 (1973).

146. A.M. Felix and G. Terkelson, Anal. Biochem., 56:610 (1973).

147. H. Nakamura and Z. Tamura, Anal. Chem., 52:2087 (1980).

148. J.D.H. Cooper and D.C. Turnell, J. Chromatogr., 227:158 (1982).

149. P. Kucera and H. Umagat, J. Chromatogr., 255:563 (1983).

150. M.H. Joseph and P. Davies, J. Chromatogr., 227:125 (1983).

151. J.R. Cronin, S. Pizzarello, and W.E. Gandy, Anal. Chem., 93:174 (1979).

152. Y. Ishida, T. Fujita, and K. Asai, J. Chromatogr., 204:143 (1981).

153. G.J. Huges, K.J. Winterhalten, E. Boller, and K.T. Wilson, J. Chromatogr., 235: 417 (1982).

154. M. Sato and K. Yagi, J. Chromatogr., 242:185 (1982).
155. J.D.H. Cooper, M.T. Lewis, and D.C. Turnell, J. Chromatogr., 285:490 (1984).
156. S.J. Wassner and J.B. Li, J. Chromatogr., 227:497 (1982).
157. A.T. Davies, S.T. Ingalls, and C.L. Hoppel, J. Chromatogr., 306:79 (1984).
158. T.P. Davies, C.W. Gehrke Jr., C.H. Williams, C.W. Gehrke, and K.O. Gerhardt, J. Chromatogr., 228:113 (1982).
159. L. Essers, J. Chromatogr., 305:345 (1984).
160. D.G. Drescher and K.S. Lee, Anal. Biochem., 84:559 (1979).
161. M. Roth and A. Hampai, J. Chromatogr., 83:353 (1973).
162. A. Himuro, H. Nakamura, and Z. Tamura, Anal. Chim. Acta, 147:317 (1983).
163. H. Maeda, N. Ishida, H. Kawauchi, and K. Tuzimura, J. Biochem., 65:777 (1969).
164. J.E. Sinsheimer, D.D. Hong, J.T. Stewart, M.L. Fink, and J.H. Burckhalter, J. Pharm. Sci., 60:141 (1971).
165. H. Ichikawa, T. Tanimura, T. Nakajima, and Z. Tamura, Chem. Pharm. Bull., 18: 1493 (1970).
166. J.J. L'Italien and S.B.H. Kent, J. Chromatogr., 283:149 (1984).
167. J.A. Shah and D.J. Weber, J. Chromatogr., 309:95 (1984).
168. G. Gubitz, R. Wintersteiger, and A. Hartinger, J. Chromatogr., 218:51 (1981).
169. J.H. Wolfram, J.I. Feinberg, R.C. Doerr, and W. Fiddler, J. Chromatogr., 132:37 (1977).
170. G.J. Krol, J.M. Banovsky, C.A. Mannan, R.E. Pickering, and B.T. Kho, J. Chromatogr., 163:383 (1979).
171. K. Imai, and Y. Watanabe, Anal. Chim. Acta, 130:377 (1981).
172. Y. Watanabe and K. Imai, J. Chromatogr., 239:723 (1982).
173. Y. Watanabe and K. Imai, J. Chromatogr., 309:279 (1984).
174. Y. Yamamoto, T. Manji, A. Saito, K. Maeda, and K. Ohta, J. Chromatogr., 162: 327 (1979).
175. M.D. Baker, H.Y. Mohammed, and H. Veening, Anal. Chem., 53:1658 (1981).
176. J. Goto, S. Komatsu, M. Inada, and T. Nambara, Anal. Sci., 2:585 (1986).
177. J. Goto, N. Goto, F. Shamsa, M. Saito, S. Komatsu, K. Suzaki, and T. Nambara, Anal. Chim. Acta, 147:397 (1983).
178. J. Goto, M. Saito, T. Chikai, N. Goto, and T. Nambara, J. Chromatogr., 276:289 (1983).
179. J. Goto, T. Chikai, and T. Nambara, J. Chromatogr., 415:45 (1987).
180. J. Goto, S. Komatsu, N. Goto, and T. Nambara, Chem. Pharm. Bull., 29:899 (1981).
181. A. Takadate, M. Irikura, T. Suehiro, H. Fujino, and S. Goya, Chem. Pharm. Bull., 33:1164 (1985).
182. F. Lankmayr, K.W. Budna, K. Mueller, F. Nachtmann, and F. Rainer, J. Chromatogr., 222:249 (1981).
183. K. Murayama and T. Kinoshita, J. Chromatogr., 205:349 (1981).
184. K. Murayama and T. Kinoshita, Anal. Lett., 15:123 (1982).
185. Y. Kanaoka, M. Machida, M.I. Machida, and T. Sekine, Biochim. Biophys. Acta, 317:563 (1973).
186. H. Takahashi, T. Yoshida, and H. Meguro, Bunseki Kagaku, 30:339 (1980).
187. N. Anzai, T. Kimura, S. Chida, T. Tanaka, H. Takahashi, and H. Meguro, Yakugaku Zasshi, 101:1002 (1981).

188. Y. Kanaoka, M. Machida, K. Ando, and T. Sekine, Biochim. Biophys. Acta, 207: 269 (1970).

189. J.O. Miners, I. Faernley, K.J. Smith, and D.J. Birkett, J. Chromatogr., 275:89 (1983).

190. B. Kagedal and M. Kallberg, J. Chromatogr., 229:409 (1982).

191. M. Machida, N. Ushijima, M.I. Machida, and Y. Kanaoka, Chem. Pharm. Bull., 23:1385 (1975).

192. C.-W. Wu, L.R. Yarbrough, and F.Y.-H. Wu, Biochemistry, 15:2863 (1976).

193. B. Jarrot, A. Anderson, R. Hooper, and W.J. Louis, J. Pharm. Sci., 70:665 (1981).

194. T. Toyooka and K. Imai, J. Chromatogr., 285:495 (1983).

195. K. Imai, T. Toyooka, and Y. Watanabe, Anal. Biochem., 128:471 (1983).

196. E. Grushka, S. Lam, and J. Chassin, Anal. Chem., 50:1398 (1978).

197. K. Hayashi, J. Kawase, K. Yoshimura, K. Ara, and K. Tsuji, Anal. Biochem., 136: 314 (1984).

198. W. Dunges and N. Seiler, J. Chromatogr., 145:483 (1978).

199. M.S. Gandelman, and J.W. Birks, Anal. Chim. Acta, 155:159 (1983).

200. S. Yoshida, S. Hirose, and M. Iwamoto, J. Chromatogr., 383:61 (1986).

201. S. Goya, A. Takadate, H. Fujino, and M. Irikura, Yakugalu Zasshi, 100:744 (1980).

202. R. Farinotti, Ph. Siard, J. Bourson, S. Kirkiacharian, B. Valeur, and G. Mahuzier, J. Chromatogr., 269:81 (1983).

203. H. Tsuchiya, T. Hayashi, H. Naruse, and N. Takagi, J. Chromatogr., 309:43 (1984).

204. S. Kamada, M. Maeda, and A. Tsuji, J. Chromatogr., 272:29 (1983).

205. R.D. Toothaker, G.M. Sundaresan, J.P. Hunt, T.J. Goehl, K.S. Rotenberg, V.K. Prasad, W.A. Craig, and P.G. Welling, J. Pharm. Sci., 71:573 (1982).

206. W. Distler, J. Chromatogr., 192:240 (1980).

207. W.D. Watkins and B.M. Peterson, Anal. Biochem., 125:30 (1982).

208. A. Takadate, T. Tahara, H. Fujino, and S. Goya, Chem. Pharm. Bull., 30:4120 (1982).

209. M. Hatsumi, S.-I. Kimata, and K. Hirosawa, J. Chromatogr., 253:271 (1982).

210. S. Imaoka, Y. Funae, T. Sigumoto, N. Hayahara, and M.M. Maekawa, Anal. Biochem., 128:459 (1983).

211. S. Goya, A. Takadate, and H. Fujino, Yakugaku Zasshi, 102:63 (1982).

212. Y. Tsuruta and K. Kohashi, J. Chromatogr., 309:309 (1984).

213. J. Goto, N. Goto, A. Hikichi, T. Nishimaki, and T. Nambara, J. Chromatogr., 239: 559 (1982).

214. H. Lingeman, A. Hulshoff, W.J.M. Underberg, and F.B.J.M. Offerman, J. Chromatogr., 290:215 (1984).

215. M. Ikeda, K. Shimada, T. Sakaguchi, and U. Matsumoto, J. Chromatogr., 305:261 (1984).

216. T. Kawasaki, M. Maeda, and A. Tsuji, J. Chromatogr., 233:61 (1982).

217. T. Hayashi, H. Tsuchiya, H. Todoriki, and H. Naruse, Anal. Biochem., 122:173 (1982).

218. T. Hayashi, H. Tsuchiya, and H. Naruse, J. Chromatogr., 273:245 (1983).

219. A.J. Speek, J. Schrijver, and W.H.P. Scheurs, J. Chromatogr., 305:53 (1984).

220. K. Tsuji, J.F. Goetz, W. van Meter, and K.A. Gusciora, J. Chromatogr., 175:141 (1979).

221. P. Helboe and S. Kryger, J. Chromatogr., 235:215 (1982).
222. D.M. Barends, J.S. Blauw, C.W. Mijnsbergen, C.J.L.R. Govers, A. Hulshoff, J. Chromatogr., 322:321 (1985).
223. D.M. Barends, C.L. Zwaan, and A. Hulshoff, J. Chromatogr., 182:201 (1980).
224. D.M. Barends, C.L. Zwaan, and A. Hulshoff, J. Chromatogr., 222:316 (1981).
225. D.M. Barends, C.L. Zwaan, and A. Hulshoff, J. Chromatogr., 225:417 (1981).
226. L.T. Wong, A.R. Beaubien, and A.P. Pakuts, J. Chromatogr., 231:145 (1982).
227. D.M. Barends, J.S. Blauw, H.M. Smits, and A. Hulshoff, J. Chromatogr., 276:385 (1983).
228. P.M. Kabra, P.K. Bhatnagar, M.A. Nelson, J.H. Wall, and L.J. Marton, Clin. Chem., 29:672 (1983).
229. P.M. Kabra, P.K. Bhatnagar, and M.A. Nelson, J. Chromatogr., 307:224 (1984).
230. B.P. Spragg and A.D. Hutchings, J. Chromatogr., 258:289 (1983).
231. C.R. Clark and M.M. Wells, J. Chromatogr. Sci., 16:322 (1978).
232. S.L. Wellons and M.A. Carey, J. Chromatogr., 154:219 (1978).
233. J.A.P. Meulendijk, and W.J.M. Underberg, in Detection-Oriented Derivatization Techniques in Liquid Chromatography (H. Lingeman, W.J.M. Underberg, Eds.), Marcel Dekker, Inc., New York, p. 267 (1990).
234. B. Bjorkqvist, J. Chromatogr., 204:109 (1981).
235. D. Tocksteinova, J. Churacek, J. Slosar, and L. Skalik, Microchim. Acta, 1:507 (1978).
236. Z. Chen, Microchim. Acta, 1:343 (1980).
237. S. Ohkuma, J. Pharm. Soc., 75:1124 (1955).
238. H.D. Durst, M. Milano, E.J. Kikta, Jr., S.A. Conelly, and E. Grushka, Anal. Chem., 47:1797 (1975).
239. E. Grushka, H.D. Durst, and E.J. Kikta, Jr., J. Chromatogr., 112:673 (1975).
240. I. Roorda, C. Gonnet, and J.L. Rocca, Analyst, 18:409 (1982).
241. R. Alric, M. Cociglio, J.P. Blayac, and R. Puech, J. Chromatogr., 224:289 (1981).
242. W.F. Kline, D.P. Enagonio, D.J. Reeder, and W.E. May, J. Liq. Chromatogr., 5:1697 (1982).
243. W.D. Watkins and M.B. Peterson, Anal. Biochem., 125:30 (1982).
244. L. Nagels, C. Debeuf, and E. Esmans, J. Chromatogr., 190:411 (1980).
245. R.F. Borch, Anal. Chem., 47:2437 (1975).
246. H.C. Jordi, J. Liq. Chromatogr., 1:215 (1978).
247. N.E. Bussell and R.A. Miller, J. Liq. Chromatogr., 2:697 (1979).
248. R.A. Miller, N.E. Bussell, and C. Ricketts, J. Liq. Chromatogr., 1:291 (1978).
249. P.H. Zoutendam, P.B. Bowman, T.M. Ryan, and J.L. Rumph, J. Chromatogr., 283:273 (1984).
250. P.H. Zoutendam, P.B. Bowman, J.L. Rumph, and T.M. Ryan, J. Chromatogr., 283:281 (1984).
251. F. Stellaard, D.L. Hachey, and P.D. Klein, Anal. Biochem., 87:359 (1978).
252. S. Lam and E. Grushka, J. Liq. Chromatogr., 1:33 (1978).
253. A. Hulshoff, H. Roseboom, and J. Renema, J. Chromatogr., 186:535 (1979).
254. D. Westerlund, J. Carlqvist, and A. Theodorsen, Acta Pharm. Suec., 16:187 (1979).
255. J. Carlqvist and D. Westerlund, J. Chromatogr., 164:373 (1979).

256. J.W. Munson and R. Bilous, J. Pharm. Sci., 66:1403 (1977).

257. R. Horikawa and T. Tanimura, Anal. Lett., 15:1629 (1982).

258. F.A. Fitzpatrick, M.A. Wynalda, and D.G. Kaiser, Anal. Chem., 49:1932 (1977).

259. J. Lehrfeld, J. Chromatogr., 120:141 (1976).

260. C.A. White, J.F. Kennedy, and B.T. Golding, Carbohydr. Res., 76:1 (1979).

261. C.A. White, S.W. Vass, J.F. Kennedy, and D.G. Large, J. Chromatogr., 264:99 (1983).

262. B. Bjorkqvist and H. Toivonen, J. Chromatogr., 153:265 (1978).

263. J. Nishiyama, and T. Kuninori, Anal. Biochem., 138:95 (1984).

264. L.G. Butler, Enzyme Microb. Technol., 1:253 (1979).

265. G.G. Guilbault, in Analytical Uses of Immobilized Enzymes, Modern Monographs in Analytical Chemistry, Vol. 2, (G.G. Guibault, Ed.), Marcel Dekker, New York (1984).

266. L.D. Bowers and W.D. Bostick, in Chemical Derivatization in Analytical Chemistry (R.W. Frei and J.F. Lawrence, Eds.), Plenum Press, New York (1981).

267. L. Dalgaard, Trends Anal. Chem., 5:185 (1986).

268. L.D. Bowers, J. Chromatogr. Sci., 34:195 (1986).

269. J.P. Cravedi and G. Delous, J. Chromatogr., 564:461 (1991).

270. L.D. Bowers and P.R. Johnson, Anal. Biochem., 116:111 (1981).

271. L.D. Bowers and P.R. Johnson, Clin. Chem., 27:1554 (1981).

272. P.R. Johnson and L.D. Bowers, Anal. Chem., 54:2247 (1983).

273. L.L. Klopf and T.A. Nieman, Anal. Chem., 57:46 (1985).

274. L. Dalgaard and L. Nordholm, J. Chromatogr., 265:183 (1983).

275. V.K. Boppana, K.L. Fong, J.A. Ziemniak, and R.K. Lynn, J. Chromatogr., 353:231 (1986).

276. M.Y.K. Ho and G.A. Rechnitz, Anal. Chem., 59:536 (1987).

277. A.T. Rhys Williams, S.A. Winfield, and R.C. Belloli, J. Chromatogr., 235:461 (1982).

278. M. Uihlein and E. Schwab, Chromatographia, 15:140 (1982).

279. R. Verbeke and P. Vanhee, J. Chromatogr., 265:239 (1983).

280. C.M. Selavka, I.S. Krull, and K. Bratin, J. Pharm. Biomed. Anal., 4:83 (1986).

281. C. de Ruiter, J. Bohle, G.J. de Jong, U.A.Th. Brinkman, and R.W. Frei, Anal. Chem., 160:666 (1988).

22

Separation

Following extraction and cleanup, the analytes of interest must be separated from the myriad individual compounds usually present in the biological extracts. During the 1970s, most chemical separations were carried out using a variety of chromatographic and other techniques including open-column chromatography, paper chromatography, thin-layer chromatography, and classic electrophoresis. However, these techniques were often inadequate to provide resolution between structurally similar compounds. In the last two decades, high-performance liquid chromatography, capillary gas chromatography, high-performance thin-layer chromatography, supercritical fluid chromatography, and capillary electrophoresis have matured into popular separation techniques.

    In general, chromatography is used to separate mixtures of chemicals into individual components. Chromatographic processes can be defined as separation techniques involving mass transfer between a stationary and a mobile phase. In all chromatographic modes, separation occurs when the sample mixture is introduced into a mobile phase that may be a gas, a liquid, or a supercritical fluid. The mobile phase is then forced through an immobile, immiscible stationary phase. The phases are chosen such that components of the sample have differing solubilities in each phase. A component that is quite soluble in a stationary phase will take longer to travel through it than a component that is not very soluble in this stationary phase but very soluble in the mobile phase. As a result of these differences in mobility, sample components will become separated from each other as they travel through the stationary phase. Those that travel the fastest will elute from the column first. Those that travel slowest will exit the column last. By changing characteristics of the mobile and stationary phases, different mixtures of chemicals can be separated. Further refinement to this separation process can be made by changing a variety of other physicochemical parameters including temperature, flow rate, counter ions, among others.

Electrophoresis is another separation process that, however, is based on the mobility of ions in an electric field. The different modes of modern capillary electrophoresis with its different separation mechanisms have paid more and more attention during the last decade.

22.1 LIQUID CHROMATOGRAPHY

Initially, pressure was selected as the principal criterion of this type of chromatography and thus the name was high-pressure liquid chromatography (HPLC). This was, however, an unfortunate term because it seems to indicate that the improved performance is primarily due to the high pressure, which is not true. Naturally, pressure is needed to permit a given flow rate of the mobile phase; otherwise, pressure is a negative factor not contributing to the improvement in separation. In fact high performance is the result of many factors including the narrow and uniform pore size and distribution of the very small particles comprising the stationary phases, the efficient high-pressure column slurry packing techniques, and the good injection and pumping systems. Recognizing this, most experienced chromatographers today refer to the technique as high-performance liquid chromatography or simply liquid chromatography (LC), still permitting use of the abbreviation HPLC.

During the past two decades, innovative LC techniques have been perfected that improved separation, purification, identification, and quantification far above early techniques (1–7). The last decade, in particular, has seen a vast development of micro- and other specialized columns as well as a variety of detectors, computers, and automation to interface with the LC to arrive at optimal analysis of the analytes (8–13).

In general, LC instrumentation includes a pump, injector, column, detector, and recorder or data system. Most commercially available instruments are constructed of stainless steel, a material that represents the best compromise of corrosion resistance, workability, strength, and cost, since it is inert to all bases and organic liquids and to most nonhalogenated acids at pH values higher than 2.0. Stainless steel is, however, extremely vulnerable to contact with halogenated acids, such as HCl, even at 0.01 N concentrations. Thus, when attempting to convert a conventional thin-layer or glass-column chromatographic method to modern LC, substitution for halogens with another acid such as nitric, boric, or acetic is strongly recommended.

The heart of any LC system is the column where separation occurs. A high-pressure pump is also required to move the mobile phase through the column since the stationary phase, which is composed of porous particles of a few micrometers, resists the mobile phase motility. Smaller bed particles require higher pressures. There are many advantages to using smaller particles, but they may not be essential for all separations. The most important advantages are higher resolution, faster analysis, and increased sample load capacity. However, only the most demanding separations require these advances in significant amounts. Many separation problems can be resolved with larger particle packings that require less pressure.

The chromatographic process begins by injecting the solute onto the top of the column. The solvent need not be the mobile phase, but frequently it is appropriately chosen to avoid detector interference, column/analyte interference, loss in efficiency, or all of these. Sample introduction can be accomplished in various ways. The simplest method is to use an injection valve. In more sophisticated LC systems, automatic sampling devices are incorporated where sample introduction is done with the help of autosamplers and microprocessors. It is always best to remove particles from the sample by filtering, or centrifuging since continuous injections of particulate material will eventually cause blockage of injection devices or columns.

Separation of components occurs as the analytes and mobile phase are pumped through the column. Eventually, each component elutes from the column as a narrow band or peak on the recorder. Detection of the eluting components is important, and this can be either selective or universal, depending upon the detector used. The response of the detector to each component is displayed on a chart recorder or computer screen and is known as a chromatogram. To collect, store, and analyze chromatograms, computers, integrators, and other data processing equipment are frequently used.

Typical LC columns are 15 or 25 cm in length and contain particles of 3, 5, or 10 μm diameter. The internal diameter of the columns is usually 4 or 4.6 mm; this is considered the best compromise among sample capacity, mobile phase consumption, speed, and resolution. Packing of the column tubing with the smaller-diameter particles requires higher skill and specialized equipment. Hence, it is generally recommended that all but the most experienced chromatographers purchase prepacked columns, since it is difficult to match the high performance of professionally packed LC columns without a large investment in time and equipment.

LC columns are fairly durable unless they are used in some manner that is intrinsically destructive, as, for example, with highly acidic or basic eluents, or with continual injections of inadequately purified biological samples. It is wise to inject some test mixture into a column when new, and to retain the chromatogram. If questionable results are obtained later, the test mixture can be injected again under the specified conditions. The two chromatograms may be compared to establish whether the column is still useful.

The nature of the stationary phase within an LC column is of critical importance for determining the separation process. Normal-phase adsorption, normal-phase partition, reversed-phase, ion-pair, ion-exchange, and size-exclusion are all liquid chromatographic modes covering most LC applications.

In normal-phase adsorption chromatography, the stationary phase is composed of strongly polar silica particles whereas the mobile phase is composed of nonpolar solvents such as n-hexane. Analytes are separated due to their varying degree of adsorption onto the solid surface. Polar samples are thus retained on the polar surface of the column packing longer than less polar materials.

Normal-phase partition chromatography also uses a polar stationary phase and an nonpolar mobile phase such as n-hexane, methylene chloride, or chloroform. In this LC mode, however, the stationary phase is a bonded siloxane with a polar functional group, which in order of increasing polarity may be the cyano ($-C_2H_4CN$), diol($-C_3H_6OCH_2CHOHCH_2OH$), amino ($-C_3H_6NH_2$), or dimethylamino ($-C_3H_6N(CH_3)_2$) group.

In reversed-phase chromatography, the stationary phase is hydrophobic in nature, while the mobile phase is a polar solvent mixture of water and methanol or acetonitrile. In this mode of chromatography, the more nonpolar the analyte the longer will be retained. Some analytes, however, might behave unexpectedly due to interactions with residual silanols or with active groups of attached ligands (14–17). Trimethylchlorosilane is the most commonly used reagent to cover accessible residual silanols. Because the molecule of this endcapping reagent is relatively small, it can penetrate to the silica surface and cover some unreacted silanols. After this treatment, silica-based stationary phases contain almost 50% of their original silanols, which, however, are not generally accessible for analytes.

Ion-pair chromatography is a popular form of chromatography in which analyte ions can be paired and separated as ion-pairs on a column (14–17). Ion-pairing agents are usually ionic compounds that contain a hydrocarbon chain that enhances the hydrophobicity of the analyte, so that the ion pair can be retained on a reversed-phase column.

Ion-exchange chromatography (IEC) is a mode of chromatography in which ionic substances are separated on cationic or anionic sites of the packing. The sample ion and usually a counterion will exchange with ions already on the ionogenic group of the packing. The operating mechanism of IEC is reversible binding of charged molecules. The stronger the charge on the sample, the stronger the attraction to the ionic surface and, thus, the longer it will take to elute. Binding strength is governed by the degree of charge on the substrate, and the pKa of the ion exchange matrix. Key features of IEC methodology are its high capacity, resolving power, and straightforward scale-up.

Column packings for IEC are ion-exchange resins bonded to inert polymeric particles (typically 10 μm diameter). Two exchanger types are differentiated: basic (positively charged) and acidic (negatively charged). They in turn can be classified into those with weakly basic or acidic character or strongly basic or acidic character. With strongly basic or acidic materials all functional groups are always present in ionized form vastly independent from the pH value in the specified operating range. For example, the quaternary amino groups (R_3N^+) are positively charged, while the sulfonic acid groups (SO_2^-) are negatively loaded. The pK values of the quaternary amino groups are around 14, while those of the sulfonate residues below 1. In addition, weakly basic types with pK values between 8 and 11, and weakly acidic types with pK values between 4 and 6 exist. The weakly basic types consist of secondary and tertiary amino functional groups, while the weakly acidic types consist of carboxyl functional group. Thus, a weakly basic exchanger should only be used at pH values below 8.5, whereas weakly acidic exchangers should be used at pH values above 6. Outside these ranges, strongly basic or strongly acidic exchangers should be used.

In IEC, mobile phases are aqueous buffers in which both pH and ionic strength are used to control elution time. With cation exchangers, increasing the pH value shortens the retention times, whereas with anion exchangers lowering the pH value shortens the retention time. Increasing the ionic strength of the counter ion shortens the retention time with both anion and cation exchangers. As a rule, short columns with a large diameter should be used in IEC. Most ion-chromatography instruments use two mobile phase reservoirs containing buffers of different pH, and a programmable pump that can change the pH of the mobile phase during the separation.

In size-exclusion chromatography (SEC) the column is filled with material having precisely controlled pore sizes. Separation is achieved by the differential exclusion or inclusion within the packing particles of the sample molecules passing through the porous stationary phase. Molecules larger than the pore size cannot enter the pores and elute first. This condition is called total exclusion. On the other hand, molecules that can enter the pores will have an average residence time in the particles that depends on the molecules size and shape. Different molecules, therefore, have different total transit times through the column. This portion of a chromatogram is called the selective permeation region. Molecules that are smaller than the pore size can enter all pores, and have the longest residence time on the column and elute together as the last peak in the chromatogram. This last peak in the chromatogram determines the total permeation limit. Mainly for historical reasons, this technique is also called gel-filtration or gel-permeation chromatography although, presently, the stationary phase is not restricted to a gel.

In any of its different modes, LC behaves as a dynamic adsorption process. Analyte molecules, while moving through the porous packing bead, tend to interact with the surface adsorption sites. Depending on the LC mode, different types of adsorption forces may be included in the retention process. Hydrophobic (nonspecific) interactions are the main ones in reversed-phase separations. Polar interactions including dipole-dipole, and dipole-induced dipole forces dominate in the normal-phase mode, whereas ionic interactions are responsible for the retention in ion-exchange chromatography. All these interactions are competitive as analyte molecules are competing with the eluent molecules for the adsorption sites. The stronger analyte molecules interact with the surface and the weaker the eluent interaction, the longer analytes are retained on the surface. However, SEC constitutes a special case since the molecular size of the components governs the separation of a mixture. In this mode, eluent molecules should have much stronger interaction with the surface than analyte molecules.

Most popular bonded phases in LC are the octyl (C_8) and octadecyl (C_{18}) modified adsorbents. Other popular bonded phases are the cyano-modified adsorbents that are very slightly polar; columns with this phase are useful for fast normal- or reversed-phase separations of mixtures consisting of very different components. Amino-modified phases are weak anion-exchangers; columns with this phase are mainly used in the normal-phase mode, especially for selective retention of aromatic compounds. Propylphenylsilane ligands attached to silica particles show weak dipole-induced dipole interactions with polar analytes; this type of bonded phase is used for group separations of complex mixtures, particularly of amino compounds that show some specific interactions with phenyl-modified adsorbent. Diols are slightly polar adsorbent for normal-phase separations; these are useful for separation of complex mixtures of compounds with different polarity that usually show a strong retention on unmodified silica. In addition, synthetic crosslinked organic polymers have been found beneficial mainly for size-exclusion chromatography and ion-exchange chromatography; in normal- or reversed-phase LC, however, polymers have limited application.

Eluent polarity is most critical in all LC modes. There are two elution types, isocratic and gradient. In the former, constant eluent composition is pumped through the column during the whole analysis. In the latter, eluent composition and, thus, strength is steadily changed during the run. The main purpose of gradient elution is to move strongly retained components of the mixture faster, but having the least retained component well resolved. Starting with the low content of the organic component in the eluent, the least retained components can be separated, while strongly retained components will sit on the adsorbent surface on the top of the column or will move very slowly. By increasing the amount of organic component in the eluent, the strongly retained components will move faster, because of the steady increase of the competition for the adsorption sites.

Gradient elution further increases the efficiency of the column. In isocratic elution, the longer a component is retained the wider its peak. In gradient elution, the tail of the peak is always under the influence of the stronger mobile phase when compared to the peak front. Thus, molecules on the tail of the chromatographic zone will move faster. This will tend to compress zone and narrow the resultant peak. Gradient elution may be considered as an analogy to the temperature programming in gas chromatography.

Liquid chromatography in its various modes is the most frequently used separation technique for the analysis of drug residues in edible animal products. Its popularity is largely due to the variety of mobile phases, the extensive library of column packings, and the variation in modes of operation. It can be most readily applied to a wide range of drugs, combining rapid sample throughput, high sensitivity, and selectivity. A major advantage of the technique is that there is a better control over separation conditions compared with thin-layer chromatography. Thus, LC can deal with various classes of antibacterials, even with high-molecular-weight compounds, providing the means to increase the selectivity for specific analytes to the desired degree. This results in a precision much better than that of microbiological assays and comparable to immunochemical and GC assays. Furthermore, the mild conditions employed in LC separations offer also the possibility to proceed to further confirmation of the separated analytes; fractions of column effluents can be readily collected and submitted to supplementary identification procedures. All these advantages have advanced the acceptance of LC both as a research tool and for routine analysis in the field of drug residues.

Over the years, numerous LC methods have been described, and in many instances quite different procedures have been suggested for the same drug in the same matrix due possibly to the large number of analytical possibilities that LC affords. Today, commercially available equipment allows fully automated and selective isolation of drug residues of a wide range of physicochemical properties from tissues, milk, eggs, and honey. Automated off-line and column-switching on-line SPE procedures are increasingly used for sample preparation, offering both convenience and versatility. A good example of automated off-line SPE is the LC assay of penicillin G in animal tissues (18). Using a commercially available sample preparation unit, unattended conditioning of SPE cartridges, loading of sample extracts, and elution with defined solvents, addition of derivatizing agents and automatic injections into an LC system could be readily realized. Online SPE and column-switching procedures have been successfully utilized in analyzing sulfonamides (19), carbadox and its metabolites (20), oxolinic acid and flumequine (21–23), and enrofloxacin (24) in various matrices. As an alternative to SPE, size-exclusion chromatography has been also applied to remove coextracted proteins in the LC analysis of swine tissues for residues of sulfonamides, and trimethoprim and its metabolites (25, 26).

Despite their distinct advantages, on-line SPE and column-switching procedures do not always represent ideal separation techniques. In many cases, only a small number of samples can be analyzed before contamination of the precolumn by proteins occurs. Alternative techniques that prevent the adsorption of macromolecules onto column packings and allow direct injection of sample extracts are those based on use of specific LC columns. Shielded hydrophobic phase (27), small pore reversed-phase (28), and internal surface reversed-phase (29, 30) columns can be used to elute proteins in the excluded volumes, allowing small molecules, such as antibacterials and metabolites, to interact with the stationary phase for separation. Wide pore reversed-phase (31) columns can be used to elute small molecules while selectively allowing proteins to permeate through the large pores without being hindered. By direct injection of sample extracts, sample handling is greatly simplified, the speed of analysis is enhanced, and the cost may be reduced. On the other hand, shortening of column life, the requirement for special columns, and the complexity of the LC column-switching system are some of the drawbacks of the direct injection procedures. The small sample volumes that should be injected ($\leq$20 μl), and the relatively high cost and low efficiency of these columns compared to the conventional columns, are major disadvantages that have, until now, hampered the application of direct-injection procedures to the analysis of drug residues in edible animal products.

Direct injection of biological samples onto a conventional LC column can be also made possible using a micellar mobile phase (32, 33). Micellar mobile phases are able to solubilize proteins present in the sample matrix and thus prevent their precipitation. Aqueous anionic and nonionic surfactants such as sodium dodecyl sulfate at concentrations above the critical micelle concentration are normally used to prepare micellar mobile phases. When the surfactant concentration is varied, reversals in the retention order may occur. Micellar mobile phases exhibit hydrophobic and electrostatic interactions with the analytes and stationary phases, which can provide additional selectivity. Major advantage is of the use of micellar mobile phases are the elimination of all sample preparation steps and the complete release of protein-bound antibacterials. There are, however, sensitivity limitations since injection volumes larger than 20 μl can cause column plugging. Low detection limits and larger injection volumes may be realized using column switching techniques. However, column switching with micellar mobile phases is a relatively new and untested technique and further investigations are needed before the full range of its applicability and limitations will be known (34).

Automatic sequential trace enrichment of dialyzates (ASTED) is another promising alternative for fully automated LC analysis of analytes that do not significantly bind to proteins. This on-line dialysis procedure utilizes both dialysis and trace enrichment to isolate analytes selectively in a form suitable for subsequent LC. In this versatile approach, an aqueous extract of the sample is introduced into the dialysis block and the injected volume is air-segmented to prevent contamination of subsequent samples and also to improve the mass transfer of the analyte to the cellulose dialysis membrane. Proteins and other macromolecules remain in the donor stream whereas the analytes pass the membrane and enter the acceptor stream. The analytes in the dialyzate are trapped on a preconcentration column while more polar coextractives are washed out. Following loading, the analytes are backflushed through column-switching technique into the analytical column and are analyzed by LC. Acceptor flow rate, temperature, hydrophobicity of the analytes, pH, ionic strength, and viscosity of the sample are all critical parameters on the performance of the analysis. Major advantages are the very limited contamination of the LC column and the high sample throughput. Compared to other methods making use of chromatographic techniques such as HPTLC, LC, or GC, ASTED is simple, efficient, and economical because it requires only minimal sample handling. Nevertheless, ASTED has not been still widely applied in residue analysis. Applications include the determination of flumequine and oxolinic acid in fish muscle (35, 36), and sulfonamides (37) and nitrofurans (38) in eggs, meat, and milk.

22.2 GAS CHROMATOGRAPHY

Gas chromatography is another powerful separation technique for resolving closely related drug residues that are sufficiently stable to be brought to a temperature at which they are appreciably volatile. However, many drugs are not sufficiently volatile and thus have to be converted to volatile derivatives before GC analysis.

The first GC methods for the residue analysis of antibacterials date back to the 1970s. Residues of chloramphenicol in animal tissues (39) and of isoxazolyl penicillins in milk (40) could be detected with reasonable accuracy by analyzing the corresponding methylated derivatives on GC columns. However, since the added steps necessary for derivatization were time-intensive and introduced analytical problems, these methods did not gain wide acceptance in the field of residues analysis in spite of being very specific and sensitive. Since that time, GC technology has undergone considerable development and a plethora of specific and sensitive methods for the analysis of drug residues, particularly chloramphenicol and sulfonamides, in edible animal products have been developed. However, GC is a technique that still deserves more utilization in veterinary drug analysis.

Gas chromatographic systems consist, in general, of a flowing mobile phase, an injection port, a separation column containing the stationary phase, and a detector. Sample components are separated due to differences in their boiling points and relative affinity for the stationary phase. For optimum column efficiency, the sample should not be too large, and should be introduced onto the column as a plug of vapor; slow injection of large samples causes band broadening and loss of resolution. The injection port is maintained at a higher temperature than the boiling point of the least volatile component in the sample mixture. The temperature of the sample port is usually about 50 °C higher than the boiling point of the least volatile component of the sample. Nowadays, autosamplers with up to several hundred sample tube holders are readily available on the market.

The injector can be used in split or splitless mode. The injector contains a heated chamber containing a glass liner into which the sample is injected through the septum. The carrier gas enters the chamber and the sample vaporizes to form a mixture of carrier gas, and vaporized solvent and solutes. A proportion of this mixture passes onto the column, but most exits through the split outlet. The septum purge outlet prevents septum bleed components from entering the column.

Since the partitioning behavior is dependent on temperature, column temperature must be electronically controlled to within tenths of a degree. The optimum column temperature is dependent upon the boiling point of the analyte. As a rule of thumb, a temperature slightly above the average boiling point of the sample results in an elution time of 2–30 mins. Minimal temperatures give good resolution, but result in increased elution times. Separating components with a wide range of boiling points is accomplished by starting at a low oven temperature and increasing the temperature over time to elute the high-boiling point components. The column temperature may be increased either continuously or in steps as separation proceeds. After the components of a mixture are separated, they must be detected as they exit the column.

Mobile phases are generally inert gases such as helium, argon, or nitrogen. The choice of carrier gas is often dependent upon the type of detector used. Gas is obtained from a tank, or sometimes from an electrolysis cell, and is passed through a series of reductors, equalizing valves, and traps to ensure constancy of pressure or flow and elimination of impurities as well.

Gas chromatography was originally a technique for nonpolar analytes, and for such analytes nonpolar packed columns prevailed. Packed columns are typically a glass or stainless steel coil, 1–5 m total length and 2–5 mm internal diameter, which is filled with the stationary phase, or a packing coated with the stationary phase. Early packed columns had low plate numbers and in the majority of instances separation could not be obtained on the basis of the differences in volatility alone. The solution was selective stationary phases, and in the 1960s there were more than 200 different stationary phases available (41).

A major improvement in column technology has been the introduction of capillary columns. Capillary columns have an internal diameter of a few tenths of millimeter, and they can be of the wall-coated open tubular (WCOT) or the support-coated open tubular (SCOT) type. Wall-coated columns consist of a capillary tube whose walls are coated with liquid stationary phase. In support-coated columns, the inner wall of the capillary is lined with a thin layer of support material such as diatomaceous earth, onto which the stationary phase has been adsorbed. SCOT columns are generally less efficient than WCOT columns. Both types of capillary column are more efficient than packed columns. In 1979, a new type of WCOT column was devised, the so-called the fused silica open tubular (FSOT) column. These have much thinner walls than the glass capillary columns, and are given strength by the polyimide coating. These columns are flexible, typically 10–100 m in length and 250 µm internal diameter, and can be wound into coils. They have the advantages of physical strength, flexibility, and low reactivity.

With capillary columns, quite high plate numbers can be achieved. Their separation power is unrivaled by any other chromatographic technique and their most prominent advantages are the inertness of surface, chemical and thermal stability, very low bleeding, and ease of instrument interchangeability (42). Improved surface deactivation permits elution of moderately polar to polar analytes. The most common stationary phases are polysiloxanes, which contain various substituent groups to change the polarity of the phase. The nonpolar end of the spectrum is polydimethyl siloxane, which can be made more polar by increasing the percentage of phenyl groups on the polymer. For very polar analytes, polyethylene glycol is commonly used as the stationary phase. After the polymer coats the column wall or packing material, it is often cross-linked to increase the thermal stability of the stationary phase and prevent it from gradually bleeding out of the column (43).

Modern GC instruments represent high resolution systems that are fully automated from sample injection to final data reduction. Utilization of new injection devices has provided the means to enhance the performance level significantly. Studies have shown, for example, that injection of the tranquilizer propionylpromazine and its sulfoxide into a hot injection port gave much poorer results than on-column injection at low temperature (44). In the latter case, however, nonvolatile sample components could enter the column. This disadvantage of classic sample injection can be eliminated through use of a programmed temperature vaporization (PTV) injector.

When a PTV instead of a classic injector was utilized in the analysis of penicillin residues, the sensitivity and the precision of the analysis were markedly improved (45). With the cooled PTV injector, some microliters could be injected, and the split–splitless mode allowed solvent venting at low injector temperatures with open slit in a first step, and quantitative transfer of volatile or derivatized drugs by a freely selected linear heat-up rate between 2–12 °C/s in the splitless mode in the second step. Sensitivity could be enhanced by multiple injections before heat-up. Nonvolatile components of a sample did not contaminate the chromatographic system, since they accumulated in the glass vaporization tube, which could be changed easily.

Technological development has not been equally intensive over the entire GC field. An area in which surprisingly little has happened during recent years is the further development of the separation columns where there are still some problems. A major problem concerns the properties of modern columns. Because of the presence of silanol groups, the surface of the fused-silica tubing is acidic. Such surface silanols have to be more or less entirely removed to be able to elute basic compounds from the column. In a recent comparison of commercially available columns, it was shown that these are not entirely satisfactory concerning elution of primary amines (46). This type of adsorptivity is evident only for users who have to separate basic compounds. Adsorption problems can also arise from the stationary phase itself in instances when the synthesis has not been appropriately performed.

Besides adsorption of analytes, active sites on the supporting surface and in the stationary phase can trigger catalytic decomposition of unstable analytes such as trimethylsilyl derivatives (47). A further source of adsorptive and catalytic activities are the residues of additives often used to deactivate the surface and to catalyze the immobilization of the stationary phase.

With the advent of improved column deactivation, elution of more polar analytes has become possible. For this type of analytes, columns coated with selectively separating stationary phases may provide the most rapid analysis. This is the background to the increasing demand for moderately polar and polar stationary phases. Users want universal columns, that is, columns that can solve a number of analytical tasks. For that purpose, the new generation of stationary phases should include phases in which different types of functional groups such as phenyl and cyanopropyl are present simultaneously (48).

22.3   THIN-LAYER CHROMATOGRAPHY

Thin-layer chromatography (TLC), sometimes also called planar chromatography, employ a stationary phase immobilized on a glass or plastic plate and an organic mobile phase. It is a rather old technique whose application in residue analysis has been limited in the past by poor chromatographic resolution, inadequate selectivity, and insufficient sensitivity (49). This was due to inherent problems in the quality of the available stationary phase materials and in the uniformity of the layers prepared. Today, the availability of affordable, precoated plates with acceptable performance and consistency has led to the general acceptance of TLC as an efficient procedure for residue analysis (50). The method is used preferentially when analysts must process large numbers of samples in a short period of time (51).

In its conventional mode, capillary action TLC is a simple but versatile procedure that does not require expensive equipment. Therefore, TLC has a particular potential as a reliable technique for laboratories with very limited resources for instrumental equipment. The sample, either liquid or dissolved in a volatile solvent, is deposited as a spot on the stationary phase. Standards are also applied on the layer to be simultaneously run with the unknown sample for identification purposes. Volume precision and exact positioning are ensured by the use of a suitable instrument. The bottom edge of the plate is placed in a solvent reservoir, and the mobile phase moves up the plate by capillary action for a predetermined distance. In this process, the different components of the sample migrate up the plate at different rates due to differences in their partitioning behavior between the mobile and the stationary phase and, thus, the sample is separated into fractions. Then the plate is removed from the solvent reservoir and, after evaporation of the mobile phase, the separated compounds are detected on the layer by their natural color, natural fluorescence, quenching of fluorescence, or as colored, UV-absorbing, or fluorescent spots after reaction with an appropriate reagent. Examples of derivatizing agents include fluorescamine and the Bratton-Marshall diazotization reagent, which have been extensively used for the detection of sulfonamide residues in meat (52). Depending on the instruments used and the sample properties, analytical results with relative standard deviation of 1–2% can be achieved.

Two-dimensional TLC uses the same liquid chromatographic procedure twice to separate spots that are unresolved by only one process. After a sample is run in one solvent, the TLC plate is removed, dried, rotated 90 degrees, and run in another solvent. Any of the spots from the first run that contain mixtures can now be separated. The finished chromatogram is a two-dimensional array of spots.

Normal-phase adsorption on silica gel with a relatively less polar mobile phase is the most widely used mode in conventional TLC. To improve separations, silica gel may be impregnated with various solvents, buffers, and selective reagents. Other commercial precoated layers include alumina, florisil, polyamide, cellulose, and ion exchangers.

Conventional TLC should be considered for applications in which many samples are to be analyzed because it is cost-effective and environmentally friendly. On a per sample basis, it uses typically 5% of the solvent consumption of LC. Sample cleanup is usually simple or not required at all. Because stationary phases are used only once, it is often possible to apply relatively crude samples including those containing irreversibly sorbed impurities. However, impurities that comigrate with the analyte can adversely affect its detection and thus should be removed prior to TLC (53).

In its modern high-performance version, thin-layer chromatography (HPTLC) is a fully instrumental technique differentiated from conventional TLC in several important respects. It is highly flexible and selective because of the great variety of the available layers. Silica gel remains the dominant stationary phase but a wide variety of chemically bonded hydrocarbon-, amino-, cyano-, diol-, and phenylphases may be also used. HPTLC is carried out on layers slightly thinner than the conventional layers and thus need less sample loading. Moreover, HPTLC layers have a smaller mean particle size and in particular a closer particle size distribution than conventional layers. This results in less diffusion and hence improved resolution, with a migration distance about 50% shorter (50 mm compared with 100–120 mm). In addition, HPTLC layers exhibit improved optical properties over conventional layers, a characteristic that gives better accuracy during densitometric evaluation. Documentation of HPTLC chromatograms can be performed by instant or conventional film cameras and associated lighting accessories for photography of colored, fluorescent, and quenched spots in UV and visible light.

HPTLC involves, in general, precise control over all operations including sample application, chromatographic development, and chromatogram recording. It offers high sample throughput with a low cost to performance ratio. HPTLC is capable of producing fast, high-resolution separations and provides accurate and precise quantifications that may compete with LC and GC (54–57). Its coupling with a different chromatographic technique can significantly enhance the selectivity because of the dual chromatographic mode, as has been demonstrated in the determination of 4-chlorotestosterone acetate in bovine urine by TLC-LC (58).

HPTLC plates are usually developed by capillary flow of the mobile phase in ascending or horizontal modes, but forced flow methods in which the mobile phase is driven through the layer by pumping under pressure or by centrifugal force are also used. In general, HPTLC applications on chemically bonded hydrocarbons are far less numerous than in LC; reversed-phase layers with a high degree of silanization cannot be developed with highly aqueous mobile phases since the hydrophobic repulsive forces are stronger than the capillary forces moving the solvent thorough the layer unless forced-flow development occurs (59). In its most common form, forced-flow development is performed in an overpressure development chamber. The layer is sealed by applying hydraulic pressure to a polymeric membrane in intimate contact with the sorbent surface, and the mobile phase is forced through the layer by using an external pump (60).

An approach complementary to forced-flow development is the automated multiple development (AMD) that can increase the separation performance through mobile phase gradients (61). The chromatogram is developed repeatedly in the same direction. Each developing run is longer than the previous one. Unlike in LC, the gradient elution starts with the most polar solvent. Between partial runs (up to 25), the solvent is completely removed from the developing chamber and the layer dried under vacuum. Mixtures containing up to 40 analytes can be separated by AMD on one chromatogram, the analytes migrating different distances according to their polarities as sharply focused zones. Detection limits are improved because of the highly concentrated zones that are produced, as has been clearly exemplified in the analysis of furazolidone in animal tissues (62). Other approaches to forced-flow development include high-pressure planar chromatography (63), rotation planar chromatography (64), vacuum planar chromatography (65), and electromigration TLC (66). These approaches can significantly enhance the separation potential but the equipment needed has not been yet sufficiently developed for routine use.

The method is unequaled for analyzing samples in quantity. The ability to separate many samples simultaneously in parallel lanes is very useful for screening purposes and applications requiring large sample throughput, as has been exemplified in the analysis of tranquilizers (67), macrolides (68), and sulfon-amides (69). Densitometric scanning of individual or all fractions can be repeated with the same or different parameters, since all fractions remain stored on the plate.

22.4 SUPERCRITICAL FLUID CHROMATOGRAPHY

Supercritical fluid chromatography (SFC) is a relatively recently developed chro-matographic technique. Because of its ability to deal with compounds that are either polar or of high molecular weight, much attention has recently focused on applications of SFC to the analysis of different analytes using a variety of fluids or fluid mixtures to provide differing solvent capabilities and selectivities. As a result there is a large amount of research currently underway both in SFC method development and in hardware development.

Supercritical fluid chromatography has several main advantages over other chromatographic methods. Compared with LC, SFC provides rapid separations without the use of organic solvents. Because SFC generally uses carbon dioxide, it contributes no new chemicals to the environment. In addition, SFC separations can be done faster than LC separations because diffusion of solutes in supercritical fluids is about 10 times higher than that in liquids. This results in a decrease in resistance to mass transfer in the column and allows for fast high-resolution separations. In addition, the ability to manage supercritical mobile phase density with temperature and pressure adjustments provides a wider range of possible conditions in which to perform separations than the LC. Compared with GC, SFC offers high resolution without the need to apply high, often very destructive temperatures, and thus allows fast analysis of thermally labile compounds.

Supercritical fluid chromatography can most easily be described as an adap-tation of either LC or GC, in which the major modification is the replacement of either the liquid or gas mobile phase with a supercritical fluid mobile phase. In general, there are two hardware setups: the LC-setup and the GC-setup. The former consists of two reciprocating pumps designed to provide a packed analyti-cal column placed in an LC oven, with a mixed mobile phase followed by an optical detector in which the pressure and flow rates can be independently con-trolled. The latter is composed of a syringe pump followed by a capillary column placed in a GC oven with a restrictor followed by a flame ionization detector, where the pressure is controlled by the flow rate of the pump. Reciprocating pumps allow easier mixing of the mobile phase or introduction of modifier fluids, whereas syringe pumps provide consistent pressure for a neat mobile phase.

Packed columns are conventional stainless steel columns that contain small deactivated particles to which the stationary phases adheres. Capillary columns are open tubular columns of narrow internal diameter made of fused silica, with the stationary phase bonded to the wall of the column. Conventional packed columns for SFC offer more rapid analysis and higher efficiency with time unit than open tubular capillary SFC, which suffers from a limited choice of stationary phases and selectivity parameters (70). For packed columns a typical LC injection valve is commonly used, whereas for capillary columns small sample volumes must be quickly injected into the column and, therefore, pneumatically driven valves are used.

In SFC, the mobile phase is initially pumped as a liquid and is brought into the supercritical region by heating it above its supercritical temperature before it enters the analytical column. It passes through an injection valve where the sample is introduced into the supercritical stream and then into the analytical column. It is maintained supercritical as it passes through the column and into the detector by a pressure restrictor placed either after the detector or at the end of the column. The restrictor is a vital component: it keeps the mobile phase supercritical throughout the separation and often must be heated to prevent clogging; both variable- and fixed-restrictors are available.

Part of the theory of separation in SFC is based on the density of the supercritical fluid, which corresponds to its solvating power. As the pressure in the system increases, the supercritical fluid density also increases and correspondingly its solvating power becomes higher. Therefore, the chromatographic efficiency and rate of separation will depend on the pressure drop across the column. This is similar to the temperature programming in GC or to the solvent gradient in LC. For this reason, the high-packing-density and high-surface-area columns developed for LC will produce a large density change resulting in poor chromatographic efficiency. Recent developments in packed SFC tend towards loosely packed low-surface-area stationary phases that show reasonable resolution and rapid elution. A detailed discussion of theoretical aspects of SFC is beyond the scope of this book, but several comprehensive reviews are available in literature (71–73).

Capillary SFC is particularly useful for compounds that are difficult to detect using LC and too unstable for GC. Nevertheless, at present there have not been enough applications to justify an investment (74, 75). In contrast, packed-column SFC has undergone a renaissance thanks to evaporative light-scattering detection (ELSD). Packed-column SFC-ELSD is a suitable method for analyzing various compounds, with or without chromophores, and with diverse polarities, as found in drug, steroid, and ionophore complex mixtures (76–79).

In addition, SFC permits the use of a flame ionization detector instead of the classic UV detector. Because the response factor of the former detector is much less dependent on the compounds to be analyzed, this is a very important advantage when analyzing compounds, which, for calibration purposes, are not available as pure substances (80).

A preliminary investigation of SFC coupled to MS/MS for the analysis of trimethoprim, diethylstilbestrol, hexestrol, and dienestrol has demonstrated the considerable potential of this separation technique (81). Packed-column SFC has been also evaluated for the analysis of nine sulfonamides in swine kidney extracts (82). Separations were performed on either silica- or amino-bonded stationary phase columns, using carbon dioxide with various modifiers as mobile phases. Each column exhibited distinctly different selectivities to the examined sulfonamides, the amino-bonded column being much more sensitive to modifier variations. In a continuation of the sulfonamide study, packed-column SFC was further evaluated for possible application to the analysis of furazolidone, chloramphenicol, and lincomycin residues (82). Separation was effected on an amino-bonded stationary phase using carbon dioxide with methanol modifier as the mobile phase, whereas detection was accomplished by MS.

22.5 CAPILLARY ELECTROPHORESIS

Electrophoresis is a technique based on the mobility of ions in an electric field. An electrode apparatus consists of a high-voltage supply, electrodes, buffer, and a support for the buffer such as filter paper, cellulose acetate strips, or a capillary tube. Positively charged ions migrate towards the negative electrode and negatively charged ions migrate toward the positive electrode. For safety reasons, one electrode is usually at ground and the other is biased positively or negatively. Ions present different migration rates depending on their total charge, size, and shape, and can therefore be separated.

In traditional electrophoresis, separation efficiency is limited by thermal diffusion and convection. Owing to long analysis times and low efficiencies, these procedures never enjoyed wide usage. Problems have arisen when trying to differentiate between structurally related drug residues such as streptomycin and dihydrostreptomycin, tetracyclines, lincomycin and clindamycin, and erythromycin and oleandomycin (83, 84). To overcome these problems, anticonvective media, such as polyacrylamide or agarose gels, have also been used.

In modern designs, electrophoretic separation is performed in narrow capillaries that are themselves anticonvective and, therefore, gel media are not essential to perform that function. Performing electrophoresis in small-diameter capillaries allows the use of very high electric fields because the small capillaries efficiently dissipate the heat produced. Increasing the electric fields produces very efficient separations and reduces separation times. Capillaries are typically of 25–75 μm inner diameter and 0.5–1 m in length, which are usually filled only with buffer. The applied potential is 20–30 kV.

The surface of the silicate glass capillary contains negatively charged functional groups that attract positively charged counterions. The positively charged ions migrate towards the negative electrode and carry solvent molecules in the same direction. This overall solvent movement is called electroosmotic flow. Due to the electroosmotic flow, all sample components migrate towards the negative electrode when a 10 nl volume of sample is injected at the positive end of the capillary.

Acidic (-COOH, -SH) or basic (NR_2) functional groups are indicators of the appropriate pH range for separating multiple analytes. Also, hydrophobic functionality is an indication that organic solvents should be added to the separation buffer. This addition can enhance the solubility of the analytes in the separation buffer, decreasing analyte–wall interactions and enhancing resolution of such components (85).

During a separation, uncharged molecules move at the same velocity as the electroosmotic flow, with very little separation. Positively charged ions move more quickly and negatively charged ions move more slowly. Peak efficiency, often in excess of 10^5 theoretical plates, is due in part to the plug profile of the electroosmotic flow that enables the simultaneous analysis of all solutes, regardless of charge. Ideally, these characteristics make CE particularly well suited for the separation and analysis of drug residues in food matrices.

CE detection is similar to detectors in, and include absorbance, fluorescence, electrochemical, and mass spectrometric detectors. The capillary can also be filled with a gel, which eliminates the electroosmotic flow. Separation is accomplished as in conventional gel electrophoresis but the capillary allows higher resolution, greater sensitivity, and on-line detection. In CE, low picogram amounts of analytes can be detected using glass fiber optics. However, this does not mean low limits of detection since only a few nanoliters can be injected.

CE is a rapidly growing separation technique and significant advances have already been made. These include improvements in migration time and peak area reproducibility, methods for on-capillary sample preconcentration to improve sensitivity, and development of capillary coatings to control electroosmotic flow and to limit solute–wall interactions. Nevertheless, the technique is still in a development and growth stage. The versatility of CE in the analysis of drug residues is partially derived from its numerous modes of operation including capillary zone electrophoresis (CZE), micellar electrokinetic chromatography (MEKC), and capillary isotachophoresis (CITP).

CZE is the most widely used mode due to its simplicity of operation and its versatility. Selectivity can be most readily altered through changes in running buffer pH or by use of buffer additives such as surfactants or chiral selectors. The major drawback with CZE is that it deals with aqueous electrolytic systems, whereas components can only be separated if they are charged and soluble in water. CZE separation of various antibacterials including penicillins, tetracyclines, and macrolides has been reported (86). Determination of cefixime, an oral cephalosporin antibiotic, and its metabolites in human urine has been also successfully carried out with CZE (87).

MEKC is a hybrid of electrophoresis and chromatography (88). In MEKC, both charged and uncharged compounds and compounds that are almost insoluble in water can be separated. The separation of neutral species is accomplished by the use of surfactants in the running buffer. Individual surfactant molecules form micelles with the hydrophobic tails of the surfactant molecules oriented towards the center, avoiding thus interaction with the hydrophobic buffer. The charged heads are oriented towards the buffer. The interaction between the micelle and the neutral solutes causes the separation. During migration, the micelles can interact with solutes in a chromatographic manner, through both hydrophobic and electrostatic interactions. The technique has been successfully applied to separate penicillin and cephalosporin antibiotics using sodium dodecyl sulfate as surfactant (88, 89).

CITP is a moving-boundary electrophoretic technique. A combination of two buffer systems is used to create a state in which the separated zones all move at the same velocity. The zones remain sandwiched between leading and terminating electrolytes. In a single CITP application, either cations or anions can be analyzed. For anion analysis, the buffer must be selected so that the leading electrolyte contains an anion with an effective mobility higher than that of the solutes. Similarly, the terminating anion must have a lower mobility than that of the solutes. When the electric field is applied, the anions start to migrate towards the anode. Since the leading anion has the highest mobility, it moves more quickly, followed by the anion with the next highest mobility, and so on. A difficulty often arises with finding buffer systems that contain both leading and trailing ions and also form the desired pH. An additional limitation is that only cations or anions can be sharpened, but not both simultaneously. The technique has been successfully used to separate penicillin and cephalosporin antibiotics and their precursors (90).

Until now, CE technology has not been widely used in biological applications, but its high resolving power presents obvious advantages in research for separating drug residues of a wide range of polarities and solubilities in aqueous and nonaqueous solvents. CE is still in its infancy and, thus, an active area of research.

22.6 MULTIDIMENSIONAL SEPARATION

Multidimensional separation involves techniques in which fractions from a primary separation system are transferred on-line to a secondary separation system. These techniques can utilize combinations of different chromatographic columns and has been practiced using LC, GC, SFC, CZE, and combinations of these methods (91).

Multidimensional GC, for example, involves coupling of GC columns of different selectivities so that the primary column isolates the fraction of interest whereas the secondary column accomplishes the final separation of the analytes within the isolates fraction. By combining two GC capillary columns with completely different selectivities, peak capacity can be increased tremendously. Since a normal GC capillary column offers about 100,000 theoretical plates, the total number of peaks than can be separated on such a column is approximately 700–800. By combining two such columns, the maximum number of compounds to be separated becomes 700×700, which is almost half a million compounds. It is, therefore, hardly surprising that multidimensional GC is a technique that will become increasingly important.

Another exciting development in multidimensional separation involves coupling of LC to GC or even to CE. In these coupling systems, LC can play a role as a high-resolution procedure for preliminary separation and/or trace enrichment. LC-GC can thereby be carried out in the column-switching and in the precolumn-analytical column mode. Although on-line LC-GC has not yet advanced widely into routine analysis, this powerful technique holds promise for the future.

REFERENCES

1. L.R. Snyder and J.J. Kirkland, in Introduction to Modern Liquid Chromatography (L.R. Snyder and J.J. Kirkland, Eds.), 2nd ed., Wiley, New York (1979).
2. A. Pryde and M.T. Gilbert, in Applications of High Performance Liquid Chromatography (A. Pryde and M.T. Gilbert, Eds.), Wiley, New York (1979).
3. J.F. Lawrence, in Organic Trace Analysis by Liquid Chromatography (J.F. Lawrence, Ed.), Academic Press, New York (1981).
4. R.J. Hamilton and P.A. Sewell, in Introduction to High-Performance Liquid Chromatography (R.J. Hamilton and P.A. Sewell, Eds.), 2nd Edition, Chapman and Hall, London (1982).
5. A.M. Krstulovic and P.R. Brown, in Reversed-Phase HPLC: Theory, Practice and Biomedical Applications (A.M. Krstulovic and P.R. Brown, Eds.), Wiley-Interscience, New York (1982).
6. R. Macrae, in HPLC in Food Analysis (R. Macrae, Ed.), Academic Press, London (1982).
7. H. Engelhardt, in Practice of High Performance Liquid Chromatography (H. Engelhardt, Ed.), Springer-Verlag, Berlin (1986).
8. L.M.L. Nollet, in Food Analysis by HPLC (L.M.L. Nollet, Ed.), Marcel Dekker, Inc., New York (1992).
9. B.A. Bidlingmeyer, in Practical HPLC Methodology and Applications (B.A. Bidlingmeyer, Ed.), Wiley, New York (1992).
10. R.P.W. Scott, in Liquid Chromatography Column Theory (R.P.W. Scott, Ed.), Wiley, New York (1992).
11. V.R. Meyer, in Practical High-Performance Liquid Chromatography (V.R. Meyer, Ed.), 2nd Edition, Wiley, New York (1994).

12. R.P.W. Scott, in Techniques and Practices of Chromatography (R.P.W. Scott, Ed.), Marcel Dekker, Inc., New York (1995).
13. L.M.L. Nollet, in Handbook of Food Analysis (L.M.L. Nollet, Ed.), Marcel Dekker, Inc., New York (1996).
14. D.J. Fletouris, J.E. Psomas, and A.J. Mantis, Chromatographia, 32:436 (1991).
15. N.A. Botsoglou, D.J. Fletouris, I.E. Psomas, and V.N. Vassilopoulos, J. Liq. Chromatogr., 17:4229 (1994).
16. N.A. Botsoglou, D.J. Fletouris, I.E. Psomas, and A.I. Mantis, Anal. Chim. Acta, 354:115 (1997).
17. N.A. Botsoglou, D.J. Fletouris, E.J. Simeonidou, and I.E. Psomas, Chromatographia, 46:477 (1997).
18. J.O. Boison, J. Chromatogr., 624:171 (1992).
19. J. Abian, M.I. Churchwell, and W.A. Korfmacher, J. Chromatogr., 629:267 (1993).
20. M.M.L. Aerts, W.M.J. Beek, H.J. Keukens, and U.A.Th. Brinkman, J. Chromatogr., 456:105 (1988).
21. N. Haagsma, C. Schreuder, and E.R.A. Rensen, J. Chromatogr., 363:353 (1986).
22. L. Larocque, M. Schnurr, S. Sved, and A. Weninger, J. Assoc. Off. Anal. Chem., 74:608 (1991).
23. S. Sved, L. Larocque, A. Weninger, M. Schnurr, and D. Vas, in Residues of Veterinary Drugs in Food, Proc. Euroresidue Conf., Noordwijkerhout, May 21–23, 1990 (N. Haagsma, A. Ruiter, and P.B. Czedik-Eysenberg, Eds.), Fac. Vet. Med., Univ. Utrecht, The Netherlands, p. 356 (1990).
24. J.A. Tarbin, D. Tyler, and G. Shearer, in Residues of Veterinary Drugs in Food, Proc. Euroresidue II Conf., Veldhoven, May 3–5, 1993 (N. Haagsma, A. Ruiter, and P.B. Czedik-Eysenberg, Eds.), Fac. Vet. Med., Univ. Utrecht, The Netherlands, p. 659 (1993).
25. M.J.B. Mengelers, J.F. Staal, M.M.L. Aerts, H.A. Kuiper, and A.S.J.P.A.M. van Miert, in Residues of Veterinary Drugs in Food, Proc. Euroresidue Conf., Noordwijkerhout, May 21–23, 1990 (N. Haagsma, A. Ruiter, and P.B. Czedik-Eysenberg, Eds.), Fac. Vet. Med., Univ. Utrecht, The Netherlands, p. 276 (1990).
26. M.J.B. Mengelers, A.M.M. Polman, M.M.L. Aerts, H.A. Kuiper, and A.S.J.P.A.M. van Miert, J. Liq. Chromatogr., 16:257 (1993).
27. D.J. Gisch, B.T. Hunter, and B. Feibush, J. Chromatogr., 433:264 (1988).
28. Y. Yoshida, I. Morita, T. Masujima, and H. Imai, Chem. Pharm. Bull., 30:2287 (1982).
29. H. Hagestam and T.C. Pinkerton, Anal. Chem., 57:1757 (1985).
30. H. Hagestam and T.C. Pinkerton, J. Chromatogr., 351:239 (1986).
31. Z.K. Shihabi, J. Liq. Chromatogr., 11:1579 (1988).
32. M.G. Khaledi, BioChromatography, 3:20 (1988).
33. M.F. Borgerding and W.L. Hinze, Anal. Chem., 57:2183 (1985).
34. M.J. Koenigbauer, J. Chromatogr., 531:79 (1990).
35. N. Haagsma, L.M.J. Mains, W. van Leeuwen, and H.W. van Gend, in Residues of Veterinary Drugs in Food, Proc. Euroresidue Conf., Noordwijkerhout, May 21–23, 1990 (N. Haagsma, A. Ruiter, and P.B. Czedik-Eysenberg, Eds.), Fac. Vet. Med., Univ. Utrecht, The Netherlands, p. 206 (1990).

36. H.H. Thanh, A.T. Andresen, T. Agasoster, and K.E. Rasmussen, J. Chromatogr., 532:363 (1990).
37. M.M.L. Aerts, W.M.J. Beek, and U.A.Th. Brinkman, J. Chromatogr., 435:97 (1988).
38. M.M.L. Aerts, W.M.J. Beek, and U.A.Th. Brinkman, J. Chromatogr., 500:453 (1990).
39. W.C. Jacobson, E.H. Allen, and H.G. Wiseman, in Determination of Chroramphenicol in Liver, Kidney, Muscle, and Whole Blood, 88th Annual Meeting of AOAC, Oct. 14–17, Washington, DC (1974).
40. J. Hamman, A. Tolle, A. Bluthgen, and W. Heeschen, Milchwissenschaft, 30:1 (1975).
41. G.E. Baiulescu, and V.A. Ilie, in Stationary Phases in Gas Chromatography (G.E. Baiulescu and V.A. Ilie, Eds.), Pergamon Press, Oxford, UK (1975).
42. M. Petz, in Residues of Veterinary Drugs in Food, Proc. Euroresidue Conf., Noordwijkerhout, May 21–23, 1990 (N. Haagsma, A. Ruiter, and P.B. Czedik-Eysenberg, Eds.), Fac. Vet. Med., Univ. Utrecht, The Netherlands, p. 53 (1990).
43. L.G. Blomberg, Trends Anal. Chem., 36:41 (1987).
44. W. Arneth, Fleischwirtschaft, 66:922 (1986).
45. U. Meetschen and M. Petz, J. Assoc. Off. Anal. Chem., 73:373 (1990).
46. M. Abdel-Rehim, M. Bielenstein, and T. Arvidsson, J. Microcol. Sep., in press (1998).
47. M. Donike, Chromatographia, 6:190 (1973).
48. L.G. Blomber, LC-GC Int., 11:760 (1998).
49. W. Horwitz, J. Assoc. Off. Anal. Chem., 64:104 (1981).
50. N.A. Botsoglou and D.J. Fletouris, in Handbook of Food Analysis, Vol. 2 (L.M.L. Nollet, Ed.), Marcel Dekker, Inc., New York, p. 1171 (1996).
51. J.P. Abjean, Chromatographia, 36:359 (1993).
52. D. Guggisberg, A.E. Mooser, and H. Koch, J. Chromatogr., 624:425 (1992).
53. J. Sherma, J. AOAC Int., 77:297 (1994).
54. H. Schuett and J. Hoelzl, Pharmazie, 49:206 (1994).
55. D.M. Bliesner, J. Planar Chromatogr., 7:197 (1994).
56. A.N. Abdelrahman, E.I.A. Karim, and K.E.E. Ibrahim, J. Pharm. Biomed. Anal., 12: 205 (1994).
57. P. Vuorela, E.L. Rahko, R. Hitunen, and H. Vuorela, J. Chromatogr., 670:191 (1994).
58. Y. Nakagawa, Lipids, 28:1033 (1993).
59. C.F. Poole and S.K. Poole, Anal. Chem., 66:27A (1994).
60. C.F. Poole and S.K. Poole, Anal. Chem., 61:1257A (1989).
61. H. Jork, G. Keller, and U. Kocher, J. Planar Chromatogr., 5:246 (1992).
62. J.P. Heotis, J.L. Mertz, R.J. Herrett, J.R. Diaz, D.C. VanHart, and I. Olivard, J. Assoc. Off. Anal. Chem., 63:720 (1980).
63. R.E. Kaiser and R.I. Reider, J. Assoc. Off. Anal. Chem., 66:79 (1983).
64. S. Nyiredy, L. Botz, and O. Sticher, J. Planar Chromatogr., 2:53 (1989).
65. P. Delvondre, C. Regnault, and E. Postaire, J. Liq. Chromatogr., 15:1673 (1992).
66. M. Procek and M. Pukl, in Abstracts of Papers, 7th Int. Symp. on Instrumental Planar Chromatography, Brighton 1993, The Chromatographic Society, Nottingham, UK, p. 9 (1993).

67. N. Haagsma, E.R. Bathelt, and J.W. Engelsma, J. Chromatogr., 436:73 (1988).
68. M. Petz, R. Solly, M. Lymburn, and M.H. Clear, J. Assoc. Off. Anal. Chem., 70: 691 (1987).
69. B.W. de Bukanski, J.-M. Degroodt, and H. Beernaert, Z. Lebensm. Unters. Forsch., 187:242 (1988).
70. M. Dreux and M. Lafosse, LC-GC Int., 10:382 (1997).
71. T.L. Chester, J. Chromatogr. Sci., 24:226 (1986).
72. C.M. White and K.R. Houck, J. High Resol. Chromatogr. Commun., 9:4 (1986).
73. C.F. Poole and S.K. Poole, Anal. Chim. Acta, 216:109 (1989).
74. M.J. Drews, K. Ivey, and J. Helvey, in Abstracts of Papers, 7th Int. Symp. on SFC and SFE, Indianapolis 1996, Indiana, USA (1996).
75. J.D. Pinkston, R. Hentschel, and T.L. Chester, in Abstracts of Papers, 7th Int. Symp. on SFC and SFE, Indianapolis 1996, Indiana, USA (1996).
76. M. Dreux and M. Lafosse, Spectra 2000, 153:24 (1990).
77. M. Dreux and M. Lafosse, J. High Resol. Chromatogr., 15:312 (1992).
78. J.L. Perrin and A. Prevot, Rev. Franc. Cops. Gras., 35:485 (1988).
79. A.J. Berry, J. Chromatogr. Sci., 34:245 (1996).
80. R. Smits, LC-GC Int., 7:505 (1994).
81. E.D. Ramsey, J.R. Perkins, D.E. Games, and J.R. Startin, J. Chromatogr., 464:353 (1989).
82. J.R. Perkins, D.E. Games, J.R. Startin, and J. Gilbert, J. Chromatogr., 540:239 (1991).
83. J. Stadhouders, F. Hassing, and T.E. Galesloot, Neth. Milk Dairy J., 35:23 (1981).
84. A.F. Lott, R. Smither, and D.R. Vaughan, J. Assoc. Off. Anal. Chem., 68:1018 (1985).
85. A.J. Tomlinson, L.M. Benson, and S. Naylor, LC-GC Int., 8:210 (1995).
86. S.K. Yeo, H.K. Lee, and S.F.Y. Li, J. Chromatogr., 585:133 (1991).
87. S. Honda, A. Taga, K. Kakehi, and Y. Okamoto, J. Chromatogr., 590:364 (1992).
88. S. Terabe, Trends Anal. Chem., 8:129 (1989).
89. H. Nishi, N. Tsumagari, and S. Terabe, Anal. Chem., 61:2434 (1989).
90. H. Nishi, N. Tsumagari, T. Kakimoto, and S. Terabe, J. Chromatogr., 477:259 (1989).
91. R. Smits, LC-GC Int., 7:505 (1994).

23

Detection

Numerous detection systems for screening, identifying, and quantifying drug residues in edible animal products have been developed over the years. They represent almost all kinds of known analytical approaches including microbiological, immunochemical, and physicochemical techniques. Each of the existing techniques has its own advantages and drawbacks that must be carefully considered in the selection of the most convenient detection/confirmation system for a particular analyte in a particular matrix. Veterinary drugs show large variation in molecular structure and, consequently, in physicochemical properties and biological activity.

Application of microbiological or immunochemical techniques offers the advantage of screening drug residues in foods with little or no previous sample preparation. Application, on the other hand, of physicochemical techniques, allows quantification and more tentative identification of residues in those samples found positive. The problem of analyzing for drug residues is complicated by the fact that it is not known whether residues exist, and if they exist, the type and quantity are not known.

23.1 MICROBIOLOGICAL TECHNIQUES

Because the aim of the control of residues is to prevent residues in food exerting an undesirable effect on humans, it would be elegant to use this biological effect as the detection principle. Hence, the detection of drug residues in edible animal products has traditionally been performed by microbiological techniques.

The earliest methods for detecting antibacterial residues in food appeared in 1945–1948, soon after microbiological assays for the evaluation of antibiotics in pharmaceutical products were first developed. The ability of a strain of *Streptococcus agalactiae* (1) or of a commercial starter culture (2) to produce acid during growth, and also the ability of *Staphylococcus aureus* (3–5), *Bacillus subtilis* (6), and group A *Streptococcus* (7) to produce haziness in agar media during growth, served as the bases for the first microbiological assays of penicillin residues in milk.

Concurrent but independent work by many investigators led to development of a plethora of methods based on inhibition of the bacterial growth by the antibacterials present in livestock products. Microorganisms such as *Bacillus cereus* (8–11), *Bacillus mesentericus* (12), *Bacillus stearothermophilus* (13, 14), *Bacillus subtilis* (6, 11, 14–24), *Brucella anthracis* (25), *Brucella bronchiseptica* (11, 26), *Brucella suis* (25), *Candida tropicalis* (11), *Escherichia coli* (11, 23, 24), *Lactobacillus bulgaricus* (27–29), *Micrococcus flavus* (11, 26), *Pseudomonas syringae* (11), *Micrococcus luteus* (11, 21, 26, 30, 31), *Staphylococcus aureus* (13–5, 9, 28, 29, 32–34), *Staphylococcus epidermidis* (11), *Streptococcus cremoris* (35), *Streptococcus faecalis* (23, 24), *Streptococcus lactis* (33, 36), and *Streptococcus thermophilus* (37–41) have all been employed with varying success for determining the presence of various antibacterials in milk. The *Bacillus subtilis* disc assay procedure (22) with modifications (17, 26, 42–47) has been used more extensively than the cylinder assay procedures (11, 48, 49), but disc and tube diffusion assays that use *Bacillus stearothermophilus* (45, 50) or *Streptococcus thermophilus* (37–41) as the test organism have gained in popularity.

Investigations into performance characteristics have shown that various factors affect the accuracy and sensitivity of the microbiological assays; their relative influence depends upon the kind of antibacterials assayed and, especially, the test organism (51). The vegetative test organism must be resistant to spontaneous change and easily cultured, maintained, and standardized; spore suspensions have similar criteria except that the spores must be capable of germinating with reasonably synchrony. Some assays are slow and labor-intensive, requiring overnight incubations and multiple platings and measurements to achieve a questionable ±35% precision at the ppb level (52). The sensitivity of microbial inhibition assays is also most influenced by the concentration of inoculum (53, 54), the quantity and pH of the assay medium on the plate (51), and sample size. The majority of original research in this area was done during the period from about 1945 to 1961. Later studies were devoted primarily to perfecting existing methods by testing their accuracy and precision and to incorporating factors into the assay to improve the rapidity and ease of performance.

Owing to the variability in results of the early developed microbiological procedures, standardized materials were introduced and are currently used for routine quality control. Depending on the format of the test, the presence of an inhibitory substance is indicated by zones of growth inhibition or a change in the color of the medium with pH and redox indicators. Examples of commercial microbial inhibition assays commonly used for milk or tissue include the Delvotest P, disk assay for milk, swab test on premises (STOP test), brilliant black reduction test (BR test), calf antibiotic sulfa test (CAST test), live animal swab test (LAST test), and the CHARM farm test (CFT) (55–63).

23.2 IMMUNOCHEMICAL TECHNIQUES

Although microbiological tests are used worldwide, most modern tests that are commercially produced for screening drug residues in foods are immunochemical procedures. They are based on the highly specific binding between the analyte (antigen) and antibodies raised against it.

A wide variety of elegant procedures have been developed for visualizing the primary antibody–antigen reaction. Precipitation and agglutination techniques represent types of reactions in which the primary antibody–antigen interaction is observed directly without use of any tagged reagent for amplification. These techniques are based on the fact that all antibodies and many antigens are multivalent and can thus form large crosslinked complexes. When soluble antigens are mixed directly with the corresponding antibodies (antiserum), large macromolecule complexes are formed and precipitates visible to the naked eye are created. If the antigen or the antibody is presented in particulate rather than soluble form, a visible agglutination can be observed (64). Latex particles can be coated with antibody or antigen to enable an agglutination reaction to be performed, as in the case of the Spot test that can detect benzylpenicillin, cephapirin, and cloxacillin residues in raw milk within 6 min (65). Gentamicin residues in milk can be also detected with an agglutination technique (66). This assay is based upon the least amount of soluble antigen necessary to inhibit agglutination or the clumping of cells that occurs after the binding of antigen to antibody. In practice, this is the amount of antigen in the last tube of a dilution series that will give a wide-ring agglutination pattern. Tubes containing less antigen than this tube allow agglutination to occur. The procedure is relatively rapid and specific but not particularly sensitive and its accuracy is dependent on the dilution sequence used.

Higher-sensitivity immunochemical assays can be obtained through amplification of the binding reaction by means of radio tags. The principles and applications of radioimmunoassays to the detection of drug residues in foods of animal origin have been recently reviewed (67). A fixed amount of radiolabeled antigen is added to the sample, and, following competitive binding to an antibody, free and antibody-bound antigen fractions are separated and the amount of labeled antigen in one of the fractions is determined. The separation of bound and unbound labeled antigens is the most critical parameter. Quantitation is based on the nonlinear inhibition of the binding reaction when increasing amounts of unlabeled antigen are successively added. Examples of separation methodology include precipitation using ethanol, ammonium sulfate, or polyethylene glycol, the use of an antiglobulin reagent or attachment of antibodies to a solid phase, and subsequent removal of the unbound labeled antigen by a washing step (68).

Radiolabeled immunoassays have been used extensively for the quantification of drug residues, particularly chloramphenicol. These assays do not generally require extensive sample cleanup. The possibility, however, that matrix components such as lipids and proteolytic enzymes may interfere with the interaction of the antigen to antibodies cannot be excluded (69, 70). Thus, whenever extremely low drug residue levels have to be detected, extensive purification of the sample may be indispensable to eliminate nonspecific interference. Radioimmunoassays are generally sensitive and specific procedures and lend themselves readily to automation. However, they necessitate the use of hazardous radioactive reagents with short shelf lives and require counting equipment, and the cost of analysis is frequently high. Nevertheless, radioimmunoassays still make up a significant portion of current immunochemical methods for the detection of drug residues, particularly chloramphenicol (71–78) and gentamicin (79), in edible animal products.

Over the years, radioimmunoassays have increasingly been replaced by nonisotopic procedures that differ in terms of the label used, endpoint detection, and the separation step. Although the use of enzyme labels as a means of amplifying and visualizing the primary antibody–antigen binding reaction is the most rapidly growing and most widely used immunoassay technology, immunoassays based on fluorescent and chemiluminescent labels are also of interest in residue analysis. Included in the former category are competitive binding fluoroimmunoassays and immunoassays based on fluorescence polarization (80, 81).

Fluorescence polarization immunoassays depend on detection of the increase in effective molecular size when a small fluorescent-labeled antigen is bound by specific antibody. The principle of this type of immunoassay (82) is based on the fact that when plane-polarized light falls on a fluorophor-labeled antigen, molecules having their long axes parallel to the plane of light are preferentially excited, and if they can rotate between excitation and emission the resultant fluorescence is nonpolarized. The degree of polarization depends on the rate of rotation and this, in turn, is inversely proportional to molecular size. The binding of a low-molecular-weight labeled antigen to antibody results in a large chemical moiety that, unlike the native antigen, is rotating at a slower rate so that much of the emitted fluorescence is still polarized. In this technique, the unlabeled antigen present in the sample competes with the added fluorescent-labeled antigen for the available antibody-binding sites, so that the extent of depolarization of the emitted fluorescence is proportional to the concentration of the analyte. No separation step is required in polarization fluorescence immunoassays, which results in to technical simplicity and ease of automation. However, the detection limits achievable by this technique cannot compare with those of radio- and enzyme immunoassays, which incorporate separation steps and have end-points with greater sensitivity.

Labels used in fluorescence immunoassays are mostly based on fluorescein (83), but fluorescein–peptide conjugates (84) and aluminum phthalocyanine-labeled streptavidin may also be used (85). Merits of fluorescence immunoassays can be considered the stability and freedom from hazards of fluorescent labels, the moderate cost of analysis, the wide availability of the equipment needed, and the high potential sensitivity (86).

Because of the dependence on molecular size, fluorescence polarization immunoassay is particularly suited to the assay of small antigens such as drugs, and it has found wide application in clinical diagnostics for therapeutic drug monitoring and screening of drugs of abuse (87). However, its applicability in drug residue analysis in foods is still very limited. Known applications concern the determination of gentamicin in tissue extracts using commercially available fluorescence polarization kits (88, 89), and development and characterization of fluorescence polarization reagents for the antibiotics sulfamethazine, chloramphenicol, and benzylpenicillin (90).

Methods based on chemiluminescent and bioluminescent labels are another area of nonisotopic immunoassays that continue to undergo active research. Most common approaches in this category are the competitive binding chemiluminescence immunoassays and the immunochemiluminometric assays. Chemiluminescence and heterogenous chemiluminescence immunoassays have been the subject of excellent reviews (91, 92). Detection in chemiluminescence immunoassays is based on either the direct monitoring of conjugated labels, such as luminol or acridinium ester, or the enzyme-mediated formation of luminescent products. Preparation of various derivatives of acridinium esters has been reported (93, 94), whereas a variety of enzyme labels including firefly or bacterial luciferase (70), horseradish peroxidase (86, 98), and alkaline phosphatase are commercially available.

Immunochemical methods based on enzyme labels make up the most popular type of immunoassay technology used in the field of veterinary drug residues (98–100). Enzyme labels are generally easier to handle, they can be readily obtained in a highly purified form, and are relatively inexpensive and stable. Moreover, they can be readily coupled to proteins and act on substrates that produce easily measured colored products. Choices for enzyme labels include horseradish peroxidase, alkaline phosphatase, glucose oxidase, pyruvate dehydrogenase, and recombinant β-galactosidase (101–103). These enzymes catalyze reactions that cause colorless substrates to degrade and form, depending on the substrate and the method used to terminate the reaction, different colors with an intensity that can be visually estimated or measured with a spectrophotometer. Most of the commonly used enzyme labels can convert at least 10^6 molecules of substrate into product, per molecule of enzyme per minute, at ambient temperature.

Substrate products can be classified as either soluble or precipitating. Soluble peroxidase substrates include o-phenylenediamine, which is converted into a yellow product; 2,2'-azino-(3-ethyl)-benzothiazoline-sulfonic acid, which is converted into a green product; and tetramethylbenzidine, which is converted into a blue product. Precipitating substrates for peroxidase include 4-chloronaphthol, which yields a blue precipitate; and aminoethylcarbizole, which forms a red precipitate. Alkaline phosphatase is most frequently used with p-nitrophenyl phosphate to give a yellow–orange soluble product, or with 5-bromo-4-chloro-3-indolyl-phosphate p-toluidine salt to yield an insoluble blue product.

Many types of mono-, bi-, and multifunctional coupling reagents are available for labeling antibodies or antigens with an enzyme. Glutaraldehyde, carbodiimide, N-succinimidyl-3-(2-pyridyldithio)propionate, and periodate oxidation of carbohydrate moieties to form active dialdehydes are several commonly used approaches in the preparation of enzyme conjugates (104–106).

Enzyme immunoassays fall into two general categories: homogenous and the heterogenous assays. The former require no separation of bound and free material because they are actually based on monitoring a change in enzyme activity. Homogenous assays are convenient for residue analysis, but their sensitivity is relatively low and their accuracy, although acceptable, can be affected by the sample matrix. Heterogenous assays, on the other hand, are more sensitive and specific because they involve separation steps that require washing between steps to remove unreacted components.

The most popular heterogenous assay in drug residue analysis is the competitive enzyme-linked immunosorbent assay (ELISA) in which one of the binding elements is attached to a solid support. The use of the solid support allows for easy separation of the unbound from the bound fraction. Immobilization of antibodies or antigens to the solid support is accomplished either in a passive manner through hydrophobic interaction or in an active manner through covalent bonding of proteins to suitable sites on the solid surface. Nonspecific interactions can be reduced by inclusion of high concentration of an unrelated protein, a detergent, and/or salt (107, 108).

Materials commonly use as solid supports include polystyrene, polyvinyl, nylon, glass, nitrocellulose, silica, polyacrylamide, or polystyrene beads. Separation of the bound from the free reagents can be achieved through either filtration for particulate solid supports such as agarose, polyacrylamide, and polystyrene beads, or centrifugation. For disposable forms of solid supports such as multiwell plates, plastic tubes, cuvettes, balls, and dipsticks, separation can be performed through simple rinsing steps.

Within ELISAs, both direct and indirect modes of performance are possible. The former are based on competition between the analyte and an enzyme-labeled analyte for a place on an immobilized antibody. The latter is based on competition between the analyte and an immobilized analyte for a place on an enzyme-labeled antibody. After washing, the amount of the enzyme-label bound (which is inversely proportional to the concentration of the analyte) is visualized by means of a substrate incubation.

A disadvantage of both competitive assays is that the enzyme conjugate solution has to be mixed with the sample solution. A sample solution, however, may contain inhibitory substances such as proteases that can alter the activity of the antibody and/or the enzyme-label used. Where enzyme-labeled antibodies are employed, such problems may be circumvented by using an unlabeled antibody in the competition phase, followed by incubation with an enzyme-labeled second antibody that is directed against the primary antibodies (109).

Competitive ELISAs are used for both qualitative and quantitative purposes. The minimum of sample preparation required, the availability of the equipment needed, and the possibility for automation make ELISAs particularly suitable for screening a large number of samples. Problems may arise, however, with respect to sensitivity when extremely low concentrations have to be detected.

Apart from concentrating the analyte prior to immunoassay, several other possibilities exist for enhancing the sensitivity of the procedure. These constitute introduction of various amplification systems, such as the peroxidase–antiperoxidase system (110), the streptavidine–biotine system (111, 112), and the substrate amplification system (113, 114), which favor the enhancement of the signal per ligand.

Problems may also arise with respect to specificity when ELISAs are applied for trace residue analysis, because any compound whose molecule is in part identical with or closely similar to the antigenic determinant of the analyte can compete for antibody-binding sites. Therefore, immunochemical methods are valuable for screening and testing purposes but cannot be considered as definitive from a regulatory perspective. For legal enforcement use, these methods should be used as part of an analytical system that consists of additional methods capable of definitively identifying the compounds of interest.

Currently, a number of immunochemical tests are commercially available in a kit format for many drugs. The 96-well plastic plate is one of the more commonly used formats of polystyrene and polyvinyl sold supports. It is well suited to automation and high throughput uses due to the wide variety of equipment that has been developed to simplify reagent transfer, rinsing steps, and interpretation of results.

A variety of on-site assay formats have been also developed that considerably simplify the training needed to perform the assay. Card formats have been developed that require no instrumentation, thus making the tests ideal for quick field screening of veterinary residues. The card has small windows through which reagents and sample extracts or standard solutions are added. Following reaction of the sample with the antibody, which is absorbed onto a fiber glass matrix support, the solution of antigen–enzyme conjugate is added. If analyte is present in the sample, some of the binding sites will have been blocked while free sites will react with the antigen–enzyme conjugate. Addition of substrate produces a color whose intensity is inversely proportional to the analyte concentration. These tests are quick and easy to perform as a check on the presence or absence of residues.

In addition, membrane-based test devices in either a dipstick or a flow-through immunofiltration format have been described (115–117). In the dipstick format, the antibody or antigen is immobilized to the end of a plastic stick or to a membrane adhered to the end of a stick. Performing the assay simply requires transferring the stick through the sample, the enzyme conjugate, and into the substrate. Rinsing can be done under tap water or with rinse solutions provided with the kit. Precipitation substrates can be used to form an insoluble color reaction over the active area of the dipstick. The test gives qualitative or semiquantitative results in less than 1 h. Compared to the corresponding microtiter plate tests, visual checks such as in the dipstick assay show a loss of sensitivity of up to orders of magnitude. However, many dipstick assays are also considerably less subject to matrix interferences and less affected by the solvent composition of the extract (118).

Several factors contribute to the higher detection limits of many on-site assay formats, probably the most important and self-explanatory being the fact that visual evaluation is less precise and sensitive than measuring absorbance with a photometer. This is particularly important in competitive immunochemical assays, in which the negative control has the most intense color and a relatively great reduction in color intensity is required between the negative control and positive samples to avoid misinterpretation by an untrained user. Therefore, the amount of antibody for coating the membrane as well as the concentration of the enzyme-labeled antigen have to be relatively high. However, this also reduces the sensitivity of a competitive immunochemical assay.

Considerable reduction of the assay time has been recently achieved by employing a membrane-based flow-through immunochemical device in which unbound reagents and sample matrices are removed by adsorption through use of a cellulose pad (119). This competitive enzyme-linked immunofiltration assay (ELIFA) is performed in an 8-well plastic test device into which antibody-coated nylon membranes have been pressed tightly to an adsorbent cellulose layer. Sample extract solution, enzyme–conjugate, and enzyme substrate–chromogen solution are sequentially added onto the membrane. The test can be evaluated visually by comparing the intensity of the resulting blue color to that of a negative control. Qualitative results can be obtained within 10 min. This type of assay finds its ideal application as an on-site test to detect the presence of the target molecule at a defined threshold level.

Today, immunochemical techniques have gone well beyond those originally employed. The area is growing quickly and new kits are increasingly appearing on the market. The range of applications seems almost endless, from those involved in ultrasensitive detection to zeptomole (10^{-21} moles) and even to yoctomole (10^{-24} moles) concentrations (120) to on-line immunoaffinity chromatography with coupled-column LC/MS detection starting with a crude extract (121).

Examples exist of different types of immunobased technology being interfaced to produce an effective analytical system. In a variety of recent methods, immunoaffinity chromatography has been employed for purification, chemiluminescence enzyme immunoassay has been used for quantification of salbutamol and clenbuterol in tissue and plasma from calves and pigs (122), clenbuterol in cattle hair (123), and monensin in chicken tissues (124). In these methods, quantification at sub-ppb levels has been demonstrated.

23.3 PHYSICOCHEMICAL TECHNIQUES

A literature survey shows that a great variety of physicochemical techniques are applied for analyzing drug residues in food. Unfortunately, no presently available physicochemical technique is as versatile or as universal as might be desired, nor is it likely that any such technique will be developed. Which type of detection principle should be used for a particular application depends on the physicochemical properties of the analyte, the sensitivity and selectivity required, and the convenience and versatility requested.

When evaluating detectors, several features should be considered to obtain optimum use of these devices. Detector noise is such a major feature that can be defined as the maximum amplitude of the combined high-frequency and short-term noise arising from instrument electronics, temperature fluctuations, line voltage surges, and other effects not directly attributable to the analyte. Detector noise is often given as the random baseline variation in units of detector response at a specified sensitivity, and it becomes most critical for sensing small peaks. The high-frequency noise appears as a fuzz and widens the baseline, while the short-term noise causes random baseline fluctuations appearing as random peaks and/or valleys on the baseline. Detector noise cannot be accurately determined unless the detector drift is small in relation to the magnitude of the noise. Detector drift is defined as a continuous up-scale or down-scale excursion of the baseline, which tends to hide both noise and small peaks.

Another feature of major interest is the detector sensitivity. This is the total change in a physical parameter required for a full-scale deflection at maximum detector sensitivity and at specified noise level. Detector sensitivity can be considered as a measure of the ability of the detector to differentiate between small differences in analyte concentration. Modern detectors have usually high sensitivities, often allowing detection of nanograms of analytes.

Selectivity is another highly desirable property of a detector. As a rule of thumb, the more selective the detection, the lower signal noise and the higher the sensitivity. A selective detector allows detection of only the analyte of interest in a chromatographic solute despite the potential copresence of many other compounds that coelute from the column. Eluted compounds are usually identified by comparing their retention time with those of reference compounds processed in an identical manner. However, retention behavior alone is not sufficient for positive identification since several compounds can frequently elute with the same retention time, constituting a chromatographic peak made up of several components. By rechromatographing the sample on a different packing material and/or using a different detection system, more convincing evidence can be obtained.

For a detector to be of use in quantitative analysis, the signal output should be linear with concentration for a concentration-sensitive detector and with mass for a mass-sensitive detector. Some detectors have an additional time constant purposely introduced to remove the high-frequency noise. This should always taken into consideration, since a slow detector response can significantly broaden and attenuate chromatographic peaks relative to those actually sensed. Moreover, a versatile detector should have a wide linear dynamic range so that major and trace components can be determined in a single analysis, over a wide concentration range.

Therefore, specific information is required on the characteristics of detectors to allow one to be selected for a particular application. In many cases, however, major performance characteristics of detectors such as noise, sensitivity, response, and linearity, are not presented in a standard format by suppliers. To complicate matters further, there are no published reference values for many of the properties utilized by different detectors for most analytes. Therefore, to determine whether a particular detector is adequate for a particular application, a similar analysis in the pertinent literature has to be found. Ultimately, the analyst will often have to test the detector under consideration on the analyte of interest itself.

23.3.1   Ultraviolet/Visible Photometric Detectors

The single most useful and versatile physicochemical detectors in drug residue analysis are probably those based on ultraviolet-visible (UV-Vis) spectrophotometry. These detectors allow a wide selection of detection wavelengths, thus offering high sensitivity for analytes that exhibit absorbance in either the ultraviolet or the visible region of the electromagnetic radiation.

Depending on its frequency, the electromagnetic radiation can interact with electrons, causing their excitation and transfer onto a higher energetical level; or can excite molecular bonds, causing their vibration or rotation of the functional groups. The UV region of the electromagnetic radiation corresponds to the excitation of the relatively low energy electrons such as π-electrons, or nonpaired electrons of some functional groups. For example, n-alkanes absorb in the UV region below 180 nm because σ-electrons require high-energy radiation to get excited and to show absorption of the radiation. On the other hand, any compounds having a benzene ring will show absorbance at 205–225 and 245–265 nm; the last absorbance corresponds to the excitation of conjugated π-electrons of the benzene ring.

The intensity of the radiation whose energy corresponds to the possible transitions decreases while it is passing through the detection cell. According to the Lambert-Bear law, absorbance of the radiation is proportional to the compound concentration and the length of the detection cell.

Most drugs used in animal production exhibit relatively high molar absorptivity within the UV absorption range, so that UV detection permits trace analysis to be made with high sensitivity. UV detectors are also ideal for use with LC gradient elution, and many common UV-transmitting solvents of varying solvent strength are available as LC mobile phases. A potential problem in using UV detectors operated at high sensitivity is distinguishing between sample peaks and pseudopeaks due to refraction effects that affect the detector signal. If the refractive index within the cell changes during an LC gradient elution, the amount of energy reaching the detector can change, because of refractive effects at the cell wall. Special designs, such as tapered cells or collimating and masking the light entering the cell, can reduce or eliminate such refractive effects.

Even though detection at the absorption maximum provides maximum sensitivity, it is sometimes more important to use the wavelength providing the highest selectivity, that is, maximum freedom from interferences. Despite revolutionary advances in LC technology, its complexity is too great for guaranteed chromatographic resolution of analytes from interfering components. Variable-wavelength UV spectrophotometric and diode-array detectors have been designed to allow for the best wavelength(s) to be selected for actual analysis. This is particularly important when no information is available on molar absorptivities at different wavelengths.

23.3.2 Fluorescence Spectroscopic Detectors

Drug residues in foods that strongly fluoresce can be more efficiently detected by fluorescence detectors. Typically, fluorescence sensitivity is 10–1000 times higher than that offered by a UV detector for strong UV-absorbing materials (125). Using a fluorescence detector, it has been possible to detect the presence of even a single analyte molecule in an LC flow cell. This type of detection is very versatile because of its ability to measure the intensity of the fluorescent radiation emitted from analytes excited by UV.

Compounds that are symmetrically conjugated and not strongly ionic often fluoresce. Most unsubstituted aromatic hydrocarbons fluoresce with quantum yield increasing with the number of rings, the degree of condensation, and the structural rigidity. The presence of conjugated π-electrons, especially in the aromatic components, gives the most intense fluorescent activity. Aliphatic and alicyclic compounds with carbonyl groups, and compounds with highly conjugated double bonds, also fluoresce but usually to a lesser degree.

Fluorescence detection has been proven to be a particularly valuable tool for analyzing drug residues in food. This is due to the fact that very few naturally occurring compounds exist that exhibit inherent fluorescence; only about 15% of all compounds exhibit natural fluorescence. Furthermore, selective fluorescence detection of the analytes can be made possible by suppressing the emission of interfering sample components, since the fluorescence intensity depends on both the excitation and emission wavelengths.

The general lack of inherent fluorescence in existing compounds, although it helps in eliminating interferences, frequently causes, application problems because there are not too many fluorescent drug residues. A possible solution to this problem is the preparation of fluorescent derivatives of the nonfluorescing analytes by specific fluorescence-labeling reactions.

Because of their high sensitivity, fluorescence detectors are particularly useful in trace analysis when either the sample size is small or the analyte concentration is extremely low. Although fluorescence detectors can become markedly nonlinear at concentrations where absorption detectors are still linear in response, their linear dynamic range is more than adequate for most trace analysis applications. Unfortunately, fluorometric detectors are often susceptible to background fluorescence and quenching effects that can plague all fluorescence measurements.

Currently available spectrofluorometers allow maximum flexibility in fluorometric detection. For example, fast switching of the excitation and emission wavelengths during an LC run offers the possibility to detect more than one analyte with different physicochemical properties in the same sample without need to repeat the analysis. Fluorescence line-narrowing spectroscopy (126) of analytes extracted from scraped TLC spots can help in determining their purity. Recent advantages in fluorometer technology, such the laser-induced fluorescence approach, hold great promise for extremely sensitive analytical applications in the future.

23.3.3   Electrochemical Detectors

Electrochemical detection is based on measurement of the current resulting from oxidation/reduction reactions of analytes at a suitable electrode as a function of the applied voltage. Since the level of the current is directly proportional to the analyte concentration, these detectors are used for both qualitative and quantitative purposes (127).

Electrochemical detection has become a popular LC choice that should be considered by the residue analyst because of the additional selectivity and sensitivity offered for some compounds. The areas of application of electrochemical detection are not large, but the compounds for which it does apply represent some of the most important drug classes.

An interesting feature of the electrochemical detection is its relatively small variation in sensitivity for various substances for which it responds. This relatively constant molar response is due to the small number of electrons, usually two or three, involved in electrochemical reactions. This feature is very convenient in trace analysis, because the analyst can predict the sample size, dilutions, and other manipulations that must be used to produce the desired analytical sensitivity.

The applicability of electrochemical detection in LC is frequently limited by the fact that the mobile phase must always be electrically conductive. In many cases, it is feasible to add a salt such as a buffer at suitable concentration in the mobile phase without affecting the separation. As an alternative, this problem can be circumvented by postcolumn addition of a suitable high-dielectric-constant solvent plus supporting electrolyte. An additional limitation that stems out from the electroactivity or not of the analyte can be overcome by pre- or postcolumn derivatization.

Detection is usually performed by connecting an electrochemical potentiostat to an electrochemical cell. Unlike potentiometry measurements, which employ only two electrodes, electrochemical measurements utilize a three-electrode electrochemical cell. The three-electrode system, comprising a working electrode, a reference electrode, and an auxiliary electrode, allows accurate application of potential functions and the measurement of the resultant current. Special electronic circuitry within the potentiostat permits the working electrode potential to be controlled with respect to the reference electrode without any appreciable current flowing at the reference electrode; rather, the current is forced to flow between the working electrode and the auxiliary electrode. By this unusual arrangement, the reference electrode is protected from internal electrochemical changes caused by current flow, whereas measurement errors related to the resistance of the test solution are kept to a minimum.

Several types of electrodes have been successfully used with electrochemical detectors including carbon-paste, glassy carbon, platinum, mercury, and gold. Most widely used is the carbon-paste electrode, which is inexpensive and has low residual current. All analytes that oxidize or reduce at the selected electrode potential can be detected. However, this electrode must be frequently standardized to maintain precise calibration because of changes that occur in its surface (128).

Although the carbon-paste electrode is quite effective for readily oxidizable analytes, a full range of electrochemical response is only available with the mercury electrode, particularly the versatile version called dropping mercury electrode. With this electrode, analyses are conducted at a frequently renewed mercury drop every second so that the electrochemical reactions always occur at a fresh surface. The flow pattern around the drop apparently eliminates many of the inherent problems that appeared with the conventional mercury electrodes.

There are a number of limitations in approaching maximum sensitivity with the dropping mercury electrode in the reductive mode. These include background currents from oxygen reduction and the reduction of trace metals originating mainly from LC mobile phases. Therefore, both oxygen and trace metals should be efficiently eliminated from the mobile phase prior to electrochemical detection; oxygen can be removed by rigorous degassing, whereas metals can be removed by adding ethylenediaminetetracetic acid complexing agent to the mobile phase. There is also a substantial contribution from capacitive current because the current is continuously measured during the growth of the mercury drop. As such, the typical signal to noise ratio allows detection limits of only approximately 10^{-5} or 10^{-6} M. Better discrimination against the capacitive current can be obtained using pulse polarographic techniques (129).

Pulse polarographic techniques are electrochemical measurements that try to minimize the background capacitive contribution to the current by eliminating the continuously varying potential ramp and replacing it with a series of potential steps of short duration. In normal-pulse polarography, each potential step begins at the same value, and the amplitude of each subsequent step increases in small increments. When the mercury drop is dislodged from the capillary, the potential is returned to the initial value in preparation for a new step. The normal-pulse polarography method increases the analytical sensitivity by 1–3 orders of magnitude reaching limits of detection of 10^{-7} to 10^{-8} M.

Many of the experimental parameters for normal-pulse polarography are the same as with differential-pulse polarography. Differential-pulse polarography is a technique that uses a series of discrete potential steps rather than a linear potential ramp to optimize specific applications (130). Unlike normal-pulse polarography, each potential step has the same amplitude, whereas the return potential after each pulse is slightly negative of the potential prior to the step. In this manner, the total waveform applied to the dropping mercury electrode is very much like a combination of a linear ramp with a superimposed square wave.

The differential-pulse polarogram is obtained by measuring the current immediately before the potential step, and then again just before the end of the drop lifetime. The analytical current in this case is the difference between the current at the end of the step and the current before the step that is the differential current. This differential current is then plotted against the average of the potential to obtain the differential-pulse polarogram. Because this is a differential current, the polarogram in many respects is like the differential of the sigmoidal normal-pulse polarogram. As a result, the differential-pulse polarogram is peak-shaped. Differential pulse polarography has even better ability to discriminate against capacitive current because it helps to subtract any residual capacitive current that remains prior to each step. Limits of detection with differential-pulse polarography are 10^{-8}–10^{-9} M.

Recent developments have led to a number of other electrochemical techniques. Each differs in the precise manner that the working electrode potential is changed during the measurement. Cyclic voltammetry is an electrolytic technique used to study electroactive species. It simultaneously generates and scans redox species over a wide potential range. In cyclic voltammetry, the working electrode potential is swept back and forth across the formal potential of the analyte. Repeated reduction and oxidation of the analyte causes alternating cathodic and anodic currents flow at the electrode. The solution is not stirred. The potential of the working electrode is controlled with respect to the reference electrode. The controlling potential applied across the two electrodes is called the excitation signal. This signal is a linear potential scan with a triangular waveform. The two values that this triangular potential excitation signal sweeps are called the switching potential. The current measured at the working electrode during the potential scan is the response signal (131). The voltammogram exhibits two asymmetrical peaks: one cathodic and the other anodic.

Anodic stripping voltammetry is another electrolytic method in which the mercury electrode is held at a negative potential to reduce metal ions in solution and form an amalgam with the electrode. The solution is stirred to carry as much of the analyte to the electrode as possible for concentration into the amalgam. After reducing and accumulating the analyte for some period of time, the potential on the electrode is increased to reoxidize the analyte and generate a current signal. The ramped potential usually uses a step function, such as in normal-pulse polarography (NPP) or differential-pulse polarography (DPP). The main advantage of stripping analysis is the preconcentration of the analyte into the electrode before making the actual current measurement. Limits of detection are as low as 10^{-10} M.

For the time being, applications of voltammetric techniques in the analysis of drug residues in edible animal products are very limited. Adsorptive-stripping voltammetry, which generally is a sensitive quantitative technique for the analysis of electroactive species, has been recently applied for rapid determination of sulfamethazine residues in milk (132). In this method, sulfamethazine is extracted from milk and diazotized at its primary amine group. The diazotized sulfamethazine is electrochemically adsorbed at pH 12 on a hanging mercury electrode to be further desorbed and monitored by applying a differential-pulse cathodic stripping potential. As the adsorption step on the electrified electrode preconcentrates the analyte that is to be subsequently desorbed, a detection limit as low as 3.8 ppb can be readily realized. Differential-pulse polarography has been also used for the determination of furaltadone in milk (133). After a simple deproteinization and extraction procedure, quantification of furaltadone in the acidified extract was made possible on the basis of the appearance of the first well-defined reduction-wave appeared.

23.3.4 Polarimetric Detectors

Substances that can rotate the orientation of plane-polarized light are said to have optical activity. Measurement of this change in polarization orientation is called polarimetry, and the measuring instrument is called a polarimeter.

The simplest polarimeter consists of a monochromatic light source, a polarizer, a sample cell, a second polarizer (which is called the analyzer), and a light detector. The analyzer is oriented 90 degrees to the polarizer so that no light reaches the detector. When an optically active substance is present in the beam, it rotates the polarization of the light reaching the analyzer so that there is a component that reaches the detector. The angle that the analyzer must be rotated to return to the minimum detector signal is the optical rotation.

Optical rotation occurs because optically active samples have different re-fractive indices for left- and right-circularly polarized light. Another way to make this statement is that left- and right-circularly polarized light travel through an optically active sample at different velocities. This condition occurs because a chiral center has a specific geometric arrangement of four different substituents, each of which has a different electronic polarizability. Light travels through matter by interacting with the electron clouds present. Left-circularly polarized light therefore interacts with an anisotropic medium differently than does right-circularly polarized light.

Linearly or plane-polarized light is the superposition of equal intensities of left- and right-circularly polarized light. As plane-polarized light travels through an optically active sample, the left- and right-circularly polarized components travel at different velocities. This difference in velocities creates a phase-shift between the two circularly polarized components when they exit the sample. Summing the two components still produces linearly polarized light, but at a different orientation from the light entering the sample.

The amount of optical rotation depends on the number of optically active species through which the light passes, and thus depends on both the sample path length and the analyte concentration. The optical rotatory dispersion is the optical rotation as a function of wavelength. It is recorded using a spectropolarimeter, which has a tungsten lamp and a scanning monochromator as the light source. A motorized mount rotates the analyzer to maintain a minimum signal at the detector. Usually a modulation is introduced into the polarization angle of the light beam, so that a DC signal to the analyzer motor then keeps the detector signal centered at the minimum value.

Polarimetric detectors have demonstrated significant advantages for identification of optically active drug residues because optical activity is an extremely rare characteristic usually associated with biological activity. Specific rotation measurements on drug residues as they elute from the LC column have the potential to identify closely related structural analogues even when present in a complicated food matrix. Laser-based polarimetric detection has been successfully applied to analyze milk samples containing erythromycin (134) or the four gentamicin analogues without prior derivatization (135). However, these systems have not been widely applied to the analysis of food materials since they are narrow in their application and cannot provide the unique structural information given by MS detectors.

23.3.5 Specific GC Detectors

The suite of gas chromatography detectors used in drug residues analysis includes, roughly in order from most common to the least, the flame ionization detector, electron capture detector, flame photometric detector, and nitrogen/phosphorus detector. All of these produce an electrical signal that varies with the amount of analyte exiting the chromatographic column. Different detectors will give different types of selectivity. The requirements of a GC detector depends on the separation application one analysis might require, for example, a detector that is selective for nitrogen-containing molecules; while another analysis might require a detector that is nondestructive so that the analyte can be recovered for further spectroscopic analysis.

GC detectors can be grouped into concentration-sensitive detectors and mass-sensitive detectors. The signal from a concentration-sensitive detector is related to the concentration of solute in the detector, which does not usually destroy the sample. Mass sensitive detectors usually destroy the sample, and the signal is related to the rate at which solute molecules enter the detector. The response of a mass-sensitive detector is unaffected by make-up gas, while that of a concentration-sensitive detector will lower with make-up gas. A summary of some important characteristics of the GC detectors specifically used in drug residue analysis is presented in Table 23.1.

The most common detector on commercial GC instruments is the flame-ionization detector (FID). This is a useful general detector for the analysis of organic compounds since it responds to any molecule with a carbon-hydrogen bond. FID consists of a hydrogen/air flame and a collector plate. The effluent from the GC column passes through the flame that breaks down organic molecules and produces ions and electrons that can conduct electricity through the flame. A collector electrode that located above the flame attracts the negative ions to the electrometer–amplifier, producing an analogue signal that is connected to the data system.

FID is mass-sensitive rather than concentration-sensitive detector; this gives the advantage that changes in mobile phase flow rate do not affect detector response. It offers high sensitivity, a large linear response range, and low noise. Its precision is high and is not susceptible to contamination from dirty samples

TABLE 23.1 Some Important Characteristics of the Gas Chromatography Detectors Specifically Used in Drug Residue Analysis

Type of detector	Category	Support gases	Selectivity	Detectability	Dynamic range
Flame ionization	Mass-sensitive	Hydrogen and air	Most organic compounds	100 pg	10^7
Electron capture	Concentration-sensitive	Make-up gas	Halides, nitrates, nitriles, peroxides, anhydrides, organometallics	50 fg	10^5
Nitrogen/phosphorus	Mass-sensitive	Hydrogen and air	Nitrogen or phosphorus-bearing compounds	10 pg	10^6
Flame photometric	Mass-sensitive	Hydrogen and air	Sulphur or phosphorus-bearing compounds	100 pg	10^3

or column bleed. FID is also robust and easy to use but, unfortunately, it destroys the sample.

The electron-capture detector (ECD) is as sensitive as the FID but has a limited dynamic range and finds its greatest application in analysis of organic molecules that contain electronegative functional groups, such as halogens, phosphorous, and nitro groups. It consists of a sealed stainless steel cylinder containing radioactive ^{63}Ni. This radioactive material emits electrons that collide with the carrier molecules, ionizing them in the process. This forms a stable cloud of free electrons in the ECD cell. When organic molecules that contain electronegative functional groups, such as halogens, phosphorous, and nitro groups, pass by the detector, they immediately capture some of the electrons, temporarily reducing the number remaining in the electron cloud. The detector electronics, which maintain a constant current of about 1 nanoampere through the electron cloud, are forced to pulse at a faster rate to compensate for the decreased number of the cloud electrons. The pulse rate is converted to an analogue output connected to the data system.

The flame-photometric detector (FPD) is similar to the FID except that the detector body is completely light-tight and a second flow of hydrogen purges the optical path between the photomultiplier tube and a hydrogen-rich flame. FPD can achieve selective and highly sensitive detection of sulfur or phosphorus-bearing compounds since it uses chemiluminescent reactions of these compounds in a hydrogen/air flame as a source of analytical information that is relatively specific for substances containing these two kinds of atoms. The phosphorous response is linear, but the sulfur response is exponential: twice the sulfur yields four times the peak area.

The emitting species for sulfur compounds is excited S_2. The lambda maximum for emission of excited S_2 is approximately 394 nm. The emitter for phosphorus compounds in the flame is excited HPO with a lambda maximum equal to doublet 510–526 nm. In order to detect one or the other family of compounds selectively as it elutes from the GC column, the suitable band-pass filter should be placed between the flame and the photomultiplier tube to isolate the appropriate emission band. In addition, a thermal infrared filter is mounted between the flame and the photomultiplier tube to isolate only the visible and UV radiation emitted by the flame. Without this filter, the large amounts of infrared radiation emitted by the combustion reaction of the flame would heat up the photomultiplier tube, thus increasing its background signal.

The nitrogen/phosphorus detector (NPD) features a new generation in source technology. This detector is similar in design to the FID, except that the hydrogen flow rate is reduced to about 3 ml/min. An electrically heated ceramic thermionic source embedded with an alkali metal catalyst is positioned near the jet orifice; nitrogen or phosphorus-containing molecules exiting the column collide with the hot source and undergo a catalytic surface chemistry reaction. The ions created in this reaction are attracted to a collector electrode, which are then amplified and output to the data system.

NPD gives a linear response, has a wide dynamic range, and provides sensitivity at picogram levels that is stable over time, producing more reliable results. The detector offers greater stability and ease of operation with a self-aligning source.

23.3.6   Mass Spectrometric Detectors

Among the available detectors, mass spectrometric (MS) ones are probably the most powerful for providing structural information about molecules. MS detectors use the difference in mass-to-charge ratio (m/z) of ionized atoms or molecules to separate them from each other. Molecules have distinctive fragmentation patterns that provide structural information to allow one to identify structural components.

In general, all mass spectrometers share at least three distinct structures: the source, the analyzer, and the detector. Differences in these three structures identify the multitude of MS systems. The source is perhaps the most crucial element of the mass spectrometer. Therefore, the selection of the source primarily differentiates the various MS systems. Although specific analyzers or detectors may be preferable for a particular MS application, mass spectrometrists will often refer to different systems solely by the source. Only occasionally, when a time-of-flight mass analyzer is used, for example, analysts refer to the method by the type of the mass analyzer.

MS operation is based on magnetic and electric fields that exert forces on charged ions in a vacuum. Therefore, a compound must be charged or ionized in the source to be introduced in the gas phase into the vacuum system of the MS. This is easily attainable for gaseous or heat-volatile samples. However, many thermally labile analytes may decompose upon heating. Such samples require either desorption or desolvation methods if they are to be analyzed by MS. Although ionization and desorption/desolvation are usually separate processes, the term "ionization method" is commonly used to refer to both ionization and desorption or desolvation methods.

The choice of the ionization method depends on both the nature of the sample and the type of information required from the analysis (Table 23.2). A great variety of ionization methods exists that can be classified into six major categories: gas-phase ionization, field desorption and ionization, particle bombardment, atmospheric pressure ionization, and the laser desorption.

Ionization methods such as electron impact, chemical ionization, desorption chemical ionization, and negative-ion chemical ionization are all based on ionization of gas-phase samples and, thus, fall within the first category of gas-phase ionization.

TABLE 23.2 Ionization Methods Commonly Used in Mass Spectrometry

Method	Sample introduction	Advantages	Limitations	Mass range (daltons)
Electron impact	Heated batch inlet Heated direct insertion probe GC LC (particle-beam interface)	Application to all volatile compounds Reproducible mass spectra Fragmentation provides structural information Mass spectra libraries can be searched for EI "fingerprint"	Samples thermally volatile and stable Molecular ion weak or absent for many compounds	Low (<1000)
Chemical ionization	Heated batch inlet Heated direct insertion probe GC LC (particle-beam interface)	Gives molecular weight information even when EI would not produce a molecular ion Simple mass spectra, fragmentation reduced compared to EI	Samples thermally volatile and stable Less fragmentation that EI, fragment pattern not informative or reproducible enough for library search Results depend on reagent gas type and pressure, or reaction time and nature of sample	Low (<1000)
Desorption chemical ionization	Sample deposition onto a filament wire Filament rapidly heated inside the CI source	Reduced thermal decomposition Rapid analysis Relatively simple equipment	Not particularly reproducible Rapid heating requires fast scan speeds Fails for large or labile compounds	Low (<1500)

(continued)

TABLE 23.2 Continued

Method	Sample introduction	Advantages	Limitations	Mass range (daltons)
Negative-ion chemical ionization	Heated batch inlet Heated direct insertion probe GC LC (particle-beam interface)	Efficient ionization, high sensitivity Less fragmentation than positive-ion EI or CI Greater selectivity for certain biologically important compounds	Not all volatile compounds produce negative ions Poor reproducibility	Low (<1000)
Field desorption	Direct insertion probe Deposition of the sample by dipping the emitter into an analyte solution Deposition of the sample onto the emitter with a microsyringe	Simple mass spectra Little or no chemical background Works well for small organic molecules, and low-molecular-weight polymers	Sensitive to alkali metal contamination and sample overloading Emitter is relatively fragile Relatively slow analysis as the emitter current is increased Samples thermally volatile to some extent to be desorbed	Low-moderate (2000–3000) Some examples with masses >1000
Field ionization	Heated direct insertion probe Gas inlet Gas chromatograph	Simple mass spectra Little or no chemical background Works well for small organic molecules and some petrochemical fractions	Samples thermally volatile	Low (<1000)

Fast atom bombardment	Direct insertion probe LC-MS (frit FAB or continuous-flow FAB)	Rapid and simple Relatively tolerant of variations in sampling Suitable for a large variety of compounds Strong ion currents—suitable for high-resolution measurements	High chemical background Difficult to distinguish low-molecular-weight compounds from chemical background Analyte soluble in the liquid matrix Not suitable for multicharged compounds with more than 2 charges	Moderate (300–6000)
Liquid secondary ion mass spectrometry	Direct insertion probe LC-MS (frit FAB or continuous-flow FAB)	Rapid Simple More sensitivity than FAB for higher masses (3000–13000 Da) Relatively tolerant of variations in sampling Works well for a large variety of compounds Strong ion currents—good for high-resolution measurements	High chemical background Difficult to distinguish low-molecular-weight compounds from chemical background Analyte soluble in the liquid matrix Not suitable for multicharged compounds with more than 2 charges Target can get hotter than in FAB, due to more energetic primary beam High-voltage arcs more common than FAB Ion source requires more maintenance than FAB	Moderate (300–13,000)

(continued)

TABLE 23.2   Continued

Method	Sample introduction	Advantages	Limitations	Mass range (daltons)
Electrospray ionization	Flow injection LC-MS Typical flow rates range from ,<1 μl/min to 1ml/ min	Suitable for charged, polar or basic compounds Detection of high-mass compounds at mass-to-charge ratios <2000–3000 Best method for analyzing multicharged compounds Very low chemical background Can control presence or absence of fragmentation by controlling the interface lens potentials Compatible with MS-MS methods	Multiply charged species require interpretation and mathematical transformation Complementary to APCI. No good for uncharged, nonbasic, low-polarity compounds Very sensitive to contaminants (alkali metals or basic compounds) Relatively low ion currents Relatively complex hardware compared to other ion sources	Low-high (<200,000)

	Sample introduction	Advantages	Limitations	Mass range
Atmospheric pressure chemical ionization	Flow injection LC-MS Typical flow rates range from <1 μl/min to 1ml/min	Works well for less-polar compounds Excellent LC-MS interface Compatible with MS-MS methods	Multicharged species require interpretation and mathematical transformation Complementary to APCI. No good for uncharged, non-basic, low-polarity compounds Very sensitive to contaminants (alkali metals or basic compounds) Relatively low ion currents Relatively complex hardware compared to other ion sources	Low-moderate (<2000)
Matrix-assisted laser desorption ionization	Direct insertion probe Continuous-flow introduction	Rapid and convenient molecular weight determination	MS-MS difficult Requires a mass analyzer compatible with pulsed ionization techniques Not easily compatible with LC-MS	Very high (<500,000)

Electron impact (EI), also referred to as electron ionization, is the oldest and best characterized of all the ionization techniques. A beam of electrons, usually generated from a tungsten filament, passes through the gas-phase sample. An electron that collides with a neutral analyte molecule can knock off another electron, resulting in a positively charged ion. The ionization process can either produce a molecular ion that will have the same molecular weight and elemental composition of the starting analyte, or it can produce a fragment ion that corresponds to a smaller piece of the analyte molecule.

Chemical ionization (CI) uses a reagent ion to react with the analyte molecules to form ions by either a proton or hydride transfer. Reagent ions are produced by introducing a large excess of gas, such as methane, into an EI ion source. Electron collisions produce CH_4^+ and CH_3^+, which further react with methane to form CH_5^+ and $C_2H_5^+$.

Desorption chemical ionization (DCI) is a variation on chemical ionization in which the analyte is placed on a filament that is rapidly heated in the CI plasma. The direct exposure to the CI reagent ions, combined with the rapid heating, acts to reduce fragmentation. Some samples that cannot be thermally desorbed without decomposition can be characterized by the fragments produced by pyrolysis desorption chemical ionization.

In negative-ion chemical ionization (NCI), a buffer gas such as methane is used to slow down the electrons in the electron beam until some of the electrons have just the right energy to be captured by the analyte molecules. The buffer gas can also help in stabilizing the energetic anions and reduce fragmentation. This is really a physical process and not a true CI process.

In NCI, negative ions can be produced by a number of processes. Resonance electron capture refers to the capture of an electron by a neutral molecule to produce a molecular anion. The electron energy is very low, and the specific energy required for electron capture depends on the molecular structure of the analyte. Electron attachment is an endothermic process, so the resulting molecular anion will have excess energy. Some molecular anions can accommodate the excess energy. Others may lose the electron or fall apart to produce fragment anions. Not all compounds will produce negative ions. However, many important compounds of biological interest can produce negative ions under the right conditions. For such compounds, NCI is more efficient, sensitive, and selective than positive-ion mass spectrometry.

Ionization methods such as field desorption and field ionization tend to produce mass spectra with little or no fragment-ion and, thus, fall within the second category of field desorption and ionization.

In field desorption (FD), the sample is deposited onto the emitter, a high voltage is applied, and a current is passed through the emitter to heat up the filament. Mass spectra are acquired as the emitter current is gradually increased and the sample is evaporated from the emitter into the gas phase. The analyte molecules are ionized by electron tunneling at the tip of the emitter "whiskers" and characteristic positive ions are produced.

In field ionization (FI), a very high electric field is created by applying a high voltage between a cathode and an anode called a field emitter. The sample is evaporated from a direct insertion probe, gas chromatograph, or gas inlet, and as the gas molecules pass near the emitter, they are ionized by losing an electron.

Fast-atom bombardment (FAB) and liquid secondary-ion mass spectrometry (LSIMS) methods make up the category of the particle bombardment ionization. In both methods the analyte is dissolved in a liquid such as glycerol, thioglycerol, m-nitrobenzyl alcohol, or diethanolamine and about 1 μl is placed on a target that is bombarded with atoms, neutrals, or ions.

In FAB a high-energy beam of neutral atoms such as Xe or Ar strikes a solid sample, causing desorption and ionization. It is used for large biological molecules that are difficult to get into the gas phase. FAB causes little fragmentation and usually gives a large molecular ion peak, making it useful for molecular weight determination.

LSIMS is nearly identical to FAB except that the primary particle beam is an ion beam, usually cesium ions, rather than a neutral beam. The ions can be focused and accelerated to higher kinetic energies than are possible for neutral beams, and sensitivity is improved for higher masses.

Ionization methods such as electrospray, ionspray, and atmospheric pressure chemical ionization, in which the analyte is sprayed at atmospheric pressure into an interface to the vacuum of the MS ion source, constitute the category of the atmospheric pressure ionization.

In electrospray ionization (ESI) a solution containing the analyte is sprayed at atmospheric pressure from a narrow-bore capillary into an orifice in the interface to the vacuum of the mass spectrometer ion source. Nebulization is due to the action of a high electric field resulting from a potential difference between the capillary and a surrounding counter electrode. The solvent emerging from the capillary breaks into fine threads that subsequently disintegrate in small droplets. The formed droplets carry charge and, as the solvent evaporates, the droplets disappear leaving highly charged analyte molecules. A combination of thermal and pneumatic means is used to desolvate the ions as they enter the ion source. In some designs, the electrospray nebulization is assisted by pneumatic nebulization. Such an approach is the so-called ionspray ionization (ISP).

In atmospheric pressure chemical ionization (APCI) a similar interface to that used for ESI is used. A corona discharge is used to ionize the analyte in the atmospheric pressure region. The gas-phase ionization in APCI is more effective than ESI for analyzing less polar species. Both ESI and APCI are complementary methods that are well-suited for LC/MS techniques.

The fifth category of ionization includes the laser ionization mass spectrometry (LIMS) methods. Matrix-assisted laser desorption ionization (MALDI) uses a pulsed laser to desorb species from a target surface. The analyte is dissolved in a solution containing an excess of a matrix such as sinapinic acid or dihydroxybenzoic acid that has a chromophore that absorbs at the laser wavelength. A small amount of this solution is placed on the laser target. The matrix absorbs the energy from the laser pulse and produces a plasma that results in vaporization and ionization of the analyte. The mechanism of ion formation within MALDI generally is considered to be analogous to that of FAB and LSIMS processes, except that a high-energy photon impinges on the sample-containing matrix rather than a high-energy atom or ion. The exact mechanism of ion formation is not fully understood. MALDI has become extremely popular as a method for the rapid determination of high-molecular-weight compounds.

After the analytes are ionized in the source of the MS, ions of discrete m/z ratios are separated and focused in the mass analyzer. Many types of mass analyzers are available, including the quadrupole, ion-trap, magnetic sector, time-of-flight (TOF), and Fourier-transform ion cyclotron resonance (FTICR) devices. The major differences between these mass analyzers are the degree of resolution and the upper mass range, which follow, generally, the order Fourier-transform (about 10^6 Da full width at half maximum form (FWHM) > magnetic sector (about 10^4 Da FWHM) > quadrupole and Ion-trap (about 1 Da FWHM) > TOF (about 0.1% FWHM of m/z) and TOF (no upper limit) > magnetic sector (about 10^4 Da) > Fourier-transform (about 8000 Da) > quadrupole (1000–4000Da) > ion-trap (850 Da), respectively.

The most commonly used mass analyzers are the Ion-trap, quadrupole, and TOF. The ion-trap uses a three-electrode system consisting of a ring electrode separating two hemispherical electrodes to trap the ionized fragments for a short period after their formation. Then the ions are ejected from the ion-trap one mass at a time. Sweeping the electrode voltages to select a range of sequential masses produces a mass spectrum in the electron-multiplier detector. The advantages of the ion-trap include compact size and the ability to trap and accumulate ions to increase the signal to noise ratio of a measurement.

In the quadrupole mass analyzer, focusing electrodes direct and accelerate the ionized fragments into a mass filter consisting of four cylindrical electrodes in a vacuum. The cylindrical electrodes establish a combination radio-frequency and direct-current electrical field that permits only those ions with a specific, selected mass-to-charge ratio to pass all the way through the filter. The rest of the ions impact the electrodes and do not travel to the exit. Varying the electrical field allows ions with other masses to pass through the filter.

The TOF mass analyzer uses the differences in transmit time through a drift region to separate ions of different masses. It operates in a pulsed mode, so ions must be produced or extracted in pulses. An electric field accelerates all ions into a field-free drift region, and lighter ions have a higher velocity than heavier ions and reach the detector at the end of the drift region sooner.

As with mass analyzers, many types of mass detectors equipped with an electron multiplier are available. Most common mass detectors are the channeltron, Daly detector, electron multiplier tubes, and the Faraday cup. All generate a current when charged analytes generated in the source and separated in the analyzer impinge on them. This current is recorded as a function of the masses selected by the electrical-field settings.

In the selective ion monitoring (SIM) mode, the mass spectrometer detector monitors only one mass value. This selectivity is sufficient to detect one compound or group of compounds that shares a common molecular fragment. By rapidly jumping the selected mass from one value to another repeatedly during analyte elution, the mass spectrometric detector provides abundance information for more than one mass across the peak width. This multiple-ion monitoring mode produces a number of selected-ion chromatograms simultaneously that may be very useful when two peaks in a chromatogram overlap. Monitoring masses unique to each peak deconvolutes the peaks and makes the independent determination of their areas possible. If the chromatogram includes unknown peaks or if peaks must be identified unambiguously, repeated scanning of the mass analyzer over a range of masses will acquire a series of complete mass spectra during analyte elution.

In the case of full-range mass spectral acquisition, the recorder records a mass spectrum at regular intervals throughout the chromatogram. The sum of the mass intensities across one mass spectrum represents the total ion current during the interval in which the mass spectrum was recorded. A series of total-ion currents displayed as a function of the elution time produces a total-ion chromatogram that is analogous to the signal of a common general detector.

MS sensitivity depends on both the type of instrumentation and the nature of the analytes, but, typically, a minimum sample size of 5–10 ng is in most cases sufficient. Limited sensitivity in a certain application is often not due to the inherent sensitivity of the MS but rather the level of background impurities that are in the isolate. It is not always appreciated that very slowly eluting LC solutes from previous separations can create substantial MS background peaks that obscure analyte identification. Thus, it is important to use a blank sample to ensure that the background of the trapped fraction is adequately free of possible interferences to the desired identification.

REFERENCES

1. P.S. Watts and D. McLeod, J. Comp. Pathol. Ther., 56:170 (1946).
2. S. Jorgensen, Nord. Mejeri Tdsskr., 14:141 (1948).
3. F.J. Weirether, D.E. Jasper, and W.E. Petersen, Proc. Soc. Exp. Biol. Med., 59: 282 (1945).
4. C.A.V. Barker, and H.P. Dussault, Can. J. Comp. Med. Vet. Sci., 9:332 (1945).

5. W.T.S. Thorp, I.J. Uhrik, and E.J. Straley, Am. J. Vet. Res., 8:157 (1947).
6. M. Welsh, P.H. Langer, R.L. Burkhardt, and C.R. Schroeder, Science, 108:185 (1948).
7. G. Slavin, Proc. Soc. Med., 39:793 (1946).
8. I.A. Schipper and W.E. Petersen, Vet. Med., 46:222 (1951).
9. J. Jacquet and L. Steeg, Ann. Falsi Fraudes, 46:5 (1953).
10. J.E. Grady and W.L. Williams, Antibiot. Chemother. 3:158 (1953).
11. J. Kramer, G.G. Carter, B. Arret, J. Wilner, W.W. Wright, and A. Kirshbaum, in Antibiotic Residues in Milk, Dairy Products, and Animal Tissues: Methods, Reports, and Protocols, Food and Drug Administration, Government Printing Office, Washington, D.C., Item 344-837 (4008) (1968).
12. I.A. Schipper and W.E. Petersen, Am. J. Vet. Res., 15:475 (1954).
13. R.T. Igarashi, R.W. Baughman, F.E. Nelson, and P.A. Hartman, J. Dairy Sci., 43: 841 (1960).
14. A.T. Johns, F.H. McDowall, and W.A. McGillivray, N.Z. J. Agr. Res., 2:62 (1959).
15. P.C. Trussel, and W.G. Stevenson, Can. J. Comp. Med. Vet. Sci., 13:209 (1949).
16. A.R. Drury, Conv. Proc. Milk Ind. Foundation, 1951:62 (1951).
17. J. Cerny and R.L. Morris, J. Milk Food Technol., 18:281 (1955).
18. W. Gogas and A.K. Bicknell, Milk Plant Monthly, 42:26 (1953).
19. C.K. Johns, J. Milk Food Technol., 23:266 (1960).
20. F.V. Kosikowski and R.A. Ledford, J. Dairy Sci., 43:842 (1960).
21. D. Levowitz, Am. Milk Rev., 22:17 (1960).
22. G.J. Silverman and F.V. Kosikowski, J. Milk Food Technol., 15:120 (1952).
23. A.G. Wolin and F.V. Kosikowski, J. Dairy Sci., 38:597 (1955).
24. A.G. Wolin and F.V. Kosikowski, J. Dairy Sci., 41:34 (1958).
25. A. Pital, D.T. Disque, and J.M. Leise, Antibiot. Chemother. 6:351 (1956).
26. D.C. Grove, and W.A. Randall, in Assay Methods of Antibiotics—A Laboratory Manual (D.C. Grove, and W.A. Randall, Eds.), Medical Encyclopedia, Inc., NY (1955).
27. V. Trecanni, Ann. Microbiol., 5:93 (1953).
28. K.M. Shahani and M.C. Badami, J. Dairy Sci., 40:602 (1957).
29. K.M. Shahani and M.C. Badami, J. Dairy Sci., 41:1510 (1958).
30. F.V. Kosikowski, Science, 126:844 (1957).
31. A.G. Mathews and N.D. Hesketh, Aust. J. Dairy Technol., 10:158 (1955).
32. C.R. Smith, W.E. Petersen, and R.W. Brown, Proc. Soc. Exptl. Biol. Med., 68:216 (1948).
33. J. Pien, J. Lignac, and P. Claude, Ann. Falsi Fraudes, 46:258 (1953).
34. L.R. Mattick, E.O. Anderson, and H.L. Williams, J. Dairy Sci., 38:829 (1955).
35. H.R. Whitehead and G.A. Cox, J. Appl. Bact., 19:247 (1956).
36. P. Dopter, Lait, 37:20 (1957).
37. N.J. Berridge, J. Dairy Sci., 23:336 (1956).
38. E.B. Collins, Milk Prod. J., 48:48 (1957).
39. T.E. Galesloot, Milk Dairy J., 9:158 (1955).
40. C.E. Neal and H.E. Calbert, Milk Prod. J., 47:14 (1956).
41. L. Kotter and H. Muspack, Milchwissenschaft, 134:122 (1958).

42. B. Arret and A. Kirshbaum, J. Milk Food Technol., 22:329 (1959).
43. C.K. Johns and I. Berzins, J. Milk Food Technol., 19:14 (1956).
44. F.V. Kosikowski, R.W. Henningson, and G.F. Silverman, J. Dairy Sci., 35:533 (1952).
45. E.H. Marth, F.J. Alexander, and R.V. Hussong, J. Milk Food Technol., 26:150 (1963).
46. O.W. Parks and F.J. Doan, J. Milk Food Technol., 22:7414 (1959).
47. F.A. Siino, R.B. Czarnecki, and W.K. Harris, J. Milk Food Technol., 21:211 (1958).
48. F.V. Kosikowski, J. Dairy Sci., 46:95 (1963).
49. W.W. Wright, J. Assoc. Off. Anal. Chem., 45:301 (1962).
50. R.T. Igarashi, R.W. Baughman, and F.E. Nelson, J. Milk Food Technol., 24:143 (1961).
51. J.J. Gavin, Appl. Microbiol., 5:25 (1956).
52. A. Carlsson and L. Bjorck, Milchwissenschaft, 42:282 (1987).
53. F.V. Thompson, Acta Pathol. Microbiol. Scand., 61:303 (1964).
54. W.W. Wright, J. Assoc. Off. Anal. Chem., 53:219 (1970).
55. J. Kraack and A. Tolle, Milchwissenschaft, 22:669 (1967).
56. J.L. Van Os, S.A. Lameris, J. Doodewaard, and J.G. Oostendorn, Neth. Milk Dairy J., 29:16 (1975).
57. R. Gudding, Acta Vet. Scand., 17:458 (1976).
58. R.W. Johnston, R.H. Reamer, E.W. Harris, H.G. Fugate, and B. Schwab, J. Food Prot., 44:828 (1981).
59. G.A. Korsrud, J.M. Naylor, C.D. Salisbury, and J.D. MacNeil, J. Agric. Food Chem., 35:556 (1987).
60. G.O. Korsrud and J.D. MacNeil, J. Food Prot., 51:43 (1988).
61. S.F. Sundlof, Bovine Pract., 25:15 (1990).
62. J.D. MacNeil, G.O. Korsrud, J.O. Boison, M.G. Papich, and W.D.G. Yates, J. Food Prot. 54:37 (1991).
63. G.O. Korsrud, J.M. Naylor, C.D. Salisbury, A.C.E. Fesser, and J.D. MacNeil, J. Food Prot., 58:1129 (1995).
64. H.N. Eisen, in Immunology (H.N. Eisen, Ed.), Harper and Row Publishers, Maryland, USA, p. 391 (1974).
65. J.J. Ryan, E.E. Wildman, A.H. Duthie, and H.V. Atherton, J. Dairy Sci., 69:1510 (1986).
66. S.J. Steiner, Ph.D. Thesis, Rutgers University, New Brunswick, N.J. (1981).
67. S.J. Steiner and J.N. Harris, in Analysis of Antibiotic/Drug Residues in Food Products of Animal Origin (V.K. Agarwal, Ed.), Plenum Press, New York, p. 23 (1992).
68. D. Catty, G. Murphy, in Antibodies Volume II—A Practical Approach (D. Catty, Ed.), IRL Oxford University Press, Oxford, England (1989).
69. R.J. Heitzman, in Analysis of Food Contaminants (J. Gilbert, Ed.), Elsevier Applied Science Publishers, Ltd., London (1984).
70. A.C. Hoek and P.R. Beljaars, Ware(n)-Chem. 19:37 (1989).
71. D. Arnold, D. vom Berg, A.K. Boertz, U. Mallick, and A. Somogyi, Arch. Lebensmittelhyg., 35:131 (1984).
72. D. Arnold and A. Somogyi, J. Assoc. Off. Anal. Chem., 68:984 (1985).

73. C. Hock and F. Liemann, Arch. Lebensmittelhyg., 36:138 (1985).
74. A.K. Boertz, D. Arnold, and A. Somogyi, Z. Ernahrungswiss., 24:113 (1985).
75. F. Scherk and O. Agthe, Arch. Lebensmittelhyg., 37:146 (1986).
76. O. Agthe and F. Scherk, Arch. Lebensmittelhyg., 37:97 (1986).
77. M. Beck, E. Martlbauer, and G. Terplan, Arch. Lebensmittclhyg., 38:99 (1987).
78. J. Pohlschmidt, I. Ulbrich, and A. Wissel-Monkemeyer, Arch. Lebensmittelhyg., 43:3 (1992).
79. N.S. Haddad, W.R. Ravis, W.M. Pedersoli, and R.L. Carson, Am. J. Vet. Res., 48: 21 (1987).
80. S.G. Schulman, G. Hochhaus, and H.T. Karnes, Pract. Spectrosc., 12:341 (1991).
81. T.M. Li and R.F. Parrish, Top. Fluoresc. Spectrosc., 3:273 (1992).
82. A.T.R. Williams and D.S. Smith, in Methods of Immunological Analysis, Vol. I (W.H.W. Albert and N.A. Staines, Eds.), VCH, Wolnheim (1992).
83. E. Koller, Appl. Fluoresc. Technol., 3:26 (1991).
84. R. Bredehorst, G.A. Wemhoff, A.W. Kusterbeck, P.T. Charles, R.B. Thompson, F.S. Ligler, and C.W. Vogel, Anal. Biochem., 193:272 (1991).
85. T.A. Kelly, C.A. Hunter, D.C. Schindele, and B.V. Pepich, Clin. Chem., 37:1283 (1991).
86. J.A.F. de Silva, J. Chromatogr., 340:3 (1985).
87. M.E. Jolley, S.D. Stroupe, K.S. Schwenzer, C.J. Wang, M. Lu-Steffes, H.D. Hill, S.R. Popelka, J.T. Holen, and D.M. Kelso, Clin. Chem., 27:1575 (1981).
88. S.A. Brown, D.R. Newkirk, R.P. Hunter, G.S. Smith, and K. Sugimoto, J. Assoc. Off. Anal. Chem., 73:479 (1990).
89. A. Vlietstra, D. Masman, and O. Steijger, in Residues of Veterinary Drugs in Food, Proc. Euroresidue II Conf., Veldhoven, May 3–5, 1993 (N. Haagsma, A. Ruiter, and P.B. Czedik-Eysenberg, Eds.), Fac. Vet. Med., Univ. Utrecht, The Netherlands, p. 670 (1993).
90. S.A. Eremin, J. Landon, D.S. Smith, and R. Jackman, in Food Safety and Quality Assurance: Applications of Immunoassay Systems (M.R.A. Morgan, C.J. Smith, and P.A. Williams, Eds.), Elsevier Applied Science, London, p. 119 (1992).
91. M. Maeda, and A. Tsuji, Farumashia, 27:1149 (1991).
92. Y. Tatsu, Bio. Ind., 9:454 (1992).
93. G. Zomer, J.F.C. Stavenuiter, R.H. van de Berg, and E.H.J.M. Jansen, Pract. Spectrosc., 12:505 (1991).
94. S. Batmanghelich, R.C. Brown, J.S. Woodhead, I. Weeks, and K. Smith, J. Photochem. Photobiol., 12:193 (1992).
95. C. Lindbladh, K. Mosbach, and L. Buelow, J. Immunol. Methods, 137:199 (1991).
96. L.J. Kricka and X. Ji, Anal. Sci., 7:1501 (1991).
97. B.B. Kim, V.V. Pisarev, and A.M. Egorov, Anal. Biochem., 199:1 (1991).
98. S.E. Katz, in Agricultural Uses of Antibiotics (W.A. Moats, Ed.), ACS Symposium Series 320, American Chemical Society, Washington, DC, p. 142 (1986).
99. N. Haagsma and C. van de Water, in Analysis of Antibiotic/Drug Residues in Food Products of Animal Origin (V.K. Agarwal, Ed.), Plenum Press, New York, p. 81 (1992).
100. D.E. Dixon-Holland, in Analysis of Antibiotic/Drug Residues in Food Products of Animal Origin (V.K. Agarwal, Ed.), Plenum Press, New York, p. 57 (1992).

101. G. Ragupathi, P. Prabhasankar, P.C. Sekharan, K.S. Annapoorani, and C. Damodaran, Hind. Antibiot. Bull., 34:13 (1992).
102. S. Sarkar, K.B. De, G.M. Bhopate, and S.R. Nalk, Hind. Antibiot. Bull., 34:16 (1992).
103. A.I. MacLean and L.G. Bachas, Anal. Biochem., 195:303 (1991).
104. K. Tateishi, H. Yamamoto, T. Ogihara, and C. Hayashi, Steroids, 30:25 (1977).
105. J. Carlsson, H. Drevin, and R. Axen, Biochem. J., 173:723 (1978).
106. C. Blake and B.J. Gould, Analyst, 109:533 (1984).
107. C.J. van Oss and J.M. Singer, Res. J. Reticuloendothel. Soc., 3:29 (1966).
108. S. Kochwa, M. Brownell, R.E. Rosenfield, and L.R. Wasserman, J. Immunol., 99: 981 (1967).
109. C. van de Water, in Development of Immunochemical Procedures for the Analysis of Chloramphenicol Residues in Food of Animal Origin, Thesis, University of Utrecht, The Netherlands (1990).
110. T. Porstmann, B. Porstmann, and R. Seifert, Clin. Chim. Acta, 129:107 (1983).
111. J. Guesdon, T. Ternynck, and S. Avrameas, J. Histochem. Cytochem., 27:1131 (1979).
112. M. Wilchek and E.A. Bayer, Anal. Biochem., 171:1 (1988).
113. C.J. Stanley, A. Johannsson, and C.H. Self, J. Immunol. Methods, 83:89 (1985).
114. R.I. Carr, M. Mansour, D. Sadi, H. James, and J.V. Jones, J. Immunol. Methods, 98:201 (1987).
115. E. Schneider, E. Usleber, R. Dietrich, E. Martlbauer, and G. Terplan, in Residues of Veterinary Drugs in Food, Proc. Euroresidue II Conf., Veldhoven, May 3–5, 1993 (N. Haagsma, A. Ruiter, and P.B. Czcdik-Eysenberg, Eds.), Fac. Vet. Med., Univ. Utrecht, The Netherlands, p. 627 (1993).
116. E. Schneider, E. Usleber, S. Ostermaier, R. Dietrich, E. Martlbauer, and G. Terplan, Abstracts of the 107th Annual AOAC Meeting, AOAC, Washington, DC, Abstr. 49 (1993).
117. E. Schneider, E. Martlbauer, R. Dietrich, E. Usleber, and G. Terplan, Arch. Lebensmittelhyg., 45:43 (1994).
118. E. Schneider, E. Usleber, and R. Dietrich, Arch. Lebensmittelhyg., 43:36 (1992).
119. E. Martlbauer, E. Usleber, E. Schneider, and R. Dietrich, Analyst, 119:2543 (1994).
120. L.J. Lricka, J. Clin. Immunoassay, 16:267 (1993).
121. G. Rule, A.V. Mordehai, and J. Henion, Anal. Chem., 66:230 (1994).
122. K. Pou, H. Ong, and A. Adam, Analyst, 119:2659 (1994).
123. M.A.J. Godfrey, S.P.L. Anderson, B. Julicher, P. Kwasowski, and M.J. Sauer, in Residues of Veterinary Drugs in Food, Proc. Euroresidue III Conf., Veldhoven, 1996 (N. Haagsma and A. Ruiter, Eds.), Fac. Vet. Med., Univ. Utrecht, The Netherlands, p. 421 (1996).
124. M.A.J. Godfrey, M.F. Luckey, and P. Kwasowski, in Residues of Veterinary Drugs in Food, Proc. Euroresidue III Conf., Veldhoven, 1996 (N. Haagsma and A. Ruiter, Eds.), Fac. Vet. Med., Univ. Utrecht, The Netherlands, p. 426 (1996).
125. D.J. Fletouris, N.A. Botsoglou, I.E. Psomas and A.I. Mantis, Anal. Chim. Acta, 345:111 (1997).
126. J.W. Hofstraat, M. Engelsma, and R.J. van de Neese, Anal. Chem., 193:193 (1987).

127. A.D. Skoog and J.J. Leary, in Principles of Instrumental Analysis (A.D. Skoog, and J.J. Leary, Eds.), 4th Edition, HBJ College Publisher, Orlando (1992).

128. P.B. Sweetser, and D.G. Swartzfager, Plant Physiol., 61:254 (1978).

129. B. De Backer and L.J. Nagels, LC-GC Int., 8:498 (1995).

130. D.G. Swartzfager, Anal. Chem., 48:2189 (1976).

131. T.P. Kissinger and W.R. Heineman, J. Chem. Education, Sept.:702 (1983).

132. W-Y. Ng and S-K. Wong, J. AOAC Int., 76:540 (1993).

133. G. Diaz, A.G. Cabanillas, L.L. Martinez, and F. Salinas, Anal. Chim. Acta, 273: 351 (1993).

134. Y.Y. Shao, P.D. Rice, and D.R. Bobbitt, Anal. Chim. Acta, 221:239 (1989).

135. K. Ng, P.D. Rice, and D.R. Bobbitt, Microchem. J., 44:25 (1991).

24

Confirmation

Microbiological or immunochemical techniques offer the advantage to screen rapidly and at low cost a large number of food samples for potential drug residues but cannot provide definitive information on the identity of the specific drug residues found. Unlike microbiological and immunochemical techniques, physicochemical techniques actually aim at the identification, quantification, and/or confirmation of the presence of violative residues in suspected samples.

For samples found positive by screening assays, residues can be tentatively identified and quantified by means of the combined force of an efficient chromatographic separation and a selective detection system such as ultraviolet (UV), fluorescence, or electrochemical. The potential of pre- or postcolumn derivatization can further enhance the selectivity and sensitivity of the analysis.

Nevertheless, unequivocal identification is not possible by such classic methods because identification is based on comparison of the retention time of the analyte with that of a reference standard that has been analyzed using the same protocol. Retention time alone fails to identify a substance positively because interfering compounds and many other substances in the sample having similar properties may be eluted from the chromatographic column at the same time. Appearance of a peak only signifies that something has been eluted from the column and that the detector responds to it; this peak could represent more than one substance. Most physicochemical detectors merely screen out analytes that do not fit the criteria for detector response and, therefore, narrow the field of candidates but still cannot identify target analytes unequivocally. Hence, more information is usually required before an analyst can proceed with the identification of an unknown drug residue in a sample containing unknown components.

A certain amount of qualitative information can be obtained by means of so-called multidimensional chromatography (1). This is a combination of different chromatographic techniques in which fractions from a primary separation step are transferred online to a secondary separation step. Multidimensional gas chromatography (GC), for example, involves coupling of GC columns of different selectivities so that the primary column isolates the fraction of interest, and the secondary column takes care of the final separation of that fraction. Using multidimensional liquid chromatography (LC), determination of androgen hormone residues in cattle liver has been possible (2).

A very exciting development in multidimensional separation involves the coupling of LC to GC or other techniques, such as capillary electrophoresis (CE). Online coupling of LC with multidimensional GC has allowed efficient determination of the stilbene hormones in corned beef (3), whereas LC–GC coupling permitted determination of levamisole residues in milk (4). With these hyphenated techniques, the potential of selective separation is becoming increasingly apparent.

Although multidimensional separation generally offers enhanced selectivity and discrimination of solutes, application of more than one hyphenated techniques is usually required for complete and unequivocal identification of the analytes. A recent report states that "two widespread misconceptions about mass spectroscopy (MS) are that GC–MS is a specific method and that GC–MS is 100% accurate" (5). The 1989 Forensic Urine Drug Confirmation Study by the American Association for Clinical Chemistry/College of American Pathologists confirmed this concern about overreliance on GC–MS as a confirmation method (5).

Over the last few years, interest in such hyphenated methods has grown enormously. The successful hyphenation of various separation procedures such as capillary GC, high-performance thin-layer chromatography (HPTLC), and LC, with one or more sophisticated detection devices including diode-array, mass spectrometric, and Fourier transform infrared spectroscopic detectors, has led to development of highly flexible, computer-aided analytical methods that offer the required possibility for unambiguous identification of drug residues in food. These fully integrated hyphenated techniques constitute a distinct step forward if large numbers of samples have to be analyzed in a routine fashion. This is especially true because in many samples a variety of analytes must be identified and/or quantified at, typically, the ppb level. A brief overview of the most important hyphenated techniques in drug residue analysis is given below.

24.1 LIQUID CHROMATOGRAPHY/CAPILLARY ELECTROPHORESIS–DIODE ARRAY TECHNIQUES

For detecting the presence of coeluting impurities in LC or CE, peak purity testing should be performed (6). With this test, a reasonable degree of confidence on the analytical results can be reached. Peak purity testing is particularly important when violative residues are found since in that case the quality of the results are most critical.

A proper peak purity testing requires access to a large portion of the ultraviolet-visible (UV-vis) spectrum of the eluting analyte without interrupting the separation. The traditional variable-wavelength UV-vis detectors are not suitable for this purpose because they examine only a single wavelength of the analyte spectrum, providing insufficient information for peak purity testing. Several attempts have been made to generate a broader range of spectral information using variable-wavelength detectors in a scanning mode, but they all proved to be laborious and destroyed the chromatographic or electrophoretic separation because they necessitated stop-flow conditions prior to the wavelength scanning. Depending on the equipment, the peak trapped in the cell was mechanically scanned over the desired wavelength spectrum and absorption was measured at several selected wavelengths. The ratio of a selected absorption reading to each of the others is highly specific for a single compound and serves to monitor the purity of the solute eluting from the column in the case of the analysis of furazolidone in eggs (7).

In contrast, modern diode array detectors (PDA) are particularly suitable for peak purity testing because they provide almost instantaneous acquisition of spectral data that can be processed to identify peaks and assess purity, without interrupting the separation. These detectors illuminate the sample with the entire spectrum of wavelengths emitted by the light source. Light transmitted by the sample is then broken into its component wavelengths by a diffraction grating and directed to a bank of photodiodes, each of which is dedicated to measuring a narrow band of the spectrum. Because no mechanical scanning is required, spectral acquisition can be accomplished in as short time as 12 ms (8). The high spectral acquisition rate of PDA during elution provides a matrix of absorbance wavelength/time data that can be computer-processed to provide more information regarding the identity of the solute.

For coeluting compounds, PDA makes it possible to differentiate both compounds even when their spectral absorption overlap in the entire range of captured spectral data. Since the introduction of diode-array detectors for monitoring LC or CE effluents, various techniques have been developed to identify and access the purity of chromatographic peaks. These include three-dimensional wavelength−time−absorbance plots (9), spectral overlays (10), derivative transformation of spectra (11, 12), isoabsorbance plots (13), peak purity parameters (14), absorbance ratioing (15, 16), and modeling for accessing interference (17). A characteristic application example is the identification of nitrofurantoin and furaltadone LC peaks in milk by first and second order derivative transformation (18).

Diode-array is currently a routinely applied technique for confirming the purity of the eluting LC peaks in residue analysis. It is a simple to perform and highly selective technique but requires approximately 25–50 ng of the analytes for proper scanning and evaluation (19).

24.2 GAS CHROMATOGRAPHY–MASS SPECTROMETRY TECHNIQUES

Mass spectrometry detection can provide more structural information about a molecule than any other analytical technique. A major advantage of GC-based procedures for analyzing drug residues in foods is that coupling with MS is in a mature state.

MS detectors are unique among GC detectors because they deliver better quantitation of partially resolved peaks as well as improved confidence in peak identification. By their use, even chlorinated compounds like the coccidiostat clopidol can be determined with improved sensitivity and selectivity compared with traditional electron capture detection (20). The amount of the time needed to conduct GC–MS varies, depending upon confirmation or identification tasks. Sample preparation may take between 10 min and 24 h; actual testing time may range from 30 min to 8 h, and evaluation between 1 and 40 h.

Most MS detectors combined with GC are compact bench-top units that operate in a mass range corresponding to the working range of most GC systems. The interface between GC and MS is critical in obtaining acceptable system performance. A fundamental problems in GC–MS interfacing is that more carrier gas may exit the column than the MS detector vacuum-pumping system can remove. In addition, establishing a vacuum at the end of the column may change the chromatographic separation. As much of the mass of the chromatographic peak as possible should enter the detector for highest sensitivity.

Two principal GC–MS interfaces are available for open-tubular GC columns. The so-called direct interface provides the highest possible detector sensitivity, whereas the open-split interface offers the least possible interference with chromatographic separation. With the direct interface, the column exit is routed from the GC oven through a heated transfer line directly into the ionization chamber. As long as the vacuum-pumping system can remove the carrier gas and maintain a sufficiently low pressure, the MS detector will function. Also, little chance exists for adsorptive loses of solute because the analytes contact only the GC column.

However, a direct interface subjects the exit of the column to vacuum conditions. The vacuum may lower the inlet pressure required to obtain the desired mass-flow rate of the carrier gas and also changes its linear-velocity profile across the column. These conditions can cause poor retention-time and peak-area precision and can even make the inlet system stop delivering carrier gas to the column. Thus, analysts should use direct interfaces only with long, narrow-bore columns for analyzing trace residue levels or samples that are sensitive to non-column-surface exposure.

The open-split interface dilutes eluted analytes with additional makeup gas and then splits the mixture into two fractions. An inert, fused-silica restrictor routes a portion of the sample-carrier gas mixture from the interface into the MS ionization chamber, whereas the remainder is vented to atmosphere. An open-split interface can affect the shapes and areas of peaks because solutes make contact with several items including the interface liner, the outer surfaces of the fused-silica column, and the restrictor, which can adsorb trace-level analytes if they are not properly deactivated (21).

For ionization of the analytes, electron-impact is the most common type of ion formation, but chemical ionization is also often used. For electron impact ionization, a collimated beam of electrons makes an impact on the sample molecules, causing loss of an electron from the molecule. When the resulting peak from this molecular ion is seen in a mass spectrum, it gives the molecular weight of the compound.

Chemical ionization begins with ionization of methane or other gas, creating a radical that in turn will have an impact on the sample molecule to produce MH^+ molecular ions, some of which will fragment into smaller daughter ions and neutral fragments; both positive and negative ions are formed but only positively charged species will be detected. In general, less fragmentation occurs with chemical ionization than with electron-impact ionization. Hence the former yields less information about the detailed structure of a molecule but does yield the molecular ion; sometimes the molecular ion cannot be detected by electron-impact ionization. The two techniques usually complement each other.

The specificity is highest when full spectral scans are used for comparison of sample and standard peaks at, however, the expense of sensitivity. Compromise between sensitivity and specificity can be achieved by scanning a limited number of characteristic fragment ions (22), in the selective ion monitoring mode (SIM). The number and relative abundance of characteristic ions are both influenced by the ionization mode applied. However, fragmentation often results in formation of various low-molecular-weight nonspecific fragments, each having a low abundance (23), while the most characteristic molecular ion may be only marginally present in the spectrum.

For ionization of the analytes, soft ionization procedures such as fast atom bombardment (FAB) and field desorption (FD) can also be used, yielding a limited number of high-molecular-weight specific fragments (24, 25) but the sensitivity of the detection is decreased. Exceptions are the negative-ion chemical ionization (NCI) and the pulsed positive ion–negative ion–chemical ionization (PPINICI) procedures, which allow selective and sensitive detection of analytes containing functional groups with electron-capturing properties. Thus, accurate quantitation of chloramphenicol (26, 27) even at ppt levels, nicarbazin (28, 29), and detomidine

(30) has been made possible by GC–NCI–MS. Moreover, analytical results obtained independently by applying four different methods on milk samples containing chloramphenicol residues have shown fascinating agreement; all GC–NCI–MS, GC–ECD, GC–EI–MS, and radioimmunoassay procedures gave results ranging from 11.1 to 11.7 ppb (31). Reliable quantification of sulfonamides at the sub-ppb level has been also made possible using GC–PPINICI–MS (32).

Commercially available GC–MS systems present major differences in their detection and recording system. Many quadrupole instruments use SIM for the determination of analytes at trace levels. With this type of instrumentation, more than 1–10 ng of the analyte is required to record a full-scan mass spectrum. In contrast, instruments based on ion-trap technology can record a full-scan mass spectrum on an analyte at pg level. With SIM, a limited number of ions are monitored during a selected time interval of the chromatogram. The presence of the analyte is determined by the presence of these diagnostic ions at the correct retention time and in the correct abundance ratio (33).

When quadrupole instruments are used for analyzing drug residues in extracts of urine, meat, or feces, limited interferences are observed as a result of the high selectivity of the detector. Using, however, an ion-trap instrument, high concentrations of coeluting molecules may influence the ionization time of the analytes and thus the detection limit. This may cause false-positive and -negative results and incorrect quantification, as has been demonstrated in the case of nortestosterone analysis by GC–MS (34). Thus, when GC–MS is used for the determination of drug residues, particularly illegal growth promoters at the ppb level, the possibility of interference should always be kept into mind.

Caution and investing time and money in the analysis may prevent wrong results. False-negative results arising from loss of the analyte during extraction/ cleanup, derivatization, or injection must be addressed by using internal standards (35–37). Synthesized stable isotopes are ideal internal standards since they behave as closely similar to the analytes as possible, while still allowing a separate detection (38–40). Unfortunately, in most cases such isotopes are not commercially available and isomers or close analogues of the analytes are used instead (41). In cases where derivatization of the analytes is not required, reliable quantitative information can be obtained even without internal standards as in the analysis of nitroimidazoles (42), levamisole (43), clenbuterol (44), and penicillin (45) residues.

False-negative results arising from disturbance of normal peak ratios of the analyte ions may be overcome by a variety of means including reinjection of the same derivative on another column, application of an alternative derivatization technique, and/or performing a second analysis with a different method. Thus, the identity, for example, of an illegal hormone residue in a suspect sample has been given by a series of different events including two values for the ratio to the front in two-dimensional HPTLC, a characteristic fluorescence after sulfuric acid induction, a retention window in LC, a retention time in capillary GC, and MS data. Although each technique on its own does not exactly fulfill the quality criteria, the combination may result in sufficient analytical accuracy. This has been realized in the LC–GC–tandem MS determination of levamisole in milk (46), and in LC–GC–MS analysis of swine tissues for sulfamethazine (47) and carbadox-related residues (48). It was also achieved in the TLC–GC–MS analysis of eggs and meat for chloramphenicol residues (49) in which the collected LC peaks and the scraped-off TLC spots were injected after appropriate processing into the GC–MS. Advantages of these approaches over direct GC–MS include extra cleanup through the additional chromatographic separation, possibility for tentative confirmation by means for example of a diode array detector, and the feasibility of limiting the use of expensive MS to only those samples in which maximum residue limits (MRLs) are exceeded. It may seem attractive to use the selective and sensitive GC–MS methods for screening, but in practice this method is still too vulnerable to be used on a routine basis.

A more powerful alternative in cases where the analytical results offered by conventional low-resolution GC-MS are not clear enough, is to resort to GC–MS–MS. This can be best exemplified in the analysis of β-agonists. Since the commonly used trimethylsilyl (TMS) derivatives of some β-agonists show only low abundance for the most specific ions, in many cases identification has to be based on the results of two independent GC–MS methods with different derivatives and/or ionization techniques, each producing two or three diagnostic ions. Thus, in the electron impact (EI) ionization mode, the spectrum of the mono–TMS–derivative of clenbuterol shows five diagnostic ions at 86, 243, 262, 264, and 277 with relative intensity values of 100.0, 3.0, 7.0, 4.7, and 1.3, respectively. At residue levels, however, the relatively low intensities of the ions, except for 86, are intefered with by matrix components. In order to obtain the necessary evidence, one is often obliged to perform a second supplementary run using a chemical ionization (CI) mode or another derivative such as boronic acid. In the CI mode, the diagnostic ions with higher masses are much more abundant than in EI, but the stability of the spectra is much decreased, again causing identification problems in one single run. With boronic acid derivatization, on the other hand, abundant ions in the high-mass range are produced, but again problems are encountered in obtaining four diagnostic ions at residue levels. In contrast, application of GC–MS–MS results in significant reduction of the background noise, leading directly to completely comparable full-scan spectra of standard and the analyte at residue levels (50).

24.3 THIN LAYER CHROMATOGRAPHY–MASS SPECTROMETRY TECHNIQUES

Acceptable agreement between the migration distance of standards and sample components, and application of specific derivatizing reagents are commonly used identification procedures in thin-layer chromatography (TLC). None of these procedures is, however, sufficiently specific for structural elucidation. Use of derivatizing reagents can provide functional group identity but that is far from structural identity.

Of more immediate interest are approaches that permit offline TLC–MS in which the spots are scraped out from the layer and the analytes are either extracted from the sorbent to be transferred to the mass spectrometer as discrete samples or are introduced without sorbent removal into the spectrometer on a direct insertion probe (51). TLC–MS quantification and confirmation efficiency can be further enhanced by submitting the TLC extract to an additional chromatographic separation using a different technique prior to the final MS analysis. Advantages of this approach over direct TLC–MS include extra cleanup through the additional chromatographic separation (52). This has been realized in the TLC–GC–MS analysis of eggs and meat for chloramphenicol residues (49).

The manual sampling approach used in offline TLC–MS procedures is very simple and can be carried out without using any complex interfacing system. However, manual sampling can be tedious, if a very large number of analytes must be identified, and can lead to loss of sample during subsequent handling. Another potential limitation concerns the selection of the ionization technique. Electron impact ionization is only really suitable for use in TLC-MS if the analytes are volatile and stable enough to be volatilized off the sorbent by heating the insertion mass probe. For analytes that do not meet these requirements, soft ionization techniques such as FAB, liquid secondary-ion mass spectrometry (LSIMS), or matrix-assisted laser desorption ionization (MALDI) have to be employed (53). However, these soft ionization techniques only provide molecular ion information on the analyte and little fragmentation. In this instance, MS–MS, which provides a fragmentation pattern, can be used to identify compounds unambiguously while differentiating among those having similar Rf values and the same molecular mass.

A simpler means for unequivocal identification of substances by TLC or HPTLC combined with MS, can be provided by online procedures (54, 55). The ability to perform MS on analytes directly on the chromatographic plate removes the need to recover them prior to identification. This greatly reduces the amount of work needed to confirm identity. The determination of midazolam in serum (56) and the identification of tetracycline residues in honey (57) are examples of TLC coupled in situ with FAB–MS.

Coupling of TLC with MS–MS provides further advantages by giving more detailed information on particular ions and eliminating interferences from ions derived from either interferences with similar retention time or the general background. Compared with TLC–MS, TLC–MS–MS is superior because the fragmentation provides diagnostic ions that allow unambiguous identification and structure determination to be readily performed.

Several types of MS–MS instrumentation are available, most common being the triple quadrupole and the magnetic sector/quadrupole hybrid. Both these tandem spectrometers can be operated to perform production scanning, precursor ion scanning, and neutral loss scanning. Product ion scanning is probably the most common mode for structural identification. In product ion scanning, the ion representing the molecular species is selected and transmitted into the collision cell for fragmentation. The resulting fragment ions are focused and detected by scanning in the second mass spectrometer to give the mass spectrum. These fragments are derived solely from the original ion, thereby enabling specific structural identification to be achieved for this ion.

In its own right, tandem mass spectrometry a very powerful analytical tool, and this has led to the suggestion that chromatographic separations are redundant. MS–MS techniques without prior chromatography have already shown the potential to quantitate samples with little or no cleanup. Such techniques have been successfully applied for the residue analysis of oxytetracycline (58), sulfonamides (59), danofloacin (60), β-lactams (61), clenbuterol (62), metoprolol (63), and betamethasone and clenbuterol (64). Tandem MS approaches generally provide sub-ppb detection limits, more or less independent of the biological matrix analyzed. In an MS–MS method for the determination sulfonamides in pig kidney (65), 400 extracts could be analyzed before MS source cleaning became necessary.

However, tandem mass spectrometry, as a separation technique, does have limitations. It cannot easily differentiate between isomeric and isobaric species, and, in complex matrices, the presence of components with a high surface activity can suppress the ionization of components with a lower surface activity, leading to the nondetection of analytes (66). Therefore, the combination of MS–MS with a readily available chromatographic separation method such as TLC affords analysts real benefits.

TLC–MS–MS has been developed using either manual or instrumental approaches for sample introduction into the MS–MS section. For manual TLC–MS–MS, the spot or zone containing the analyte is removed from the plate after suitable concentration and, if FAB or LSIMS is going to be the ionization technique, it is suspended in a liquid matrix such as glycerol. The resulting mixture is then applied to the probe tip to be introduced into the spectrometer in the usual way. Although this approach involves manipulation of the sample and thus the potential for loss of some of the spatial resolution obtained by the TLC separation, it is readily implemented and requires no additional equipment or interface.

The instrumental approach uses a dedicated probe onto which a segment of the TLC plate can be fixed. With this probe, the plate is gradually moved through the ion source, allowing mass chromatograms to be generated and mass spectra to be obtained for each of the analytes present on the selected track. Aluminum-backed plates have to be used to ensure good electrical contact with the probe. As with the manual approach, the surface of the plate has to be impregnated with the matrix prior to spectrometry if FAB or LSIMS is to be used.

Despite the resolving power of TLC–MS–MS, few applications in drug residuc analysis have been reported. One application concerns the HPTLC–MS–MS analysis of a number of nonsteroidal anti-inflammatory drugs, including salicylic acid and its glycine conjugate salicylhippuric acid, diclofenac, indomethacin, naproxen, phenacetin, and ibuprofen (67). Another application describes the detection and identification of some of these compounds or their metabolites in urine by TLC–MS–MS (67).

24.4 LIQUID CHROMATOGRAPHY–MASS SPECTROMETRY TECHNIQUES

The online coupling of LC with MS for the determination of drug residues in food of animal origin has been under investigation for almost two decades. LC–MS is now in a mature state, but it still cannot be considered routine in the field of drug residue analysis. Possible reasons are the high initial cost, which is two to four times higher than that of GC–MS; and the poor detection limits, which are approximately 100 times higher than in GC–MS. Coupling of LC with tandem MS may be a solution for improving detection limits by reducing the background noise, but this combination is two or three times more expensive than its LC–MS analogue.

Three major difficulties have been generally met in directly combining LC with MS. The first concerns the ionization of nonvolatile and/or thermolabile analytes. The second is related to the mobile-phase incompatibility as result of the frequent use of nonvolatile mobile-phase buffers and additives in LC. The third is due to the apparent flow rate incompatibility as expressed in the need to introduce a mobile phase eluting from the column at a flow rate of 1 ml/min into the high vacuum of the MS.

The ionization of the analytes is no longer considered a problem in LC–MS applications. Considerable progress has been made in the development of powerful ionization techniques, particularly the soft ionization atmospheric pressure procedures, electrospray (ESP) and ionspray ionization (ISP). For the second difficulty, however, no technical and general solution is available; a routine, long-term use of nonvolatile mobile phase constituents, such as phosphate buffers and ion-pairing agents, is prohibited by all current LC–MS methods. However, some interfaces, such as the atmospheric pressure chemical ionization (APCI) with countercurrent drying gas, exhibit a higher tolerance than others. As for the third difficulty, a wide range of different LC–MS interfaces has been developed. Owing to the flow rates of the highly polar solvents, the presence of buffer salts, and the volatilization characteristics of the analytes, several different interfacing mechanisms are required to provide broad analytical coverage. Hence, the choice of a suitable interface for a particular application has always to be related to the analytes considered, especially their polarity and molecular mass, and the specific analytical problem as well.

One of the main problems of the currently available interfaces is the lack of fragmentation data provided for structure determination. All modern interfaces operate in a basically CI mode, providing mild ionization and making identification of unknowns difficult or impossible. However, techniques producing abundant molecular or pseudomolecular ions are ideally suited to MS–MS, which can produce characteristic full-scan spectra rich in fragmentation detail. In a method reported on the separation and identification of 21 sulfonamides by LC–MS–ISP, positive-ion mass spectra yielded only abundant protonated molecular ions. However, using tandem MS, more structural information through daughter ion spectra could be obtained (68). It is in the direction of LC–MS–MS that further progress towards the elusive universal combination of LC and MS will be made (69).

At present, the most powerful and promising interfaces for drug residue analysis are the particle-beam (PB) interface that provides online EI mass spectra, the thermospray (TSP) interface that works well with substances of medium polarity, and more recently the atmospheric pressure ionization (API) interfaces that have opened up important application areas of LC to LC–MS for ionizable compounds. Among the API interfaces, ESP and ISP appear to be the most versatile since they are suitable for substances ranging from polar to ionic and from low to high molecular mass. ISP, in particular, is compatible with the flow rates used with conventional LC columns (70). In addition, both ESP and ISP appear to be valuable in terms of analyte detectability. These interfaces can further be supplemented by preanalyzer collision-induced dissociation (CID) or tandem MS as realized with the use of triple quadrupole systems. Complementary to ESP and ISP interfaces with respect to the analyte polarity is APCI with a heated nebulizer interface. This is a powerful interface for both structural confirmation and quantitative analysis.

24.4.1 Particle–Beam Interface

The particle–beam interface is an analyte-enrichment interface in which the column effluent is pneumatically nebulized into a near atmospheric-pressure desolvation chamber connected to a momentum separator, where the high-mass analytes are preferentially directed to the MS ion source while the low-mass solvent molecules are efficiently pumped away (71, 72). With this interface, mobile phase flow rates within the range 0.1–1.0 ml/min can be applied (73). Since the mobile phase solvent is removed prior to introduction of the analyte molecules into the ion source, both EI and CI techniques can be used with this interface.

PB–MS appears to have high potential as an identification method for residues of some antibiotics in foods, since it generates library-searchable EI spectra and CI solvent-independent spectra. Limitations of the PB–MS interface, as compared with other LC–MS interfaces, include lower sensitivity, difficulty in quantification, and lower response with highly aqueous mobile phases. In addition, this method suffers a limited application range in terms of analyte volatility, polarity, and molecular mass.

The low sensitivity can be attributed in part to chromatographic band broadening during the transmission of the sample through the interface and in part to nonlinearity effects that appear at low analyte concentrations (74). Nevertheless, PB–MS signal enhancement can be made possible through addition of a carrier to the mobile phase, a phenomenon known as a carrier effect (75). Carriers such as ammonium acetate (76), malic acid (77), phenoxyacetic acid (78), phenylurea (79), or the isotopically labeled analogue of the analyte (80) have been shown to improve the transfer efficiency through the PB interface, resulting in increase of sensitivity and restoration of the linearity. This effect, dependent as it is on the analyte, carrier, and interface hardware, is not predictable.

LC–PB–MS has been investigated as a potential confirmatory method for the determination of malachite green in incurred catfish tissue (81); and of cephapirin, furosemide, and methylene blue in milk, kidney, and muscle tissue, respectively (82). Results showed that the mobile-phase composition, nebulization–desolvation, and source temperature all play an important role in the sensitivity of the method. The sensitivity increases with decreasing heat capacity of the mobile phase in the order methanol > acetonitrile > isopropanol > water and with decreasing flow rate. A comparison of the PB with the thermospray interface showed that less structural information was provided by the latter, whereas the sensitivity was generally lower with the thermospray interface.

LC–PB–MS has been also investigated for the analysis of ivermectin residues in bovine liver and milk (83). The specificity required for regulatory confirmation was obtained by monitoring the molecular ion and characteristic fragment ions of the drug under NCI–selective ion monitoring (SIM) conditions. Coeluting matrix components were found to alter the abundance pattern of the analyte, thus enhancing the total response. As a result, concentrations as low as 2 ppb and 15 ppb of the drug could be readily quantified in milk and liver, respectively. The enhancement was attributed to improved transmission through the PB interface in a kind of carrier effect. To compensate for the variation in the relative abundance produced by coeluting compounds, control milk was spiked with ivermectin standard for the abundance matching requirement of regulatory confirmation.

Quantification and confirmation of tetracycline, oxytetracycline, and chlortetracycline residues in milk (84) as well as chloramphenicol residues in calf muscle (85) have been also carried out using LC–PB–NCI–MS. Use of an SIM mode allowed a detection limit of about 100 ppb for the tetracyclines and 2 ppb for chloramphenicol residues.

24.4.2 Thermospray Interface

The TSP interface is widely used for the determination of drug residues in foods (86). TSP is typically used with reversed-phase columns and volatile buffers.

In the thermospray interface, aqueous mobile phases containing an electrolyte such as ammonium acetate are passed at flow rates of 1–2 ml/min through a heated capillary prior entering a heated ion source. The end of the capillary lies opposite a vacuum line. Nebulization takes place as a result of the disruption of the liquid by the expanding vapor formed at the capillary wall upon evaporation of part of the liquid in the capillary. This results in formation of a supersonic jet of vapor containing a mist of fine, electrically charged droplets.

As the droplets move through the hot source area, they continue to vaporize. The electric field at the liquid surface increases until ions present in the eluent are ejected from the droplet. Ions are sampled through a conical exit aperture in the mass analyzer. The ionization of the analytes takes place by means of direct ion evaporization of the sample ion or by solvent-mediated CI reactions: an ion of the electrolyte ejected from a droplet reacts with a sample molecule in the gas phase and generates a sample ion that is mass analyzed. In addition, fragment ions can be observed due to the high temperatures associated with TSP; negative ions are also produced by TSP, and negative ion detection is recommended for acidic compounds.

With TSP, ammonium acetate has emerged as the best general-purpose electrolyte for ionizing neutral samples. Improved ionization can be obtained by the use of a filament or discharge electrode to generate reactive ions for CI (87, 88). The processes involved in filament or discharge-assisted ionization must be used when operating in the absence of a buffer with nonaqueous eluents. With ionic analytes, the mechanism of ion evaporation is supposed to be primarily operative since ions are produced spontaneously from the mobile phase (89). Ion evaporation often yields mass spectra with little structural information; in order to overcome this problem, other ionization modes or tandem MS have been applied (90).

The TSP interface is typically combined with quadrupole MS, but coupling with ion-trap (91) or magnetic sector MS (92) has been also reported. Drawbacks of LC–TSP–MS are the requirements for volatile modifiers and the control of temperature, particularly for thermolabile compounds. Lack of structural information from LC–TSP–MS applications can be overcome by the use of LC–TSP–MS–MS. Use of this tandem MS approach provides enhanced selectivity, generally at the cost of a loss of sensitivity as a consequence of a decreased ion transmission.

LC–TSP–MS has been successfully applied for confirmation of nicarbazin residues in chicken tissues using negative-ion detection and SIM at three characteristic ions in the TSP mass spectrum of the drug (93). LC–TSP–MS in the SIM mode has been also used for quantification of several sulfonamides in meat (94), residues of moxidectin in cattle tissues and fat (95), and nitroxynil, rafoxanide, and levamisole in muscle (96).

Confirmatory methods based on LC–TSP–MS have further been developed for the determination of various penicillin derivatives, penicillin G, and cephapirin and its metabolite in milk. In the assay for penicillin derivatives (97), ammonium acetate buffer replaced the ion-pair reagents used in the mobile phase, whereas the positive-ion TSP mass spectra of penicillins displayed both MH^+ and MNa^+ ions, which provided unequivocal proof of the suspected drug residue. The detection limits in this assay were estimated to be in the range of 100–200 ppb. A detection limit of 100 ppb was also observed in one of the assays of penicillin G in milk (98), although another assay (99) offered a detection limit of only 3 ppb. This was probably due to the fact that only ultrafiltration was employed for milk cleanup in the former assay, while both protein precipitation and solid-phase cleanup were used in the latter. In the case of the cephapirin analysis (100), the principal metabolite in milk was identified as deacetylcephapirin by both LC–PDA detection and LC–TSP–MS. In the LC–MS method, the detection limits for cephapirin and deacetylcephapirin were 100 and 50 ppb, respectively.

Apart from LC–MS, TSP has been also used in LC–MS–MS systems. With such a tandem system, residues of chloramphenicol have been detected in milk and fish by CID on the basis of the mass spectrum of the chloramphenicol protonated molecule (101). In both food commodities, chloramphenicol residues could be identified unequivocally at the 500 ppb level.

Comparative evaluation of the confirmatory efficiency of LC–TSP–MS and LC–TSP–MS–MS in the assay of maduramicin in chicken fat showed the former approach to be marginally appropriate (102). In contrast, LC–TSP–MS–MS was found to be highly efficient since it could adequately resolve the analyte from tissue coextractives, providing reproducible MS data that are useful for identification purposes.

24.4.3 Electrospray Interface

An alternative sample-introduction approach is the electrospray (ESP) interface that also constitutes a widely applicable soft ionization technique (103). ESP operates at the low μl/min flow rate, necessitating use of either capillary columns or postcolumn splitting of the mobile phase (104–106).

For ESP ionization, the analytes must be ionic, or have an ionizable functional group, or be able to form an ionic adduct in solution; the analytes are commonly detected as deprotonated species or as cation adducts of a proton or an alkali metal ion. When using positive ion ESP ionization, use of ammonium acetate as a mobile-phase modifier is generally unsuitable. Instead, organic modifiers, such as heptafluorobutyric or trifluoroacetic acid, usually at a concentration of 0.1% are strongly recommended. For negative ion applications, the choice of the modifier is even more limited; triethylamine is currently the only suitable compound.

LC–ESP–MS has been successfully used simultaneously to determine and confirm β-lactam antibiotics in food of animal origin. Multiresidue assay of penicillin G, ampicillin, amoxicillin, cloxacillin, and cephapirin in milk ultrafiltrate was carried out at the 100 ppb level with LC–ESP–MS after postcolumn splitting of the eluent and recording under SIM conditions in the positive-ion mode (107, 108). By varying the voltage between the capillary and the skimmer in the ESP interface, structurally relevant CID fragments ions could be formed for all five analytes. The ESP response was found to be dependent on both the solvents and the additives used for preparation of the mobile phase; the greater the participation of the organic solvent in the mobile phase, the higher the ESP response. The response could be considerably increased by the addition of formic or acetic acid in the mobile phase.

Significantly lower detection limits were reported by other workers who described an LC–ESP–MS confirmatory procedure for the simultaneous determination of five penicillins in milk and meat (108). Using highly sophisticated instrumentation, all the LC effluent could be provided for the ESP–MS; in this way, limitations, such as the low flow rate and the use of a postcolumn splitter, that restricted the practicability of the previous method could be overcome. Acquisition of penicillin signals was carried out under SIM conditions in the negative-ion mode.

In addition, determination of a variety of sulfonamides has been carried out by coupling capillary LC with quadrupole MS through an ESP interface; induced dissociation of the analytes by increasing the skimmer voltage could allow confirmation at the low-picomole range (110). LC–ESP–MS has been also found suitable for the determination of four coccidiostats in poultry products (111).

ESP has been further shown to be useful as a generic screening method for some classes of veterinary drugs, such as sulfonamides and tetracyclines, which exhibit spectra with four common ions; however, this was not possible for the group of β-agonists because of their more diverse chemical structure (112). Negative-ion ESP–MS has been found useful for the detection and identification of a number of nonsteroidal anti-inflammatory drugs, including phenylbutazone, flunixin, oxyphenbutazone, and diclofenac, after their reversed-phase LC separation. In general, fragmentation increased at higher cone voltages, whereas the molecular ion peaks were more intensive at lower cone voltages (113).

24.4.4 Ionspray Interface

The ionspray (ISP) interface is closely related to the ESP. Unlike the ESP interface, ISP allows higher flow rates by virtue of pneumatically assisted vaporization

(114–116). Like ESP, ISP is suitable for analytes that are ionic or have an ionizable functional group or are able to form an ionic adduct in solution.

Since both ESP and ISP produce quasimolecular ions, more sophisticated techniques, such as LC–MS–MS are required to obtain diagnostic fragment ions and, thus, analyte structure elucidation (117, 118). Identification can often be achieved by using daughter ion MS–MS scans and collisionally induced dissociation (CID), most commonly on a triple quadrupole MS; in this way, dissociation of the quasimolecular ion occurs and diagnostic structural information can be obtained (119).

LC–ISP–MS proved to be an attractive approach for the determination of semduramicin in chicken liver (120). Tandem MS using CID of the molecular ions could further enhance the specificity, providing structure elucidation and selective detection down to 30 ppb under SRM conditions.

LC–ISP–MS has been also successfully applied for the assay of 21 sulfonamides in salmon flesh (121). Separation was achieved in a reversed-phase LC system with gradient elution. Simple positive-ion spectra with an intense protonated molecule and no fragment ions of relevant abundance were displayed by all analytes by operating in the full-scan acquisition and SIM modes. Further application of tandem MS using SRM for increased sensitivity could overcome the lack of structural information presented by the ISP mass spectra.

Coupling of LC with either ISP–MS or ISP–MS–MS has been also investigated as an attractive alternative for the determination of erythromycin A and its metabolites in salmon tissue (122). The combination of these methods permitted identification of a number of degradation products and metabolites of erythromycin, including anhydroerythromycin and N-demethyerythromycin at the level of 10–50 ppb.

Tandem MS with CID has been also applied for the specific monitoring of danofloxacin and its metabolites in chicken and cattle tissues at levels down to 50 ppb (123). LC separation was carried out on a microbore column with a mobile phase of acetonitrile–0.1% trifluoroacetic acid.

Both ISP–MS in the SIM mode and pulsed amperometric detection were found to be suitable for the determination of aminoglycoside antibiotics in bovine tissues (124). Various stationary and mobile phases, and several ion-pairing reagents, were examined for efficient LC separation and optimum LC–MS sensitivity.

24.4.5 Atmospheric Pressure Chemical Ionization Interface

In order to combine reversed-phase LC with atmospheric pressure chemical ionization (APCI)–MS (125), a commercially available heated nebulizer interface that can handle pure aqueous eluents at flow rates up to 2 ml/min in addition to nonvolatile buffers has been used (126). The heated nebulizer inlet probe consists of a concentric pneumatic nebulizer and a large-diameter heated quartz tube. The nebulized liquid effluent is swept through the heated tube by an additional gas flow that circumvents the nebulizer. The heated mixture of solvent and vapor is then introduced in the ionization source, where a corona discharge electrode initiates APCI (127). The spectra and chromatograms from APCI are somewhat similar to those from TSP, but the technique is more robust, especially with gradient LC, and is often more sensitive. APCI is particularly useful for heat-labile compounds and for low-mass as well as high-mass compounds.

In contrast to TSP interface, no extensive temperature optimization is needed with APCI. For systems providing a countercurrent drying gas, it is claimed that volatile as well as nonvolatile buffers can be used. Uncharged volatile material is swept away from the nozzle by the countercurrent drying gas, whereas nonvolatile contamination deposited in the source chamber can readily be wiped away without the need to switch off the vacuum system.

The applicability of the APCI interface is restricted to the analysis of compounds with lower polarity and lower molecular mass compared with ESP and ISP. An early demonstration of the potential of the APCI interface is the LC–APCI–MS–MS analysis of phenylbutazone and two of its metabolites in plasma and urine (128). Other applications include the LC–APCI–MS analysis of steroids in equine and human urine and plasma (129–131), the determination of six sulfonamides in milk samples after a simple solid-phase extraction and LC separation (132), of tetracyclines in muscle at the 100 ppb level (133), of fenbendazole, oxfendazole, and the sulfone metabolite in muscle at the 10 ppb level, and of five thyrcostats in thyroid tissue at the 1 ppm level (134).

24.5 GAS CHROMATOGRAPHY–INFRARED SPECTROSCOPY TECHNIQUES

Infrared spectroscopy can fill some of the current gaps in testing methodology and allow analysts to cope with a wider range of analytical problems (135). Combining MS with infrared (IR) data creates a highly complementary identification system.

Most organic compounds have a large number of relatively narrow absorption bands in the midinfrared spectral region. These absorptions are highly specific and can give detailed structural information about a particular compound because the frequencies at which they appear are directly correlated to the bonds of the analyzed compound. The greater the masses of attached atoms, the lower the IR frequency at which the bond will absorb. Because each interatomic bond may vibrate in several different motions, such as stretching or bending, individual bonds may absorb at more than one IR frequency. Stretching absorptions usually produce stronger peaks than bending. However, the weaker bending absorptions can be useful in differentiating similar types of bonds. IR spectroscopy involves collecting absorption information and analyzing it in the form of a spectrum.

By itself, the entire IR spectrum of an organic compound provides a unique fingerprint, which can be readily differentiated from the absorption patterns of other compounds. This means that when reference spectra are available, most compounds can be unambiguously identified on the basis of their IR spectra.

Upon first inspection, a typical infrared spectrum can be divided visually into two regions. The left half, which is above $2000 \, cm^{-1}$, usually contains relatively few peaks, but some very diagnostic information can be found here. First, alkane C–H stretching absorptions just below $3000 \, cm^{-1}$ demonstrate the presence of saturated carbons, and signals just above $3000 \, cm^{-1}$ demonstrate unsaturation. A very broad peak in the region between 3100 and $3600 \, cm^{-1}$ indicates the presence of exchangeable protons, typically from alcohol, amine, amide, or carboxylic acid groups. The frequencies from 2800 to $2000 \, cm^{-1}$ are normally void of other absorptions, so the presence of alkene or nitrile groups can be easily seen here. In contrast, the right half of the spectrum, which is below $2000 \, cm^{-1}$, normally contains many peaks of varying intensities, many of which are not readily identifiable. Two signals that can be seen clearly in this area is the carbonyl group, which is a very strong peak around $1700 \, cm^{-1}$, and the C-O bond with can be one or two strong peaks around $1200 \, cm^{-1}$.

These features make IR spectrometry a potentially strong technique for the characterization of chromatographic peaks. However, compared with UV-vis absorbance, extinction coefficients in IR are rather low, and the amount of analyte needed for IR detection therefore is often larger that the amounts usually injected into a GC or LC. Nevertheless, enhanced sensitivity can be achieved by the Fourier transform (FT) version of the infrared spectroscopy (FTIR) (136).

In FTIR, a continuum light source is used to produce light over a broad range of infrared wavelengths. Light coming from this continuum source is split into two paths using a half-silvered mirror; this light is then reflected from two mirrors back onto the beamsplitter, where it is recombined. One of these mirrors is fixed, and the second is movable. If the light intensity is measured and plotted as a function of the position of the movable mirror, the resultant graph is the Fourier transform of the intensity of light as a function of the wavelength. Advantages of FTIR include small sample size, detailed chemical bonding information, analysis of liquids and solids, nondestructive analysis, molecular-specific identification, and recording of a complete spectrum within 1 s. The later feature enables IR detection to be performed in an online mode, allowing thus GC–FTIR to become a well established technique.

In the various GC–FTIR systems that are commercially available, three essentially different types of GC–FTIR interfaces can be identified (137). With the most commonly used interface, the GC column effluent flows through a heated light-pipe, and vapor-phase spectra are collected in real time at 1 s intervals. This light-pipe-based system is relatively simple but presents an inherent sensitivity limitation that has been addressed by the use of alternative interfaces in which the analytes are stored on a low-temperature substrate prior to IR detection. In the most promising type of these storage interfaces, the so-called cryotrapping interface, the GC eluates are condensed at 77 K on a moving IR transparent window and the trapped compounds are subsequently scanning by FTIR microscopy (138). A unique feature of the system is the possibility of performing extended postrun scanning of the previously condensed solutes. Thus, considerable improvement of the signal-to-noise ratio of the IR spectra is obtained, facilitating identification and increasing the limit of detection to the picogram range. The technique has been successfully applied to detect and identify the trimethylsilyl derivatives of clenbuterol, mabuterol, and salbutamol in samples extracted from urine and liver of veal calves and cattle with a detection limit of 1–2.5 ppb in the original sample (139).

24.6 LIQUID CHROMATOGRAPHY–INFRARED SPECTROSCOPY TECHNIQUES

Progress in the field of hyphenation during the past decade has brought LC–FTIR to a stage of real analytical utility (140). In the earliest systems, flow cells were used in a fashion analogous to LC with online UV absorption detection. Flow-through IR detectors would be desirable except for a fundamental limitation: the mobile phases used in LC applications are invariably strong absorbers in the IR spectral region and mask the spectra of solutes. This has greatly delayed the widespread use of the technique.

Since the major part of LC involves reversed-phase separations, more recent work in the field of LC–FTIR has concentrated on the development of interfaces suitable for the elimination of aqueous eluents. Solvent-elimination interfaces with which the eluent is eliminated prior to IR detection have shown to be much more versatile and to yield interference-free spectral information for considerably smaller amounts of analytes, which is the primary objective of LC–FTIR.

Solvent-elimination approaches include evaporative spray deposition onto infrared-transparent surfaces (141) or reflective surfaces and powders (142, 143). Other approaches include partial evaporation of the mobile phase before spray deposition (144, 145), and continuous liquid–liquid extraction systems that transfer solutes from LC mobile phases to solvents possessing an infrared window (146). Spray systems include both pneumatic and ultrasonic nozzles (147).

Attributes of commercially available reversed-phase LC–FTIR systems in which the column effluent is either sent directly to the solvent elimination interface or is mixed online with a reagent, prior to solvent evaporation, to facilitate the elimination of the aqueous solvent, are summarized in Table 24.1. Systems based on thermospray, particle beam, and ultrasonic nebulization can handle relatively high flows of aqueous eluents (0.3–1 ml/min) and allow the use of conventional size LC, which evidently is an advantage. However, due to diffuse spray characteristics and/or a low efficiency of the analyte transfer to the substrate, these systems often exhibit identification limits that are at best moderate (100 ng) and often unfavorable (1–10 μg). Best results (0.05–5 ng injected) are obtained with pneumatic and electrospray nebulizers, but considerable more attention has been devoted to the former approaches. Pneumatic interfaces combine rapid solvent elimination with a relatively narrow spray. The latter aspect allows analytes to be deposited on ZnSe in a narrow trace, so that transmission detection by FTIR microscope can be applied to achieve mass sensitivities in the low- or even subnanogram range (148).

However, systems based on pneumatic nebulization are limited with regard to the LC flow rate, the water content, and the type of buffer salts in the eluent. The flow rates that can be handled directly by these systems are 2–50 μl/min, which means that micro- or narrow-bore LC has to be applied. On the other hand, the water content of the eluent that can be tolerated depends on the flow rate. If flow rates of 2–5 μl/min are used as in micro-LC, even pure water can be eliminated efficiently by a pneumatic nebulizer. However, if the flow rate is in the 20–50 μl/min range, as in narrow-bore LC, rapid evaporation of highly aqueous eluents will cause problems. In these instances, further enhancement of the solvent evaporation efficiency is required by either mixing the effluent with nitrogen gas before it enters the nebulizer (149) or by placing both the nebulizer and the deposition substrate inside a vacuum chamber (150). As far as buffer salts are concerned, even volatile salts are not completely eliminated by a pneumatic nebulizer and can therefore cause interfering absorbances in the analyte spectra. Buffer salts can, however, be removed by using a phase-switching technique such as online liquid–liquid extraction.

Despite the distinct advantages of pneumatic nebulizers, ultrasonic nebulizers may alternatively be used, in some instances, with success. In a recent application, a variation of ultrasonic nebulizer called spray nozzle-rotating disk FTIR interface was successfully applied to confirm the presence of methyltestosterone, testosterone, fluoxymesterone, epitestosterone, and estradiol and testosterone cypionate in urine, after solid-phase extraction and reversed-phase LC separation (151). Using a commercial infrared microscopy spectrometer, usable spectra from 5 ng steroid deposits could be readily obtained. To achieve success with this interface, phosphate buffers in the mobile phase were not used because these nonvolatile salts accumulate on the collection disk and their spectra tend to swamp out small mass deposits. Another limitation of the method was that only nonvolatile analytes could be analyzed because volatile compounds simply evaporated off the collection-disk surface prior to scanning.

TABLE 24.1 Attributes of Reversed-Phase Liquid Chromatography–Fourier Transform Infrared Systems Using Direct or Indirect Eluent Elimination

Interface type	LC flow-rate (µl/min)	Substrate	Infrared mode	Identification limit Mass (ng)	Concentration (mg/L)	Ref.
Direct						
Thermospray	50	Diamond powder	Diffuse reflectance	10	—	152
	1000	Stainless steel tape	Reflection-absorption	1000	25	153
Particle beam	300	KBr window	Transmission	1000	200	154, 155
Ultrasonic nebulizer	500	Ge disk	Reflection-absorption	100	20	156
Electrospray	4	ZnSe window	Transmission with FTIR microscope	1	10	157
Pneumatic nebulizer	30	Aluminum mirror	Reflection-absorption	30	30	158
	2	ZnSe window	Transmission with FTIR microscope	0.5	8	159
	50	ZnSe window	Transmission with FTIR microscope	1	17	160
	20	ZnSe window	Transmission with FTIR microscope	5	3	161, 162
Indirect						
Online liquid–liquid extraction/concentrator	800	KCl powder	Diffuse reflectance	100	10	163
Online liquid–liquid extraction/pneumatic nebulizer	200	ZnSe window	Transmission with FTIR microscope	30	0.2	164
	200	ZnSe window	Transmission with FTIR microscope	50	0.001	165
Makeup/pneumatic nebulizer	2	ZnSe window	Transmission with FTIR microscope	20	0.02	166

REFERENCES

1. R. Smits, LC-GC Int., 7:505 (1994).
2. G.W.F. Stubbings and M.J. Shepherd, J. Liq. Chromatogr., 16:241 (1993).
3. C.G. Chappell, C.S. Creaser, and M.J. Shepherd, J. High Resol. Chromatogr., 16: 479 (1993).
4. C.G. Chappell, C.S. Creaser, and M.J. Shepherd, J. Chromatogr., 626:223 (1992).
5. K.S. Kalasinsky, B. Levine, and M. Smith, Crit. Rev. Anal. Chem., 23:441 (1993).
6. A. Kohn, LC-GC Int., 7:652 (1994).
7. N.A. Botsoglou, J. Agric. Food Chem., 36:1224 (1988).
8. L. Huber, S.A. George, in Diode-Array Detection in HPLC (L. Huber and S.A. George, Eds.), Marcel Dekker, Inc., New York (1993).
9. B.F.H. Drenth, R.T. Ghijsen, and R.A. de Zeeuw, J. Chromatogr., 238:113 (1982).
10. J.C. Miller, S.A. George, and B.G. Willis, Science, 218:241 (1982).
11. A.F. Fell, Anal. Proc., 17:512 (1980).
12. A.F. Fell, H.P. Scott, R. Gill, and A.C. Moffat, Chromatographia, 16:68 (1982).
13. B.J. Clark, A.F. Fell, H.P. Scott, and D. Westerlund, J. Chromatogr., 286:261 (1984).
14. T. Alfredson, T. Sheehan, T. Lenert, S. Aamodt, and L. Correia, J. Chromatogr., 385:213 (1987).
15. P.C. White and T. Catterick, J. Chromatogr., 280:376 (1983).
16. P.C. White and B.B. Wheals, J. Chromatogr., 303:211 (1984).
17. M.H. Kroll, M. Ruddel, D.W. Blank, and R.J. Elin, Clin. Chem., 23:1121 (1987).
18. P.C. White, Analyst, 113:1625 (1988).
19. T.G. Diaz, L.L. Martinez, M.M. Galera, and F. Salinas, J. Liq. Chromatogr., 17: 457 (1994).
20. G. Mildau and S. Maixner, Lebensmittelchemie, 44:19 (1990).
21. J.V. Hinshaw, LC-GC Int., 8:22 (1995).
22. W.G. de Ruig, R.W. Stefany, and G. Dijkstra, J. Assoc. Off. Anal. Chem., 72:487 (1989).
23. W.J. Morris, G.J. Nandrea, J.E. Roybal, R.K. Munns, W. Shimoda, and H.R. Skinner, J. Assoc. Off. Anal. Chem., 70:630 (1987).
24. D.R. Newkirk and C.J. Barnes, J. Assoc. Off. Anal. Chem., 72:581 (1989).
25. J.E. Matusik, C.G. Guyer, J.N. Geleta, and C.J. Barnes, J. Assoc. Off. Anal. Chem., 70:546 (1987).
26. P. Furst, C. Kruger, H.A. Meemken, and W. Groebel, Dtsch. Lebensm. Rundsch., 84:108 (1988).
27. E. van der Heeft, A.P.J.M. de Jong, L.A. van Ginkel, H.J. van Rossum, and G. Zomer, Biol. Mass Spectrom., 20:763 (1991).
28. G.S.F. Bories, J.C. Peleran, and J.M. Wal, J. Assoc. Off. Anal. Chem., 66:1521 (1983).
29. J.J. Lewis, T.D. Macy, and D.A. Garteiz, J. Assoc. Off. Anal. Chem., 72:577 (1989).
30. L. Vuorilehto, J.S. Salonen, and M. Antilla, J. Chromatogr., 530:137 (1990).
31. G. Balisz and D. Arnold, Chromatographia, 27:489 (1989).
32. A.E. Mooser, and H. Koch, J. AOAC Int., 76:976 (1993).
33. Official Journal of the European Communities, No. L351, Brussels, p. 39 (1989).

34. H.F. De Brabander, P. Batjoens, D. Courtheyn, and K. de Wasch, LC-GC Int., 9: 534 (1996).
35. R. Malisch, Z. Lebensm. Unters. Forsch., 182:385 (1986).
36. R. Malisch, Z. Lebensm. Unters. Forsch., 183:253 (1986).
37. R. Malisch, Z. Lebensm. Unters. Forsch., 184:467 (1987).
38. F.B. Suhre, R.M. Simpson, and J.W. Shafer, J. Agric. Food Chem., 29:727 (1981).
39. Official Journal of the European Communities, No. L351, Brussels, p. 32 (1989).
40. W.A. Garland, B.J. Hobson, G. Chen. G. Weiss, N.R. Felicito, and A. MacDonald, J. Agric. Food Chem., 28:273 (1990).
41. H.J. Keukens, M.M.L. Aerts, W.A. Traag, J.F.M. Nouws, W.G. de Ruig, W.M.J. Beek, and J.M.P. den Hartog, J. Assoc. Off. Anal. Chem., 75:245 (1992).
42. W.J. Morris, G.J. Nandrea, J.E. Roybal, R.K. Munns, W. Shimoda, and H.R. Skinner, J. Assoc. Off. Anal. Chem., 70:630 (1987).
43. S. Porter, R. Patel, S. Neate, and P. Osso, in Residues of Veterinary Drugs in Food, Proc. Euroresidue II Conf., Veldhoven, May 3–5, 1993 (N. Haagsma, A. Ruiter, and P.B. Czedik-Eysenberg, Eds.), Fac. Vet. Med., Univ. Utrecht, The Netherlands, p. 548 (1993).
44. W. Haasnoot, M.P. Ploum, R.J.A. Paulussen, R. Schilt, and F.A. Huf, J. Chromatogr., 519:323 (1990).
45. G. Langeloh, and M. Petz, in Residues of Veterinary Drugs in Food, Proc. Euroresidue II Conf., Veldhoven, May 3–5, 1993 (N. Haagsma, A. Ruiter, and P.B. Czedik-Eysenberg, Eds.), Fac. Vet. Med., Univ. Utrecht, The Netherlands, p. 433 (1993).
46. C.G. Chappell, C.S. Creaser, J.W. Stygall, and M.J. Shepherd, Biol. Mass Spectrom., 21:688 (1992).
47. G. Carignan and K. Carrier, J. Assoc. Off. Anal. Chem., 74:479 (1991).
48. M.L. Lynch, F.R. Mosher, R.P. Schneider, and H.G. Fouda, J. Assoc. Off. Anal. Chem., 74:611 (1991).
49. L.A. van Ginkel, H.J. van Rossum, P.W. Zoontjes, H. van Blitterswijk, G. Ellen, E. van der Heeft, A.P.J.M. de Jong, and G. Zomer, Anal. Chim. Acta, 237:61 (1990).
50. D. Courtheyn, H. de Brabander, J. Vercammen, P. Batjoens, M. Logghe, and K. de Wasch, in Residues of Veterinary Drugs in Food, Proc. Euroresidue III Conf., Veldhoven, May 6–8, 1996 (N. Haagsma and A. Ruiter, Eds.), Fac. Vet. Med., Univ. Utrecht, The Netherlands, p. 75 (1996).
51. K.L. Busch, J. Planar Chromatogr., 5:72 (1992).
52. C. Weins and H.E. Hauck, LC-GC Int., 9:710 (1996).
53. K. Rogers, J. Milnes, and J. Gormally, Int. J. Mass Spectrom. Ion Processes, 123: 125 (1993).
54. K.L. Busch, Trends Anal. Chem., 11:314 (1992).
55. G. Somsen, W. Morden, and I.D. Wilson, J. Chromatogr., 703:613 (1995).
56. D. Ghosh, N.K. Mathur, and C.K. Narang, Chromatographia, 37:543 (1993).
57. H. Oka, Shokuhin Eiseigaku Zasshi, 34:517 (1993).
58. P. Traldi, S. Daolio, B. Pelli, R. Maffei Facino, and M. Carini, Biomed. Mass Spectrom., 12:493 (1985).
59. W.C. Brumley, Z. Min, J.E. Matusik, J.A.G. Roach, C.J. Barnes, J.A. Sphon, and T. Fazio, Anal. Chem., 55:1405 (1983).

60. R.P. Schneider, J.F. Ericson, M.J. Lynch, and H.G. Fouda, Biol. Mass Spectrom., 22:595 (1993).

61. R.F. Straub and R.D. Voyksner, J. Chromatogr., 647:167 (1993).

62. J. van der Greef, C.J.M. Arts, M. van Baak, and E.R. Verheij, in Residues of Veterinary Drugs in Food, Proc. Euroresidue II Conf., Veldhoven, May 3–5, 1993 (N. Haagsma, A. Ruiter, and P.B. Czedik-Eysenberg, Eds.), Fac. Vet. Med., Univ. Utrecht, The Netherlands, p. 35 (1993).

63. A. Walhagen, L.E. Edholm, C.E.M. Heeremans, R.A.M. van der Hoeven, W.M.A. Niessen, U.R. Tjaden, and J. van der Greef, J. Chromatogr., 474:257 (1989).

64. J. Henion, G.A. Maylin, and B.A. Thomson, J. Chromatogr., 271:107 (1983).

65. E.M.H. Finlay, D.E. Games, J.R. Startin, and J. Gilbert, Biomed. Environm. Mass Spectrom., 13:633 (1986).

66. I.D. Wilson and W. Morden, LC-GC Int., 12:72 (1999).

67. W. Morden and I.D. Wilson, Rapid Comm. Mass Spectrom., 10:1951 (1996).

68. S. Pleasance, P. Blay, and M.A. Quilliam, J. Chromatogr., 558:155 (1991).

69. J. van der Greef, C.J.M. Arts, M. van Baak, and E.R. Verheij, in Residues of Veterinary Drugs in Food, Proc. Euroresidue II Conf., Veldhoven, May 3–5, 1993 (N. Haagsma, A. Ruiter, and P.B. Czedik-Eysenberg, Eds.), Fac. Vet. Med., Univ. Utrecht, The Netherlands, p. 35 (1993).

70. R.K. Boyd, J. High Resol. Chromatogr., 14:573 (1991).

71. R.C. Willoughby and R.F. Browner, Anal. Chem., 56:2626 (1984).

72. T.D. Behymer, T.A. Bellar, and W.L. Budde, Anal. Chem., 62:1686 (1990).

73. P.C. Winkler, D.D. Perkins, W.K. Williams, and R.F. Browner, Anal. Chem., 60: 489 (1988).

74. A.P. Tinke, R.A.M. van der Hoeven, W.M.A. Niessen, U.R. Tjaden, and J. van der Greef, J. Chromatogr., 554:119 (1991).

75. M. Careri, A. Mangia, and M. Musci, J. Chromatogr., 727:153 (1996).

76. T.A. Bellar, T.D. Behymer, and W.L. Budde, J. Am. Soc. Mass Spectrom., 1:92 (1990).

77. I.S. Kim, F.I. Sasinos, R.D. Stephens, and M.A. Brown, J. Agric. Food Chem., 38: 1223 (1990).

78. M.J. Incorvia Mattina, J. Chromatogr., 542:385 (1991).

79. M.J. Incorvia Mattina, J. Chromatogr., 549:237 (1991).

80. D.R. Doerge, M.W. Burger, and S. Bajic, Anal. Chem., 64:1212 (1992).

81. S.B. Turnipseed, J.E. Roybal, H.S. Rupp, J.A. Hurlbut, and A.R. Long, J. Chromatogr., 670:55 (1995).

82. R.D. Voyksner, C.S. Smith, and P.C. Knox, Biomed. Environ. Mass Spectrom., 19:523 (1990).

83. D.N. Heller and F.J. Schenck, Biol. Mass Spectrom., 22:184 (1993).

84. P.J. Kijak, M.G. Leadbetter, M.H. Thomas, and E.A. Thompson, Biol. Mass Spectrom., 20:789 (1991).

85. B. Delepine and P. Sanders, J. Chromatogr., 582:113 (1992).

86. C.R. Blakley and M.L. Vestal, Anal. Chem., 55:750 (1983).

87. P. Arpino, Mass Spectrom. Rev., 9:631 (1990).

88. P. Arpino, Mass Spectrom. Rev., 11:3 (1992).

89. B.A. Thomson, J.V. Iribarne, and P.J. Dziedzic, Anal. Chem., 54:2219 (1982).

90. W.M.A. Niessen, and J. van der Greef, in Liquid Chromatography–Mass Spectrometry, Principles and Application (W.M.A. Niessen, and J. van der Greef, Eds.), Marcel Dekker, New York (1992).

91. R.E. Kaiser, J.D. Williams, S.A. Lammert, R.G. Cooks, and D. Zackett, J. Chromatogr., 562:3 (1991).

92. W.C. Davidson, R.M. Dinallo, and G.E. Hansen, Biol. Mass Spectrom., 20:389 (1991).

93. J.L. Lewis, T.D. Macy, and D.A. Garteiz, J. Assoc. Off. Anal. Chem., 72:577 (1989).

94. M. Horie, K. Saito, Y. Hoshino, N. Nose, M. Tera, T. Kitsuwa, H. Nakazawa, and Y. Yamane, Eisei Kagaku, 36:283 (1990).

95. A. Khunachak, A.R. Dakunha, and S.J. Stout, J. AOAC Int., 76:1230 (1993).

96. A. Cannavan, W.J. Blanchflower, and D.G. Kennedy, Analyst, 120:331 (1995).

97. R.D. Voyksner, K.L. Tyczkowska, and A.L. Aronson, J. Chromatogr., 567:389 (1991).

98. K.L. Tyczkowska, R.D. Voyksner, and A.L. Aronson, J. Chromatogr., 490:101 (1989).

99. J.O.K. Boison, L.J.-Y. Keng, and J.D. MacNeil, J. AOAC Int., 77:565 (1994).

100. K.L. Tyczkowska, R.D. Voyksner, and A.L. Aronson, J. Vet. Pharmacol. Ther., 14:51 (1991).

101. E.D. Ramsey, D.E. Games, J.R. Startin, C. Crews, and J. Gilbert, Biomed. Environ. Mass Spectrom., 18:5 (1989).

102. S.J. Stout, L.A. Wilson, A.I. Kleiner, A.R. Dacunha, and T.J. Francl, Biomed. Environ. Mass Spectrom., 18:57 (1989).

103. A.P. Bruins, Mass Spectrom. Rev., 10:53 (1991).

104. A.P. Bruins, Trends Anal. Chem., 13:37 (1994).

105. A.P. Bruins, Trends Anal. Chem., 13:81 (1994).

106. L. Voress, Anal. Chem., 66:481A (1994).

107. R.F. Straub and R.D. Voyksner, J. Chromatogr., 647:167 (1993).

108. K.L. Tyczkowska, R.D. Voyksner, R.F. Straub, and A.L. Aronson, J. AOAC Int., 77:1122 (1994).

109. W.J. Blanchflower, S.A. Hewitt, and D.G. Kennedy, Analyst, 119:2595 (1994).

110. J.R. Perkins, C.E. Parker, and K.B. Tomer, J. Am. Soc. Mass Spectrom., 3:139 (1992).

111. W.J. Blanchflower and D.G. Kennedy, Analyst, 120:1129 (1995).

112. J. Harris and J. Wilkins, in Residues of Veterinary Drugs in Food, Proc. Euroresidue III Conf., Veldhoven, May 6–8, 1996 (N. Haagsma, and A. Ruiter, Eds.), Fac. Vet. Med., Univ. Utrecht, The Netherlands, p. 476 (1996).

113. P. Gowik, and B. Julicher, in Residues of Veterinary Drugs in Food, Proc. Euroresidue III Conf., Veldhoven, May 6–8, 1996 (N. Haagsma and A. Ruiter, Eds.), Fac. Vet. Med., Univ. Utrecht, The Netherlands, p. 431 (1996).

114. A.P. Bruins, T.R. Covey, and J.D. Henion, Anal. Chem., 59:2642 (1987).

115. G. Hopfgartner, T. Wachs, K. Bean, and J.D. Henion, Anal. Chem., 65:439 (1993).

116. C. Molina, M. Honing, and D. Barcelo, Anal. Chem., 66:4444 (1994).

117. V. Katta, A.L. Rockwood, and M.L. Vestal, Int. J. Mass Spectrom. Ion Processes, 103:129 (1991).

118. M. Mann, Org. Mass Spectrom., 25:575 (1990).

119. S.A. McLuckley, J. Am. Soc. Mass Spectrom., 3:599 (1992).

120. R.P. Schneider, M.J. Lynch, J.F. Ericson, and H.G. Fouda, Anal. Chem., 63:1789 (1991).

121. S. Pleasance, P. Blay, M.A. Quilliams, and G. O'Hara, J. Chromatogr., 558:155 (1991).

122. S. Pleasance, J. Kelly, M.D. Leblanc, M.A. Quilliams, R.K. Boyd, D.D. Kitts, K. McErlane, M.R. Bailey, and D.H. North, Biol. Mass Spectrom., 21:675 (1992).

123. L.G. McLaughlin and J.D. Henion, J. Chromatogr., 591:195 (1992).

124. R.P. Schneider, J.F. Ericson, M.J. Lynch, and H.G. Fouda, Biol. Mass Spectrom., 22:595 (1993).

125. E.C. Horning, M.G. Horning, D.I. Carroll, I. Dzidic, and R.N. Stillwell, Anal. Chem., 45:936 (1973).

126. J.D. Henion, B.A. Thomson, and P.H. Dawson, Anal. Chem., 54:451 (1982).

127. I. Dzidic, D.I. Carroll, R.N. Stillwell, and E.C. Horning, Anal. Chem., 48:1763 (1976).

128. T.R. Covey, E.D. Lee, and J.D. Henion, Anal. Chem., 58:2453 (1986).

129. P.O. Edlund, L. Bowers, and J.D. Henion, J. Chromatogr., 487:341 (1989).

130. P.O. Edlund, L. Bowers, J.D. Henion, and T.R. Covey, J. Chromatogr., 497:49 (1989).

131. W.M. Muck, and J.D. Henion, Biomed. Environ. Mass Spectrom. 19:37 (1990).

132. D.R. Doerge, S. Bajic, and S. Lowes, Rapid Commun. Mass Spectrom., 7:1126 (1993).

133. R.J. McCracken, W.J. Blanchflower, S.A. Haggan, and D.G. Kennedy, Analyst, 120:1763 (1995).

134. W.J. Blanchflower, A. Cannavan, R.J. McCracken, S.A. Hewitt, P.J. Hughes, S.A. Haggan, and D.G. Kennedy, in Residues of Veterinary Drugs in Food, Proc. Euroresidue III Conf., Veldhoven, May 6–8, 1996 (N. Haagsma and A. Ruiter, Eds.), Fac. Vet. Med., Univ. Utrecht, The Netherlands, p. 253 (1996).

135. R.N. Jones, in Chemical, Biological, and Industrial Applications of Infrared Spectroscopy (J.R. Durig, Ed.), John Wiley and Sons, Chichester, UK (1985).

136. P.R. Griffiths, and J.A. de Haseth, in Fourier Transform Infrared Spectrometry (P.R. Griffiths and J.A. de Haseth, Eds.), Wiley, New York (1986).

137. P. Jackson, G. Dent, D. Carter, D.J. Schofield, J.M. Chalmers, T. Visser, and M. Vredenbregt, J. High Resol. Chromatogr., 16:515 (1993).

138. S. Bourne, A.M. Haefner, K.L. Norton, and P.R. Griffiths, Anal. Chem., 62:2448 (1990).

139. T. Visser, M.J. Vredenbregt, A.P.J.M. de Jong, L.A. van Ginkel, H.J. van Rossum, and R.W. Stephany, Anal. Chim. Acta, 275:205 (1993).

140. G.W. Somsen, C. Gooijer, N.H. Velthorst, and U.A.Th. Brinkman, J. Chromatogr., 811:1 (1998).

141. K. Jinno and C. Fujimoto, J. High Resol. Chromatogr. Communic., 4:532 (1981).

142. J.J. Gagel and K. Biemann, Anal. Chem., 58:2184 (1986).

143. J.J. Gagel and K. Biemann, Anal. Chem., 59:1266 (1987).
144. D. Keuhl and P.R. Griffiths, J. Chromatogr. Sci., 17:471 (1979).
145. D. Keuhl and P.R. Griffiths, Anal. Chem., 52:1394 (1980).
146. J.W. Hellgeth and L.T. Taylor, Anal. Chem., 59:295 (1987).
147. A.H. Dekmezian and T. Moriojka, Anal. Chem., 61:458 (1989).
148. C.L. Putzig, M.A. Leugers, M.L. McKelvy, G.E. Mitchell, R.A. Nyquist, R.R. Papenfuss, and L. Yurga, Anal. Chem., 66:26R (1994).
149. J.J. Gagel and K. Biemann, Anal. Chem., 59:1266 (1987).
150. P.R. Griffiths and A.J. Lange, J. Chromatogr. Sci., 30:93 (1992).
151. J.L. Dwyers, A.E. Chapman, and X. Liu, LC-GC Int., 8:704 (1995).
152. P.R. Griffiths and C.M. Conroy, Adv. Chromatogr., 25:105 (1986).
153. A.M. Robertson, D. Littlejohn, M. Brown, and C.J. Dowle, J. Chromatogr., 588: 15 (1991).
154. R.M. Robertson, J.A. de Haseth, J.D. Kirk, and R.F. Browner, Appl. Spectrosc., 42:1365 (1988).
155. R.M. Robertson, J.A. de Haseth, and R.F. Browner, Appl. Spectrosc., 44:8 (1990).
156. M.X. Liu and J.L. Dwyer, Appl. Spectrosc., 50:348 (1996).
157. M.W. Raynor, K.D. Bartle, and B.W. Cook, J. High Resol. Chromatogr., 15:361 (1992).
158. J.J. Gagel and K. Biemann, Anal. Chem., 59:1266 (1987).
159. A.J. Large, P.R. Griffiths, and D.J.J. Fraser, Anal. Chem., 63:782 (1991).
160. P.R. Griffiths and A.J. Large, J. Chromatogr. Sci., 30:93 (1992).
161. G.W. Somsen, R.J. van de Nesse, C. Gooijer, U.A.Th. Brinkman, N.H. Velthorst, T. Visser, P.R. Kootstra, and A.P.J.M. de Jong, J. Chromatogr., 552.635 (1991).
162. G.W. Somsen, L.P.P. van Stee, C. Gooijer, U.A.Th. Brinkman, N.H. Velthorst, and T. Visser, Anal. Chim. Acta, 290:269 (1994).
163. C.M. Conroy, P.R. Griffiths, P.J. Duff, and L.V. Azaragga, Anal. Chem., 56:2636 (1984).
164. G.W. Somsen, E.W.J. Hooijschuur, C. Gooijer, U.A.Th. Brinkman, N.H. Velthorst, and T. Visser, Anal. Chem., 68:746 (1996).
165. G.W. Somsen, I. Jagt, C. Gooijer, N.H. Velthorst, U.A.Th. Brinkman, and T. Visser, J. Chromatogr., 756:145 (1996).
166. T. Visser, M.J. Vredenbregt, G.J. den Hove, A.P.J.M. de Jong, and G.W. Somsen, Anal. Chim. Acta, 342:151 (1997).

25

Validation

Method validation is the process of confirming that the analytical procedure employed for a specific analysis is suitable for its intended use. Analytical methods need to be validated or revalidated before their introduction into routine use, or whenever the conditions for which the methods have been validated change.

The process of method development and validation has a direct impact on the quality of the final method. Performing a thorough method validation can be a tedious process, but the quality of the data generated with the method is directly linked to the quality of this process. Time constraints often do not allow for sufficient method validation. However, many researchers have experienced the consequences of invalid methods and realized that the amount of time and resources required to solve problems discovered later exceeded what would have been expended initially if the validation studies had been performed properly (1).

Although a thorough validation cannot rule out all potential problems, the process of method development and validation would address the most common ones. Examples of typical problems that can be minimized or avoided include interferences that coelute with the analyte in liquid chromatography (LC), a particular type of column that no longer produces the separation needed because the supplier of the column has changed the manufacturing process, an assay method that is unable to achieve the same detection limit after a few weeks, or a quality assurance audit of a validation report that finds no documentation on how the validation was performed.

Problems increase as additional analysts and laboratories apply the method or different equipment is used to perform the method. When the method is used in the laboratory where it was first developed, a small adjustment is usually enough to make the method work, but this flexibility is lost once the method is transferred to other laboratories and used for official product testing. This is especially true in the field of drug residue analysis, in which methods are submitted to regulatory agencies and changes may require formal approval before they can be implemented for official testing.

Method validation becomes of more crucial importance as requests for drug residue determinations are constantly being pushed to lower limits of detection. Under such conditions, analytical reproducibility becomes more difficult to attain and precision becomes poorer; performing replicate analyses improves the reliability, but for regulatory monitoring programs, this reduces the actual number of samples that can be analyzed and increases the analytical cost for each reported analytical result. In addition, confidence of scientific credibility and disposition of product is lessened, and may be seriously challenged by producers, meat processing establishments, consumers, consumer action groups, or other regulatory control agencies, as analytical determinations are pushed to lower limits.

Validation procedures and key analytical parameters usually examined in common validation practice for both inhouse-developed and standard methods in the field of drug residue analysis are briefly discussed below.

25.1   PARAMETERS FOR METHOD VALIDATION

Detailed guidelines on what parameters should be validated have been described by working groups of many national and international committees (2–11). Unfortunately, definitions given for some parameters vary between different authorities. Recently, an attempt at harmonization was made through an international conference at which representatives from the industry and regulatory agencies from the United States, Europe, and Japan defined parameters, requirements and, to some extent, methodology for the validation of analytical methods (3).

Typical parameters that are generally considered most important for validation of analytical methods are specificity, selectivity, precision, accuracy, extraction recovery, calibration curve, linearity, working range, detection limit, quantification limit, sensitivity, and robustness.

25.1.1   Specificity and Selectivity

Specificity and selectivity are often used interchangeably. A detailed discussion of these terms, as defined by some standard-setting organizations, has been recently reported (12).

Specificity, in general, is the ability of a method to respond only to the substance being measured. This characteristic is often a function of the measuring principle and the function of the analyte under study. A key consideration of specificity is that it must be able to differentiate a compound quantitatively from homologues, analogues, or metabolic products of the residue of interest under the experimental conditions employed.

Selectivity refers to a method that provides responses for a number of chemical entities that may or may not be differentiated from each other. If the response is differentiated from all other responses, the method is said to be selective. Since very few methods respond to only one analyte, the term selectivity is usually more appropriate than specificity.

A selective method must provide for the identification of the compound being measured. Suitable identification tests should be able to discriminate between compounds of closely related structures that are likely to be present. In addition, the identification test may be applied to materials structurally similar or closely related to the analyte to confirm that a positive response is not obtained. The choice of such potentially interfering materials should be based on sound scientific judgment with a consideration of the interferences that could occur. Since it is not always possible to demonstrate that an analytical procedure can completely discriminate for a particular analyte, additional supporting analytical procedures should be available to demonstrate overall selectivity.

The techniques used to demonstrate selectivity will depend on the intended objective of the analytical procedure. The selectivity of a procedure may be confirmed by obtaining positive results from samples containing the analyte, while obtaining negative results from blank samples. For chromatographic procedures, representative chromatograms should be used to demonstrate selectivity and individual components should be appropriately labeled. Similar considerations should be given to other separation techniques.

Critical separations in chromatography should be investigated at an appropriate level. For critical separations, selectivity can be demonstrated by the resolution of the two components that elute closest to each other. Peak purity tests using diode array or mass spectrometric detectors may be useful to show that the analyte chromatographic peak is not attributable to more than one component.

25.1.2 Precision

Precision together with accuracy is one of the most important criteria for judging the performance of an analytical method. It expresses the closeness of agreement or the degree of scatter between a series of measurements obtained from multiple sampling of the same homogeneous sample under the prescribed conditions (13–19). Precision determines random errors that are revealed when replicate measurements of a single quantity are made and cause the individual readings to fall on either side of the mean value.

Precision is usually expressed as a standard deviation, variance, or percentage relative standard deviation of a series of measurements. The most useful term is the percentage relative standard deviation (RSD%) or coefficient of variation

(CV%), because it is relatively constant over a considerable concentration range that ideally covers the level of interest.

Acceptance criteria for precision depend very much on the type of analysis. For pharmaceutical quality control, precision of better than 1% RSD is easily attained, while for biological samples the precision is more like 16% at the detection limit and 10% at higher concentration levels. For environmental and food samples, the precision is very much dependent on the sample matrix, the level of the analyte, and on the analytical method, being in the range of 2% to more than 20% RSD. Acceptable precision values as a function of the analyte concentration have been suggested (11) by the Association of Official Analytical Chemists (AOAC) peer-verified methods program (Table 25.1).

Precision may be considered at three levels: repeatability, intermediate precision, and reproducibility (2, 3). Repeatability expresses the precision obtained by repeatedly analyzing, in one laboratory on the same day by one operator using one piece of equipment, aliquots of a homogeneous sample, each of which has been independently prepared according to the method procedure. Repeatability is also termed intra-assay or within-day precision. It is assessed using a minimum of nine determinations. Repeatability can help in determining the sample preparation procedure, the number of replicate samples to be prepared, and the number of injections required for each sample in the final method setting.

Intermediate precision is defined as the long-term variability of the measurement process and is determined by comparing the results obtained when a method is run within a single laboratory over a number of days. Intermediate precision may reflect discrepancies in the results obtained by different operators, from different instruments, with different sources of reagents, with multiple lots of

TABLE 25.1   Analyte Precision and Recovery at Different Concentrations

Analyte concentration	Precision (RSD %)	Mean recovery (%)
100%	1.3	98–102
10%	2.8	98–102
1%	2.7	97–103
0.1%	3.7	95–105
100 ppm	5.3	90–107
10 ppm	7.3	80–110
1 ppm	11	80–110
100 ppb	15	80–110
10 ppb	21	60–115
1 ppb	30	40–120

Source: From Ref. 11.

columns, or a combination of these factors. Hence, intermediate precision is also termed intra-assay or between-day precision.

The extent to which intermediate precision should be established depends on the circumstances under which the procedure is intended to be used. The developing analyst should establish the effects of random events on the precision of the analytical procedure and identify which of the above factors contributes significant variability to the final result. The objective of intermediate precision validation is to verify that in the same laboratory the method will provide the same results once the developmental phase is over.

Reproducibility is defined as the precision obtained between laboratories. The objective is to verify that the method will provide the same results when it is applied in different laboratories. It is determined by analyzing aliquots from homogeneous lots in different laboratories with different analysts and by using operational and environmental conditions that may differ from, but are still within, the specified parameters of the method, often as part of interlaboratory crossover studies.

The evaluation of reproducibility results often focuses more on measuring bias in results than on determining differences in precision alone. Statistical equivalence is often used as a measure of acceptable interlaboratory results. An example of reproducibility criteria for an assay method could be that the assay results obtained in multiple laboratories will be statistically equivalent or the mean results will be within 2% of the value obtained by the primary testing laboratory.

Intermediate precision and reproducibility studies form much of what historically has been called ruggedness. The variability obtained in the developing laboratory, after considerable experience with the method, is usually less than that achieved by less-experienced laboratories who may later use the method. For this reason, if a method cannot achieve a suitable level of repeatability in the developing laboratory, it cannot be expected to do any better in other laboratories.

25.1.3 Accuracy and Extraction Recovery

The accuracy of an analytical method is estimated as the percentage difference (bias) between the mean values generated by the method and the true or known concentrations. Accuracy is usually synonymous with systematic errors. Systematic errors cause all the results in a series of replicates to deviate from the true value of the measured quantity in a particular sense (i.e., all the results are too high or all are too low) (20). Accuracy has also been used in recent years to refer to any error causing a single measurement to deviate from the true value (i.e., to encompass elements of random and systematic errors) (21).

Accuracy can be assessed in several ways. Since for real samples the true value is not known, one approach is to compare test results from the method with results from an existing, alternative, well-characterized method, the accuracy of which is defined. Another approach is to analyze a sample of known concentration (for example, a certified reference material) and compare the measured value with the true value as supplied with the material. Table 25.2 presents a list of reference materials available or under preparation by the Standards, Measurement and Testing program of the European Union for drug residue analysis in food (22).

If a certified material is not available, as is usually the case in drug residue analysis, an approximation can be obtained by spiking the blank sample matrix to a nominal concentration. The accuracy of the method is then determined by assessing the agreement between the measured and nominal concentrations of the analytes in the spiked drug-free matrix sample. The spiking levels should cover the range of concern and should include one concentration close to the quantitation limit.

Since the spiking-based approach also measures the effectiveness of the sample preparation procedure, care should be taken to mimic the actual sample preparation as closely as possible. It should be always considered that in many cases the analyte added to a sample may not behave in the same manner as the same analyte biologically incurred; at relatively high concentrations, and particularly with methods involving a large number of sample preparation steps, percentage recoveries may be lower.

Accuracy, in general, is assessed using a minimum of nine determinations over a minimum of three concentration levels covering a range of 50–150% of the target concentration (e.g., three concentration levels with three replicates each). The criteria for acceptable accuracy of the assay results cannot be generalized because accuracy depends on the concentrations of the analytes being evaluated and the acceptable criteria depend on the purpose of the analysis (23).

A literature survey shows that the concentration of the analyte found when analyzing a spiked blank sample matrix is often expressed as the percentage of the known or true drug concentration and is called recovery. By this definition, recovery is the same as accuracy, which is why accuracy is reported as recovery in many scientific reports. The difference is that the recovery, as defined, should be close to 100%, while the accuracy close to 0%.

Recovery experiments are usually performed during the developmental phase of the assay method. The extraction recovery can be determined by processing a spiked blank matrix and calculating its response as a percentage of the response of a pure standard that has not been subjected to sample preparation (24). It is best established by comparing the responses of extracted samples at low, medium, and high spiked matrix concentrations in replicates of at least six with those of nonextracted standards that represent 100% recovery. The effect of coextracted endogenous sample components may be studied by comparing the response of extracted samples spiked before extraction with the response of extracted blank matrix samples to which analyte has been added at the same

TABLE 25.2 Reference Materials Available or Under Preparation

Reference material	Current situation	Status	Availability
Diethylstilbestrol in urine	Ready	Certified	Available (BCR)[a]
Hexestrol in urine	Ready	Certified	Available (BCR)
Dienestrol in urine	Ready	Indicative value	Available (BCR)
Chloramphenicol in muscle	Ready	Certified	Available (BCR)
Chloramphenicol in milk and eggs	Ready	Not certified	Available (BCR)
Diethylstilbestrol in muscle	Ready	Not certified	Available (BCR)
β-Agonists in urine	Ready	Certified	Available (BCR)
Oxytetracycline in milk	Ready	Certification under discussion	Available (BCR)
Ampicillin in milk	Under evaluation	Not certified	To be determined
Neomycin in milk	Ready	Certification under discussion	Available (BCR)
Zeranol in urine, liver and muscle	Ready	Certification under discussion	Available (BCR)
Sulphadimidine in muscle, liver and kidney	Ready	Not certified	Available (BCR)
Nortestosterone	Ready	Certified	Available (BCR)
Trenbolone in urine	Ready	Certified	Available (BCR)
Clenbuterol, salbutamol and terbutaline in liver	Ready	Certified	Available (BCR)
Trenbolone in liver	Ready	Certified	Available (BCR)
Chlortetracycline in pig liver, kidney and muscle	In preparation	Certification planed 1997–98	Available 1998–99
Ronidazole in poultry muscle	In preparation	Certification planed 1997–98	Available 1998–99
Dimetridazole in poultry muscle	In preparation	Certification planed 1997–98	Available 1998–99
Clenbuterol in eye	In preparation	Certification planed 1998	Available 1998–99

[a] European Communities Bureau of Reference.
Source: From Ref. 22.

nominal concentration just before the final measurement (25). The extraction recovery, defined as above, is sometimes also called absolute recovery.

Although it is desirable to attain recoveries as close to 100% as possible in order to maximize the efficiency of the method, it may be equally desirable intentionally to sacrifice high recovery in order to achieve better selectivity with some sample preparation procedures. It is unlikely that recoveries at around 50% will compromise the integrity of a method that has adequate selectivity and, hence, good precision. Acceptable recovery data as a function of analyte concentration have been suggested (11) by the AOAC peer-verified methods program (Table 25.1).

25.1.4 Calibration, Linearity, and Working Range

A calibration curve is a graph on which concentration is plotted along the x-axis and analytical response is plotted along the y-axis. The line connecting the points represents the calibration curve. The calibration curve study is generally performed by preparing standard solutions at five concentration levels, from 50 to 150% of the target analyte concentration. A minimum of five levels is required to allow detection of curvature in the plotted data.

In addition, or as an alternative, to the visual evaluation of the linearity of the calibration curve, frequently the linearity is evaluated mathematically by calculation of a regression line with the method of least squares (26). Data from the regression line, such as the correlation coefficient, y-intercept, slope of the regression line, and residual sum of squares, help greatly in providing mathematical estimates of the degree of linearity. Acceptability of linearity data is often judged by examining the correlation coefficient and y-intercept of the linear regression line for the response versus concentration plot. A correlation coefficient higher than 0.999 is generally considered evidence of an acceptable fit of data to the regression line, while the y-intercept should be less than a few percent of the response obtained for the analyte at the target level.

In some instances, calibration test data may need to be subjected to some kind of mathematical transformation, prior to the regression analysis, in order to obtain linear calibration plots. In some cases, however, such as in immunochemical assays, linearity cannot be demonstrated even after any transformation. The use of nonlinear calibration curves for analysis has been discussed (27).

Nevertheless, in most cases calibration plots exhibit linearity within a certain concentration range. This range of concentrations is referred to as the linear dynamic range of the analysis. If we analyze a sample in the linear dynamic range, we can calculate the regression line equation and use it to solve for concentration rather than using pencil and ruler. If the sample concentration is outside of that range, we can either dilute it or concentrate it further by evaporating some of the solvent.

When an assay method is performed repeatedly to analyze a high volume of samples, the instability of the calibration curves or an apparent change in response factor often indicates that some conditions of the assay are drifting, are no longer stable, and need to be evaluated. Reasons for the instability of the calibration curves can include variation of the extraction procedures, deterioration of the efficiency of a chromatographic column, or decline of the efficiency of the detection system (28).

The linearity of an analytical method is its ability to elicit test results that are directly, or by means of well-defined mathematical transformations, proportional to the concentration of the analyte in the sample within a given range. It is determined by analyzing a series of three to six replicates of five or more blank samples, each spiked with the analyte at a different concentration within the examined concentration range. Analytical response should be proportional to the concentrations of the analytes in spiked samples. A linear regression equation applied to the results should have an intercept not significantly different from zero. If a significant nonzero intercept is obtained, it should be demonstrated that there is no effect on the accuracy of the method. Linearity verifies that the sample extracts are in a concentration range where analyte response is linearly proportional to concentration.

The working range of an analytical method is the interval between the upper and lower concentrations of the analyte in the sample for which it has been demonstrated that the method has acceptable precision, accuracy and linearity. This interval is normally derived from linearity studies and depends on the intended application of the method. However, validating over a range wider than actually needed provides confidence that the routine standard levels are well removed from nonlinear response concentrations, and allows quantitation of crude samples in support of process development. The range is normally expressed in the same units as the test results obtained by the analytical method.

In practice, the working range of an analytical method is determined using data from the linearity and accuracy studies. Assuming that acceptable linearity and accuracy results were obtained, the only remaining factor to be evaluated is precision. Precision may change as a function of the analyte level. In general, the percentage RSD values increase significantly as the concentration decrease. Higher variability is expected as the analyte levels approach the detection limit for the method. The developer must judge at what concentration the imprecision becomes too great for the intended use of the method. An example of range criteria for an assay method is that the acceptable range will be defined as the concentration interval over which linearity and accuracy are obtained per previously discussed criteria and that, in addition, yields a precision of better than 10% RSD.

25.1.5   Limit of Detection, Limit of Quantification, and Sensitivity

These terms have been defined in different ways, thus giving rise to a great deal of confusion (29–42). The limit of detection has been described as the lowest concentration or quantity of an analyte that an analytical method can detect with reasonable certainty (31) or can reliably detect (29). Such descriptions based on definition of the terms "reasonable certainty" and "reliable detect" allow considerable freedom to define the limit of detection.

In the field of analytical chemistry, the limit of detection is commonly defined as the concentration of an analyte that gives a measured signal equal to the mean blank signal plus three times the standard deviation of the blank signal (43). Thus, in chromatography, the detection limit is the injected amount that results in a peak with a height typically three times as high as the baseline noise level. On the other hand, the concentration of an analyte that gives a measured signal equal to the mean blank signal plus 10 times the standard deviation of the blank is defined as the limit of quantification (41, 44, 45).

Estimate of the standard deviation of the blank can be carried out in a variety of ways. One way is to measure the magnitude of the analytical background response by analyzing an appropriate number of blank samples and calculating the standard deviation of these responses. Another way is to construct a specific calibration curve using samples containing the analyte in the range of the detection limit and calculating the residual standard deviation of the regression line or the standard deviation of the y-intercepts of multiple regression lines. The latter approach has been considered as a more accurate measure of the blank signal to define the limit of detection and the limit of quantification (44).

Both the limit of detection and the limit of quantification have been also defined as ratios of the analyte signal to the background signal (S/N). Thus, an S/N ratio of 3 has been used to define the detection limit, whereas a S/N ratio of 10 has been used to define the limit of quantification. Determination of the signal-to-noise ratios is performed by comparing measured signals from samples with known low concentrations of analyte with those of blank samples.

The limit of quantification is more relevant than the limit of detection in the analysis of drug residues in foods. In these applications, the limit of quantification can be more practically defined as the lowest drug concentration in food samples that can be measured with a desired level of accuracy and precision. It is usually determined by reducing the analyte concentration until a level is reached where the precision of the assay becomes unacceptable. If the required precision of the method at the limit of quantification has been specified, a number of samples with decreasing amounts of the analyte are analyzed 6 times at minimum, and the calculated RSD% of the precision is plotted against the analyte amount; the amount that corresponds to the previously defined required precision is equal to the limit of quantification.

Both the detection limit and the limit of quantification, as defined, are often not very stable characteristics of an analytical method, because the blank signal and the signal generated by the very low concentrations of the analyte are frequently dependent on certain analytical parameters, including the purity of reagents, sample matrices, environmental conditions, instrumentation, and the analysts themselves. Sensitivity is a measure of the ability of an analytical method to discriminate between small differences in analyte concentration. It is defined as the analyte signal per unit concentration of the analyte. Despite the apparent simplicity of the sensitivity concept, a degree of confusion surrounds its use. This confusion stems from the perception that the sensitivity of a method is the same as the limit of detection.

However, one principle on which all authorities agree is that the sensitivity is simply the slope of the calibration plot. It is common practice to define sensitivity as the slope of the calibration curve; an ideal situation would be afforded by a linear curve. In practice, the concept of the limit of detection is of limited value in comparing methods, since it depends so much on experimental conditions; for example, the limit of detection of a spectrophotometric determination can be simply increased by increasing the optical path length.

25.1.6 Robustness

Robustness is the ability of a method to remain unaffected by small changes in operational parameters and provides an indication of its reliability during normal usage.

For determining the robustness of a method a number of parameters, such as extraction time, mobile-phase pH, mobile-phase composition, injection volume, source of column lots and/or suppliers, temperature, detection wavelength, and the flow rate, are varied within a realistic range and the quantitative influence of the variables is determined. If the influence of a parameter is within a previously specified tolerance, this parameter is said to be within the robustness range of the method. These method parameters may be evaluated one factor at a time or simultaneously as part of a factorial experiment.

Obtaining data on the effects of these parameters may allow one to judge whether a method needs to be revalidated when one or more parameters are changed. For example, if column performance changes over time, adjusting the mobile-phase strength to compensate for changes in the column may be allowed if such data are included in the validation.

The evaluation of robustness should be considered during the developmental phase of a method and depends on the type of procedure under study. If measurements are susceptible to variations in analytical conditions, the analytical conditions should be suitably controlled or a precautionary statement should be included in the procedure. Once the robustness of a method has been established, data on system suitability criteria, which are required prior to routine use of the method to ensure that it is performing appropriately, can be collected. Typically, the process involves making five injections of a standard solution and evaluating several chromatographic parameters such as resolution, number of theoretical plates, and tailing factor.

25.2 PROCEDURES FOR METHOD VALIDATION

Frameworks for performing method validation are provided by international organizations and conferences on harmonization (2–11). However, validation requirements vary widely, depending on the intended use of the method, the regulatory agency, and the type of the drug being tested. Moreover, in practice, there is great diversity in how the validation studies are performed, although there has been general agreement about what types of validation studies should be used. As a result, virtually every laboratory and organization has problems when it comes to establishing methods developed elsewhere. In fact, establishing a method developed elsewhere could be viewed as more difficult than developing a method from first principles (1).

The validity of a specific method should be demonstrated in laboratory experiments using test samples or standards that are similar to the unknown samples analyzed in the routine. For example, control tissue samples from non-treated animals, control tissue samples spiked with the analyte at several known concentrations, and dosed or incurred tissue samples from animals that have been treated with the drug, should all be available to the analyst before starting a validation process. All these samples will enable the analyst to define the background noise, to identify the amounts of the analyte added to the control tissue, and demonstrate that the method can satisfactorily recover the biologically incurred residue.

The preparation and execution should follow a validation protocol, in which the scope of the method and its validation criteria should first be defined (46). The scope of the analytical method should be clearly understood since this will govern the validation characteristics that need to be evaluated. For example, if the method is to be used for qualitative trace residue analysis, there is no need to examine and validate its linearity over the full dynamic range of the equipment. The scope of the method should also include the different types of equipment and the locations where the method will be run. In this way, experiments can be limited to what is really necessary. For example, if the method is intended for use in one specific laboratory, there is no need to include other laboratories and different equipment in the validation experiments.

On the other hand, a complete list of validation criteria should be agreed on by the developer and the end users before the method is developed, so that expectations are becoming clear. During the actual studies and in the final validation report, these criteria will allow clear judgment about the acceptability of the analytical method.

Satisfactory results for a method can only be obtained with well-performing equipment. Therefore, before an instrument is used to validate a method, its performance should be verified using universal standards (47). Special attention should be paid to the equipment specifications that are critical for the performance of the method. For example, if detection limit is critical for a specific method, the detector specifications for baseline noise and the response to the specified compounds should be checked. Furthermore, any reagent or reference standard used to determine critical validation parameters should be double-checked for accurate composition and purity.

The suitability of a method for its intended use should be proven in initial experiments. These introductory studies should include the approximate precision, accuracy, detection limit, and working range. If these preliminary validation data appear to be inappropriate, either the method itself or the acceptance limits should be changed. The developer does not know whether the method conditions are acceptable until validation studies are performed. Results of validation studies may indicate that a change in the procedure is necessary, which may then require revalidation. In this way, method development and validation seems to be an iterative process; during each developmental phase, key method parameters are determined and then used for all subsequent validation steps.

Apart from establishing analytical validation parameters, other activities should include experimental optimization of each procedural step or method manipulation to determine the critical control steps that have a substantial impact on method performance. The ruggedness or process variability that may be employed in any particular method step, without reducing method performance, should be determined. It should be identified, for example, whether an analytical method may be stopped without adversely affecting the result.

In a well-designed validation procedure, the periodicity of quality-control checks should also be defined. For example, it is often essential, for routine testing, that solutions be stable enough to allow for delays such as instrument breakdowns or overnight analyses using autosamplers. At this point, the limits of stability should be tested. Samples and standards should be tested over at least a 48 h period, and quantification of components should be determined by comparison with freshly prepared standards. If the solutions are not stable over 48 h, storage conditions or additives should be identified that can improve stability. Criteria should be defined to indicate when the method and system are out of statistical control. The target is to optimize these experiments so that, with a minimum number of controls, the method will provide long-term results that will meet the objectives defined in the scope of the method.

Besides the development and the optimization of the analytical method itself, the most important factor in defining performance characteristics is the multilaboratory validation study. The principles of conducting either a validation or collaborative study of a method are the same. Methods with high reliability for residue testing should be able to undergo successfully a collaborative study involving at least eight different laboratories. Considerations include informing participants of the study and involving them in the study design. Laboratories should be chosen with as wide a distribution as possible, and should include regulatory control agency, international authority, industry, and academic laboratories. Sample shipment techniques should be prearranged and should include practice samples. This is particularly important when studies are conducted internationally. Prudent and thorough planning are essential for these studies because of their expense.

Subjecting methods to different residue-testing environments may place some additional requirements on methods. Warmer environments require reagents to be more thermally stable, solvents to be less volatile, and tissue sample considerations to be more tolerant. Cooler environments may require reagents and solvents with physical properties such as lower freezing points and higher solvating properties to ensure effective extraction of an analyte. Environmental temperatures may also influence the time required to perform an analysis, as well as such phenomena as reaction rates for derivatization and color development. These considerations may strain efforts to standardize methods in broadly differing environments, because of the need to adapt methods to different environmental factors.

Methods intended for regulatory residue control should be designed with as much simplicity as possible to limit the variety, size, and type of glassware and equipment needed; to minimize the potential for analytical error; and to reduce costs. Reagents and standards must be readily available while specific instrumentation should be based on performance characteristics rather than a particular manufacturer.

Residue methods should further be portable and capable of running many samples in a reasonable period of time. The capability for simultaneous analyses aids in method efficiency by allowing sets or batches of samples to be analyzed at the same time. This attribute is particularly important when large numbers of samples must be analyzed within 1 working day.

Finally, the method must be written in thorough, concise, unambiguous language. A list of the reagents and supplies, as well as their commercial sources, must be included. Instrument parameters, and procedures to test instrument performance, need to be described as part of the method. Detailed conditions on how the experiments were performed, including sample preparation, must be presented. Method performance parameters and conditions have to be documented. Critical parameters indicated from robustness testing must be addressed. Procedures for quality control in the routine and statistical calculations must be summarized. These factors will facilitate method transfer into a regulatory monitoring program.

REFERENCES

1. R.D. McDowall, LC-GC Int., 11:648 (1998).
2. EURACHEM Guidance Document No. WGD 2, Accreditation for chemical laboratories: Guidance on the interpretation of the EN 45000 series of standards and ISO/IEC Guide 25, EURACHEM, Middlesex, UK (1993).
3. VICH, Guideline on Validation of Analytical Procedures: Methodology, Veterinary International Cooperation on Harmonization, EMEA/CVMP/590/98-Final, London, UK (1998).
4. US EPA, Guidance for Methods Development and Methods Validation for the Resource Conservation and Recovery Act Program, Washington, USA (1995).
5. US FDA Technical Review Guide, Validation of Chromatographic Methods, Center for Drug Evaluation and Research, Rockville, MD, USA (1993).
6. US FDA, General Principles of Validation, Center for Drug Evaluation and Research, Rockville, MD, USA (1987).
7. US FDA, Guidelines for Submitting Samples and Analytical Data for Method Validation, Center for Drugs and Biologics, Department of Health and Human Services, Rockville, MD, USA (1987).
8. G. Szepesi, M. Gazdag, and K. Mihalyfi, J. Chromatogr., 464:265 (1989).
9. J.M. Green, Anal. Chem., 68:305A/309A (1996).
10. W. Wegscheider, in Validation of Analytical Methods (H. Guenzler, Ed.), Springer Verlag, Berlin, Germany (1996).
11. AOAC Peer Verified Methods Program, Manual on Polices and Procedures, Arlington, VA, USA (1993).
12. J. Vessman, J. Pharm. Biomed. Anal., 14:867 (1996).
13. D.M. Holland, and F.F. McElroy, Environ. Sci. Technol., 20:1157 (1986).
14. D.H. Besterfield, in Quality Control (D.H. Besterfield, Ed.), 2nd Edition, Prentice-Hall, Englewood Cliffs, NJ (1986).
15. B. Kratochvil and N. Motkosky, Anal. Chem., 59:1064 (1987).
16. L.C. Alwan and M.G. Bissell, Clin. Chem., 34:1396 (1988).
17. J.F. Wilson, J. Williams, L.M. Tsanaclis, J.E. Tedstone, and A. Richens, Ther. Drug Monit., 10:438 (1988).
18. J.F. Wilson, L.M. Tsanaclis, J. Williams, J.E. Tedstone, and A. Richens, Ther. Drug Monit., 11:185 (1989).
19. J.F. Wilson, L.M. Tsanaclis, J. Williams, J.E. Tedstone, and A. Richens, Ther. Drug Monit., 11:196 (1989).
20. J.C. Miller and J.N. Miller, Analyst, 113:1351 (1988).
21. G.T. Wernimont, and W. Spedley, in Use of Statistics to Develop and Evaluate Analytical Methods (G.T. Wernimont, and W. Spedley, Eds.), Association of Official Analytical Chemists, Arlington, VA, USA (1985).
22. L.A. van Ginkel and C. Dirscherl, in Residues of Veterinary Drugs in Food, Proc. Euroresidue III Conf., Veldhoven, May 6–8, 1996 (N. Haagsma, and A. Ruiter, Eds.), Fac. Vet. Med., Univ. Utrecht, The Netherlands, p. 143 (1996).
23. M. Thompson, Analyst, 113:1579 (1998).
24. R. Causon, J. Chromatogr., 689:175 (1997).

25. S. Braggio, R.J. Barnaby, P. Grossi, and M. Cugola, J. Pharm. Biomed. Anal., 14: 375 (1996).
26. M. Mulholland, and D.B. Hibbert, J. Chromatogr., 762:73 (1997).
27. F. Cverna and C.R. Hamlin, Clin. Chem., 32:1307 (1986).
28. J. Masse, P. Leclerc, and M. Pouliot, Clin. Chem., 34:599 (1988).
29. G.H. Morrison, Anal. Chem., 52:2241 (1980).
30. J.B. Philips, Anal. Chem., 58:2091 (1986).
31. IUPAC, Spectrochim. Acta B, 33B:242 (1987).
32. C.A. Clayton, J.W. Hines, and P.D. Elkins, Anal. Chem., 59:2508 (1987).
33. Analytical Methods Committee, Analyst, 112:199 (1987).
34. J. Vogelgesang, Fresenius. Z. Anal. Chem., 328:213 (1987).
35. G. Bergmann, B. Von Oepen, and P. Zinn, Anal. Chem., 59:2522 (1987).
36. L.A. Currie, in Detection in Analytical Chemistry (L.A. Currie, Ed.), American Chemical Society, Washington, DC, USA (1988).
37. T.W. Williams and E.D. Salin, Anal. Chem., 60:725 (1988).
38. S.G. Weber and J.T. Long, Anal. Chem., 60:903a (1988).
39. G.W. Peng and W.L. Chiou, J. Chromatogr., 531:3 (1990).
40. J.N. Miller, Analyst, 116:3 (1991).
41. G.C.C. Su, J. AOAC Int., 81:105 (1998).
42. M. Thompson, Analyst, 123:405 (1998).
43. D.L. Massart, B.G.M. Vandeginste, S.N. Deming, Y. Michotte, and L. Kaufman, in Chemometrics: A Textbook (D.L. Massart, B.G.M. Vandeginste, S.N. Deming, Y. Michotte, and L. Kaufman, Eds.), Elsevier, Amsterdam (1988).
44. D.G. Mitchell and J.S. Garden, Talanta, 29:921 (1982).
45. A.C. Mehta, Talanta, 34:355 (1987).
46. L. Huber, LC-GC Int., 11:96 (1998).
47. L. Huber, LC-GC Int., 9:794 (1996).

26

Analytical Strategy

The demand for reliable, sensitive, automated, fast, low-cost methods for residue analysis that are also applicable to a wide range of drugs and matrices is growing fast, especially in the field of food inspection. A universal analytical scheme that could simultaneously quantify all compounds of interest in the edible animal products, correctly identify the molecular structure of the analytes, and, at the same time, produce very few false-negative and -positive results to protect the consumer, producer and international trade, would provide the most desirable approach. A unified procedure would eliminate the need for using separate multi-residue methods to screen food commodities for potential drug residues, and combinations of suitable single- or multianalyte methods to identify and quantify residues of individual analytes.

However, such ideal methods are not encountered in the real world. Therefore, it is necessary to combine a number of different methods, each making use of appropriate separation and detection principles, into an integrated system that will be applied according to the analytical objectives (1). For regulatory purposes, this integrated system should include a screening phase, an intermediate phase, and a confirmation phase (2).

Methods used in the screening phase should prevent false-negative results and provide an acceptable percentage of false-positive results with a high sample throughput at low cost. Methods used in the confirmation phase should prevent false-positive results; such methods usually have low sample throughput and a high cost, but enable the surveillance to be spread more comprehensively than would be the case if all samples had to be initially analyzed by time-, labor- and cost-intensive laboratory methods. Finally methods used in the intermediate phase should tentatively identify and, sometimes, quantify the type of residues.

26.1   CLASSIFICATION OF METHODS FOR REGULATORY PURPOSES

Regulatory, control, and standard-setting bodies have used different terminology to describe regulatory methods in the field of drug residues analysis. Most often, methods used for surveillance testing are classified according to their intended purpose. Terms such qualitative, quantitative, semiquantitative, multiresidue, single-residue, screening, pre- or postslaughter screening, confirmatory, routine, and reference methods have all been used to characterize regulatory analytical methods. An alternative to the potential difficulty of categorizing methods and the stigma associated with these descriptive terms is to define regulatory methods according to their attributes of method performance.

26.1.1   Classification According to the Intended Use

Methods for residue analysis are classified as qualitative, quantitative, or semiquantitative. Qualitative methods employ a predetermined cutoff value to classify samples as positive or negative relative to an established drug concentration. Quantitative methods require that positive samples covering a wide range of drug concentrations be tested with each sample test, thus permitting residue quantification by extrapolation from a standard curve; such methods are usually based on specific instrumentation to measure the test response and determine the standard curve (3, 4). Semiquantitative methods are similar to quantitative methods except that test results are interpreted relative to a range of positive controls run with test samples (e.g., low-positive, high-positive, or negative samples).

Most residue methods used in field applications are qualitative or semiquantitative and are classified as screening methods. Quantitative methods require much more technical expertise, and, therefore, their primary use is in laboratory applications primarily for confirmation purposes. Both screening and confirmation methods can be subclassified into multiresidue methods aiming at the detection of groups of compounds having similar analytical characteristics, and single-residue methods applicable to only one specific analyte.

Screening methods are the first procedures applied in a regulatory residue program, the purpose being to establish the presence or absence of residues above their established maximum residue limits (MRL). A screening method may be defined as an assay that gives a reliable and accurate indication that the analyte of interest is not present in the sample at unsafe or violative levels (1, 5). This requires that screening assays provide a detection limit optimized below the tolerance or MRLs levels so that a violative sample will have a high probability of causing a positive test result (1).

Methods used in the screening phase should be able to detect the presence of as many drug residues as possible at the established for each drug level of interest, with a high sample throughput at low cost. Most microbiological methods are excellent screening procedures because they generally lack specificity, and therefore are able to detect many different antibacterials simultaneously. These methods can detect all substances that are inhibitory to growth of added microorganisms, but noninhibitory metabolites of antibacterials or conjugated residues that have not been previously hydrolyzed cannot be detected. They offer versatility, simplicity, high sample capacity, low cost, and often better sensitivity than many physicochemical instrumental methods. However, offered sensitivity varies strongly with each specific antibacterial, and in some cases may be inadequate for residue control. Special expertise and/or sophisticated equipment is not generally required, but imprecision and inaccuracy can be a serious problem when there is a deviation from the assay protocol. In addition, certain compounds that occur naturally in food of animal origin are frequently inhibitory to the growth of the assay microorganism interfering with the analysis.

On the other hand, it has to be realized that a microbiological inhibition-free food commodity does not necessarily describe a residue-free sample. Since not all veterinary drugs and/or their metabolites exhibit antimicrobial activity, immunochemical and chromatographic methods have to be also applied for screening purposes. These methods also help in identifying individual compounds within a group of antimicrobial residues in samples found positive by microbiological screening tests. As a rule, these methods are very sensitive and selective but they are expensive and cannot be considered as definitive from a regulatory perspective because they may yield false-positive results. Screening tests based on immunochemical reactions, in particular, provide several exciting capabilities to drug residue detection.

Since they do not require complicated instrumentation, screening tests are usually very rapid in performance, with analytical results being achieved in minutes. Not only can more tests be performed in a given time period, but many screening tests can be used outside the laboratory. This capability is an advantage in residue control and public health protection, because an initial analysis is a real possibility at the level of drug use. The importance of these screening tests in residue detection can be exemplified by the number of different tests commercially available for milk testing.

Since the problem of drug residues in food supplies and manufactured products originates at the farm level, quick and reliable preslaughter screening tests that can be used at the farm gate level have been also developed to ensure that any live animal that has been treated with veterinary drugs and is to be shipped to slaughter is residue-free. Examples of such tests include agar diffusion tests for preslaughter field screening of antibacterial residues in urine (6, 7); immunochemical tests for rapid field screening for residues of the β-agonist clenbuterol in cattle hair (8, 9); residues of clenbuterol, mabuterol, and cimaterol in bovine urine (10); residues of estrogenic anabolics in urine from veal calves (11) and residues of nandrolone in swine urine (12); and physicochemical methods for screening of tranquilizers in porcine urine (13) and dexamethasone in cattle urine (14). Quick postslaughter screening tests such as the agar diffusion tests for examination of slaughtered animals for the presence of antibacterial residues in renal pelvis fluid (15, 16) have been also developed. Hence, screening methods may be subclassified into preslaughter and postslaughter tests.

Postslaughter screening tests for antibiotic residues, in general, have to cope with thousands of samples. Simplicity, low cost, and nonspecificity are advisable to detect a wide range of antibacterials. Samples that give a presumptive positive reading have then to be examined further by confirmatory and/or determinative methods that, generally, have a low sample throughput at high cost, to establish unequivocally the concentration and identity of the residue, thus enabling the surveillance to be spread more comprehensively than if all samples had to be initially analyzed by time-, labor- and cost-intensive laboratory methods.

For reliable identification of a residue, detailed information about the molecular structure of the analyte is essential. The total information about the molecular structure of the analyte is the sum of the information derived from each individual analytical step of the method. Frequently used selective analytical steps based on chromatography or immunoaffinity, provide more or less general indirect information. For example, solid-phase extraction (SPE) cleanup followed by liquid chromatography/ultraviolet detection (LC/UV) has been suggested for screening and quantification of ivermectin residues in liver, but presumptive positive samples can be confirmed by derivatizing an aliquot of the SPE eluate and reanalyzing the fluorescent derivative of ivermectin in an LC-fluorescence system (17).

For complete identification, relevant direct information on the molecular structure of the analyte is always more specific and hence more reliable than indirect information. Analytical steps based on molecular spectroscopy all provide direct more or less detailed information on the structure of the analyte. This is particularly true for fourier-transform infrared (FTIR) and mass spectroscopy (MS), where the spectra have a very high information content.

The European Union also follows a classification system according to the intended use. In this system, methods for drug residue analysis are grouped as routine and reference. Because the European Union does not recommend official methods of analysis, this distinction, originally aimed at differentiating the methods into two categories, should be applied in the National Programs of the individual European Union members for monitoring the illegal use of hormonal growth promoters in slaughtered animals. Routine methods are used for screening while reference methods are used for confirming positive residue findings. However, no sharp definition for each category has been given, although it was generally accepted that reference methods should supply more reliable results for the intended purpose than the routine methods.

26.1.2 Classification According to Performance Attributes

During the last decade, minimum quality criteria for routine (18) and reference (19) methods have been set within the European Union. With the introduction of these criteria, a scientific base was founded in European Union that could help in better specifying the suitability of the regulatory methods. Since setting the minimum quality criteria for a method does not tell anything about its actual validation and practicability status, in 1988 an EU expert group started to draft a performance status list for analytical methods, ranking the validation status of each method in one of the seven categories presented in Table 26.1. A summary of status for residue reference methods for growth promoting and antimicrobial agents was prepared at that time (Table 26.2). This most promising classification system, providing sharp definition for each category of regulatory methods on the basis of their performance attributes, has not been completed yet.

An alternative interesting classification approach has been proposed within the Codex Committee for Residues of Veterinary Drugs in Foods (20). In this approach, methods are classified according to their performance attributes. This alternative approach defines methods by the level of analytical detail or information provided concerning the amount and nature of the analyte of interest, and identifies three levels.

Level I methods incorporate the ability to quantify the amount of a specific analyte or class of analytes and positively identify the presence of an analyte in a single analytical procedure. These are assays with the highest level of credibility,

TABLE 26.1 Classification of Analytical Methods in the European Union According to their Validation Status

Category	Status
a	Method under research and development.
b	Method suitable for screening purposes.
c	Published method from a single laboratory.
d	Published method EC Peer Reviewed as potential reference method.
e	Method satisfactory for reference method but not EC ring tested. Method already has been tested in more than one laboratory or/and may already be officially used in an EC member state.
f	Method successfully used and/or demonstrated at an EC analytical workshop.
g	Method ring tested and EC approved as reference method.

Source: From Ref. 81.

TABLE 26.2 Summary of Status in 1989 for Potential EC Residue Reference Methods for Growth-Promoting and Antimicrobial Agents

Analyte method	Thyreostatics AC/TLC	Chloramphenicol		Trenbolone HPLC/EIA Img	Anabolic agents IAC or HPLC/GC-MS	Antimicrobial agents GC-MS
		RIA	HPLC-UV			
Category						
a. Research/develop.	+	+	+	+	+	+
b. Screen/routine	+	+	+	+	+	+
c. Published (1 lab)	+	+	+	+	+	+
ISO-SOP	+	+	+	+	+	?
d. EC Peer reviewed	+	+	+	+	+	
e. Potent. ref. method	+	+	+	+	+	
National ring tested	+	+	+	+	+	
f. Check/demo EC Workshop	+[a]	+	+	+	+	
g. EC ring tested			+		+	
Approved ref. method						
Ring test material	Urine lyophilized	Urine lyophilized	Frozen muscle and milk	Urine lyophilized	Urine lyophilized	
Reference material (in preparation)	Urine	Urine	Muscle	–	Urine	
Certified ref. material	no	no	no	no	no	

[a] Partially ring tested in 1977.

IAC, immunoaffinity chromatography; RIA, radioimmunoassay; EIA Img, enzyme immunoassay immunogram.

Source: From Ref. 81.

and are unequivocal at the level of interest. They may be single procedures that determines both the concentration and identity of the analyte, or combinations of methods for determining and confirming a residue for definitive identification. They frequently employ a chromatographic technique combined with mass spectrometry.

Level II methods are those that are not unequivocal but are used to determine the concentration of an analyte at the level of interest, and to provide some structural information. For example, these methods may employ molecular, functional-group, or immunochemical properties as the basis of the analytical scheme. Hence, these methods are often reliable enough to be used as reference methods. Level II methods commonly separate the determinative from the identification procedures, and may also be used to corroborate the presence of a compound or class of compounds. Thus, a combination of two level II methods may provide attributes suitable for a level I method. The majority of analytical methods presently available and used by regulatory control agencies are level II methods.

Level III methods are those that generate imperfect, although useful, information. These testing procedures detect the presence or absence of a compound or class of compounds at some designated level of interest, and often are based on noninstrumental techniques for analytical determination. Results on a given sample are not as reliable as level I or II methods without corroborating information. Level III methods may provide reasonably good quantitative information but poor compound or class specificity or identity, or may provide strong identification with very little quantitative information.

Many of the microbiological and immunochemical procedures fall into the level III category. They are commonly used because of their greater sample capacity, portability, convenience, and potential suitability to nonlaboratory environments. The hallmark of level III methods is action based on individual positive results that require verification using level I or II methods, as required by the uncertainty of an individual result. To a regulatory control program, these methods may offer substantial advantages, including analytical speed, sample efficiency through batch analysis, portability to nonlaboratory environments, sensitivity, and the ability to detect classes of compounds. Even though level III methods may not detect specific compounds at regulatory limits on all samples, they are able to test larger numbers of samples with a limited level of resources.

Two key characteristics of the level III methods that require further definition are the percentage false-positive and false-negative results when measured against a validated quantitative assay in a statistically designed protocol. The percentage false-negative results must be quite low at the levels of interest, while slightly more flexibility may be acceptable for false-positive findings. A minimum residue detection limit can be described based on these two parameters. Reliability for level I methods must be restrictive. False-positive and false-negative results should be at or near zero. For level II methods, false-positive and false-negative results should approach level I methods, particularly for those methods that are used in regulatory control programs having evidence of residue violations. Level III methods can produce a low percentage of false-positive findings, because a level I or II method will commonly be used to verify and quantify results.

26.2 QUALITY CRITERIA FOR SELECTING AN ANALYTICAL METHOD

The quality of analytical data is a key factor in the success of a residue monitoring program. Analytical results from methods with performance standards provide the necessary information for developing and managing programs that are responsive to public health protection needs. Regulatory authorities want effective and practical analytical methods that can routinely detect, reliably quantify, and unambiguously identify residues of any drug that may be present in meat, milk, or eggs at the appropriate level of interest. Unfortunately, methods with these attributes are not available for all drugs, in part because of the extensive number of potential residues that may find their way into the food chain.

The amount of information in scientific papers is generally less than is needed to establish effectively the methods described within them. There are some exceptions to this statement, but these depend initially on how the author wishes to describe the method and how the paper is reviewed before being accepted by the journal. Some methods may only have a relatively small number of samples analyzed on 1 or 2 days before publication of the manuscript. In contrast, other methods may have examined several thousand samples before the manuscript is written and submitted. The methods in the former case have virtually no robustness data and knowledge of operation compared with the latter. Some analysts develop more complex methods that are necessary to demonstrate their scientific expertise at the expense of their colleagues.

The performance of an analytical method and its inherent reliability are characterized by a set of quality parameters that determine its applicability and its usefulness. For a quantitative method, the most notable parameters are its precision, accuracy, and limit of detection. For a qualitative method, the most important characteristic is its reliability in the identification of the analyte. Since there may be found in the literature an enormous set of different methods for analyzing a particular analyte in a particular matrix, it must be decided which method is the most appropriate for the analysis.

Quality criteria for quantitative analytical methods, in general, have been proposed or are to be proposed by several international organizations including the Association of Official Analytical Chemists, the Food and Drug Administration, the Codex Committee for Residues of Veterinary Drugs in Food, the International Dairy Federation, and the European Union. The European Union, in particular, has laid down minimum quality criteria for quantitative drug residue methods,

TABLE 26.3 Numerical Requirements for Accuracy and Repeatability of Analytical Methods in the European Union

True content (T) of reference sample (μg/kg)	Accuracy as % deviation of mean from T	Repeatability as coefficient of variation of mean
T ≤ 1	−50 to +20	0.30[a]
1 < T ≤ 1	−30 to +10	0.20[a]
T > 10	−20 to +10[a]	0.15[a]

[a] Values also suitable for reference methods.
Source: From Ref. 18.

which, for accuracy and precision, use the numerical values presented in Table 26.3.

Information on quality criteria for qualitative methods is rare, especially in the field of the unambiguous identification of drug residues in foods. Most interesting appear to be the general requirements laid down by the European Union (21) in the field of qualitative residue analysis of some anabolic steroids at moderately low concentrations by immunochemical, gas chromatographic (GC), liquid chromatographic (LC), thin-layer chromatographic (TLC), fourier-transform infrared (FTIR), and low-resolution mass spectroscopic (MS) techniques (Table 26.4). Research, however, has shown that strict application of these criteria can readily lead to false-negative results when GC–MS is used (22). This risk becomes particularly high when residues of anabolics occur at concentrations lower or equal to the action level of 2 ppb and/or their MS spectra contain only a limited number of high abundant ions, as is actually the case for many important β-agonists. In both cases, the relative intensities of the ions are easily influenced by the GC background noise and coeluting substances (23).

Unlike with GC–MS, quality criteria for identification of drug residues by LC–MS have not been yet defined within the European Union, but this is currently under review. Criteria for GC–MS stipulate the measurement of preferably at least four diagnostic ions. However, this is not always possible with LC–MS because most compounds will only produce an M^+ ion in positive mode or a M^- ion in negative mode, with little fragmentation when using thermospray (TSP), electrospray (ESP), or atmospheric pressure chemical ionization (APCI). Even where the ions and ratios are in agreement, there will be still possibility of misidentification. For this reason, mass spectra data are often interpreted with additional supporting data such as the LC retention times, as, for example, in the LC–MS analysis of sulfadimethoxine and sulfadoxine that present identical mass spectra (24).

TABLE 26.4 Requirements for the Various Analytical Techniques Used for Routine Residue Analysis in the European Union

Immunoassay
- Quality control samples at zero, low, mid, and high T range
- CV control samples at limit of detection ≤0.15 (15%)
- Quality control data in line with preceding assays

Gas and Liquid Chromatography
- Cochromatography is mandatory (for confirmatory purposes)
- Nearest peak maximum should be separated from analyte peak by at least one full width at half maximum peak height

Thin-Layer Chromatography
- Cochromatography is mandatory (for confirmatory purposes)
- Two-dimensional TLC is mandatory (for confirmatory purposes)

Low-Resolution-Mass Spectrometry
- At least two, preferably four, diagnostic ions should be scanned
- Relative intensities as % of base peak should be within ≤20% in CI mode and ≤10% in EI mode with respect to standard analyte

Fourier Transform Infrared Spectrometry
- Adequate peaks in between 1800 and 500 cm^{-1}
- Minimum of six adequate peaks for standard analyte
- % score of adequate peaks ≥50% in sample

Source: From Refs. 18, 21.

Apart from the European Union quality criteria, uncertainty factors may be used for defining the reliability of a qualitative method. The European Union criteria lay down standards that have to be fulfilled only in the detection step of the method (18). However, every method is a combination of many analytical steps, including sample extraction, sample cleanup, and detection. Uncertainty factors simply represent qualitative values for the remaining uncertainty after use of a well-defined analytical method (25).

Even using uncertainty factors, the problem of determining the reliability of qualitative methods has not be solved because the usual statistical approaches are often not applicable. In residue analysis, this problem is often amplified because concentrations frequently are in the low or even sub-ppb range. Most promising appears to be a model that helps in estimating, in arbitrary units, the overall selectivity of an analytical method on the basis of partial selectivity indices. Selectivity indices are nothing more than a combination of the above-mentioned tools with the experience obtained within the European Union from recognized laboratory experts (26).

The model was tested on a set of 12 different combinations of qualitative selective analytical steps using experimental chemometrics based on the personal judgment of 25 analytical experts, together representing the European Union Member States National Reference Laboratories, during a desk-top peer review (27). For each of the individual steps used in the methods tested, a partial selectivity index was estimated as based on, among others, the uncertainty factors. For each of the methods the selectivity index was calculated, subsequently, by summation of the partial indices. This calculated selectivity index was divided by the highest value obtained from the set of the 12 methods to obtain a theoretical relative selectivity index (Table 26.5). This model suggests that highly selective cleanup procedures can increase the selectivity of the complete method, allowing use of less selective detection systems. On the basis of the data in Table 26.5, it appears that an optimal approach for residue Analysis is the combination of the highly selective immunoaffinity chromatography with a relative simple low-resolution MS detection.

TABLE 26.5 Theoretical Selectivity Indices for Selected Analytical Steps

Analytical steps	Index
Extraction from the sample matrix	
Simple extraction (e.g., liquid–liquid or liquid–solid partition)	0
Specific extraction (e.g., pH adjustment and/or ion-pair extraction)	1
Solid-phase extraction	2
Immunoaffinity chromatography	3
Purification of primary extract	
Solid-phase extraction	1
High-performance liquid chromatography	2
Immunoaffinity chromatography	3
Detection/identification	
UV absorbance (e.g., single wavelength, HPLC)	1
UV spectrum matching (e.g., full-spectrum PDA, HPLC)	3
Detection of a spot at the right R_f value	1
Detection of a spot at the intersection of R_f values	2
Low-resolution mass spectrometry	
Detection of (pseudo-) molecular ion	4
Detection of molecular ion minus (e.g. CH_3 or HF)	3
Detection of other diagnostic ion	2
Detection of additional but non-diagnostic ion	1
High-resolution mass spectrometry: Peak match of molecular ion	8

Source: From Ref. 27.

Apart from confirmatory analytical methods, quality criteria have been also defined for screening tests. Screening tests must be demonstrated as having been performed with acceptable figures of merit for accuracy, specificity, and reproducibility. Although no esoteric performance requirements are peculiar to screening tests, some particular points are especially useful in the evaluation of screening tests.

In order to be accepted by the US Food and Drug Administration (FDA), an immunochemical screening test has to meet two standards: one related to its sensitivity rate and the other to its selectivity rate. The sensitivity rate is defined as the proportion of reference positive samples that are test-positive while the selectivity rate is the proportion of reference negative samples that are test-negative. In both cases, it is critical that the definitions of reference positive and negative be clarified (28). The sensitivity standard requires the tests to detect samples containing residues of claimed drugs at their established tolerance/safe levels 90% of the time with 95% confidence. The selectivity standard requires tests to identify correctly, with 95% confidence, samples containing no drug residues in 90% of the samples.

A test can meet these standards by correctly identifying 30 of 30 zero control samples and 30 of 30 samples containing each claimed drug at its tolerance/safe level. With this selectivity standard for acceptance, the probability is low that an accepted screening test would produce a positive result on a sample that does not contain any of the drug it is designed to detect.

Nevertheless, screening tests can give positive results at drug concentrations below the tolerance/safe level. A number of comments have inferred that tests should not have been accepted by the FDA since they were to have been evaluated exactly at the safe level or tolerance. However, had FDA not accepted tests that give a positive result at drug concentrations below the tolerance/safe level, none of the tests would have been accepted. The FDA recognizes that screening tests for detecting antimicrobial drugs in food are neither drug-specific nor quantitative in their performance.

An ideal test would differentiate between positive and negative samples 100% of the time, but it could be difficult to achieve both excellent sensitivity and selectivity in the same test. Unfortunately, a gain in one is often made at the expense of the other (29). As shown in a schematic example of a frequency distribution curve that might be obtained during field evaluations of a qualitative competitive enzyme-linked immunosorbent assay (ELISA) (Fig. 26.1), there is an area of uncertainty or overlap between high-negative and low-positive samples (B + C). Knowledge of the magnitude of this overlap area and at what concentrations it occurs is essential when evaluating method performance and determining critical cutoff points. For example, if one were to move the cutoff point to the left from 1 to 3, the area represented by C would decrease while B would increase in size. In other words, there would be a decrease in the number of false-negative

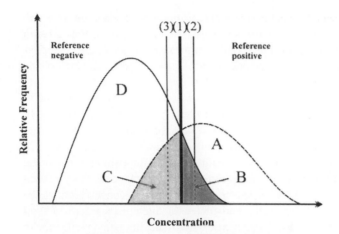

FIG. 26.1   Relative frequency distribution curves obtained during field evaluation of a competitive ELISA for drug residues; the area represented by (A) contains the true-positive results; (D) true-negative results; (B) false-positive results; (C) false-negative results.

test results and an increase in the number of false-positive test results. A test with low sensitivity will lead to more false-negative results while a test with low selectivity will lead to more false-positive results. Conversely, if the cutoff point was shifted from 1 to 2, the opposite would occur; a corresponding decrease in sensitivity or more false-negative results, and an increase in selectivity or fewer false-positive results.

Apart from sensitivity and selectivity, another important performance parameter is the predictive value of the screening test, which reflects the fraction of positive or negative results that are true positives or negatives, respectively (30, 31). To give an example, assume that we get 10% false-positive and 10% false-negative results and that the true percentage of positives in the population is 1%. If 1000 samples are measured, the pool should contain 10 positives (1%), but only 9 are detected because 1 is a false-negative result. In addition, we have 990 true negatives, but of these 99 (10%) are false-positive findings. We report 100 positives when actually we have only 10. So, the predictive value of a positive test is only 10%. But we have 990 true negatives and report 891, that is, 990 minus 99, so the predictive value for negatives is about 90%. These estimates depend highly on the true frequencies in the population. Using the same false-positive and false-negative rates of 10%, but increasing the number of true positives to 10% makes the test more useful. In the population of 1000 we now have 100 true positives and therefore we report 90. Thus, the predictive value of a positive test is 90%, which is a far better performance than when the true frequency was lower. Our certainty has been increased by a factor of 9 as a result of the situation in the population, which is a circumstance outside of the characteristics of the test itself. This is a dramatic demonstration of the influence of the intended use on evaluating test suitability (32).

Once the test selectivity, sensitivity, and predictive values are known, decisions can be made as to the suitability of the test. The cost of false-negative results from drug residue screening tests is difficult to estimate. The direct cost of false-positive results to producers can be substantial, however, since positive results may trigger the disposal of the commodity and the imposition of penalties. False-positive results may also have some indirect costs such as the early culling of diseased cattle to avoid risks associated with treatment, concerns about the accuracy of drug withdrawal periods, and increased anxiety in regard to food safety among consumers (33, 34). In such cases, due to the uncertain public health implications of drug residues in foods, it may be more appropriate to use a test with a higher selectivity and a lower sensitivity or to use two assays in combination. Initial screening with a high-sensitivity assay followed by confirmatory testing with a high-selectivity assay that can quantify the drug residue present, especially when large volumes of a commodity are involved. If the quantitative assay detects a concentration greater than the tolerance/MRL, only then should the commodity be disposed of and penalties imposed.

The US Center for Veterinary Medicine is presently working with a new test kit evaluation program recently established by the Association of Official Analytical Chemists. The purpose of this program is to provide an independent evaluation of proprietary test kits and a verification of the sponsor's performance claims. It is expected that all mentioned concepts and ideas about acceptable and feasible error probabilities for regulatory or forensic results of residue analyses (35, 36), experimental chemometrics based on professional experience rather than statistics (27), minimum quality performance criteria for residue analyses (18, 27, 37–39), uncertainty factors for analytical techniques (25), and the balance of false-negative and false-positive analytical results in inspection procedures based on a multistep system (40) will contribute to a new kind of approach for matching the current and future increasing demands for chemical residue analyses and the available human resources, laboratory facilities, and budgets, which in general have shown no parallel increase.

26.3 INTERPRETATION OF ANALYTICAL RESULTS

Correct interpretation of the analytical results in the field of residue analysis is a matter of major importance. Truly positive, false-violative, false-positive, false-negative, and truly negative are all types of test results that may be produced during food monitoring for drug residues. Truly positive is a positive test result on a sample in which the actual drug concentration is at or above the established safe level, tolerance or MRL; false-violative is a positive test result on a sample in which the actual drug concentration is at or above the detection limit of the test, but below the established safe level, tolerance or MRL; false-positive is a positive test result on a sample that actually contains no drug residues at a detectable concentration; false-negative is a negative test result on a sample that contains drug residues at a detectable concentration; truly negative is a negative test result on a sample that actually contains no drug residues at a detectable concentration.

A different method of interpretation is frequently observed between inspection services and analytical laboratories. This is because inspection services are interested mainly in a yes/no answer to questions, such as "Has the animal been treated with anabolics?" or "Does the food commodity contain residues above their MRL?", in order to proceed to such action as rejection of the food commodity or removal of the test-positive animals from the farm. On the other hand, laboratories mainly use quality criteria to convert analytical results into yes/no answers. This conversion, however, is often obscured by inherent analytical difficulties including estimation of the impact of systematic and random errors and the way of sampling.

Many screening tests, for example, are dichotomous yes/no tests. If this is the case and the test is designed to indicate the presence or absence of an analyte, the limit of detection must be known so that the lower concentration level of what will be detected is known. A negative result, however, does not prove that the analyte is absent from the sample, because its concentration might be below the limit of detection.

False-negative results may be obtained because of a partial loss of the analyte during sample preparation including extraction, cleanup and concentration steps; in that case, only an unknown fraction of the true content of the analyte will be available for final detection and/or quantification. To prevent such false-negative results, either the recovery of the method must be known or a standard addition technique should be applied. The usual approach in standard addition (41, 42) is to add a known amount of the analyte to an aliquot of the sample and to analyze this spiked test portion in parallel with the original sample. From this experiment, the true concentration of the analyte can be calculated without explicit knowledge of the recovery of the method, assuming that the recovery of the analyte originally present in the sample is equal to the recovery for the standard analyte added to the sample.

If the purpose of the test is to establish whether the analyte exceeds or meets some established level, the limit of detection becomes of minor importance, whereas the performance of the test at the level of interest determines actually the reliability of the results. Ideally, screening tests should give no positive results when there are drug residues below the tolerance/MRL level. Equally desired is for the tests to give a positive result 100% of the time when the drug concentration is exactly at or above the tolerance/MRL level. Unfortunately, most screening tests do not perform in this manner. Due to limitations of screening test technology, tests cannot turn on or off at precisely the established level for each drug. This can be best illustrated with the immunochemical in which where the antibody titration curve is sigmoidal rather than linear.

Useful information about the characteristics of screening tests can be obtained by development of the characteristic operating curve (32). In this technique, a panel of test samples is produced by fortifying control matrix at several levels with the analyte of interest. The test is run on each sample with 15–20 replicates at each concentration level. For rapid screening tests this should not represent an undue analytical burden. The results are plotted as the percentage of samples that are positive at each concentration level.

The data from this curve will indicate the concentrations of drug residues that can be detected, the confidence associated with each level, and the false-positive samples that will be expected. As drug concentration increases, there is also a corresponding increase in percentage positive until a concentration plateau is reached after which all samples will be positive. Samples that are in the false-violative area of the curve will read positive, despite the fact that the drug concentration is below the safe/tolerance level. This is a concern to veterinarians and their producer clients. Samples, on the other hand, that are in the false-negative area of the curve will read negative, even though the drug is present at violative levels; this is the area of potential concern to consumers.

In cases where quantitative analyses give concentration values much lower than the specified MRL for a certain analyte, positive quantitative errors do not play a role in the "no" answer. However, negative quantitative errors may be important; if a screening test such as the four-plate test for antibiotics or an enzyme-immunosorbent assay for β-agonists is used, some specific analytes for which the test has no or very low response may slip through the holes (43).

When the results obtained lie above the MRL, both qualification and quantification are becoming very important. Immunochemical tests that are often used for surveillance of registered drugs are prone to cross-reactions that may influence the result. It is therefore important to confirm and quantify the results of immunochemical methods with an independent physicochemical method.

For values obtained in the neighborhood of the MRL, quantitative accuracy and precision are of extreme importance. Thus, a laboratory should take a safety measurement zone depending upon the validation performance of the used method. Questions may also sometimes arise as to which way some numerical concentration values (such as 1.56 ppb) would be rounded to be converted into a "yes" or "no" answer when the action level is, for example, 2 ppb. In that case, caution should be exercised with regard to the number of significant values to reflect the precision of the applied analytical method.

Attention should also be paid in the interpretation of the sensitivity figures quoted for the various microbiological screening tests because they are generally susceptible to influences by factors outside the test system itself, such as those arising from the nature of the matrix being tested. Milk samples, for example, exhibit considerable compositional variation. The variation in bacteriological quality, somatic cell content, and content of natural antimicrobial substances, such as lysozyme and lactoferrin, will occasionally affect the result. Because the influence of these factors is proportionally greater when the antibiotic concentration is close to the limit of detection of the test, decisive interpretation should be avoided close to those limits (44).

Another issue of relevant importance to the interpretation of analytical results is the analytical specificity of the test, particularly when in an immunobased assay. Specificity is exquisite in immunochemical assays but, at the same time, it can be exquisitely troublesome. For example, when an immunochemical assay for the penicilloyl group is used to monitor the pharmacokinetics of penicillin elimination from the serum of treated animals, the measured levels remain high for at least several weeks, although the antibacterial activity was all eliminated from bovine serum within 24 h after injection. This is because the immunochemical assay measured not only the free drug but also the penicilloyl groups covalently bound to proteins in serum. The half-life of these bound residues is roughly equal to the half-life of the proteins in the circulation.

The interpretation of test results is sometimes further complicated by the problem of antibiotic stability in the organs and tissues. Caution should be exercised in interpreting the results of inhibition tests applied to animal tissues remote from the place and time of slaughter. For example, the concentrations of penicillin G, ampicillin, amoxycillin, and the cephalosporins in the kidney decrease rapidly upon storage at 4°C, due probably to release of autolytic enzymes (45), whereas the aminoglycosides and oxytetracycline remain essentially unchanged. These findings may be linked in part to the strong affinity of the latter antibiotics to tissue components (46), since it has been established that extensively bound drugs are less likely to be metabolized or degraded enzymatically (47). Antibiotic stability in the meat is considerably greater than in the kidney upon cold storage for 4 days, whereas heating considerably influences the stability of certain antibiotics. Heating, for example, pork in cans at 65°C for 60 min, reduces chlortetracycline and oxytetracycline concentrations to 20% of their original value, while heating at 110–120°C destroys these antibiotics within 1 min (48). Therefore, application of ancillary tests would seem advisable before rejecting meat on the basis of "presumed" antibiotic residues (49).

Whether a small but nonzero probability of false-negative results in regulatory, legislative, or forensic residue control is acceptable or not, was in the Netherlands, been decided in 1981 in the Court of Justice. Jurisprudence was established that a zero probability is not feasible in practice (35), but no indication was given on what probability could be considered as acceptable, although 5% was judged as unacceptably high. After years of discussions in the Netherlands between those involved in regulatory residue control including state inspectors, prosecutors, lawyers, administrators, and residue chemists, a compromise was found between acceptable reliability and required analytical effort. In economic offenses for forensic, purposes from 1988, a probability of false-positive results smaller than 1 : 10000 (0.01%) or even 1 : 1000 (0.1%) appears to be acceptable and defensible in the Court.

26.4   STRATEGIES FOR MONITORING FOOD SUPPLY FOR DRUG RESIDUES

Strategies for the analysis of food supply for drug residues differ in detail between laboratories and are to some extent governed by factors such as sample number, submission rate, type of analyte, and variety of matrices. Sampling, quality, cost, and accreditation are just a few of other important issues normally considered.

Different demands may be placed on analytical strategies for different purposes. In case of international dispute, for example, different methods are needed from those normally used in national surveillance and monitoring programs. A high degree of certainty is required in establishing the identity and quantity of a drug residue in meat, milk, or eggs if the intent is to assess penalties against individuals or organizations for violation of law or regulations. In public health monitoring, definitive identification of specific drug entities is desirable but not strictly necessary in order to take effective action. It is necessary that the analytical result indicate that there is a high probability that a food safety problem may exist in the sample and that further action is warranted to determine the disposition of the food commodity. Food control related directly to public health or international trade must be performed rapidly and with high reliability, and should be based on professional consensus within a limited budget. For the most part, however, there will be a progression from high-capacity screening methods to much lower-volume confirmatory methods.

Screening methods generate imperfect but useful data, designed to filter out samples containing no residues. Microbiological inhibition tests are still the most convenient screening test for large-scale antibiotic residue monitoring. They are easy to perform, inexpensive, and have the added advantage of detecting multiple residues with very different chemical structures. This vastly reduces the number of samples requiring more detail analysis, but care must be taken to ensure that the number of false-negative results is kept to a minimum. For these reasons, microbial inhibition tests will always keep their importance.

In monitoring food supply for drug residues, any efficient microbiological procedure can be used as an initial screen to detect the presence of a wide range of substances that are inhibitory to the growth of microorganisms. Some information on the nature of antimicrobials found positive in the screening test can be obtained by reanalyzing the samples with different microbial-inhibitor assays, such as the three- or six-plate test (50), the German *Bacillus subtilis* BGA test (51), or the EC four-plate test (52), which have the potential to differentiate between specific groups of antimicrobials. These screening tests can provide presumptive information on the existence of a drug residue in a test sample, but they do not provide definitive information on the identity of specific drug residues. An example of a receptor assay test is the Charm II test designed to test for multiple β-lactam residues in milk. This test can give an initial alert that β-lactam residues may be present in milk, but identification of the specific β-lactam residue requires verification by more specific analytical methods.

Additional analyses will normally be required in order to identify and quantify individual residues within a group of antimicrobials to determine whether a positive result exceeds the MRL level. For suspect penicillin residues, identification can be made by repeating the microbiological assay in the presence of β-lactamase. If the inhibition zone disappears by this addition, penicillin residues are present in the sample. If not, no conclusion can be drawn because several new-generation β-lactams are less sensitive to inactivation by β-lactamase.

Since not all veterinary drugs and/or their metabolites exhibit antibacterial activity, immunochemical assays are also widely used for screening and testing purposes. Class-specific multiresidue immunochemical tests are preferentially employed since they can recognize several compounds within a group of drugs; for example, a corticosteroid screening test that simultaneously detects dexamethasone, betamethasone, flumethasone, triamcinolone, and prednisolone; or a β-agonists test that can simultaneously detect clenbuterol, salbutamol, mabuterol, mapenterol, and terbutaline residues (53).

Like the microbiological tests, immunochemical tests, although very sensitive, cannot be considered as definitive from a regulatory perspective because they may yield false-positive results. Therefore, for legal enforcement use, they should be used as part of an analytical system that consists of additional methods capable of definitively identifying the analytes of interest. Immunochemical tests can also greatly help in identifying individual residues within a group of antibacterials in samples found positive by a microbiological screening test. They thereby facilitate selection of the most appropriate physicochemical method for subsequent quantification. A number of factors need to be considered, including knowledge of the common antibacterial drugs, ability to subclassify the potential residues into analytical target groups, and identification of the individual compounds within those groups.

Methods combining principles of both microbiological and physicochemical procedures have been traditionally used to obtain an indication of the identity of growth-inhibiting residues found in samples by classic microbiological tests. High-voltage electrophoresis in agar gel (54–57) followed by bioautography detection with different microorganisms has been employed with considerable success for identification purposes. This offers the advantage that all antibacterials detectable by bioautography can be classified on the basis of their electrophoretic mobility.

Further testing may be required for the separation and quantification of compounds with similar electrophoretic behavior, unless more than one buffer is used (54). High-voltage electrophoresis allows analysis of concentrated sample extracts, thus, favoring low detection limits. Natural microbial inhibitors found in some animal tissues such as lysozymes either do not interfere or can be eliminated by applying a semipermeable dialysis membrane between sample and agar (58, 59). It has been reported, however, that antibacterial residues confirmed by high-voltage electrophoresis and bioautography in kidney and muscle could account for only 50% and 37%, respectively, of those detected by the EU four-plate test (57). Apart from this, the procedure is very laborious, time-consuming, and provides results that are neither quantitative nor informative about molecular structure.

Procedures relying on thin-layer chromatography in combination with bioautography can also be elaborated for identification purposes (60–63). Following chromatographic separation of the analytes, the developed plate can be placed upon an agar layer inoculated with suitable microorganisms, thus enabling, diffusion of the antibacterials onto the agar. The location of zones of inhibition can be used to identify individual residues within a class of antibacterials; using a series of appropriate liquid–liquid partitions of the sample extracts prior to chromatography and a series of different thin-layer chromatographic (TLC) plates, 14 commonly used antimicrobial drugs have been positively detected by this procedure (64).

TLC–bioautography has been used in Canada since 1984 for the confirmation of tetracycline-positive in plant tests (65). However, TLC–bioautography is not quantitative and only gives direction to the analyst as to what confirmatory method of analysis should be used. Therefore, presumptive positives must be confirmed by physicochemical techniques that have been validated in terms of detection limit, precision, and accuracy.

The diversity of the methods that can be used for identification/confirmation is great. When an interlaboratory study was organized in 1995 within Europe for the determination of chloramphenicol in bovine urine and plasma, GC/electron capture detection (ECD), LC/MS, GC/MS/negative-ion chemical ionization (NCI), GC/MS/MS/NCI, LC/UV, LC/diode array detection (PDA), GC/MS/electron impact (EI), LC/radioimmunoassay (RIA)/immunogram (IMG), LC/MS/MS, and GC/high resolution MS/NCI were all used, at varying levels of success, for identification/confirmation (66). Normal-phase, reversed-phase, size-exclusion, and ion-exchange are all examples of chromatographic conditions that operate on different physicochemical principles and, when use with appropriate standards, can give a good insight into the identity of a test analyte. Different detectors such as diode array, ultraviolet, fluorescence, and electrochemical detectors can be also used to exploit the different chemical features characteristic of a given analyte.

Coupling chromatographic procedures with immunochemical techniques can also provide a very sensitive and specific analytical system for either determinative or confirmatory analysis. If the antibody used is very specific for the analyte of interest and the antibody reactivity is known to be sensitive to small variations in the structure of the analyte tested, positive reactions with the method are strongly indicative that an analyte of defined structural characteristics is present in the sample. Full rigorous confirmation, however, would depend on further analysis by mass spectrometry, which is the method of choice in confirmatory analysis. Mass spectrometry gives specific information on the identity and structure of the compound of interest. Coupled with chromatographic techniques it becomes a very powerful confirmatory tool for both quantitative and qualitative assessment of drug residues in foods.

Analytical methods for residue monitoring programs must be evaluated within a context of use. At each stage of the analytical strategy, not always the theoretically or proven very best method must be selected but also the method most suitable for a particular purpose. To ask if a method is good is to ask only half a question; one must ask if it is good for a particular purpose. A method ideal for one purpose may be totally inadequate for another. Thus, for nearly every analytical problem, in general, a whole series of analytical solutions must be available that can be ranked, among others, in order of reliability, suitability, and feasibility. This results in a hierarchy of methods.

Before a decision is made on the methods to be adopted, a number of questions in key areas need to be asked (Table 26.6). In seeking answers to these questions, an analytical strategy that fits the requirements of the customer is more likely to be achieved. Careful planning at the start will ensure that the analytical strategy is truly fit for its intended purpose.

This approach has been successfully applied to a number of areas within the field of drug residue analysis in many laboratories all over the world. For example, the analytical strategy followed by the Food Production and Inspection Branch of Agriculture Canada for detecting antibacterial residues in shell and processed eggs is an integrated approach that involves application of rapid screening tests allowing detection of multiple drug residues at relatively low cost. Only presumptive positives are then examined, enabling expensive resources to be targeted most usefully. In order to cover as wide a range of drugs as possible, samples are screened for general inhibition using the Brilliant black reduction test (67), which detects antibiotics and sulfonamides with limited sensitivity. Attempts are also made to narrow the search to possible groups of compounds by using other available rapid tests kits such as the CITE Probe tetracycline or β-lactam test kits (68), and the IDS gentamicin and neomycin Microtiter well

TABLE 26.6 Questions to be Asked in Developing an Analytical Strategy for Drug Residues in Food

---

General information
- Will the analyte be qualified or quantified or both?
- How accurate and precise the analytical result need to be?
- How soon are the results required?
- What will be the cost?
- What is the budget?

Information on samples
- How many samples are to be analyzed?
- What is the expected concentration range of the analyte(s) in the samples?
- What size of sample is available?
- Will they arrive in one shipment or spread over a period of time?
- What matrix will the analyte be likely to be found in?
- What storage conditions do samples require?

Information on the analyte(s)
- What are the physicochemical properties of the analyte?
- Is the analyte a member of a larger chemical group?
- How stable is the analyte?
- What storage conditions does the analyte require?
- What are the biological properties of the analyte?
- Can the analyte be metabolized further?
- Are there any MRL or action limits?

Information on the analytical method
- What analytical equipment is available?
- How sensitive does the detection need to be?
- How many samples should be analyzed simultaneously?
- What analytical methods are available?
- What sample treatment will be required?
- What interferences are possible?
- What separation procedure will be required?
- How much skill will be required by the operator?
- What is the preamble cost?

Information on quality assurance
- Can a proven method be validated inhouse?
- What does the customer/task require (Good Laboratory Practice)?
- What does the laboratory require (Quality Control)?
- Are there any performance assessment schemes?

---

test kits (69). In addition, EZ-Screen tests are applied for sulfamethazine, sulfadimethoxine, and chloramphenicol at the lower detection limit required for residue control (70). Charm II tests are used for the qualitative detection of macrolides and streptomycin residues (71). These rapid tests would cover the majority of expected positives based on the experience of Agriculture Canada for drug residues in foods.

If the identity of the detected drug residue is still unknown after these tests have been performed, a TLC–bioautography procedure is then applied to isolate and tentatively identify the residues (64, 72). This method is not quantitative and only gives direction to the analyst as to what determinative/confirmatory method of analysis should be used. Following this tentative identification, presumptive positives are then quantified and confirmed by validated physicochemical methods. A TLC method (73) is applied for analyzing presumptive sulfonamide residues, a GC–ECD method (74) followed by a GC–MS NCI method (75) for analyzing chloramphenicol, and LC/UV methods (76, 77) for analyzing β-lactams and tetracyclines.

In the United Kingdom, nearly 34,000 kidney samples were submitted to the State laboratories in 1995 for analysis of a range of antimicrobials including penicillins, tetracyclines, streptomycin, chloramphenicol, and sulfonamides. The turnaround time was 28 days from receipt of samples. The selected analytical strategy started with an initial screening phase using the microbiological four-plate test, followed by application of selective enzyme-linked immunosorbent assay (ELISA), and ended up with determinative/confirmatory LC methods (78). The four plate test was selected because it is not expensive, can handle a large sample throughput, and does not require a high degree of analytical skill. The impact of this initial screening was to reduce the number of samples requiring further analysis from 34,000 samples to only 170. While this test screens out large numbers of negatives, it gives little information concerning which of the many possible inhibitory substances are present. Thus, the 170 samples were then submitted to selective ELISA assays (79) in order to identify the particular drugs tentatively, thus enabling a focused confirmatory analysis by specific physicochemical methods.

Another characteristic example of analytical strategy is that followed in the United Kingdom for the analysis of tranquilizers and β-blockers (78). A total of 180 samples distributed over a whole year (15 samples per month) should be analyzed within a turnaround time of 28 days from receipt of sample. In that case, the expense of developing a two-tier analytical strategy was not justified by the sample throughput. Thus, the selection was direct application of a multiresidue LC/PDA confirmatory method (80).

In the Netherlands, about 40,000 urine samples from groups of calves and cattle in the farmhouse are screened every year for the presence of β-agonists, corticosteroids, and estrogenic and androgenic compounds. For screening purposes, immunochemical assays and receptor-binding techniques are used. Suspected samples are further analyzed by GC–MS methods using either low or high-resolution EI and CI techniques.

In Belgium, 0.1% of the slaughtered cattle and swine are screened for antibiotic residues each year. In the analytical strategy applied, meat samples are screened with a modified four-plate test followed by screening with a group-specific ELISA for the identification of the antibiotics and confirmation by specific LC methods.

REFERENCES

1. R.W. Stephany, in Residues of Veterinary Drugs in Food, Proc. Euroresidue Conf., Noordwijkerhout, May 21–23, 1990 (N. Haagsma, A. Ruiter, and P.B. Czedik-Eysenberg, Eds.), Fac. Vet. Med., Univ. Utrecht, The Netherlands, p. 76 (1990).
2. W.H. Heeschen and G. Suhren, Milchwissenschaft, 51:154 (1996).
3. W.A. Moats, J. Assoc. Off. Anal. Chem., 73:343 (1990).
4. B. Shaikh, J. Chromatogr., 643:369 (1993).
5. J.J. O'Rangers, in Residues of Veterinary Drugs in Food, Proc. Euroresidue II Conf., Veldhoven, May 3–5, 1993 (N. Haagsma, A. Ruiter, and P.B. Czedik-Eysenberg, Eds.), Fac. Vet. Med., Univ. Utrecht, The Netherlands, p. 75 (1993).
6. Handbook No. 601, How to Perform the Live Animal Swab Test for Antibiotic Residues, United States Department of Agriculture, Food Safety and Inspection Service, Washington, DC (1984).
7. J.P. Tritschler, R.T. Duby, S.P. Oliver, and R.W. Prange, J. Food Prot., 50:97 (1987).
8. M.A.J. Godfrey, S.P.L. Anderson, B. Julicher, P. Kwasowski, and M.J. Sauer, in Residues of Veterinary Drugs in Food, Proc. Euroresidue III Conf., Veldhoven, May 6–8, 1996 (N. Haagsma and A. Ruiter, Eds.), Fac. Vet. Med., Univ. Utrecht, The Netherlands, p. 421 (1996).
9. A. Gleixner, H. Sauerwein, and H.H.D. Meyer, in Residues of Veterinary Drugs in Food, Proc. Euroresidue III Conf., Veldhoven, May 6–8, 1996 (N. Haagsma and A. Ruiter, Eds.), Fac. Vet. Med., Univ. Utrecht, The Netherlands, p. 411 (1996).
10. V. Helbo, M. Vandenbroeck, and G. Maghuin-Rogister, in Residues of Veterinary Drugs in Food, Proc. Euroresidue II Conf., Veldhoven, May 3–5, 1993 (N. Haagsma, A. Ruiter, and P.B. Czedik-Eysenberg, Eds.), Fac. Vet. Med., Univ. Utrecht, The Netherlands, p. 362 (1993).
11. C.J.M. Arts, M.J. van Baak, G.R.M.M. Haenen, and J. van der Greef, in Residues of Veterinary Drugs in Food, Proc. Euroresidue II Conf., Veldhoven, May 3–5, 1993 (N. Haagsma, A. Ruiter, and P.B. Czedik-Eysenberg, Eds.), Fac. Vet. Med., Univ. Utrecht, The Netherlands, p. 143 (1993).
12. G. Alfredsson, A. Lundstrom, and B.-G. Osterdahl, in Residues of Veterinary Drugs in Food, Proc. Euroresidue II Conf., Veldhoven, May 3–5, 1993 (N. Haagsma, A. Ruiter, and P.B. Czedik-Eysenberg, Eds.), Fac. Vet. Med., Univ. Utrecht, The Netherlands, p. 129 (1993).

13. M.L. Macho and P. Munoz, in Residues of Veterinary Drugs in Food, Proc. Euroresidue II Conf., Veldhoven, May 3–5, 1993 (N. Haagsma, A. Ruiter, and P.B. Czedik-Eysenberg, Eds.), Fac. Vet. Med., Univ. Utrecht, The Netherlands, p. 465 (1993).

14. K. Vanoosthuyze, E. Daeseleire, A. van Overbeke, and C. van Peteghem, in Residues of Veterinary Drugs in Food, Proc. Euroresidue II Conf., Veldhoven, May 3–5, 1993 (N. Haagsma, A. Ruiter, and P.B. Czedik-Eysenberg, Eds.), Fac. Vet. Med., Univ. Utrecht, The Netherlands, p. 669 (1993).

15. J.F.M. Nouws, N.J.G. Broex, and J.M.P. den Hartog, Tijdschr. Diergeneeskd., 113: 243 (1988).

16. F.K. Stekelenburg, in Residues of Veterinary Drugs in Food, Proc. Euroresidue II Conf., Veldhoven, May 3–5, 1993 (N. Haagsma, A. Ruiter, and P.B. Czedik-Eysenberg, Eds.), Fac. Vet. Med., Univ. Utrecht, The Netherlands, p. 650 (1993).

17. Th. Reuvers, R. Diaz, J. Gomez, and M. Ramos, in Residues of Veterinary Drugs in Food, Proc. Euroresidue II Conf., Veldhoven, May 3–5, 1993 (N. Haagsma, A. Ruiter, and P.B. Czedik-Eysenberg, Eds.), Fac. Vet. Med., Univ. Utrecht, The Netherlands, p. 567 (1993).

18. Official Journal of the European Communities, No. L223, Brussels, p. 18 (1987).

19. Official Journal of the European Communities, No. L351, Brussels, p. 39 (1989).

20. FAO/WHO Codex Alimentarius Commission, Alinorm 89/31A, Rome, Italy (1989).

21. Official Journal of the European Communities, No. L118, Brussels, p. 64 (1993).

22. D. Courtheyn, H. de Brabander, J. Vercammen, P. Batjoens, M. Logghe, and K. de Wasch, in Residues of Veterinary Drugs in Food, Proc. Euroresidue III Conf., Veldhoven, May 6–8, 1996 (N. Haagsma and A. Ruiter, Eds.), Fac. Vet. Med., Univ. Utrecht, The Netherlands, p. 75 (1996).

23. H. de Brabander, P. Batjoens, C. van den Braembussche, P. Dirinck, F. Smets, and G. Pottie, Anal. Chim. Acta, 275:9 (1993).

24. S. Porter, R. Patel, and I. Kay, in Residues of Veterinary Drugs in Food, Proc. Euroresidue III Conf., Veldhoven, May 6–8, 1996 (N. Haagsma and A. Ruiter, Eds.), Fac. Vet. Med., Univ. Utrecht, The Netherlands, p. 795 (1996).

25. W.G. de Ruig, G. Dijkstra, and R.W. Stephany, Anal. Chim. Acta, 223:277 (1989).

26. R.W. Stephany, Belg. J. Food Chem. Biotechnol., 139:153 (1989).

27. L.A. van Ginkel and R.W. Stephany, in Residues of Veterinary Drugs in Food, Proc. Euroresidue II Conf., Veldhoven, May 3–5, 1993 (N. Haagsma, A. Ruiter, and P.B. Czedik-Eysenberg, Eds.), Fac. Vet. Med., Univ. Utrecht, The Netherlands, p. 303 (1993).

28. S.W. Martin, A.H. Meek, and P. Willeberg, in Veterinary Epidemiology (S.W. Martin, A.H. Meek, and P. Willeberg, Eds.), Iowa State University Press, Ames, USA, p. 48 (1987).

29. J.M. Mitchell, M.W. Griffiths, S.A. McEwen, W.B. McNab, and A.J. Yee, J. Food Prot., 61:742 (1998).

30. R. Gudding, Acta Vet. Scand., 17:458 (1976).

31. W.M. Sischo, J. Diary Sci., 79:1065 (1996).

32. J.J. O'Rangers and D.B. Berkowitz, in Veterinary Drug Residues (W.A. Moats and M.B. Medina, Eds.), American Chemical Society, Washington, DC (1995).

33. J.S. Cullor, J. Chem. Vet. Med., 8:845 (1991).

34. I.A. Gardner, J.S. Cullor, F.D. Galey, W. Sischo, M. Salman, B. Slenning, H.N. Erb, and J.W. Tyler, J. Am. Vet. Med. Assoc., 209:46 (1996).
35. R.W. Stephany, E.H.J.M. Jansen, and J. Freudenthal, Tijdschrift Diergeneesk., 110: 654 (1985).
36. R.W. Stephany, J. Chromatogr., 489:3 (1989).
37. Official Journal of the European Communities, No. L286, Brussels, p. 33 (1990).
38. W.G. de Ruig, R.W. Stephany, and G. Dijkstra, J. Assoc. Off. Anal. Chem., 72:487 (1989).
39. W.G. de Ruig and J.M. Weseman, J. Chemometrics, 4:61 (1990).
40. W.G. de Ruig and A.A.M. Jansen, in Criteria to Limit the Number of False Positive and False Negative Results for Analyses Near the Limit of Determination, WHO/ FAO Codex Alimentarius Commission, Document CX/MAS 92/15/7, Rome, Italy (1992).
41. H.E. Solberg, J. Clin. Chem. Clin. Biochem., 25:645 (1987).
42. M.G. Bagur, D. Gazquez, and M. Sanchez-Vinas, Analusis, 24:374 (1996).
43. H.F. de Brabander, G. Pottie, D. Courtheyn, and F. Smets, in Residues of Veterinary Drugs in Food, Proc. Euroresidue III Conf., Veldhoven, May 6–8, 1996 (N. Haagsma and A. Ruiter, Eds.), Fac. Vet. Med., Univ. Utrecht, The Netherlands, p. 283 (1996).
44. International Dairy Federation, Bull. Int. Dairy Fed., 258 (1991).
45. J.F.M. Nouws and G. Ziv, Tijdschr. Diergeneesk., 101:1145 (1976).
46. C.M. Kunin, J. Inf. Dis., 121:55 (1970).
47. M.C. Meyer and D.E. Guttman, J. Pharm. Sci., 57:895 (1968).
48. K.O. Honikel, U. Schmidt, W. Woltersdorf, and L. Leistner, J. Assoc. Off. Anal. Chem., 61:1222 (1978).
49. R. Smither, J. Appl. Bact., 45:267 (1978).
50. International Dairy Federation, Bull. Int. Dairy Fed., 220 (1987).
51. A. Ab, Z. Lebensm. Unters. Forsch., 155/156:6 (1974).
52. R. Bogaerts and F. Wolf, Fleischwirtschaft, 60:672 (1980).
53. W. Haasnoot, S.M. Ezkerro, and H. Keukens, in Residues of Veterinary Drugs in Food, Proc. Euroresidue II Conf., Veldhoven, May 3–5, 1993 (N. Haagsma, A. Ruiter, and P.B. Czedik-Eysenberg, Eds.), Fac. Vet. Med., Univ. Utrecht, The Netherlands, p. 347 (1993).
54. R. Smither and D.R. Vaughn, J. Appl. Bacteriol., 44:421 (1978).
55. J. Stadhouders, F. Hassing, and T.E. Galesloot, Neth. Milk Dairy J., 5:23 (1981).
56. A.F. Lott and D.R. Vaughn, Soc. Appl. Bacteriol. Tech. Ser., 18:331 (1983).
57. S.H. Tao and M. Poumeyrol, Recl. Med. Vet., 161:457 (1985).
58. W.W.B. Engel, F.W. Van Leusden, and J.F.M. Nouws, in Antimicrobials and Agriculture Proc. 4th Int. Symp. on Antibiotics in Agriculture (W. Woodbrine, Ed.), Butterworth Publ. London, p. 491 (1984).
59. K. Koenen-Dierick, L. de Zutter, and J. van Hoof, Arch. Lebensmittelhyg., 38:128 (1987).
60. J.D. MacNeil, G.O. Korsrud, J.M. Naylor, and W.D.G. Yates, Am. J. Vet. Res., 50: 72 (1989).
61. R. Bossuyt, R. van Renterghem, and G. Waes, J. Chromatogr., 124:37 (1976).
62. D.V. Herbst, J. Pharm. Sci., 69:616 (1980).

63. A.B. Barbiers and A.W. Neff, J. Assoc. Off. Anal. Chem., 59:849 (1976).

64. E. Neidert, P.W. Saschenbrecker, and F. Tittiger, J. Assoc. Off. Anal. Chem., 70: 197 (1987).

65. G.O. Korsrud and J.D. MacNeil, J. Food Prot., 51:43 (1988).

66. Ch. Wolf, D. Behrendt, and B. Julicher, in Residues of Veterinary Drugs in Food, Proc. Euroresidue III Conf., Veldhoven, May 6–8, 1996 (N. Haagsma and A. Ruiter, Eds.), Fac. Vet. Med., Univ. Utrecht, The Netherlands, p. 169 (1996).

67. The Brilliant Black Reduction Test, Enterotox Labs., Krefeld, Germany.

68. CITE Probe Tetracycline and CITE Probe Beta-Lactam Test kits, IDEXX Laboratories, INC., Westbrook, Maine, USA.

69. IDS Gentamicin and IDS Neomycin One-step ELISAs, International Diagnostic Systems Corp., St. Joseph, MI, USA.

70. EZ-Screen test, Chloramphenicol in Milk, Sulfamethazine in Milk, Sulfadimethoxine in Milk, Environmental Diagnostics, Inc., Burlington, NC, USA.

71. Charm II test, Charm Sciences, Inc., Malden, MA, USA.

72. C.D.C. Salisbury, C.E. Rigby, and W. Chan, J. Agric. Food Chem., 37:105 (1989).

73. K. Helrich, AOAC, Official Methods of Analysis (K. Helrich, Ed.), 15th Edition, Association of Official Analytical Chemists, Arlington, VA, Sec. 983.31 (1990).

74. Food Safety and Inspection Service (FSIS), in Chemistry Laboratory Guide Book, US Department of Agriculture, Washington, DC (1983).

75. L.A. van Ginkel, H.J. van Rossum, P.W. Zoontjes, H. van Blitterswisk, G. Ellen, E. van der Heeft, A.P.J.M. de Jong, and G. Zomer, Anal. Chim. Acta, 237:61 (1990).

76. J.O. Boison, C.D.C. Salisbury, W. Chan, and J.D. MacNeil, J. Assoc. Off. Anal. Chem., 74:497 (1991).

77. H. Oka, H. Matsumoto, K. Uno, K.-I. Harada, S. Kadowaki, and M. Suzuki, J. Chromatogr., 325:265 (1985).

78. R. de La Haye, R. Patel, and S. Porter, in Residues of Veterinary Drugs in Food, Proc. Euroresidue III Conf., Veldhoven, May 6–8, 1996 (N. Haagsma and A. Ruiter, Eds.), Fac. Vet. Med., Univ. Utrecht, The Netherlands, p. 481 (1996).

79. R. Jackman, in Residues of Veterinary Drugs in Food, Proc. Euroresidue III Conf., Veldhoven, May 6–8, 1996 (N. Haagsma and A. Ruiter, Eds.), Fac. Vet. Med., Univ. Utrecht, The Netherlands, p. 99 (1996).

80. S. Porter, R. Patel, and N. Johnston, in Residues of Veterinary Drugs in Food, Proc. Euroresidue II Conf., Veldhoven, May 3–5, 1993 (N. Haagsma, A. Ruiter, and P.B. Czedik-Eysenberg, Eds.), Fac. Vet. Med., Univ. Utrecht, The Netherlands, p. 543 (1993).

81. R.W. Stephany and L.A. van Ginkel, Workshop on Screening Methods for Veterinary Drugs and Natural Contaminants in Food Animal production (S.C. Fitzpatrick, J.O. Rangers, A. MacDonald, and D. Newkirk, Eds.), Animal Health Institute Foundation, Center for Veterinary Medicine Food and Drug Administration, Food Safety and Inspection Services US Department of Agriculture, Association of Official Analytical Chemists, Food and Agriculture Organization, Washington, DC, p. 60 (1989).

27

Microbiological Methods

Under the pressure of an increasing number of drugs with fixed tolerance or maximum residue limits (MRLs), demands on methods to detect antimicrobial residues in edible animal products have changed markedly during recent decades (1). To satisfy these demands and prevent contaminated products from entering the food chain, many microbiological tests with sufficient detection sensitivity of as many analytes as possible in animal tissues, milk, eggs, honey, and fish have been developed or modified.

27.1 ASSAY FORMATS

Assays for detection of antimicrobial residues in foods are based on the microbial growth inhibition, microbial receptor, and enzymatic colorimetric formats.

27.1.1 Microbial Growth Inhibition Assays

The earliest methods used for the detection of antimicrobial residues in foods were based on the detection of growth inhibition of various sensitive bacterial stains. These methods, originally developed for use in clinical medicine, were based on microbial agar diffusion tests, or the inhibition of acid production or coagulation by starter organisms. Other growth inhibition methods such as conductance and ATP bioluminescence measurements have not been well received in current regulatory programs (2, 3).

The basic microbial inhibition assay format involves a standard culture of a test organism, usually *Bacillus stearothermophilus, Bacillus subtilis, Bacillus cereus, Micrococcus luteus, Escherichia coli, Bacillus megatherium,* or *Strepto-*

coccus thermophilus seeded in an agar or liquid growth medium. This is then inoculated with milk, urine, tissue, egg, or honey sample and incubated for periods up to several hours. Sample can be applied directly to the medium, in stainless steel cylinders or on a paper disc impregnated with the liquified sample. During incubation, the liquid diffuses into the medium and, if the sample contains sufficient amounts of inhibitory compounds, the growth of the test organism will be reduced or inhibited. Depending on the particular test, the presence of an inhibitory compound in the test sample is indicated by zones of growth inhibition or a change in the color of the medium.

Owing to the variability in results of the early developed microbiological procedures, standardized tests were introduced and are currently used for routine quality control. Examples of commercially available microbial tests for food analysis include the Delvotest-P, Brilliant black reduction (BR) test, CHARM farm test, swab test on premises (STOP) live animal swab test (LAST), and the calf antibiotic and sulfa test (CAST). The primary advantages of these tests are that they are inexpensive, easy to perform, and adaptable to screening of large numbers of samples. Their major disadvantage is that they are not intended to provide definitive information on the identity of specific drug residues. Instead, these tests can be very effectively used to give an indication that a residue problem may exist in the sample tested.

Microbial inhibition tests are extremely sensitive for β-lactam antibiotics, primarily penicillin, but mostly are more than 100-fold less sensitive for other commonly used antibacterials such as macrolides, sulfonamides, tetracyclines, or chloramphenicol (4, 5). Therefore, inhibition tests usually classify residues as belonging to the β-lactam group. Antibiotics other than β-lactams and sulfonamides can be detected by use of the enzyme penicillinase and aminobenzoic acid, respectively (1, 6).

Investigations into performance characteristics have shown that various factors affect the efficiency of the microbiological assays; their relative influence depends upon the kind of antibacterials assayed and, especially, the test organism (7). Agar composition and pH, type of test strain, incubation temperature, depth of the agar, and the manner of incubation are all parameters of critical importance (7–9).

The efficiency of a test system depends also on the matrix used for examination. Many reports have stated that growth-inhibition tests are subject to the effect of several natural inhibitory food components such as lysozyme, lactoferrin, lactoperoxidase, somatic cells, long-chain fatty acids, bile, and lactic acid. These compounds may give rise to false-positive results, particularly when mastitic milk from individual cows, kidneys from pigs, and urine samples are tested (10–17). Some of these effects can be overcome by use of paper discs, heat treatment of samples prior to testing, or use of dialysis membranes to separate high-molecular-weight proteins from the low-molecular-weight antibiotics (15, 16, 18).

27.1.2 Microbial Receptor Assays

More versatile than the growth-inhibition assays and potentially applicable to determining the presence of different antibiotic residues in different matrices are the microbial receptor CHARM I and II test assays (19, 20). The Charm I test, developed exclusively for β-lactams in milk, constitutes the first rapid test recognized by The Association of Official Analytical Chemists (AOAC) with a test time of 15 min (19). The speed and sensitivity of this test permitted testing of milk tankers before they unloaded at the processing plant (21). In 1984–1985, the CHARM I test was further developed to test for antibiotics beyond β-lactams to include tetracyclines, sulfonamides, aminoglycosides, chloramphenicol, novobiocin, and macrolides. The extended version has been referred to as CHARM II test.

The CHARM II test is a general screening and identification test for members of different groups of antibacterial residues in milk in a rapid 15 min procedure (22–24). The test has been also applied to the analysis of other animal products, but a simple 30 min extraction with an aqueous buffer is usually required for tissue and eggs.

The CHARM II test is based on the irreversible binding reaction between functional groups of antibacterials and receptor sites on or within the cell of added microorganisms. For example, β-lactams bind to D-alanine carboxypeptidase on the cell wall, whereas other binding sites are found on ribosomes. Cells from two different organisms provide the binding sites for seven groups of antibacterials, which include aminoglycosides, β-lactams, chloramphenicol, macrolides, novobiocin, sulfonamides, and tetracyclines. The test employs ^{14}C-labeled or ^{3}H-labeled antibacterials to compete for the binding sites. This competition for receptor sites prevents the radiolabeled antibacterial from binding. Thus the more radiolabeled compound bound, the less analyte in the sample. A control point, established by spiking the most common family member into the matrix at a predetermined level, identifies contaminated samples.

Although analogous in test principle to the radioimmunoassays, the CHARM II test cannot be classified by strict definition as immunochemical assay. In addition, it may be considered that inhibition tests also bind antibiotics to microbial receptors. In this case, the results of antibiotic binding is measured by growth inhibition and lack of acid production. In cases where the initial binding and final mode of action take place on the same site as with sulfonamides and β-lactams, there is excellent correlation between receptor and inhibition assays. On the other hand, macrolides/lincomycin and aminoglycosides that have additional subsites (25) give less correlation. In some cases, weak binding of the antibiotic to the receptor limits the sensitivity. When this happens an antibody binder may be better, especially in a drug family with few members.

The procedure for detecting residues in milk is relatively simple and rapid. For the detection of β-lactams, for example, a 5 ml milk sample is incubated with a mixture of the ^{14}C-labeled β-lactam and the microbial receptor sites for 4 min at 85°C, and centrifuged. The supernatant is discarded; the precipitate is resuspended in water to be mixed further with scintillation fluid. For screening purposes the sample is counted for 1 min, while for quantitation purposes it is counted for 5 min. The reported limits of detection in milk range from less than 5 ng/ml for β-lactams and sulfonamides to 500 ng/ml for tetracyclines (20, 24, 26). The test can be regarded as a sensitive, rather complex screening method complementary to conventional microbiological methods.

When the CHARM II test was applied on kidney, liver, and muscle tissue samples, the detection limits obtained for penicillin G, sulfamethazine, streptomycin, and erythromycin were 5, 15, 100, and 150 ppb, respectively (27). The degree of response obtained with the β-lactam assay varied among equimolar amounts of eight β-lactams. The sulfa assay was positive, with varying response, to equimolar amounts of four different sulfonamides and negative for trimethoprim. The streptomycin assay also detected dihydrostreptomycin, but was negative for gentamicin and neomycin. The erythromycin assay was negative for oleandomycin but positive for tilmicosin and tylosin. No evidence of cross-reactivity was detected among the compounds targeted by the four assays.

The CHARM II test for tissues is relatively fast, easy to perform, and requires limited laboratory equipment. However, for antibacterials with established tolerance levels, it can serve only as a screening test because the results are not quantitative and therefore should be supported by additional quantitative chemical methods. The microbial receptor assay, with its broad-spectrum capability, can enhance any existing monitoring system as a first-line monitoring test or as a confirmation for any program using microbial inhibition tests.

27.1.3 Enzymatic Colorimetric Assays

The enzymatic colorimetric format is followed by the Penzyme test. This test is a qualitative enzymatic assay for rapid detection of β-lactam residues in milk (28–30). The detection principle of the Penzyme test is based on measurement of the degree of inactivation of the enzyme DD-carboxypeptidase is involved in the synthesis of the bacterial cell wall by β-lactam antibiotics. These residues bind specifically with the enzyme and inactivate it, thus interfering with bacterial cell wall formation.

In the Penzyme test, freeze-dried *Streptomyces* DD-carboxypeptidase is placed in sealed vials to which the milk sample is added. A preliminary incubation is carried out for 5 min at 47°C to cause some inactivation of the enzyme molecules. The degree of inactivation is dependent on the amount of β-lactams presumed to be present in the milk sample. Subsequent addition of a reagent tablet containing synthetic D-alanine oligopeptide and D-amino acid oxidase followed by reincubation at 47°C for 15 min results in the release of D-alanine, its amount depending on the remaining active enzyme. D-Alanine is oxidized in turn to pyruvic acid with simultaneous formation of hydrogen peroxide, and the latter is measured by use of a redox color indicator that is oxidized to a white–yellow color if the test result is positive, reduced to a pink color if the test result is negative. A coloration midway between the pink and the white–yellow allows semiquantitative estimation of β-lactams present in milk in the range 0–0.017 IU/ml.

27.2 APPLICATIONS

Applications of microbiological methods in the field of drug residues analysis include all types of food matrices: milk, meat, eggs, and honey.

27.2.1 Milk Analysis

The focus of testing for antibiotic residues in milk is changing from that of preventing manufacturing problems to more of an emphasis on food safety. The significance of using methods that detect inhibitors solely because they suppress starter cultures in dairy products is taking a secondary role to methodology that detects antibiotic residues at established levels of concern.

In the context of residue control, antibiotic residues in milk are the easiest and most practical to accommodate. In the past, inhibitor tests sensitive primarily to β-lactam antibiotics were used to control drug residues in milk. More recently, other drugs have become the focus of concern, and new concepts for the detection of antibiotics in milk are repeatedly being reported (31).

In 1989, an experimental study designed by the International Dairy Federation in 53 laboratories of 22 different countries to achieve deeper insight into state of proficiency of routinely applied tests showed that the most frequently used microbial inhibitor screening tests were the disc assays with *Bacillus stearothermophilus,* Delvotest-P, Brilliant black reduction test, acidification test, CHARM II test, and the Penzyme test (32). Currently available microbial inhibitor tests for screening of residual antibacterials in milk and milk products are presented in Table 27.1.

In the disc assay plate tests, a paper disk impregnated with the milk sample is placed on the surface of an agar medium inoculated with either *Bacillus stearothermophilus* var. *calidolactis* ATCC 10149 (Disc assay for penicillin and disc assay with indicator) or *Bacillus subtilis* ATCC 6633 (*Bacillus subtilis* field test). During incubation, growth of the test organisms causes the agar to become cloudy if inhibitory substances are not present. Presence of inhibitory substances causes a clear zone around the disc, the zone size depending on both the type and concentration of the inhibitory substances. Therefore, any clear zone surrounding a disc prepared from a heat-treated milk is considered to show a positive result.

TABLE 27.1 Microbiological Methods for Screening Residual Antibacterials in Milk

Type of test	Sample treatment	Test organism	Incubation conditions	Indicator	Confirmation agent	Ref.
SCREENING ASSAYS						
Accusphere test (Intervet Lab. Ltd.)	Heating at 95°C	*S. thermophilus* in sphere form	4 h at 45°C into tube	Bromocresol purple (visual check of colour change)	Penicillinase	34
Acidification test	Heating at 100°C for 5 min	*S. thermophilus* T.J.	2.5 h at 45°C into tube	Bromocresol purple (visual check of color change	Penicillinase or p-amino benzoic acid and trimethoprim	34
Arla microtest (Arla, Sweden)	Heating at 80°C for 2 min	*B. subtilis* ATCC 6633 in tablet form	6 h at 40°C in micro-titre plate	Triphenyltetrazolium chloride (visual check of color change)	Trimethoprim	127, 128
Bioluminescence test (Biosys SA)	Heating at 100°C for 2 min	*S. thermophilus* T.J.	20, 40 and/or 60 min at 45°C into tube	Luciferin–luciferase (use of luminometer)	Penicillinase or p-amino benzoic acid and trimethoprim	42
B. subtilis field test	Direct assay	*B. subtilis* ATCC 6633	14–24 h at 32°C or 5–7 h at 35°C or 3–4 h at 37°C on agar plate	None (visual check of inhibition zone)	None	129

Method	Treatment	Test organism	Conditions	Indicator	Inhibitor	Ref.
BR-test/AS/Blue Star/6/7 (Enterotox Lab., Germany)	Direct assay	*B. stearothermophilus* var. *calidolactis* ATCC 10149	2.5–3.5 h at 60–70°C on microtitre tablets	Brilliant Black B (visual or by microplate reader-check of color change)	Penicillinase or p-amino benzoic acid and trimethoprim	36, 39
Charm farm test (Penicillin Assays, USA)	Heating at 100°C for 6 min	*B. stearothermophilus* in tablet form	3.8 h at 67°C into tube	Bromocresol purple (visual check of color change)	Penicillinase or p-amino benzoic acid	34
Charm inhibition assay (Penicillin Assays, USA)	Direct assay	*B. stearothermophilus* var. *calidolactis* ATCC 10149	2.3 h at 64°C on agar plate	Bromocresol purple (visual check of color change)	Penicillinase or p-amino benzoic acid	34
Disc assay for penicillin	Direct assay	*B. stearothermophilus* var. *calidolactis* ATCC 10149	2.5–5 h at 55°C on agar plate	None (visual check of inhibition zone)	Penicillinase	21
Disc assay with indicator	Direct assay	*B. stearothermophilus* var. *calidolactis* ATCC 10149	3–4 h at 55°C or 2–3 h at 64°C on agar plate	Bromocresol purple (visual check of color change)	Penicillinase or p-amino benzoic acid and trimethoprim	34
Delvotest P/SP/multi (Gist-Brocades NV, Netherlands)	Direct assay	*B. stearothermophilus* var *calidolactis* ATCC 10149	2.5 h at 64°C into ampules or cups of a polystyrene plate	Bromocresol purple (visual check of color change)	Penicillinase	130
Inhibitor test with Sarcina lutea	Direct assay	*Sarcina lutea* (*M. luteus*) ATCC 9341	16–18 h at 30°C in cylinder plate	None (visual check of inhibition zone)	Penicillinase	41, 129

(continued)

TABLE 27.1 Continued

Type of test	Sample treatment	Test organism	Incubation conditions	Indicator	Confirmation agent	Ref.
Lumac test (Lumac B.V., NL)	Direct assay	*S. thermophilus* OL 1010.59	35 min at 41°C into Lumacuvettes	3-(4,4-dimethylthiazolyl-2-)2,5-diphenyl-tetrazolium bromide	—	34
Tube diffusion test	Direct assay	*B. stearothermophilus* var. *calidolactis* ATCC 10149	2.5–2.75 h at 64°C into tube	Bromocresol purple (visual check of color change)	Penicillinase or p-amino benzoic acid and trimethoprim	34
Valio T101 test (Valio Dairies Association, Finland)	Heating at 95°C for 5 min	*S. thermophilus* T101	4.5 h at 42°C into vials or microwells	Bromocresol purple (visual check of color change)	—	131

TENTATIVE CONFIRMATION ASSAYS

Test	Treatment	Organism	Incubation	Detection	Identification	Ref.
Three-plate test:	Heating at 80°C for 10 min	B. stearothermophilus var calidolactis ATCC 10149	2.5 h at 55°C on agar plate	None (visual check of inhibition zone)	Penicillinase and trimethoprim	34
		B. subtilis ATCC 6633	16–18 h at 30°C on agar plate	None (visual check of inhibition zone)	—	
		B. megaterium ATCC 9885	5 h at 37°C on agar plate	None (visual check of inhibition zone)	Trimethoprim and p-amino benzoic acid	
Six-plate test	Direct assay	B. cereus var mycoides ATCC 9634	18–24 h at 30°C on agar plate	None (visual check of inhibition zone)	Penicillinase or p-amino benzoic acid and trimethoprim (provisional)	34
		B. stearothermophilus var calidolactis ATCC 10149	4 h at 63°C after 4 h diffussion at 20°C on agar plate	None (visual check of inhibition zone)		
		B. subtilis BGA	18–24 h at 30°C on agar plate	None (visual check of inhibition zone)		
		B. subtilis BGA	18–24 h at 30°C on agar plate	None (visual check of inhibition zone)		
		Escherichia coli 28 PR 271	18–24 h at 37°C on agar plate	None (visual check of inhibition zone)		
		M. luteus ATCC 9341	18–24 h at 37°C on agar plate	None (visual check of inhibition zone)		

In assays in which bromocresol purple indicator is incorporated into the medium (disc assay for penicillin, disc assay with indicator), a clear bluish zone around the disk appears if samples contain inhibitory substances. When addition of penicillinase to positive milk samples eliminates the zone, the inhibitors can be roughly identified as β-lactams. Among these tests, the 3 h *Bacillus stearother-mophilus* disc assay was selected in 1981 as the regulatory test for detecting antibiotic residues in milk. Although particularly sensitive to β-lactams, this test is relatively insensitive to a number of commonly used antibiotics (20).

In the Accusphere test a freeze-dried sphere containing the test organism *Streptococcus thermophilus* and bromocresol purple as indicator disperses into the test milk sample. The acidification test is very similar: the milk sample is heated to be further inoculated with a *Streptococcus thermophilus* culture containing yeast extract, bromocresol purple indicator, and trimethoprim. It is then incubated for 2.5 h at 45°C (33). In the presence of inhibitory substances, the organism growth is suppressed, acid production is reduced or eliminated, and the color of the indicator remains unchanged. Addition of penicillinase to a positive milk sample results in change of the color of the indicator from purple to yellow when only β-lactams are present.

The Arla test is a routine assay in which a heat-treated milk sample is added to a well of a microtiter plate containing a freeze-dried tablet containing *Bacillus subtilis* ATCC 6633, nutrients, and triphenyltetrazoliumchloride as redox indicator (33). Following incubation, the normal growth of the organism is inhibited if antibacterials are present, and the uncolored indicator is not reduced into its red form. Detection of sulfonamides requires prior addition of trimethoprim in the milk samples analyzed.

The CHARM inhibition assay (CIA), Charm farm test (CFT), and Valio T101 test are all simple multiresidue screening tests based on microbial inhibition (34, 35). The CIA test is actually a disc assay using *Bacillus stearothermophilus* and specially formulated agar media to increase the sensitivity to sulfonamides. The CFT is a tube assay using the same test organism in a specific formulation, which, along with the nutrients, is in a tablet form. To roughly identify penicillins and sulfonamides with the CIA and CFT tests, positive samples should be reanalyzed after the addition of penicillinase and p-aminobenzoic acid.

In contrast to the previous multiresidue tests, the Valio T101 test uses a freeze-dried *Streptococcus thermophilus* T101-strain dispersed into the milk. During incubation, the test organisms grow and produce acid, which causes the pH indicator to change color from blue to yellow. In the presence of any inhibitory substances, the indicator remains blue or turns to a greenish color depending on the concentration of inhibitors.

The BR-test constitutes a nonspecific screening assay for the systematic control of raw milk, which combines principles of both agar diffusion and color reduction procedures (36). In this test, the sample is introduced into a microtiter tablet filled with agar containing *Bacillus stearothermophilus* and is incubated. During the incubation period, the microorganisms multiply and cause reduction of the incorporated redox indicator to the yellow form. If the sample contains inhibitory substances, the growth of the microorganism is restrained and the medium retains the blue color of the oxidized form of the brilliant black indicator. Addition of penicillinase in positive samples causes reduction of the indicator to its yellow color form if only β-lactams are present in the sample.

The BR-test has been modified several times (37, 38). One of its versions, known as the BR-test AS, contains antifolates that make it possible to detect sulfones and sulfonamides in addition to the usual inhibitory substances. Another version, which is called BR-test "Blue Star," has been officially accepted and used in Canada. By decreasing the spore concentration in the detection medium, a sensitivity of less than 40 ng sulfamethazine/ml milk is possible with this test (38).

In an effort to improve further the detection limits for tetracyclines, sulfonamides, and aminoglycosides, additional versions of the BR-test have been developed. Using the BR-tests 6 and 7 in which the pH value of the medium was reduced from 8.0 to 6.0 or 7.0, respectively, the detection limits of tetracyclines, sulfonamides, and aminoglycosides were significantly improved (39). Although lactoferrin and lysozyme in combination presented an enhanced inhibitory effect in both of these tests, their physiological concentrations in milk were not sufficient to induce positive test results. Nevertheless, storing the milk samples pending analysis at refrigerated temperatures has been strongly recommended for minimizing false-positive results (40). Rough classification of detected inhibitors into penicillins, sulfonamides, and other inhibitory substances is possible by these tests through use of penicillinase and p-aminobenzoic acid.

The *Sarcina lutea* test is the official US Food and Drug Administration (FDA) test for detecting penicillin residues in milk and dairy products (41). In this test, milk samples are placed in stainless steel cylinders on an agar plate seeded with *Sarcina lutea* ATCC 9341. As milk diffuses into the agar, inhibitors prevent the growth of the organism, causing a zone the width of which is a measure of the antibiotic concentration. The test is sensitive to about 0.006 μg/ml penicillin G, and confirmation of positive results can be performed by the addition of penicillinase.

The ATP test is a bioluminescence procedure based on the reaction between adenosine-5-triphosphate (ATP) and a luciferin–luciferase enzymatic system (42, 43). The principle of the test relies on the fact that after a certain incubation period the intracellular ATP level, which gives a reliable indication of the state of development of a suitable bacterial culture (44), will remain low relative to a control, when antimicrobial residues are present. In its first version the ATP test employed *Bacillus subtilis* ATCC 6633 as the test organism, but a current version is based on the use of *Streptococcus thermophilus* T.J. culture.

In the current version, the milk sample is slightly heated to be mixed further into a tube with yeast extract, trimethoprim, apyrase, and *Streptococcus thermophilus* T.J. culture in the exponential phase of the growth. Following incubation for 20 min, 40 min, and/or 60 min, a bacterial extractor, a stabilizer, and a luciferin–luciferase reagent are all added. The bioluminescence emitted after addition of the luciferin–luciferase reagent is measured with an appropriate photometer. The ratio of the values obtained at 40 and 20 min, and/or at 60 and 20 min, indicates the presence of inhibitors when it is lower than those obtained with inhibitor-free milk samples. Presence of penicillin or sulfonamides can be roughly confirmed in positive samples through the addition of penicillinase or p-amino-benzoic acid, respectively.

The Lumac test is a rapid detection procedure for a wide range of antibiotic residues in milk. It is based on measurement of the inhibition of the metabolic activity of a specially developed strain of *Streptococcus thermophilus* after a 30 min incubation time (33). In absence of inhibitory substances, the organism grows and enzymes are produced. In presence of the chromogen 3-(4,4-dimethylthiazo-lyl-2-)2,5-diphenyltetrazolium bromide, a color change from greenish to purple occurs because of oxidation of the chromogen by the produced enzymes. When antibiotic residues are present in samples, production of enzymes is suppressed and therefore less color change is observed. With this test, a slight color difference between test samples and control milk is enough to denote the presence of antibiotic residues in the tested milk samples. However, application of this test in milk from cows with mastitis may lead to false-negative results because high concentrations of somatic cells can counteract with the activity of the antibiotics.

Since yogurt cultures are about 10 times more sensitive to penicillin than other starters, a yogurt inhibitor test has been also developed to detect this drug in milk (45, 46). In this test, the milk is heated and inoculated with a yogurt culture. Following incubation, inhibitory substances are considered to be present when the increase of the Soxhlet-Henkel acidity of the test sample is lower than half the increase of acidity of an inhibitory-free control milk sample.

Another widespread and simple-to-handle tube diffusion assay is the Del-votest-P test (47). In this test, the milk sample and a tablet containing nutrients and a pH-indicator are added to an ampoule containing agar seeded with spores of *Bacillus stearothermophilus*. Following incubation, the organism produces enough acid to change the color of the incorporated pH-indicator from purple to yellow when inhibitory substances are absent. When antibacterials are present, the normal growth of the organism is inhibited, acid production is delayed, and the incorporated pH-indicator does not change its color. In this test, all inhibitory substances have to diffuse down into the agar to affect the growth of the test organism. Although antibacterials readily penetrate the whole agar layer, natural inhibitory substances, such as lactoferrin and lysozyme, diffuse only a small distance and therefore do not affect the growth of the organism. This is due to the fact that the diffusion of those positively charged proteins into the agar medium is inhibited by their interaction with the sulfate groups of the agar (48).

However, when both lactoferrin and lysozyme are present in considerably higher concentrations than in normal milk, as in mastitis milk, a complex may be formed in which the basic functions of the compounds are masked and therefore diffusion of the complex into the agar occurs. This diffusion can be further enhanced when lactoferrin is in excess, due to neutralization of the electrical charge of the agar (11). Fortunately, the raw farm milk does not show such inhibition because any affected milk is too diluted by unaffected milk. Appearance, therefore, of a narrow, purple, upper layer above yellow-colored agar indicates a negative test result. Rough identification of penicillin or sulfonamides in positive samples is possible through the addition of penicillinase or p-aminobenzoic acid, respectively, in the tested milk samples (49).

The Delvotest-P-Multitest is a modification of the original Delvotest-P test (50). This is not an ampoule test but a polystyrene plate-based test with cups similar in principle to the original version. Its main advantage is that it permits up to 96 test cups to be used at one time. Following a collaborative study (51), both tests have been adopted by the Association of Official Analytical Chemists (AOAC) as official tests for the detection of β-lactams in milk and milk products.

A more recent ampoule-based version with quite different test principle has been also available in the market as Delvo-X-Press test (52). This is a qualitative enzyme-linked receptor-binding assay in which residues of β-lactam antibiotics are captured by a penicillin-binding protein conjugated to the enzyme horseradish peroxidase. Although analogous in principle to immunochemical assays, the Delvo-X-Press test does not use antibodies specifically to bind the β-lactams, and therefore cannot be classified as immunochemical test. In the first step of this test, calibrated amounts of milk and conjugate are mixed and incubated. The enzyme conjugate will bind with β-lactams that may be present in the milk sample. This mixture is then transferred to a tube coated with β-lactam antibiotic. If a plastic unit containing sample and control spots on a filter paper is used instead of tubes, the test although similar in principle is called Snap test (53).

Only free enzyme conjugate will bind to the coating. Addition of an enzyme substrate results in formation of a blue color, the intensity of which is inversely proportional to the amount of β-lactam in the sample. Absence of β-lactams in a sample results in all of the enzyme conjugate remaining unbound and available for binding to the immobilized β-lactam. Presence of β-lactams results in a portion of the enzyme conjugate being bound and unavailable to bind with the immobilized β-lactam. The Delvo-X-Press test uses an optical density reader to compare the optical density of a standard set at a cutoff level of 5 ppb penicillin G, with that of each sample tube in total assay time of about 10 min.

Apart from detection, some microbial inhibitor tests including the three-plate and the six-plate tests are further suitable for tentative confirmation of antibacterial residues in milk samples found positive by other microbial inhibitor screening tests (Table 27.1). In the three-plate test, a paper disc impregnated with the milk sample is placed on each of the three test plates (33). One plate has been inoculated with *Bacillus stearothermophilus*, the other with *Bacillus subtilis*, and the third with *Bacillus megatherium*, respectively. In this way, detection and presumptive identification of antibiotic substances that may be present in milk can be made possible, since *Bacillus stearothermophilus* is particularly suitable, apart from penicillins, for the detection of penicillins and tetracyclines, whereas *Bacillus subtilis* is suitable for aminoglycosides and macrolides, and *Bacillus megatherium* for chloramphenicol and sulfonamides.

In the six-plate test, the sample is brought in a punch hole or a paper disc on each of the six test plates that have been inoculated with *Bacillus cereus*, *Bacillus subtilis* (pH 6), *Bacillus subtilis* (pH 8), *Sarcina lutea*, *Escherichia coli*, and *Bacillus stearothermophilus*, respectively (33). Once the samples have been introduced, the plates are incubated for the required time at the required temperature. If, on one of the plates, a zone of inhibition of 1.0 mm is observed around the disks or holes, the result of the test is considered positive, provided that interferences have been excluded.

Detectable concentrations of various antibacterials in milk attained by different microbiological tests are presented in Table 27.2. Milk constitutes a matrix that, apart from heating to destroy natural inhibitory substances, does not generally necessitate further sample treatment. Some antibiotics, however, exhibit some instability to heat treatment (54–56) and, therefore, if further confirmation is required reference frozen samples should always be available. When raw milk is directly analyzed, critical evaluation is generally required because natural inhibitors such as somatic cells, immunoglobulins, and metabolites may cause zones of inhibition (56, 57). Furthermore, several factors including marked pH-deviations, use of paper disks that contain inhibitory substances, and work with forceps that are too hot or have not been cleaned properly can readily lead to false-positive readings (56, 58).

Application of some kind of sample treatment may have the potential to improve substantially the detection of certain antibacterials in milk by microbial routine methods (59). Treatment, for example, of milk samples with ammonium oxalate solution prior to analysis can lead to lower limits of detection of tetracyclines by both microbial inhibition and microbial receptor assays. This is due to the fact that tetracycline residues tend to form chelates with divalent cations and bind to proteins, which reduce their antibacterial efficacy. However, the oxalate treatment causes splitting of complex and/or protein bonds without increasing the detection limits of other antibacterials commonly used in dairy cows.

27.2.2 Meat, Egg, and Honey Analysis

Muscle, liver, and kidney constitute the target tissues used for inspection of the whole carcass for the presence of antibacterial residues. A major advantage in

TABLE 27.2 Detectable Concentrations (ppm) of Various Antibacterials in Milk by Different Microbiological Tests

Type of test	Aminoglycosides	β-Lactams	Macrolides	Tetracyclines	Sulfonamides	Chloramphenicol
Accusphere test	5.0–10.0	0.006–0.2	0.1–5.0	0.5	200.0	0.5
Acidification test	5.0	0.003–0.2	0.06	0.4	0.1–1.0	1.2
Arla microtest	2.5–5.0	0.004	0.6	0.1	0.1–1.0	0.6
ATP test	3.0	0.002–0.1	0.02	0.04	3.0–30.0	0.5
BR-test	13–28	0.005–0.035	2.25	0.4–0.5	0.1–1.0	15.0
BR-test AS/Blue star	0.3–12.5	0.002–0.03	C.02–2.5	0.1–0.2	0.005–1.5	2.75
BR-test 6	0.175–7.0	0.0009–0.013	0.025–2.25	0.05–0.09	–	1.5
BR-test 7	0.125–4.25	0.0015–0.015	C.02–1.0	0.075–0.15	–	1.5
CHARM farm test	0.04–0.125	0.003–0.05	2.25	0.06–0.1	0.01–0.015	–
CHARM inhibition assay	0.5	0.004–0.1	0.25	0.2–0.25	0.005–0.01	–
CHARM test II	0.01	0.003–0.03	C.01–0.02	0.08–0.1	0.0005–0.003	0.08
Disc assay (*B. stearothermophilus*)	13–28	0.004–0.035	2.25	0.4–0.5	0.1–1.0	15.0
Delvotest P multi	0.5–15	0.0025–0.015	0.4–5	0.25–0.7	–	8.0
Lumac test	0.5–10.0	0.001–0.05	1.25	0.25–0.3	–	1.0
Penzyme test	n.d.	0.003–0.04	n.d.	n.d.	n.d.	n.d.
Tube diffusion test	13.0–28.0	0.004–0.035	2.25	0.4–0.5	0.1–1.0	15.0
Valio T101 test	0.5–1.0	0.003–0.2	0.05	0.2	1.0	1.0
Three-plate test	0.3–20	0.003–0.03	0.1	0.4	0.1–1.0	2.0
Six-plate test	13–28	0.004–0.035	2.25	0.4–0.5	1–1.2	15.0

Source: From Refs. 34, 39, 130.

analyzing muscle is that this tissue constitutes primarily the edible part of the animal for which maximum residue limits have been established. A disadvantage is that a variety of different microbiological methods have to be used in order to meet the low tolerance/maximum residue limits (MRLs) established for this matrix. Test systems using liver or kidney as target tissue do not necessitate use of different test microorganisms from those for muscle because they usually contain the drug residues at much higher levels, thus offering greater sensitivity. Drawbacks for liver and kidney analyses are, on one hand, the false-positive results frequently obtained because of the presence in these samples of many endogenous inhibiting compounds and, on the other hand, the varying ratios of residue levels between liver or kidney and muscle tissues when animals are not healthy.

Unlike milk, tissues have to be generally submitted to some kind of extraction procedure prior to undergoing microbiological assay. Extraction is generally carried out by blending a weighed portion of tissue with a predetermined ratio of a solvent, preferably an aqueous buffer solution. The homogenized mixture is then analyzed either directly or after centrifugation or other cleanup manipulation. Concentration of sample extracts as a means of increasing the sensitivity of the assay is not usually carried out, since interferences are increased as well. In cases, however, where volatile organic solvents are used for extraction, concentration of the extract and subsequent partitioning into a suitable aqueous buffer is indispensable. Thus, for bacitracin analysis, the tissue is blended with aqueous pyridine and centrifuged. An aliquot of the supernatant is diluted with methanol, centrifuged, and the supernatant is evaporated to dryness to be further reconstituted with a pH 6.5 buffer. Whenever binding of the analytes to tissue components may occur, specific extraction procedures are usually employed. Extraction, for example, with a pH 4.5 phosphate buffer or ethyl acetate can minimize the binding of tetracyclines or novobiocin, respectively, to tissue components (60).

When working with concentrated chicken and pork muscle extracts, nonspecific inhibition zones are occasionally produced. The pH value of the concentrated extract and its lactic acid content are considered major causes for this effect (61). Buffering of the extract with a pH 7 phosphate buffer can greatly reduce, but does not always eliminate, these nonspecific inhibition zones (62). Substances produced in the muscle postmortem, contaminants of the solvents employed in the extraction, and insufficient heat inactivation of contaminated glassware have all been also considered as partly responsible for appearance of these nonspecific zones (61, 62). Development of inhibitory substances at refrigeration temperatures can also cause failures in simple tests designed to detect antibiotic residues, even when the meat is organoleptically acceptable. Therefore caution should be exercised in interpreting the results of inhibition methods applied to animal tissues remote from the place and time of slaughter (16).

Over the years, numerous methods have been developed for detecting antibacterial residues in animal tissues. Most of these methods are agar diffusion procedures using paper disks or steel cylinders to apply samples to the agar plates. The sensitivity of the disk assay methods is generally relatively lower because drug residues in samples bind to filter papers (63), whereas the sensitivity of the cylinder plate assay methods is compromised by sample debris plugging the cylinder bottom (64). Unlike with meat, very few microbiological methods have been developed for eggs and honey. The high frequency of false-positive results caused by the lysozyme present in eggs may be a major reason for this general lack of methods (65–68). Table 27.3 summarizes microbiological methods specifically developed for screening residual antibacterials in animal tissues, eggs and honey.

Apart from those methods, a variety of test assays primarily derived from modifications of the existing fast milk testing procedures have been also developed and widely used for testing animal tissues, eggs, and honey for antibacterial residues. Sound examples are the CHARM II test and the CHARM farm test (CFT), which have been successfully used since 1987 in many animal-derived products and matrices such as swine and cattle tissues, eggs, and honey.

The CHARM II microbial receptor assay, with its broad-spectrum capability, can enhance any existing monitoring system as a first-line screening or confirmation test for any program using microbial inhibition tests. A simple 30 min extraction procedure using an aqueous buffer is performed for tissue and eggs. Extracts may be assayed for several common antibiotic families simultaneously, including β lactams, sulfonamides, tetracyclines, aminoglycosides, macrolides, novobiocin, chloramphenicol and spectinomycin. With CFT, a low incidence of false-positive kidney results and a high incidence of false-positive muscle results have been observed for cattle and swine diagnostic samples, with false-negative kidney results being more frequent than false-negative muscle results (69). When extracts from incurred swine muscle and kidney samples were assayed by CFT for sulfamethazine, chlortetracycline, and penicillin G residues, not too many false-positive results were obtained (70).

An adaptation of the CFT for use with 96-well microtiter plates is the so-called antimicrobial inhibition monitor (AIM-96). This test has been recently evaluated for potential application in muscle analysis (71). Unfortunately, its sensitivity for most antimicrobials, with the exception of penicillin G, was not found sufficient to monitor at MRLs and, thus, the manufacturer of the test is continuing developmental work.

Since 1974, *Bacillus subtilis* BGA has been officially employed as the test organism in the German Hemmstoff test to detect residues of tetracyclines, β-lactams and aminoglycosides in kidney and muscle tissues with high sensitivity (72). Macrolides can be also detected, but to a lesser extent, whereas chloramphenicol and sulfonamides are difficult to detect. For better detection of sulfonamides, a modification of this test, the German three-plate inhibition test, was developed. This test is based on the same test organism but uses three pH values (6, 8, and 7.2), with the addition of trimethoprim. The pH relationship between the three

TABLE 27.3 Microbiological Methods for Screening Residual Antibacterials in Animal Tissues, Eggs, and Honey

Antibacterial	Matrix	Sample preparation	Test organism	Ref.
Bacitracin	Animal tissues	Blending with aqueous pyridine, MeOH addn, centrgn, evapn, and reconstitution in pH 6.5 buffer	*M. flavus* ATCC 10240	132
Cephalexin	Chicken tissues	TCA extn, macroreticular resin (Diaion HP-20) column cleanup, aqueous MeOH elution, evapn, and reconstitution in H₂O/MeOH (2:1)	*B. stearothermophilus* C953 NIZO	133
Chloramphenicol	Animal tissues	Blending with buffered saline and centrgn	*M. luteus* ATCC 9341 and *B. cereus* ATCC 11778	134
	Animal tissues	EtOAc extn, centrgn, evapn, and reconstitution in pH 6 buffer	*M. luteus* ATCC 9341	135
Chlortetracycline, oxytetracycline	Animal tissues	Blending with MeOH/pH 6.5 buffer, centrgn, evapn, and reconstitution in pH 6.5 buffer	*B. cereus* ATCC 11778	136
Colistin	Animal tissues	Blending with pH 6 buffer	*Bordetella bronchiseptica* ATCC 4617	132
	Animal tissues	Extraction by acid hydrolysis at pH 3.5	*Bordetella bronchiseptica* ATCC 4617	137
Erythromycin, oleandomycin, penicillin, tylosin	Animal tissues	Blending with pH 6 buffer	*M. luteus* ATCC 9341	132

Flumequine	Eggs	Direct assay	*Escherichia coli* 14 Bayer	138
	Animal tissues	Punching of cylindrical tissue pieces	*Escherichia coli* 14 Bayer	139
	Animal tissues	Punching of cylindrical tissue pieces	*Escherichia coli* 14 Bayer	140
Hygromycin	Animal tissues	Blending with H_2O	*Pseudomonas syringae* ATCC 12885	132
Neomycin	Eggs	Blending with a surfactant pH 8 buffer, heating at 85°C for 15 min, and centrgn	*B. stearothermophilus* ATCC 12980	141
Nosiheptide	Animal tissues and eggs	DMF/acetone extn, centrgn	*S. aureus* ATCC 6538P	142
Novobiocin	Animal tissues	Blending with EtOAc, pH 10 buffer extn	*S. epidermidis* ATCC 12228	132
Oxytetracycline	Honey	Diln with pH 7 buffer	*B. cereus* ATCC 11778	143
	Animal tissues	Blending with H_2O	*B. stearothermophilus* ATCC 10149 (Delvotest P)	84
Penicillin	Animal tissues	Blending with pH 7 buffer	*M. luteus* ATCC 9341	144
	Animal tissues	Blending with ACN/pH 6 buffer, centrgn, and evapn of the supernatant	*M. luteus* ATCC 9341	61
	Animal tissues	Blending with pH 6 buffer, and centrgn	*M. luteus* ATCC 9341	145

(continued)

Table 27.3 Continued

Antibacterial	Matrix	Sample preparation	Test organism	Ref.
Penicillin, tetracyclines	Animal tissues	Extraction with oxalate/EDTA/acetone soln, evapn, and reconstitution in pH 7 buffer	M. luteus ATCC 9341	62, 146
Spectinomycin	Animal tissues	Blending with acidic ammonium sulfate, purification over Charcoal/Celite column, evapn to dryness, and reconstitution with pH 8 buffer	Escherichia coli	132
Streptomycin	Animal tissues	Blending with pH 1.5 buffer, pH 8.5 adjustment, centrgn	B. subtilis ATCC 6633	132
	Eggs	Blending with a surfactant pH 8 buffer, heating at 85°C for 15 min, and centrgn	B. subtilis ATCC 6633	147
Tetracyclines	Animal tissues	Blending with pH 4.5 buffer	B. cereus ATCC 11778	132
Various antibacterials	Animal tissues	Punching of cylindrical tissue pieces	B. subtilis BGA	148
Various antibacterials	Animal tissues	Blending with an appropriate buffer, centrgn	B. stearothermophilus BBL 12018	149
Various antibacterials	Animal tissues	Centrgn or ACN extn of tissue paste	M. luteus ATCC 9341 and B. cereus ATCC 11778	150

Addn, addition; centrgn, centrifugation; evap, evaporation; diln, dilution.
Other abbreviations as in Table 20.2.

results for each sample can give an incidence to groups of antibiotics contained in the sample. A comparative evaluation study has shown that this test, which is the official test in Germany, apart from a low sensitivity for bacitracin, is identical in performance with the EU four-plate test (73).

The four-plate test was initially based on the German Hemmstoff-test with an additional plate of *Sarcina lutea* at pH 8.0, designed for the detection of lower levels of macrolides, and a fourth plate of *Escherichia coli* at pH 7.2 for the detection of sulfonamides (74,75). The modified version adopted by the European Community for screening carcasses is based on three plates with *Bacillus subtilis* BGA at pH values of 6.0, 8.0, and 7.2 with added trimethoprim, respectively, and a fourth plate with *Micrococcus luteus* NCTC 8340 at pH 8.0 (74). This test as described elsewhere (76) is intended to detect residues of β-lactams, tetracyclines, aminoglycosides, sulfonamides, and macrolides in muscle tissue of slaughtered animals, without any prior extraction or cleanup.

In the four-plate test, the sample is applied in the form of a sliced deep-frozen tissue disk directly on each of the four plates, and incubation is carried out at 30°C for 18–24 h. The test is sensitive and reasonably easy to standardize but it is time-consuming and thus rather expensive. Its performance has been found to be affected, at least in part, by the composition and the properties of the test medium, and the nature of antibiotics being tested (77–80).

However, recent investigations on the effect of the tissue matrix on the detection limits attained by this test have indicated that ceftiofur, sulfonamides, streptomycin, and some macrolide antibiotics cannot be detected in intact meat with the plates and the bacterial strains prescribed in the European four-plate test (81, 82). Two plates of this system were not found suitable for screening sulfamethazine or streptomycin at levels far above the MRL; the third plate detected tetracyclines and β-lactams up to the MRL levels; whereas the fourth was sensitive to β-lactams and some but not all macrolides. Detection, on the other hand, of the fluoroquinolones enrofloxacin and ciprofloxacin could only be made possible by an additional *Escherichia coli* plate not included in the four-plate test.

Another test that has been adapted by the Center for Veterinary Drug Residues, Saskatoon, Canada, to screen muscle samples from imported carcasses is the cube inhibition test (CIT) (83). Tissue preparation is similar to that in the German three-plate test in that tissue cubes are placed on seeded media. The organism is *Bacillus subtilis,* two different agar plates are used, and incubation is carried out at 37°C for 18–24 h.

The Delvotest-P test (84), which was originally designed for rapid detection of penicillins in milk, has also been successfully employed for the detection of oxytetracycline residues in chicken tissues. In this method samples of liver, kidney, and muscle tissue are homogenized with distilled water, and the homogenates are analyzed with the Delvotest as earlier described. The method provides results in 3 h, it is easy to perform, and has a detection limit of 0.62 ppb.

A similar fast color-change test, adapted to screen antibacterials in meat, is the BR-test (85) which has not been widely used by the meat industry until now. A version of this test, the BR AS test, which detects with limited sensitivity residues of antibiotics and sulfonamides, has been also employed to screen eggs for general inhibition. In this test, egg samples are homogenized, combined with Bacto-FA buffer, mixed thoroughly and inactivated at 71–72°C for 20 min. An aliquot of the sample is then analyzed using the BR AS test. If a sample is found to be positive, it is reanalyzed with the addition of the antifolate para-aminobenzoic acid for canceling the bactericide effect of sulfonamides. If the sample still remains positive, the inhibitor is not a sulfonamide. The test works well with normal eggs but it is not applicable to dried albumen or to powdered egg mix containing salt or sugar.

For very rapid on-farm screening of antibiotic residues in animal tissues, the swab test on premises (STOP) has been widely employed (86). This test involves inserting a cotton swab directly into meat tissues, allowing it to absorb tissue fluids. The swab is the removed and placed on a test plate to be incubated with *Bacillus subtilis* ATCC 6633 spores at 29°C overnight for evidence of inhibition around the swab.

Detectable concentrations of various antibacterials in animal tissues by different microbiological tests are presented in Table 27.4. Although the microbiological tests mentioned are generally well suited for screening edible animal products, they cannot cover all needs of a regulatory residues program. For example, some antibiotics, such as chloramphenicol, cannot be readily traced in meat because 6 h after administration of the antibiotic, kidney and liver, the usual target organs, no longer contain detectable amounts of the drug. Since chloramphenicol spreads all over the body as an inactive glucuronide and is constantly eliminated in the urine, a delay in sampling may result in consumption of a carcass for which the residue status may not actually be known.

To overcome this problem, an agar diffusion test has been developed to detect chloramphenicol residues in the urine of slaughtered animals (87). The principle of the test is based upon incorporation of β-glucuronidase in an agar medium shown with *Bacillus subtilis*. With this test, the glucuronide of chloramphenicol, which is the major metabolite in urine, is hydrolyzed and the antibacterial activity is demonstrated according to the usual microbiological detection assays.

In addition, a number of other assays have been developed for screening antibiotic residues in body fluids of animals at slaughter. They include an agar plate assay for detecting tilmicosin in bovine serum (88), modified CFT and BR-test assays for screening penicillin G residues in plasma of healthy steers (89), a modified CFT for screening plasma and urine samples from healthy market

TABLE 27.4 Detectable Concentrations (ppm) of Various Antibacterials in Tissues by Different Microbiological Tests

Antibacterial	German three-plate test	EEC four-plate test	CHARM II test	New Dutch kidney test	STOP	CAST	FAST	CHARM farm test	ATP test
Ampicillin	0.01	0.01	0.04	0.025	0.01	0.1	—	0.008	0.08
Bacitracin	250.0	2.5	—	—	100.0	0.5	—	—	—
Chloramphenicol	1.0	1.0	—	5.0	0.5	0.5	—	—	4.0
Chlortetracycline	0.005	—	0.1	0.25	0.01	0.05	0.3	0.3	—
Colistin	10.0	50.0	—	500.0	50.0	10.0	—	—	—
Erythromycin	0.025	0.05	0.4	0.5	0.1	0.1	0.05	0.3	1.0
Gentamicin	0.1	0.5	0.4	10.0	0.01	0.1	0.05	0.25	5.0
Kanamycin	0.1	50.0	—	25.0	0.025	0.05	—	—	12.5
Neomycin	0.1	0.5	0.8	50.0	0.1	0.1	0.1	0.3	10.0
Oleandomycin	0.1	—	—	10.0	0.25	0.5	—	—	—
Oxytetracycline	0.05	—	0.5	1.0	0.1	0.1	0.7	0.3	0.3
Penicillin	0.025	—	0.02	0.025	0.01	0.1	0.1	0.005	0.06
Spiramycin	0.25	0.1	—	100.0	0.5	1.0	—	—	12.5
Streptomycin	0.1	—	0.15	50.0	0.025	0.5	1.0	1.5	25.0
Sulfadimethoxine	0.1	—	0.01	0.05	10.0	0.1	4.0	0.06	0.15
Sulfaguanidine	2.5	—	—	10.0	—	2.5	—	—	—
Sulfamethazine	0.05	—	0.025	0.5	50.0	0.25	3.0	0.1	—
Tetracycline	0.05	—	0.05	1.0	0.05	0.1	0.7	0.2	—

Source: From Refs. 43, 73, 151.

pigs (70), and a disc assay for detecting antibiotics in urine from livestock (90). The live animal swab test (LAST) has been also described (91, 92) for screening urine from live animals, but its performance is easily affected by the pH of the substrate (93); a high percentage of false-positive results was observed when LAST was used to screen urine from cull dairy cows (91).

Since the highest residue concentration in animal carcasses is generally found in kidney, a variety of rapid prescreening tests have been also developed to facilitate selection of slaughtered animals suspected of antimicrobial residues as soon as possible. Most of these test use the urine present in the renal pelvis as a matrix, because only aminoglycosides preferentially occur in the renal cortex (94–96). A disadvantage is that the high level of residues in the urine is not always related to the residue status of the carcass meat; it may be higher in urine by a factor varying between 10 and 1000. Particularly in diseased animals, no correlation can be established between muscle and kidney or urine concentrations. Therefore, any final judgment of the residue status of the carcass meat should be based on additional muscle tests performed with suitable methods.

The calf antibiotic and sulfa test (CAST), the fast antimicrobial screen test (FAST), and the swab test on premises (STOP) are all bacterial inhibition tests developed at the US Department of Agriculture Food Safety and Inspection Services to screen kidneys for antimicrobial drug residues at slaughter (97–101). For CAST and FAST, an incision is made with a knife, whereas for STOP the tissue is macerated with the shaft of the swab. For all three tests, cotton swabs are inserted into kidney tissue to soak up fluids. Swabs are then incubated on inoculated medium with a disc containing an antibiotic standard used to monitor the viability of the organism and its growth inhibition.

The CAST uses *Bacillus megatherium* and a 16–24 h incubation at 44–45°C, whereas STOP employs *Bacillus subtilis* and a 16–24 h incubation at 27–29°C. A zone of inhibition around the swab suggests the presence of a microbial inhibitor in the sample. In the US, bob veal calf carcasses are condemned on the basis of a positive CAST without further confirmation. For FAST, the organism and temperature are the same as those for the CAST, but the CAST medium is supplemented with dextrose and bromocresol purple. The faster growth rate of bacteria with FAST, allows reduction of minimum incubation from 16 to 6 h.

All three tests lack the sensitivity to detect chloramphenicol and sulfa drugs. The CAST is more sensitive to sulfa drugs than STOP but lacks the sensitivity to enforce an MRL of 100 ppb. CAST and FAST are less rugged than STOP, requiring a higher temperature and more precise temperature control. The advantages of FAST compared with CAST are minimal, unless the slaughter plant is running two shifts per day (71).

Another kidney prescreening procedure or emergency slaughtered animals is the *Sarcina lutea* kidney test (102), which has been in use in Netherlands since

1973. In this test, an incision is made in sample kidneys into which paper discs are inserted and left for 30–60 min. The moistened discs are placed on agar plates seeded with *Sarcina lutea* ATCC 9341. The test is highly sensitive for penicillin but shows moderate sensitivity to sulfonamides, tetracyclines, macrolides, and aminoglycosides (103). It is insensitive to chloramphenicol (104).

In April 1988, the new kidney Dutch test (NKDT) replaced the *Micrococcus* (formerly *Sarcina*) *luteus* kidney test. The NKDT is an one-plate test based on examination of the urine present in the renal pelvis by means of paper discs inserted in the renal pelvis (104). The test organism is *Bacillus subtilis* BGA and incubation is performed for 13–18 h at 37°C. The kidney is incised, and four paper discs are inserted and left there for 30 min. Two paper disks are placed diagonally on the surface of the test plate, and three control disks containing 0.5 μg oxytetracycline, 0.05 μg sulfamethazine, and 0.5 μg tylosin are also placed in the middle of the plate. If both sample inhibition diameters are equal to or higher than 20 mm, the whole carcass is condemned.

The NKDT test is sensitive to residues of β-lactams, tetracyclines, and macrolides. It is more sensitive to sulfonamides than the German three-plate test or the EU four-plate test, but it is relatively insensitive to aminoglycosides. With respect to MRLs set for liver or kidney, the NKDT is too insensitive for aminogly-cosides, sulfonamides, and macrolides. One analyst can complete 150–200 tests per day. Due to the high ratio of residue levels in preurine and muscle, a negative result of this test implies that residue levels in muscle are below the limit of detection.

A one-plate screening assay is also the official test used in Belgium for monitoring antimicrobial residues in kidney and muscle tissues of slaughtered animals. This test is based on the growth inhibition of *Bacillus subtilis* at pH 7 in an agar medium containing trimethoprim for better detection of sulfonamides (105). In addition, β-glucuronidase is added to the samples to enable the detection of chloramphenicol residues.

A rapid test based on ATP/bioluminescence (106) is also available for kidney prescreening. In this test, a paper filter disc is inserted for 30 min into the renal pelvis of the kidney sample. It is then transferred to a cuvette and incubated with a commercially available test culture *Bacillus subtilis* BGA at 40°C for 3 h in presence of trimethoprim. The amount of ATP is estimated on the basis of the light released after addition of luciferin/luciferinase reagent. In a variation of this test (107), small cubes of kidney tissue are excised and frozen to be placed directly upon four agar plates, each seeded with a different microorganism. The plates are refrigerated for approximately 4 h, and then are incubated overnight at 37°C.

To determine the group of compounds or specific compounds present in tissues of animals found positive by screening tests, a seven-plate test is often employed (108). This test is based on the susceptibility or resistance of four microorganisms against various drugs, including three strains of *Micrococcus luteus*. The test organism *Micrococcus luteus* ATCC 9341a is susceptible to penicillin and erythromycin but resistant to streptomycin. The test organisms *Micrococcus luteus* ATCC 9341 and 15957 are resistant to neomycin and streptomycin, respectively. *Staphylococcus epidermidis* is susceptible to neomycin but resistant to tetracycline. *Bacillus subtilis* is susceptible to streptomycin, and *Bacillus cereus* var. *mycoides* is susceptible to tetracycline. These drugs show characteristic patterns of results with these assays.

The presence of β-lactam antibiotics can be confirmed by digestion with Penase, a type I penicillinase, or with a β-lactamase (109). In the seven-plate assay, Penase is incorporated in all but one plate to differentiate β-lactam antibiotics from other types. However, β-lactams such as cloxacillin and the cephalosporins are resistant to degradation by Penase (110–112). Thus, they may not be identified as β-lactams by this procedure and are classified as unidentified microbial inhibitors. However, these Penase-resistant compounds can be degraded by other β-lactamases.

It has been recently reported (109) that use of both Penase and lactamase II hydrolysis and screening assays prior to chromatographic analysis can tentatively classify β-lactams into three subgroups: the first group includes a ceftiofur metabolite represented by desfuroyl-ceftiofur-cysteine; the second, cephapirin; and the third, penicillin G, ampicillin, amoxicillin, and cloxacillin. In this approach, portions of aqueous extracts of tissues are treated separately with Penase and lactamase II, and results are compared with those of untreated samples and positive controls. Bioactive ceftiofur metabolites are present, provided that the extracts retain inhibitory activity after Penase treatment but lose activity after lactamase II treatment and are positive in response to the immunochemical Lac-Tek-Cef test but negative to the Lac-Tek-B1 test (113). This approach can eliminate a large number of negative samples and, therefore, increases the efficiency of the assay.

27.2.3   Fish Analysis

Several microbiological methods have been reported for analyzing residues within the groups of sulfonamides, tetracyclines, macrolides, and β-lactams in fish tissues; however, references for these groups of compounds are limited to sulfadiazine and trimethoprim, oxytetracycline and chlortetracycline, erythromycin, and ampicillin, respectively.

Initial studies on sulfonamides (114) were limited to qualitative assessment of the occurrence of sulfamerazine residues in muscle and interior organs of rainbow trout using *Sarcina lutea* (ATCC 9341) and *Staphylococcus aureus* (ATCC 6538P) as test organisms. The method involved application of fish fluids to discs placed on the agar, or direct application of core samples of tissue to the agar plate.

Later studies concerned the detection of both sulfonamides and sulfonamide potentiators in fish tissues. Mixtures containing ethyl acetate, sodium sulfate, and sodium hydroxide (80), or ethyl acetate and sodium hydroxide (115), have been all used for extracting residues of sulfadiazine and trimethoprim from trout and salmon tissues. In the former approach, para-aminobenzoic acid was employed to neutralize sulfadiazine prior to the microbiological assay of trimethoprim, whereas in the latter approach *Bacillus subtilis* (ATCC) was directly used for sulfadiazine detection. The limit of detection for sulfadiazine using *Bacillus subtilis* was found to be 0.04 ppm. The test indicator organism used in both approaches to detect trimethoprim down to 0.1 ppm was *Bacillus pumilus* (CN60 Welcome Research Laboratories, London) (115,116).

For detection of oxytetracycline residues in serum and tissue samples of various trout species, plate diffusion methods with *Bacillus cereus* var. *mycoides* (ATSS 11778) (115,117) or *Bacillus subtilis* (ACTC 6633) (118) as the test organisms have been employed. Using *Bacillus cereus,* the limit of detection for muscle tissue was found to be 0.25 ppm. *Bacillus cereus* has been also successfully employed in a disc assay for the quantification of residues of oxytetracycline in serum of adult sockeye salmon (119). With this method, linear standard curves over a concentration range of 0.07–2.24 ppm oxytetracycline could be established. In addition, a cylinder diffusion assay has been used for determining oxytetracycline residues in young rainbow trout (120). Extraction of oxytetracycline from muscle tissues was performed using a mixture of methanol and hydrochloric acid at a ratio of 98/2. Tissue extracts were reconstituted in a phosphate buffer of pH 4.5 and diffused through a pH-6 agar seeded with *Bacillus cereus* for 3 h at room temperature; incubation was carried out overnight at 30°C.

Most sensitive and specific determination of tetracyclines in fish has been offered, however, by a hybrid analytical procedure that couples bacterial growth inhibition with the separating power of a chromatographic technique (121). Paper chromatography followed by bioautography with *Bacillus cereus* var. *mycoides* as the test organism, could efficiently separate oxytetracycline and chlortetracycline, thus offering the possibility to identify specifically the type of tetracycline that contributed to the bacterial growth inhibition in muscle samples derived from cod, haddock, and flounder. Other antibiotics potentially present did not interfere with the assay because neomycin, streptomycin, kanamycin, and penicillin G either were not recovered in the tissue extract or were inactivated by the butanol that participated in the mobile phase solvent. The migration, on the other hand, of other antibiotics such as erythromycin and chloramphenicol during the chromatographic development differed from that of the tetracyclines.

Microbiological methods reported for detection of erythromycin in fish are based either on a cylinder plate assay using *Sarcina lutea* (ATCC 9341) (122), or on the swab test on premises (STOP) that uses *Bacillus subtilis* (ACTC 6633) as the test organism (123). However, both of these methods lack specificity and sensitivity; they cannot differentiate between different antimicrobials. An alternative approach that can provide higher sensitivity and is relatively less prone to interference is TLC followed by bioautography (124). Using this approach, erythromycin was detected in nonsalmonid tissue down to 0.08 ppm completely separated from other antibiotics.

Ampicillin residues in cultured fish muscle have been detected by a disk diffusion assay using *Bacillus stearothermophilus* (ATCC 10149) as the test organism (125). In this method, fish sample was homogenized with phosphate buffer, pH 6.0, and centrifuged. The supernate was heated at 82°C for 2 min, and *analyzed* according to the AOAC assay including the confirmatory β-lactamase step. Recoveries of ampicillin ranged from 99 to 104%, whereas the limit of determination was 0.025–1.00 μg/g. This method has also been successfully applied for the determination of amoxicillin residues in catfish muscle (126).

REFERENCES

1.   G. Suhren, and W. Heeschen, Nahrung, 40:1 (1996).
2.   J.M. Hawronsky, M.R. Adams, and A.L. Kyriakides, J. Soc. Dairy Technol., 46: 31 (1993).
3.   H.C. Chen, and T.C. Chang, J. Dairy Sci., 77:1515 (1994).
4.   L.A. Ouderkirk, J. Assoc. Off. Anal. Chem., 62:985 (1979).
5.   J.R. Bishop, and C.H. White, J. Food Prot., 47:647 (1984).
6.   A.E.M. Vermunt, J. Stadhouders, G.F.M. Loeffen, and R. Baker, Neth. Milk Dairy J., 47:31 (1993).
7.   J.J. Gavin, Appl. Microbiol., 5:25 (1956).
8.   F.V. Thompson, Acta Pathol. Microbiol. Scand., 61:303 (1964).
9.   W.W. Wright, J. Assoc. Off. Anal. Chem., 53:219 (1970).
10. F.F. Busta, J. Dairy Sci., 49:751 (1966).
11. A. Carlsson, L. Bjorck, and K. Persson, J. Dairy Sci., 72:3166 (1989).
12. J.S. Cullor, Vet. Clin. North Am. Food Anim. Pract., 9:609 (1993).
13. L.W. Halbert, R.J. Erskine, P.C. Bartlett, and G.L. Johnson, J. Food Prot., 59:886 (1996).
14. H. Korkeala, O. Sorvettula, O. Maki-Petays, and J. Hirn, Meat Sci., 9:291 (1983).
15. F.V. Kosikowsky, J. Dairy Sci., 46:96 (1963).
16. R. Smither, J. Appl. Bacteriol., 45:267 (1978).
17. J.W. Tyler, J.S. Cullor, R.J. Erskine, W.L. Smith, J. Dellinger, and K. McClure, J. Am. Vet. Med. Assoc., 201:1378 (1992).
18. J.M. Booth, In. Pract., 4:100 (1982).
19. S.E. Charm and C.K. Ruey, J. Assoc. Off. Anal. Chem., 65:1186 (1982).
20. S.E. Charm and R. Chi, J. Assoc. Off. Anal. Chem., 71:304 (1988).
21. J.W. Messer, J.E. Leslie, G.A. Houghtby, J.T. Peeler, and J.E. Barnett, J. Assoc. Off. Anal. Chem., 65:1208 (1982).

22. G. Suhren and W. Heeschen, Milchwissenschaft, 42:493 (1987).
23. D.L. Collins-Thompson, D.S. Wood, and I.Q. Thompson, J. Food Prot., 51:632 (1988).
24. A. Carlsson and L. Bjorck, Milchwissenschaft, 44:7 (1989).
25. L.E. Bryan and H.M. van den Elzen, Antimicrob. Agents Chemother., 12:163 (1977).
26. G. Suhren and W. Heeschen, Dtsch. Molkerei-Ztg., 48:1566 (1987).
27. G.O. Korsrud, C.D.C. Salisbury, A.C.E. Fesser, and J.D. MacNeil, in Analysis of Antibiotic/Drug Residues in Food Products of Animal Origin (V. K. Agarwal, Ed.), Plenum Press, New York, p. 75 (1992).
28. S.A. Thorogood, and A. Ray, J. Soc. Dairy Technol., 37:38 (1984).
29. A.H. Knight, N. Shapton, and G.A. Prentice, J. Soc. Dairy Technol., 40:30 (1987).
30. G. Suhren, J. Reichmuth, and H.G. Walte, 51:269 (1996).
31. G. Suhren, J. Reichmuth, and W. Heeschen, Milch. Dtsch. Milchwirtschaft, 26:812 (1991).
32. G. Suhren, Bull. Int. Dairy Fed., 283:15 (1993).
33. International Dairy Federation, Bull. Int. Dairy Fed., 220 (1987).
34. International Dairy Federation, Bull. Int. Dairy Fed., 258 (1991).
35. International Dairy Federation, Bull. Int. Dairy Fed., 283 (1993).
36. J. Kraack and A. Tolle, Milchwissenschaft, 22:669 (1967).
37. A. Ebrecht, Dtsch. Milchwissenschaft, 36:14 (1985).
38. F.J. Muller, Dtsch. Milchwissenschaft, 41:15 (1990).
39. F.J. Muller and A. Jones, Bull. Int. Dairy Fed., 283:24 (1993).
40. A.P. Schifmann, M. Schutz, and H.U. Wiesner, Milchwirtschaft, 47,770 (1992).
41. G.G. Carter, National Center for Antibiotic and Insulin Analysis, Food and Drug Administration, Washington, D.C. (1974).
42. D.C. Westhoff and T. Engler, J. Milk Food Technol., 38:537 (1975).
43. F.K. Stekelenburg, in Residues of Veterinary Drugs in Food, Proc. Euroresidue II Conf., Veldhoven, May 3–5, 1993 (N. Haagsma, A. Ruiter and P.B. Czedik-Eysenberg, Eds.), Fac. Vet. Med., Univ. Utrecht, The Netherlands, p. 650 (1993).
44. P.E. Stanley, J. Biolum. and Chemilum., 4:375 (1989).
45. K. Fleischmann, Deut. Mokeri-Ztg., 75:534 (1954).
46. A.D. Adamse, Neth. Milk Dairy J., 9:121 (1955).
47. J.L. Van Os, S.A. Lameris, J. Doodewaard, and J.G. Oostendorn, Neth. Milk Dairy J., 29:16 (1975).
48. A.E.M. Vermunt, J. Stadhoulders, G.J.M. Loeffen, and R. Bakker, Neth. Milk Dairy J., 47:31 (1993).
49. G. Suhren and R. Beukers, J. AOAC Int., 81:978 (1998).
50. J.L. Van Os, S.A. Lameris, J. Doodewaard, and J.G. Oostendorn, J. Food Prot., 43:510 (1980).
51. W.N. Kelley, J. Assoc. Off. Anal. Chem., 65:1193 (1982).
52. M. Mitchell, B. Bodkin, and J. Martin, J. Food Prot., 58:577 (1995).
53. C. Bell, J.R. Rhoades, P. Neaves, and D. Scannella, Neth. Milk Dairy J., 49:15 (1995).
54. E.M. Rutczynska-Skonieczna and M. Nikonorow, Mitt. Lebensm. Unters. Hyg., 31:377 (1966).

55. M. van Schothorst, in Residuen van Antibiotica in Slachtdieren, Thesis, University of Utrecht, The Netherlands (1969).
56. H. Mol, in Antibiotic and Milk, Thesis, University of Utrecht, The Netherlands (1975).
57. R.T. Igarashi, R.W. Boughman, F.E. Nelson, and P.A. Hartman, J. Milk Food Tech., 4:143 (1961).
58. Th.E. Galesloot and F. Hassing, Ned. Melk Zuivel Tijdschr., 16:89 (1962).
59. G. Suhren and W. Heeschen, in Residues of Veterinary Drugs in Food, Proc. Euroresidue Conf., Noordwijkerhout, May 21–23, 1990 (N. Haagsma, A. Ruiter, and P.B. Czedik-Eysenberg, Eds.), Fac. Vet. Med., Univ. Utrecht, The Netherlands, p. 351 (1990).
60. W.W. Wright, J. Assoc. Off. Anal. Chem., 53:219 (1970).
61. G. Loftsgaard, E.J. Briskey, and C. Olson, Am. J. Vet. Res., 28:167 (1967).
62. B. Moreno, A. Calles, and V. Diez, J. Food Prot., 43:558 (1980).
63. L.A. Ouederkirk, J. Assoc. Off. Anal. Chem., 59:112 (1976).
64. S.E. Katz, in Agricultural Uses of Antibiotics (W.A. Moats, Ed.), ACS Symposium series 320, American Chemical Society, Washington, DC, p. 142 (1986).
65. G. Schelhaas, Fortschr. Veter. Med., 20:272 (1974).
66. G. Anhalt, S. Wenzel, and P. Conrad, Arch. Lebensmittelhyg., 27:201 (1976).
67. M. Yoshida, D. Kubota, S. Yonezawa, H. Nogawa, H. Yoshimura, and O. Ito, Jpn. Poult. Sci., 13:129 (1976).
68. W.E. Meredith, H.H. Weiser, and A.R. Winter, Appl. Microbiol., 1:86 (1965).
69. G.O. Korsrud, M.G. Papich, A.C.E. Fesser, C.D.C. Salisbury, and J.D. MacNeil, J. Food Prot., 58:1129 (1995).
70. G.O. Korsrud, M.G. Papich, A.C.E. Fesser, C.D.C. Salisbury, and J.D. MacNeil, J. Food Prot., 59:161 (1996).
71. G.O. Korsrud, J.O. Boison, J.F.M. Nouws, and J.D. MacNeil, J. AOAC Int., 81: 21 (1998).
72. A. AB, Z. Lebens. Unters. Forsch., 155/156:6 (1974).
73. G. Schramm. L. Ellerbroek, E. Weise, and G. Reuter, in Residues of Veterinary Drugs in Food, Proc. Euroresidue II Conf., Veldhoven, May 3–5, 1993 (N. Haagsma, A. Ruiter, and P.B. Czedik-Eysenberg, Eds.), Fac. Vet. Med., Univ. Utrecht, The Netherlands, p. 632 (1993).
74. R. Bogaerts and F. Wolf, Fleischwirtschaft, 60:672 (1980).
75. M. van Schothorst, and G. Peelen-Knol, J. Vet. Sci., 3:85 (1970).
76. R.J. Heitzman, in Veterinary Drug Residues—Residues in Food-producing Animals and their Products: Reference Materials and Methods (R.J. Heitzman, Ed.), Blackwell Scientific Publications, Oxford, p. Sg3/1–8 (1994).
77. M.L. Bates, D.G. Lindsay, and D.H. Watson, J. Appl. Bacteriol., 55:495 (1983).
78. G.O. Korsrud, J.O. Boison, J.F.M. Nouws, and J.D. MacNeil, J. AOAC Int., 81: 21 (1998).
79. L. Ellerbroek, C. Schwartz, G. Hildebrandt, E. Weise, E.-M. Bernoth, H.-J. Pluta, and G. Arndt, Arch. Lebensmittelhyg., 48:3 (1997).
80. L. Ellerbroek, Arch. Lebensmittelhyg., 49:7 (1998).
81. L. Okerman, K. de Wasch, and J. van Hoof, Analyst, 123:2361 (1998).

82. L. Okerman, J. van Hoof, and W. Debeuckelaere, J. AOAC Int., 81:51 (1998).

83. C.D.C. Salisbury, C.E. Rigby, and W. Chan, J. Agric. Food Chem., 37:105 (1989).

84. K. Bugyei, W. Black, S. Mcewen, and A.H. Meek, J. Food Prot., 57:141 (1994).

85. D.N. Loyd and D. van der Merwe, J. S. Afr Vet Assoc., 183:35 (1987).

86. R.W. Johnston, R.H. Reamer, E.W. Harris, H.G. Fugate, and B. Schwab, J. Food Prot., 44:828 (1981).

87. R. Bogaerts, D. de Vos, and J.-M. Degroodt, Fleischwirtsch., 64:185 (1984).

88. M.R. Coleman, J.S. Peloso, and J.W. Moran, J. AOAC Int., 78:659 (1995).

89. J.O. Boison, G.O. Korsrud, M.G. Papich, and J.D. MacNeil, J. AOAC Int., 78:1144 (1995).

90. W.G. Huber, M.B. Carlson, and M.H. Lepper, J. Am. Vet. Med. Assoc., 154:1590 (1969).

91. J.P. Tritschler, R.T. Duby, S.P. Oliver, and R.W. Prange, J. Food Prot., 50:97 (1987).

92. Handbook No. 601, How to Perform the Live Animal Swab Test for Antibiotic Residues, United States Department of Agriculture, Food Safety and Inspection Service, Washington, DC (1984).

93. T.N. TerHune and D.W. Upson, J. Am. Vet. Med. Assoc., 194:918 (1989).

94. J.F.M. Nouws, N.J.G. Broex, J.M.P. Hartog, F. Driessens, and W.M.D. Driessen-van Lankveld, Tijdschr. Diergeneeskd., 113:247 (1988).

95. N.J.G. Broex, J.M.P. Hartog, and J.F.M. Nouws, Tijdschr. Diergeneeskd., 113:254 (1988).

96. R. Bogaerts and F.A. Wolf, Fleischwirtschaft, 60:672 (1980).

97. R.W. Johnston, R.H. Reamer, E.W. Harris, H.C. Fugate, and B. Schwab, J. Food Prot., 44:828 (1981).

98. S.A. Bright, S.L. Nickerson, and N.H. Thaker, Poster presented at the Association of Official Analytical Chemists's Annual Meeting, St. Louis, MO (1989).

99. J.D. MacNeil and R.L. Ellis, in Chemical Analysis for Antibiotics Used in Agriculture (H. Oka, H. Nakazawa, K. Harada, and J.D. MacNeil, Eds.), AOAC International, Arlington, VA, p. 1 (1995).

100. Technical Report, Performing the Calf Antibiotic and Sulfa Test, United States Department of Agriculture, Food Safety and Inspection Service, Washington, DC (1984).

101. Food Safety Update, J. Am. Vet. Med. Assoc., 200:886 (1992).

102. M. van Schothorst and G. Peelen-Knol, Neth. J. Vet. Sci., 3:85 (1970).

103. J.F.M. Nouws and G. Ziv, Arch. Lebensmittelhyg., 30:197 (1979).

104. J.F.M. Nouws, Arch. Lebensmittelhyg., 32:97 (1981).

105. K. Koenendierick, L. Okerman, L. Dezutter, J.M. Degroodt, J. Van Hoof, and S. Srebrnik, Food Addit. Contam., 12:77 (1995).

106. F.K. Stekelenburg, in Residues of Veterinary Drugs in Food, Proc. Euroresidue II Conf., Veldhoven, May 3–5, 1993 (N. Haagsma, A. Ruiter, and P.B. Czedik-Eysenberg, Eds.), Fac. Vet. Med., Univ. Utrecht, The Netherlands, p 650 (1993).

107. J. Takacs and S. Kovaes, Acta Vet. Acad. Sci. Hung., 19:11 (1969).

108. H.G. Fugate, Microbiology Laboratory Guidebook, FSIS, USDA, Sec. 6 (1974).

109. M.B. Medina, D.J. Poole, and M.R. Anderson, J. AOAC Int., 81:963 (1998).

110. V.W. Gedek and C. Baath, Arch. Lebensmittelhyg., 27:170 (1976).
111. D.J. Fletouris, J.E. Psomas, and A.J. Mantis, J. Agric. Food Chem., 40:617 (1992).
112. W.A. Moats, J. AOAC Int., 76:535 (1993).
113. W.A. Moats, R.D. Romanowski, and M.B. Medina, J. AOAC Int., 81:1135 (1998).
114. L. Silven, N. Johansson, and O. Lyngberg, Bull. Off. Int. Epizoot., 69:1465 (1968).
115. R. Salte and K. Liestol, Acta Vet Scand., 21:18 (1980).
116. D.H. McCarthy, J.P. Stevenson, and A.W. Salisbury, Aquaculture, 4:299 (1974).
117. R.I. Herman, D. Collis, and T.I. Bullock, Bur. Sports. Fish Wildl., 37:3 (1969).
118. J.I. Grondel, J.F.M. Nouws, A.R. Schutte, and F. Driessens, J. Vet. Pharmacol. Ther., 12:157 (1989).
119. G.A. Strasdine and J.R. McBride, J. Fish Biol., 15:135 (1979).
120. A. McCracken, S. Fidgeon, J.J. O'Brien, and D. Anderson, J. Appl. Bacteriol., 40: 61 (1976).
121. J. Blackely, J. Kramer, and G.B. Selzer, J. Assoc. Off. Anal. Chem., 52:935 (1969).
122. D.C. Grove and W.A. Randall, in Assay Methods of Antibiotics (D.C. Grove, and W.A. Randall, Eds.), Medical Encyclopedia, New York (1955).
123. R.W. Johnston, R.M. Reamer, E.W. Harris, H.E. Fugate, and B. Schwab, J. Food Prot., 44:828 (1981).
124. E. Neidert, P.W. Saschenbrecker, and F. Tittiger, J. Assoc. Off. Anal. Chem., 70: 197 (1987).
125. S.M. Plakas, A. De Paola, and M. Moxey, J. Assoc. Off. Anal. Chem., 74:910 (1991).
126. C.Y.W. Ang, W. Luo, C.R. Kiessling, K. McKim, R. Lochmann, C.C. Walker, and H.C. Thompson, Jr, J. AOAC Int., 81:33 (1998).
127. J. Palmer and F. Kosikowski, J. Dairy Sci., 50:1390 (1967).
128. R. Fonden, L. Adler, L. Jonesson, and S. Lindwall, International Dairy Federation Congress XXI, Moscow, Vol. 1, Book 1, p. 170 (1982).
129. J.C. Bruhn, R.E. Ginn, J.W. Messer, and E.M. Mikolajcik, In Standard Methods for the Examination of Dairy Products (G. A. Richardson, ed.), 15th Edition, American Public Health Association, Washington, D.C., p. 265 (1985).
130. J.L. van Os and R. Beukers, J. Food Prot., 43:510 (1980).
131. A. Mayra-Makinen, Bull. Int. Dairy Fed., 283:29 (1993).
132. J. Kramer, G.G. Carter, B. Arret, J. Wilner, W.W. Wright, and A. Kirshbaum, Antibiotic Residues in Milk, Dairy Products, and Animal Tissues: Methods, Reports, and Protocols, Food and Drug Administration, Government Printing Office, Washington, D.C., Item 344–837 (4008) (1968).
133. J. Okada, I. Higuchi, S. Kondo, and B.-I. Saito, J. Assoc. Off. Anal. Chem., 71: 337 (1988).
134. G.A. Korsrud, J.M. Naylor, C.D. Salisbury, and J.D. MacNeil, J. Agric. Food Chem., 35:556 (1987).
135. C.J. Singer and S.E. Katz, J. Assoc. Off. Anal. Chem., 68:1037 (1985).
136. K.O. Honikel, U. Schmidt, W. Woltersdorf, and L. Leistner, J. Assoc. Off. Anal. Chem., 61:1222 (1978).
137. M. Hamm, A. Ebrecht, and S. Wenzel, Arch. Lebensmittelhyg., 41:109 (1990).
138. I. Samaha, A. Ebrecht, L. Ellerbroek, S. Matthes, and S. Wenzel, Arch. Lebensmittelhyg., 42:37 (1991).

139. L. Ellerbroek, in Residues of Veterinary Drugs in Food, Proc. Euroresidue II Conf., Veldhoven, May 3–5, 1993 (N. Haagsma, A. Ruiter, and P.B. Czedik-Eysenberg, Eds.), Fac. Vet. Med., Univ. Utrecht, The Netherlands, p. 280 (1993).

140. I. Samaha, L. Ellerbroek, A. Ebrecht, S. Matthes, and S. Wenzel, Arch. Lebensmittelhyg., 42:32 (1991).

141. S.E. Katz and P.R. Levine, J. Assoc. Off. Anal. Chem., 61:1103 (1978).

142. C. Pascal, C. Gaillard, and M. Moreau, J. Assoc. Off. Anal. Chem., 62:976 (1979).

143. L.A. Roth, S. Kwan, and P. Sporns, J. Food Prot., 49:436 (1986).

144. W.A. Moats, E.W. Harris, and N.C. Steele, J. Agric. Food Chem., 34:452 (1986).

145. S.E. Katz, C.A. Fassbender, A. Depaolis, and J.D. Rosen, J. Assoc. Off. Anal. Chem., 61:564 (1978).

146. H. Pedersen, in Royal Veterinary and Agricultural College Yearbook, Copenhagen, Denmark, p. 33 (1965).

147. J.M. Inglis and S.E. Katz, J. Assoc. Off. Anal. Chem., 61:1098 (1978).

148. M. Zavanella, P. Aureli, and A.M. Ferrini, Arch. Lebensmittelhyg., 37:118 (1986).

149. M. Bielecka, J.D. Baldock, and A.W. Kotula, J. Food Prot., 44:194 (1981).

150. R. Smither, J. Appl. Bact., 38:235 (1975).

151. S.E. Charm, in Analysis of Antibiotic/Drug Residues in Food Products of Animal Origin (V.K. Agarwal, Ed.), Plenum Press, New York, p. 31 (1992).

28

Immunochemical Methods

Immunochemical methods provide a powerful tool in the field of drug residue analysis. The exquisite specificity that can be obtained with immunochemical reagents provides new analytical opportunities that were previously not possible with classic analytical methods and can greatly reduce the amount of sample cleanup required prior to analysis.

Immunoassays were first developed around 1960 primarily for use in the field of clinical chemistry (1). Their application in food analysis has lagged due to a general lack of familiarity with the principles of immunology. These assays are based on the primary antibody–antigen binding reaction to identify specific analytes. Antigens are substances that cause a defensive immune response when introduced into the host animal body. The ability of an antigen to stimulate an immune response is called immunogenicity, while its ability to combine with an antibody is called antigenicity.

Probably the most important parameter of any immunochemical assay is the specificity of the antibody to the analyte, which is largely determined by the immunogen introduced into the host animal to elicit antibody formation. Antibodies have a specificity to the antigen comparable to that exhibited by enzymes to their substrate. Antibodies are proteins, specifically immunoglobulins, formed by the host animal in response to invasion by antigens. Immunoglobulins (Ig), can be classified into five groups: IgA, IgD, IgE, IgG, and IgM. The most common immunoglobulin capable of binding with antigens to inactivate them is IgG. Binding forces involved in the antibody–antigen reaction are weak molecular interactions like Coulomb and Van der Waals forces as well as hydrogen bonding and hydrophobic binding (2).

Essential elements of any immunochemical method are the antigens, antibodies, other chemicals used in visualizing the primary antibody–antigen reaction, and the format into which the reagents are placed to perform the assay. The antibody as a substance may have different stability and handling characteristics than a standard chemical reagent, but, if the singular attributes and liabilities of the antibody are understood, it should pose no greater problem of handling than any other delicate reagent. Understanding exactly what the antibody detects is a key issue in selecting the most appropriate immunochemical method for the intended application.

A wide variety of reagent and format configurations have been devised to simplify handling and visualization of the end point, with the different formats reflecting solutions to different end-user requirements.

28.1 ANTIGEN DEVELOPMENT

Characteristics of the target analyte such as molecular weight, three-dimensional structural complexity, and solubility properties all play an important role in the development or selection of useful antigens. Identifying exactly what the assay should and should not detect is another critical piece of information that needs to be taken into account in antigen development or selection.

Although molecules with molecular mass greater than 5000 da, such as proteins, glycoproteins, and carbohydrates, can readily elicit a potent antibody formation, molecules such as drugs that have low molecular masses cannot stimulate an immunogenic response. These molecules, widely known as haptens, will bind with preformed antibodies but will not cause antibodies to be produced.

To become immunogenic, a hapten has to be linked with a large molecule, such as a protein, prior to its introduction into the host animal. Several proteins can act as such carrier molecules including bovine serum albumin, human serum albumin, ovalbumin, thyroglobulin, poly-L-lysine, and hemocyanin. Among these proteins, bovine serum albumin is most commonly used because it is inexpensive, readily available, very soluble, highly immunogenic, and, in addition, resists denaturation (3).

Several types of reactions can be used to link a hapten to a carrier protein molecule. Functional groups on protein carriers that are used to form a suitable bond include the amino group of lysine, the free carboxyl of aspartate or glutamate, the imidazo group of histidine, the indole group of tryptophan, the sulfhydryl group of cysteine, and the guanidine group of arginine. Albumin provides approximately 60 free amino groups for linkage while thyroglobulin has about 400 sites available for binding (4).

Functional groups on haptens that are mostly used for linkage are the amino and carboxyl groups. As a result, the most common linkages are peptide bonds between a carboxyl and an amino group. Other groups that can be also used for coupling are the hydroxyl and carbonyl groups of ketone and aldehydes. If reactive groups are not present, haptens must be properly derivatized in order to create a site for attachment to the carrier protein. Use of structural analogues is another approach to the production of the hapten–carrier link. Commonly used coupling procedures include *N*-hydroxysuccinimide (5), carbodiimide (6), periodate (7), glutaraldehyde (8, 9), diazotization (10), and the mixed anhydride (11) reactions.

The chemistry and orientation used in attaching the hapten to the carrier molecule have a great impact on the specificity of the antibodies subsequently elicited. Specificity is lost to the region of the hapten molecule involved in the protein linkage because this is sterically shielded from interaction with the immune system. Therefore, the structure of an analyte should be carefully considered in order to design an appropriate antigen based upon the reactivity spectrum desired in the final assay.

The ratio of the hapten to the carrier molecules is also very important for the success of an immunochemical assay. Too few or too many hapten molecules linked to a carrier molecule will inevitably lead to poor immunogenicity. Desirable ratios of hapten to carrier molecules are in the range 10–100:1 (3).

Since many soluble antigens are rapidly metabolized and/or excreted and, therefore, can be cleared from the circulation by routes that usually bypass the lymph nodes and spleen, production of antibodies is rarely stimulated by these antigens unless adjuvants are used. Adjuvants are substances that provide a long-lasting antigen reservoir that releases antigen slowly into the body. In this way, macrophages become activated by the antigen and in turn stimulate lymphocytes (12, 13).

Most popular adjuvants are the incomplete and the complete forms of Freund. The incomplete adjuvant is a water-in-oil emulsion by which the antigen is slowly released, providing a long period of contact between antigen and immune system. The complete adjuvant contains heat-killed *Mycobacteria* that causes a local injury and granuloma formation, thus providing a nonspecific stimulus.

28.2 ANTIBODY DEVELOPMENT

A variety of approaches and choices should be considered in the process of antibody development. The target is to immunize host animals with a specific antigen carrying a number of antigenic determinants and to obtain antibodies that have the specificity and sensitivity required for the intended application. To accomplish this target, one must first decide whether to develop polyclonal or monoclonal antibodies.

Serum from immunized animals contains a large number of antibodies of varying isotype, affinity, and specificity, called polyclonal because they are products of different cell types. Different clones respond to different antigenic sites on the hapten to create a mixture of antibodies. Some of these antibodies will have a strong affinity for and bind readily to the selected antigen. Monoclonal antibodies, on the other hand, are derived from a single clone and produce a homogenous population of antibodies.

Although both polyclonal and monoclonal antibodies have been effectively used in immunochemical assays, only the latter can provide the high specificity required in some applications. Antibody specificity, on the other hand, is both a major advantage and disadvantage for immunochemical methods. It allows for highly selective detection of analytes but at the same time may complicate the development of multiresidue methods. Moreover, production of monoclonal antibodies requires special expertise and it is much more expensive than polyclonal antibodies. Thus, in cases where a range of analytes similar in molecular structure are required to be determined, a polyclonal may be more suitable than a monoclonal antibody.

The choice of the host animal into which the antigen is introduced is based on the amount of antisera and the type of antibodies required, species response to the introduced antigen, and genetic makeup of the animal. Polyclonal antibodies can be raised in many different animals; however rabbits, guinea pigs, sheep and goats are most frequently used. Use of sheep and goats enables larger quantities of sera to be rapidly collected with a minimum amount of pooling. These animals are often chosen for producing commercial quantities of polyclonal antibodies. If monoclonal antibodies are required, the host animals most commonly employed are mice.

The route of antigen administration depends on the nature of the antigen itself, the animal species, the use of an adjuvant, and the immunological response. When producing antisera from rabbits, subcutaneous and intradermal administration are the most popular routes. Intramuscular injections can be used in the presence of Freund adjuvants because this route provides rapid access to the lymphatic system. The intravenous route is used with particulate antigens because injection can produce a response, which, although rapid, is not sustained.

To elicit an antibody response, host animals are administered the antigen periodically according to an immunization schedule. The first dose primes the animal as the developing immunological response is short-lived, with the resulting antibodies produced for only a few weeks. During this period, memory cells are produced, which, when stimulated by another injection of antigen, produce antibody more rapidly for a longer period of time and at higher titers. The antisera should be collected 1–2 weeks after a booster injection (14). During the course of the immunization schedule, test bleeds from the animal must be screened against a panel of target and nontarget analytes to identify the presence and quantity of antibodies specific to the target analyte.

To produce monoclonal antibodies, the first antigen injection in mice is followed a few weeks later by a booster of the same antigen. When polyclonal antibodies are detected in the serum of mice a few days after the booster injection, the spleen is removed and the mouse lymphocytes are fused in the presence of polyethylene glycol with cultured mouse myeloma cells deficient in the enzyme hypoxanthineguanine ribosyltransferase (HAT). The fused cells, called heterokaryons, are cultured in a medium containing HAT that prevents the growth of the myeloma cells.

The mouse lymphocytes normally die after a week, leaving only heterokaryon colonies that possess the combined traits of the lymphocytes and the myeloma cells. These cells are called hybridomas. Hybridomas are screened for production of the specific antibody by using microtiter plates or a similar immunoassay. Cells that produce the desired antibody are cloned to produce a cell line that is stable. The antibody that is expressed by the cell line can be produced through growth of ascites tumors in mice or by cell culture systems (15, 16). The latter technique involves growth of the cell lines in flasks using an artificial growth medium. Since yields of monoclonal antibodies range from 10 to 100 μg/ml, many flasks are necessary to produce large quantities of monoclonal antibodies, but the antibody contains only a small amount of nonspecific IgG.

A normal outgrowth of the batch procedure is the use of stirred reactors that have been used for propagation of suspended animal cells. A variation of this approach is the perfusion system of propagating hybridoma cells to produce large amounts of antibody. In perfusion systems, the fresh culture medium is added on a continuous or incremental basis, while equivalent amounts of cell-free culture fluid are removed. Perfusion systems can be used for extended periods of time, producing large quantities of uniform antibody harvested from the effluent (17). Therefore, monoclonal antibodies possess the advantage of a continuous supply of constant quality, besides their high specificity against a single antigen or a specific segment of the antigenic molecule.

Although immunochemical assays can employ crude antisera, purification helps in improving assay sensitivity and specificity, reduces analysis time, and aids in standardization of the assay. Various degrees of antibody purification can be performed prior to incorporation of an antibody into the assay format.

A classic preliminary step in antibody purification is precipitation with ammonium sulfate. With the use of this reagent, most immunoglobulins are precipitated at 35–40% saturation. Concentrations greater than this level seldom increase the yield of immunoglobulins but, instead, result in further increase of antibody contamination by other proteins. Following immunoglobulin precipitation, ammonium sulfate is eliminated commonly with dialysis.

One of the simplest methods for further antibody purification is application of ion-exchange chromatography based on diethylaminoethylcellulose resin. Since antibodies are basic serum proteins with isoelectric points between 6 and 8, they carry a negative charge at pH 8 while the resin has a strong positive charge. Thus, binding can occur under such conditions at low ionic strengths. Elution of the antibodies can be effected, with increasing strength of the competing anions usually provided by a gradient elution system. Since antibodies are very basic proteins, they will elute from the column first (18). Antibodies can likewise be eluted in the order of their isoelectric point by lowering the pH of the eluent.

If higher purification of the antibody is required, gel-permeation chromatography is usually employed. This procedure is used more as an adjunct to other methods than as a primary purification method. Affinity chromatography can be also used for purifying the antibody by immobilizing the antigen on a solid support such as agarose and binding the antibody from solution. Elution of the antibody from the solid support can be accomplished with a relatively small volume of eluent.

28.3   REAGENT FORMATTING

Once antibodies and antigens have been developed, they must be incorporated into an assay system for visualization of the primary antibody–antigen reaction. To accomplish this task effectively, an assay format and procedures to visualize the antibody–antigen reaction must be first selected, the necessary reagents must then be prepared, and the final immunochemical method including sample preparation must be optimized for the intended application.

The wide variety of format and reagent configurations currently being available for visualization of the end point have been already discussed in Chapter 23. In selecting the most suitable format, one must thoroughly understand the end-user requirements. The matrix into which the assay will be applied, throughput and time requirements, and the level of quantification needed are some of the most common variables to consider in selecting format selection. In addition, sensitivity, precision, accuracy, and the ruggedness of the assay must equal or exceed the limits for the particular application. Equipment, personnel, and expertise needed to perform the assay, as well as the length of time it takes to apply the assay, must fit the application. In general, the value of the information offered must be greater than the cost of performing the assay.

Common immunochemical assay formats to select from include the 96-well microtiter plates, dipsticks, coated test tubes, and membrane-based flow through devices. If the end-user is a trained technician working in a well-equipped laboratory and needs to detect and tentatively identify, for example, antimicrobial residues in hundreds of meat samples per day, a multiwell or other high-throughput format should be chosen. If, on the other hand, the end user is a quality control inspector at a milk factory who has limited time to find out whether the penicillin residues in the milk waiting to be unloaded exceed a certain level, the same reagents used in the first instance may require a more user-friendly format such as dipstick or membrane-based flow through device.

28.4 APPLICATIONS

In recent years, many immunochemical assays within the groups of aminoglyco-sides, β-lactams, chloramphenicol, sulfonamides, tetracyclines, anthelminthics, anticoccidials, anabolic hormonal-type growth promoters, β-agonists, and other drugs have been developed. Immunochemical assays make up some of the most powerful techniques that can be used advantageously in many drug residue appli-cations to achieve rapid, economical, and sensitive results.

Generic immunochemical assays with broad specificity toward several members within a group of drugs allow the targeting of more specific analyses for the final identification of the contaminating residue. Compound-specific im-munochemical assays also have a part to play in this process, as well as plugging some of the gaps not filled by the generic assays.

Apart from home-made methods, a number of quick, sensitive, and easy-to-perform immunochemical tests are currently available in a kit format. Table 28.1 gives an example of the detection limits attainable by some commercially

TABLE 28.1 Detection Limits (ppb) of Various Immunochemical Kits Commonly Used by the Dairy Industry

Antibacterial	CTII test	CITE test	LacTek	EZ Screen	Spot test
Amoxicillin	5	10	5		
Ampicillin	5	10	10		
Ceftiofur	5	10	>100		
Cephapirin	5	5	10		15
Chlortetracycline	5	30			
Cloxacillin	20	100	10		62.5
Erythromycin	50				
Gentamicin	30	30	30	30	
Neomycin	500	500	500	10	
Novobiocin	100				
Oxytetracycline	30	30			
Penicillin G	2.5	5	5		3.7
Spectinomycin	30	>1000	>1000		
Streptomycin	10	>1000	>1000		
Sulfadiazine	5		>1000	>1000	
Sulfadimethoxine	5	10	100	5	
Sulfamerazine	5		100	>1000	
Sulfamethazine	5	5	10	10	
Sulfathiazole	5	10	>1000	>1000	
Tetracycline	5	30			
Tylosin	150				

Source: From Refs. 170, 171.

available immunochemical kits. The area is growing quickly and new kits appear increasingly frequently.

28.4.1 Aminoglycosides

Since aminoglycosides are a diverse group of chemicals, a generic immunobased analytical scheme for this group of compounds has not been yet developed. Instead, a number of drug-specific immunoassays are available for several aminoglycosides including streptomycin, dihydrostreptomycin, gentamicin, and spectinomycin.

Streptomycin and dihydrostreptomycin are closely related aminoglycosides that have been widely used in veterinary practice. They differ structurally at only a single substituent, with the carbonyl group in the streptose moiety of streptomycin being reduced to an alcohol to give dihydrostreptomycin. Therefore, construction of an antigen employing conjugation to a carrier protein through the point of difference between the two compounds would allow the resultant sera to be utilized in an immunoassay with complete cross reactivity (19). For this conjugation, direct Schiff's base formation with primary amino groups cannot readily be performed, so the stronger reaction of carbonyl groups with hydrazides is employed. Since modification of the hapten is contraindicated, an alternative procedure involving the derivatization of the carrier protein, ovalbumin has been applied. This was realized by introducing adipic dihydrazide into the protein through carbodiimide activation. In this way, a stable reagent was formed that is promising for facile crosslinking of a number of different carbonyl-containing haptens including streptomycin. Using a streptomycin–horseradish peroxidase conjugate prepared in the same way and tetramethylbenzidine as substrate, a direct enzyme-linked immunosorbent assay (ELISA) has been developed that allows rapid testing of milk samples for streptomycin and dihydrostreptomycin residues down to 1.5 ppb (20).

Instead of derivatizing the protein prior to its conjugation with the hapten, other workers preferred to derivatize the hapten itself using carboxymethoxylamine to convert streptomycin to its oxime derivative. This was subsequently conjugated to bovine serum albumin in the presence of water-soluble carbodiimide (21). The specificity and sensitivity of the produced antibodies were tested in a competitive assay using a streptomycin–horseradish peroxidase conjugate in a double-antibody solid-phase technique (22). In this enzyme immunoassay, the wells of the microtiter plates are coated with anti-rabbit IgG (23), and the milk sample, the streptomycin–enzyme conjugate, and the antibody are subsequently added and incubated for 2 h at room temperature. Using a suitable substrate, both streptomycin and dihydrostreptomycin could be quantified in milk samples at levels as low as 6 and 0.8 ppb, respectively (21). Prior to the assay, milk samples were defatted by centrifugation at 4°C and used either undiluted or after dilution with Tween/phosphate buffer at a ratio of 1:10.

An indirect competitive ELISA has been also developed for the determination of streptomycin and dihydrostreptomycin in milk (24). Prior to the analysis, the milk sample was skimmed and treated with oxalic acid. The antiserum was raised in rabbits using streptomycin linked to a bacterial protein as the antigen. To perform the test, microtiter plates were coated with streptomycin, and antiserum and milk samples were mixed to be added in the wells where they were incubated for 1 h. Depending on the amount of residues in the sample, more or less antibody remained available for binding to the streptomycin coat. A pig antirabbit antibody–enzyme conjugate was subsequently added and incubated for 90 min. Using a suitable substrate, streptomycin and dihydrostreptomycin could be detected down to 1.6 ppb, whereas quantification could be made possible up to 100 ppb when samples were used undiluted.

Drug-specific immunoassays have been described for gentamicin residues as well. However, 2 weeks soaking of tissue homogenates in glycine-buffered saline followed by repeated soakings and rinsing of the tissue precipitates has been found indispensable for extraction and quantification of gentamicin residues from bovine tissue using a commercially available radioimmunoassay test kit (25).

The usefulness of an automated fluorescence polarization immunoassay test kit originally developed to quantify gentamicin in serum has been also demonstrated in the analysis of gentamicin in kidney and muscle extracts, and milk (26, 27). Sodium hydroxide digestion of the nonhomogenized samples at 70°C for 20 min was found to be a superior procedure for extracting gentamicin from tissues compared with direct homogenization, or trichloroacetic acid precipitation, or sodium hydroxide digestion of homogenized samples. For all types of samples, detection limits in the range of 10–39 ppb gentamicin could be readily attained.

Spectinomycin, a major member of the aminocyclitol antibiotics, has been analyzed in chicken plasma by a competitive indirect enzyme-linked immunosorbent assay (28). In this assay, spectinomycin 4-carboxymethyloxime was synthesized to be used as a hapten. Coupling of the hapten to bovine serum albumin that was used as a carrier protein was carried out at the C-4 position by means of a reaction with tri-n-butylamine and isobutyl chloroformate. Spectinomycin 4-carboxymethyloxime was also coupled to ovalbumin by a mixed anhydride procedure for preparing the spectinomycin 4-carboxymethyloxime-ovalbumin conjugate employed to coat the wells of the microtiter plate used in the assay. Since the antiserum raised against the spectinomycin 4-carboxymethyloxime–bovine serum albumin conjugate could recognize functional groups of spectinomycin remote from C-4 that was linked to the carrier protein, dihydrospectinomycin and tetrahydrospectinomycin exhibited significant cross-reactivity, although acetylated compounds and other aminoglycosides did not. The detection limit of the assay in undiluted chicken plasma was estimated at 40 ppb.

Apart from those homemade methods, a large number of commercial kits have been developed and are currently available in the market. The area is fast growing and a complete list cannot be presented. Examples of such kits include the LacTek gentamicin test (IDETEK, Inc., Sunnyvale, CA), the gentamicin test (TRANCIA, Lyon, France), the IDS gentamicin and neomycin one-step ELISAs (International Diagnostics Systems Corp., St. Joseph, MI), the CHARM II streptomycin and dihydrostreptomycin test (Charm II Test, Charm Sciences, Inc., Malden, MA), the EZ-screen neomycin and gentamicin card tests (Environmental Diagnostics, Inc., Burlington, NC), the CITE gentamicin, neomycin, and streptomycin tests (IDEXX Laboratories, Inc., Westbrook, ME), the neomycin and kanamycin tests (Cortecs Diagnostics, Ltd., Deeside, UK), the neomycin and streptomycin tests (Euro-Diagnostica, Apeldoorn, The Netherlands), and the Signal gentamicin and neomycin tests (SmithKline Beecham Animal Health, Exton, PA).

28.4.2 β-Lactam Antibiotics

Penicillin G is by far the most common β-lactam antibiotic used in veterinary medicine; however, cloxacillin, ampicillin, amoxicillin, cephalexin, and cefuroxime also share a high proportion of the market. As a result of this rather wide use, a generic β-lactam immunochemical assay that can detect several different β-lactam residues by a single test assay would be highly desirable. However, such a generic assay is not available at present. Attempts to produce penicillin antisera through use of the primary amino group of cephalexin, ampicillin, and aminopenicillanic acid did not result in the required specificity for the intact antibiotic (29). Produced antisera exhibited, moreover, a cross-reactivity for penicilloic acid of many hundred percent. To fill this gap in analytical capability, drug-specific antisera and immunochemical methods have been developed. The requirement in this area is for very specific ELISAs that would not cross-react with others members within this group nor with penicilloic acid, the major hydrolytic breakdown product, which is much more immunogenic than the intact β-lactam ring (30).

Because the β-lactam ring is highly susceptible to hydrolysis in aqueous solutions, traditional methods for the production of antigens often result in extensive hydrolysis of the hapten. Ring-opening accompanied by degradation of the β-lactam molecule to small fragments makes preparation of antigens difficult. Hence, preferred reactions for producing penicillin and cephalosporin antisera are those proceeding under mild conditions.

Mild conjugation reactions have been used in an enzyme-linked immunoassay for detecting cephalexin residues in milk, hen tissues, and eggs. The assay was a double-antibody separation procedure based on use of a rabbit antiserum to cephalexin, and β-D-galactosidase-labeled cephalexin (31). The antigen was prepared by coupling the amino group of cephalexin to thiol groups introduced into bovine serum albumin by the use of N-(m-maleimidobenzoyloxy)succinimide as a cross-linker. Highly titered antiserum to cephalexin was produced in rabbits immunized with the antigen. Enzyme labeling of cephalexin with β-D-galactosidase was performed using N-(γ-maleimidobutyryloxy)succinimide as a cross-linker.

In this assay, milk samples could be analyzed without dilution, but tissue and egg white samples should be homogenized in 5% trichloroacetic acid, centrifuged, and brought to pH 7 prior to analysis. Egg yolks required a separate treatment involving mixing with a pH 7.4 phosphate–EDTA buffer, incubation for 3 h at 25°C with cephalexin antiserum and enzyme-label cephalexin, and centrifugation. The assay could detect cephalexin down to 30 ppb in milk, 60 ppb in egg yolk, and 400 ppb in hen tissue.

Instead of using mild conjugation reactions, some workers have concentrated on procedures that minimize the contact of the water-labile haptens with aqueous solvents prior to injection to the host animal (19). For preparing penicillin G antigens, a mixed anhydride procedure was used to provide a leaving group on the carboxylic acid of the thiazolidine ring and was carried out in dioxane at 4°C (32). Several moles excess of the isobutyl chloroformate activation reagent allowed rapid coagulation and precipitation of the antigen when the solution of activated penicillin was mixed with carrier protein. The insoluble antigen was washed rapidly to remove excess reagents and used within 30 min to inoculate sheep. In this way, specific antisera with crossreactivity less than 4% for penicilloic acid were obtained and successfully used in a method for analyzing penicillin G in milk (33).

Antisera to cloxacillin/oxacillin/dicloxacillin and cefuroxime were also produced by similar procedures and successfully utilized in methods for the detection of these antibiotics in milk (34). Unfortunately, a number of other β-lactams including aminopenicillins and some cephalosporins were not amenable to this mixed anhydride procedure. Thus, a carrier protein derivatization procedure was used to allow cross-linking of cephalosporins, such as cephataxime that has an acetoxy side chain, to ovalbumin. Because acetoxy groups react readily with the heterocyclic nitrogen atoms, the latter were introduced into ovalbumin through the carbodiimide-mediated derivatization of protein carboxyl groups with aminomethylpyridine (34).

Beyond polyclonal antibodies, monoclonal antibodies to isoxazolyl penicillins were recently produced by immunization of mice with a cloxacillin–human serum albumin conjugate prepared by a mixed anhydride procedure (35). Sensitivity and specificity of these antibodies were tested in an indirect ELISA in which a cloxacillin–glucose oxidase conjugate prepared by an activated ester procedure served as a coating agent. It was found that the prepared antibodies could be classified, on the basis of their cross-reactivity with the other isoxazolyl penicil-lins, into two groups representing different clones. Antibodies within the first clone showed major cross-reactivity only to dicloxacillin, whereas antibodies within the second clone had a marked crossreactivity with both dicloxacillin and oxacillin. Application of the latter monoclonal antibodies in milk analysis by an indirect ELISA showed that cloxacillin, dicloxacillin, and oxacillin could be read-ily detected in milk at concentrations of 0.9, 0.4, and 8.2 ppb, respectively.

Apart from those homemade methods, numerous commercial kits including the EZ-screen β-lactam card tests (Environmental Diagnostics, Inc., Burlington, NC), the CITE probe β-lactam test (IDEXX Laboratories, Inc., Westbrook, ME), the LacTek β-lactam test (IDETEK, Inc., Sunnyvale, CA), and the spot test for benzylpenicillin, cephapirin, and cloxacillin (Angenics, Inc., Cambridge, MA) are also available.

28.4.3   Chloramphenicol

Despite the fact that the preparation of chloramphenicol-specific antibodies was reported as early as in 1966 (36), it was 1984 before the first immunoassay was published for the determination of chloramphenicol residues in swine muscle, eggs, and milk (37). This first-published method was a radioimmunoassay that required an extraction procedure and special laboratory facilities to attain a quanti-fication limit of 1 ppb. Employed polyclonal antibodies showed insignificant crossreactivity with structurally related compounds, except that thiamphenicol that did not interfere with the analysis. However, cross-reactivity was significant for metabolites deviating from the parent compound in the acyl side chain.

All radioimmunoassays published thereafter, except those described by Hock and Liemann (38), Freebairn and Crosby (39), and Pohlschmidt et al. (40), were based on a similar procedure (Table 28.2). However, Hock and Liemann (38) applied a more simplified extraction/cleanup procedure for the analysis of chloramphenicol residues in animal tissues, milk, urine, and plasma. In this assay, competitive inhibition between chloramphenicol labeled with ^{14}C and antibody has been demonstrated.

Freebairn and Crosby (39) used polyclonal antibodies produced following conjugation of chloramphenicol to keyhole limpet hemocyanin. Tissue samples were freeze-dried, defatted, and homogenized. Following centrifugation, C_{18} solid-phase extraction columns were used to purify the extracts further. Dextran-coated charcoal was used for separation of the bound from the unbound labeled chloramphenicol. Due to the efficient sample cleanup, the sensitivity of the assay was as low as 0.2 ppb. However, the recovery of the method ranged from 15% to 90%, the variation being attributed to inhomogeneity of the fat content of the sample. Instead of using charcoal for the separation of bound and free chloram-

TABLE 28.2 Immunochemical Methods for Chloramphenicol Residues

Matrix	Sample preparation	Type of immunoassay	Antibody	Sensitivity	Ref.
Swine muscle, eggs	ACN extn, liq–liq partns	Radioimmunoassay	Polyclonal	0.2 ppb	37
Milk	CHCl₃/isooctane extn				37
Bovine muscle	Buffered saline (pH 7.2) extn	Indirect competitive enzyme-linked immunoassay	Polyclonal	1 ng/ml of extract	11
Meat, eggs, milk	Analogous to Ref. 37	Radioimmunoassay	Polyclonal	0.2 ppb	172
Urine, plasma	Dilution	Radioimmunoassay	Polyclonal	10^{-12} mol/	38
Milk	ACN, DCM, and EtOAc extns			L of final extract	38
Rabbit tissues	Buffered saline homogenization, ether/EtOAc extn				38
Swine tissues	Analogous to Ref. 37	Radioimmunoassay	Polyclonal	1–5 ppb	173
Eggs	Analogous to Ref. 37	Radioimmunoassay	Polyclonal	1 ppb	174
Swine, bovine, and veal muscle	Analogous to Ref. 37	Radioimmunoassay	Polyclonal	1 ppb	175
Animal tissues, eggs	Analogous to Ref. 37 followed by LC purification of extract	Radioimmunoassay	Polyclonal	1 ppb	176

(continued)

TABLE 28.2 Continued

Matrix	Sample preparation	Type of immunoassay	Antibody	Sensitivity	Ref.
Milk	Buffered saline diln	Enzyme-linked immunosorbent assay	Polyclonal	<0.5 ppb	43
Eggs	Analogous to Ref. 37	Radioimmunoassay Enzyme-linked immunosorbent assay	Polyclonal	0.5 ppb	44
Swine muscle	EtOAc extn, SPE cleanup, liq–liq partn	Indirect competitive enzyme-linked immunosorbent assay	Monoclonal	5 ppb	45
Swine muscle	H_2O extn, cleanup of blanks on immunoaffinity gel	Indirect streptavidin–biotin enzyme-linked immunosorbent assay	Monoclonal	10 ppb	46
Milk	Centrgn, filtn, cleanup of blanks on immunoaffinity gel	Indirect streptavidin–biotin enzyme-linked immunosorbent assay	Monoclonal	1 ppb	47

Milk, eggs, meat	Analogous to Ref. 37	Radioimmunoassay using antibody-coated microtiter-plates		1–10 ppb	40
Urine	Buffered saline diln or enzymatic digestion and EtOAc extn	Indirect enzyme-linked immunosorbent assay	Polyclonal	1.3–2.2 ppb	48
Milk	Centrgn at 4°C or centrgn and EtOAc extn			0.6 or 0.03 ppb	48
Tissues, eggs	EtOAc extn, liq–liq partn			0.045 ppb	48
Milk	Direct assay	Membrane-based direct enzyme-linked immunoassay techniques: Immunofiltration Dipstick assay		0.7 ppb 1 ppb	53

liq–liq, liquid–liquid; partn, partition; filtn, filtration; extn, extraction.
Other abbreviations as in Tables 20.2 and 27.3.

phenicol, Pohlschmidt et al. (40) utilized antibody-coated microtiter plates as a means to reduce the number of analytical steps by nearly one-half.

A critical study of reference standards for residue analysis of chloramphenicol in meat and milk was also carried out using a radioimmunoassay and gas chromatography (GC) equipped with electron capture and mass detectors (41). Although the concentration of chloramphenicol was only 1 ppb in milk and 10 ppb in meat, approximately 70% of the antibiotic could be recovered by the assay. A stability study of chloramphenicol in milk samples stored at -30 to $-80°C$ showed that stability decreases with increasing drug concentration when the sample is stored at $-30°C$.

Apart from radioimmunoassays, various enzyme-linked immunosorbent assays have been described as well. Campbell et al. (42) first reported a sensitive and specific ELISA using polystyrene tubes and a polyclonal antibody. However, the performance of this method was not evaluated with real samples but only with standards and aqueous muscle tissue extracts. Sensitive ELISAs were also developed for the determination of chloramphenicol in milk (43) and eggs (44); the results drawn by the latter assay correlated well with those obtained by application of a radioimmunoassay.

Monoclonal antibodies were first produced in 1987 and used in an ELISA format for the determination of chloramphenicol in swine muscle tissue (45). The results drawn by this method correlated well with those obtained using liquid chromatography (LC). Later, the sensitivity of the ELISA assay was significantly improved by the introduction of a streptavidin–biotin system and by using a coating agent with lower chloramphenicol incorporation (46, 47). Analysis time was also largely shortened by omitting the cleanup step, which made the procedure rather time-consuming; to correct, however, for variable matrix interferences, part of the crude aqueous extract was purified though use of an immobilized monoclonal antibody preparation prior to analysis.

An indirect enzyme immunoassay suitable for the determination of chloramphenicol and its glucuronide was developed for the analysis of urine, milk, tissue, and eggs as well (48). In this assay, chloramphenicol succinate was coupled to both bovine serum albumin and horseradish peroxidase by a mixed anhydride procedure. Unlike tissue and egg samples, urine and defatted milk could be directly analyzed, but when an ethyl acetate extraction was employed in milk analysis, the limit of detection was lowered at least 10 times.

In general, most of published immunochemical methods on chloramphenicol assay are based on antibodies particularly specific for the aromatic ring and the propanediol moiety of chloramphenicol. This is due to the fact that the main chloramphenicol analogues such as thiamphenicol differ from chloramphenicol in one of these parts of the chloramphenicol molecule. To obtain such antibodies, chloramphenicol was linked to the carrier bovine serum albumin at the acyl chain of the molecule by mixed anhydride or carbodiimide reactions (49, 50). In both procedures, terminal carboxyl groups of the hapten were linked to the terminal ε-amino groups of the protein. The acyl side chain of chloramphenicol, however, does not possess a carboxyl group or active group to which a carboxyl group can be easily attached. For this reason, an alternative conjugation procedure in which sulfydryl groups were introduced in the protein carrier by means of a reaction with S-acetyl-mercaptosuccinic anhydride has been employed (51, 52).

Rapid and simple visual read-out alternatives for the detection of chloramphenicol in raw milk have also been described recently (53). These tests employ membrane-based immunochemical procedures based on either enzyme-linked immunofiltration or dipstick enzyme immunoassay format. In both test systems, a nylon membrane coated with polyclonal antibodies was either mounted on a plastic dipstick or fixed in a plastic test device with close contact to an integrated filter layer. Dipsticks or plastic test devices were incubated in a test tube containing the sample and chloramphenicol-enzyme conjugate solution for 30 min, washed, and finally incubated in an enzyme substrate–chromogen solution. In the enzyme-linked immunofiltration assay, enzyme conjugate and developing solution were subsequently added waiting for about 30 s between additions to allow absorption of the liquid by the filter layer.

Several commercial kits including the EZ-quant chloramphenicol test (EDI-TEK, Inc., Burlington, NC), the chloramphenicol test (Euro-Diagnostica, Apeldoorn, The Netherlands), the Ridascreen chloramphenicol test (Riedel-de Haen, AG, Seelze, Germany), the EZ screen chloramphenicol test (Environmental Diagnostics, Inc., Burlington, NC), and the chloramphenicol test (TRANCIA, Lyon, France) are available commercially.

28.4.4 Sulfonamides

Most immunochemical methods published for the determination of sulfonamides in edible animal products, serum, and urine concern sulfamethazine analysis (Table 28.3). Early methods for screening sulfamethazine in swine blood (54) necessitated extraction of the antibiotic from the sample and application of long assay protocols that rendered them impractical for routine analysis in hog slaughterhouses. Later methods developed for the detection of sulfamethazine residues in swine serum (55), urine and muscle (8), and in milk (9) addressed the extraction and assay problems of previous methods.

In each of these methods, undiluted serum, urine, acid-deproteinized milk, or a buffered saline extract of muscle was mixed with sulfamethazine–horseradish peroxidase and added to antibody-coated wells of a microtiter plate. A sulfamethazine–bovine serum albumin conjugate prepared by the glutaraldehyde procedure (56) was used for antibody production. Results showed that screening of serum was of value since sulfamethazine concentrations in serum directly correlated with those in swine tissues. Thus, for example, a level of 100 ppb of sulfamethazine in

TABLE 28.3 Immunochemical Methods for Sulfonamide Residues Using Polyclonal Antibodies

Antibacterial	Matrix	Sample preparation	Type of immunoassay	Sensitivity (ppb)	Ref.
Sulfadiazine	Swine bile and urine	Direct assay	Direct competitive enzyme-linked immunosorbent assay	32–36	67
Sulfamethazine	Swine urine	Direct assay	Direct competitive enzyme-linked immunosorbent assay	10	177
	Swine muscle	Buffered saline (pH 7.2) extn	Direct competitive enzyme-linked immunosorbent assay	20	177
	Milk	Acidification, centrgn, pH adjustment, centrgn,	Direct competitive enzyme-linked immunosorbent assay	1	178
	Swine liver and muscle	Matrix solid-phase dispersion (MSPD) cleanup	Direct competitive enzyme-linked immunosorbent assay	5	59
	Swine plasma and serum	Direct assay	Direct competitive enzyme-linked immunosorbent assay	10	65
	Swine plasma	Direct assay	Direct competitive enzyme-linked immunosorbent assay	10	60
	Swine serum	Direct assay	Direct competitive enzyme-linked immunosorbent assay	13	55
	Milk	Direct assay	Indirect competitive enzyme-linked immunoassay	0.05	66
Sulfathiazole	Honey	H_2O diln	Indirect competitive enzyme-linked immunoassay	300	179
Sulfonamides	Milk	Direct assay	Eight-well strip competitive enzyme-linked immunoassay	0.02	68

Abbreviations as in Table 28.2.

the serum corresponds in 100 ppb in the liver and 25 ppb in the muscle (57, 58). The possibility to test for residue levels in the liver and tissue without having to sample tissue is a real advantage.

In another method for the determination of sulfamethazine in muscle and liver tissues (59), the extraction problem was successfully addressed by applying a matrix solid-phase dispersion procedure for rapid and efficient purification of the tissue extracts. Determination was made by ELISA on the basis of antibodies raised against sulfamethazine-diazo–bovine serum albumin conjugates.

Excellent performance characteristics have been reported in an ELISA method developed for screening sulfamethazine in swine plasma (60). In this method, a sulfamethazine-diazo–bovine thyroglobulin conjugate was used for antibody production whereas immobilization of the antibodies on the surface of the wells was carried out through use of protein-A molecules. Since protein-A binds through the Fc portion of immunoglobulin, it may not as easily disassociate as the case may be with the direct antibody adsorption to the surface (61). This special immobilization procedure helped in highly improving the precision of the assay because it eliminated batch differences in the physical structure of the microtiter plates (62). It also reduced lateral surface interaction of the adsorbed antibody that could distort the molecule (63). Besides, it eliminated interaction of the lipophilic moieties of the antibody with the solid matrix, which might either concern the antigen binding site or contribute to steric binding hindrance for optimal antigen access and/or binding (64).

This assay was later modified to a high-volume test system suitable for screening sulfamethazine-treated hogs in a slaughterhouse environment where the speed of the assay should be able to keep up with the kill speed (65). By incorporating a robotics liquid handling system, approximately 2400 plasma samples could be analyzed in a normal working day. Thus, a slaughterhouse with a turnover rate of 10,000 pigs per day would be able to test 5–10% of the pigs and reach a decision the same day about the wholesomeness of the carcass using the full capacity of the high-volume system.

Sulfamethazine has been further detected in milk without prior sample treatment (66). Using antibodies raised against sulfamethazine-ovalbumin C, an indirect ELISA was developed that allowed a detection limit of 0.05 ppb to be readily attained.

A semiautomated enzyme immunoassay was recently developed as a means to investigate the use of urine and bile as potential matrices for screening residues of sulfamethazine and sulfadiazine in swine (67). Urine was chosen as the screening matrix because sulfonamides are mainly excreted through this body fluid; compared with urine, the levels of sulfonamides in plasma, serum, and bile drop relatively sharply after withdrawal. An extensive investigation was followed to compare the efficiency of sulfonamide-positive bile and urine at predicting sulfonamide-positive kidneys. Bile was found to be an extremely efficient predictor of sulfonamide-positive kidneys. Using an 700 ppb cutoff level, bile was found to be 17 times more efficient than urine at predicting sulfamethazine-positive kidney and 11 times more efficient at predicting sulfadiazine-positive kidney.

Molecular modeling studies of the sulfonamides and their derivatives has indicated a much greater diversity of shape than would be expected from a superficial examination of the structure. As a result, attempts to raise antibodies capable of recognizing the sulfonamido structure common to sulfonamides have so far proved unsuccessful. In the absence of immunoreagents capable of recognizing the sulfonamido group, a series of drug-specific antisera and immunoassays have been developed for screening sulfamethazine, sulfadiazine, sulfadoxine, sulfamerazine, sulfapyridine, sulfanilamide, sulfamethoxypyridazine, sulfachlorpyridazine, sulfadimethoxine, sulfaguanidine, sulfaquinoxaline, and sulfathiazole (68). On the basis of these antisera, a multiresidue method was developed for kidney analysis using a microtiter plate format. In this method (68), each column of wells was coated with a different specific antiserum, enabling six kidney homogenates, one negative control, and one mixed positive control to be assayed on each plate. Using the corresponding specific sulfonamide-peroxidase enzyme conjugate for each column, identification of each sulfonamide could be readily achieved.

A compromise between absolute specificity and generic detection of sulfonamides has been the basis for a reduction in the immunoreagents and complexity of the immunoassays required to produce a sulfonamide screen for a limited range of such compounds. Antisera raised to particular sulfa drugs comprise minor antibody populations capable of exhibiting recognition of different or heterologous sulfonamide–enzyme conjugates. These properties have been used to develop an immunoassay utilizing a single mixed-hapten enzyme conjugate of sulfathiazole, sulfadoxine, and sulfadimethoxine to detect sulfadiazine, sulfamerazine, sulfachlorpyridazine, and sulfaquinoxaline but not straight-chain compounds such as sulfaguanidine and sulfanilamide. An ELISA for the detection of sulfamethazine, sulfamerazine, sulfadiazine, and sulfadimethoxine has also been developed by introducing a carboxylic group into sulfaguanidine after reaction with dioxoheptanoic acid (34). Antigens prepared by cross-linking this product to ovalbumin through the carbodiimide or the mixed anhydride procedures resulted in antisera capable of recognizing mentioned sulfonamides.

Antisera to sulfamethazine have been raised using hapten conjugates prepared by diazotization of the aromatic amino group. Although successful, titers have often been low, and, more importantly, the preparation of standardized and reproducible enzyme conjugates by this method is difficult to attain, probably due to the highly colored side products obtained during the diazotization procedure (34). An alternative method is to prepare succinyl sulfamethazine and utilize the introduced carboxyl residue for cross-linking to protein with soluble carbodiimide. Traditionally, succinylation with succinic anhydride is carried out in pyridine, but recoveries are as low as 4–12%. A sixfold improvement was obtained with anhydrous ethanol as the solvent, which also allowed rapid crystallization of the product.

Apart from homemade methods, a large number of commercial test kits based on ELISAs and other "state of the art" immunoassays have been developed. Examples include the Signal sulfamethazine detection test (SmithKline Beecham Animal Health, Exton, PA), the IDS sulfadimethoxine one-step ELISA (International Diagnostics Systems Corp., St. Joseph, MI), the CITE sulfa trio test for sulfadimethoxine, sulfamethazine, and sulfathiazole (IDEXX Laboratories, Inc., Westbrook, ME), the EZ-screen sulfadimethoxine (Environmental Diagnostics, Inc., Burlington, NC), the sulfamethazine test (RANDOX Laboratories, Ltd., Ardmore, UK), the sulfamethazine and sulfadimethoxine tests (TRANCIA, Lyon, France), the Sulfamethazine test (Novo Food Diagnostics, Ltd., Copenhagen, Denmark), the LacTek sulfamethazine (IDETEK, Inc., Sunnyvale, CA), the Agri-screen sulfamethazine (Neogen, St. Louis, MO), the sulfamethazine and sulfadiazine tests (Euro-Diagnostica, Apeldoorn, The Netherlands), and the sulfamethazine, sulfadiazine, sulfamerazine, sulfamethoxazole, sulfaquinoxaline, sulfadimethoxine, sulfamonomethoxine tests (Cortecs Diagnostics, Ltd., Deeside, UK).

28.4.5 Tetracyclines

An indirect enzyme immunoassay for the detection of tetracycline in milk has been described (69). A tetracycline–bovine serum albumin conjugate was used for antibody production, a homologous tetracycline-β–casein conjugate served as coating agent, whereas goat antirabbit IgG–horseradish peroxidase was used as second antibody. When milk samples were defatted by centrifugation, diluted at least 1:30 in phosphate-buffered saline, and directly assayed by the method, a detection limit of 5 ppb could be readily achieved. Although not generic, the assay could also detect as low as 5 ppb of chlortetracycline due to the strong cross-reactivity of the used antibody to this drug as well.

Strong crossreactivity to chlortetracycline has been also observed when a commercialized kit (70) was applied to analyze tetracycline, chlortetracycline, and oxytetracycline residues in honey (71). The detection limit for both tetracycline and chlortetracycline was at 15 ppb, but for oxytetracycline at 250 ppb due to the low crossreactivity of the used antibodies to this analyte. Experiments using honey free of tetracyclines showed that dilution of honey with buffer at a ratio of a 1:50 was sufficient to eliminate matrix interferences.

The same test kit has been also applied to detect all members of the tetracycline group of antibiotics in kidney and meat tissue (72), although its crossreactivity varied from 4–5% for oxytetracycline and doxycycline to 100% for tetracycline and chlortetracycline. However, the applied sample preparation procedure was rather complex, necessitating homogenization of the samples with McIlvaine extraction buffer, centrifugation, filtration, and solid-phase extraction cleanup prior to the final immunoassay.

Key to the successful production of generic antisera for the tetracycline antibiotics has been the synthesis of the hapten 4-hydrazino-4-dedimethylamino-tetracycline and its subsequent conjugation to protein (73). The immunochemical method developed from this sera could detect tetracycline, chlortetracycline, and oxytetracycline residues in meat and milk, with adequate sensitivity (19).

A number of commercial kits including the CITE probe tetracycline test (IDEXX Laboratories, Inc., Westbrook, ME), the Ridascreen tetracycline test (Riedel-de Haen, AG, Seelze, Germany), the LacTek oxytetracycline test (IDE-TEK, Inc., Sunnyvale, CA), and the CHARM II test for tetracyclines are available on the market. A more widely used test is the CHARM II test (74), which uses antibody binders and works well with samples containing more than 30 ppb of tetracycline but misclassifies a substantial number of samples with less than 30 ppb. While some disagreement in results near the cutoff point is inevitable, the results with low level samples suggest that the CHARM II test may be responding to substances other than tetracyclines as well (74). It has been reported, for example, that fatty acids interfere with the CHARM II test for tetracyclines (75).

28.4.6 Anthelminthics

Since all members of the benzimidazole anthelminthics except thiabendazole contain a benzimidazole carbamate moiety, attempts have been made to produce antibodies recognizing this structure (19). Most successful was an approach in which a carboxylated analogue of albendazole was used as hapten and coupling to the carrier protein was performed using N-hydroxysuccinimide and morpholi-noethyl isocyanide in the presence of dimethylamino pyridine.

Antisera to this antigen showed a high degree of cross-reactivity to many compounds within the benzimidazole group of drugs including oxfendazole, oxfendazole sulfone, cambendazole, fenbendazole, flubendazole, mebendazole, and oxibendazole, with only triclabendazole and thiabendazole being unrecognized. On the basis of this antiserum, a generic ELISA for benzimidazole anthelminthics has been developed that is used as part of the immunoassay screening program for residues in meat within the United Kingdom (19). The limits of detection, expressed as the concentration of the analyte producing a depression of the end-point signal greater that three standard deviations from the mean of replicate negative tissue determinations, ranged with the particular benzimidazole from 5 to 55 ppb.

Using 2-methylbenzimidazolecarbamate as a hapten, monoclonal antibodies that specifically bind fenbendazole, fenbendazole sulfone, oxfendazole, albendazole sulfone, and albendazole sulfoxide have been also produced (76). On the basis of these antibodies, a rapid enzyme immunoassay was developed for screening benzimidazole residues in bovine liver. When samples were homogenized in water and clarified by centrifugation, the assay exhibited detection limits that ranged from 50 to 400 ppb for the individual analytes (77).

Unlike other benzimidazole anthelminthics, thiabendazole cannot be assayed by the previously mentioned procedures because it is structurally very different to the other members of this group of drugs. For this compound, monoclonal antibody-based ELISAs suitable for bovine liver analysis have been reported (78). The haptens selected to ensure specificity of the prepared antisera were 2-succinamidothiabendazole and 5-succinamidothiabendazole (79, 80). These substances were synthesized by condensation of thiourea and bromopyruvic acid to yield aminocarboxythiazole followed by reaction with phenylenediamine (81). Succinic anhydride was used to introduce a terminal carboxyl group on the amino substituent of the aminothiazolyl benzimidazoles. Both haptens were coupled to amino groups of bovine serum albumin and horseradish peroxidase using soluble carbodiimide as carboxyl group activating reagent. Prepared antigens were used for antibody and hybridoma production using spleen cells from responding mice (82). The monoclonal antibodies elicited with the conjugate of the former hapten had high affinity for thiabendazole, while those elicited with the latter hapten bound strongly to thiabendazole, 5-hydroxythiabendazole, and cambendazole. The two competitive ELISA methods developed on the basis of these two antibodies permitted quantification of thiabendazole down to 20 ppb, following a 10 min aqueous sample extraction.

Apart from benzimidazoles, avermectins and other anthelminthics can be also analyzed by immunochemical methods. Ivermectin, a member of the avermectin group, is the compound for which most methods have been developed. Schmitt et al. (83) first reported the production of the ivermectin hemisuccinate derivative formed through the oxygen on C-5 and its potential use in ivermectin antiserum production. The monoclonal antibodies produced by these workers and used to develop an immunoassay for serum were raised against 4-O-succinoylivermectin. Cross-reactivity of the monoclonals was not determined, although the unique structure of the avermectins would limit cross-reactivity to only the parent drugs and their metabolites. Mitsui et al. (84) also reported production of ivermectin antisera raised to a conjugate at C-5, but using an oxime rather than a hemisuccinate derivative. The produced antibodies, although polyclonal, were highly specific to the ivermectin oxime derivative with no cross-reactivity to moxidectin. Unfortunately, neither of these antibodies was used in immunoassay procedures for analyzing edible animal tissues.

A competitive enzyme immunoassay for the quantification of ivermectin residues in bovine liver has also been reported recently (85). This method uses a polyclonal antiserum raised in rabbits against 5-O-succinoylivermectin-transferrin conjugate. Cross-reactivity was demonstrated with doramectin, a member of the avermectins group, but not with moxidectin. As low as 1.6 ppb can be readily detected in liver by this method, but samples have to be extracted with acetonitrile, defatted by liquid–liquid partitioning with hexane, evaporated to dryness, reconstituted in water, extracted with ethyl acetate, submitted to solid-phase cleanup, evaporated to dryness, reconstituted in ethanol twice, and mixed with sodium acetate solution prior to the endpoint assay.

The anthelminthic hygromycin B is another compound for which immuno-chemical studies have been carried out, probably due to the zero tolerance level set by the Food and Drug Administration (FDA) in swine and poultry products. For preparing monoclonal antibodies against the drug, three conjugation methods were examined, each of which used a reactive amine group on hygromycin B to conjugate the hapten to the carrier protein (86). In the first method (87), hygro-mycin B was conjugated directly to the carrier protein using carbodiimide. In the second method (88), the carrier protein was modified with glutaraldehyde to introduce reactive aldehyde groups into the protein. In the third method (89), the carrier protein was modified with 2-iminothiolane to introduce reactive free sulfydryl groups into the protein. After removal of the excess modifier, hygro-mycin B and the heterobifunctional cross-linker sulfosuccinimidyl 4-(p-maleido-phenyl)butyrate were added to the modified protein. Results showed that only the third method could result in a positive immune response to free hygromycin B. Following conjugation, splenocytes from mice immunized with the hygromycin B–ovalbumin conjugate were fused with myeloma cells, and hybridomas secret-ing antibodies against hygromycin B were selected and cloned. The selected antibody was highly specific to hygromycin B, with no cross-reactivity with structurally similar aminoglycoside antibiotics. Using this antibody, a competitive indirect ELISA was developed to screen swine kidney samples rapidly for the presence of hygromycin B residues (86). In this assay, kidney samples were minced, digested with NaOH solution for 45 min, neutralized to pH 6.5–7.0, and centrifuged prior to the ELISA assay.

28.4.7 Anticoccidials

Among anticoccidials, polyether antibiotics have been most widely used in veteri-nary practice. This was possibly the reason why the first immunoassay reported for anticoccidials concerned monensin, a widely used drug within the group of polyether antibiotics. In this assay, treatment of monensin with bromoacetyl bro-mide produced a monobromoacetate ester, presumably of the hydroxyl group at C-26 position. This compound reacted with bovine serum albumin to produce the antigen that allowed production of monensin-specific rabbit antisera, and also with keyhole limpet hemocyanin protein to produce the coating antigen. Follow-ing hapten coupling to the proteins, 73% and 22% of the total amino groups available for reaction in bovine serum albumin and keyhole limpet hemocyanin, respectively, remained unreacted. This is equivalent to 17 molecules of hapten per molecule of bovine serum albumin, a value in the optimum range for an immune response (50). The lack of cross-reactivity of this indirect ELISA with lasalocid or narasin demonstrated the specificity of the produced polyclonal antibodies to monensin. The limit of detection attained by this method in equine serum and urine was as low as 2 ppb (90).

In 1993, another immunoassay for the detection of monensin was developed but, unfortunately, was never applied to biological material (91). Quite recently a competitive ELISA and a compatible extraction procedure suitable for screening monensin in poultry liver samples was described (92). In this assay, a polyclonal antiserum raised against a monensin–transferrin conjugate and prepared via an acid anhydride intermediate (93) was used. Significant cross-reactivity with other polyethers commonly used by the broiler industry, such as maduramicin, lasalocid, salinomycin, and narasin, was not found. A detection limit of 3 ppb could be readily attained when liver samples were submitted to extraction with aqueous acetonitrile, partitioning between aqueous sodium hydroxide solution and a hexane–diethyl either mixture, evaporation of the organic phase, and reconstitution in ethanol/sodium acetate solution.

A more sophisticated sample preparation procedure has been described in another method developed for the determination of monensin residues in chicken tissues by means of a competitive chemiluminescence ELISA (94). Using an active ester synthetic route (95), monensin was conjugated with both the carrier protein, keyhole limpet hemocyanin, to produce the antigen used to elicit the immune response, and thyroglobulin to produce the coating agent. The produced antisera were used for both immunoaffinity chromatography (IAC) and ELISA system development. In this method, fat, kidney, liver, muscle, and skin tissue samples were homogenized in alcohol to be incubated first at 37°C for 16 h in presence of papain and dithioerythritol pH 9.1 solutions and finally for 1 h at 60°C. Digests were centrifuged and applied on IAC solid-phase cleanup columns containing aminoactivated porous silica coated with monensin antiserum. This IAC/ELISA process resulted in a detection limit of 0.22 ppb and an overall analytical limit of quantification for all chicken tissues less than 2 ppb.

Other anticoccidials for which immunoassays have been developed include the polyethers salinomycin and lasalocid, and the quinazoline drug halofuginone. Concern over the potential toxicity of salinomycin has led to development of two competitive ELISAs for detecting and measuring salinomycin residues in poultry tissues. In the first ELISA (96), 16 monoclonal antibodies were prepared and evaluated for their ability to produce a rapid and low-cost screening procedure for residues of salinomycin in poultry liver. In the second (97), the antibodies produced showed cross-reactivity with narasin but not with lasalocid, maduramycin, or monensin. The sensitivity of the latter assay allowed detection of salino-mycin at levels as low as 0.2 ppb.

For lasalocid assay, polyclonal antibodies were raised in sheep (98). These antisera were applied in an ELISA validated for chicken serum, liver, and muscle. Bridge homology in the ELISA was overcome by absorbing unspecific antisera onto a conjugate between salinomycin and chicken serum albumin, which was immobilized onto Biosilon beads. The assay was highly specific for lasalocid and was capable of detecting it at concentrations less than 0.15 ppb.

Halofuginone can be also analyzed in chicken serum by a competitive ELISA developed on the basis of monoclonal antibodies (99). In this study, a serum matrix effect that afforded a higher sensitivity for the detection of halofugi-none in chicken serum than in assay buffer or in highly diluted serum was observed. The sensitivity of the ELISA improved when used in more concentrated serum.

28.4.8   Anabolic Hormonal-Type Growth Promoters

Use of hormonal-type substances for growth promotion and fattening purposes in food-producing animals is prohibited or restricted in many countries. Adminis-tration of diethylstilbestrol, in particular, has been totally banned worldwide. This implies that adequate analytical methods should be available for regulatory control. Due to its sensitivity, radioimmunoassay has have become most important in diethylstilbestrol analysis and represents the final detection step in the EU reference method for stilbene residues analysis (100).

Diethylstilbestrol is particularly difficult to quantitate below 1.0 ppb in bovine tissues, especially in liver, which is among the last tissues to contain diethystilbestrol after cattle are withdrawn from receiving the drug (101, 102). Interferences from tissue matrix constitute a major problem that might be due to nonspecific interference of lipids and fatty compounds (103, 104). In addition, problems with false-positive results often appear in urine analysis unless a chro-matographic step such as a solid-phase extraction cleanup (105, 106) is intro-duced. Simple sample preparation procedures such as those based on solvent extraction and liquid–liquid partitioning do not usually give satisfactory results (107, 108).

The inherent tendency of diethylstilbestrol to form isomers can also influ-ence the analytical results unless the applied extraction and purification proce-dures can recover both isomers or selectively recover the *trans*-diethystilbestrol isomer, which is the biologically active form of diethystilbestrol (109). Measure-ment of both free diethystilbestrol and its glucuronides is important since most diethystilbestrol in biological samples normally occurs in form of glucuronides (110, 111).

Since many interferences with diethylstilbestrol analysis are caused by undefined sources, use of a highly specific antibody would probably not correct the problem. Nevertheless, several attempts to prepare a drug-specific antibody have been made without success. Thus, more emphasis was finally placed on developing more efficient extraction and cleanup procedures to ensure selectivity. Current methods combine several cleanup steps based on different isolation principles to provide adequately purified sample extracts for the determination of diethystilbestrol by radioimmunoassays (Table 28.4).

Apart from diethylstilbestrol, several other anabolics including nortestosterone, methyltestosterone, hexestrol, trenbolone, zeranol, and medroxyprogesterone have also gained importance from a regulatory point of view. Examples of immunochemical methods applied in the analysis of edible animal products for residues of these anabolics are presented in Table 28.4.

Results of residue monitoring programs are increasingly indicating that 19-nortestosterone and its esters are still the most frequently used anabolizing agents in cattle production, probably as a direct consequence of the ban on diethylstilbestrol administration (112). As a result of this use, urine and bile samples are routinely screened by immunoassays for nortestosterone residues.

Immunochemical methods employing either radioactive (113) or chemiluminescent (114) labels have long been available for urine analysis but they were limited to the determination of 17β-19-nortestosterone. Injection, however, of 19-nortestosterone or its esters into veal calves results in formation of 17α-19-nortestosterone as the predominant metabolite in urine (115). Therefore, efficient regulatory control is not possible unless the latter metabolite can be also determined (116).

A competitive enzyme immunoassay capable of screening 17α-19-nortestosterone in urine has been described (117). In order to elicit an immune response to 17α-19-nortestosterone with low affinity to the 17β-stereoisomer, the 3-position of the steroid moiety was chosen as the site of attachment. To obtain a homologous immunoassay, both the antigen and the enzyme conjugate were coupled at the 3-position. Using antibodies raised in rabbits against 17α-19-nortestosterone-3-carboxymethyloxime-bovine serum albumin conjugate, an immunoassay based on the competitive incubation of 17α-19-nortestosterone and 17α-19-nortestosterone-3-carboxymethyloxime–horseradish peroxidase conjugate was developed that allowed a limit of detection as low as 0.1 ppb. Prior to the assay, urine samples were hydrolyzed by incubation for 1 h at 37°C in presence of *Helix pomatia* juice pH 7, and purified by solid-phase extraction on C_{18} columns.

A test strip enzyme immunoassay that could not discriminate between the 17α- and 17β-stereoisomers but allowed on-site screening of urine samples within 45–60 min was also reported (118). In this assay, 17β,19-nortestosterone was coupled to bovine serum albumin through a hemisuccinate bridge at the 17-position (119). This conjugate was used to raise polyclonal antibodies that would

TABLE 28.4 Immunochemical Methods Commonly Used for Screening Residues of Anabolics in Edible Animal Products

Analyte	Matrix	Sample preparation	Type of immunoassay	Tracer	Ref.
Diethylstilbestrol (DES)	Animal tissues	Ether extn, liq–liq partns	Radioimmunoassay	[3H]-DES	180
	Bovine tissues	Ether extn, liq–liq partns, Silica gel column cleanup	Radioimmunoassay	[3H]-DES	181
	Muscle	Enzymatic digestion, ether extn, Sephadex LH-20 column cleanup, LC fractionation	Radioimmunoassay	[3H]-DES	182
	Muscle	Ether extn, liq–liq partns, Sephadex LH-20 or RP-C_{18} column cleanup	Radioimmunoassay	[3H]-DES	183
Diethylstilbestrol and metabolite	Bovine liver	MeOH extn, enzymatic deconjugation, liq–liq partn, Sephadex LH-20 column cleanup,	Radioimmunoassay	[3H]-DES	184
Hexestrol	Bovine and ovine tissues	Ether extn, deconjugation, liq–liq partns, Silica gel column cleanup	Radioimmunoassay	[3H]-Hexestrol	185
Medroxyprogesterone acetate (MPA)	Adipose tissue	Pet. ether extn, SPE cleanup, LC fractionation	Radioimmunoassay	[3H]-MPA	186
Methyltestosterone (MT)	Muscle	Enzymatic digestion, ether extn, Lipidex-5000 or RP-C_{18} column cleanup	CLIA	MT-ABEI	187

Analyte	Matrix	Sample preparation	Method	Label	Ref.
Nortestosterone (NT)	Animal tissues	Enzymatic digestion, ether extn, Lipidex-5000 column cleanup	CLIA	NT-ABEI	125
19-Nortestosterone	Kidney fat	MeOH extn, liq–liq partn, SPE cleanup, LC fractionation	Enzyme immunoassay	NT-Alkaline phosphatase	188
Trenbolone (TB)	Animal tissues	EtOH extn, liq–liq partns	Radioimmunoassay	^{3}H-TB	189
	Bovine muscle	Ether extn, enzymatic deconjugation, liq–liq partn, magnesia column cleanup	Radioimmunoassay	^{3}H-TB	190
	Bovine tissues	Enzymatic deconjugation, ether extn, liq–liq partns, Sephadex LH-20 column cleanup	Radioimmunoassay	^{3}H-TB	191
Zeranol	Bovine tissues	Ether extn, liq–liq partns	Radioimmunoassay	^{3}H-Zeranol	192
19-Nortestosterone and methyltestosterone	Meat	Enzymatic digestion, SPE cleanup, LC fractionation	Radioimmunoassay	^{3}H-NT ^{3}H-MT	124
Acetylgestagens	Kidney fat	MSPD cleanup, SPE cleanup	Enzyme immunoassay	–	193
Steroids	Meat	t-Butyl-methyl ether extn, liq–liq partn, SPE cleanup	Radioimmunoassay and enzyme immunoassay	Various	194

ABEI, N-(4-aminobutyl)-N-ethyl isoluminol; CLIA, chemiluminescence immunoassay; SPE, solid-phase extraction; MSPD, matrix solid-phase dispersion; RP, reversed phase. Other abbreviations as in Table 28.2.

also react with steroids having a comparable structure, especially those with similar A and B rings. The conjugate was chosen to give antibodies that would react strongly with 17α,19-nortestosterone and 19-norandrostene-3,17-dione, which can be formed by oxidation of 17α- and 17β-19-nortestosterone in urine samples. Further, such antibodies might be used to determine directly the glucuronic and sulfuric acid conjugates at the 17-position of the steroid, since most of nortestosterone is excreted under these forms in the urine (120–122). In this assay, urine samples were incubated together with enzyme-labeled analyte and a nitrocellulose test strip with immobilized antibodies. Following incubation, the strip was placed in a chromogen-containing substrate solution for color reaction.

Bile analysis for 19-nortestosterone residues has been carried out by combining an immunoaffinity cleanup with a chemiluminescence immunoassay (123). In order to maximize possible crossreactivity of the antisera to both 17α- and 17β-isomers and to the glucuronide conjugates as well, the antigen employed to produce antisera was 19-nortestosterone coupled to bovine serum albumin at the 17-position via a hemisuccinate linkage. For preparing the immunoaffinity column, the produced antibodies were covalently immobilized to activated controlled pore glass. The competitive ELISA plates were coated with 19-nortestosterone–thyroglobulin conjugate.

Screening of meat samples for 19-nortestosterone can be performed by a variety of immunochemical methods including radio-, chemiluminescence-, and enzyme-labeled procedures. The main characteristic of these methods is that the tissue sample is purified and fractionated so that only the fraction containing 17β-19-nortestosterone is subjected to the endpoint immunoassay (Table 28.4). Thus, one method combines liquid chromatographic purification and radioimmunoassay (124), whereas other methods combine liquid chromatography and chemiluminescence (125) or enzyme-linked (126) immunoassay. When certified blank meat samples were submitted to the chemiluminescence immunoassay (125), luminescence signals suggested that all samples contained a certain amount of nortestosterone background indistinguishable from 62.5 pg 19-nortestosterone. This background actually determines the quantification limit of the assay, which was estimated at about 0.6 ppb.

For screening of 19-nortestosterone, a number of commercial kits are also available on the market. Examples of such kits are the zeranol, stilbenes, 19-nortestosterone, trenbolone tests (Genego SPA, Gorizia, Italy), the hormones tests (Laboratoire d'Hormonologie, Marloie, France), the trenbolone and 19-nortestosterone tests (RANDOX Laboratories, Ltd., Ardmore, UK), and the nortestosterone and progesterone tests (Euro-Diagnostica, Apeldoorn, The Netherlands).

28.4.9 β-Adrenergic Agonists

Different sample materials including urine, feces, cattle feed, tissues, hair, eyes, and bile are offered for monitoring the illegal use of β-agonists. In determining illegal use, there are obvious advantages in selecting tissues that accumulate residues. Of the edible tissues, liver appears to contain the highest concentrations throughout the withdrawal period (127). Among blood, urine, and feces samples that can be taken from the live animal, urine, which can be taken in both farm and slaughterhouses, may contain the highest β-agonists concentrations postwithdrawal and therefore is still the most frequently analyzed material. Bile also suits the requirements of a screening assay since there is a high correlation between liver and bile levels (128) and, therefore, it will reflect for a much longer time than other edible tissues or urine that illegal compounds have been given to animals as withdrawal proceeds (129). Furthermore, this matrix is easy to collect on a routine basis just after slaughter of the animal and before carcass evisceration, without disruption of the throughput of the cattle being killed at the abattoir. It has also recently been indicated (127) that the eye may achieve concentrations an order of magnitude higher than in liver, providing evidence for the value of this organ in screening for abuse in the slaughter population.

For screening, two types of immunochemical methods are generally used: radioimmunoassays and enzyme immunoassays. A number of sophisticated analytical schemes have been devised that allow low concentrations of β-agonists to be detected even after long withdrawal periods have been observed before slaughter. Table 28.5 presents the immunochemical methods commonly used for screening residues of β-agonists in biological materials.

The first radioimmunoassay of β-agonists appears in 1976 (130). It was used for studying the pharmacokinetics of clenbuterol after its administration to dogs and cats. Later radioimmunoassays have been targeted to the determination of clenbuterol in urine (131), liver (132), and biological specimen (133) of treated cattle. They were all based on antisera raised in rabbits by immunization against a clenbuterol-diazo derivative coupled to human serum albumin. Their assay principle was based on competition between the clenbuterol residues present in samples and tritium-labeled clenbuterol; bound and free radioactivity was separated using dextran-coated charcoal. Sample cleanup was not required prior to the assay of urine (131), although it was necessary for liver samples (132) in order to achieve determinations at the sub-ppb level.

In 1982, the first enzyme immunoassay of clenbuterol was described (134). It was used to determine clenbuterol levels in plasma of human patients treated by oral route with this drug. It was a highly sensitive double-antibody and heterologous immunoassay based on a competition for binding to a clenbuterol-specific antibody between a diazotized clenbuterol analogue labeled with β-galactosidase and unlabeled standard or sample clenbuterol. The antibody-bound enzyme hapten was separated from free hapten by anti-rabbit IgG immobilized to a polystyrene ball. The assay could detect levels as low as 0.5 pg clenbuterol per tube.

The first applications of enzyme immunoassay for animal screening appeared in the early 1990s and concerned mainly urine analysis. Later, an enzyme

TABLE 28.5 Immunochemical Methods Commonly Used for Screening Residues of β-Adrenergic Agonists in Biological Materials with Polyclonal Antibodies

Analyte	Matrix	Sample preparation	Type of immunoassay	Sensitivity (ppb)	Ref.
Clenbuterol	Animal tissues	Enzymatic digestion, IAC cleanup	Enzyme-linked immunosorbent assay	0.5	142
	Bovine bile	Direct IAC cleanup	Double antibody chemiluminescence immunoassay	0.1	143
	Bovine hair	Enzymatic digestion, IAC cleanup	Competitive chemiluminescence immunosorbent assay	0.04	144
	Bovine liver	HCl homogenization, liq–liq partn	Enzyme-linked immunosorbent assay	0.3	89
	Urine	0.1 N NaOH diln, liq–liq partn	Enzyme-linked immunosorbent assay	0.15	89
	Bovine liver	MSPD cleanup	Radioimmunoassay	0.5	132
	Bovine liver	H_2O homogenization, immobilized antibody preincubation	Enzyme-linked immunosorbent assay	0.25	140
	Bovine urine	Direct assay	Radioimmunoassay	0.24	131
			Enzyme-linked immunosorbent assay	0.15	131
	Bovine liver	Buffer homogenization	Enzyme-linked immunosorbent assay	<0.5	135

Analyte	Matrix	Sample preparation	Method		Ref.
	Bovine eye	Enzymatic digestion		0.2	135
	Bovine urine	SPE cleanup		0.2	135
	Poultry tissues	HCl homogenization, IAC cleanup		0.5	141
Ractopamine	Bovine Urine	Centrgn, enzymatic digestion, H$_2$O diln	Enzyme-linked immunosorbent assay	1.9–2.1	147
Salbutamol	Animal liver	Enzymatic digestion, concn HCl clarification, SPE cleanup	Enzyme-linked immunosorbent assay	1	146
Clenbuterol, salbutamol, cimaterol	Bovine Urine	SPE cleanup	Enzyme-linked immunosorbent assay	1	136
β-Agonists	Urine	5-fold diln in buffer, centrgn, pH adjustment, or pH adjustment, liq–liq partn	Enzyme-linked immunosorbent assay	0.05	195
β-Agonists	Urine	5-fold diln in buffer, pH adjustment	Enzyme-linked immunosorbent assay	0.05	137
		Enzymatic digestion, pH adjustment, liq–liq partn			137
β-Agonists	Urine	Direct assay	Test tube enzyme-linked immunosorbent assay	1	138

Abbreviations as in Table 28.2.

immunoassay for the determination of clenbuterol in bovine urine and tissues was developed using an antiserum raised in rabbits by immunization against a clenbuterol-diazo derivative coupled to human serum albumin (89). Horseradish peroxidase coupled to the clenbuterol-diazo derivative was selected as a label. Simple butyl methyl ether extraction of the samples under alkaline conditions proved adequate to eliminate background interference effectively.

Instead of using human serum albumin as a carrier protein, other workers (135) utilized ovalbumin for preparing the diazotized clenbuterol antigen in an enzyme immunoassay developed for screening of clenbuterol residues in bovine urine, liver, and eye. Alkaline phosphatase rather than β-galactosidase was also used as an enzyme label in the preparation of the enzyme–clenbuterol conjugate.

In a screening assay for clenbuterol, salbutamol, and cimaterol residues in urine, solid-phase extraction cleanup has been recommended as a means to prevent false-positive results (136). The antigen used in this assay was clenbuterol-diazo–bovine serum albumin, whereas salbutamol–carboxymethyl ether–biocytin was employed as a label; the labeled conjugate was prepared by heating salbutamol and monochloroacetic acid under alkaline conditions to produce salbutamol-4-carboxymethyl ether, which was linked to biocytin via a peptide bond. Without this cleanup, procedural blanks of negative samples inconsistently contained 0.2–1.9 ppb clenbuterol equivalents, whereas, after cleanup, procedural blanks always contained less than 0.02 clenbuterol equivalents if stored properly at $-24°C$. Storage of urine samples for 1–4 weeks at a higher temperature could cause elevated background levels up to -0.22 ppb.

A generic immunoassay based on a mixture of two polyclonal antibodies raised against salbutamol and clenbuterol, respectively, has been also described (137). In the Netherlands, this competitive microtiter plate method has been used by the national Inspection Services for screening samples at the laboratory level. In this assay, the cross-reactivity of antibodies raised against different β-agonist conjugates to the carrier protein has been independently exploited. Salbutamol hemisuccinate–horseradish peroxidase was used as the enzyme conjugate. Due to the antibody mixture, this immunoassay could simultaneously detect salbutamol, clenbuterol, bromobuterol, cimbuterol, mapenterol, mabuterol, tulobuterol, clenpenterol, terbutaline, carbuterol, and cimaterol in urine samples. Urine samples could be analyzed without cleanup but blank urine samples showed background values that differed with the age of the sampled animals; blank calf urine samples showed background values of less than 0.5 ppb whereas blank values of bovine urine samples were as high as 3 ppb. However, these background values could be reduced by applying cleanup procedures. In addition, an enzymatic hydrolysis prior to the assay ensured measurements of the glucuronidated and/or sulfated forms of basic β-agonists such as salbutamol, terbutaline, and carbuterol.

The principle of this generic immunoassay was further exploited to develop a tube enzyme immunoassay test for on-site screening of urine samples (138).

Apart from the format, changes were made in sample preparation, sample volume, and interpretation of the results. In the Netherlands, this tube test is used by the General Inspection Service as prescreening for urine samples at farmhouses to detect animals treated with β-agonists. Due to the low sensitivity of the tube test, all samples are reanalyzed by laboratory methods. The tube test results are used to locate treated animals directly at the farm and, if suspected samples are found, to increase sampling.

Methods originally developed for determination of clenbuterol in urine might be suited tissue analysis if suitable modifications are made. Such a possibility was investigated by some workers (140) who subjected an ELISA for urine analysis (139) to several modifications and optimizations to suit liver analysis. In an attempt to decrease assay time, a horseradish peroxidase enzyme label was substituted for the alkaline phosphatase label. Utilizing the 4% cross-reactivity of the clenbuterol antibody with salbutamol, salbutamol–horseradish peroxidase was prepared by the conjugation of salbutamol hemisuccinate to ammoniated horseradish peroxidase and substituted for the clenbuterol–horseradish peroxidase conjugate. In this way, assay sensitivity was further improved owing to the lower affinity of antibodies for salbutamol than for the clenbuterol in the test sample. By increasing, on the other hand, sample volume and sample concentration, sensitivity was doubled without significantly increasing background color. This optimized procedure permitted determination of clenbuterol residues in bovine liver at the MRL of 0.5 ppb with a confidence higher than 99%, although prior sample enrichment was not carried out.

Since immunoassays for the determination of clenbuterol in kidney and liver samples often give unreliable results due to matrix effects, an enzyme immunoassay has been developed in which clenbuterol is extracted from poultry tissue samples by 0.01 N HCl and the extracts are purified with immunoaffinity chromatography prior to the end-point immunoassay (141). In this method, diazotized clenbuterol bound to bovine serum albumin was used as antigen, whereas salbutamol–hemisuccinate coupled with horseradish peroxidase, according to the procedure of Kyrein (119), was used as enzyme conjugate. Immunoaffinity chromatography combined with ELISA has also been suggested for screening of clenbuterol residues in liver, kidney, and muscle samples (142).

Novel rapid screening tests have recently appeared for the detection of clenbuterol in bovine bile (143) and hair (144). Extraction and purification of clenbuterol from bile were performed using immunoaffinity chromatography, whereas end-point determination was carried out by a double-antibody chemiluminescence immunoassay capable of giving results of 37 samples in 120 min, with sequential assays being run every 30 min (143). Hence, it was possible to run up to 777 samples in a 14 h time period. A significant contributing factor to the effectiveness of this assay was the choice of the bile as a target matrix. Bile required minimal sample preparation before assay, while it mirrored the levels of residues present in edible tissue. For screening of cattle hair for residues of clenbuterol (144), on the other hand, samples were enzymatically digested, the digest was purified by immunoaffinity chromatography, and the purified extracts were quantified by competitive chemiluminescence ELISA.

Unlike clenbuterol, salbutamol is a difficult compound to analyze due to its particular chemical attributes. It is a basic compound subjected to protein binding; poor recoveries are obtained especially when protein precipitation techniques are used to prepare the extracts (145). In addition, salbutamol is charged at all pH values and does not readily lend itself to simple, specific back-extracting procedures. This severely restricts the options of sample cleanup. However, a Subtilisin protease digestion step followed by acid clarification and solid-phase extraction has been suggested (146) as an adequate extraction and cleanup procedure prior to the end-point determination of salbutamol by an enzyme immunoassay (139) based on the cross-reactivity of anticlenbuterol antibodies.

Ractopamine, a phenethanolamine member of the class of β-agonists, can be also analyzed in bovine urine samples by an ELISA procedure employing a polyclonal antibody raised in goat to detect ractopamine residues (147). For preparing the antigen, ractopamine was coupled to human serum albumin and to horsradish peroxidase using the coupling agent, butane-1,4-diol diglycidyl ether (148, 149).

Apart from the above-mentioned methods, a number of commercial kits are also available in the market. ELISAs and other ''state of the art'' immunoassays are utilized in these kits that allow for rapid, efficient, cost-effective food monitoring. Examples include the RIDASCREEN Clenbuterol test (Riedel-de Haen, AG, Seelze, Germany), the β-agonists tests (Laboratoire d'Hormonologie, Marloie, France), the clenbuterol and β-agonists tests (Euro-Diagnostica, Apeldoorn, The Netherlands), and the β-agonists tests (Genego SPA, Gorizia, Italy).

28.4.10 Miscellaneous

28.4.10.1 Bovine Somatotropin

Application of recombinant DNA technology to clone and express the gene for bovine somatotropin has made it possible to obtain an unlimited amount of the hormone and provides further an opportunity to investigate benefits that may be derived from controlling milk production through supplemental administration of bovine somatotropin on a commercial scale. Central to studies conducted to investigate the safety and efficacy of recombinant-derived bovine somatotropin is the need for a sensitive analytical method that could be used to estimate bovine somatotropin levels in various biological fluids.

A rapid avidin/biotin ELISA has been developed for the determination of bovine somatotropin in blood and milk (150). The method uses affinity-purified polyclonal antisera raised in rabbits to immobilize bovine somatotropin from blood or milk samples on the wells of microtiter plates. Bound bovine somato-tropin was quantified by adding biotinylated antibovine somatotropin antibody during the sample incubation step, followed by incubations with horseradish per-oxidase-labeled avidin D. Since a high-affinity antibovine somatotropin antibody was used, and the biotinylated antibody was added directly to the sample, the assay could be performed in less that 4 h while sensitivities of 0.2 and 2 ppb in milk and blood, respectively, were maintained. This method offers advantages of speed and sensitivity compared to a previous ELISA method (151).

28.4.10.2 Corticosteroids

Since dexamethasone, a synthetic glucocorticosteroid, is sometimes used illegally in animal production, screening methods to detect its presence in animal products are of value. Several immunoassays based on either radio or enzyme labels have been developed, all based on the same commercially available antigen, dexameth-asone-21-hemisuccinate-bovine serum albumin, to produce the antidexametha-sone antibodies. In the radioimmunoassays (152, 153), the tracer commonly used was tritium-labeled dexamethasone and the detection limit was as low as 0.4 ppb in urine, whereas in the ELISAs (154) the drug was conjugated to horseradish peroxidase for detection in urine at a limit of 10 ppb. The assays do not require cleanup steps for urine and milk samples, but their inherent cross-reactivity with endogenous corticosteroids may affect the validity of the analytical results.

To overcome this problem, a radioimmunoassay method was developed (155) in which urine is enzymatically hydrolyzed to be subsequently purified by C_{18} solid-phase extraction. Elution was carried out using ethyl acetate, and the extract was analyzed by reversed-phase LC. The fraction containing the analyte was collected, evaporated, and submitted to radioimmunoassay. In this way, dexa-methasone separated from natural corticosteroids and other synthetic corticoste-roids that could cross-react in the assay.

A generic enzyme immunoassay for the determination of several synthetic corticosteroids including dexamethasone, betamethasone, flumethasone, triam-cinolone, prednisolone, and methylprednisolone in milk, liver, kidney, and muscle samples was recently developed (156). Antibodies raised against dexamethasone-21-hemisuccinate-bovine serum albumin were used in this assay, whereas dexa-methasone–horseradish peroxidase was the label conjugate. Skimmed milk could be directly screened for the presence of corticosteroids at limits of detection of 0.1 ppb for dexamethasone, betamethasone, and flumethasone, 0.3 ppb for triamcinolone and 0.5 ppb for prednisolone. Tissue samples were submitted, prior to the immunoassay, to an extraction/cleanup procedure involving liquid–liquid partitions with acetonitrile–water followed by hexane–chloroform. Background values for bovine liver, swine kidney, and calf muscle were determined to be 0.26, 0.26, and 0.07 ppb, respectively, of dexamethasone equivalents.

28.4.10.3   Macrolides

An enzyme immunoassay for the determination of spiramycin in raw milk has been developed (157). Hens were immunized using a spiramycin–bovine serum albumin conjugate and specific antibodies were extracted from egg yolk by precipitation with polyethylene glycol (158). The ELISA was carried out as an indirect competitive assay with antigen coating and antichicken immunoglobulin linked to alkaline phosphatase. It allowed a clear positive-negative classification of raw milk samples containing spiramycin at the quantification limit of 5.6 ppb. Sample preparation was limited to defatting and dilution in buffer. Since 1995, this method has been routinely applied in an integrated system for the detection of antimicrobials at the MRL level in Germany.

28.4.10.4   Nitrofurans

A common structural moiety is exhibited by all the compounds within this group and from which the group name is derived. Furazolidone, nitrofurazone, furaltadone, nitrovin, nitrofurantoin, and nitrofuroxazide all contain a five-membered furan ring with a nitro substituent at position C-2. A synthetic hapten, 5-nitro-2-furaldehyde, was used to derivative the carrier protein ovalbumin by direct Schiff's base condensation with primary amino groups. Antisera raised to this antigen enabled an generic immunochemical method to be developed that detects all mentioned nitrofurans in liver tissue except nitrovin (19).

28.4.10.5   Peptide Antibiotics

Colistin, a peptide antibiotic, has been determined in rainbow trout tissue by a double-antibody enzyme immunoassay (159). Polyclonal antibodies against colistin were produced in rabbits immunized with a colistin conjugate. The conjugate was produced by a procedure devised to couple an amino group of colistin to thiol groups of bovine serum albumin introduced by thiol exchange reduction of its disulfide bonds with dithiothreitol, using N-(m-maleimidobenzoyloxy)succinimide as a cross-linker (160, 161). Enzyme labeling of colistin with β-D-galactosidase was performed by utilizing another cross-linker, N-(γ-maleimidobutyryloxy)-succinimide, by means of a convenient labeling method (162, 163). With this assay, as little as 30 ppb of colistin could be determined using labeled colistin and colistin antiserum. Sample preparation procedure was limited to homogenization of the fish tissue with trichloroacetic acid, centrifugation, and pH-adjustment of the supernate at 7.2.

28.4.10.6   Quinolones

A substituted quinolone structure is common to the group of quinolone antimicrobials, many of which are also fluorinated. There is sufficient similarity of structure as well as molecular shape to suggest that, with the appropriate antigen, a generic antibody for the whole class of these compounds could be produced. Using as hapten norfloxacin linked to a carrier protein through the secondary amine of the piperazine side group, a group-specific immunochemical assay was developed that could screen for 10 quinolones including norfloxacin, naladixic acid, enrofloxacin, flumequine, ciprofloxacin, ofloxacin, oxolinic acid, pipedimic acid, and enoxacin, at or below 25 ppb levels in meat, poultry, and fish (19). Specific immunochemical methods for naladixic acid, enrofloxacin, and flumequine have been also developed and applied to the analysis of kidney tissue.

28.4.10.7 Sedatives and β-Blockers

Benzodiazepines are an important group of drugs with tranquilizing properties. Available immunochemical methods include radioimmunoassays (164, 165), a radioreceptor assay (166), and nonseparation immunoassays such as the widely used enzyme-monitored immunotest (EMIT) and fluorescent polarization immunoassays (167, 168). Such assays generally require sophisticated apparatus and dedicated laboratories. However, a relatively simple enzyme-linked immunosorbent assay was recently described for screening benzodiazepines in urine (169).

The assay employs a mouse antioxazepam antibody highly specific for benzodiazepines. The antigen oxazepam hemisuccinate–keyhole limpet hemocyanin and the oxazepam–porcine thyroglobulin coating conjugate were prepared via the corresponding N-hydroxysuccinamidyl esters. N-Desmethyldiazepam showed equal cross-reactivity to oxazepam, 11 benzodiazepines cross-reacted weakly, whereas flurazepam and chlordiazepoxide did not cross-react at levels reported to be found in urine. No cross-reactivity was also observed for a range of therapeutic drugs commonly found in urine. The limit of detection was 0.3 ppm. The total assay time for a full 96 well plate was typically 120 min for assay of 22 samples per plate.

REFERENCES

1. R.S. Yalow and S.A. Berson, Nature, 184:1643 (1959).
2. E. Kuss, J. Clin. Chem. Clin. Biochem., 22:851 (1984).
3. J.W. Goding, in Monoclonal Antibodies, Principles and Practice (J.W. Goding, Ed.), 3rd Edition, Academic Press, New York, NY (1996).
4. S.E. Katz and M.S. Brady, J. Assoc. Off. Anal. Chem., 73:557 (1990).
5. D.J. Schmidt, C.E. Clarkson, T.A. Swanson, M.L. Egger, R.E. Carlson, J.E. van Emon, and A.E. Karu, J. Agric. Food Chem., 38:1763 (1990).
6. A.H.M. Schotman, Receil des Travax Chim. des Pays. Bas., 110:319 (1991).
7. D.B. Berkowitz and S.E. Katz, J. Assoc. Off. Anal. Chem., 69:437 (1986).
8. D.E. Holland and S.E. Katz, J. Assoc. Off. Anal. Chem., 71:1137 (1989).
9. D.E. Holland and S.E. Katz, J. Assoc. Off. Anal. Chem., 72:447 (1989).
10. J.R. Fleeker and L.J. Lovett, J. Assoc. Off. Anal. Chem., 68:172 (1985).

11. G.S. Campbell, R.P. Mageau, B. Schwab, and R.W. Johnston, Antimicrob. Agents Chemother., 25:205 (1984).

12. P.L. Carpenter, in Immunology and Serology (P.L. Carpenter, Ed.), 3rd Edition, W.B. Saunders Co, Philadelphia, PA (1975).

13. S. Sell, in Immunology, Immunopathology and Immunity (S. Sell, Ed.), 3rd Edition, Harper and Row, Hagerstown, MD (1980).

14. J.G. Tew and T.E. Mandel, Immunology, 37:69 (1979).

15. G. Kohler and C. Milstein, Nature, 256:495 (1975).

16. J.W. Goding, J. Immunol. Meth., 39:285 (1985).

17. J. van Brunt, Biotechnology, 4:505 (1986).

18. Affinity Chromatography Handbook, Pharmacia Fine Chemical Co., Piscataway, NJ (1985).

19. R. Jackman, in Residues of Veterinary Drugs in Food, Proc. Euroresidue III Conf., Veldhoven, 1996 (N. Haagsma, and A. Ruiter, Eds.), Fac. Vet. Med., Univ. Utrecht, The Netherlands, p. 99 (1996).

20. S.J. Mitchell, R. Jackman, M.P. Dibb-Fuller, D.P. Moswetsi, and A.J. Brown, in Food Safety and quality Assurance: Applications of Immunoassay Systems (M.R.A. Morgan, C.J. Smith, and P.A. Williams, Eds.), Elsevier Applied Science, London, p. 181 (1992).

21. P. Schnappinger, E. Usleber, E. Martlbauer, and G. Terplan, Food Agric. Immunol., 5:67 (1993).

22. H. Arakawa, M. Maeda, A. Tsuji, and A. Kambegawa, Steroids, 38:453 (1981).

23. E. Martlbauer, M. Gareis, and G. Terplan, Appl. Environ. Microbiol., 54:225 (1988).

24. P. Hammer, H. Kirchoff, and G. Hahn, Anal. Chim. Acta, 275:313 (1993).

25. N.S. Haddad, W.R. Davis, W.M. Pedersoli, and R.L. Carson, Am. J. Vet. Res., 48: 21 (1987).

26. S.A. Brown, D.R. Newkirk, R.P. Hunter, G.S. Smith, and K. Sugimoto, J. Assoc. Off. Anal. Chem., 73:479 (1990).

27. A. Vlietstra, D. Masman, and O. Steijger, in Residues of Veterinary Drugs in Food, Proc. Euroresidue II Conf., Veldhoven, May 3–5, 1993 (N. Haagsma, A. Ruiter and P.B. Czedik-Eysenberg, Eds.), Fac. Vet. Med., Univ. Utrecht, The Netherlands, p. 670 (1993).

28. T. Tanaka, H. Ikebuchi, J.-I. Sawada, M. Okada, and Y. Kido, J. AOAC Int., 79: 426 (1996).

29. T. Kitagawa, K. Uchihawa, W. Ohtani, Y. Gotoh, Y. Kohri, and T. Kinoue, in Immunoassays for Veterinary and Food Analysis–1 (B.A. Morris, M.N. Clifford, and R. Jackman, Eds.), Elsevier Applied Science Publishers, London, p. 37 (1988).

30. P. Rohner, M. Schallibaum, and J. Nicolet, J. Food Prot., 48:59 (1985).

31. T. Kitagawa, Y. Gotoh, K. Uchihara, Y. Kohri, T. Kinoue, K. Fujiwara, and W. Ohtani, J. Assoc. Off. Anal. Chem., 71:915 (1988).

32. B.F. Erlanger, Methods Enzymol., 70:85 (1980).

33. R. Jackman, J. Chesham, S.J. Mitchell, and S.D. Dyer, J. Soc. Dairy Technol., 43: 93 (1990).

34. R. Jackman, in Food Safety and Quality Assurance: Applications of Immunoassay Systems (M.R.A. Morgan, C.J. Smith, and P.A. Williams, Eds.), Elsevier Applied Science, London, p. 215 (1992).

35. R. Dietrich, E. Usleber, and E. Martlbauer, in Residues of Veterinary Drugs in Food, Proc. Euroresidue III Conf., Veldhoven, 1996 (N. Haagsma, and A. Ruiter, Eds.), Fac. Vet. Med., Univ. Utrecht, The Netherlands, p. 382 (1996).

36. R.N. Hamburger, Science, 152:203 (1966).

37. D. Arnold, D. vom Berg, A.K. Boertz, U. Mallick, and A. Somogyi, Arch. Lebensmittelhyg., 35:131 (1984).

38. C. Hock, and F. Liemann, Arch. Lebensmittelhyg., 36:138 (1985).

39. K.W. Freebairn, and N.T. Crosby, in Immunoassays for Veterinary and Food Analysis (B.A. Morris, M.N. Clifford, and R. Jackman, Eds.), Elsevier Applied Science, New York (1988).

40. J. Pohlschmidt, I. Ulbrich, and A. Wissel-Monkemeyer, Archiv. Lebensmittelhyg., 43:3 (1992).

41. G. Balizs and D. Arnold, Chromatographia, 27:489 (1989).

42. G.S. Campbell, R.P. Mageau, B. Schwab, and R.W. Johnston, Antimicrob. Agents Chemother., 25:205 (1984).

43. E. Martlbauer and G. Terplan, Arch. Lebensmittelhyg., 38:3 (1987).

44. M. Beck, E. Martlbauer, and G. Terplan, Arch. Lebensmittelhyg., 38:99 (1987).

45. C. van de Water, N. Haagsma, P.J.S. van Kooten, and W. van Eden, Z. Lebensm. Unters. Forsch., 185:202 (1987).

46. C. van de Water and N. Haagsma, J. Assoc. Off. Anal. Chem., 73:534 (1990).

47. C. van de Water and N. Haagsma, Food Agric. Immunol., 2:11 (1990).

48. G. Cazemier, W. Haasnoot, and P. Stouten, in Residues of Veterinary Drugs in Food, Proc. Euroresidue III Conf., Veldhoven, 1996 (N. Haagsma and A. Ruiter, Eds.), Fac. Vet. Med., Univ. Utrecht, The Netherlands, p. 315 (1996).

49. B.F. Erlanger, Pharmacol. Rev., 25:271 (1973).

50. B.F. Erlanger, in Methods in Enzymology, Vol. 70 (B.F. Erlanger, Ed.), Academic Press, New York, NY, p. 85 (1980).

51. I.M. Klotz and R.E. Heiney, Arch. Biochem. Biophys., 96:605 (1962).

52. C.N. Pang and D.C. Johnson, Steroids, 23:203 (1974).

53. E. Schneider, E. Martlbauer, R. Dietrich, E. Usleber, and G. Terplan, Arch. Lebensmittelhyg., 45:25 (1994).

54. J.R. Fleeker and L.J. Lovett, J. Assoc. Off. Anal. Chem., 68:172 (1985).

55. D.E. Dixon-Holland, in Analysis of Antibiotic/Drug Residues in Food Products of Animal Origin (V.K. Agarwal, Ed.), Plenum Press, New York, p. 57 (1992).

56. S. Avrameas, Immunochemistry, 6:43 (1969).

57. R.B. Ashworth, R.L. Epstein, M.H. Thomas, and L.T. Frobish, Am. J. Vet. Res., 47:2596 (1985).

58. V.W. Randecker, J.A. Reagan, R.E., Engel, D.L. Soderberg, and J.E. McNeal, J. Food Prot., 50:115 (1987).

59. C. Renson, G. Degand, and G. Maghuin-Rogister, Anal. Chim. Acta, 275:323 (1993).

60. P. Singh, B.P. Ram, and N. Sharkov, J. Agric. Food Chem., 37:109 (1989).

61. J. Deisenhofer, Biochemistry, 20:2363 (1981).

62. I.C. Shekarachi, J.L. Sever, and Y.J. Lee, J. Clin. Microbiol., 19:89 (1984).

63. B.M. Morrissey, Ann. N.Y. Acad. Sci., 283:50 (1977).

64. W. Schramm, T. Yang, and A.R. Midgley, Clin. Chem., 33:1338 (1987).
65. B.P. Ram, P. Singh, L. Martins, T. Brock, N. Sharkov, and D. Allison, J. Assoc. Off. Anal. Chem., 74:43 (1991).
66. V. Kolar and M. Franek, in Residues of Veterinary Drugs in Food, Proc. Euroresidue III Conf., Veldhoven, 1996 (N. Haagsma and A. Ruiter, Eds.), Fac. Vet. Med., Univ. Utrecht, The Netherlands, p. 620 (1996).
67. T.L. Fodey, S.R.H. Crooks, C.T. Elliott, and W.J. McCaughey, Analyst, 122:165 (1997).
68. R. Jackman, A.J. Brown, A.N. Dell, and S.J. Everest, in Residues of Veterinary Drugs in Food, Proc. Euroresidue II Conf., Veldhoven, May 3–5, 1993 (N. Haagsma, A. Ruiter and P.B. Czedik-Eysenberg, Eds.), Fac. Vet. Med., Univ. Utrecht, The Netherlands, p. 391 (1993).
69. B. Lang, E. Martlbauer, and G. Terplan, Arch. Lebensmittelhyg., 43:77 (1992).
70. Ridascreen Tetracycline, R-Biopharm GmbH, Darmstadt, Germany.
71. E. Usleber, R. Dietrich, E. Martlbauer, and W. Unglaub, in Residues of Veterinary Drugs in Food, Proc. Euroresidue III Conf., Veldhoven, 1996 (N. Haagsma and A. Ruiter, Eds.), Fac. Vet. Med., Univ. Utrecht, The Netherlands, p. 948 (1996).
72. S. Croubels, L. Okerman, K. Vanoosthuyze, J. van Hoof, and C. van Peteghem, in Residues of Veterinary Drugs in Food, Proc. Euroresidue III Conf., Veldhoven, 1996 (N. Haagsma, and A. Ruiter, Eds.), Fac. Vet. Med., Univ. Utrecht, The Netherlands, p. 362 (1996).
73. S.J. Everest, A.L. Cobb, G.M. Courboin, and R. Jackman, Food Agric. Immunol., 6:55 (1994).
74. W.A. Moats, K.L. Anderson, J.E. Rushing, and D.P. Wesen, in Residues of Veterinary Drugs in Food, Proc. Euroresidue II Conf., Veldhoven, May 3–5, 1993 (N. Haagsma, A. Ruiter, and P.B. Czedik-Eysenberg, Eds.), Fac. Vet. Med., Univ. Utrecht, The Netherlands, p. 495 (1993).
75. A. Carlsson and L. Bjorck, J. Food Prot., 55:374 (1992).
76. D.L. Brandon, R.G. Binder, A.H. Bates, and W.C. Montague, J. Agric. Food Chem., 42:1588 (1994).
77. D.L. Brandon, K.P. Holland, J.S. Dreas, and A.C. Henry, J. Agric. Food Chem., 46:3653 (1998).
78. D.L. Brandon, R.G. Binder, A.H. Bates, and W.C. Montague, J. Agric. Food Chem., 40:1722 (1992).
79. D.L. Brandon, R.G. Binder, A.H. Bates, and W.C. Montague, Food Agric. Immunol., 7:99 (1995).
80. R.J. Bushway, D.L. Brandon, A.H. Bates, L. Li, and K.A. Larkin, J. Agric. Food Chem., 43:1407 (1995).
81. W.H. Newsome, and P.G. Collins, J. Assoc. Off. Anal. Chem., 70:1025 (1987).
82. D.L. Brandon, S. Haque, and M. Friedman, J. Agric. Food Chem., 35:195 (1987).
83. D.J. Schmitt, C.E. Clarkson, T.A. Swanson, M.E. Egger, R.E. Carlson, J.M. van Emon, and A.E. Karu, J. Agric. Food Chem., 38:1763 (1990).
84. Y. Mitsui, H. Tanimori, T. Kitagawa, Y. Fujimaki, and Y. Aoki, Am. J. Trop. Med. Hyg., 54:243 (1996).
85. S.R.H. Crooks, A.G. Baxter, I.M. Traynor, C.T. Elliott, and W.J. McCaughey, Analyst, 123:355 (1998).

86. C. Kamps-Holtzapple, L.H. Stanker, and J.R. DeLoach, J. Agric. Food Chem., 42: 822 (1994).
87. J.I. Azcona-Olivera, M.M. Abouzied, R.D. Plattner, and J.J. Pestka, J. Agric. Food Chem., 40:531 (1992).
88. A.A.G. Candlish, W.H. Stimson, and J.E. Smith, J. Assoc. Off. Anal. Chem., 71: 961 (1988).
89. G. Degand, A. Bernes-Duyckaerts, and G. Maghuin-Rogister, J. Agric. Food Chem., 40:70 (1992).
90. M.E. Mount and D.L. Failla, J. Assoc. Off. Anal. Chem., 70:201 (1987).
91. S. Paulliac, T. Halmos, H. Labrousse, K. Antonakis, and S. Avrameas, J. Immunol. Methods, 164:165 (1993).
92. S.R.H. Crooks, I.M. Traynor, C.T. Elliot, and W.J. McCaughey, Analyst, 122:161 (1997).
93. B.F. Erlanger, F. Borek, S.M. Beiser, and S. Lieberman, J. Biol. Chem., 228:713 (1957).
94. M.A.J. Godfrey, M.F. Luckey, and P. Kwasowski, in Residues of Veterinary Drugs in Food, Proc. Euroresidue III Conf., Veldhoven, 1996 (N. Haagsma and A. Ruiter, Eds.), Fac. Vet. Med., Univ. Utrecht, The Netherlands, p. 426 (1996).
95. H. Hosoda, Y. Sakai, S. Miyrairi, K. Ishi, and T. Nambara, Chem. Pharm. Bull., 27:742 (1979).
96. M.H. Elissalde, R.C. Beier, L.D. Rowe, and L.H. Stanker, J. Agric. Food Chem., 41:2167 (1993).
97. D.G. Kennedy, W.J. Blanchflower, and B.C. Odornan, Food Addit. Contam., 12: 93 (1995).
98. D.G. Kennedy, W.J. Blanchflower, and B.C. Odornan, Food Addit. Contam., 12: 83 (1995).
99. R.C. Beier, L.D. Rowe, M.I.A.E. Nasr, M.H. Elissalde, and L.H. Stanker, Food Agric. Immunol., 8:11 (1996).
100. Commission of the European Communities, Directorate-General for Agriculture, Document No 2526/IV/84-EN, File No 6.21 II-4 (1984).
101. A.L. Donoho, W.S. Johnson, R.F. Sieck, and W.L. Sullivan, J. Assoc. Off. Anal. Chem., 56:785 (1973).
102. P.W. Aschbacher, J. Toxicol. Environ. Health. Suppl. 1:45 (1976).
103. W. Shaw, I.L. Hubert, and F.W. Spierto, Clin. Chem., 22:673 (1976).
104. J.M. Rash, I. Jerkunica, and D.S. Sgoutas, Clin. Chem., 26:84 (1980).
105. E.H.J.M. Jansen and R.W. Stephany, Vet. Q., 7:35 (1985).
106. P. Gaspar and G. Maghuin-Rogister, J. Chromatogr., 328:413 (1985).
107. B. Hoffman, J. Assoc. Off. Anal. Chem., 61:1263 (1978).
108. R.M. Gutierrez-Cernosek and S.F. Cernosek, Ann. Clin. Lab. Sci., 7:35 (1977).
109. C.H. van Peteghem, M.F. Lefevere, G.M. van Haver, and A.P. de Leenheer, J. Agric. Food Chem., 35:228 (1987).
110. P.W. Aschbacher, E.J. Thacker, and T.S. Rumsey, J. Anim. Sci., 40:530 (1975).
111. T.S. Rumsey, R.R. Oltjen, F.L. Daniels, and A.S. Kozak, J. Anim. Sci., 40:539 (1975).
112. M. Rapp and H.H.D. Meyer, Arch. Lebensmittelhyg., 38:60 (1984).

113. E.H.J.M. Jansen, R.H. van den Berg, G. Zomer, and R.W. Stephany, J. Clin. Chem. Clin. Biochem., 23:145 (1985).

114. E.H.J.M. Jansen, G. Zomer, R.H. van den Berg, and R.W. Stephany, Vet. Q., 6: 101 (1984).

115. H.H.D. Meyer, M. Rapp, and P. Funcke, Labor-Medizin, 10:127 (1987).

116. M. Rapp, P. Funcke, and H.H.D. Meyer, Arch. Lebensmittelhyg., 39:114 (1988).

117. L.J. van Look, E.H.J.M. Jansen, R.H. van den Berg, G. Zomer, K.E. Vanoosthuyze, and C.H. van Peteghem, J. Chromatogr., 564:451 (1991).

118. M.E. Ploum, W. Haasnoot, R.J.A. Paulussen, G.D. van Bruchem, A.R.M. Hamers, R. Schilt, and F.A. Huf, J. Chromatogr., 564:413 (1991).

119. H.J. Kyrein, Z. Lebensm.-Unters.-Forsch., 177:426 (1983).

120. C.H.L. Shackleton, J. Chromatogr., 379:91 (1986).

121. M.C. Dumasia, E. Houghton, and S. Sinkins, J. Chromatogr., 377:23 (1986).

122. E. Houghton, M.C. Dumasia, P. Teale, M.S. Moss, and S. Sinkins, J. Chromatogr., 383:1 (1986).

123. P. Kwasowski, I.M.M. Ruutel, J.M. Vernon, and M.A.J. Godfrey, in Residues of Veterinary Drugs in Food, Proc. Euroresidue III Conf., Veldhoven, 1996 (N. Haagsma and A. Ruiter, Eds.), Fac. Vet. Med., Univ. Utrecht, The Netherlands, p. 634 (1996).

124. E. Daeseleire, A. de Guesquiere, and C. van Peteghem, J. Chromatogr., 564:445 (1991).

125. C. van Peteghem, J. Chromatogr., 369:253 (1986).

126. H.H.D. Meyer, F.-X. Hartmann, and M. Rapp, J. Chromatogr., 489:173 (1989).

127. H.H.D. Meyer and L. Rinke, J. Anim. Sci., 69:4538 (1991).

128. M.J. Sauer, R.J. Pickett, S. Limer, and S.N. Dixon, J. Vet. Pharmacol. Ther., 18: 81 (1995).

129. M. Gibaldi, in Biopharmaceutics and Clinical Pharmacokinetics (M. Gibaldi, Ed.), 4th Edition, Lea & Febiger, Philadelphia, PA (1991).

130. Z. Kopitar and A. Zimmer, Arzneim.-Forsch., 26:1450 (1976).

131. P. Delahaut, G. Degand, M. Dubois, P. Schmitz, and G. Maghuin-Rogister, in Residues of Veterinary Drugs in Food, Proc. Euroresidue Conf., Noordwijkerhout, May 21–23, 1990 (N. Haagsma, A. Ruiter, and P.B. Czedik-Eysenberg, Eds.), Fac. Vet. Med., Univ. Utrecht, The Netherlands, p. 149 (1990).

132. D. Boyd, P. Shearan, J.P. Hopkins, M. O'Keefe, and M.R. Smyth, Anal. Chim. Acta, 275:221 (1993).

133. P. Delahaut, M. Dubois, I. Pri-Bar, O. Buchman, G. Degand, and F. Ectors, Food Addit. Contam., 8:43 (1991).

134. I. Yamamoto and K. Iwata, J. Immunoassay, 3:155 (1982).

135. M.J. Sauer, R.J.H. Pickett, and A.L. MacKenzie, Anal. Chim. Acta, 275:195 (1993).

136. H.H.D. Meyer, L. Rinke, and I. Dursch, J. Chromatogr., 564:551 (1991).

137. W. Haasnoot, G. Cazemier, P. Stouten, and A. Kemmers-Voncken, in Residue Analysis in Food Safety: Applications of Immunoassay Methods (R.C. Beier and L.H. Stanker, Eds.), American Chemical Society, Washington, DC, p. 60 (1996).

138. W. Haasnoot, L. Streppel, G. Cazemier, M. Salden, P. Stouten, M. Essers, and P. van Wichen, Analyst, 121:1111 (1996).

139. R.J.H. Pickett and M.J. Sauer, Anal. Chim. Acta, 275:269 (1993).
140. S.D. Bucknall, A.L. MacKenzie, M.J. Sauer, D.J. Everest, R. Newman, and R. Jackman, Anal. Chim. Acta, 275:227 (1993).
141. W. Haasnoot, A.R.M. Hamers, R. Schilt, and C.A. Kan, in Food Safety and Quality Assurance: Applications of Immunoassay Systems (M.R.A. Morgan, C.J. Smith, and P.A. Williams, Eds.), Elsevier Applied Science, London, p. 185 (1992).
142. R.I. McConnell, J.V. Lamont, J. Campbell, and S.P. Fitzerald, in Residues of Veterinary Drugs in Food, Proc. Euroresidue II Conf., Veldhoven, May 3–5, 1993 (N. Haagsma, A. Ruiter, and P.B. Czedik-Eysenberg, Eds.), Fac. Vet. Med., Univ. Utrecht, The Netherlands, p. 485 (1993).
143. R. Sayers, P. Kwasowski, and M. O'Connor, in Residues of Veterinary Drugs in Food, Proc. Euroresidue III Conf., Veldhoven, 1996 (N. Haagsma and A. Ruiter, Eds.), Fac. Vet. Med., Univ. Utrecht, The Netherlands, p. 848 (1996).
144. M.A.J. Godfrey, S.P.L. Anderson, B. Julicher, P. Kwasowski, and M.J. Sauer, in Residues of Veterinary Drugs in Food, Proc. Euroresidue III Conf., Veldhoven, 1996 (N. Haagsma and A. Ruiter, Eds.), Fac. Vet. Med., Univ. Utrecht, The Netherlands, p. 421 (1996).
145. M.D. Osselton, I.C. Shaw, and H.M. Stevens, Analyst, 103:1160 (1978).
146. L. Howells, M. Sauer, R. Sayer, and D. Clark, Anal. Chim. Acta, 275:275 (1993).
147. C.T. Elliott, C.S. Thompson, C.J.M. Arts, S.R.H. Crooks, M.J. van Baak, E.R. Verheij, and G.A. Baxter, Analyst, 123:1103 (1998).
148. A. Lommen, W. Haasnoot, and J.M. Weseman, Food Agric. Immunol., 7:123 (1995).
149. C.T. Elliott, A. Baxter, W. Haasnoot, A. Lommen, and W.J. McCaughey, Food Agric. Immunol., 8:219 (1996).
150. C.M. Zwickl, H.M. Smith, and P.H. Bick, J. Agric. Food Chem., 38:1358 (1990).
151. C. Secchi, P.A. Biondi, A. Berrini, T. Simonic, and S. Ronchi, J. Immunol. Methods, 110:123 (1988).
152. A.W. Meilke, L.G. Lagerquist, and F.H. Tyler, Steroids, 22:193 (1973).
153. L.E. Sing, G. Huttinot, M. Fein, and T.B. Cooper, J. Pharm. Sci., 78:1040 (1989).
154. W. Haasnoot, S. Morais Ezkerro, and H. Keukens, in Residues of Veterinary Drugs in Food, Proc. Euroresidue II Conf., Veldhoven, May 3–5, 1993 (N. Haagsma, A. Ruiter, and P.B. Czedik-Eysenberg, Eds.), Fac. Vet. Med., Univ. Utrecht, The Netherlands, p. 347 (1993).
155. P.H. Delahaut, Y. Colemonts, and M. Dubois, in Residues of Veterinary Drugs in Food, Proc. Euroresidue II Conf., Veldhoven, May 3–5, 1993 (N. Haagsma, A. Ruiter, and P.B. Czedik-Eysenberg, Eds.), Fac. Vet. Med., Univ. Utrecht, The Netherlands, p. 262 (1993).
156. P. Stouten, W. Haasnoot, G. Cazemier, P.L.M. Berende, and H. Keukens, in Residues of Veterinary Drugs in Food, Proc. Euroresidue III Conf., Veldhoven, 1996 (N. Haagsma and A. Ruiter, Eds.), Fac. Vet. Med., Univ. Utrecht, The Netherlands, p. 902 (1996).
157. U. Albrecht, P. Hammer, and W. Heeschen, in Residues of Veterinary Drugs in Food, Proc. Euroresidue III Conf., Veldhoven, 1996 (N. Haagsma and A. Ruiter, Eds.), Fac. Vet. Med., Univ. Utrecht, The Netherlands, p. 194 (1996).

158. M. Gassmann, P. Thommes, T. Weiser, and U. Hubscher, FASEB J., 4:2528 (1990).
159. T. Kitagawa, W. Ohtani, Y. Maeno, K. Fujiwara, and Y. Kimura, J. Assoc. Off. Anal. Chem., 68:661 (1985).
160. T. Kitagawa, T. Kawasaki, and H. Munechika, J. Biochem., 92:585 (1982).
161. K. Fujigawa, M. Yasuno, and T. Kitagawa, J. Immunol. Methods, 45:195 (1981).
162. T. Kitagawa, H. Fujitake, H. Taniyama, and T. Aikawa, J. Biochem., 83:1493 (1978).
163. H. Tanimori, H. Ishikawa, and T. Kitagawa, J. Immunol. Methods, 62:123 (1983).
164. D. Altunkaya and R.N. Smith, Forensic Sci. Int., 39:23 (1988).
165. R. Dixon, Methods Enzymol., 84:490 (1982).
166. J. Lund, Scan. J. Clin. Lab. Invest., 41:275 (1981).
167. O. Beck, P. Lafolie, P. Hjemdahl, S. Borg, G. Odelius, and P. Wirbing, Clin. Chem., 38:271 (1992).
168. A. Fraser, A.F. Isner, and W. Bryan, J. Anal. Toxicol., 17:427 (1993).
169. D. Laurie, A.J. Mason, N.H. Piggot, F.J. Rowell, J. Seviour, D. Strachan, and J.D. Tyson, Analyst, 121:951 (1996).
170. J.R. Bishop, S.E. Duncan, G.M. Jones, and W.D. Whittier, In Report from Virginia Polytechnic Institute and State University, Blackburn, VA (1991).
171. J.J. Ryan, E.E. Wildman, A.H. Duthie, and H.V. Atherton, J. Dairy Sci., 69:1510 (1986).
172. D. Arnold and A. Somogyi, J. Assoc. Off. Anal. Chem., 68:984 (1985).
173. A.K. Boertz, D. Arnold, and A. Somogyi, Z. Ernahrungswiss., 24:113 (1985).
174. F. Scherk and O. Agthe, Arch. Lebensmittelhyg., 37:146 (1986).
175. O. Agthe and F. Scherk, Arch. Lebensmittelhyg., 37:97 (1986).
176. G. Knupp, G. Bugl-Kreickmann, and C. Commichau, Z. Lebensm. Unters. Forsch., 184:390 (1987).
177. D.E. Dixon-Holland and S.E. Katz, J. Assoc. Off. Anal. Chem., 71:1137 (1988).
178. D.E. Dixon-Holland and S.E. Katz, J. Assoc. Off. Anal. Chem., 72:447 (1989).
179. H.B. Sheth and P. Sporns, J. Assoc. Off. Anal. Chem., 73:871 (1990).
180. K. Vogt, Arch. Lebensmittelhyg., 31:117 (1980).
181. B. Hoffmann and W. Laschutza, Arch. Lebensmittelhyg., 31:77 (1980).
182. C.H. van Peteghem and G.H. van Haver, Anal. Chim. Acta, 182:293 (1986).
183. M. O'Keeffe and J.P. Hopkins, J. Chromatogr., 489:199 (1989).
184. J.C. Gridley, E.H. Allen, and W. Shimoda, J. Agric. Food Chem., 31:292 (1983).
185. D.J. Harwood, R.J. Heitzman, and A. Jouquey, J. Vet. Pharmacol. Therap., 3:945 (1980).
186. M. Rapp and H.H.D. Meyer, Food Addit. Contam., 6:59 (1989).
187. C.H. van Peteghem, L. van Look, and A. de Guesquiere, J. Chromatogr., 489:219 (1989).
188. H.H.D. Meyer, F.-X. Hartman, and M. Rapp, J. Chromatogr., 489:173 (1989).
189. K. Vogt, Arch. Lebensmittelhyg., 35:136 (1984).
190. J.P. Duchatel, P. Evrard, and G. Maghuin-Rogister, Ann. Med. Vet., 126:147 (1982).
191. M. O'Keeffe, Brit. Vet. J., 140:592 (1984).
192. S.N. Dixon and K.L. Russell, J. Vet. Pharmacol. Therap., 9:94 (1986).

193. J. Rosen, K.-E. Hellenas, P. Tornqvist, and P. Shearan, Analyst, 119:2635 (1994).
194. H.H.D. Meyer, Arch. Lebensmittelhyg., 41:4 (1990).
195. W. Haasnoot, A.R.M. Hamers, G.D. van Bruchen, R. Schilt, and L.M.H. Frijns, in Food Safety and Quality Assurance: Applications of Immunoassay Systems (M.R.A. Morgan, C.J. Smith, and P.A. Williams, Eds.), Elsevier Applied Science, London, p.237 (1992).

:

29

Physicochemical Methods

Microbiological and immunochemical procedures are designed for screening purposes, whereas physicochemical methods are used primarily for the isolation, separation, quantification, and confirmation of the presence of violative residues in samples. This requires that the sensitivity of the screening method and the determinative or confirmatory method be compatible. To reach this target, numerous physicochemical procedures based on almost any aspect of analytical principle have been developed. Although the chemical structure of a drug largely dictates the most suitable method for its determination, different procedures have been suggested for the same analyte because of the large number of possibilities that physicochemical procedures afford. Available methods within the groups of aminoglycosides and aminocyclitols, amphenicols, β-lactam antibiotics, macrolides and lincosamides, nitrofuran antibacterials, quinolones, sulfonamides and diaminopyrimidine potentiators, tetracyclines, miscellaneous antibacterials, anthelminthic drugs, anticoccidial and other antiprotozoal drugs, antimicrobial growth promoters, anabolic hormonal-type growth promoters, β-adrenergic agonists, dye drugs, sedatives and β-blockers, corticosteroids, diuretic and nonsteroidal anti-inflammatory drugs, and thyreostatic drugs, are discussed below.

29.1 AMINOGLYCOSIDES AND AMINOCYCLITOLS

Aminoglycosides are water-soluble, not volatile, heat-resistant, and highly polar compounds. Structurally, aminoglycosides are polybasic cations consisting of two or more sugars, usually aminosugars, attached to an aminocyclitol ring with glycoside linkages. They are stable at both high and low pH values, but should be handled in plastic lab ware since they have the tendency to bind onto glass surfaces.

Most aminoglycosides consist of several almost identical components differing either in the degree of methylation of one amino sugar unit, as in the case of gentamicin, or in the stereochemistry of the disaccharide unit, as in the case of neomycin. Owing to this structure, any aminoglycoside contains more than one closely related component in its formulations. Another complicating factor in the analysis of aminoglycosides is that the molecules of these compounds lack useful chromophore or fluorophor functions. Detection by modern instrumental techniques requires often suitable derivatization. These inherent characteristics have made aminoglycosides a particularly difficult group of antibiotics to analyze by physicochemical methods.

For liquid matrices such as milk, a pretreatment step for fat removal that is accomplished by centrifugation (1–3) or hexane extraction (4) may be required. Solid samples such as muscle, kidney, and liver necessitate usually more intensive sample pretreatment through use of a mincing and/or a homogenizing apparatus. In some cases, as in the analysis of apramycin in swine kidney tissue, protein digestion with concentrated ammonium hydroxide may be needed to achieve better recovery of the analyte from the matrix (5).

In general, an efficient extraction procedure of aminoglycoside residues from food matrices must be able to remove most if not all of the proteins from the sample extract, rendering, concurrently, residues that are bound to proteins soluble, and providing high yields for all analytes. High or low pH conditions have all been successfully employed to free aminoglycoside residues from proteins and keep them in solution. Extraction/deproteinization has been performed by either vortexing liquid samples or homogenizing solid samples with trichloroacetic acid (1–3, 6–8), trifluoroacetic acid (9), perchloric acid (10, 11), trichloroacetic acid/ citrate buffer (12, 13), or methanol/hydrochloric acid (14). Extraction under alkaline conditions has also been employed for the determination of apramycin in swine kidney using methanol/ammonium hydroxide as an extraction solvent (5). Extraction of food samples with alkaline buffers followed by heat deproteinization has been suggested as another effective means to extract and purify extracts for aminoglycoside analysis (15–17).

In most published methods, the primary sample extracts are subjected to various types of cleanup procedures including conventional liquid–liquid partitioning, solid-phase extraction, matrix solid-phase dispersion, and online trace enrichment. In many cases, some of these procedures are used in combination in order to help obtaining highly purified extracts.

Liquid–liquid partitioning cleanup is generally directed to the transfer of the matrix components from the aqueous into the organic immiscible phase (3, 5–7). Owing to their high polarity, aminoglycosides cannot be recovered into the organic phase at any pH value, remaining in the aqueous phase. There has been, however, a case in which a 90% recovery of apramycin into the ethyl acetate phase was noted when octanesulfonic acid, an ion-pairing reagent, was added in the extraction medium (5).

Removal of proteins and other matrix constituents from sample extracts can also be accomplished using solid-phase extraction columns. The highly polar nature of the aminoglycosides dictates that use of cation-exchange sorbents should be the best choice for such a procedure. Hence, solid-phase extraction columns packed with cation-exchange materials such as CM-Sephadex C-25 (8, 17), Amberlite CG-50 (18), aromatic sulfonic acid (10), and carboxylic acid (12, 13) have all been widely used for isolation and/or cleanup of these antibiotics. Cleanup and concentration of aminoglycosides from coextracted materials have also been accomplished using normal- (17) or reversed-phase (2, 6, 7) sorbents, the later being especially applied under ion-pairing conditions using heptanesulfonic acid as the ion-pairing reagent to enhance the retention of the analytes onto the hydrophobic C_{18} materials (6, 7).

Matrix solid-phase dispersion techniques have also been suggested for the determination of aminoglycoside residues in bovine tissues (19, 20). The solid-phase material employed in these methods was a cyanopropylsilyl (CN) sorbent.

More convenient online trace enrichment techniques have further been described for purification of aminoglycoside residues from matrix constituents (10, 11). These techniques involve trapping of the streptomycin and dihydrostreptomycin residues onto a liquid chromatographic (LC) precolumn (Inertsil C_8) under ion-pair conditions, rinsing of the coextracted materials to waste, and, finally, flushing of the concentrated analytes onto the analytical column. In a somewhat different approach, an initial acidic mobile phase has been suggested to trap the coextracted materials on a cation-exchange precolumn; the nonretained spectinomycin residues were directed to the analytical column using a second mobile phase (13).

Following extraction and cleanup, aminoglycoside residues must be submitted to some kind of chromatographic separation followed by fluorometric, electrochemical, polarimetric, or mass spectrometric detection. By combining a thin-layer chromatographic (TLC) separation with a bioassay (*B. subtilis*) detection, a TLC/bioautographic technique was developed that was capable to identify several antibiotic residues, including aminoglycosides, in animal tissues (14). However, this technique lacked the sensitivity required to detect aminoglycosides at the low ppb residues levels likely to occur in tissues and milk.

LC separations of aminoglycosides have been generally carried out using both cation-exchange and nonpolar reversed-phase columns (Table 29.1). Owing to their high polarity, aminoglycosides can be easily separated on cation-exchange columns, but are poorly retained on reversed-phase columns. However, addition of ion-pairing reagents such as alkyl sulfonates (1–3, 6–8, 10, 11, 15, 16) or pentafluoropropionic acid (19, 20) in the mobile phase, can increase the retention

TABLE 29.1 Physicochemical Methods for Aminoglycoside and Aminocyclitol Antibacterials in Edible Animal Products

Antibacterial(s)	Matrix	Sample preparation	Steps	Stationary phase	Mobile phase	Detection/Identification	Sensitivity/Recovery	Ref.
THIN-LAYER CHROMATOGRAPHIC METHODS								
Four amino-glycosides	Animal tissues	MeOH cleanup, MeOH/HCl extn	15	Silica gel or cellulose	BuOH/MeOH/HOAc/H$_2$O or Acetone/CHCl$_3$/PrOH/0.01N phthalate buffer/glycerine	B. subtilis bioautography	30–200 ppm/ NR	14
LIQUID CHROMATOGRAPHIC METHODS								
Apramycin	Swine kidney	NH$_4$OH digestion, MeOH extn, ion-pair extn, liq–liq partns, on-line precolumn derivatization with OPA	13	Nova-Pak C$_{18}$, 5 μm	H$_2$O/ACN/HOAc (60:40:2) contg 5mM octanesulfonic acid	Fluorometric, ex: 230 nm, em: 389 nm/ MS-ISP after mobile phase modification	500 ppb/ 76–86%	5
Dihydro-streptomycin	Kidney and meat	TCA extn, liq–liq partn, SPE cleanup, liq–liq partn, 1-heptanesulfonic acid addn	27	Supelcosil LC-ABZ, 5 μm, analytical and guard column	0.04M octanesulfonic acid in 0.4mM NQS, pH 3.24/ ACN (68:32), at 31°C	Fluorometric, postcolumn derivatization with NQS, ex: 375 nm, em: 420 nm	40 ppb/ 73–83%	7

Milk	TCA extn, liq–liq partn, SPE cleanup, liq–liq partn, 1-heptanesulfonic acid addn	17	Supelcosil LC-ABZ, 5 μm, analytical and guard column	Solvent A: 0.04M octanesulfonic acid, 0.02M ethanedsulfonic acid, 0.005M ninhydrin, pH 3.2 Solvent B: 0.3% TEA in ACN Solvent C: MeOH (63:19:18)	Fluorometric, postcolumn derivatization with ninhydrin, ex: 305 nm, em: 500 nm	25 ppb/ 83 ± 1.2%	6
Gentamicin Bovine tissues	Phosp. buffer, pH 8.8, extn, heat deprtn, CM-Sephadex C-25 column cleanup, SPE cleanup, precolumn derivatization with OPA	32	Ultremex C$_{18}$, 5 μm	Solvent A: MeOH/H$_2$O/HOAc (70:29:1) contg 0.5% heptanesulfonic acid Solvent B: MeOH Concave gradient from (80:20) to (40:60)	Fluorometric, ex: 340 nm, em: ?	200 ppb/ 69–107%	17

(continued)

TABLE 29.1 Continued

Antibacterial(s)	Matrix	Sample preparation	Steps	Stationary phase	Mobile phase	Detection/ Identification	Sensitivity/ Recovery	Ref.
	Bovine tissues	TCA/EDTA extn, CM-Sephadex C-25 column cleanup, camphorsulphonate addn	11	LiChrospher 100 RP-18, 5 μm analytical and guard column	0.05M sodium dl-camphor-10-sulfonate in 0.1mM EDTA, pH 2.2/MeOH (45:55), at 45°C	Fluorometric, postcolumn derivatization with OPA, ex: 340 nm, em: 440 nm	50–100 ppb/ 68–98%	8
	Milk	Centrgn, TCA extn, SPE cleanup, pentanesulfonic acid addn	11	Spherisorb ODS-2, 5 μm, analytical and guard column	H_2O/MeOH (82:18), contg 5.6mM Na_2SO_4, 0.1% HOAc, and 11 mM pentanesulfonic acid	Fluorometric, postcolumn derivatization with OPA, ex: 340 nm, em: 430 nm	15 ppb/ 72–88%	2
	Milk	TFA extn	3	RP C_{18}, 10 μm	0.4M TFA, pH 5.5/MeOH (80:20)	Laser-based polarimetric	NR/>90%	9

Milk	Phosp. buffer, pH 6.5, diln, liq–liq partn, SPE cleanup, on-line precolumn derivatization with OPA	10	Novapak C$_{18}$, 4 µm	Solvent A: 15mM sodium heptane-sulfonate/ MeOH, pH 3.7 (35:65) Solvent B: 15mM sodium heptane-sulfonate/ MeOH, pH 3.7 (25:75) Gradient from (100:0) to (0:100)	Fluorometric, ex: 365 nm, em: 415 nm	20 ppb/ 64%	4
Neomycin	Animal tissues	Buffer, pH 8.0, extn, heat deprtn, acidfn, centrgn	10	Supelcosil LC-8-DB or LC-18-DB, or Spherisorb ODS-2, 5 µm, with Supelguard LC-8-DB, 5 µm, or LiChrosorb RP-18, 10 µm, guard column	H$_2$O/MeOH (98.5:1.5 or 97:3), contg 0.056M Na$_2$SO$_4$, 0.007M HOAc, and 10 mM 1-pentane-sulfonate	Fluorometric, postcolumn derivatization with OPA, ex: 340 nm, em: 455 nm/ Peak height ratios	1 ppm/ 60–110%	15

(continued)

TABLE 29.1 Continued

Antibacterial(s)	Matrix	Sample preparation	Steps	Stationary phase	Mobile phase	Detection/ Identification	Sensitivity/ Recovery	Ref.
	Milk	Centrgn, TCA extn, 1-pentanesulfonic acid addn	4	Supelcosil LC-8-DB, 5 μm, with supelguard LC-8-DB, 5 μm guard column	H_2O/MeOH (98.5:1.5), contg 0.056M Na_2SO_4, 0.007M HOAc, and 10 mM 1-pentane-sulfonate, at 32.5°C	Fluorimetric, postcolumn derivatization with OPA, ex: 340 nm, em: 455 nm	150 ppb/ 76–110%	1
	Milk	CG-50 Amberlite column cleanup, precolumn derivatization with OPA	6	Hisep, 5 μm	Solvent A: MeOH/0.2% EDTA (70:30) Solvent B: MeOH Concave gradient from (100:0) to (40:60)	Fluorometric, ex: 340 nm, em: ?	50 ppb/ 87–109%	18

Analyte	Matrix	Sample preparation		Column	Mobile phase	Detection	LOD/recovery	Ref.
	Bovine kidney	Buffer, pH 8.0, extn, heat deprtn, acidfn, centrgn, 1-pentanesulfonic acid addn	11	Spherisorb 5 ODS-2, analytical and guard column	H_2O/MeOH/HOAc (88.4:11.5:0.1) contg 0.01M Na_2SO_4 and 10 mM 1-pentane-sulfonate, at 35°C	Fluorometric, postcolumn derivatization with OPA, ex: 340 nm, em: 440 nm	500 ppb/80–115%	16
Spectinomycin	Animal tissues, eggs	Citrate/TCA/DCM extn, SPE cleanup, on-line cleanup on Spherisorb SCX, 5 μm, (eggs) or Ionospher C, 5 μm, (tissues) column and switching to analytical column	14	Spherisorb SCX, 5 μm	0.15M, pH 3.5, phosp. buffer/ACN (80:20)	Fluorometric, postcolumn derivatization with OPA, ex: 340 nm, em: 460 nm	50 ppb/74–97%	13
	Bovine tissues	Citrate/TCA/DCM extn, SPE cleanup	12	Crompack Ionosphere C	Na_2SO_4/ACN (80:20) Ionic gradient from 80% 0.05M Na_2SO_4 to 55% 0.05M/25% 0.05M Na_2SO_4 0.5M Na_2SO_4	Fluorometric, postcolumn derivatization with OPA, ex: 340 nm, em: 455 nm	100 ppb/81–94%	12
				Zorbax SB C_{18}	1% HOAc/MeOH (92:8)	MS-MS-APCI		

(continued)

TABLE 29.1 Continued

Antibacterial(s)	Matrix	Sample preparation	Steps	Stationary phase	Mobile phase	Detection/ Identification	Sensitivity/ Recovery	Ref.
	Milk	Centrgn, TCA extn, liq–liq partns, 1-decanesulfonic acid addn	15	Ultracarb ODS-2, 5 μm, analytical and guard column	0.02M citric acid contg 2mM 1-decanesulfonic acid, pH 6.1/ ACN (84:16), at 30°C	Electro-chemical	50 ppb/ 76–80%	3
Streptomycin, dihydro-streptomycin	Animal tissues	HClO$_4$ extn, SPE cleanup, 1-hexanesulfonic acid addn, on-line trace enrichment on Inertsil C$_8$, 5 μm, preconcn column and switching to analytical column	7	Supelcosil LC-8-DB, 5 μm	H$_2$O/ACN (83:17) contg 10 mM 1-hexanesulfonic acid and 0.4 mM NQS, pH 3.3	Fluorometric, postcolumn derivatization with NQS, ex: 347 nm, em: 418 nm	10–20 ppb/ 46–72%	10
	Milk	HClO$_4$ extn, 1-hexanesulfonic acid addn, on-line trace enrichment on Inertsil C$_8$, 5 μm, preconcn column and switching to analytical column	3	Supelcosil LC-8-DB, 5 μm	H$_2$O/ACN (83:17) contg 10 mM 1-hexanesulfonic acid and 0.4 mM NQS, pH 3.3	Fluorometric, postcolumn derivatization with NQS, ex: 365 nm, em: 418 nm	10–20 ppb/ 33–65%	11

Analyte	Matrix	Sample preparation		Column	Mobile phase	Detection	Limits/recovery	Ref.
Streptomycin, dihydro-streptomycin, spectinomycin, hygromycin B	Bovine tissues	MSPD extn/ cleanup	10	Spherisorb ODS-2, 3 or 5 μm with 3 μm guard column	H$_2$O/ACN (92:8) contg 20 mM pentafluoro-propionic acid, pH 1.9	Electro-chemical, or MS-ISP	2.5 ppm/ NR	19
Six amino-glycosides	Bovine kidney	MSPD extn/ cleanup, pentafluoro-propionic acid addn	12	Spherisorb ODS-2, 5 μm with 3 μm guard column	Solvent A: H$_2$O/ ACN (40:60) contg 20 mM pentafluoro-propionic acid Solvent B: H$_2$O/ ACN (95:5) contg 20 mM pentafluoro-propionic acid Step gradient from (0:100) to (100:0)	MS-MS-ISP	30–520 ppb/ 46–75%	20

OPA, o-phthalaldehyde; NQS, β-naphthoquinone-4-sulfonate; ex, excitation; em, emission; ISP, Ionspray; APCI, atmospheric pressure chemical ionization; MSPD, matrix solid-phase dispersion; SPE, solid-phase extraction; deprtn, deproteinization; acidfn, acidification; RP, reversed phase; NR, not reported. Other abbreviations as in Table 20.2.

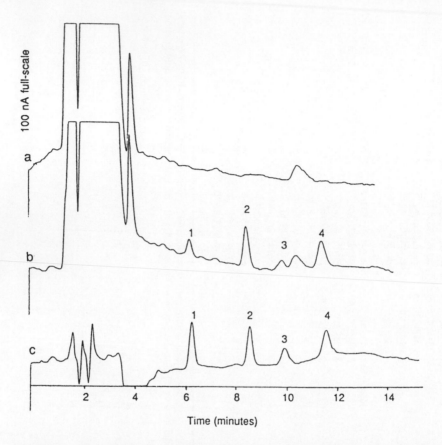

FIG. 29.1   HPLC-PDA of (a) MSPD extract of control bovine kidney, (b) MSPD extract of bovine kidney fortified at the 20 ppm level, and (c) synthetic mixture of standards at levels of 15 ng per component injected. Peaks: 1, spectinomycin; 2, hygromycin B; 3, streptomycin; 4, dihydrostreptomycin. (Reprinted from Ref. 19 with permission from Elsevier Science.)

of aminoglycosides, thus allowing use of reversed-phase columns (Fig. 29.1). Precolumn derivatization of aminoglycosides, on the other hand, can produce lower-polarity compounds that are easily separated on reversed-phase columns, without the addition of ion-pairing reagents. Nevertheless, ion-pairing reagents have often been employed in order to alter the retention and improve the peak shape of the derivatized compounds (4, 5, 17).

A protein exclusion column (Hisep) that separates proteins from the analyte has also been proposed to analyze neomycin residues in milk (18). Using this column, neomycin penetrated into the polymeric surface during elution, while proteins passed through the column unretained.

The separation mechanism in the LC analysis of aminoglycosides is usually highly dependent on the applied derivatization technique, either precolumn or postcolumn. This is due to the fact that a prerequisite of aminoglycosides analysis is most often suitable derivatization to produce fluorescent derivatives; the presence of primary amine groups in most of the aminoglycoside antibiotics enables a number of derivatives to be readily formed.

The most common derivatizing reagent in aminoglycosides analysis is *o*-phthaladehyde (OPA). This reagent can be used either in the precolumn or postcolumn mode, with the derivative monitored by fluorescence detection. For precolumn derivatization, the reaction can be conducted in solution (4, 5), or oncolumn if the analytes have previously been trapped to ion-exchange (18) or silica (17) solid-phase materials during sample cleanup. Postcolumn derivatization requires a postcolumn reaction unit or a separate reagent pump, a mixing tee, and a reaction coil (1, 2, 8, 12, 13, 15, 16). For the streptidine-based aminoglycosides including streptomycin and dihydrostreptomycin, derivatization takes place at the guanidino functions, so standard primary amine-derivatizing reagents are not suitable in that case. Thus, β-naphthoquinone-4-sulfonate (NQS) (7, 10, 11) or ninhydrin (6) reagents have been used in the postcolumn mode to produce fluorescent derivatives of those residues in milk and tissue samples.

A promising fluorescence method in terms of simplicity, selectivity, and sensitivity has been described by Kijak et al. (2) for screening and even confirmation of the four major components of gentamicin in milk. According to this method, milk sample (10 ml) is centrifuged at 4°C, the top fat layer is removed, and the defatted sample is deproteinized by mixing with 1 ml 30% trichloroacetic acid. After centrifugation, the supernatant is passed through a C_{18} solid-phase extraction column. Following successive column washing with water, water/methanol (1:1) and methanol, gentamicin is eluted with 16% ammonium hydroxide in methanol. The eluate is evaporated to near dryness and taken up with water. An aliquot of the sample is then mixed with the ion-pairing pentanesulfonic acid to be further analyzed by liquid chromatography. Separation is performed on a 15-cm Spherisorb ODS2 (5 μm) analytical column protected by a guard column with the same packing material. Using a water-methanol (82:18) mobile phase that contained 0.1% acetic acid, 5.6 mM sodium sulfate, and 11 mM pentanesulfonic acid, total concentrations of the four components down to 15 ppb could be determined after postcolumn derivatization with *o*-phthalaldehyde and fluorometric detection.

Electrochemical detection has also been suggested for determination of underivatized aminoglycosides in edible animal products (3, 19), while laser-based polarimetric detection has also been used in the analysis of underivatized gentamicin in milk (9). Liquid chromatography combined with mass spectrometry has been reported to be particularly suited for analyzing aminoglycoside residues in foods. Typical applications of mass spectrometric detection in confirming the presence of aminoglycoside residues in edible animal products include interfacing liquid chromatography with mass spectrometry via ionspray (5, 19, 20) or atmospheric-pressure chemical ionization (12).

A different approach was followed by McLaughlin et al. (20) in a liquid chromatographic multiresidue method for the determination of streptomycin, dihydrostreptomycin, neomycin B, the four major components of the gentamicin complex, hygromycin B, and spectinomycin in bovine kidney, using ionspray mass spectrometric detection. According to this confirmatory method, the tissue homogenate (0.5 g) is mixed with 2 g cyanopropyl packing material (Bondesil cyanopropyl, 40 μm) and the resulting mixture is transferred onto a solid-phase extraction column. The column is successively washed with hexane, ethyl acetate, methanol, and methanol/water (1 : 1), and the analytes are eluted with water followed by 0.1 M formic acid or 0.1 N sulfuric acid. The eluate is filtered, concentrated, and a solution containing 100 mM pentafluoropropionic acid is then added. The resulting mixture is filtered, and an aliquot is analyzed by liquid chromatography. Separation is performed under the conditions shown in Table 29.1, on a 10 cm Spherisorb ODS2 (5 μm) analytical column protected by a guard column with the same packing material. Concentrations as low as 60 ppb for neomycin B, 30 ppb for the gentamicin complex, 100 ppb for dihydrostreptomycin, 130 ppb for streptomycin, 340 ppb for hygromycin B, and 520 ppb for spectinomycin could be readily detected using ionspray tandem mass spectrometric detection.

29.2 AMPHENICOLS

Major drugs within the group of amphenicols are chloramphenicol, thiamphenicol, and florfenicol. They are all synthetic, highly polar compounds with comparable chemical structures. In thiamphenicol, the *p*-nitro group on the benzene ring of chloramphenicol is replaced with a methyl sulfonyl group. In florfenicol, the hydroxyl group on the side chain of thiamphenicol is replaced with a fluorine. Amphenicols are light-stable compounds that also exhibit remarkable stability upon storage.

For analyzing amphenicol residues in liquid samples such as milk, a pretreatment centrifugation step for fat removal is usually required (21, 22). Dilution of milk samples with water prior to solid-phase extraction cleanup is also often needed (23, 24). Semisolid samples such as muscle, kidney and liver, require, however, more intensive sample pretreatment. The most popular approach for tissue break-up is through use of a mincing and/or a homogenizing apparatus.

Following pretreatment, samples can be further treated with β-glucuronidase (25–27) to achieve hydrolysis of conjugated chloramphenicol residues. It has been reported (28) that more than one-half of the total chloramphenicol residues present in liver and kidney from treated swine occur in conjugated form. However, conjugated residues are not detected in muscles of swine, chicken, and calf (26).

Sample extraction/deproteinization is usually accomplished by vortexing liquid samples or homogenizing semisolid samples with ethyl acetate (23, 25–27, 29–46). Extraction of amphenicols with acetonitrile (47–57) or water (22, 26, 58–61) has been also reported, but the recoveries observed in those instances were not as high as with ethyl acetate, making the latter solvent most suitable for extracting all three amphenicols. Additionally, organic and inorganic solvents including acetone (62), methanol (14), diethyl ether (63), isopentyl acetate (64), trichloroacetic acid (22), pH-7.8 phosphate buffer (65), and urea solution (46) have all been successfully used for extraction of amphenicols from edible animal products.

Following initial sample extraction, the primary extract must frequently be subjected to some kind of further cleanup including liquid–liquid partitioning, diphasic dialysis, solid-phase extraction, matrix solid-phase dispersion, immunoaffinity chromatography cleanup, liquid chromatography cleanup, or online trace enrichment. In some instances, some of these procedures are used in combination in order to attain higher purification levels.

Liquid–liquid partitioning targets either to extract the drugs from their aqueous solutions with an organic solvent or to wash out interfering substances from organic or aqueous drug solutions. Ethyl acetate has been found more effective than any other organic solvent tested in extracting all three drugs from their aqueous solutions (21, 31–33, 35, 36, 40, 45, 48, 50, 53, 59). Occasionally, addition of sodium chloride in the aqueous drug solution at a final concentration of 3–4% is sufficient to increase the extraction efficiency of the ethyl acetate, especially for the more polar thiamphenicol and florfenicol (33, 35, 45, 50).

To remove lipids, sample extracts are frequently also partitioned with n-hexane (25, 33–35, 37, 40, 43, 45, 47, 49, 50, 53–57, 62), petroleum ether (31, 38, 63), isooctane (36, 41, 48), or toluene (26, 58, 59, 61). Use of n-toluene is not recommended, however, in chloramphenicol and florfenicol analysis, because these drugs have the tendency to transfer into toluene to some extent during the partitioning process. As an alternative to the classic liquid–liquid partitioning cleanup, some workers in the field (24, 26, 34, 58, 59) have suggested use of diatomaceous earth columns as another option of a liquid–liquid partitioning process that offers substantial reduction in emulsification problems and, thus, allows a high recovery increase.

Direct elimination of proteins and other matrix constituents from food samples can also be accomplished with matrix solid-phase dispersion or diphasic dialysis membrane techniques. A matrix solid-phase dispersion technique was used for the determination of chloramphenicol in meat (66) and milk (67) using

C_{18} derivatized silica as the sorbent, while a diphasic dialysis membrane procedure was employed for the isolation of chloramphenicol residues from milk constituents using ethyl acetate as the extraction solvent (68).

Solid-phase extraction techniques that are based mostly on reversed-phase (C_{18}) sorbents, have been also widely used for cleanup and concentration purposes (23, 25, 27, 31, 34, 37, 46, 51, 52, 55, 65). However, many applications have indicated that cleanup using these nonpolar materials may not be very effective in removing interfering substances from sample extracts. Hence, polar sorbents such as silica (23, 26, 29, 30, 32, 40, 42, 44, 52, 53) or Florisil (45) have been also suggested as more powerful alternatives for the isolation and/or cleanup of amphenicols.

Higher-specificity techniques such as immunoaffinity chromatography have been also found widespread acceptance for the determination of chloramphenicol residues in edible animal products. The first pertinent reports concerned the determination of chloramphenicol residues in swine muscle (60) and milk and eggs (21). Alternative immunoaffinity chromatography procedures were suggested later for extraction/preconcentration of chloramphenicol residues from swine tissues (50), or for online immunoaffinity extraction for the determination of chloramphenicol in milk and swine muscle by an automated column-switching system (22).

Liquid chromatography cleanup on a LiChrosorb Diol column has been further proposed for the offline purification of chloramphenicol residues from bovine muscle and eggs (32). An online approach based on reversed-phase principles has also been described for isolation of chloramphenicol residues from swine kidney by an automated column switching system (63). Use of a protein exclusion column (Hisep) has been also suggested in an online trace-enrichment method for the determination of chloramphenicol in animal tissues (52). By employing a column-switching system, all chloramphenicol that eluted from the protein exclusion column was trapped at the entry of a 5 μm Supelcosil LC-18 preconcentration column, to be subsequently back-flashed into the analytical column.

Following extraction/cleanup, amphenicols can be separated by thin-layer, liquid, or gas chromatography and measured by spectrophotometric, electron capture, or mass spectrometric detectors (Table 29.2).

In thin-layer chromatographic methods, chloramphenicol is separated using various mobile phases to be subsequently detected visually on the basis of either its yellow–green native color, or the fluorescent derivative formed after spraying with fluorescamine and examining the plate under 366 nm UV light (29, 30). Detection of the chloramphenicol spots can also be carried out by bioautography using *Bacillus subtilis* as the test organism (14). These methods, in general, do not offer the accuracy, reproducibility, and sensitivity characteristics required to detect the low ppb levels likely to occur in food of animal origin.

TABLE 29.2 Physicochemical Methods for Amphenicol Residues in Edible Animal Products

Antibacterial(s)	Matrix	Sample preparation	Steps	Stationary phase	Mobile phase	Detection/ Identification	Sensitivity/ Recovery	Ref.
THIN-LAYER CHROMATOGRAPHIC METHODS								
Chloram- phenicol	Animal tissues	MeOH extn, liq–liq partns	14	Silica gel	CHCl₃/MeOH/ acetone/ glycerine	*B. subtilis* bioauto- graphy	1–2 ppm/ NR	14
	Meat	EtOAc extn, SPE cleanup	10	HPTLC silica gel	EtOAc/hexane	UV-Vis 366 nm after fluorescamine reduction	10 ppb/NR	29
	Swine muscle	EtOAc extn, SPE cleanup	9	Silica gel	PrOH/hexane	UV-Vis 366 nm after fluorescamine reduction	10 ppb/NR	30
GAS CHROMATOGRAPHIC METHODS								
Chloram- phenicol	Animal tissues	EtOAc extn, liq–liq partns, SPE cleanup, TMS derivative	16	Gas-Chrom Q with 3% OV-1	Nitrogen	ECD/CI-MS	<5 ppb/ 52–68%	31
	Bovine muscle	β-Glucuronidase hydrolysis, EtOAc extn, liq–liq partn, SPE cleanup, TMS derivative	24	25 m capillary coated with OV-1	Helium	ECD/NICI- MS	0.6 ppb/ NR	25

(continued)

TABLE 29.2 Continued

Antibacterial(s)	Matrix	Sample preparation	Steps	Stationary phase	Mobile phase	Detection/ Identification	Sensitivity/ Recovery	Ref.
	Bovine muscle, eggs	EtOAc extn, SPE cleanup, liq–liq partns, LC purification on LiChrosorb Diol, 5 μm, column, TMS derivative	16	CP-Sil-19CB, 25 m, capillary	Helium	NICI-MS	0.1 ppb/ NR	32
	Eggs	EtOAc extn, liq–liq partns, TMS derivative	27	DB-1701, 30 m, capillary	Argon/methane	ECD	0.5 ppb/ 73–92%	33
	Eggs	ACN extn, liq–liq partns, Carbopack BHT column cleanup, di-TMS derivative	16	HP, 25 m, capillary, coated with methyl silicone	Hydrogen	ECD	0.1 ppb/ 80%	47
	Milk	EtOAc extn, Kieselguhr column cleanup, liq–liq partn, SPE cleanup, TMS derivative	14	DB-1, 30 m, capillary, coated with methyl silicone	Helium	NICI-MS	0.5 ppb/ NR	34
	Milk	ACN extn, liq–liq partns, HFBA derivative	16	Supelcoport AW DMCS with 3% Dexsil 300	Nitrogen	ECD	50 ppb/ 81%	48
	Milk, meat, eggs	ACN extn, liq–liq partns, Kieselgel-SC column cleanup, TMS derivative	17	DB17, 50 m, capillary coated with Se-30 or Se-30:Se-52	Nitrogen	ECD	1 ppb/NR	49

	Matrix	Sample preparation		Column	Carrier gas	Detection	LOD/Recovery	
	Shrimp	EtOAc extn, liq–liq partns, TMS derivative	24	Supelcoport with 3% OV-7 or HP-5, 25 m, capillary coated with 5% phenyl methyl silicone	Argon/methane or helium	ECD	1–5 ppb/92–116%	35
	Swine tissues	ACN-4% NaCl extn, liq–liq partns, IAC cleanup, liq–liq partns, TMS derivative	19	CB-5, 25 m, capillary	Argon/methane	ECD	0.2–2 ppb/54–96%	50
	Swine tissues	Isopentyl acetate extn, TMS derivative	5	Chromosorb W AW DMCS with 3% OV-1	Nitrogen	ECD	10 ppb/NR	64
Chloramphenicol, florfenicol, thiamphenicol	Milk	ACN extn, SPE cleanup, TMS derivatives	13	HP-5, 25 m, capillary coated with 5% phenyl methyl silicone	Helium	ECD	5 ppb/92–104%	51
LIQUID CHROMATOGRAPHIC METHODS								
Chloramphenicol	Animal tissues	EtOAt extn, liq–liq partns	12	Spherisorb C_{18} CDS, 5 μm	H_2O/MeOH (65:35)	UV 280 nm/GC-EI-MS	10 ppb/68–81%	36
	Animal tissues	β-Glucuronidase hydrolysis, EtOAc extn, liq–liq partn, SPE cleanup	14	Merck RP-18, 5 μm	H_2O/MeOH (60:40) or (65:35), contg 0.01% K_2HPO_4, at 35°C	UV 278 nm	10 ppb/45–68%	27

(continued)

TABLE 29.2 Continued

Antibacterial(s)	Matrix	Sample preparation	Steps	Stationary phase	Mobile phase	Detection/ Identification	Sensitivity/ Recovery	Ref.
	Animal tissues	*Screening:* H_2O extn, Kieselguhr column cleanup, liq–liq partn	8	Cp™Spher C_{18}, 8 μm, with Bondapak C_{18} guard column	0.01M, pH 4.3, acetate buffer/ ACN (71:29)	UV 278 nm/ PDA (225–400 nm)	5 ppb/ 58 ± 6%	26
		Confirmation: β-Glucuronidase hydrolysis, EtOAc extn, SPE cleanup, liq–liq partns	12				10 ppb/ 85 ± 5%	
	Animal tissues	60°C drying, ACN extn, two SPE cleanups, online cleanup on LC-HISEP, 5 μm, column, trace enrichment on Supelcosil LC-18, 5 μm, preconcn column and switching to analytical column	21	Supelcosil LC-18, 5 μm,	H_2O/ACN/THF (18:80:2)	UV 278 nm	2 ppb/ 74–113%	52
	Animal tissues	EtOAc extn, liq–liq partn, SPE cleanup	12	Supelcosil LC-18-DB, 5 μm, with Supelguard LC-18-DB column	0.2M acetate buffer/ACN (75:25), pH 3.0, at 40°C	UV 280 nm/ PDA	5 ppb/ 90–100%	37

Matrix		Sample preparation	Column	Mobile phase	Detection	Limit/Recovery	Ref.
Animal tissues, milk	10	*Tissues:* Piperonyl butoxide addn, EtOAc extn, SPE cleanup	LiChrosorb RP-18, 5 μm	H₂O/ACN (65:35), contg 0.1M ammonium acetate	NICI-MS-TSP	1 ppb/ 80–102%	23
	3	*Milk:* H₂O diln, SPE cleanup				2 ppb/ 81–90%	
Animal and fish muscle	9	EtOAc extn, liq–liq partns	Two ChromSpher C₈ analytical columns in tancem, with Perisorb RP-8, 30–40 μm, guard column	0.01M, pH 4.3, acetate buffer/ ACN (80:20)	UV 280 nm/ PDA (200–400 nm)	2 ppb/ 71–78%	38
Calf muscle	7	EtOAc extn, liq–liq partn	LiChrospher RP18, 5 μm, with RP18e guard column	0.2% formic acid/MeOH (57:43)	NICI-MS-PB	2 ppb/ ≈100%	39
Chicken tissues	6	Phosp. buffer, pH 7.8, extn, SPE cleanup	LiChrosorb RP-18, 7 μm, with C₁₈, 40 μm, guard column	H₂O/ACN (78:22), at 35°C	UV 280 nm	10 ppb/ 90–92%	65
Chicken muscle	19	ACN extn, liq–liq partns, SPE cleanup, liq–liq partns	Nova-Pak C₁₈, 4 μm	0.01M, pH 4.8, acetate buffer/ ACN (70:30)	UV 278 nm/ PDA (220–340 nm)	10 ppb/ 75–81%	53
Eggs	13	ACN extn, liq–liq partns	LiChrosorb RP-18, 5 μm	H₂O/MeOH (70:30)	UV 280 nm	10 ppb/ 75–84%	54

(continued)

TABLE 29.2 Continued

Antibacterial(s)	Matrix	Sample preparation	Steps	Stationary phase	Mobile phase	Detection/ Identification	Sensitivity/ Recovery	Ref.
	Foie gras	ACN extn, liq–liq partn, SPE cleanup	8	Spherisorb ODS-2, 5 μm	0.01M, pH 4.3, acetate buffer/ ACN (78:22)	UV 280 nm	2.5 ppb/ 56 ± 8.7%	55
	Goose and duck liver	H$_2$O addn, hexane defattening, EtOAc extn, SPE cleanup, liq–liq partns	18	Nova-Pak C$_{18}$, 4 μm, with reversed-phase guard column	0.005M, pH 7.9, ammonium phosp. buffer/ ACN (81:19)	UV 278 nm/ PDA (220–320 nm)	0.8 ppb/ 69–73%	40
	Meat	H$_2$O extn, Kieselguhr column cleanup, liq–liq partns	10	ChromSpher C$_8$ or C$_{18}$, 5 μm, with Perisorb C$_8$, 30 μm, guard column	0.01M, pH 4.3, acetate buffer/ ACN (75:25)	UV 285 nm/ PDA (220–400 nm) & GC-EI-MS	1.5 ppb/ 55 ± 18%	58, 59
	Meat	MSPD extn/ cleanup	6	Spherisorb C$_{18}$ ODS2, 5 μm	Solvent A: 0.01M, pH 5.2, acetate buffer Solvent B: ACN/ MeOH (70:30) Gradient from (56:44) to (36:64), at 35°C	UV 290 nm/ PDA (200–450 nm)	5 ppb/ 72–75%	66

Sample	Extraction		Column	Mobile phase	Detection	Limit/recovery	Ref.
Meat, milk, eggs	ACN extn, liq–liq partns	6	MOS-Hypersil, 3 μm, analytical and guard column	0.01M, pH 4.6, acetate buffer/ACN (75:25)	UV 275 nm	20 ppb/88–104%	56, 57
Milk	EtOAc extn, liq–liq partns	12	Spherisorb C$_{18}$ ODS, 5 μm	H$_2$O/MeOH (70:30)	UV 280 nm	10 ppb/68–104%	41
Milk	MSPD extn/cleanup	8	Varian MCH-10, 10 μm	0.017M H$_3$PO$_4$/ACN (65:35), at 35°C	UV 278 nm/PDA (200–350 nm)	62.5 ppb/61–79%	67
Milk	Diphasic dialysis using EtOAc	5	Nova-Pak C$_{18}$, 4 μm	H$_2$O/ACN (80:20)	UV 270 nm	5 ppb/61–82%	68
Milk, eggs	Centrgn, filtn, IAC cleanup	7	ChromSpher C$_8$, 5 μm, with reversed-phase guard column	0.01M, pH 5.4, acetate buffer/ACN (75:25)	UV 280 nm	1 ppb/80–100%	21
Milk, swine muscle	Centrgn, TCA (milk) or H$_2$O (muscle) extn, online IAC cleanup on SelectiSpher-10 column and switching to analytical column	5	ChromSpher C$_8$, 5 μm, with reversed-phase guard column	0.01M, pH 5.4, acetate buffer/ACN (75:25)	UV 280 nm	1–10 ppb/64–70%	22
Swine muscle	EtOAc extn, liq–liq partn, SPE cleanup	14	ChromSpher C$_8$, 5 μm with reversed-phase guard column	0.01M, pH 4.3, acetate buffer/ACN (75:25)	UV 280 nm	10 ppb/77–85%	42

(continued)

TABLE 29.2 Continued

Antibacterial(s)	Matrix	Sample preparation	Steps	Stationary phase	Mobile phase	Detection/ Identification	Sensitivity/ Recovery	Ref.
	Swine muscle	H_2O extn, IAC cleanup	7	ChromSpher C_8, 5 μm, with reversed-phase guard column	0.01M, pH 5.4, acetate buffer/ ACN (75:25)	UV 280 nm	10 ppb/ 66–75%	60
	Swine kidney	Ether extn, liq–liq partn, LC on PRP-1, 5 μm, column and switching to analytical column	4	Chromsep C_{18}, 5 μm	H_2O/ACN (10:90)	UV 280 nm/ PDA (230–330 nm)	<10 ppb/ 41 ± 2.8%	63
Thiamphenicol	Bovine muscle	EtOAc extn, liq–liq partns	12	Nucleosil 120, C_{18}, 5 μm	H_2O/MeOH (75:25), at 40°C	UV 224 nm	10 ppb/ 65–76%	43
	Milk	EtOAc extn, SPE cleanup	13	Nucleosil 120, C_{18}, 5 μm	H_2O/MeOH (70:30), at 35°C	UV 224 nm	30 ppb/ 71–90%	I44
	Milk	H_2O diln, Kieselguhr column cleanup	4	Wakosil-II 5C18 HG, 5 μm	H_2O/ACN (60:40)	UV 224 nm/ MS-APCI	100 ppb/ 92 ± 4.4%	24
Florfenicol and metabolite	Fish tissues	Acetone extn, liq–liq partns	9	Supelcosil LC-18-DB, 5 μm, analytical and guard column	0.025, pH 3.85, phosp. buffer, contg 20 mM heptane-sulfonate/ MeOH contg 0.1% TEA (68:32)	UV 220 nm	20–50 ppb/ 94–107%	62

Analyte	Matrix	Sample prep		Column	Mobile phase	Detection	LOD/Recovery	Ref
Chloramphenicol, thiamphenicol	Gamebird meat	H_2O extn, SPE cleanup, liq–liq partns	11	Hypersil RP-18, 5 μm	0.05M, pH 3, TEA-phosp. buffer/ACN (79:21) for chloramphenicol or (86:14) for thiamphenicol	UV 278 & 224 nm/ PDA (210–350 nm) & first order derivatization	2 ppb/ 67–72%	61
Chloramphenicol, thiamphenicol, florfenicol	Animal and fish muscle	EtOAc extn, liq–liq partns, SPE cleanup	14	Chromatorex CDS, 5 μm	H_2O/MeOH (85:15), at 55°C	UV 225 and 270 nm	10 ppb/ 68–83%	45
Chloramphenicol and metabolites	Chicken tissues	Urea extn, SPE cleanup	9	LiChrosorb RP-18, 5 μm, analytical and precolumn	0.005M $(NH_4)_2HPO_4$/ MeOH (73:27), pH 7.98	UV 278 nm	15–80 ppb/ 61–94%	46
		EtOAc extn, liq–liq partn	8		0.2% H_2SO_4, contg 0.002 M sodium octylsulfate/ ACN/MeOH (71:14.5:14.5)		10–25 ppb/ 68–99%	

TMS, trimethylsilane; HFBA, heptafluorobutyric anhydride; IAC, immunoaffinity chromatography; TSP, thermospray; PB, particle beam; EI, electron impact; CI, chemical ionization; NICI, negative ion chemical ionization; ECD, electron-capture detector; PDA, photodiode array.
Other abbreviations as in Tables 20.2 and 29.1.

In liquid chromatographic methods, reversed-phase columns are usually employed due to hydrophobic interaction of the amphenicols molecules with the C_8 or C_{18} stationary phases. Ion-pairing liquid chromatography has been also described for the separation of florfenicol and florfenicol amine (62) or chloramphenicol and deacetylchloramphenicol residues (46) using heptanesulfonate or octylsulfate-pairing ions, respectively.

Since amphenicols exhibit strong ultraviolet absorption, they are ideal for direct determination by liquid chromatography, without any need for derivatization (Fig. 29.2.1). Their detection wavelengths have been set at 224 nm for thiamphenicol, 220 or 225 nm for florfenicol, and 270–290 nm for chloramphenicol (Table 29.2). Use of photodiode array detectors has been suggested for tentative confirmation of the identity of chloramphenicol residues analyzed by liquid chromatography (26, 37, 38, 40, 53, 58, 59, 61, 63, 66, 67).

Although confirmation with a photodiode array detector is a relatively simple procedure, the specificity and sensitivity features of this detector are not usually sufficient to determine or identify trace levels of residual chloramphenicol in edible animal products. Only the coupling of liquid chromatography with mass spectrometry can provide unequivocal on-line spectrometric identification of individual amphenicols at the very low residue levels required by regulatory agencies. On-line mass spectrometry offers the added advantage of allowing identification of polar nonvolatile compounds without the need for derivatization. Typical applications describe coupling of liquid chromatography with mass spectrometry via thermospray (23) or particle-beam (39) interfaces and use of negative-ion detection. An atmospheric-pressure chemical–ionization interface has been also suggested for identification of thiamphenicol residues in bovine milk (24).

Gas chromatography on capillary or conventional columns has been also widely employed for separation of amphenicol residues. Chloramphenicol molecule contains two chlorine atoms, thiamphenicol two chlorine atoms and an aromatic methylsulfonyl group, while florfenicol contains an aromatic methylsulfonyl group and a fluorine atom, all of which exhibit a high electron affinity. Therefore, detectors based on electron capturing are particularly useful for the determination of chloramphenicol (25, 31, 33, 35, 47–50, 64) or all three amphenicols simultaneously (51), with good sensitivity and specificity. To confirm the presence of chloramphenicol residues in edible animal products, mass spectrometric detectors are also frequently employed. Typical examples of such applications are those coupling gas chromatography with mass spectrometry via a chemical ionization interface (25, 31, 32, 34).

Gas chromatographic separation of amphenicols is further complicated by the need for derivatization of their polar functional groups. Silyl derivatives formed by treating sample extracts with N,O-bis(trimethylsilyl)acetamide (49), trimethylsilyl N,N-dimethyl carbamate (47), N,O-bis(trimethylsilyl)trifluoroacetamide/trimethylchlorosilane (99:1) mixture (32, 51), or mixture of

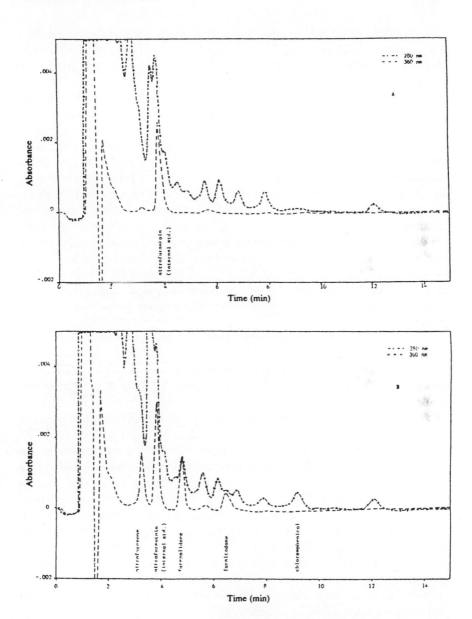

FIG. 29.2.1 Chromatograms of a blank meat sample containing 10 ppb nitrofu-rantoin (A); and a spiked meat sample (B) containing 5 ppb chloramphenicol, furaltadone, furazolidone, and nitrofurazone; internal standard: nitrofurantoin. Detection at 280 (—.—.—.—) and 360 nm (-----). (From Ref. 38.)

hexamethyldisilazone and trimethylchlorosilane in pyridine, have been most commonly employed (25, 31, 33–35, 50, 64). Heptafluorobutyric anhydride (48) was also used for derivatization of chloramphenicol residues isolated from milk samples.

Pfenning et al. (51) have proposed a promising gas chromatographic method for the simultaneous determination of amphenicols residues in milk, using meta-nitrochloramphenicol as the internal standard. In this method, milk is extracted with acetonitrile. After centrifugation, the supernatant is evaporated to dryness, and the residue is dissolved with water to be further purified using C_{18} solid-phase extraction cartridge. Elution of the drugs is effected with 60% methanol, and the eluate is evaporated to dryness and derivatized with Sylon BFT [N,O-bis(trimethylsilyl)trifluoroacetamide/trimethylchlorosilane 99/1]. Following derivatization, toluene is added directly to the sample, followed by water to quench the derivatization process. The mixture is centrifuged, and the organic layer is used for gas chromatographic analysis on a OV-1 fused-silica capillary column (30 m × 0.25 mm internal diameter [i.d.]) with helium as the carrier gas (Fig. 29.2.2). Using electron capture detection, chloramphenicol, thiamphenicol and florfenicol residues could be readily determined in milk samples at concentrations as low as 5 ppb.

A different approach was suggested van Ginkel et al. (32) for the identification and quantification of chloramphenicol residues in eggs and bovine muscle. According to this method, homogenized sample is extracted with ethyl acetate in presence of sodium sulfate. After centrifugation, the supernatant is evaporated to dryness, and the residue is dissolved with dichloromethane to be further applied to a Sep-Pak silica cartridge. Following cartridge washing with dichloromethane, chloramphenicol is eluted with water/acetonitrile (8:2), and the eluate is extracted with ethyl acetate. Following a water washing, the extract is evaporated to dryness and reconstituted in isooctane/ethanol (97:3) to be further purified by liquid chromatography using a LiChrosorb Diol (5 μm) analytical column. The fraction of the eluate corresponding to chloramphenicol is collected and evaporated to dryness. The residue is derivatized with N,O-bis(trimethylsilyl)trifluoroacetamide/trimethylchlorosilane (99/1) mixture, and analyzed on a CP-Sil-19CB fused-silica capillary column (25 m × 0.25 mm i.d.) with helium as the carrier gas. Using a mass spectrometric detector operating in the negative-ion chemical ionization mode and [$^{37}Cl_2$] chloramphenicol as the internal standard, concentrations as low as 0.1 ppb in eggs and bovine muscle could be determined.

A specific cleanup procedure based on immunoaffinity chromatography with polyclonal antibodies has been described by Gude et al. (50) for the gas chromatographic determination of chloramphenicol in swine tissues. In this method, tissue sample is extracted with acetonitrile/4% sodium chloride (1:1) Following centrifugation, the supernatant is purified with n-hexane, and chloram-

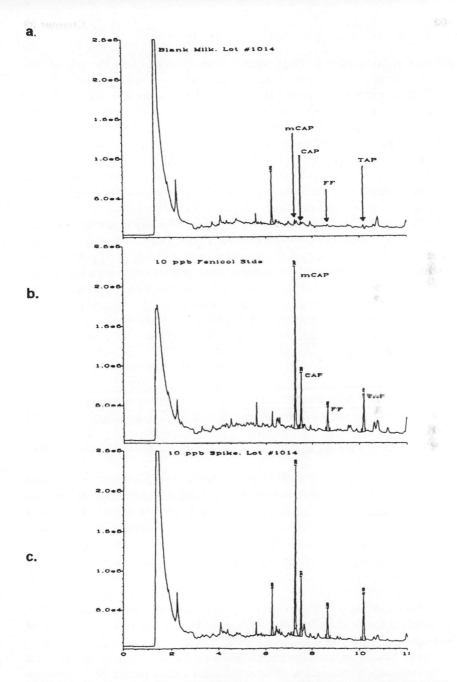

FIG. 29.2.2 Representative chromatograms of a blank milk sample (a), a 10 ppb amphenicol standard solution (b), and a milk sample (c) spiked at 10 ppb. (Reprinted from Ref. 51. Copyright, (1998), by AOAC INTERNATIONAL.)

phenicol is extracted with ethyl acetate. After evaporation of the solvent, the residue is dissolved with 10% ethanol and applied to an immunoaffinity column. Following column washing with phosphate-buffered saline and water, chloramphenicol is eluted with ethanol, and the eluate is evaporated to dryness and derivatized with a mixture of hexamethyldisilazone and trimethylchlorosilane in pyridine. After evaporation of the solvent, the residue is dissolved immediately in *n*-hexane and analyzed on a DB-5 capillary column (25 m × 0.25 mm i.d.) with argon/methane (95:5) as the carrier gas. Using monochloro-chloramphenicol as internal standard, concentrations as low as 0.2 ppb in muscle and 2 ppb in liver and kidney could be determined by electron capture detection.

Nagata and Saeki (45) described a multiresidue liquid chromatographic method for the determination of amphenicols in animals and cultured fish muscle. According to this method, minced muscle is extracted with ethyl acetate. After centrifugation, the supernatant is evaporated to dryness and the residue is dissolved with 3% sodium chloride. Following fat removal with *n*-hexane, the analytes are extracted with ethyl acetate, the solvent is evaporated, and the residue is dissolved with *n*-hexane to be further applied to a Sep-Pak Florisil cartridge. Following cartridge washing with *n*-hexane and ethyl acetate, amphenicols are eluted with ethyl ether/methanol (7:3), and the eluate is evaporated to dryness. The residue is reconstituted in 1 ml methanol to be further analyzed by liquid chromatography. Separation is performed on a 15 cm Chromatorex ODS (5 μm) analytical column, with water/methanol (85:15) as the mobile phase, at a flow-rate of 1.2 ml/min and a column temperature of 55°C. Under these conditions, concentrations as low as 2 ppb could be determined using an ultraviolet spectrophotometer at 225 nm for thiamphenicol and florfenicol and at 270 nm for chloramphenicol.

A different approach was followed by Blanchflower et al. (23) in a liquid chromatographic–mass spectrometric method for the determination of chloramphenicol residues in milk and animal tissues, using deuterated chloramphenicol as internal standard. For milk analysis, the sample is diluted with 1 volume of water and purified by loading the diluted milk onto a C_{18} Sep-Pak extraction column. Following column washing with water, chloramphenicol is eluted with methanol. The eluate is evaporated to dryness, and the residue is dissolved in water/acetonitrile (7:3).

For tissue analysis, the sample is extracted with ethyl acetate in the presence of sodium chloride and piperonyl butoxide. After centrifugation, the supernatant is evaporated to dryness, and the residue is dissolved with dichloromethane/hexane (1:1) to be applied onto a Bond-Elut silica cartridge. Following successive cartridge washing with petroleum ether and ethyl acetate/hexane (4:6), chloramphenicol is eluted with ethyl acetate/hexane (7:3) and the eluate is evaporated to dryness. The residue is dissolved in 0.05 M Tris/hydrochloric acid buffer pH 10.4, extracted with diethyl ether, and the extract is evaporated to dryness. The residue is reconstituted in water/acetonitrile (7:3) to be further analyzed by liquid chromatography. Separation is performed on a 12.5-cm LiChrosorb RP18 (5 μm) analytical column, with a mobile phase of water/acetonitrile (65:35) containing 0.1 M ammonium acetate. Under these conditions, concentrations as low as 1 ppb in tissue and 2 ppb in milk could be determined using thermospray mass spectrometric detection in the negative-ion chemical ionization mode.

29.3 β-LACTAM ANTIBIOTICS

β-Lactam antibiotics are natural or semisynthetic compounds whose basic nuclear structure consists of a β-lactam ring coupled to a thiazolidine (five-membered) or a dihydrothiazine (six-membered) ring to form the penicillin or cephalosporin nucleus, respectively. To those nuclei, various side chains that determine most of the properties of the different β-lactams are attached. All members of this group of antibiotics are readily attacked at the β-lactam nitrogen by nucleophilic reagents such as hydroxyl ions, alcohols, and primary amines, as well as by secondary amines. They are also susceptible to electrophilic attack at both the β-lactam nitrogen and the sulfur atom of the thiazolidine ring.

β-Lactams are fairly polar, nonvolatile, but somewhat heat-sensitive compounds. Owing to the presence of a free carboxyl group in their molecule, β-lactam antibiotics are fairly strong organic acids with a pKa value of about 2.6–2.7. On the other hand, β-lactams, such as ampicillin (pK_{COO^-} = 2.7 and p$K_{NH_3^+}$ = 7.2) carrying an amino group in the side chain are amphoteric compounds. Their sensitivity in acids or bases varies with the nature of the side chain. Thus, maximum stability for the monobasic compounds is exhibited in the pH range 6–7, whereas for the amphoteric compounds the maximum stability coincides with the isoelectric point.

Prior to analysis of β-lactam residues in liquid foods such as milk, a pretreatment step for fat removal, accomplished by centrifugation (69–71), is usually required. In instances where milk is to be submitted to ultrafiltration, dilution with water/acetonitrile (72–76) or water/acetonitrile/methanol (77–79) is often needed. Milk filtration (80) or dilution with acetate (81, 82) or phosphate buffers (83) is sometimes essential prior to solid-phase extraction. Unlike milk, semisolid food samples such as muscle, kidney, and liver require normally more intensive sample pretreatment. Tissue break-up is mostly carried out by the combined use of a mincing apparatus and a tissue homogenizer.

Extraction of β-lactam antibiotics from edible animal products should render residues that are bound to proteins soluble, remove most if not all of the sample proteins, and provide high yields for all analytes. Sample extraction/deproteinization may be carried out with organic solvents and/or organic and inorganic acids, or even with ultrafiltration. Organic solvents including acetonitrile (70, 84–94), acidified acetonitrile (95–100), methanol (14, 101, 102), acetone (103, 104), and dichloromethane at acidic conditions (105), have all been used with varying success to free the noncovalently bound residues. Use of acetonitrile in the presence of an ion-pairing reagent has also been reported to work extremely well in the extraction of β-lactam residues from milk (106–110) and tissues (110, 111).

Organic and inorganic acids such as sulfuric acid/sodium tungstate mixture (69, 83, 112–116) and trichloroacetic acid (117–119) have also been extensively used, although some penicillins can be readily degraded at such acidic conditions. As an alternative, ultrafiltration has been occasionally applied for removing proteinaceous material from milk samples (72–79, 120). With this technique, milk ultrafiltrate can be analyzed either directly or following further purification. Ultrafiltration involves the use of cut-off filters of 10000 da molecular mass to remove proteinaceous material. With use of this technique, however, not all low-molecular-mass proteins are removed, whereas many other endogenous compounds that interfere with the analysis may remain in the sample extract.

Using mentioned extraction/deproteinization procedures, the obtained aqueous or organic extracts often represent very dilute solutions of the analyte(s). These extracts may also contain coextractives that, if not efficiently separated prior to analysis of the final extract, will increase the background noise of the detector making it impossible to determine the analyte(s) at the trace residue levels likely to occur in the analyzed samples. Hence, to reduce potential interferences and concentrate the analyte(s), the primary sample extracts are often subjected to some kind of additional sample cleanup such as liquid–liquid partitioning, solid-phase extraction, or online trace enrichment and liquid chromatography. In many instances, more than one of these cleanup procedures may be applied in combination to allow higher purification of the analyte(s).

Liquid–liquid partitioning constitutes the most popular cleanup approach used for purification of residues of monobasic β-lactam antibiotics. Such residues are generally extracted from the primary aqueous sample extracts by dichloromethane or chloroform under acidic conditions in which the ionization of their carboxylate moiety is suppressed, and then back-extracted into pH 7 phosphate buffers (84, 85, 89, 92, 95, 97, 99). In these instances, however, all analytical steps involving contact of the analytes with acids should be performed in a highly reproducible fashion and for a minimum length of time due to the instability of these compounds, especially penicillin G, in the acidic media employed.

Liquid–liquid partitioning at neutral conditions can be only performed using the ion-pair extraction techniques suggested by Fletouris et al. (105) and Berger and Petz (96). By adjusting the pH of the aqueous extracts at 7.0 (pH of maximum stability) and using tetrabutylammonium (105) or 18-crown-6 ether (96) as pairing ions, these workers succeeded in readily extracting the formed penicillin ion-pairs into chloroform or dichloromethane, respectively, in developing methods for the determination of monobasic penicillins in milk. Although suitable for monobasic β-lactams, the above-described liquid–liquid partitioning cleanup procedures are not, however, effective for amphoteric compounds such as ampicillin and amoxicillin.

Solid-phase extraction seems to be more suitable for multiresidue cleanup. This procedure has become the method of choice for isolation and/or cleanup of β-lactam antibiotics from biological matrices, because it requires low solvent consumption, it is generally less time-consuming and labor-intensive, and offers a variety of alternative approaches that allow better extraction of the more hydrophilic β-lactam antibiotics such as ampicillin. It is usually performed using reversed-phase C_{18} (69–71, 80–83, 90, 92–94, 99, 107, 112–116, 121–125) or C_8 (103), anion-exchange (95, 124), and polar diol (95) or alumina (101, 113) sorbents. In recent applications, some workers demonstrated the potential of online solid-phase extraction in the determination of monobasic penicillins in bovine muscle tissues using a reversed-phase C_{18} 5 μm cartridge and an automated column-switching system (92, 99).

Online trace enrichment has also been described for the isolation/purification of penicillin G residues from bovine tissues (113). This technique involved trapping of the analyte onto an LC preconcentration column (LiChrosorb RP-18, 5 μm), rinsing of coretained material to waste, and flushing of the concentrated analytes onto the analytical column. In a somewhat similar but seemingly different approach, liquid chromatographic cleanup was successfully employed in the determination of β-lactam antibiotics in milk and animal tissues (69, 86–88, 106–111). This approach involved loading of the sample extract onto a reversed-phase column, elution with a suitable mobile phase, collection of predetermined fractions of the chromatographic effluents containing the analytes, and their reanalysis by liquid chromatography.

Following their extraction and cleanup, residues of β-lactam antibiotics in sample extracts can be detected by either direct nonchromatographic methods, or thin-layer, gas, or liquid chromatographic methods (Table 29.3).

Direct nonchromatographic methods target screening of either ampicillin residues in milk extracts by fluorometric detection (126) or β-lactam residues in kidney extracts by photometric detection (120). These methods are rapid but cannot differentiate among particular β-lactams and are less sensitive than other screening tests usually employed for regulatory purposes.

In thin-layer chromatographic methods, penicillin residues were first separated using various solvent mixtures as mobile phase, and subsequently detected by bioautography using *Bacillus subtilis* (14) or *Sarcina lutea* (102, 104) as the test organisms. For a laboratory not having access to sophisticated instrumentation, these technique will generally allow detection of penicillin residues at levels higher than 50–100 ppb and provide some measure of analytical support for a

TABLE 29.3 Physicochemical Methods for β-Lactam Antibacterials in Edible Animal Products

Antibacterial(s)	Matrix	Sample preparation	Steps	Stationary phase	Mobile phase	Detection/ Identification	Sensitivity/ Recovery	Ref.
SPECTROMETRIC METHODS								
Ampicillin	Milk	Acetate buffer extn, filtn, derivatization with 1,2,4-triazole-mercuric chloride	3	—	—	Fluorometric ex: 342 nm, em: 410 nm	40 ppb/ 95–103%	126
β-Lactams	Kidney	Phosp. buffer, pH 7, extn, ultrafiltn, CPase inhibition	5	—	—	Vis 510 nm	50 ppb/ NR	120
THIN-LAYER CHROMATOGRAPHIC METHODS								
Penicillin G	Animal tissues	MeOH extn, liq–liq partns	14	Silica gel or cellulose	CHCl$_3$/MeOH/ acetone/ glycerine or Acetone/ CHCl$_3$/PrOH/ 0.01N phthalate buffer/glycerine	B. subtilis bioauto-graphy	50–100 ppb/ NR	14
Ampicillin, penicillin G	Animal tissues	MeOH extn	2	Silica gel	EtAOc/MeOH/ H$_2$O	S. lutea bioauto-graphy	NR	102
Ampicillin, cloxacillin, oxacillin	Milk	Acetone/ACN extn, liq–liq partns	7	Silica gel	MeOH/CHCl$_3$	S. lutea bioauto-graphy	0.1–1 ppm/ NR	104

GAS CHROMATOGRAPHIC METHODS

Seven penicillins	Bovine tissues, milk	48	ACN extn, liq–liq partns, SPE cleanup, liq–liq partn, CH_2N_2 methylation, SPE cleanup for liver and kidney extracts	DB-1, 30 m, capillary coated with methyl silicone	Nitrogen	NSTD	0.1–2.5 ppb/ 46–83%	95
Seven penicillins	Milk	40	Phosp. buffer, pH 2.2, addn, ACN extn, liq–liq partns, CH_2N_2 methylation	Ultra-1, 25 m, capillary coated with methyl silicone	Nitrogen	NSTD	0.1–0.4 ppb/ 41–92%	97

LIQUID CHROMATOGRAPHIC METHODS

Amoxicillin	Catfish and salmon tissues	26	Phosp. buffer, pH 4.5, extn, TCA addn, SPE cleanup, liq–liq partn, precolumn derivatization with formaldehyde, liq–liq partn	Spherisorb S5 ODS2	0.05M, pH 5.6, KH_2PO_4/ACN (80:20)	Fluorometric, ex: 358 nm, em: 440 nm	1.2–2 ppb/ 67–82%	117
Ampicillin	Animal muscle	10	Phosp. buffer, pH 4.5/TCA extn, precolumn derivatization with formaldehyde	Prodigy ODS-3, 5 μm	0.02M, pH 3.5, KH_2PO_4/ACN (75:25)	Fluorometric, ex: 346 nm, em: 422 nm	1.5 ppb/ 85–98%	118
	Bovine muscle	12	Ammonium acetate buffer, pH 8.5, extn, SPE cleanup	Merck RP 18e with guard column	0.2% formic acid/MeOH (55:45)	PICI-MS-ESP	25 ppb/ NR	125

(continued)

TABLE 29.3 Continued

Antibacterial(s)	Matrix	Sample preparation	Steps	Stationary phase	Mobile phase	Detection/ Identification	Sensitivity/ Recovery	Ref.
	Fish tissues	MeOH extn, SPE cleanup	11	Nucleosil C_{18}	Buffer, pH 6.0/ MeOH (85:15), at 30°C	UV 222 nm	30 ppb/ 56–78%	101
	Milk	ACN/TCA extn, precolumn derivatization with formaldehyde	9	Prodigy ODS-3, 5 μm	0.01M, pH 5.6, KH_2PO_4/ACN (76:24)	Fluorometric, ex: 346 nm, em: 422 nm	1.2 ppb/ 85–96%	100
	Milk	ACN extn, liq–liq partns, LC purification on PLRP-S, 5 μm, column, decanesulfonate and H_3PO_4 addn	8	PLRP-S, 5 μm	0.01M H_3PO_4/ ACN (76:24) contg 10 mM sodium decanesulfonate	UV 210 nm/ Penicillinase	5 ppb/ 60–70%	87
Ceftiofur	Milk	ACN/H_2O diln, ultrafiltn	2	Ultremex phenyl, 3 μm	H_2O/ACN (80:20) contg 0.25% H_3PO_4, 0.25% TEA, 2.5 mM octanesulfonate and 2.5 mM dodecanesulfonate, at 40°C	UV 289.6 nm/ PDA (200–350 nm) & MS-TSP after LC conditions modification	50 ppb/ 87–100%	73

	Matrix	Sample prep		Column	Mobile phase	Detection	LOD/Recovery	Ref
	Milk	0.1M Ammonium acetate diln, SPE cleanup	10	Supelcosil LC-C_{18} DB, 5 μm, analytical and guard column	0.1M, pH 3.3, acetate buffer/ACN (80:20), at 35°C	UV 293 nm	7 ppb/80–100%	82
	Milk	ACN/H_2O diln, ultrafiltn	2	Nova-Pak C_{18}	H_2O/ACN contg 1% HOAc and 25 mM heptafluorobutyric acid Gradient from (95:05) to (05:95)	MS-ESP	25 ppb/95 ± 6.8%	74
Cephapirin	Milk	Acetate buffer diln, SPE cleanup	8	Ultrasphere-ODS, 5 μm, with RP-18 Spheri-10 guard column	0.01M NaOAc/ACN/MeOH (85:11.25:3.75)	UV 254 nm	10 ppb/61–81%	81
	Milk	Ion pair/ACN extn, LC purificationn on Supelcosil LC-18, 5 μm, column	7	PLRP-S, 5 μm	0.02M, pH 2.26, phosp. buffer/ACN (80:20), contg 10mM decane-sulfonate	UV 290 nm/Penicillinase	2 ppb/91–98%	106
Cloxacillin	Milk	HCl addn, ACN extn, liq-liq partns	8	Nova-Pak C_{18}, 4 μm	0.02M KH_2PO_4/ACN (79:21), pH 5	UV 225 nm	10–50 ppb/75–93%	98

(continued)

TABLE 29.3 Continued

Antibacterial(s)	Matrix	Sample preparation	Steps	Stationary phase	Mobile phase	Detection/ Identification	Sensitivity/ Recovery	Ref.
Penicillin G	Animal tissues	H_2SO_4/sodium tungstate extn, SPE cleanup, precolumn derivatization with 1,2,4-triazole-mercuric chloride	14	Nova-Pak C_{18}, 4 μm	0.1M phosp. buffer, contg 0.0157M sodium thiosulfate/ ACN (75:25)	UV 325 nm	5 ppb/ 85–94%	112
	Bovine tissues	H_2SO_4/sodium tungstate extn, alumina column cleanup, SPE cleanup, on-line trace enrichment on LiChrosorb RP-18, 5 μm, preconcn column and switching to analytical column	8	LiChrosorb RP-18, 5 μm, with Permaphase ETH guard column	H_2O/MeOH/0.2M, pH 5.0, phosp. buffer (60:35:5), at 40°C	UV 210 nm	50 ppb/ 75–93%	113
	Bovine and swine tissues	Ion pair/ACN extn, LC purification on Supelcosil LC-18, 5 μm, column	9	Inertsil ODS-2, 5 μm	0.0067M KH_2PO_4, 0.0033M H_3PO_4/ACN (68:32)	UV 215 nm/β-Lactamase	5 ppb/ 66–95%	111

Matrix	Extraction/cleanup		Column	Mobile phase	Detection	LOD/Recovery	Ref
Eggs	H_2SO_4/sodium tungstate extn, SPE cleanup, precolumn derivatization with 1,2,4-triazole-mercuric chloride	12	Inertsil C_8	0.05, pH 6.5, phosp. buffer/ACN (72:28)	UV 325 nm	NR/56–85%	115
Milk	Acetone extn, liq–liq partns, SPE cleanup	19	Supelcosil LC-C_{18} DB, 5 μm, analytical and guard column	0.01M, pH 2.15, phosp. buffer, contg 20mM heptane-sulfonate/ACN (64:34), at 35°C	UV 200 nm	4 ppb/82 ± 0.8%	103
Milk	H_2SO_4/sodium tungstate extn, SPE cleanup, precolumn derivatization with 1,2,4-triazole-mercuric chloride	10	Nova-Pak C_{18}, 4 μm	0.1M phosp. buffer, contg 0.0157M sodium thiosulfate/ACN (75:25)	UV 325 nm/MS-TSP after LC conditions modification	3 ppb/70–89%	115
Milk	ACN/MeOH/H_2O diln, ultrafiltn	2	Brownlee Microbore Phenyl Spheri-5, 5 μm	H_2O/ACN (75:25), contg 2.5 mM octane-sulfonate, 2.5 mM dodecane-sulfonate, 0.5% H_3PO_4, and 0.5% TEA, at 40°C	UV 210 nm/PDA (200–360 nm) & PPINICI–MS–TSP after LC conditions modification	10 ppb/76–90%	78

(continued)

TABLE 29.3 Continued

Antibacterial(s)	Matrix	Sample preparation	Steps	Stationary phase	Mobile phase	Detection/ Identification	Sensitivity/ Recovery	Ref.
	Milk	Centrgn, H_2SO_4/ sodium tungstate extn, SPE cleanup, LC purification on Kromasil 5C$_8$, 5 μm, column	13	Kromasil 5C$_8$, 5 μm	Solvent A: 0.01M H_3PO_4 Solvent B: 0.01M H_3PO_4/ACN (20:80) Isocratic (100:0) for 5 min and gradient to (0:100)	UV 320 nm, postcolumn derivatization with imidazole– mercury chloride	2 ppb/ 70 ± 7.6%	69
	Milk	ACN extn, liq–liq partn, LC purification on PLRP-S, 5 μm, column	8	PLRP-S, 5 μm	0.01M, pH 1.96, phosp. buffer/ ACN (66:34)	UV 210 nm/ Penicillinase	2 ppb/ 92 ± 9%	86
Ampicillin, amoxicillin	Milk	Ion pair/ACN extn, LC purification on Supelcosil LC-18, 5 μm, column, sodium decanesulfonate addn	7	Supelcosil LC-18, 5 μm	0.01M phosp. buffer/ACN (67:33), contg 5 mM sodium dodecylsulfate, for ampicillin. 0.015M H_3PO_4/ ACN (70:30), contg 7.5	UV 210 nm/ Penicillinase	2–5 ppb/ 62–102%	107

Analyte	Matrix		Sample preparation	Column	Mobile phase	Detection	LOD/Recovery	Ref.
	Milk	12	Phosp. buffer, pH 4.5, diln, H₂SO₄/sodium tungstate extn, SPE cleanup, precolumn derivatization with salicylaldehyde	Prodigy ODS-3, 5 μm	mM sodium dodecylsulfate, for amoxicillin, 0.02M, pH 5.5, phosp. buffer/ACN (68:32) for 12 min and (50:50) for 10 min	Fluorometric, ex: 354 nm, em: 445 nm	1.7–2.4 ppb/82–87%	83
Ampicillin, cephapirin	Milk	15	Centrgn, ACN extn, SPE cleanup	Luna C₈, 5 μm, with Symmetry C₈ guard column	H₂O/0.5M, pH 3.75, acetate buffer/ACN (76:20:4), at 30°C	Integrated pulsed electro-chemical	5–10 ppb/67–80%	70
Cephapirin, ceftiofur	Milk	16	ACN extn, SPE cleanup	Supelcosil LC-18, 5 μm, analytical and guard column	Solvent A: 0.033M H₃PO₄, contg 9 mM SDS/ACN (90:10) Solvent B: ACN Solvent C: MeOH Step gradient from (75:25:0) to (35:45:20), at 40°C	UV 290 nm	2–4 ppb/76–87%	94

(continued)

TABLE 29.3 Continued

Antibacterial(s)	Matrix	Sample preparation	Steps	Stationary phase	Mobile phase	Detection/ Identification	Sensitivity/ Recovery	Ref.
Cephapirin, desacetyl-cephapirin	Milk	ACN/MeOH/H$_2$O diln, ultrafiltn	2	Brownlee Microbore Phenyl Spheri-5, 5 μm	H$_2$O/ACN/MeOH/ H$_3$PO$_4$ (74.9:20:5:0.1), contg 5 mM dodecane-sulfonate, at 40°C	UV 291 nm/PDA (200–360 nm) & PPINICl-MS–TSP after LC conditions modification	10–50 ppb/ 79–90%	77
Cloxacillin, penicillin V	Milk	ACN extn, liq–liq partn, LC purification on PLRP-S, 5 μm, column	8	PLRP-S, 5μ	0.01M H$_3$PO$_4$/ ACN (62:38) for penicillin V, (58:42) for cloxacillin	UV 210 nm/ Penicillinase	1 ppb/ 75–111%	88
Penicillin G, cloxacillin	Animal tissues	ACN extn, SPE cleanup, precolumn derivatization with 1,2,4-triazole-mercuric chloride	16	Nova-Pak C$_{18}$	0.1M phosp. buffer, contg 0.0157M sodium thiosulfate/ ACN (77.5:22.5)	UV 325 nm	5 ppb/ 75–100%	90
	Bovine and swine tissues	ACN extn, liq–liq partns	18	Varian MCH-10 C$_{18}$, 10 μm	0.01M or 0.02M H$_3$PO$_4$/ACN Gradient from (80:20) to (40:60)	UV 220 nm	50–500 ppb/ 90–98%	85

Analyte	Matrix	Sample preparation		Column	Mobile phase	Detection	LOD/Recovery	Ref.
Ampicillin, amoxicillin, cloxacillin	Milk	ACN/MeOH/H$_2$O diln, ultrafiltn	2	Brownlee Microbore Phenyl Spheri-5, 5 μm	Different for each β-lactam antibiotic	UV 220 nm/PDA (200–340 nm) & PPINICI-MS–TSP after LC conditions modification	50–100 ppb/ 66–96%	79
Oxacillin, cloxacillin, dicloxacillin	Bovine muscle	ACN extn, liq-liq partns, on-line SPE cleanup	12	LiChrospher 100 RP-18, 5 μm, with LiChroCART guard column	0.2M, pH 3, phosp. buffer/ACN (60:40); at 35°C	UV 225 nm	75 ppb/ 71–104%	92
	Milk	Phosp. buffer, pH 4–4.5, extn, SPE cleanup, precolumn derivatization with 1,2,4-triazole-mercuric chloride	12	Symmetry C$_8$, 5 μm	0.1M, pH 6.5, phosp. buffer contg 15 mM thiosulfate and 30 mM tetrabutylammonium hydrogen sulfate/ACN/MeOH (58:37:5)	UV 340 nm	2–5 ppb/ 65–84%	123
	Milk, meat, cheese	H$_2$SO$_4$/sodium tungstate (milk, meat), phosp. buffer, pH 6.5, (cheese) extn, SPE cleanup, precolumn derivatization with 1,2,4-triazole-mercuric chloride	11–16	Nova-Pak C$_{18}$, 4 μm	0.1M, pH 6.5, phosp. buffer contg 50 mM thiosulfate/ACN Gradient from (75:25) to (55:45), at 40°C	UV 345 nm	5–7 ppb/ 75–93%	116

(continued)

TABLE 29.3 Continued

Antibacterial(s)	Matrix	Sample preparation	Steps	Stationary phase	Mobile phase	Detection/ Identification	Sensitivity/ Recovery	Ref.
Penicillin G, penicillin V, ampicillin	Milk	Filtn, SPE cleanup	5	LiChrosorb RP-18, 5 μm	H_2O/MeOH/0.2M, pH 4.0, phosp. buffer (65:25:10), contg 11 mM sodium heptanesulfonate, at 45°C	UV 210 nm/ Penicillinase	30 ppb/ 87–101%	80
Penicillin G, penicillin V, cloxacillin	Bovine and swine tissues	H_2O addn, ACN extn, liq–liq partns	13	PLRP-S, 5 μm	0.01M, pH 7.0, phosp. buffer/ ACN (85:15) for penicillin G, (82:18) for penicillin V, (78:22) for cloxacillin	UV 210 nm/ Penicillinase	5–100 ppb/ 67–107%	89
	Milk	ACN extn, liq–liq partns	17	Varian MCH-10 C_{18}, 10 μm	0.01M H_3PO_4/ ACN Gradient from (80:20) to (40:60)	UV 220 nm	2–5 ppb/ 88–105%	84

Ceftiofur and metabolites	Swine tissues	Dithioerythritol/ borate buffer, pH 9, extn, precolumn derivatization with iodoacetamide, three SPE cleanups,	23	BDS Hypersil C_{18}, 5 μm, analytical and guard column	H_2O/ACN, contg 0.1% TFA Gradient from (100:0) to (65:35) for muscle and kidney Isocratic (85:15) for 5 min and gradient to (75:25) for liver and fat	UV 266 nm	100 ppb/ 70–95%	124
Four penicillins	Bovine muscle	Phosp. buffer, pH 8.5, extn, SPE cleanup, precolumn derivatization with acetic anhydride and 1,2,4-triazole-mercuric chloride	20	Spherisorb ODS2, 5 μm, with Spherisorb C_{18} guard column	0.1M, pH 6.5, phosp. buffer, contg 15.7 mM sodium thiosulfate/ ACN Step gradient from (82:18) to (0:100)	UV 325 nm	10 ppb/ 72–85%	121

(continued)

TABLE 29.3 Continued

Antibacterial(s)	Matrix	Sample preparation	Steps	Stationary phase	Mobile phase	Detection/ Identification	Sensitivity/ Recovery	Ref.
Four penicillins	Bovine muscle	Phosp. buffer, pH 8.5, extn, SPE cleanup, precolumn derivatization with benzoic anhydride and 1,2,4-triazole-mercuric chloride	21	Symmetry C_8, 5 μm	0.1M, pH 6.5, phosp. buffer contg 15.7 mM sodium thiosulfate/ ACN (74:26)	UV 325 nm	2–5 ppb/ NR	122
Four penicillins	Milk	H_2SO_4 addn, DCM extn, liq–liq partns, ion-pair extn	12	Nucleosil C_{18}, 5 μm	0.02M phosp. buffer/ACN (62:38), pH 6, contg 5 mM tetrabutyl-ammonium hydrogen sulfate, at 40°C	UV 210 nm/ Penicillinase	3–4 ppb/ 79–102%	105
Four penicillins	Animal tissues	Acetone/TCA extn, liq–liq partn, SPE cleanup	13	Supelcosil LC-C_{18} DB, 5 μm, analytical and guard column	0.01M ammonium acetate/MeOH (50:50)	NICI-MS-ISP	15–100 ppb/ 58–99%	119

Analyte	Matrix	Extraction/cleanup		Column	Mobile phase	Detection	LOD/Recovery	Reference
Five penicillins	Bovine muscle	ACN extn, liq–liq partns, online SPE cleanup	25	LiChrospher 100 RP-18e, 5 μm	0.2M, pH 3.0, phosp buffer/ACN (65:35), contg 2 mM Na$_2$EDTA, at 35°C	Electro-chemical, postcolumn photochemical degradation	50 ppb/NR	99
Five penicillins	Milk	ACN extn, SPE cleanup	8	Kaseisorb LC ODS-300-5, 5 μm	0.05M KH$_2$PO$_4$/ACN/MeOH (80:20:10), contg 5 mM decanesulfonate, pH 3.5, at 40°C	UV 210 nm	30–50 ppb/80–89%	93
Five penicillins	Milk	ACN/H$_2$O diln, ultrafiltn	2	Ultremex C$_{18}$, 3 μm	H$_2$O/ACN/HOAc (59:40:1), pH 3.0	UV 230 nm/PICI-MS-ESP	100 ppb/NR	72
Six penicillins	Milk	Centrgn, H$_2$SO$_4$/sodium tungstate extn, SPE cleanup, liq–liq partn, precolumn derivatization with benzoic anhydride and 1,2,4-triazole-mercuric chloride	20	Nova-Pak C$_{18}$, 4 μm	Solvent A: 0.1M, pH 6.5, phosp. buffer/ACN (90:10) Solvent B: 0.1M, pH 6.5, phosp. buffer/ACN (70:30) Gradient from (100:0) to (0:100), at 30°C	UV 325 nm/Penicillinase	2–4 ppb/87–102%	71

(continued)

Table 29.3 Continued

Antibacterial(s)	Matrix	Sample preparation	Steps	Stationary phase	Mobile phase	Detection/ Identification	Sensitivity/ Recovery	Ref.
Six β-lactams	Milk	ACN/H$_2$O diln, ultrafiltn	2	Ultremex phenyl, 3 μm	H$_2$O/ACN (82:18) contg 0.25% H$_3$PO$_4$, 0.30% TEA, 0.25 mM octane-sulfonate and 4.75 mM dodecane-sulfonate, at 40°C	UV 210, 230, & 290 nm/PDA (200–350 nm) & PICI–MS–ESP after LC conditions modification	100 ppb/ 57–106%	75
Six β-lactams	Milk	ACN/H$_2$O diln, ultrafiltn	2	Porous II R/H, 7–8 μm, perfusion microcolumn	Solvent A: H$_2$O contg 0.5% formic acid and 25 mM hepta-fluorobutyric acid Solvent B: ACN contg 0.5% formic acid and 25 mM hepta-fluorobutyric acid Gradient from (100:0) to (50:50)	Ultraspray-MS-ESP	10 ppb/ NR	76

Seven β-lactams	Milk	Ion pair/ACN extn, LC purification on Supelcosil LC-18, 5 μm, column, sodium decanesulfonate addn (aminopenicillins)	8	Supelcosil LC-18-DB, Supelcosil LC-18, and PLRP-S, 5 μm	Different for each β-lactam antibiotic	UV 210, 214, 290, & 295 nm/ β-Lactamase	2–5 ppb/ 60–105%	108, 109
Seven penicillins	Bovine tissues	ACN extn, precolumn derivatization with mercury dichloride (for fluorometric determination of aminopenicillins), liq–liq partn	10	Wakosil-II C_{18}, 5 μm	0.01M KH_2PO_4/ ACN/MeOH (70:19:11), pH 7.1	UV 220 nm and flurometric, ex: 355 nm, em: 435 nm, for amoxicillin, ex: 340 nm, em: 420 nm, for ampicillin	NR/ 72–103%	91
Seven penicillins	Milk	ACN extn, liq–liq partns, ion-pair extn, precolumn derivatization with 4-bromomethyl-7-methoxycoumarin	8	LiChrospher RP-18, 4 μm, with 5 μm, guard column	0.05M, pH 4.5, acetate buffer/ ACN (47:53)	Fluorometric, ex: 320 nm, em: 400 nm	10 ppb/NR	96
Fifteen or more penicillins	Milk and tissues	Ion pair/ACN extn, LC purification on Supelcosil LC-18, 5 μm, column	8	Supelcosil LC-18-DB, Supelcosil LC-18, and PLRP-S, Inertsil ODS-2	Different for each β-lactam antibiotic	UV 215, 260, 290, & 270 nm/ β-Lactamase	NR	110

NSTD, nitrogen-selective thermionic detector; ISP, ionspray; TSP, thermospray; ESP, electrospray; PICI, positive-ion chemical ionization; NICI, negative-ion chemical ionization; PPINICI, pulsed positive-ion–negative ion–chemical ionization; PDA, photodiode array; SDS, sodium dodecylsulfate; CPase, carboxypeptidase. Other abbreviations as in Tables 20.2 and 29.1.

regulatory program. However, these methods generally lack the accuracy, repro-ducibility, and sensitivity required to detect the low ppb levels likely to occur in milk and animal tissues.

Gas chromatographic methods have been successfully used for the determi-nation of penicillin molecules bearing neutral side-chains in milk and tissues (95, 97), but cannot be used for amphoteric β-lactams. Gas chromatography of penicillin residues is further complicated by the necessity for derivatization with diazomethane. This derivatization step is particularly important because it not only leads to formation of the volatile penicillin methyl esters but also improves their chromatographic properties (thermal stability and decreased polarity). Using a fused-silica capillary column in connection with a thermionic nitrogen-selective detector, excellent separation and sensitivity figures were obtained.

At present, liquid chromatography is the most widely used technique for determining β-lactam antibiotics in edible animal products (Table 29.3). Chro-matographic separation is generally achieved on nonpolar reversed-phase col-umns packed with octadecyl, octyl, phenyl, or polymeric sorbents. Extensive research has been carried out to compare the chromatographic behavior of β-lactams with respect to the column type and temperature, mobile phase pH, mobile phase buffer concentration, type and concentration of ion-pairing reagents, and the organic modifier type and content in the mobile phase (127–132).

Regarding the type of organic modifier, there has not been any particular reason for selecting methanol or acetonitrile in the preparation of the mobile phase. Adjusting the mobile phase at a pH value lower than 3.0, the ionization of the carboxylate moiety is suppressed and increased retention of the analytes can be achieved. Under these conditions, however, problems may appear due to the high sensitivity of some penicillins at these pH values.

Increased retention of the analytes can also be achieved by addition of various ion-pair reagents in the mobile phase Tetrabutylammonium cations have typically been used as counter ions, at around pH 6.5, to increase retention and improve the selectivity in the analysis of monobasic penicillins (105, 123). Alkyl-sulfonic acids have been also used to improve the separation of β-lactams bearing an amine function in their side chain or having a neutral side chain. Heptanesul-fonic acid (80, 103), decanesulfonic acid (87, 93, 106), dodecanesulfonic acid (77, 107–110), or mixtures of octanesulfonic and dodecanesulfonic acids (73, 75, 78, 79) constitute the principal alkylsulfonic acids used in β-lactam analysis. In some applications, heptafluorobutyric acid (74, 76) or sodium thiosulfate (90, 112, 115, 116, 121, 122) has also been used as an ion-pairing reagent.

Although spectrophotometric, fluorometric, electrochemical, and mass spectrometric detectors have all been equally well used in liquid chromatographic analysis of β-lactam antibiotics, most popular is the ultraviolet photometric detec-tor. Penicillins do not have a specific ultraviolet chromophore and thus show an extremely weak absorption in the ultraviolet region. Greater sensitivity is exhibited at wavelengths below 200 nm, but the selectivity is becoming poor due to the appearance of high background noise that interferes with analyses at trace residue levels. Hence, most methods use the native UV absorptivity of β-lactams between 200 and 230 nm for penicillins, and 254 and 295 nm for cephalosporins (Table 29.3).

Higher specificity and selectivity can be obtained by reacting β-lactams with suitable reagents to form derivatives with improved ultraviolet chromophores. Thus, precolumn derivatization of penicillins with triazole–mercuric chloride and ultraviolet detection at 325 nm (71, 90, 112, 114, 115, 121, 122), 340 nm (123), or 345 nm (116) has become the method of choice for more selective detection and matrix interferences reduction. An alternative precolumn reaction using iodoacetamide as derivatizing reagent has been described in ceftiofur analysis (124), while imidazole–mercuric chloride has also been suggested for on-line postcolumn derivatization of penicillin G (69).

Fluorometric detection has been mainly employed for the determination of aminopenicillins such as amoxicillin and ampicillin in edible animal products because it confers the advantages of selectivity and sensitivity. Fluorometric detection of penicillins, however, necessitates their precolumn derivatization to produce the corresponding fluorescent derivatives. The most commonly used derivatizing reagents are formaldehyde (100, 117, 118), salicylaldehyde (83), and mercury dichloride (91). 4-Bromomethyl-7-methoxycoumarin has also been employed as a fluorescence label for the selective and sensitive detection of seven penicillins in milk (96).

Electrochemical detection has also been successively applied for the determination of nonderivatized β-lactam antibiotics in edible animal products (70, 99).

Confirmation of the identity of the β-lactam residues detected by liquid chromatography has been attempted through use of photodiode array detectors (73, 75, 77–79). This procedure is relatively simple, but does not offer the specificity and the sensitivity required to determine or identify trace levels of residual β-lactam antibiotics in edible animal products. Better residue confirmation can be more readily attained by treatment of the suspected samples with β-lactamase or penicillinase and their reanalysis (71, 80, 86–89, 105, 106–111). In this instance, absence of a chromatographic peak with the proper retention time provides unequivocal evidence that a given residue is not present above the detection limit of the method. Thus, use of β-lactamase provides a simple, inexpensive and sensitive confirmatory test for β-lactam residues.

Coupling of liquid chromatography with mass spectrometry provides further unequivocal online spectrometric identification of individual analytes at the very low residue levels required by regulatory agencies for confirmatory analysis of β-lactam residues in animal-derived foods. Online mass spectrometry offers the added advantage to allow analysis and identification of polar nonvolatile compounds without the need for derivatization procedures. Typical applications of mass spectrometry in confirming β-lactam residues in edible animal products are through connecting liquid chromatography with mass spectrometry via thermospray (73, 77–79, 115), electrospray (72, 74, 75, 125) or ionspray (119) interfaces, and using negative or positive-ion detection (Fig. 29.3.1).

The most promising literature methods, in terms of simplicity, selectivity, and sensitivity, for screening and even confirmation of β-lactam residues in edible animal products appear to be those reported by Boison and Keng (122), Fletouris et al. (105), Lihl et al. (99), Straub et al. (76), and Moats and Harik-Khan (108).

Boison and Keng (122) described a multiresidue liquid chromatographic method for the determination of amoxicillin, ampicillin, penicillin G, and cloxacillin residues in bovine muscle. According to this method, a 3 g sample of homogenized muscle is extracted with phosphate buffer, pH 8.5, and dilute sulfuric acid. After centrifugation, the pH of the supernatant is adjusted between 8.3 and 8.5, and the extract is applied to a t-C_{18} Sep-Pak cartridge. Following cartridge washing with 0.1M phosphate buffer, pH 8.5, penicillins are eluted with acetonitrile and the eluate is evaporated to dryness. The residue is reconstituted in 0.1M, pH 6.5, phosphate buffer/acetonitrile (6:4), derivatized with benzoic anhydride and 1,2,4-triazole-mercuric chloride, and analyzed by liquid chromatography. Separation is performed on a 15 cm Symmetry C_8 (5 μm) analytical column, with a pH 6.5 phosphate buffer/acetonitrile (74:26) mobile phase containing sodium thiosulfate, at a flow-rate of 1.2 ml/min. Under these conditions, concentrations as low as 2 ppb for amoxicillin and penicillin G, and 5 ppb for ampicillin and cloxacillin could be determined in bovine muscle using a detection wavelength of 325 nm.

Fletouris et al. (105) reported an ion-pair liquid chromatographic method for the determination of penicillin G, penicillin V, oxacillin, and cloxacillin in milk. According to this method, a 7 g milk sample is acidified at pH 3 and extracted with 30 ml dichloromethane. The extracted penicillins are partitioned into a phosphate buffer, pH 7, and, following addition of saturated ammonium sulfate solution, the extracts are purified by treatment with diethyl ether and repartitioned into acetonitrile. The acetonitrile extracts are concentrated into phosphate buffer, pH 7, and, following addition of tetrabutylammonium hydrogen sulfate, the formed penicillin ion-pairs are extracted into chloroform. The extract is evaporated to dryness, and the residue is reconstituted in 1 ml mobile phase to be further analyzed by liquid chromatography. Separation is performed on a 25 cm Nucleosil C_{18} (5 μm) analytical column using a 0.02M phosphate buffer/acetonitrile (62:38), pH 6, mobile phase containing 5 mM tetrabutylammonium hydrogen sulfate, at a flow-rate of 1 ml/min and a column temperature of 40°C

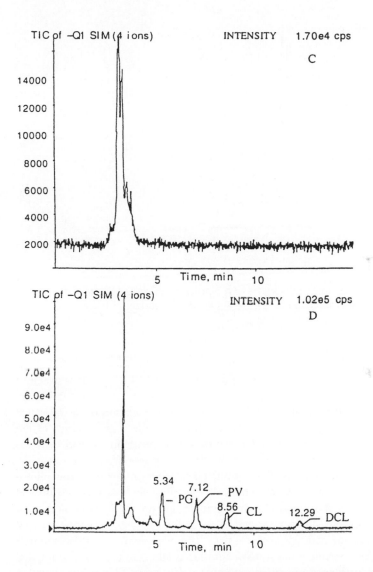

FɪG. **29.3.1**   Chromatograms of a blank meat sample (C) and a meat sample (D) spiked with penicillin G (PG), penicillin V (PV), cloxacillin (CL), and dicloxacillin (DCL) at 100 ppb level. (From Ref. 119.).

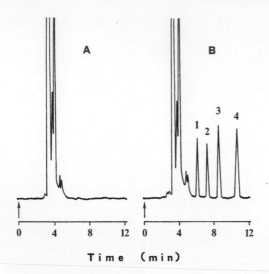

Time (min)

Fɪɢ. 29.3.2   Typical chromatograms of a blank milk sample (A) and a milk sample (B) spiked with penicillin G (1), penicillin V (2), oxacillin (3), and cloxacillin (4) at 30 ppb level. (From Ref. 105.).

(Fig. 29.3.2). Under these conditions, concentrations as low as 3 ppb for oxacillin and cloxacillin and 4 ppb for penicillin G and penicillin V could be determined in milk using a detection wavelength of 210 nm. Confirmation of the presence of penicillins in the suspected samples was based on the disappearance of the recorded peaks after treatment of the samples with penicillinase and their re-analysis.

A different approach based on automated solid-phase extraction and photo-chemical degradation with electrochemical detection was followed by Lihl and co-workers (99) for the liquid chromatographic determination of penicillin G, penicillin V, oxacillin, cloxacillin, and dicloxacillin residues in bovine muscle. According to this method, 25 g muscle tissue are homogenized with acetonitrile at pH 2.2. After centrifugation, sodium chloride is added to the supernatant, and penicillins are partitioned into dichloromethane. The organic layer is evaporated, and the concentrate is suspended in light petroleum ether to be extracted with phosphate buffer, pH 7. A 1.5 ml aliquot of the phosphate buffer is transferred to an autosampler vial to be submitted in online solid-phase extraction and liquid chromatography. Separation is performed on a 25-cm LiChrospher 100 RP-18e (5 μm) analytical column, with a pH-3 phosphate buffer/acetonitrile (65:35) mobile phase containing 2 mM sodium EDTA, at a flow-rate of 1 ml/min and a column temperature of 35°C. Under these conditions, concentrations as low as 50 ppb could be determined in bovine muscle using postcolumn photochemical degradation with electrochemical detection.

Straub et al. (76) reported a method for the identification and quantification of penicillin G, ampicillin, amoxicillin, cephapirin, cloxacillin, and ceftiofur residues in milk using perfusive-particle liquid chromatography combined with ultrasonic nebulization electrospray mass spectrometry. According to this method, a 0.5 ml milk sample is diluted with an equal volume of a solution consisting of acetonitrile/water (1:1), and ultrafiltrated in a microseparation system with a 10000 da molecular mass cut-off filter. An aliquot of the ultrafiltrate is then analyzed on a 15 cm porous II R/H LC (7–8 μm) perfusion analytical column using the chromatographic conditions shown in Table 29.3. Concentrations as low as 10 ppb could be readily determined in milk by electrospray mass spectrometric detection.

A specific cleanup procedure, based on liquid chromatography, has been described by Moats and Harik-Khan (108) for the liquid chromatographic determination of amoxicillin, ampicillin, penicillin G, penicillin V, cloxacillin, cephapirin, and ceftiofur residues in milk. In this method, a 10 ml milk sample is extracted with acetonitrile in presence of tetraethylammonium chloride. After filtration, 1 ml water is added to the filtrate, and the acetonitrile is completely removed by evaporation. The volume of the water is adjusted at a final volume of 4 ml, and a 2 ml aliquot is loaded on a Supelcosil LC-18, 5 μm, column. β-Lactams are eluted from the column with a 0.01M potassium dihydrogen phosphate/acetonitrile mobile phase, using a gradient elution program. Following collection of a narrow fraction (1.5–2 ml) centered on the retention times of the compounds of interest, the eluted analytes are reanalyzed by liquid chromatography under the conditions shown in Table 29.3. Concentrations as low as 2–5 ppb could be readily determined in milk using ultraviolet detection at 210, 214, 290, and 295 nm. Confirmation of the presence of β-lactam antibiotics in the suspected samples was based on the disappearance of the recorded peaks after treatment of the samples with β-lactamase and their reanalysis.

29.4 MACROLIDES AND LINCOSAMIDES

Macrolide and lincosamide antibiotics are weakly basic compounds slightly soluble in water but readily soluble in common organic solvents. They are most composed of several closely related components that may vary in proportion depending upon the source of the formulation. Macrolides other than oleandomycin are stated to be unstable at both acidic and basic aqueous solutions.

For the analysis of macrolide and lincosamide residues in liquid foods such as milk, a pretreatment step for fat removal carried out by centrifugation (133–135) is usually required. Semisolid food samples such as muscle, kidney, and liver require often more intensive sample pretreatment including a mincing and/or a homogenization step for breaking up tissue.

For efficient extraction of macrolide and lincosamide residues from edible animal products, bound residues should be rendered soluble, most if not all of the proteins should be removed, and high recoveries for all analytes should be provided. Since these antibiotics do not strongly bind to proteins, many effective extraction methods have been reported. Sample extraction/deproteinization is usually accomplished by vortexing liquid samples or homogenizing semisolid samples with acetonitrile (136–139), acidified (136, 140–142) or basified acetonitrile (143), methanol (14, 144, 145), acidified (145–147) or basified methanol (148), chloroform (149–151), or dichloromethane under alkaline conditions (152). However, for extraction of sedecamycin, a neutral macrolide antibiotic, from swine tissues, use of ethyl acetate at acidic conditions has been suggested (153), while for lincomycin analysis in fish tissues, acidic buffer extraction followed by sodium tungstate deproteinization has been proposed (154).

Following the primary sample extraction, the crude extract can be further subjected to various types of cleanup procedures including conventional liquid–liquid partitioning, solid-phase extraction, and liquid chromatography cleanup. In some instances, more than one of these cleanup procedures may be used in combination to obtain highly purified extracts.

In liquid–liquid partitioning cleanup, the lipophilic macrolides and lincosamides are generally extracted from the primary aqueous sample extracts with immiscible organic solvents including dichloromethane (139–143), ethyl acetate (143, 154), or chloroform (144). This extraction is usually carried out at alkaline conditions where the ionization of the basic amino sugar function of these antibiotics is suppressed. Following extraction, the organic extract is either evaporated to dryness and reconstituted in the mobile phase or back-extracted with an acidic buffer prior to analysis. Sometimes, several extraction steps are necessary to eliminate interfering substances, and cleanup may become a rather time-consuming and complicated procedure.

Cleanup of macrolides and lincosamides from coextracted material can also be accomplished with solid-phase extraction columns. Nonpolar sorbents such as XAD-2 resin (148) or reversed-phase sorbents (133, 134, 137, 141, 142) are usually employed in solid-phase extraction. In the latter case, ion-pairing with pentanesulfonic acid can also be applied for enhancing retention onto the hydrophobic C_{18} material (154). However, these sorbents are not always effective for efficient cleanup of liver and kidney extracts. The basic character of macrolides and lincosamides suggests that cation-exchange sorbents such as aromatic-sulfonic acid (145, 147), or polar sorbents such as silica (144, 152, 153), aminopropyl (139), or diol (149–151), can be powerful alternative approaches for isolation and/or cleanup of these compounds.

Liquid chromatography cleanup has been further described for purification of lincomycin residues from milk and tissue extracts (146). This procedure involves loading the sample extract onto a reversed-phase column (Supelcosil LC-

18 or LC-18-DB), elution with an ion-pairing mobile phase, collection of the narrow fraction of the eluate corresponding to lincomycin, and rechromatography by a second liquid chromatographic system.

Following extraction and cleanup, macrolides and lincosamides may be detected by spectrophotometric, electrochemical, or mass-spectrometric techniques, usually after liquid chromatographic separation. By combining thin-layer chromatographic (TLC) separation with a bioassay detection with *Bacillus subtilis* or *Microspora luteus* as the test organisms, TLC/bioautographic methods have been developed for identification of macrolide and lincosamide residues in animal tissues, milk, and eggs (14, 143, 148). A gas chromatographic–mass spectrometric method has also been reported for the determination of erythromycin in bovine and swine muscle (144). However, this method is rather complicated due to the need for derivatization (acetylation) of the analyte with pyridine/acetic anhydride.

At present, methods based on liquid chromatography are most widely used for determining macrolides and lincosamides in biological samples (Fig. 29.4).

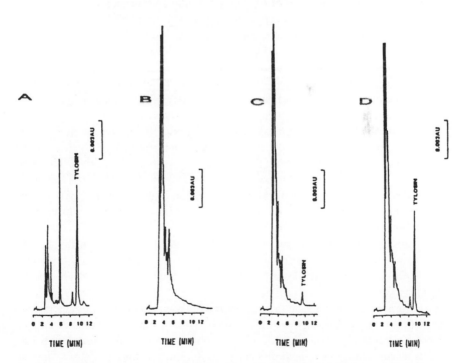

FIG. 29.4 Representative chromatograms of a tylosin standard solution (A), a blank muscle tissue (B), and a blank muscle tissue fortified with tylosin at a concentration of 50 ppb (C), and 400 ppb (D). (From Ref. 152.).

Chromatographic separation is generally carried out on octadecyl, octyl, phenyl, and polymeric reversed-phase columns, although polar stationary phases such as silica (153) or cyanopropyl (141, 142) have been also used in the analysis of sedecamycin and pirlimycin residues, respectively.

The preferred type of reversed-phase sorbents is C_{18} bonded silica (Table 29.4). Using this reversed-phase sorbent, ion-pair separation of lincomycin (154), spiramycin (138), and tylosin (145) residues has also been reported through use of octanesulfonate, heptanesulfonate, and tetrabutylammonium pairing ions, respectively. Phenyl-bonded silica or polymeric stationary phases have also been described for the separation of tilmicosin (133) and lincomycin (146) residues, respectively.

In liquid chromatographic analysis of macrolides and lincosamides, most popular is the ultraviolet detector (Table 29.4). Tylosin, tilmicosin, spiramycin, sedecamycin, and josamycin exhibit relatively strong ultraviolet absorption, but erythromycin, lincomycin, pirlimycin, and oleandomycin show extremely weak absorption in the ultraviolet region. Hence, detection at 200–210 nm has been reported for the determination of lincomycin (146). However, a combination of poor sensitivity and interference from coextractives necessitated extensive cleanup and concentration of the extract. Precolumn derivatization of pirlimycin with 9-fluorenylmethyl chloroformate has also been described to impart a chromophore for ultraviolet detection at 264 nm (140).

Electrochemical detection is better suited to the analysis of erythromycin and lincomycin. This method of detection has been applied for the determination of erythromycin A (139) and lincomycin (154) residues in salmon tissues. Liquid chromatography coupled with mass spectrometry is particularly suitable for confirmatory analysis of the nonvolatile macrolides and lincosamides. Typical applications of this technique are through thermospray mass spectrometry, which has been used to monitor pirlimycin in bovine milk and liver (141, 142), and chemical ionization, which has been applied for identification of tilmicosin (151) in bovine muscle, and for identification of spiramycin, tylosin, tilmicosin, erythromycin, and josamycin residues in the same tissue (150).

Most promising in terms of simplicity, selectivity, and sensitivity, for screening and even confirmation of macrolide residues in edible animal products, appear to be the methods described by Horie et al. (147) and Delepine et al. (150).

Horie et al. (147) has described a method allowing simultaneous determination of josamycin, kitasamycin, mirosamicin, spiramycin, and tylosin in animal tissues. According to this method, a 5 g tissue sample is homogenized with 100 ml 0.3% metaphosphoric acid/methanol (7:3), and the homogenate is filtered through Hyflo Super-Gel coated on a suction funnel. The filtrate is concentrated at 20 ml to be further applied to a cation-exchange solid-phase extraction column (Bond Elut SCX). Following column washing with water and 0.1M dipotassium

TABLE 29.4 Physicochemical Methods for Macrolide and Lincosamide Antibacterials in Edible Animal Products

Compounds(s)	Matrix	Sample preparation	Steps	Stationary phase	Mobile phase	Detection/Identification	Sensitivity/Recovery	Ref.
THIN-LAYER CHROMATOGRAPHIC METHODS								
Lincomycin	Animal tissues	MeOH/NaOH extn, liq–liq partn, XAD-2 column cleanup	16	Silica gel	H_2O/acetone/methyl ethyl ketone	M. luteus bio-autography	100 ppb/ 78–95%	148
Erythromycin, oleandomycin, tylosin	Animal tissues	MeOH extn, liq–liq partns	14	Silica gel	$CHCl_3$/MeOH/acetone-glycerine	B. subtilis bio-autography	1–20 ppm/ NR	14
Four macrolides	Milk, eggs, tissues	ACN/Na_2CO_3 extn, liq–liq partns	15	Silica gel	$BuOH/H_2O$/HOAc	Vis/Xanthydrol or B. subtilis bio-autography	20 ppb/ 51–96%	143
GAS CHROMATOGRAPHIC METHODS								
Erythromycin	Bovine and swine muscle	MeOH extn, liq–liq partns, silica gel column cleanup, HCl hydrolysis, liq–liq partns, pyridine/acetic anhydride acetylation	25	Chromosorb WHP with 5% OV-101	Helium	PICI-MS	10 ppb/ 69–88%	144

(continued)

TABLE 29.4 Continued

Compounds(s)	Matrix	Sample preparation	Steps	Stationary phase	Mobile phase	Detection/ Identification	Sensitivity/ Recovery	Ref.
LIQUID CHROMATOGRAPHIC METHODS								
Erythromycin A	Salmon flesh	ACN extn, liq–liq partns, SPE cleanup	25	Zorbax RX-C$_8$, 5 μm	0.005M sodium perchlorate/ ACN (50:50) at 40°C	Electro-chemical	200 ppb/ >90%	139
Lincomycin	Milk, and animal tissues	MeOH/NH$_4$H$_2$PO$_4$ extn, LC purification on Supelcosil LC-18 or LC-18-DB, 5 μm, column	10	PRLP-S, 5 μm, or Supelcosil LC-18 or LC-18-DB, 5 μm, analytical and guard columns	0.01M, pH 7.5 or 8.0, phosp. buffer/ACN (80:20) or (78:22) for the PLRP-S column, and (76:24) or (74:26) for the Supelco packing, at 40°C	UV 200–210 nm	20–50 ppb/ 89–99%	146
	Salmon tissues	0.01M KH$_2$PO$_4$ extn, sodium tangstate deprtn, 1-pentanesulfonic acid addn, SPE cleanup, liq–liq partns	25	Spherisorb S5 ODS2	0.02M KH$_2$PO$_4$ contg 20 mM 1-octanesulfonic acid, pH 4.5/ ACN (88:22)	Electro-chemical	17–24 ppb/ 79–96%	154

Compound	Matrix	Extraction/cleanup		Column	Mobile phase	Detection	Detection limit/recovery	Ref.
Pirlimycin	Bovine milk, and liver	ACN/HCl (milk) or ACN/TFA (liver) extn, liq–liq partns, SPE cleanup (milk)	14	CPS-Hypersil-2, 5 μm, with cyanopropyl guard column	0.1M ammonium acetate/ACN (70:30) for milk, (75:25) for liver	MS–TSP	50 ppb/ 83–113%	141
	Bovine milk, and liver	ACN/HCl (milk) or ACN/TFA (liver) extn, liq–liq partns, SPE cleanup (milk)	14	CPS-Hypersil-2, 5 μm, with cyanopropyl guard column	0.1M ammonium acetate/ACN (70:30)	MS–TSP	25–50 ppb/ 84–108%	142
	Milk	ACN/HCl extn, liq–liq partns, precolumn derivatization with Fmoc	15	Hypersil ODS, 5 μm	1% HOAc/ACN/ MeOH (40:30:30), at 35°C	UV 264 nm	50 ppb/ 89 ± 4%	140
Sedecamycin and metabolites	Swine tissues	EtOAc extn, Silica gel/Florisil column cleanup	13	μPorasil, 10 μm, analytical and guard column	n-Hexane/ isopropanol (80:20)	UV 227 nm	12–44 ppb/ 76–90%	153
Spiramycin	Bovine tissues	$CHCl_3$ extn, SPE cleanup	6	LiChrocart RP 18E, 5 μm, with RP 8E guard column	0.5% H_2SO_4/ACN (80:20)	UV 231 nm	50 ppb/ 76–97%	149
	Chicken tissues	ACN extn, liq–liq partns	13	Zorbax BP-C_8	0.4% H_3PO_4/ MeOH (30:70), contg 0.2% 1-heptanesulfonic acid, at 30°C	UV 231 nm	50 ppb/ 85–95%	138

(continued)

TABLE 29.4 Continued

Compounds(s)	Matrix	Sample preparation	Steps	Stationary phase	Mobile phase	Detection/ Identification	Sensitivity/ Recovery	Ref.
Tilmicosin	Bovine muscle	CHCl$_3$ extn, SPE cleanup	14	LiChrospher RP 18, 5 μm, with C$_{18}$ guard column	5% Formic acid/ MeOH/ACN (35:45:20)	NICI–MS	6 ppb/ NR	151
	Milk	Centrgn, SPE cleanup	15	Apex phenyl RP, 5 μm	Solvent A: H$_3$PO$_4$/ACN (50:50), pH 2.5 Solvent B: H$_3$PO$_4$, pH 2.5 Solvent C: 0.08 M dibutylammonium phosp. buffer, pH 2.5 Gradient from (100:0:0) to (34:41:25), at 35°C	UV 280 nm	20 ppb/ 80–106%	133

Tylosin	Bovine tissues	DCM extn, SPE cleanup	13	Spherisorb C$_{18}$ ODS, 5 μm	0.005M NH$_4$H$_2$PO$_4$/ ACN/MeOH (8:72:20)	UV 280 nm	15 ppb/ 85–107%	152
	Milk	Centrgn, SPE cleanup	9	LiChrospher RP 18, 5 μm, analytical and guard column	Solvent A: 0.1 M ammonium formate/ACN/ MeOH (61:29:10), pH 6.0 Solvent B: H$_2$O/ACN/ MeOH (61:29:10) Gradient from (100:0) to (0:100), at 25°C	UV 287 nm/ PDA (200–350 nm)	15 ppb/ 82–88%	134
	Swine tissues	H$_2$O/MeOH extn, SPE cleanup	8	Prodigy ODS, 5 μm	0.01 M KH$_2$PO$_4$ contg 20 mM tetrabutyl-ammonium bromide/ MeOH/ACN (50:35:15)	UV 280 nm	15 ppb/ 70–85%	145
	Swine tissues	ACN extn, liq–liq partns	11	Micro Pak MCH-10-N-Cap	0.005M NH$_4$H$_2$PO$_4$/ ACN/MeOH (10:60:30)	UV 280 nm	100 ppb/ 83–97%	136

(continued)

TABLE 29.4 Continued

Compounds(s)	Matrix	Sample preparation	Steps	Stationary phase	Mobile phase	Detection/ Identification	Sensitivity/ Recovery	Ref.
Tylosin, spiramycin	Milk	Centrgn, SPE cleanup, liq–liq partn	8	Supelcosil LC-8-DB	Phosp. buffer pH 3.0/ACN (70:30) and (60:40)	UV 232 and 280 nm	8–14 ppb/ 64–80%	135
Tylosin, tilmicosin	Animal tissues	ACN extn, SPE cleanup	13	Inertsil C_{18}, 5 μm	0.1M Ammonium formate/ACN/ MeOH (60:30:10)	UV 287 nm	10–20 ppb/ 74–97%	137
Five macrolides	Animal tissues	Metaphosphoric acid/MeOH extn, SPE cleanup	9	Puresil $5C_{18}$, 5 μm	0.025M, pH 2.5, phosp. buffer/ ACN Gradient from (60:40) to (0:100), at 35°C	UV 232 and 287 nm (wavelength programming)	50 ppb/ 71–90%	147
Five macrolides	Bovine muscle	$CHCl_3$ extn, SPE cleanup	14	LiChrospher RP 18, 5 μm, with C_{18} guard column	0.1% TFA/MeOH/ ACN Gradient from (60:20:20) to (20:55:25)	NICI-MS & PICI-MS	50 ppb/ NR	150

Fmoc, 9-fluorenylmethyl chloroformate.
Other abbreviations as in Tables 29.1 and 29.3.

hydrogen phosphate, macrolides are eluted with methanol and the eluate is evaporated to dryness. The residue is reconstituted in 1 ml 0.05M sodium dihydrogen phosphate/acetonitrile (7:3) to be further analyzed by liquid chromatography. Separation is performed on a 15 cm Puresil 5C$_{18}$ (5 μm) analytical column, using a gradient system of 0.025M, pH 2.5, with phosphate buffer–acetonitrile as mobile phase (Table 29.4). Concentrations as low as 50 ppb for each of the analytes could be readily determined by ultraviolet detection.

Liquid chromatography coupled with mass spectrometry was followed by Delepine et al. (150) in a multiresidue method for the determination of spiramycin, tylosin, tilmicosin, erythromycin, and josamycin in bovine muscle. According to this confirmatory method, a 2 g muscle sample is homogenized with 2 ml, pH 8, phosphate buffer, and 10 ml chloroform, and the homogenate is centrifuged. The chloroform layer is filtered, and the filtrate is purified on a diol solid-phase extraction column (Bond Elut diol). Following column washing with chloroform and water, macrolides are eluted with 0.1M ammonium acetate/methanol (1:1), and an aliquot is analyzed by liquid chromatography. Separation is performed on a 12.5 cm Lichrospher RP 18 (5 μm) analytical column protected by a C$_{18}$ guard column, using a gradient system of 0.1% trifluoroacetic acid–methanol–acetonitrile as mobile phase (Table 29.4). Concentrations as low as 50 ppb for each of the analytes could be readily determined using negative and positive chemical ionization mass spectrometric detection.

29.5 NITROFURANS

Nitrofuran antibacterials are synthetic compounds that are substitution products of the 5-nitrofuran nucleus, differing in the substituent at position 2. This substituent may be an azomethine group connected with other ring systems, or an alkyl, acyl, hydroxyalkyl, or carboxyl group, free or esterified. All these antibacterials are susceptible to photolysis, particularly by sunlight, and manipulations must be carried out under subdued light.

When analyzing milk samples for nitrofuran residues, dilution with sodium chloride solution (155) or lyophilization (156) prior to extraction may be required. Dilution of egg samples with water prior to their solid-phase extraction has been also reported (157). Semisolid samples such as muscle, kidney, and liver, require a more intensive sample pretreatment. This involves use of a mincing apparatus followed by sample homogenization in water (37), sodium chloride solution (155), or dilute hydrochloric acid (158).

Extraction of nitrofuran antibacterials from edible animal products should render the bound residues soluble, remove most if not all of the proteins, and provide high yields for all analytes. Sample extraction/deproteinization is usually accomplished with organic solvents capable to free the noncovalently bound residues from the endogenous macromolecules. Organic solvents including acetonitrile (56, 57, 159–167), ethyl acetate (29, 37, 38, 168, 169), dichloromethane (170–172), and dichloroethane (158) have all been used with varying success. Moreover, use of trichloroacetic acid (173), methanol/ethanol/diethyl ether (174), McIlvaine buffer/methanol (175, 176), metaphosphoric acid/methanol (177), citric acid/disodium hydrogen phosphate (178), and chloroform/ethyl acetate/dimethylsulfoxide (179) has been suggested for precipitating sample proteins and efficiently extracting the analytes.

To reduce coextractives in the primary sample extract and concentrate the analyte(s), various types of sample cleanup procedures can be applied. They include conventional liquid–liquid partitioning, solid-phase extraction, matrix solid-phase dispersion, and online dialysis and subsequent trace enrichment (Table 29.5). In many applications, more than one of these procedures is applied in combination to decrease the background noise of the detector, thus making it possible to quantify trace level residue concentrations.

Liquid–liquid partitioning is the most popular cleanup procedure employed. It is performed either to extract the analytes from their aqueous solution into an organic solvent or to wash out interfering substances from organic or aqueous extracts. Dichloromethane was proven to be more efficient than any other organic solvent tested in extracting nitrofurans from aqueous sample extracts at acidic conditions (56, 57, 165, 166, 170, 171, 175, 176). Occasionally, sodium chloride may be added to the aqueous solution to increase the extraction efficiency of dichloromethane (56, 57, 165, 166, 170). To reduce emulsification problems during the extraction process, diatomaceous earth columns can also be employed as an alternative to the classic liquid–liquid partitioning cleanup (157, 169). Sample extracts are often further subjected to a defatting procedure by partitioning with n-hexane (37, 56, 57, 159, 161, 163–172).

Cleanup of nitrofurans from coextracted substances and concentration of the extracts can also be accomplished with solid-phase extraction columns. Nonpolar sorbents such as reversed-phase (C_{18}) (37, 159–161, 170, 173, 177) or XAD-2 (178) materials are usually employed, since they provide high recovery of the analytes. However, in many cases, cleanup on these nonpolar sorbents is not effective in removing interfering substances from the extracts. Therefore, polar sorbents such as silica (29, 162), alumina (160, 179, 180), or aminopropyl (175, 176) materials are also frequently employed as a more powerful alternative for extract cleanup.

In contrast to the solid-phase extraction approach, only nonpolar C_{18}-derivatized silica has been used as the sorbent in matrix solid-phase dispersion technique. This technique has been successfully applied in the determination of furazolidone in meat (66), milk (181), and swine tissues (180).

Online dialysis followed by trace enrichment of the analytes can also be employed for the determination of nitrofurans in foods of animal origin. The efficiency of this technique has been demonstrated in a method for the determina-

TABLE 29.5 Physicochemical Methods for Nitrofuran Antibacterials in Edible Animal Products

Antibacterial(s)	Matrix	Sample preparation	Steps	Stationary phase	Mobile phase	Detection/ Identification	Sensitivity/ Recovery	Ref.
Thin-Layer Chromatographic Methods								
Furazolidone	Animal tissues	HCl/NaCl addn, DCE extn, liq–liq partns	20	HPTLC Silica gel	CHCl₃/ACN/ HCOOH	Fluorometric/ Pyridine	2 ppb/ NR	158
Furazolidone, nitrofurazone, nitrofurantoin	Meat	ACN extn, liq–liq partn, SPE cleanup	10	HPTLC Silica gel	DCM/EtOAc	Fluorometric/ Pyridine	1 ppb/ >90%	159
Four nitrofurans	Meat	EtOAc extn, SPE cleanup	10	HPTLC Silica gel	EtOAc/hexane	UV-Vis/ Pyridine	5 ppb/ NR	29
Liquid Chromatographic Methods								
3-Amino-2-oxazolidinone (furazolidone metabolite)	Swine tissues	MeOH, EtOH, ether extn, precolumn derivatization with 2-nitrobenzaldehyde, liq–liq partns	19	LiChrospher RP18, 5 μm, analytical and guard column	0.1M ammonium acetate/ACN (65:35)	MS-TSP	10 ppb/ >80%	174
Furazolidone	Turkey tissues	DCM extn, liq–liq partns, SPE cleanup, liq–liq partn	30	Ultrasphere ODS, 5 μm, with Vydac 30/44 μm guard column	0.01M, pH 5.0, acetate buffer/ MeOH (70:30)	UV-Vis 365 nm	0.5 ppb/ 76–92%	170
	Eggs, milk and meat	ACN extn, liq–liq partns	11	MOS-Hypersil, 3 μm, analytical and guard column	0.01 or 0.02M, pH 4.6, acetate buffer/ACN (75:25)	UV 275 nm, or UV-Vis 365 nm	10 ppb/ 80–90%	56,57

(continued)

TABLE 29.5 Continued

Antibacterial(s)	Matrix	Sample preparation	Steps	Stationary phase	Mobile phase	Detection/ Identification	Sensitivity/ Recovery	Ref.
	Eggs	EtOAt extn, liq–liq partns	21	CP™Spher C_{18}, 10 μm, with Bondapak C_{18}, 37–50 μm, guard column	Acetate buffer, pH 5.0/ACN (75:25)	UV-Vis 365 nm/ PDA (240–420 nm)	5 ppb/ 86 ± 4.5%	168
	Eggs	H_2O diln, Kieselguhr column cleanup	4	Wakosil-II 5C18 HG	H_2O/ACN (60:40)	UV-Vis 358 nm/ MS-APCI	100 ppb/ 87 ± 4.3%	157
	Swine tissues	EtOAt extn, liq–liq partn, Kieselguhr column cleanup	14	Hypersil ODS 5, with OD-GU RP-18 guard column	H_2O/ACN/1M acetate buffer (67.5:25:7.5)	UV-Vis 362 nm	2 ppb/ 76–102%	169
	Eggs	DCM extn, dry-ice cooled filtn, liq–liq partns	18	Perkin-Elmer C_8, 10 μm	0.01M, pH 5.0, acetate buffer/ ACN/MeOH (45.5:35:19.5), at 35°C	UV-Vis 365 nm/ online: absorbance rationing, offline: TLC	1 ppb/ 92–107%	171
	Meat	MSPD extn/ cleanup	6	Spherisorb C_{18} ODS2, 5 μm	Solvent A: 0.01M, pH 5.2, acetate buffer Solvent B: ACN/MeOH (70:30) Gradient from (56:44) to (36:64), at 35°C	UV-Vis 365 nm/ PDA (200–450 nm)	3.5 ppb/ 30–87%	66

Sample	Extraction/cleanup		Column	Mobile phase	Detection	LOD/recovery	Ref.
Milk	MSPD extn/cleanup	8	Varian MCH-10, 10 μm	0.017M H_3PO_4/ACN (60:40), at 40°C	UV-Vis 365 nm/ PDA (200–550 nm)	78 ppb/ 82 ± 8%	181
Swine tissues	Na_2SO_4 addn, DCM extn, liq–liq partn	11	Tandem Spheri-10 RP-18 and Ultrasphere C_{18}, 5 μm	0.067M, pH 5.0, acetate buffer/ ACN (75:25)	Electro-chemical	0.5 ppb/ 67–71%	172
Salmon tissues	McIlvaine buffer/ MeOH extn, liq–liq partn, SPE cleanup	14	ODS-Hypersil, 3 μm, with C_{18} pellicular, 40 μm, guard column	H_2O/ACN (84:16) contg 1 mM EDTA and 0.1M KNO_3, pH 3.2	Vis 400 nm	5 ppb/ 90–99%	175
Swine tissues	MSPD extn/ cleanup, alumina column cleanup	9	Micro Pak ODS, 10 μm	0.015M H_3PO_4/ ACN (60:40), at 45°C	UV-Vis 365 nm/ PDA (200–450 nm)	7.8 ppb/ 90 ± 8%	180
Fish tissues	Metaphosphoric acid/MeOH extn, SPE cleanup	7	Inertsil ODS, 5 μm, with RP-8 Newguard column	0.005M oxalic acid/ACN (55:45)	UV 265 nm	50 ppb/ 87–90%	177
Poultry tissues	Citric acid-Na_2HPO_4 extn, Amberlite XAD-2 column cleanup	9	LiChrospher RP18	1% H_3PO_4/ACN (75:25)	UV-Vis 360 nm/ PDA (195–380 nm)	5–10 ppb/ 55–79%	178
Shrimp	ACN extn, tandem SPE cleanup	11	Ultrasphere, 5 μm, with Adsorbcsphere C_{18}, 5 μm, guard column	0.01% H_3PO_4/ ACN (70:30)	UV-Vis 365 nm	5 ppb/ 74–80%	160

(continued)

TABLE 29.5 Continued

Antibacterial(s)	Matrix	Sample preparation	Steps	Stationary phase	Mobile phase	Detection/Identification	Sensitivity/Recovery	Ref.
Furazolidone, nitrofurazone	Swine muscle	McIlvaine buffer-MeOH extn, liq–liq partn, SPE cleanup	12	LiChrosorb RP18	H_2O/ACN (75:25), contg 0.1M ammonium acetate	PICI-MS-TSP	0.6 ppb/65–88%	176
	Poultry tissues	H_2O addn, EtOAc extn, liq–liq partn, SPE cleanup	12	Supelcosil LC-18-DB, 5 μm, with Supelguard LC-18-DB column	0.2M, pH 3.0, acetate buffer/ACN (75:25), at 40°C	UV-Vis 360 nm/PDA	3 ppb/90–100%	37
	Chicken tissues	$CHCl_3$/EtOAc/DMSO extn, alumina column cleanup	7	Supelcosil LC-18, 5 μm	0.05M, pH 6.0, phosp. buffer contg 1 mM EDTA/MeOH (57.5:72.5)	Electro-chemical	2.5 ppb/74–90%	179
	Shrimp muscle	ACN extn, liq–liq partn, SPE cleanup	12	ODS-Hypersil C_{18}, 5 μm, analytical and guard column	1% HOAc/ACN (75:25), at 40°C	UV-Vis 375 nm/PDA	4 ppb/71–78%	161
Furazolidone, furaltadone, nitrofurazone	Animal and fish muscle	EtOAc extn, liq–liq partns	9	Two ChromSpher C_8 analytical columns in tandem, with Perisorb RP-8, 30–40 μm, guard column	0.01M, pH 4.3, acetate buffer/ACN (80:20)	UV-Vis 360 nm/PDA (200–400 nm)	1–2 ppb/69–88%	38

Drug	Matrix		Extraction	Column	Mobile phase	Detection	LOD/Recovery	Ref.
	Eggs, chicken tissues	9	ACN extn, liq–liq partns	Spherisorb ODS2 S5, 5 μm with μBondapak C18 guard column	0.02M, pH 4.6, acetate buffer/ACN (79:21), at 25°C	UV-Vis 362 nm/PDA (220–550 nm) & PICI-MS-ISP after LC conditions modification	1–5 ppb/ 83–88%	166
	Eggs, poultry muscle	15	Na2SO4 addn, ACN (eggs) or DCM/EtOAc (muscle) extn, SPE cleanup	Spherisorb ODS-2, 5 μm, analytical and guard column	H2O/ACN (75:25)	UV-Vis 362 nm	1–2 ppb/ 84–128%	162
Furazolidone, furaltadone, nitrofurantoin	Milk	10	Liophylization, ACN/DMF extn	Pecosphere CR C18	0.1M, pH 3.2, acetate buffer/ACN (90:10)	UV-VIS 360 nm/ differential processing of spectra	250–500 ppb/ 79–88%	156
	Milk	5	TCA extn, SPE cleanup	Nova-Pak C18, 4 μm, with Symmetry C18 guard column	0.1M sodium perchlorate/ACN (72:28) contg 0.5% HOAc	Electro-chemical	4–5 ppb/ 85–98%	173
Furazolidone, nitrofurazone, nitrofurantoin	Catfish muscle	10	ACN extn, liq–liq partns	ODS-Hypersil, 5 μm	1% HOAc/ACN (75:25), at 40°C	UV-Vis 375 nm/PDA (220–400 nm)	5 ppb/ 71–102%	163

(continued)

TABLE 29.5 Continued

Antibacterial(s)	Matrix	Sample preparation	Steps	Stationary phase	Mobile phase	Detection/ Identification	Sensitivity/ Recovery	Ref.
Four nitrofurans	Bovine muscle	ACN extn, liq–liq partns	10	ODS-Hypersil C$_{18}$, 5 μm, with C$_{18}$, μm, guard column	0.01M, pH 4.5, sodium acetate/ACN (70:30), at 35°C	UV-Vis 365 nm/PDA (200–550 nm)	2 ppb/ 60–110%	167
Four nitrofurans	Bovine tissues	KH$_2$PO$_4$ addn, ACN extn, liq–liq partns	8	Zorbax CN, 5 μm, with pellicular RP guard column	0.01M, pH 5.0, acetate buffer/ MeOH (60:40)	UV-Vis 365 nm	1 ppb/ 52–100%	164
Four nitrofurans	Milk, meat, eggs	NaCl solution addn, purification by online dialysis and subsequent trace enrichment on Bondapak C$_{18}$/Corasil, 37–50 μm, or XAD-4, 50–100 μm, preconcn column and switching to analytical column	2	ODS-Hypersil, 5 μm	0.1M, pH 5, acetate buffer/ ACN (80:20)	UV-Vis 365 nm	1–5 ppb/ 75–89%	155
Five nitrofurans	Eggs, milk, meat	ACN extn, liq–liq partns	11	Zorbax CN, with HPLC-Sorb Vydac 201 RP guard column	0.01M, pH 5.0, acetate buffer/ ACN (70:30), at 30°C	UV-Vis 360 nm	10 ppb/ 67–100%	165

DCE, dichloroethane; DMSO, dimethylsulfoxide.
Other abbreviations as in Tables 29.1 and 29.3.

tion of four nitrofurans in meat, milk, and eggs (155). This method involved on-line isolation of the analytes through use of a diphasic dialysis membrane, trapping of the analytes onto a liquid chromatographic preconcentration column (Bondapak C_{18}/Corasil, 37–50 μm, or XAD-4, 50–100 μm), rinsing of the coextracted material to waste, and flushing of the concentrated analytes onto the analytical column.

Following extraction and cleanup, nitrofurans are separated by thin-layer or liquid chromatography and measured by spectrophotometric, fluorometric, electrochemical, or mass spectrometric detectors (Table 29.5). Thin-layer chromatography has been carried out on commercially available silica gel plates. Nitrofurans were separated using various solvent mixtures as mobile phases and subsequently detected after spraying with pyridine, using spectrophotometric (29) or fluorometric (158, 159) detectors.

In the liquid chromatographic methods, separation of nitrofurans is generally carried out on nonpolar reversed-phase columns, the preferred sorbent being octadecyl bonded silica (Table 29.5). Polar columns containing cyanopropyl-based sorbents (164, 165) have also been used for the isocratic separation of nitrofuran residues isolated from edible animal products. A literature survey shows that there exists a clear preference for acidic mobile phases containing acetonitrile as the organic modifier (Fig. 29.5.1).

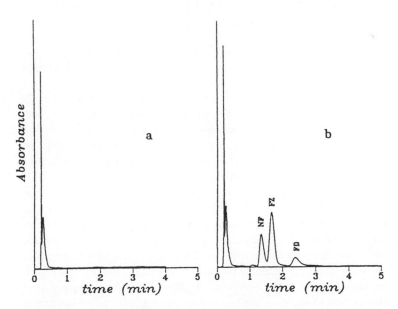

FIG. 29.5.1 Chromatograms of a blank milk sample (a) and a milk sample (b) spiked with nitrofurantoin (NF), furazolidone (FZ), and furaltadone (FD). (From Ref. 156.).

In liquid chromatographic analysis of nitrofuran antibacterials, the most popular detector is the ultraviolet visible (UV-vis) spectrophotometer. Nitrofurans exhibit strong absorption at wavelengths around 365 nm and are, therefore, ideal for direct determination (Table 29.5). Detection wavelengths of 275 nm (56, 57) and 400 nm (175) have also been suggested. Electrochemical detection is also frequently applied in liquid chromatographic methods for the determination of various nitrofuran antibacterials in edible animal products (172, 173, 179).

Confirmatory analysis of suspected liquid chromatographic peaks is usually accomplished by a photodiode array detector that continuously collects spectral data during the chromatographic separation and further compares the spectrum (200–550 nm) of the eluted suspected compound with that of a standard (37, 38, 66, 161, 163, 166–168, 178, 180, 181). Online absorbance ratio techniques combined with off-line thin-layer chromatography have been also reported (171). Although these confirmation techniques are relatively simple, their sensitivity is not generally adequate to identify trace levels of residual nitrofurans in edible animal products.

Coupling of liquid chromatography with mass spectrometry allows un-equivocal online spectrometric identification of all nitrofurans at the very low residue concentrations required by regulatory agencies for confirmatory analysis in animal-derived foods. Typical examples of mass spectrometry applications in confirming nitrofuran residues in edible animal products employ thermospray (174, 176), ionspray (166), or atmospheric pressure chemical ionization (157) interfaces.

Most promising methods in terms of simplicity, selectivity, and sensitivity appear to be those described by Degroodt et al. (38), Botsoglou (171), Diaz et al. (173), and Draisci et al. (166).

Degroodt et al. (38) developed a liquid chromatographic method for the determination of furazolidone, furaltadone, and nitrofurazone in meat and fish. According to this method, a 10 g meat sample is acidified with 1 M ammonium acetate buffer, pH 4.8, and extracted with 25 ml ethyl acetate after addition of 10 g sodium sulfate. Following centrifugation, the separated upper organic layer is evaporated, and the remaining oily residue is dissolved in mobile phase to be further defatted by partitioning with petroleum ether and n-pentane. An aliquot of the lower layer is collected and analyzed by liquid chromatography. Separation is performed on two joined 10 cm ChromSpher C_8 analytical columns, protected with a Perisorb RP-8 (30–40 μm) precolumn. The mobile phase is a mixture of pH 4.3 acetate buffer and acetonitrile (80:20). Under these conditions, concentrations as low as 1 ppb for furazolidone and nitrofurazone and 2 ppb for furaltadone could be determined in meat and fish using a photodiode array detector set at 360 nm. Confirmation of the suspected violative samples is based on continuous collection of spectral data during the analysis and checking for interfering substances by comparing the spectrum (200–400 nm) of the sample with that of the standard.

Botsoglou (171) described a liquid chromatographic method for the determination of furazolidone residues in eggs. According to this method, 8 g homogenized sample is acidified at pH 4 and extracted with 30 ml dichloromethane. Following centrifugation, the separated lower organic layer is evaporated, and the oily residue that remains is dissolved in acetone to be further cooled in dry ice/acetone and filtered. The filtrate is evaporated, and the oily residue is partitioned between hexane and water. The aqueous layer separated by centrifugation is extracted with dichloromethane. An aliquot of the lower organic layer is collected, evaporated to dryness, and the residue is reconstituted in water to be further analyzed by liquid chromatography. Separation is performed on a 25 cm Perkin-Elmer C_8 (10 μm) analytical column, with an acetate buffer, pH 5/acetonitrile/methanol (45.5:35:19.5) mobile phase, at a flow-rate of 1 ml/min and a column temperature of 35°C. Under these conditions, concentrations of furazolidone as low as 1 ppb could be determined in eggs using an ultraviolet-visible spectrophotometer set at 365 nm. Confirmation of the presence of furazolidone in suspected samples is based on both the on-line characterization of the eluted peaks by an absorbance ratio technique and the off-line thin-layer chromatography and spraying of the developed furazolidone spot with pyridine to form a characteristic fluorescent product.

A different approach was followed by Diaz et al. (173) for the liquid chromatographic determination of furazolidone, furaltadone, and nitrofurantoin residues in milk. According to this method, 50 g cow milk is deproteinized with 25 ml 20% (w/v) trichloroacetic acid. Following filtration, the pH of the extract is adjusted in the range 4.5–5, and the solution is diluted with water. An aliquot of 25 ml is passed through a C_{18} solid-phase extraction cartridge (Sep-Pak Plus C_{18}), and the analytes are eluted with 2.5 ml mobile phase to be further analyzed by liquid chromatography. Separation is performed on a 15-cm Nova-Pak C_{18} (4 μm) analytical column, protected with a Symmetry C_{18} guard column, using a 0.1 M sodium perchlorate/acetonitrile (72:28) mobile phase containing 0.5% acetic acid, at a flow rate of 1 ml/min. Under these conditions, concentrations as low as 4 ppb for furaltadone and nitrofurantoin and 5 ppb for furazolidone could be determined in milk by electrochemical detection.

Draisci et al. (166) quantified and identified furazolidone, nitrofurazone, and furaltadone residues in chicken eggs and tissues using liquid chromatography combined with photodiode array and ionspray mass spectrometry. In the suggested method, 10 g homogenized eggs, chicken liver, or muscle is extracted with 30 ml acetonitrile. After centrifugation, sodium chloride solution (10%, w/v) is added to the supernatant, and the mixture is partitioned with dichloromethane. The separated lower organic phase is filtered through anhydrous sodium sulfate and evaporated to dryness. The residue is reconstituted in acetate buffer, pH 4.6/methanol/acetonitrile (4:5:1), extracted with n-hexane, and analyzed by liquid chromatography. Separation is performed on a 15 cm Spherisorb ODS2 S5 (5 μm) analytical column protected with a μBondapak C18 guard column, using a mobile phase of pH-4 acetate buffer/acetonitrile (79:21), at a flow rate of 1 ml/min and a column temperature of 25°C. Under these conditions, concentrations as low as 2.5 ppb for furazolidone and nitrofurazone, and 5 ppb for furaltadone could be determined and tentatively identified in chicken eggs and tissues using a photodiode array detector at 362 nm and examining the spectra of the eluted compounds in the wavelength range 220–550 nm. For unequivocal online identification, nitrofurans separation is performed on a 25 cm Supelcosil L C_{18}-DB (5 μm) analytical column, with a water/acetonitrile (50:50) mobile phase containing 1 mM ammonium acetate and 0.025% acetic acid, at a flow rate of 0.6 ml/min and a column temperature of 25°C (Fig. 29.5.2). Under these conditions, concentrations as low as 3 ppb could be identified using ionspray mass spectrometric detection operating in the positive-ion chemical ionization mode.

29.6 QUINOLONES

Quinolone carboxylic acid antibacterials are synthetic compounds whose basic nuclear structure includes a quinolone ring and a carboxylic acid group. Fluoroquinolones are second-generation quinolones that contain in their molecule a fluorine and a piperazine ring. Quinolones are amphoteric compounds slightly soluble in polar solvents such as water, and insoluble in nonpolar solvents such as benzene and hexane. Most of these drugs are fluorescent and are quite stable in aqueous solution toward light, except miloxacin, which is reported to be unstable.

When analyzing quinolone residues in semisolid food samples such as muscle, kidney, and liver, a pretreatment step for tissue break-up may be required. This can be accomplished by means of a mincing and/or a homogenizing apparatus. To achieve better recovery of the analytes, drying of the tissue sample with anhydrous sodium sulfate prior to its extraction has been recommended (182–188).

Sample extraction and deproteinization is usually accomplished with organic solvents including ethyl acetate (182–187, 189–192), acetone (193–196), methanol (177, 197–200), acetonitrile (201, 202), and ethanol (188). To optimize the extraction efficiency, acidification of the sample has been suggested by many workers (177, 188, 192, 197–199). In acidic conditions (pH < 3), quinolones, being zwitterions, are fully protonated and, therefore, are becoming less bound by the matrix and more soluble in organic extraction solvents. Extraction of quinolones from food samples can also be accomplished using water (203), phosphate buffer, pH 9 (204), or trichloroacetic acid (205).

To eliminate or reduce interference and concentrate the analyte(s), the primary sample extract may further be subjected to various types of cleanup procedures including conventional liquid–liquid partitioning, solid-phase extraction, matrix solid-phase dispersion, and online dialysis and subsequent trace enrichment (Table 29.6). In most instances, more than one of these procedures is used in combination to enhance the cleanup efficiency.

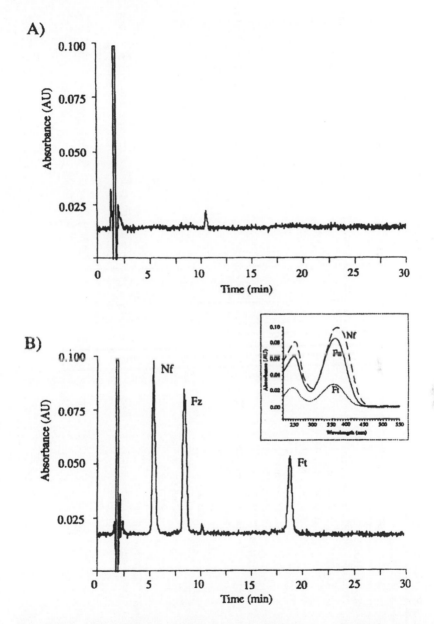

FIG. 29.5.2   HPLC–PDA chromatograms of (A) blank and (B) fortified (20 ppb) egg control samples and related UV-Vis spectra. Peaks: Nf, nitrofurazone; Fz, furazolidone; Ft, furaltadone. (Reprinted from Ref. 166, with permission from Elsevier Science.)

TABLE 29.6 Physicochemical Methods for Quinolone Antibacterials in Edible Animal Products

Antibacterial(s)	Matrix	Sample preparation	Steps	Stationary phase	Mobile phase	Detection/ Identification	Sensitivity/ Recovery	Ref
SPECTROMETRIC METHODS								
Nalidixic acid	Chicken tissues	Buffer pH 6 addn, EtOAc extn, alumina column cleanup, liq–liq partns, derivatization with H_2SO_4	17	—	—	Fluorometric	100 ppb/ 71–149%	189, 190
GAS CHROMATOGRAPHIC METHODS								
Oxolinic acid, nalidixic acid, piromidic acid	Fish muscle	Buffer pH 6 addn, EtOAc extn, liq–liq partns, sodium tetrahydroborate reduction, liq–liq partns, SPE cleanup	25	DB-5, 15 m, capillary	Helium	PICI-MS	3 ppb/ 63–116%	191
LIQUID CHROMATOGRAPHIC METHODS								
Enrofloxacin	Milk, meat	ACN extn, liq–liq partns	5–8	PLRP-S, 5 μm, analytical and guard column	Solvent A: 0.02M heptane-sulfonate, 0.002M H_3PO_4, Solvent B: ACN Solvent C: MeOH (65:27:8)	Fluorometric, ex: 278 nm, em: 440 nm	3–5 ppb/ 86–93%	201

Flumequine	Fish muscle	H2O extn, purification by online dialysis and subsequent trace enrichment on reversed phase, 40 μm, preconcn column and switching to analytical column	2	CTI™ Spher C8	0.01M, pH 3.0, KH2PO4/MeOH/TEA (40:60:0.5)	Fluorometric, postcolumn derivatization with H2SO4, ex: 240 nm, em: 370 nm	10 ppb/ 60–65%	203
Miloxacin	Fish muscle	Metaphosphoric acid/MeOH extn, SPE cleanup	7	L-column ODS	0.05M NaH2PO4/ACN (65:35)	UV 260 nm, or fluorometric, ex: 325 nm, em: 365 nm	10 ppb/ 85–88%	198
Oxolinic acid	Catfish muscle	MSPD extn/cleanup	6	Versapack C18, 10 μm, with Guard-Pak column	0.05M HOAc/MeOH Gradient from (100:0) to (0:100), at 40°C	UV 269 nm	50 ppb/ 63–100%	206
	Eggs	EtOAc extn, liq–liq partn	7	LiChrospher RP-18E, 5 μm	H2O/ACN/HOAc (72:25:3)	Fluorometric, ex: 334 nm, em: 382 μm	5 ppb/ 65–80%	192
	Mussel shell	MeOH/oxalic acid extn	8	LiChropher 100 FP-18E, 5 μm, analytical and guard column	0.02M H3PO4/ACN (76:24), pH 2.3	UV 262 nm	12 ppb/ 72 ± 11%	199
	Salmon muscle	Na2SO4 addn, EtOAc extn, liq–liq partn	8	Parisil ODS-3, 5 μm	0.01 oxalic acid/ACN/MeOH (60:30:10)	Fluorometric, ex: 327 nm, em: 369 nm	10 ppb/ 71–83%	183, 184, 185

(continued)

TABLE 29.6 Continued

Antibacterial(s)	Matrix	Sample preparation	Steps	Stationary phase	Mobile phase	Detection/ Identification	Sensitivity/ Recovery	Ref
Sarafloxacin	Catfish muscle	ACN/H$_2$0 extn, liq-liq partn	16	YMC, ODS, 120A, 5 μm, spherical	Solvent A: ACN/ MeOH (3:2) Solvent B: 0.1% TFA Step gradient from (20:80) to (90:10)	Fluorometric, ex: 280 nm, em: 389 nm	1.4 ppb/ 84–110%	202
Flumequine, hydroxy-flumequine	Fish tissues	Na$_2$SO$_4$ addn, EtOAc extn, SPE cleanup, or liq-liq partn	10	ChromSpher C$_8$, 5 μm, with RP guard column	0.035M, pH 2.2, oxalic acid/ ACN (20:80)	Fluorometric, ex: 327 nm, em: 369 nm	5 ppb/ 70–91%	182
Oxolinic acid, flumequine	Chicken liver	Acetone extn, liq-liq partns, purification by on-line dialysis and subsequent trace enrichment on PLRP-S or Hypersil ODS preconcn column and switching to analytical column	15	PLRP-S, 5 μm	0.02M, pH 5.0, Na$_3$PO$_4$/ACN/ THF (65:20:15)	Fluorometric, ex: 318 nm, em: 364 nm	2.5–5 ppb/ 94–115%	193
	Fish tissues	Na$_2$SO$_4$ addn, EOAc extn, liq-liq partn	8	LiChrosorb RP-8, 5 μm	0.025M, pH 3.2, oxalic acid/ ACN (68:32)	Fluorometric, ex: 327 nm, em: 369 nm	2–5 ppb/ 51–89%	186

	Sample	Extraction		Column	Mobile phase	Detection	LOD/Recovery	Ref.
	Fish tissues	TCA extn, liq–liq partn	7	PLRP-S, 5 μm, analytical and guard column	0.02M H_3PO_4/ACN/THF (65:20:15)	Fluorometric, ex: 325 nm, em: 360 nm	30–35 ppb/ 51–71%	205
	Salmon muscle	Buffer, pH9, extn, purification by online dialysis and subsequent trace enrichment on polymeric, 36 μm, preconcn column and switching to analytical column	4	PLRP-S, 5 μm	0.02M H_3PO_4/ACN/THF (75:20:14)	Fluorometric, ex: 325 nm, em: 365 nm	2–3 ppb/ NR	204
Oxolinic acid, nalidixic acid, piromidic acid	Fish muscle	Metaphosphoric acid/MeOH extn, SPE cleanup	7	Inertsil ODS, 5 μm, with RP-8 Newguard column	0.05M oxalic acid/ACN (55:45)	UV 265 nm	20–50 ppb/ 85–90%	177
	Fish muscle	Acetone extn, liq–liq partns, alumina column cleanup, liq–liq partns	21	Nucleosil C_{18}, with RP-2 Spher-10 guard column	H_2O/THF/ACN/H_3PO_4 (69.94:29:1:0.06)	UV 260 nm	20–80 ppb/ 75–91%	194
	Fish muscle	Metaphosphoric acid/MeOH extn, SPE cleanup	8	Kaseisorb LC ODS 300-5	0.005M NaH_2PO_4/ACN (60:40)	UV 280 nm, for piromidic acid, and fluorometric, ex: 325 nm, em: 365 nm, for the rest/ GC-MS for oxolinic acid	10 ppb/ 81–89%	197

(continued)

TABLE 29.6 Continued

Antibacterial(s)	Matrix	Sample preparation	Steps	Stationary phase	Mobile phase	Detection/ Identification	Sensitivity/ Recovery	Ref
	Fish muscle	MeOH extn, liq–liq partns	18	Nucleosil C_8, 7 μm	0.1M citric acid/ MeOH/ACN (40:40:20) contg 10 mM tetrabutyl-ammonium bromide	UV 254 nm, for oxolinic and nalidixic acid, and 280 nm for piromidic acid	50 ppb/ 83–93%	200
	Fish muscle	Hexane/EtOAc extn, SPE cleanup	8	Nucleosil 3 C_{18}, 3 μm	0.01M oxalic acid/ACN/ MeOH (60:30:10)	UV 295 nm	50 ppb/ 74–96%	187
Four quinolones	Milk	EtOH/HOAc extn, SPE cleanup	17	Inertsil, phenyl, 5 μm	2% HOAc/ACN (85:15), at 40°C	Fluorometric, ex: 278 nm, em: 450 nm	5 ppb/ 69–99%	188
Four quinolones	Catfish muscle	Acetone extn, liq–liq partns	29	PLRP-S, 5 μm	0.02M H_3PO_4/ ACN/THF (72:16:12), at 46°C	Fluorometric, ex: 325 nm, em: 365 nm/ GC-MS	5 ppb/ 78–107%	196
Four quinolones	Salmon and shrimp muscle	Acetone extn, liq–liq partns	29	PLRP-S, 5 μm	0.02M H_3PO_4/ ACN/THF (72:16:12), at 46°C	Fluorometric, ex: 325 nm, em: 365 nm/ GC-MS	10–20 ppb/ 64–108%	195

Abbreviations as in Tables 29.1 and 29.3.

Liquid–liquid partitioning is intended either to extract the drugs from an organic solvent into an aqueous solution or to wash out interfering substances from organic or aqueous solutions. In general, quinolones are extracted from chloroform or ethyl acetate sample extracts into alkaline buffers, to then be back-extracted into chloroform or ethyl acetate at acidic conditions (191, 195, 196, 200). Occasionally, sodium chloride may be added to the sample extracts in order to increase the extraction efficiency of ethyl acetate or chloroform (193–196, 200). To remove lipids, sample extracts are often also partitioned with *n*-hexane (183–186, 193–196, 202, 204), or diethyl ether (189, 190, 201).

Cleanup and concentration of quinolones from coextracted matrix constituents can also be accomplished with solid-phase extraction columns that contain either nonpolar reversed-phase (C_{18}) sorbents (177, 197, 198), or polar sorbents such as alumina (189–191, 194), aminopropyl (182, 187), and propylsulfonic acid (188). Reversed-phase C_{18} material has also been employed as the sorbent in matrix solid-phase dispersion cleanup for the determination of oxolinic acid in catfish muscle (206).

Online dialysis and subsequent trace enrichment has been further described for isolation/purification of flumequine residues from fish muscle (203), or oxolinic acid and flumequine from chicken liver (193) and salmon muscle (204). This involves online purification by diphasic dialysis membrane and trapping of the analytes onto a liquid chromatographic preconcentration column (reversed-phase C_{18} or polymeric), rinsing of the coextracted materials to waste, and finally flushing of the concentrated analytes onto the analytical column.

Following their extraction and cleanup, residues of quinolone antibiotics in sample extracts can be determined by either direct nonchromatographic methods, or gas or liquid chromatographic methods. Spectrophotometric, fluorometric, or mass spectrometric detection systems have all been successfully used in quinolone analysis (Table 29.6).

A direct spectrometric method for screening nalidixic acid in chicken tissues (189, 190) has been reported. This method was based on fluorometric detection after derivatization of the analyte with sulfuric acid. The major drawback of this method is that it cannot differentiate among the various quinolones, it is less sensitive than the screening tests usually employed for regulatory purposes, and it is complicated by the necessity for derivatization.

A gas-chromatographic mass-spectrometric method has also been described for determination of oxolinic, nalidixic, and piromidic acids in fish muscle (191). However, this method is rather complicated due to the need for derivatization (reduction) with sodium tetrahydroborate.

At present, liquid chromatography is the method of choice for determining residues of quinolone antibacterials in edible animal products (Table 29.6). Separation is generally carried out on nonpolar reversed-phase columns containing octadecyl, octyl, phenyl, or polymeric sorbents. Either methanol or acetonitrile may be used as organic modifiers in the mobile phases. Adjusting the mobile phase pH at a value lower than 3.0, the ionization of the carboxylate moiety, of the analytes is suppressed, and although increased retention and improved separation are effected, tailing chromatographic peaks are generally recorded. However, this phenomenon can be prevented by addition to the mobile phase of counter ions (201, 203), or oxalic acid (177, 182–187).

In liquid chromatographic analysis of quinolone antibacterials, most popular is the fluorometric detector due to the inherent fluorescence of these drugs and the advantages in terms of selectivity and sensitivity that this detector offers (Table 29.6). Fluorometric detection after postcolumn derivatization with sulfuric acid has also been reported (203). However, quinolones exhibit also remarkable ultraviolet absorption and are therefore ideal for direct determination without derivatization. Detection can be performed in the wavelength range of 254–295 nm.

Confirmation of the identity of the suspected liquid chromatographic peaks in quinolone analysis can be made by converting the analytes to the corresponding decarboxylated derivatives and analyzing them by gas chromatography–mass spectrometry (195, 196). Most promising screening and even confirmatory methods in terms of simplicity, selectivity, and sensitivity, are those described by Munns et al. (196), Roybal et al. (188), and Eng et al. (193).

Munns et al. (196) described a multiresidue liquid chromatographic method for the determination of flumequine, oxolinic acid, nalidixic acid, and piromidic acid in catfish muscle. According to this method, 10 g homogenized muscle is extracted twice with 50 ml acetone. Following centrifugation, the supernatant is diluted with 15 ml n-propanol, concentrated in a rotary evaporator to approximately 15 ml and, after addition of acetone and 3% sodium chloride solution, the mixture is defatted with hexane. Quinolones are extracted into chloroform, repartitioned into 0.1 M sodium hydroxide, and, following pH adjustment at 6, the drugs are back-extracted into chloroform. The extract is evaporated to dryness, and the residue is reconstituted in 1 ml mobile phase to be further analyzed by liquid chromatography. Separation is performed on a 15 cm PLRP-S (5 μm) analytical column with a pH 6 mobile phase of 0.02M phosphoric acid/acetonitrile/tetrahydrofuran (72:16:12), at a flow-rate of 1 ml/min and a column temperature of 46°C (Fig. 29.6.1). Under these conditions, concentrations as low as 5 ppb could be readily determined in catfish muscle by fluorometric detection (325 nm for excitation and 365 nm for emission). The presence of flumequine, oxolinic acid, and nalidixic acid in the suspected samples could be confirmed by analyzing the decarboxylated quinolones by gas chromatography–mass spectrometry.

Roybal et al. (188) developed another liquid chromatographic method for the determination of enrofloxacin, ciprofloxacin, sarafloxacin, and difloxacin in milk. In this method, a 5 ml milk sample is extracted twice with a mixture of

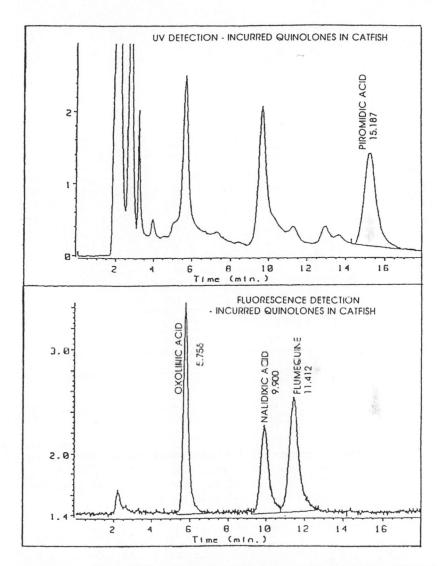

FIG. 29.6.1 Chromatograms obtained with UV and fluorescence detection from analysis of catfish tissue containing incurred quinolones. (Reprinted from Ref. 196. Copyright, (1995), by AOAC INTERNATIONAL.)

F
L
U
O
R
E
S
C
E
N
C
E

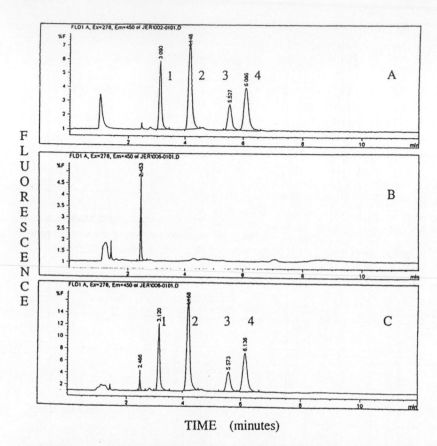

TIME   (minutes)

FIG. 29.6.2   Typical chromatograms of 10 ppb quinolones standard solution (A), a blank milk sample (B), and a milk sample (C) fortified with 20 ppb ciprofloxacin (1), enrofloxacin (2), sarafloxacin (3), and difloxacin (4). (Reprinted from Ref. 188. Copyright, (1997), by AOAC INTERNATIONAL.)

ethanol and 1% acetic acid (99:1) in the presence of sodium sulfate. Following centrifugation, the supernatant is diluted with 1% acetic acid to then be applied to a propylsulfonic acid solid-phase extraction column (Bond Elut LRC). Following successive column washing with methanol, water, and methanol, fluoroquinolones are eluted with 25% ammonium hydroxide in methanol, and the eluate is evaporated to dryness. The residue is reconstituted in 2 ml 1% acetic acid to be further analyzed by liquid chromatography. Separation is performed on a 15 cm Inertsil, phenyl (5 μm) analytical column, with a mobile phase of 2% acetic acid/

acetonitrile (85:15), at a flow-rate of 1.0 ml/min and a column temperature of 40°C (Fig. 29.6.2). Under these conditions, concentrations as low as 5 ppb could be determined using fluorescence detection (275 nm for excitation and 450 nm for emission).

A different approach based on online dialysis was followed by Eng et al. (193) in the liquid chromatographic determination of flumequine and oxolinic acid in chicken liver. According to this method, 1 g of homogenized liver tissue is extracted twice with 5 ml acetone. After centrifugation, the supernatant is diluted with acetone and 3% sodium chloride solution, and the mixture is defatted with hexane. Quinolones are extracted into chloroform, and repartitioned into pH 9.0 phosphate buffer. An aliquot of the phosphate buffer is transferred to an autosampler vial for on-line dialysis using an M_r 15000 MWCO Cuprophan (cellulose acetate) membrane and an automated column switching system. The extract is further purified on-line by loading the dialyzate onto a trace enrichment preconcentration column (PLRP-S or Hypersil ODS). Following column washing with a 0.02 M, pH 5.0, phosphate buffer, the trapped analytes are injected into the analytical column (PLRP-S, 5 μm) and analyzed under the conditions shown in Table 29.6. Concentrations as low as 5 ppb for flumequine and 2.5 ppb for oxolinic acid could be readily determined using fluorescence detection (318 nm for excitation and 364 nm for emission).

29.7 SULFONAMIDES AND DIAMINOPYRIMIDINE POTENTIATORS

Sulfonamides are synthetic compounds whose common chemical nucleus, which is essential for the exhibited antibacterial activity, comes from sulfanilamide, the simpler member of the sulfonamide group. In this nucleus, the sulfonamide ($—SO_2NH_2—$) nitrogen has been designated as N^1, and the amino ($—NH_2$) nitrogen as N^4. Most sulfonamides have been synthesized by chemical substitution at the N^1 position since substitution at the N^4 position results, with certain exceptions, in compounds with greatly reduced antibacterial activity compared to their unsubstituted counterparts.

Parent sulfonamides are relatively insoluble in water but their sodium salts have greater water solubility than the parent compounds and are commonly included in commercial preparations. These drugs have good solubility in polar solvents such as ethanol, acetone, acetonitrile, chloroform, dichloromethane, and ethyl acetate but are relatively insoluble in nonpolar solvents. They show large variations in polarity and exhibit amphoteric properties due to the acidic N–H linkage adjacent to the sulfonyl group and the basic character of the para-NH_2 group. These amphoteric properties are both a help and a hindrance in extraction and cleanup processes due to a dramatic pH-dependent variation of their partition coefficients between aqueous and organic solvents in the 7–9 pH range.

Before the extraction procedure may commence, the sample must be prepared in such a way that it is in a condition for extraction of the analyte(s). For analyzing sulfonamide residues in liquid samples such as milk, a pretreatment dilution step with water prior to direct fluorometric detection may be required (207). Dilution of milk with aqueous buffer (208) or sodium chloride solution (209) prior to sample cleanup has also been reported. For the analysis of honey a simple dissolution of the sample in water (210, 211) or aqueous buffer (212) is generally required. Semisolid samples such as muscle, kidney, and liver, require, however, more intensive sample pretreatment. The analyte(s) must be exposed to extracting solvents to ensure maximum extraction. The most popular approach for tissue break-up is through use of a mincing and/or homogenizing apparatus. Lyophilization (freeze-drying) of swine kidney has been carried out prior to supercritical-fluid extraction of trimethoprim residues (213).

Extraction of sulfonamides and diaminopyrimidine potentiators from edible animal products should render the bound residues soluble, remove most or all of the proteins, and provide high yields for all analytes. Sample extraction/deproteinization is traditionally accomplished with polar solvents including acidic aqueous solutions (211, 214–222), acetonitrile (56, 223–232), chloroform (233–240), ethyl acetate (29, 241–244), dichloromethane (204, 242, 245–247), acetone (194, 248, 249), or various combinations of them. Use of dichloromethane at pH 10 in the presence of an ion-pairing reagent (tetrabutylammonium) has also been reported to work extremely well in the extraction of sulfadimethoxine and ormetoprim residues from catfish muscle (250) and animal tissues (251). Anhydrous sodium sulfate may be added to dehydrate tissue samples to permit better exposure of the matrix to the solvent.

The aqueous or organic extract obtained at this point may be a very dilute solution containing interfering compounds and making it difficult to determine trace level concentrations of the analyte(s) of interest. To reduce interferences and concentrate the analyte(s), the primary sample extract is further subjected to various types of sample cleanup procedures such as conventional liquid–liquid partitioning, solid-phase extraction, matrix solid-phase dispersion, online trace enrichment, liquid chromatography, online dialysis and subsequent trace enrichment, and supercritical fluid extraction. In most cases some of these procedures are used in combination to obtain highly purified extracts.

Liquid–liquid partitioning has been used for many years for the purification of sulfonamides and diaminopyrimidine potentiators. When partitioning from an organic into an aqueous phase, the adjustment of the pH of the aqueous phase is critical to obtain quantitative recoveries. Sulfonamides are generally extracted from the primary organic sample extract into strong acidic (238, 239, 242, 249, 252–254) or basic (241, 248, 255) aqueous solutions. For better sample cleanup, back-extraction of the analyte(s) into dichloromethane (241, 253, 254), or ethyl acetate (256), after pH adjustment of the aqueous phase at values between 5.1

and 5.6 has also been reported. As an alternative, ion-pair extraction of sulfonamides into dichloromethane may be used; adjusting the pH of the aqueous extract at 10 (255) or 11 (257) and using tetrabutylammonium as pairing ion, the formed sulfonamides ion-pairs could be readily extracted into dichloromethane. To remove lipids, sample extracts have often been partitioned with n-hexane or diethyl ether.

Removing proteins and other matrix constituents can also be accomplished with solid-phase extraction procedure, which is more suited to multiresidue analysis. This procedure has become the method of choice in many laboratories for the isolation and/or cleanup of sulfonamides from biological matrices. It is particularly advantageous because it requires low solvent usage, is generally less time-consuming and less labor-intensive, and has a variety of special properties that allow better extraction of these hydrophobic compounds. Cleanup and concentration of sulfonamides from coextracted substances have been accomplished with nonpolar materials, such as reversed-phase (C_{18} or C_8) (177, 216, 222, 233, 237, 258–260) sorbents, since they provide high recovery of the analytes. However, in many cases, cleanup on these nonpolar materials seems not to be effective in removing interfering substances from the sample extract. Therefore, polar sorbents such as silica (29, 204, 224, 256, 261), alumina (194, 208, 210, 225, 227, 229, 257, 259, 262), or Florisil (247), and ion exchange sorbents (210, 218, 244, 258, 259, 261–263), have been reported to be a more powerful approach for the isolation and/or cleanup of these compounds. In some cases, combination of the above mentioned sorbents to obtain highly purified extracts has been reported (208, 210, 259, 261, 262).

In contrast to the solid-phase extraction approach, only nonpolar C_{18}-derivatized silica has been used as the sorbent in matrix solid-phase dispersion technique. This technique, which simplifies the overall methodology and removes most of the interfering compounds from milk and tissues, has been successfully applied in the determination of sulfonamides in fish muscle (264–267), bovine and swine muscle (66, 268, 269), and milk (270).

Online trace enrichment has also been described for the isolation/purification of nine sulfonamides residues from milk (221). This technique involved trapping of the analyte onto an LC preconcentration column (Brownlee RP-18, 10 μm), rinsing of coretained material to waste, and flushing of the concentrated analytes onto the analytical column. In another approach, combination of online liquid chromatographic cleanup on Progel-TSK gel-permeation column with online trace enrichment on PLRP-S preconcentration column was successfully employed in the determination of sulfadimethoxine, sulfamethoxazole, and trimethoprim in swine tissues (214, 215). Online liquid chromatographic cleanup on Supelcosil LC-18-DB column for the isolation/purification of sulfamethazine residues from swine tissues has also been reported (223). This approach involved loading of the sample extract onto the reversed-phase column, elution with a suitable mobile phase, collection of predetermined fraction of the chromatographic effluent containing the analyte, and reanalysis by gas chromatography.

Online dialysis followed by trace enrichment of the analytes can also be employed for the determination of sulfonamides in foods of animal origin. The efficiency of this technique has been demonstrated in a method for the determination of 13 sulfonamides in meat, milk, and eggs (209). This method involved on-line isolation of the analytes through use of a flat cellulose membrane, loading of the aqueous dialysate containing sulfonamides onto a liquid chromatographic preconcentration column (Bondapak C_{18}/Corasil, 37–50 μm, or XAD-2 or XAD-4, 50–100 μm, or Perisorb RP-2, 30–40 μm), rinsing of the coextracted material to waste, and flushing of the concentrated analytes onto the analytical column.

Supercritical fluid extraction has been used for the isolation/cleanup of trimethoprim, along with three steroid hormones, from swine kidney (213). During the period of extraction with unmodified CO_2, the extracted drugs are strongly retained at the inlet of the column, while the majority of extracted endogenous components are eluted rapidly and directed to waste. The drugs and more polar endogenous components are then eluted by adding modifier to the mobile phase. This technique, however, needs further optimization to achieve sufficiently low detection limits.

Following their extraction and cleanup, residues of sulfonamides and diaminopyrimidine potentiators in sample extracts can be detected by direct nonchromatographic methods, or thin-layer, gas, liquid, or supercritical fluid chromatographic methods (Table 29.7).

Direct nonchromatographic methods using photometric detection at 540 or 545 nm after derivatization with N-(1-naphthyl)ethylenediamine (Bratton-Marshall reagent) have been reported for screening of sulfamethazine in bovine tissues (252) and milk (262), and sulfathiazole in honey (210). In a different approach, Salinas et al. (212) described a fourth-derivative spectrophotometric method for the determination of sulfathiazole in honey. Fluorometric detection for screening for sulfacetamide and sulfaquanidine residues in milk extracts has also been described (207). Although useful, these methods cannot differentiate among individual sulfonamides.

Supercritical-fluid chromatography has been applied by Ramsey et al. (213) for the determination of trimethoprim, along with three steroid hormones, in swine kidney. Separation was performed on a Spherisorb 5 amino-bonded column, using carbon dioxide with methanol modifier as the mobile phase. Detection at levels greater than 10 ppm was accomplished by tandem mass spectrometry using thermospray interface. However, this method lacks the sensitivity required to detect the low ppb levels likely to occur in milk and tissues.

In thin-layer chromatographic methods, sulfonamide residues were first separated on commercially available silica gel plates using various solvent mixtures as mobile phase, and subsequently detected by fluorometry after spraying

TABLE 29.7 Physicochemical Methods for Sulfonamides and Diaminopyrimidine Potentiators in Edible Animal Products

Antibacterial(s)	Matrix	Sample preparation	Steps	Stationary phase	Mobile phase	Detection/ Identification	Sensitivity/ Recovery	Ref.
SPECTROMETRIC METHODS								
Sulfamethazine	Bovine tissues	CHCl$_3$/acetone extn, liq–liq partns, derivatization with N-(1-naphthyl)-ethylenediamine	18	—	—	Vis 545 nm	100 ppb/ 70–97%	252
Sulfathiazole	Honey	H$_2$O diln, tandem alumina and AG MP-1 column cleanup, derivatization with N-(1-naphthyl)-ethylenediamine	14	—	—	Vis 540 nm	1 ppm/ 76–98%	210
	Honey	Acetate buffer, pH 3.8, diln	1	—	—	Fourth-derivative spectro-photometry	3 ppm/ 81–113%	212
Sulfacetamide, sulfaguanidine	Milk	H$_2$O diln	1	—	—	Fluorometric, ex: 260 nm, em: 345 nm	20–100 ppb/ 90–102%	207

(continued)

Table 29.7 Continued

Antibacterial(s)	Matrix	Sample preparation	Steps	Stationary phase	Mobile phase	Detection/Identification	Sensitivity/Recovery	Ref.
Sulfamethazine, N⁴-acetyl-sulfamethazine	Milk	Tandem chromosorb 102, buffered anion-exchange resins, and alumina column cleanup, derivatization with N-(1-naphthyl)-ethylenediamine	10	—	—	Vis 540 nm	0.5 ppb/80–90%	262
THIN-LAYER CHROMATOGRAPHIC METHODS								
Sulfamethazine	Milk	Buffer, pH 5.7, diln, SPE cleanup, tandem alumina and AG MP-1 column cleanup	16	HPTLC Silica gel	EtOAc/toluene	Fluorometric, after fluorescamine derivatization	0.5 ppb/88–103%	208
	Swine muscle	H₂O extn, SPE cleanup, tandem alumina and AG MP-1 column cleanup	18	HPTLC Silica gel	EtOAc/toluene	Fluorometric, after fluorescamine derivatization	2 ppb/84–114%	259
Sulfathiazole	Honey	DCM extn	4	Silica gel	CHCl₃/PeOH	Fluorometric, after fluorescamine derivatization	20 ppb/>98%	245
		H₂O diln, tandem alumina and AG MP-1 column cleanup	14	HPTLC Silica gel	PrOH/NH₄OH	Vis, after N-(1-naphthyl)-ethylenediamine derivatization	100 ppb/76–96%	210

Sulfa-dimethoxine, sulfaquinoxaline	Chicken liver	CHCl₃/EtOAc extn, SPE cleanup, liq–liq partn, ion-pair extn	13	Silica gel G	CHCl₃/EtOAc/MeOH	Vis, after N-(1-naphthyl)-ethylenediamine derivatization	100 ppb/64–78%	257
Sulfamethazine, sulfathiazole	Swine liver	CHCl₃/EtOAc extn, liq–liq partn, ion-pair extn	8	Silica gel G	EtOAc/MeOH	Vis, after N-(1-naphthyl)-ethylenediamine derivatization	20 ppb/38–55%	255
Four sulfonamides	Muscle	EtOAc extn, SPE cleanup	10	HPTLC Silica gel	EtOAc/hexane	UV-Vis, after fluorescamine derivatization	100 ppb/NR	29
Five sulfonamides	Animal tissues	DCM extn, SPE cleanup	10	HPTLC Silica gel	CHCl₃/BuOH	UV-Vis after fluorescamine derivatization	50 ppb/NR	246
Five sulfonamides	Animal tissues	EtOAc extn, liq–liq partns	11	Silica gel	CHCl₃/BuOH	Fluorometric, after fluorescamine derivatization	100 ppb/79–107%	241
Five sulfonamides	Salmon muscle	MSPD extn/cleanup	7	HPTLC Silica gel	EtOAc/BuOH/MeOH/NH₃(30%)	Fluorometric, after fluorescamine derivatization	40–100 ppb/45–76%	264
GAS CHROMATOGRAPHIC METHODS								
Sulfamethazine	Swine tissues	CHCl₃/acetone extn, liq–liq partns, CH₂N₂ methylation	23	Gas-Chrom Q with 3% OV-17	Helium	SIM-MS	50 ppb/NR	253

(continued)

TABLE 29.7 Continued

Antibacterial(s)	Matrix	Sample preparation	Steps	Stationary phase	Mobile phase	Detection/Identification	Sensitivity/Recovery	Ref.
Swine tissues	Swine tissues	$CHCl_3$/acetone extn, two SPE cleanups, liq–liq partns, CH_2N_2 methylation and MSTFA silylation	29	DB-5MS, 15 m, capillary	Helium	PICI-EI-MS	50 ppb/ 91–114%	261
	Swine tissues	ACN/Na_2SO_4 extn, liq–liq partn, LC purification on Supelcosil LC-18-DB column, CH_2N_2 methylation	11	DB-5, 15 m, capillary	Helium	EI-MS	1–5 ppb/ NR	223
Sulfamethazine and metabolites	Swine and bovine tissues	$CHCl_3$/acetone extn, liq–liq partns, CH_2N_2 methylation	16	Gas-Chrom Q with 5% OV-7	Nitrogen or argon/methane	ECD/PICI-MS	10 ppb/ 75–117%	254
Four sulfonamides	Bovine and swine liver	$CHCl_3$/acetone extn, liq–liq partns, CH_2N_2 methylation	16	Gas-Chrom Q with 5% OV-7	Argon/methane	ECD/PICI-MS-MS	100 ppb/ 50–145%	271
Six sulfonamides	Animal tissues, eggs	ACN extn, SPE cleanup, CH_2N_2 methylation, silica gel column cleanup, liq–liq partn	25	DB-5, 15 m, capillary	Helium	PICI-MS	10–50 ppb/ 59–107%	224

Compound	Matrix	No.	Sample preparation	Column	Mobile phase/carrier	Detection	Sensitivity/recovery	Ref.
Thirteen sulfonamides	Animal tissues	41	Acetone extn, liq–liq partns, silica gel 60 column cleanup, liq–liq partn, CH_2N_2 methylation followed by acylation with N-methyl-bis(trifluoroacetamide), SPE cleanup	DB-5, 30 m, capillary, coated with methyl-5% phenylsilicone	Helium	PPINICI-EI-MS	Low sub-ppb level	256

LIQUID CHROMATOGRAPHIC METHODS

Compound	Matrix	No.	Sample preparation	Column	Mobile phase/carrier	Detection	Sensitivity/recovery	Ref.
Sulfadimethoxine	Catfish muscle	8	MSPD extn/cleanup	Micro Pak ODS, 10 µm	0.017M H_3PO_4/ACN (65:35), at 40°C	UV 270 nm/PDA (200–350 nm)	50 ppb/95–106%	265
	Salmon muscle	9	Acetone extn, liq–liq partn, freeze-drying concn	Supelcosil LC-18-DB, 5 µm	H_2O/ACN (65:35), contg 0.1% formic acid	UV 265 nm/PDA (200–340 nm), MS-ISP	25 ppb/60%	248
Sulfamethazine	Animal tissue	10	$CHCl_3$ extn, liq–liq partn, SPE cleanup	Spherisorb C_{18} ODS, 5 µm	0.05M NaH_2PO_4/MeOH (70:30)	UV 265 nm	2 ppb/84–96%	233
	Fish muscle	5	DCM extn, SPE cleanup	ChromSpher C_8	0.01M, pH 6.8, acetate buffer/ACN (90:10)	UV 280 nm	10 ppb/75–82%	204

(continued)

TABLE 29.7 Continued

Antibacterial(s)	Matrix	Sample preparation	Steps	Stationary phase	Mobile phase	Detection/ Identification	Sensitivity/ Recovery	Ref.
	Milk	CHCl₃ extn, liq–liq partn	5	Supelcosil LC-18-DB, 5 μm, analytical and guard column	0.1M KH₂PO₄/ MeOH (70:30), at 35°C	UV 265 nm/ GC-PICI-MS	5 ppb/ 69–88%	234, 235
Sulfathiazole	Honey	Acetone extn, liq–liq partn	7	μBondapak phenyl	Phosp. buffer, pH 3.0/ACN (90:10)	UV 254 nm	60 ppb/ 51–95%	249
Sulfisomidine	Swine tissues	ACN extn, liq–liq partn, alumina column cleanup	11	Nucleosil 5 C₁₈	0.01M, pH 5.6, phosp. buffer/ ACN (92:8), at 30°C	UV 270 nm/ PDA	10 ppb/ 83–91%	225
Trimethoprim	Bovine tissues	CHCl₃/acetone extn, liq–liq partn	9	Partisil 5 ODS 3	H₂O/ACN/HOAc (73.7:25:1.3), contg 50 mM ammonium acetate, at 45°C	PICI-MS-TSP	25 ppb/ 60–79%	277
	Meat, milk	Buffer, pH 3, (meat), or McIlvaine buffer (milk) extn, SPE cleanup	8–10	Nova-Pak C₁₈, 4 μm	0.005M, pH 3, phosp. buffer contg 5 mM pentanesulfonic acid/ACN (87.5:12.5)	UV 229 and 280 nm	5–15 ppb/ 73–98%	216

Swine tissues	5	Acetate buffer extn, online cleanup on Progel-TSK gel-permeation column, trace enrichment on PLRP-S, 15–25 μm, preconcn column and switching to analytical column	Supelcosil LC-18-DB, with RP guard column	0.05M acetate buffer, contg 0.2% TEA, pH 6.0/ACN (85:15), at 30°C	UV 240 nm	15–25 ppb/ 67–82%	215
Sulfadiazine, sulfamethazine, Milk	4	CHCl$_3$ extn	Merck RP-C$_2$, 10μm	H$_2$O/MeOH (75:25) and (60:40), contg 0.01M LiClO$_4$	Electro-chemical	10 ppb/ 94–110%	236
Sulfadimethoxine, N^4-acetyl-sulfadimethoxine, Catfish muscle	10	MSPD extn/ cleanup	Hypersil ODS, 5 μm	0.017M H$_3$PO$_4$/ACN (71:29)	UV 265 nm/ PDA (210–320 nm)	26 ppb/ 97–126%	266
Sulfamethazine, N^4-acetyl-sulfamethazine, Animal tissues	7	Metaphosphoric acid/MeOH extn, SPE cleanup	Superspher RP-18e	0.05M NaH$_2$PO$_4$/ACN (80:20)	UV 275 nm/ PDA (220–340 nm)	20 ppb/ 90–94%	260

(continued)

TABLE 29.7 Continued

Antibacterial(s)	Matrix	Sample preparation	Steps	Stationary phase	Mobile phase	Detection/ Identification	Sensitivity/ Recovery	Ref.
Sulfadi-methoxine, ormetoprim	Animal tissues	Ion pair/DCM extn	4	μPorasil Silica	$CHCl_3$/MeOH/ H_2O/conc NH_4OH (1000:28:2:05.5) for chicken, and (1000:28:2:0.6) for bovine and catfish tissues	UV 288 nm	50 ppb/ 72–128%	251
	Catfish muscle	Ion pair/DCM extn	5	μPorasil Silica	$CHCl_3$/MeOH/ H_2O/conc NH_4OH (2000:56:4:1.2), at 30°C	UV 288 nm	50 ppb/ 85–127%	250
Sulfadiazine, trimethoprim	Chicken tissues	DCM (kidney, liver, skin, fat), or EtOAc (muscle) extn, liq–liq partn	5	LiChrospher RP-18, 5 μm, analytical and guard column	0.01M KH_2PO_4/ ACN Gradient from (92:8) to (70:30)	UV 270 nm	50 ppb/ 60–85%	242
	Fish tissues	TCA/acetone/DCM extn, liq–liq partn	10	Supelcosil LC-18-DB, 5 μm, analytical and guard column	0.025M, pH 2.8, phosp. buffer, contg 20 mM hexane-sulfonate/ACN contg 0.1% TEA (80:20)	UV 270 nm	30–160 ppb/ 60–102%	275

Analyte	Sample	No.	Extraction/cleanup	Column	Mobile phase	Detection	Range/recovery	Ref.
Sulfadimethoxine, sulfamethazine	Animal tissues	16	CHCl$_3$ extn, liq–liq partn, SPE cleanup	Spherisorb C$_{18}$ ODS, 5 μm	0.05M NaH$_2$PO$_4$/ACN (72:28)	UV 265 nm/MS-TSP	10–20 ppb/75–84%	237
Sulfadimethoxine, sulfamethoxazole	Swine tissues	6	Acetate buffer extn, heat deprtn, on-line cleanup on Progel-TSK gel-permeation column, trace enrichment on PLRP-S, 15–25 μm, preconcn column and switching to analytical column	Supelcosil LC-18-DB, with RP guard column	0.05M, pH 6.0, acetate buffer/ACN (85:15), at 30°C, for sulfadimethoxine, and 0.05M, pH 4.6, acetate buffer/ACN (80:20), at 30°C, for sulfamethoxazole	UV 270 nm	10–25 ppb/63–85%	214, 215
Sulfanilamide, sulfaguanidine	Animal tissues, eggs, milk	11	ACN extn, liq–liq partns	Nucleosil 5 SA, 5 μm	0.05M, pH 2.0, phosp. buffer/MeOH (85:15)	Fluorometric, ex: 275 nm, em: 340 nm/on-line UV 275 nm	10–100 ppb/62–80%	226
Sulfaquinoxaline, N^4-acetyl-sulfaquinoxaline,	Chicken tissues	16	ACN extn, liq–liq partns, alumina column cleanup	L-column ODS	0.01M, pH 5.0, phosp. buffer/ACN (79:21), at 40°C	UV 270 nm	3 ppb/84–104%	227

(continued)

TABLE 29.7 Continued

Antibacterial(s)	Matrix	Sample preparation	Steps	Stationary phase	Mobile phase	Detection/ Identification	Sensitivity/ Recovery	Ref.
Sulfamono-methoxine, sulfadi-methoxine, sulfisozole	Fish muscle	Metaphosphoric acid/MeOH extn, SPE cleanup	7	Inertsil ODS, 5 μm, with RP-8 New-guard column	0.005M oxalic acid/ACN (55:45)	UV 265 nm	50 ppb/ 80–89%	177
Four sulfonamides	Chicken muscle	$CHCl_3$ extn, liq–liq partn, precolumn derivatization with fluorescamine	7	Nucleosil 120 C_{18}, 5 μm	0.02M, pH 4.0, phosp. buffer/ ACN (66:34), contg 20 mM octanesulfonate, at 30°LC	Fluorometric, ex: 405 nm, em: 495 nm	3–40ppb/ 78–92%	238
Four sulfonamides	Fish muscle	Acetone extn, liq–liq partns, alumina column cleanup, liq–liq partns	21	Nucleosil C_{18}, with RP-2 Spher-10 guard column	H_2O/THF/ACN/ H_3PO_4 (69,94:29:1:0.06)	UV 260 nm	40–60 ppb/ 71–92%	194
Four sulfonamides	Swine tissues	ACN extn, liq–liq partn, precolumn derivatization with fluorescamine	11	Nova-Pak C_{18}, 10 μm	0.01M KH_2PO_4/ ACN (70:30)	Fluorometric, ex: 390 nm, em: 475 nm	NR/ 59–97%	228

Five sulfonamides	Bovine and swine muscle	MSPD extn/ cleanup	10	Nova-pak C$_{18}$, 4 μm, with μBondapak C$_{18}$, 6–12 μm, guard column	0.01M, pH 5, acetate buffer/ ACN Gradient from (100:0) to (60:40)	UV 263 nm/ PDA (220–367 nm)	10 ppb/ 37–85%	268
Five sulfonamides	Chicken tissues	ACN extn, liq–liq partn, alumina column cleanup	11	Nucleosil 5 C$_{18}$	0.01M, pH 5.9, phosp. buffer/ ACN (85:15)	UV 270 nm	20–50 ppb/ 79–103%	229
Five sulfonamides	Eggs, milk, meat	ACN extn, liq–liq partns	11	MOS-Hypersil, 3 μm, analytical and guard column	0.01M, pH 4.6, acetate buffer/ ACN (75:25)	UV 275 nm	100 ppb/ 70–94%	56
Five sulfonamides	Eggs, milk, trout muscle	TCA extn	5	Spherisorb C$_{18}$ ODS2, 5 μm, analytical and guard column	H$_2$O/ACN Isocratic (97:3) for 5 min and gradient to (60:40)	Fluorometric, postcolumn derivatization with OPA, ex: 302 nm, em: 412 nm	27–340 ppb/ 95%	219
Five sulfonamides	Eggs, milk, honey	H$_2$O diln (honey), TCA extn (eggs, milk)	2–5	Spherisorb C$_{18}$ ODS2, 5 μm, analytical and guard column	H$_2$O/ACN Isocratic (97:3) for 5 min and gradient to (60:40)	UV 260 nm	30–80 ppb/ 90–110%	211

(continued)

TABLE 29.7 Continued

Antibacterial(s)	Matrix	Sample preparation	Steps	Stationary phase	Mobile phase	Detection/ Identification	Sensitivity/ Recovery	Ref.
Five sulfonamides	Salmon muscle	MSPD extn/ cleanup	10	Supelcosil LC-18-DB, 5 μm	0.01M, pH 5.5, acetate buffer/ ACN Gradient from (82:18) to (20:80)	UV 270 nm/ PDA (250–290 nm)	48–228 ppb/ 66–82%	267
Five sulfonamides	Swine tissues	CHCl$_3$/acetone extn, SPE cleanup	13	CP^{TM}Spher C$_8$, 8 μm, with Chrompack RP guard column	0.01M, pH 4.6, acetate buffer/ ACN (70:30)	UV 254 nm	50 ppb/ 82–96%	263
Six sulfonamides	Milk	ACN extn, precolumn derivatization with fluorescamine	9	Nova-Pak C$_{18}$, 10 μm	0.01M KH$_2$PO$_4$/ ACN (70:30)	Fluorometric, ex: 390 nm, em: 475 nm	1 ppb/ 63–107%	230
Six sulfonamides	Animal tissues	CHCl$_3$/acetone extn, liq–liq partns	17	μBondapak C$_{18}$, 10 μm, with Brownlee RP 18, 7 μm, guard column	Solvent A: 1% HOAc Solvent B: ACN/H$_2$O (80:20) Gradient from (90:10) to (60:40)	Vis 450 nm, postcolumn derivatization with DMBA/ GC-SIM-MS	20 ppb/ 71–104%	276

Six sulfonamides	Meat	5	EtOAc extn	Microspher C$_{18}$, 3 μm	0.05M ammonium acetate/MeOH (77:23)	MS-MS-TSP	2–10 ppb/ 40–70%	243
Eight Sulfonamides	Meat	5	MSPD extn/ cleanup	Spherisorb C$_{18}$ ODS2, 5 μm	Solvent A: 0.01M, pH 5.2, acetate buffer Solvent B: ACN/MeOH (70:30) Gradient from (86:14) to (46:54), at 35°C	UV 275 and 365 nm/ PDA (200–450 nm)	3.5–66 ppb/ 39–90%	66
Eight sulfonamides	Meat, meat products	7	CHCl$_3$ extn, liq–liq partn, precolumn derivatization with fluorescamine	Chemcosorb 5-ODS-H, 5 μm	2% HOAc/ACN (62.5:37.5), at 55°C	Fluorometric, ex: 405 nm, em: 495 nm	?/ 78–107%	239
Eight sulfonamides	Milk	7	HCl extn, precolumn derivatization with fluorescamine	Inertsil ODS–2, 5 μm	2% HOAc/ACN (62.5:37.5), at 55C	Fluorometric, ex: 405 nm, em: 495 nm	2.5–10 ppb/ 94–116%	217
Eight sulfonamides	Milk	12	Oxalic acid extn, SPE cleanup	Supersher 100 RP-18	0.01M, pH 4.6, acetate buffer/ ACN/MeOH (78:17:15), at 25°C	UV 275 nm	5–10 ppb/ 62–85%	218

(continued)

TABLE 29.7 Continued

Antibacterial(s)	Matrix	Sample preparation	Steps	Stationary phase	Mobile phase	Detection/Identification	Sensitivity/Recovery	Ref.
Eight sulfonamides	Milk	MSPD extn/cleanup	8	Supelcosil LC-18, 3 μm	0.017M H_3PO_4/ACN (90:10), at 45°C	UV 270 nm/PDA (200–350 nm)	31–62 ppb/73–94%	270
Eight sulfonamides	Milk	$CHCl_3$/acetone extn, liq–liq partn	10	Octadecyldimethylsilyl, 5 μm, analytical and guard column	0.1M KH_2PO_4/MeOH (88:12) or (70:30), at 35°C	UV 265 nm	5–20 ppb/55–87%	220
Eight sulfonamides	Swine muscle	MSPD extn/cleanup	8	Varian MCH-10, 10 μm	0.017M H_3PO_4/ACN (70:30), at 40°C	UV 270 nm/PDA (200–350 nm)	31–62 ppb/70–96%	269
Nine sulfonamides	Milk	HCl extn, liq–liq partns, online trace enrichment on Brownlee RP-18, 10 μm, preconcn column and switching to analytical column	11	Spherisorb ODS-2, 5 μm	Solvent A: 0.1M acetate buffer (1% formic acid) Solvent B: ACN/H_2O (70:30) contg 0.1M NH_4OAc (1% formic acid) Gradient from (100:0) to (25:75)	UV 254 nm online with MS–TSP	10 ppb/NR	221

Ten sulfonamides	Animal and fish muscle, eggs	EtOAc extn, SPE cleanup	8	Wakosil C$_{18}$, 5 μm	0.02M H$_3$PO$_4$/ACN (76:24)	UV 272 nm	50 ppb/74–99%	244
Ten sulfonamides	Honey	NaCl addn, DCM extn, SPE cleanup	7	LiChrosphere RP-18e, 5 μm, analytical and guard column	0.05M NaH$_2$PO$_4$/ACN (66.6:33.4)	UV 275 nm/PDA (220–360 nm)	50 ppb/62–90%	247
Ten sulfonamides	Milk	CHCl$_3$/acetone extn, liq–liq partn	6	Supelcosil LC-18-DB, 5 μm, analytical and guard column	0.1M KH$_2$PO$_4$/MeOH (88:12) or (70:30), at 35°C	UV 265 nm	1–9 ppb/44–87%	240
Twelve sulfonamides	Milk	McIlvaine/EDTA buffer extn, heat deprtn, SPE cleanup	9	LiChrosorb RP-8, 10 μm	0.01M, pH 4.6, acetate buffer/ACN (78:22)	UV 245.5 nm/LC receptorgram	1–5 ppb/NR	222
Thirteen sulfonamides	Eggs, milk, meat	Diln with NaCl solution, purification by online dialysis and subsequent trace enrichment on XAD-2 or XAD-4, 5–100 μm, or Bondapak C$_{18}$/Corasil, 37–50 μm or Perisorb RP-2, 30–40 μm preconcn column and switching to analytical column	2	LiChrosorb RP-8, 10 μm or Cp™Spher C$_{18}$, 7 μm, or μBondapak C$_{18}$, 10 μm	0.05M, pH 4.6, acetate buffer/ACN (82.5:17.5), or 0.05M, pH 6.85, acetate buffer/ACN (87.5:12.5), or H$_2$O/ACN/HOAc (97:2:1)	UV 280 nm, or postcolumn derivatization with DMAB and Vis 450 nm	5–20 ppb/85–90%	209

(continued)

TABLE 29.7 Continued

Antibacterial(s)	Matrix	Sample preparation	Steps	Stationary phase	Mobile phase	Detection/ Identification	Sensitivity/ Recovery	Ref.
Fourteen sulfonamides	Salmon tissues	ACN/HOAc extn, liq–liq partns	13	Symmetry C_{18}, 3.5 μm, with C_{18} guard column	Solvent A: 2% HOAc/MeOH/ ACN (85:10:5) Solvent B: 2% HOAc/MeOH/ ACN (65:10:25) Gradient from (100:0) to (0:100)	Fluorometric, postcolumn derivatization with fluorescamine, ex: 400 nm, em: 495 nm	1–5 ppb/ 58–94%	231
Twenty nine sulfonamides	Eggs, milk, meat	ACN/HOAc extn, liq–liq partns	17	Spherisorb ODS, 5 μm	Solvent A: 0.02M, pH 4.8, acetate buffer Solvent B: ACN/H_2O (60:40) Gradient from (92:8) to (10:90)	UV 275 and 290 nm/ PDA (245– 360 nm)	20–50 ppb/ 70–90%	232
SUPERCRITICAL-FLUID CHROMATOGRAPHIC METHODS								
Trimethoprim	Swine kidney	Lyophilization, SFE (CO_2)	6	Spherisorb 5 amino	CO_2/MeOH Isocratic (100:0) for 8 min and then gradient to (80:20)	MS-MS-TSP	10 ppm/ NR	213

SFE, Supercritical-fluid extraction; MSTFA, N-methyl-N-(trimethylsilyl)trifluoro-acetamide; OPA, o-phthalaldehyde; DMBA, p-dimethyl-aminobenzaldehyde.
Other abbreviations as in Tables 29.1 and 29.3.

with fluorescamine (208, 241, 245, 259, 264), and spectrophotometry after spraying with fluorescamine (29, 246) or Bratton-Marshall reagent (210, 255, 257). These methods have limited application and are generally used for screening or qualitative analysis since they lack the performance characteristics required to detect the low ppb levels likely to occur in edible animal products.

Gas chromatographic separation has not gained wide acceptance in spite of being quite sensitive and specific. This mode of separation is complicated by the need for derivatization of sulfonamide residues before gas chromatographic analysis. These drugs are subjected to derivatization via methylation with diazomethane (223, 224, 253, 254, 271), or double derivatization via methylation followed either by silylation with N-methyl-N-trimethylsilyltrifluoroacetamide (261) or by acylation with N-methyl-bis(trifluoroacetamide) (256). This derivatization step is required not only to form the volatile derivatives of the sulfonamides but also to improve their chromatographic properties (thermal stability and decreased polarity).

Excellent separation of sulfonamides can be achieved on conventional or fused silica capillary columns, the preferred type been the DB-5 capillary column. Following separation, electron-capture detector (254, 271) can be used for the determination of these drugs with good sensitivity and specificity. To confirm the presence of sulfonamides residues in edible animal products, mass spectrometric detectors are also frequently employed. Typical examples of such applications are those coupling gas chromatography with mass spectrometry via a chemical ionization (224, 254, 271) or electron impact (223, 256, 261) interface.

At present, liquid chromatography has become the most widely used technique for determining sulfonamides and diaminopyrimidines in edible animal products (Table 29.7). The separation of these drugs is generally done on nonpolar reversed-phase columns (octadecyl, octyl and phenyl), the preferred type being the octadecyl bonded silica. However, ion-exchange (226) and polar (250, 251) columns have also been used for the determination of sulfonamides and ormetoprim in edible animal products. Extensive research has been carried out to compare the chromatographic behavior of sulfonamides with respect to the column type and temperature, mobile phase pH, mobile phase buffer concentration, type and concentration of ion-pairing reagents, and the organic modifier type and content in the mobile phase (272–274).

There is no clear preference for either methanol or acetonitrile as organic modifier in the mobile phase. Nevertheless, addition of alkylsulfonic acids in the mobile phase has been employed to alter the retention and improve the peak shape and separation of trimethoprim and sulfonamides ion pairs. Pentanesulfonic acid (216), hexanesulfonic acid (275), or octanesulfonic acid (238) are the alkylsulfonic acids used in the analysis of these drugs.

Although spectrophotometric, fluorometric, electrochemical, and mass spectrometric detectors have all been equally well used in liquid chromatographic analysis of sulfonamides and diaminopyrimidines, most popular is the ultraviolet photometric detector. Since these drugs exhibit strong ultraviolet absorption, they are ideal for direct determination by liquid chromatography, without any need for derivatization. Their detection wavelengths have been set at 254–288 nm for sulfonamides, and 229–288 nm for diaminopyrimidines (Table 29.7). However, postcolumn derivatization with p-dimethylaminobenzaldehyde (DMAB) and spectrophotometric detection at 450 nm has been reported for the determination of 13 sulfonamides in eggs, milk and meat (209), and 6 sulfonamides in animal tissues (276).

Fluorometric detection has also been employed for the determination of sulfonamides in edible animal products, because it confers the advantages of selectivity and sensitivity. Although sulfonamides possess weak native fluorescence, their sensitive fluorometric detection necessitates use of precolumn or postcolumn derivatization producing the corresponding fluorescent derivatives. The most commonly used derivatizing reagent for precolumn derivatization is fluorescamine (217, 228, 230, 238, 239), while for postcolumn derivatization fluorescamine (231), and o-phthalaldehyde (OPA), and β-mercaptoethanol (219) are most often used.

Electrochemical detection has been successively applied (236) for the determination of sulfadiazine and sulfamethazine in milk.

To confirm sulfonamides in liquid chromatography-based methodologies, the photodiode array detector, which collects continuous spectral data during the analysis to check for interfering substances by comparing the spectrum (200–450 nm) of sample with that of the standard, has been used (66, 225, 232, 247, 248, 260, 265–270). Although confirmation with a photodiode array detector is a relatively simple procedure, the specificity and sensitivity features of this detector are not usually sufficient to determine or identify trace levels of residual sulfonamides and diaminopyrimidines in edible animal products. Only the coupling of liquid chromatography with mass spectrometry can provide unequivocal on-line spectrometric identification of these drugs at the very low residue levels required by regulatory agencies. Typical applications describe coupling of liquid chromatography with mass spectrometry via thermospray (213, 221, 237, 243, 277) or ionspray (248) interfaces.

Most promising literature methods, in terms of simplicity, selectivity, and sensitivity, for screening and even confirmation of sulfonamide residues in edible animal products appear to be those reported by Horie et al. (247), Simeonidou et al. (238), Boulaire et al. (66), and Abian et al. (221).

Horie et al. (247) described a multiresidue liquid chromatographic method for the determination of 10 sulfonamides in honey. According to this method, 5 g honey is dissolved into 50 ml 30% sodium chloride and extracted with 60 ml dichloromethane. The extract is dried with anhydrous sodium sulfate and applied to a Sep-Pak Florisil cartridge. Following cartridge washing with 10 ml

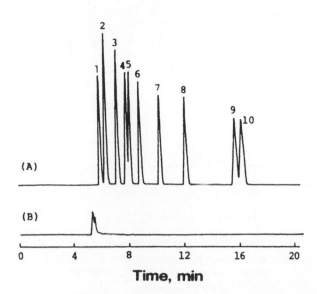

Fɪɢ. 29.7.1 Typical chromatograms of sulfonamides standard solution (A) and a blank honey sample (B). Peaks: 1, sulfathiazole; 2, sulfadiazine; 3, sulfamerazine; 4, sulfamethoxypyridazine; 5, sulfadimidine; 6, sulfamonomethoxine; 7, sulfachlorpyridazine; 8, sulfamethoxazole; 9, sulfaquinoxaline; 10, sulfadimethoxine. (Reprinted from Ref. 247. Copyright, (1992), by AOAC INTERNATIONAL.)

acetonitrile/dichloromethane (2:8), the analytes are eluted with 10 ml methanol/dichloromethane (2:8) and the eluate is evaporated to dryness. The residue is reconstituted in 1 ml mobile phase and analyzed by liquid chromatography. Separation is performed on a 25-cm LiChrosphere RP-18e (5 μm) analytical column protected by a guard column with the same packing material. Using a 0.05M sodium dihydrogen phosphate–acetonitrile (2:1) mobile phase, at a flow rate of 0.5 ml/min, concentrations of the 10 analytes down to 50 ppb could be determined in honey using an ultraviolet detector monitored at 275 nm (Fig. 29.7.1). Tentative confirmation of the presence of sulfonamides in the suspected samples can be achieved using a photodiode array detector.

Simeonidou et al. (238) reported an ion-pair liquid chromatographic method for the determination of sulfadiazine, sulfamethazine, sulfadimethoxine, and sulfaquinoxaline residues in chicken muscle. According to this method, a 3 g ground tissue sample is extracted with 30 ml chloroform. Following centrifugation the supernatant is filtered and a 10 ml aliquot is extracted with 1 ml 3N hydrochloric acid and submitted to precolumn derivatization with fluorescamine. Liquid chro-

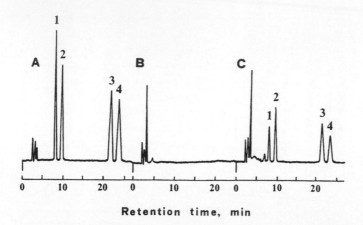

Retention time, min

FIG. 29.7.2 Typical chromatograms of sulfonamides standard solution (A), a blank muscle tissue sample (B), and a muscle tissue sample (C) fortified with 10 ppb sulfadiazine (1), 20 ppb sulfamethazine (2), 30 ppb sulfadimethoxine (3), and 100 ppb sulfaquinoxaline (4). (From Ref. 238.).

matographic separation of the fluorescent derivatives is performed on a 25 cm Nucleosil 120 C_{18} (5 μm) analytical column, with a 0.02M, pH 4, phosphate buffer–acetonitrile (66:34) mobile phase containing 20 mM sodium octanesulfonate, at a flow rate of 1.2 ml/min and a column temperature of 30°C (Fig. 29.7.2). Under these conditions concentrations as low as 3 ppb for sulfadiazine, 4 ppb for sulfamethazine, 9 ppb for sulfadimethoxine, and 40 ppb for sulfaquinoxaline could be readily determined in chicken muscle using a fluorescence detector monitored at 405 nm excitation and 495 nm emission wavelengths.

A specific cleanup procedure, based on matrix solid-phase dispersion, has been described by Boulaire et al. (66) for the liquid chromatographic determination of eight sulfonamide and six other drugs in meat. In this method, a 0.5 g ground tissue sample is blended in a mortar with C_{18} material and the resulting mixture is transferred to a 10 ml syringe barrel. After the syringe is washed with hexane, the analytes are eluted with 8 ml dichloromethane and the eluate evaporated to dryness. The residue is reconstituted in 0.25 ml 0.01M, pH5.2, ammonium acetate buffer–acetonitrile–methanol (86:10:4) mixture and analyzed by liquid chromatography. Separation is performed on a 25 cm Spherisorb C_{18} ODS II (5 μm) analytical column, with the mobile phase and the gradient elution program presented in Table 29.7, at a flow rate of 1 ml/min and a column temperature of 35°C. Under these conditions concentrations ranging from 3.5 to 66 ppb could be readily determined in meat using an ultraviolet spectrometer monitored at 275 and 365 nm. Tentative confirmation of the presence of sulfonamides in the suspected samples can be achieved using a photodiode array detector.

A different approach was followed by Abian et al. (221) for the liquid chromatographic–mass spectrometric determination of nine sulfonamide residues in milk, by means of an online trace enrichment method. In the proposed method, a 5 ml milk sample is acidified with concentrated hydrochloric acid (0.1 ml). Following centrifugation the supernatant is washed twice with hexane and evaporated to dryness. The residue is dissolved in methanol and after centrifugation the methanolic phase is concentrated to dryness. The residue is reconstituted in water and the analytes are trapped at the beginning of a 10 μm Brownlee RP-18 preconcentration column. Using an automated column switching system, the trapped analytes are back-flashed into the analytical column (Spherisorb ODS-2, 5 μm) and analyzed under the gradient elution conditions shown in Table 29.7. Under these conditions, concentrations as low as 10 ppb could be readily determined in milk using an ultraviolet detector connected on-line with a mass spectrometer via a thermospray interface.

29.8 TETRACYCLINES

Tetracycline antibiotics are closely related derivatives of the polycyclic naphthacenecarboxamide. They are amphoteric compounds with characteristic dissociation constants corresponding to the acidic hydroxyl group at position 3 (pK$_a$ about 3.3), the dimethylamino group at position 4 (pK$_a$ about 7.5), and the hydroxyl group at position 12 (pK$_a$ about 9.4). In aqueous solutions of pH 4–7, tetracyclines exist as dipolar ions, but as the pH increases to 8–9 marked dissociation of the dimethylamine cation occurs. They are soluble in acids, bases, and alcohols but are quite insoluble in organic solvents such as chloroform. Their ultraviolet spectra show strong absorption at around 270 and 360 nm in neutral and acidic solutions. Tetracyclines are readily transformed into fluorescent products in the presence of metal ions or under alkaline conditions.

Due to their extremely polar character, tetracyclines bind with proteins to form conjugates that are difficult to extract from biological matrices. Use of dilute mineral acids is of great help in dissociating tetracyclines from proteins, but once in aqueous solution, their extraction into volatile organic solvents for further concentration and cleanup is hampered by the unfavorable partition coefficients. Most of these antibiotics are photosensitive compounds, whereas all of them show poor stability under strong acidic and alkaline conditions with reversible formation of the 4-epi-tetracyclines in weakly acidic conditions (pH 3), and anhydro-tetracyclines in strong acidic conditions (below pH 2).

When analyzing liquid samples such as milk for tetracycline residues, a pretreatment centrifugation step for fat removal is usually required (278–281). Dilution of liquid samples, prior to cleanup, with acetate buffer (212), phosphate buffer (282), McIlvaine buffer (283), or McIlvaine/EDTA buffer (284, 285) is also frequently applied. Semisolid samples, such as muscle, kidney, and liver, normally require a more intensive sample pretreatment for tissue break-up. This is generally accomplished by mechanical dispersion using a mincing apparatus and a tissue homogenizer.

Isolation of the tetracycline antibiotics from edible animal products is quite a complex procedure. The main difficulty in isolating these compounds is associated with the propensity of the tetracyclines to form chelation complexes with metal ions and to bind with sample matrix constituents. For enhancing the extraction efficiency, inclusion of a competing chelating agent such as ethylenediamine tetra-acetate (EDTA), citrate, succinate, or oxalic acid, is often recommended. Consideration must also be given to providing the appropriate conditions to minimize protein binding. Strong acids and acidic deproteinizing agents are suitable for this purpose, but tetracyclines may decompose to their anhydro-forms under strong acidic conditions.

Sample extraction/deproteinization is usually accomplished with mild acidic solvents to free the noncovalently bound tetracyclines from macromolecules. McIlvaine buffer, pH 4.0 (286, 287), McIlvaine/EDTA buffer, pH 4.0 (283, 287–293), succinate buffer, pH 4.0 (278–281, 294–296), acidic acetonitrile (297–299), and acidic methanol (14, 199, 300) have all been used successfully. Moreover, trichloroacetic acid, pH 2.0 (301, 302), metaphosphoric acid (303), acetate buffer (126, 280), citrate buffer, pH 4.0 (304), citrate buffer/ethyl acetate, pH 4–5 (305), and hydrochloric acid/glycine buffer (306, 307) have all been employed with varying success to precipitate proteins from the sample homogenates.

Alternative sample extraction techniques include an approach that combines the deproteinizing efficiency of dichloromethane with the ion-pairing ability of phenylbutazone for isolating tetracyclines from eggs (308). Another approach that was employed for extracting oxytetracycline from milk (285) or swine tissues (309), and tetracycline, oxytetracycline, and chlortetracycline from milk (284), was based on ultrafiltration. With ultrafiltration, however, not all low molecular-mass proteins are retained in the cut-off filters while interfering substances pass through the filter.

The aqueous or organic extract obtained at this step of analysis may be a very dilute solution of the analyte(s) of interest. It may also contain coextractives, which if allowed in the final extract will increase the background noise of the detector, making it impossible to determine trace level concentrations of the analyte(s). To reduce interferences and concentrate the analyte(s), the primary sample extract must be subjected to cleanup procedures such as liquid–liquid partitioning, solid-phase extraction, matrix solid-phase dispersion, ultrafiltration, immunoaffinity chromatography, and online trace enrichment. In many instances, more than one of these procedures may be used in combination for increasing extract purification.

Liquid–liquid partitioning cleanup is generally directed to removal of the matrix constitutents from the aqueous extract into organic immiscible solvents (14, 298, 299, 302, 308). Unfortunately, tetracyclines cannot be quantitatively recovered into organic immiscible solvents at any pH value because of their high polarity. However, recoveries higher than 85% were reported when tetrabutylammonium ions were employed in the ion-pair extraction of oxytetracycline and tetracycline into dichloromethane at pH 8.2 (297).

Solid-phase extraction has also been widely employed for the isolation and/ or cleanup of tetracycline antibiotics from biological matrices since it does not require high volume of solvents, and it is generally less time-consuming and labor-intensive. The solid-phase extraction applications reported for tetracycline antibiotics have been mainly accomplished using reversed-phase C_{18} sorbents (281, 283, 286–293, 296, 300, 301, 304) although nonpolar sorbents such as polymeric (280) and cyclohexyl (306, 307) materials have also been employed. To avoid potential loss of the analytes during their passage through the solid-phase extraction sorbents due to the well-known binding tendency of tetracyclines, pretreatment of the reversed-phase solid-phase cartridges with EDTA has been generally employed.

Elimination of coextracted materials and concentration of tetracyclines have also been accomplished using mixed-phase extraction membranes with both reversed-phase and cation exchange properties (294, 295), or solid-phase extraction columns packed with cation-exchange materials such as CM-Sephadex C-25 (301), aromatic sulfonic acid (310), and carboxylic acid (283, 300). For the same purpose, metal chelate affinity chromatography has also been employed. In this technique, the tetracyclines are specifically absorbed on the column sorbent by chelation with copper ions bound to small chelating Sepharose fast flow column (278–281, 294–296).

A matrix solid-phase dispersion technique has been further applied for the determination of oxytetracycline, tetracycline, and chlortetracycline in milk (290, 311), using octadecylsilyl- (C_{18}) derivatized silica as the solid phase. To facilitate extraction of the tetracycline antibiotics from milk, addition of an equal ratio of EDTA to oxalic acid has been found advantageous.

Ultrafiltration (278, 279) and immunoaffinity chromatography (282) have also been described for removal of matrix components from milk extracts, while online trace enrichment has been reported for isolation/purification of tetracycline, oxytetracycline, demeclocycline, and chlortetracycline residues from animal tissues and egg constituents (305). The latter technique involves trapping of the analytes onto a metal chelate affinity preconcentration column (Anagel-TSK Chelate-5PW), rinsing of coextracted materials to waste, and finally flushing of the concentrated analytes onto the analytical column.

Following sample extraction and cleanup, tetracycline antibiotics may be separated by thin-layer or liquid chromatographic procedures, and quantified by spectrophotometric, fluorometric, or mass spectrometric detection systems. Direct spectrophotometric and capillary electrophoretic methods have also been described (Table 29.8).

Direct spectrophotometric methods using fluorometric detection have been reported for screening of tetracycline in milk extracts (126, 282), and three tetracyclines in tissues extracts (302, 310). In a different approach, Salinas et al. (212) described a fourth-derivative spectrophotometric method for the determination of oxytetracycline in honey. Although useful, these methods cannot differentiate among individual tetracycline antibiotics and are less sensitive than the screening tests used for regulatory purposes.

Capillary electrophoresis has been applied by Chen and Gu (281) for simultaneous determination of oxytetracycline, tetracycline, chlortetracycline, and doxycycline residues in bovine milk. Separation was performed on a noncoated capillary column, 57 cm total length with 50 cm effective length, 75 μm internal diameter (i.d.) and 375 μm outside diameter (o.d.), using a mobile phase containing 10 mM sodium dodecyl sulfate, 50 mM borate, and 50 mM phosphate, pH 8.5. Under these conditions, concentrations below 10 ppb could be determined in milk using an ultraviolet spectrophotometer set at 370 nm.

Thin-layer chromatography has been carried out on commercially available silica gel (14) and/or C_8 modified silica gel high-performance thin-layer chromatography (HPTLC) plates (283, 287). In the former case, the silica gel plate was predeveloped with aqueous EDTA, while in the latter the C_8-modified silica gel HPTLC plate was developed with a mobile phase containing 0.5M aqueous oxalic acid. Following separation, tetracyclines could be detected by a variety of detection systems including bioautography using *Bacillus subtilis* (14) as the test organism, fluorometry after spraying with magnesium chloride and triethanolamine (283), and spectrophotometry after spraying with Fast Blue BB and pyridine (287). These methods lack generally the performance characteristics required to detect the low ppb levels likely to occur in animal tissues. However, for a regulatory laboratory without access to sophisticated instrumentation, these methods are valuable because they allow detection of tetracyclines at levels higher than 100 ppb and can, thus, provide some analytical support for a regulatory program.

Liquid chromatography has become the most widely used separation technique for determining tetracycline antibiotics in edible animal products (Table 29.8). Separation is generally carried out on octadecyl, octyl, and polymeric reversed-phase columns using mobile phases containing appropriate modifiers. Because tetracyclines have the tendency to form chelates with metal ions, they can adsorb on free silanol groups in the reversed-phase sorbents and, therefore, are apt to appear as tailing peaks. These drawbacks have been overcome to a large degree either by column manufacturing processes such as end-capping and prepa-

TABLE 29.8 Physicochemical Methods for Tetracycline Antibacterials in Edible Animal Products

Antibacterial(s)	Matrix	Sample preparation	Steps	Stationary phase	Mobile phase	Detection/ Identification	Sensitivity/ Recovery	Ref.
SPECTROMETRIC METHODS								
Tetracycline	Milk	Phosp. buffered saline diln, IAC cleanup, derivatization with europium (III)	5	—	—	Fluorometric, ex: 394 nm, em: 616 nm	19 ppb/ 94–100%	282
	Milk	Acetate buffer extn, filtn, derivatization with europium (III)	3	—	—	Fluorometric, ex: 342 nm, em: 550 nm	125 ppb/ 93–103%	126
Oxytetracycline	Honey	Acetate buffer, pH 3.8, diln	1	—	—	Fourth- derivative spectro- photometry	3 ppm/ 81–113%	212
Tetracycline, oxytetracycline, chlortetracycline	Swine tissues	EtOAc extn, SPE cleanup	6	—	—	Fluorometric, ex: 380 nm, em: 505 nm	50–200 ppb/ 47–74%	310
	Animal tissues	Glycine buffer/TCA extn, deprtn, liq–liq partn, sodium barbital and magnesium acetate addn	8	—	—	Fluorometric, ex: 440 nm, em: 505 nm	50–300 ppb/ 30–45%	302

(continued)

TABLE 29.8 Physicochemical Methods for Tetracycline Antibacterials in Edible Animal Products

Antibacterial(s)	Matrix	Sample preparation	Steps	Stationary phase	Mobile phase	Detection/Identification	Sensitivity/Recovery	Ref.
THIN-LAYER CHROMATOGRAPHIC METHODS								
Tetracycline, oxytetracycline, chlortetracycline	Animal tissues	MeOH/HCl extn, liq–liq partns	15	Silica gel or cellulose	Various eluents	*B. subtilis* bioautography	0.5–15 ppm/ NR	14
Four tetracyclines	Animal tissues	McIlvaine buffer extn, SPE cleanup	14	HPTLC Silica gel or C_8	$CHCl_3$/MeOH/EDTA or MeOH/ACN/oxalate	UV-Vis/Fast blue, pyridine	100 ppb/ 58–93%	287
Seven tetracyclines	Honey	McIlvaine buffer diln, SPE cleanup	8	HPTLC Silica gel or C_8	$CHCl_3$/MeOH/EDTA or MeOH/ACN/oxalate	Fluorometric/$MgCl_2$ or TEA	100 ppb/ NR	283
LIQUID CHROMATOGRAPHIC METHODS								
Chlortetracycline	Swine muscle	HCl/glycine buffer extn, SPE cleanup	12	PLRP-S, 5 μm	0.1M, pH 12, glycine buffer/ACN (87.5:12.5)	Fluorometric, ex: 340 nm, em: 420 nm	50 ppb/ 86–94%	306
Oxytetracycline	Fish tissues	Citric acid/Na_2HOP_4 extn, SPE cleanup	16	Spheric C_{18}, 5 μm, analytical and guard column	0.01M oxalic acid/ACN/DMF (72:22:6), pH 2.1, at 25°C	UV-Vis 355 nm	50–100 ppb/ 88–95%	304
	Milk	McIlvaine/EDTA buffer diln, ultrafiln	2	LiChrospher 100 RP-18e, 5 μm, analytical and guard column	0.01M oxalic acid/ACN (85:15)	UV-Vis 354 nm	95 ppb/ 89–93%	285

Mussel shells	MeOH/oxalic acid extn	8	LiChroSpher 100 RP-18E, 5 μm, analytical and guard column	0.02M H_3PO_4/ACN (76:24), pH 2.3	UV-Vis 355 nm	8 ppb/ 65 ± 11%	199
Salmon muscle	TCA/phosp. buffer, pH 2, extn, two SPE cleanups	11	Ultrasphere ODS, 5 μm	0.02M, pH 2.25, phosp. buffer/MeOH (76:24)	UV-Vis 365 nm	100 ppb/ 62–82%	301
Salmon muscle	Metaphosphoric acid extn	12	Ultrasphere ODS, 5 μm with New-Guard RP-18, 7 μm, column	0.025M oxalic acid/ACN/THF (75:22.5:2.5.) contg 10 mM octanesulfonate	UV-Vis 355 nm	50 ppb/ 86–95%	303
Shrimp	Succinate buffer extn, metal chelate affinity column cleanup, SPE cleanup	17	PLRP-S, 5 μm	0.005M oxalic acid/MeOH (42:58)	NiCl-MS-PB	100 ppb/ ~50%	280
Swine tissues	ACN/imidazole/ magnesium acetate/EDTA buffer extn, ultrafiltn	4	L-column ODS, 5 μm	1M imidazole, pH 7.2, buffer contg 50 mM, magnesium acetate and 10 mM EDTA/ACN (90:10), at 40°C	Fluorometric, ex: 380 nm, em: 520 nm	50 ppb/ 58–67%	309

(continued)

TABLE 29.8 Continued

Antibacterial(s)	Matrix	Sample preparation	Steps	Stationary phase	Mobile phase	Detection/ Identification	Sensitivity/ Recovery	Ref.
Doxycycline	Turkey tissues	Succinate buffer extn, metal chelate affinity column cleanup, concn on cation-exchange extraction membrane	23	PLRP-S, 8 μm, analytical and guard column	0.01M oxalic acid/ACN/ MeOH Gradient from (80:15:5) to (40:20:40)	Fluorometric, postcolumn derivatization with zirconyl chloride, ex: 406 nm, em: 515 nm	1 ppb/ 66 ± 3%	294
Oxytetracycline, chlortetracy-cline	Animal tissues	McIlvaine/EDTA buffer/MeOH extn, two SPE cleanups	12	Asahi ODP-50, 5 μm	Sorensen, pH 12, buffer/ACN (90:10), at 40°C	Fluorometric, ex: from 350 nm to 374 nm, em: from 420 nm to 508 nm, using time programming technique	NR/ 62–87%	300
Oxytetracycline, tetracycline	Milk	H_2SO_4 addn, ACN extn, liq–liq partn, ion-pair extn, liq–liq partn	12	Nucleosil 120, C_{18}, 5 μm	0.02M H_3PO_4/ ACN (76:24), at 35°C	UV-Vis 355 nm	10 ppb/ 71–89%	297

Oxytetracycline, tetracycline, chlortetracy-cline	Animal tissues	McIlvaine/EDTA buffer extn, SPE cleanup	10	C_8, 5 or 10 μm deactivated column	0.01M oxalic acid/ACN/MeOH (60:30:10), for 5 μm LC column, 0.01M oxalic acid/ACN/MeOH (70:20:10) for 10 μm LC column	UV-Vis 350 nm	0.1–0.6 ppm/ 18–127%	288
	Bovine and swine tissues	HCl addn, ACN extn, liq–liq partn	5	PRP-1, 10 μm, or PLRP-S, 5 μm, with recommended guard column	0.01M H_3PO_4/MeOH/ACN Gradient from (80:20:0) to (30:20:50)	UV-Vis 355 nm	100 ppb/ 71–106%	298
	Bovine and swine tissues	McIlvaine/EDTA buffer extn, SPE cleanup	10	Nova-Pak C_{18}, 4 μm, with μBondapak C_{18}, guard column	0.01M citric acid-K_2HPO_4/ACN (72:28), contg 5 nM tetramethyl-ammonium chloride and 0.01% EDTA	UV-Vis 365 nm/PDA (190–367 nm)	10 ppb/ 50–70%	289
	Eggs	Ion pair/DCM extn, liq–liq partn	9	HC-ODS-SIL-X-I, 10 μm	H_2O/ACN/0.1M NaH_2PO_4 (70:20:10), pH 2.6, at 30°C	UV-Vis 361 nm	16–80 ppb/ 95–106%	308
	Milk	McIlvaine/EDTA buffer diln, ultrafiltn	3	Nova-Pak C_{18}	0.01M oxalic acid/ACN/MeOH Gradient from (100:0:0) to (70:22:8), at 30°C	UV-Vis 360 nm	14–52 ppb/ 75–106%	284

(continued)

TABLE 29.8 Continued

Antibacterial(s)	Matrix	Sample preparation	Steps	Stationary phase	Mobile phase	Detection/ Identification	Sensitivity/ Recovery	Ref.
	Milk	HCl addn, ACN extn, liq–liq partn	6	PLRP-S, 5 μm, analytical and guard column	0.05M, pH 2.0, oxalate buffer, contg 5 mM decanesulfonate/ ACN Gradient from (80:20) to (62:28)	UV-Vis 356 nm	5 ppb/ 87–99%	299
	Milk	MSPD extn/ cleanup, in presence of EDTA and oxalic acid	8	Micro Pak ODS, 10 μm	0.01M oxalic acid/ACN (70:30), at 40°C	UV-Vis 365 nm/PDA (200–450 nm)	100 ppb/ 40–98%	311
	Milk	MSPD extn/ cleanup, in presence of EDTA and oxalic acid	8	LiChrosorb RP-18, 5 μm	0.01M oxalic acid/ACN/ MeOH (65:17.5:17.5)	UV-Vis 365 nm	30 ppb/ 89–93%	290
	Milk, meat, cheese	McIlvaine/EDTA buffer extn, SPE cleanup	12–15	LiChrosorb RP-18, 5 μm	0.01M oxalic acid/ACN/ MeOH (65:17.5:17.5)	UV-Vis 365 nm	15–22 ppb/ 48–86%	290
	Muscle and kidney	HCl/glycine buffer extn, SPE cleanup	15	Prodigy ODS2 or Inertsil ODS2	Solvent A: H₂O/ ACN (90:10) contg 0.04%	PICI–MS– APCI	10–20 ppb/ 59–83%	307

Analyte	Sample	Extraction		Column	Mobile phase	Detection	Range/Recovery	Ref.
					heptafluorobutyric acid, 10 mM oxalic acid and 10 μM EDTA Solvent B: H₂O/ACN (10:90) contg 0.04% heptafluorobutyric acid, 10 nM oxalic acid and 10 μM EDTA Gradient from (90:10) to (10:90), at 25 °C			
	Salmon muscle	McIlvaine buffer extn, SPE cleanup	14	LiChroCART RP-18, 7 μm, with Brownlee RP-18 ODS guard column	0.01M oxalic acid/ACN/ MeOH (73:17:10)	UV-Vis 355 nm	80–500 ppb/ 45–100%	286
Four tetracyclines	Animal tissues and egg	Succinate buffer extn, metal chelate affinity column cleanup, concn on cation-exchange extraction membrane	23	PLRP-S, 8 μm, analytical and guard column	0.01M, pH 2.0, oxalic acid/ ACN Gradient from (85:15) to (60:40)	Fluorometric, postcolumn derivatization with zirconyl chloride, ex: 406 nm, em: 515 nm	2–5 ppb/ 40–70%	295

(continued)

TABLE 29.8 Continued

Antibacterial(s)	Matrix	Sample preparation	Steps	Stationary phase	Mobile phase	Detection/ Identification	Sensitivity/ Recovery	Ref.
Four tetracyclines	Animal tissues and egg	EtOAc/citrate buffer extn, online trace enrichment on Anagel-TSK Chelate-5PW metal chelate affinity preconen column, and switching to analytical column	11	PLRP-S, 5 μm, analytical and guard column	Solvent A: 0.1M KH_2PO_4-0.01M citric acid-0.01M EDTA Solvent B: ACN/MeOH/1M, pH 4, citrate buffer (25:10:65) Gradient from (100:0) to (0:100) for 10 min and then isocratic (0:100)	UV-Vis 350 nm	3–6 ppb/ 42–101%	305
Four tetracyclines	Bovine liver	McIlvaine/EDTA buffer extn, SPE cleanup	10	LiChrosorb RP-8, 10 μm	0.01M oxalic acid/ACN/ MeOH (54.5:27.3:18.2)	UV-Vis 350 nm	50–100 ppb/ 68–95%	291
Four tetracyclines	Bovine tissues	McIlvaine/EDTA buffer extn, SPE cleanup	14	TSK Gel Super Octyl, 2 μm	0.05% TFA/ACN (80:20)	MS-MS-ESP	100 ppb/ 56–79%	292

Analyte	Matrix	Sample preparation	No.	Column	Mobile phase	Detection	LOD/recovery	Ref.
Four tetracyclines	Bovine and swine tissues	McIlvaine/EDTA buffer extn, SPE cleanup	14	LiChrosorb RP-8, 10 μm	0.01M oxalic acid/ACN/MeOH (54.5:27.3:18.2)	UV-Vis 350 nm	10 ppb/ 59–90%	287
Four tetracyclines	Milk	McIlvaine/EDTA buffer extn, SPE cleanup	13	Bakerbond C8, 5 μm	0.01M oxalic acid/ACN/MeOH (50:30:20)	UV-Vis 350 nm/TLC-FAB-MS	10–20 ppb/ 73–93%	293
Six tetracyclines	Milk	Centrgn, acetic acid extn, metal chelate affinity column cleanup, SPE cleanup	17	PLRP-S, 5 μm	0.005M oxalic acid/MeOH (42:58)	NICI-MS-PB	30 ppb/ ≈50%	280
Seven tetracyclines	Honey	McIlvaine/EDTA buffer extn, two SPE cleanups	8	Chemcosorb 3 C8, 3 μm	0.01M oxalic acid/ACN/MeOH (76.2:14.3:9.5), pH 3.0	UV-Vis 350 nm	20–50 ppb/ 84–100%	283
Seven tetracyclines	Kidney	Succinate buffer extn, metal chelate affinity column cleanup, SPE cleanup	16	Two ChromSpher C8, 5 μm, analytical columns in tandem, with Perisorb RP-8 guard column	0.01M oxalic acid/ACN (80:20)	UV-Vis 365 nm/PDA (200–400 nm)	10–30 ppb/ 44–77%	296
Seven tetracyclines	Milk	Centrgn, succinate buffer extn, metal chelate affinity column cleanup, ultrafiltn	13	PLRP-S, 5 μm, analytical and guard column	0.01M oxalic acid/ACN/MeOH Gradient from (100:0:0) to (70:22:8)	UV-Vis 355 nm	1–2 ppb/ 63–91%	278

(continued)

TABLE 29.8 Continued

Antibacterial(s)	Matrix	Sample preparation	Steps	Stationary phase	Mobile phase	Detection/ Identification	Sensitivity/ Recovery	Ref.
Seven tetracyclines	Milk	Centrgn, succinate buffer extn, metal chelate affinity column cleanup, ultrafiltn	13	PLRP-S, 5 μm analytical and guard column	0.01M oxalic acid/ACN/ MeOH Gradient from (100:0:0) to (70:22:8)	UV-Vis 355 nm	30 ppb/ 60–110%	279
CAPILLARITY ELECTROPHORETIC METHODS								
Four tetracyclines	Milk	Centrgn, succinate buffer extn, metal chelate affinity column cleanup, SPE cleanup	17	Beckman 50 cm × 75 μm uncoated capillary, at 15 kV and 23°C	0.05M borate- 0.05M phosphate contg 10 mM sodium dodecyl sulfate, pH 8.5	UV-Vis 370 nm/PDA (200—440 nm) and first order derivatization	2–9 ppb/ 40–84%	281

IAC, immunoaffinity chromatography; PB, particle beam; APCI, atmospheric pressure chemical ionization; ESP, electrospray; FAB, fast atom bombardment.
Other abbreviations as in Tables 29.1 and 29.3.

ration of all-polymer-based solid supports or by the inclusion of citrate (289, 305), oxalate (278–280, 283–288, 290, 291, 293–296, 299, 303, 304, 307, 311), and/or EDTA (289, 305, 307, 309) in the mobile phase. Overnight treatment of the stationary phase with a mobile phase containing chlortetracycline as the blocking agent has also been suggested as a powerful means to eliminate tailing of the oxytetracycline and tetracycline peaks (297).

Since tetracyclines have several pK_a values and can exist as zwitterions, one must always consider the control of the mobile-phase pH in the development of an analytical method. The property of tetracyclines to exist in the form of ions also makes the use of ion-pairing reagents attractive, and several methods have been developed that utilize this approach (289, 299, 303, 307).

In liquid chromatographic analysis of tetracycline antibiotics, the most popular detector is the UV-Vis spectrophotometer. Since the extinction coefficients of tetracyclines are relatively large, monitoring of samples at wavelengths in the range 350–370 nm allows detection of tetracycline residues into the low ppb levels (Table 29.8).

Although tetracyclines possess the inherent ability to fluoresce, few methods exploiting this property have been reported (300, 306, 309). Instead, fluorometric methods based on the reaction of tetracyclines with suitable derivatizing agents have been developed. The use, for example, of zirconyl chloride as a fluorescence label in the postcolumn derivation of tetracyclines, has allowed highly selective and sensitive detection of these antibiotics in animal tissues (294, 295).

Confirmatory analysis of suspected liquid chromatographic peaks is usually accomplished by a photodiode array detector that continuously collects spectral data during the chromatographic separation (Fig. 29.8.1) and further compares the spectrum (200–450 nm) of the eluted suspected compound with that of a standard (281, 289, 296, 311). Although confirmation with a photodiode array detector is simple, specificity and sensitivity are not sufficient to determine or identify trace levels of residual tetracyclines in edible animal products.

Coupling of liquid chromatography with mass spectrometry provides unequivocal online spectrometric identification of tetracycline antibiotics in animal-derived foods. Typical applications of mass spectrometry in confirming tetracycline residues in edible animal products describe coupling of liquid chromatography with mass spectrometry via particle-beam (280), electrospray (292), or atmospheric pressure chemical ionization (307), using negative-ion detection interfaces.

Fletouris et al. (297), Cooper et al. (305), and Carson et al. (280) described promising methods, in terms of simplicity, selectivity, and sensitivity, for screening and even confirmation of tetracycline residues in edible animal products.

Fletouris et al. (297) described a liquid chromatographic method for the determination of oxytetracycline and tetracycline residues in milk. According to

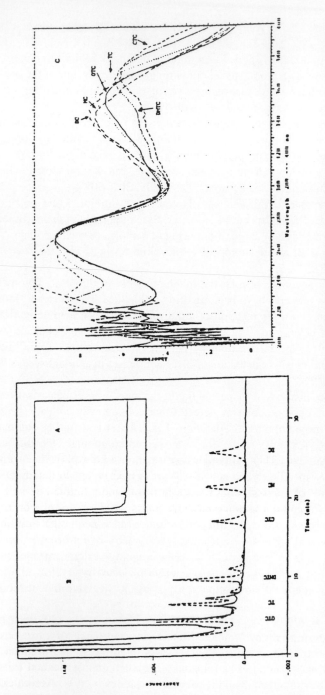

FiG. 29.8.1 Chromatograms of a blank kidney sample (A), a kidney sample (B) fortified with 4 ppm of oxytetracycline (—), and 250 ppb of each tetracycline (---), and ultraviolet spectra (C) of the corresponding tetracyclines. Peaks: OTC, oxytetracycline; TC, tetracycline; DMTC, demethylchlortetracycline; CTC, chlortetracycline; MC, methacycline; DC, doxycycline. (From Ref. 296.).

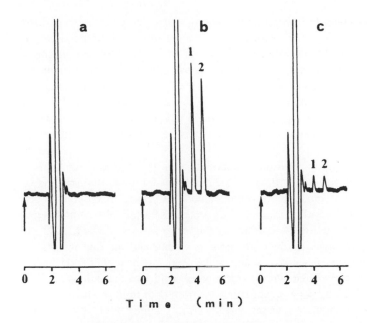

Fɪɢ. 29.8.2 Typical chromatograms of a blank milk sample (a), a milk sample (b) fortified with 93 ppb oxytetracycline (1) and 100 ppb tetracycline (2), and a sample fortified with 10 ppb of each tetracycline (c). (From Ref. 297.).

this method, a 5 g milk sample is acidified at pH 2.7 with 0.6N sulfuric acid, and extracted with 10 ml acetonitrile. The extract is partly purified by treatment with saturated ammonium sulfate solution and concentrated into 2 ml phosphate buffer, pH 8.2. Following addition of tetrabutylammonium reagent, tetracyclines are extracted as ion pairs into dichloromethane, reextracted into 0.1M perchloric acid, and analyzed by liquid chromatography. Separation is performed on a 25 cm Nucleosil 120 C_{18} (5 μm) analytical column, which has been preconditioned overnight with a solution containing chlortetracycline. Elution is effected with a mobile phase of 0.02 M phosphoric acid/acetonitrile (76:24) at a flow-rate of 1.2 ml/min and a column temperature of 35°C (Fig. 29.8.2). Under these conditions, concentrations as low as 10 ppb of oxytetracycline and tetracycline residues could be determined in milk using ultraviolet detection at 355 nm.

In a different approach, Cooper et al. (305) developed an online metal chelate affinity chromatography–liquid chromatographic method for the determination of oxytetracycline, tetracycline, demeclocycline, and chlortetracycline residues in animal tissues and egg. According to this method, a 2 g blended egg or thinly sliced tissue is homogenized with citrate buffer pH 5 (pH 4, for chicken liver) and ethyl acetate. Following centrifugation the supernatant is evaporated to dryness, and the residue is reconstituted in methanol to be trapped at the beginning of an Anagel-TSK Chelate-5PW metal chelate affinity preconcentration column. The trapped analytes are back-flashed using an automated column switching system into the analytical column (15-cm PLRP-S, 5 μm), and analyzed under the gradient elution conditions shown in Table 29.8. Concentrations as low as 3 ppb for oxytetracycline, 5 ppb for tetracycline and demeclocycline, and 6 ppb for chlortetracycline could be readily detected in tissues and egg using ultraviolet detection at 350 nm.

Liquid chromatography with mass spectrometry was suggested by Carson et al. (280) in a multiresidue method for the determination of oxytetracycline in shrimp, and oxytetracycline, tetracycline, chlortetracycline, doxycycline, demeclocycline, and minocycline in milk using a particle beam interface and negative ion chemical ionization. According to this confirmatory method, a 40 ml milk sample is centrifuged at 10°C to separate cream, and the lower "skim" layer is mixed with glacial acetic acid and centrifuged. On the other hand, shrimp tissue (10 g) is homogenized with 0.1M succinic acid and the homogenate is centrifuged at 10°C. The supernatant solutions from both milk or shrimp tissue extracts are then applied to a metal chelate affinity chromatography column. Following column washing sequentially with 0.5M sodium chloride, water, methanol, and water, tetracyclines are eluted with McIlvaine-EDTA-sodium chloride buffer to be further applied to a Supelclean ENVI-Chrom P solid-phase extraction cartridge. After column washing with water, tetracyclines are eluted with methanol and the eluate is evaporated to dryness. The residue is reconstituted in 1 ml water to be further analyzed by liquid chromatography. Separation is performed on a 15 cm PLRP-S (5 μm) analytical column, with 0.005M oxalic acid/methanol (42:58) mobile phase at a flow rate of 0.5 ml/min. Under these conditions, concentrations as low as 100 ppb of oxytetracycline in shrimp and 30 ppb of oxytetracycline, tetracycline, chlortetracycline, doxycycline, demeclocycline, and minocycline in milk could be readily confirmed by mass spectrometry using a particle-beam interface and negative ion chemical ionization.

29.9 MISCELLANEOUS ANTIBACTERIALS

This section reviews those antibacterials that do not fall into the classes discussed above. Major drugs in this section are novobiocin, colistin, and tiamulin.

Novobiocin is a weak dibasic acid with both enolic (pK_a 4.3) and phenolic (pK_a 9.2) character, which is almost insoluble in chloroform and water at pH below 7.5 but is readily soluble in other polar organic solvents such as lower alcohols, acetone, and ethyl acetate.

Determination of novobiocin in animal tissues and milk has been reported using either thin-layer chromatography–bioautography (14) or liquid chromatography (312, 313). The former method, although valuable, does not offer the sensitivity required to detect the low ppb levels likely to occur in food of animal origin. Better sensitivity is feasible by the liquid chromatographic method developed by Moats and Leskinen (312) for the determination of novobiocin in milk and tissues. A few years later this method was successfully validated by Reeves (313) for the determination of this drug in milk.

According to this method, tissue or milk samples are blended or diluted, respectively, with 3 ml 0.2M ammonium dihydrogen phosphate/g of sample. Aliquots (10 ml) of tissue homogenates or diluted milk are deproteinized by adding methanol and filtering to be further analyzed by liquid chromatography. Separation is performed on a 15 cm Supelcosil LC-18-DB (5 μm) analytical column, protected with a LC-18-DB guard column, using the mobile phase and the gradient elution program presented in Table 29.9, at a flow rate of 1 ml/min (Fig. 29.9). Under these conditions, concentrations as low as 10 ppb could be determined using an ultraviolet spectrophotometer monitored at 340 nm.

Colistin is a linear-ring peptide antibiotic. Its main components are colistin A and colistin B. It is a member of the polymyxin family of antibiotics that is stable in dry form and in water solution. The sulfate salt of colistin, which is usually administered as feed additive, is soluble in water, slightly soluble in methanol, and practically insoluble in acetone and ether. Colistin components do not have any specific fluorophore and UV chromophore, so detection by liquid chromatography at residue levels of interest is difficult without including a suitable derivatization step in the analytical method.

There is only one physicochemical method for the quantitation of colistin components in bovine muscle (314). In the proposed method a 5 g ground tissue sample is extracted with 20 ml 0.5% sulfuric acid. After centrifugation the supernatant is filtered and applied to a Bond Elut C_{18} cartridge. Following cartridge washing with water, and 0.1M trifluoroacetic acid/acetonitrile (85:15), colistin is eluted with 0.017M trifluoroacetic acid/acetonitrile (80:20) and the eluate is analyzed by liquid chromatography. Separation is performed on a 15 cm Inertsil Ph (5 μm) analytical column, using a 0.017M trifluoroacetic acid/acetonitrile (80:20) mobile phase. Following postcolumn derivatization with *o*-phthalaldehyde (OPA), concentrations as low as 200 ppb for colistin A and colistin B could be readily determined in bovine muscle using a fluorescence detector monitored at 340 nm excitation and 455 nm emission wavelengths.

Tiamulin is a semisynthetic derivative of the diterpene antibiotic pleuromutilin. Determination of residues of this drug in foods of animal origin has relied solely on gas chromatography. By now only two methods have been developed for the quantitation and/or confirmation of tiamulin in swine liver (315, 316). According to these methods, which have the same sample preparation procedure, 30 g liver homogenate is extracted twice with 300 ml 0.5N hydrochloric acid/acetone (1:60). After filtration the extract is cooled in acetone–dry ice bath, filtrated

TABLE 29.9 Physicochemical Methods for Miscellaneous Antibacterials in Edible Animal Products

Antibacterial(s)	Matrix	Sample preparation	Steps	Stationary phase	Mobile phase	Detection/ Identification	Sensitivity/ Recovery	Ref.
Thin-Layer Chromatographic Methods								
Novobiocin	Animal tissues	MeOH extn, liq–liq partns	14	Silica gel	CHCl₃/MeOH/ acetone/ glycerine	B. subtilis bioautography	2 ppm/ NR	14
Gas Chromatographic Methods								
Tiamulin	Swine liver	0.5N HCl/acetone extn, dry-ice filtration, alk hydrolysis, liq–liq partns, derivatization with pentafluoropropionic anhydride, Florisil column cleanup	27	Supercoport with 3% SP-2250	Nitrogen	ECD	200 ppb/ 89–93%	315
	Swine liver	0.5N HCl/acetone extn, dry-ice filtration alk hydrolysis, liq–liq partns, derivatization with pentafluoropropionic anhydride, Florisil column cleanup	27	Supelcoport with 3% SP-2100	Helium	MS	200 ppb/ 89–93%	316

Liquid Chromatographic Methods

Colistin A and B	Bovine musle	0.5% H_2SO_4 extn, SPE cleanup	9	Inertsil Ph, 5 μm	0.017M TFA/ACN (80:20)	Fluorometric, postcolumn derivatization with OPA, ex: 340 nm, em: 455 nm	A: 200 ppb, B: 200 ppb/ 65%	314
Novobiocin	Animal tissues, milk	0.2M $NH_4H_2PO_4$ addn, MeOH extn	4	Supelcosil LC-18-DB, 5 μm, analytical and guard column	0.01 M H_3PO_4/ ACN/MeOH Isocratic (50:0:50) for 1 min and gradient to (20:80:0)	UV 340 nm	10 ppb/ 92–103%	312
	Milk	0.2M $NH_4H_4PO_4$ addn, MeOH extn	4	Supelcosil LC-18-DB, 5 μm, analytical and guard column	0.005M H_3PO_4/ ACN/MeOH Isocratic (50:0:50) for 1 min and gradient to (20:80:0)	UV 340 nm	10 ppb/ 89–100%	313

OPA, phthalaldehyde.
Other abbreviations as in Tables 29.1 and 29.3.

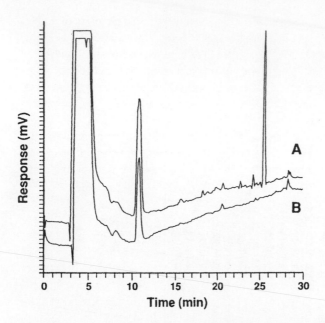

Fɪɢ. 29.9 Chromatogram of (A) novobiocin-dosed milk containing approximately 0.14 ppm novobiocin and (B) control milk. (Reprinted from Ref. 313. Copyright, (1992), by AOAC INTERNATIONAL.)

again, and concentrated to a volume of 10–15 ml. Following filtration the aqueous extract is hydrolyzed at alkaline conditions, acidified with concentrated hydrochloric acid, and extracted three times with dichloromethane. The organic layer is evaporated to an oily residue and the major hydrolytic product (8-α-hydroxymutilin) is derivatized with pentafluoropropionic anhydride and then applied to an activated Florisil column. After the column is washed four times with 4 ml acetone/hexane (1:50), the analyte is eluted with 200 ml acetone/hexane (1:50), and the eluate is evaporated to dryness. The residue is reconstituted in 20 ml toluene or benzene and analyzed by gas chromatography on a Supelcoport SP-2250 or SP-2100 column with nitrogen or helium as the carrier gas. Using electron capture (315) or mass spectrometric (316) detection, tiamulin residues could be readily determined in swine liver at concentrations greater than 200 ppb.

29.10 ANTHELMINTHIC DRUGS

Included in this group of drugs are the benzimidazoles, imidazothiazoles, tetrahydropyrimidines, salicylanilides, substituted phenols, macrocyclic lactones, sulfonamide, and pyrazino-isoquinoline derivatives. The benzimidazole class of anthelminthics is derived from the simple benzimidazole nucleus and includes the thiabendazole analogues and the benzimidazole carbamates. Substitution of side chains and radicals on the benzimidazole nucleus gives rise to the individual members of this class of drugs, including thiabendazole, albendazole, fenbendazole, oxfendazole, febantel, netobimin, oxibendazole, mebendazole, parbendazole, and luxabendazole.

Levamisole constitutes the best-known member of the class of imidazothiazoles drugs, while coumaphos, dichlorvos, and trichlorphon are organophosphates commonly used in food-producing animals. Pyrantel and its methyl analogue, morantel, constitute the group of the tetrahydropyrimidine anthelminthics. Closantel, niclosamide, oxyclozanide, rafoxanide, dibromsalan, and tribromsalan are the better-known members of the salicylanilides group of anthelminthics. A range of substituted phenols including nitroxynil, dichlorophen, hexachlorophen, niclofolan, and bithionol are still used as anthelminthics in food-producing animals.

Included in the class of macrocyclic lactones are avermectins and milbemycins, which are fermentation products possessing a 16-member cyclic lactone, a spiroketal moiety, and a disaccharide unit. Abamycin, ivermectin, doramectin, and eprinomycin are the avermectins most often available for anthelminthic treatment of livestock, whereas moxidectin is a milbemycin with worldwide acclaim as a cattle anthelminthic. Other anthelminthics currently used in food-producing animals are clorsulon, which is a benzenesulphonamide derivative; praziquantel, which is a racemate derivative of pyrazino-isoquinoline; and hygromycin B, which is an aminoglycoside antibiotic that exhibits anthelminthic properties.

In residue analysis of benzimidazoles in liver or milk, samples are often subjected to a pretreatment procedure to convert the glucuronide- and/or sulfate-conjugated metabolites to the unconjugated forms. This conversion is sometimes carried out by overnight incubation with gluculase, an enzyme mixture of β-glucuronidase and sulfatase (317). More often, however, acid hydrolysis is the preferred procedure because it can be completed at $80-110°C$ in $1-4$ h compared with the overnight reaction required by the enzymatic digestion (318–322).

When liquid samples such as serum, plasma, milk, or honey are not to be extracted using direct liquid–liquid partitions with organic solvents but through use of solid-phase extraction or matrix solid-phase dispersion techniques, dilution with water (323, 324), phosphate buffer saline (325), or phosphoric acid (326, 327) is often the only sample preparation procedure applied. Milk analysis sometimes requires further pretreatment for fat removal (328). Centrifugation at about 7000g at $4-10°C$ for 20 min is the usually applied procedure for making the fat floating on top of milk readily eliminated.

Semisolid samples such as muscle, liver, and kidney normally require a more intensive sample pretreatment for tissue break-up. This is generally accom-

plished by mechanical dispersion using a mincing apparatus and/or a tissue homogenizer to expose the analytes to the extraction solvent.

Following sample pretreatment, extraction of the analytes from the sample
matrix is mostly accomplished with ethyl acetate (317–319, 329–343) and acetonitrile (320, 344–358), but methanol (359–361), acetone (362, 363), dimethylformamide (364), acetone/dichloromethane (365), acetone/isooctane (366),
acetone/ethanol (367), acetone/acetonitrile (368), and ethyl acetate/ethanol/isooc-
tane (369) have also been used with varying success. Since most anthelminthics
are weakly basic hydrophobic compounds with appreciable solubility in polar
organic solvents, extraction, particularly with ethyl acetate, is usually performed
after alkalinizing the sample through addition of either sodium hydroxide
(336–339) and sodium carbonate (330, 331, 335, 340–342), or ammonium hydroxide (329, 333, 334, 360, 369) solution. Adjustment of the sample pH is not
needed, however, when acetonitrile is used for extraction of the analytes. Possible
reason for this behavior might be the appreciable deproteinizing ability of acetonitrile that destroys the irreversible binding of the analytes with sample constituents
and, thus, recovery losses due to binding are virtually eliminated (345).

In many applications, relatively large quantities of anhydrous sodium sulfate can be added to the sample, prior to extraction by organic solvents, in order
to enhance the partitioning process (333–336, 341, 342, 354, 365, 370). In some
instances, such as in the analysis of clorsulon in bovine liver and milk, addition
of hydroxylamine hydrochloride is often recommended prior to extraction (329,
360). The use of this agent is to prevent interactions between the analyte and
endogenous aldehydes that lead to loss of recovery.

The aqueous or organic extract obtained at this step of analysis may be a
very dilute solution of the analyte(s) of interest. It may also contain coextractives,
which, if allowed in the final extract, will increase the background noise of the
detector, making it impossible to determine trace level concentrations of the
analyte(s). To reduce interferences and concentrate the analyte(s), the primary
sample extracts are subjected to some kind of cleanup including liquid–liquid
partitioning, solid-phase extraction, matrix solid-phase dispersion, online trace
enrichment, affinity chromatography, immunoaffinity chromatography, and ultrafiltration. In many instances, more than one of these procedures may be used in
combination to increase extract purification.

Liquid–liquid partitioning cleanup is sometimes directed solely to the removal of fat from the sample extract. This can be accomplished through use of
either hexane for the removal of fat from acetonitrile (329, 332, 352, 355, 358,
363, 369) and acidified aqueous extracts (317, 322, 333, 334, 341) or cyclohexane
and isooctane from acidified aqueous (330, 331) and acetonitrile (345) extracts,
respectively. In most cases, liquid–liquid cleanup is based on pH-dependent extractions and back-extractions between organic and aqueous solvents since most
anthelminthics show a strong tendency to partition from basic aqueous solutions

into organic solvents and back-extracted into acidified aqueous solutions. This inherent property has been extensively exploited in the analysis of levamisole in cattle and swine liver (330) and milk (328), thiabendazole and its metabolite in bovine tissues (317), albendazole-2-aminosulfone in bovine liver (319), fenbendazole in bovine liver (333, 334), praziquantel in fish plasma and tissues (363), thiabendazole and levamisole in meat (336), four benzimidazoles in milk (341), and eight benzimidazoles in bovine liver (325).

Liquid–liquid partitioning cleanup on a hydrophilic matrix has also been employed for purification of the primary sample extract. This procedure was only applied in the determination of fenbendazole and four metabolites in plasma and liver using a Chem Elut disposable column to partition an alkalinized aqueous sample extract into dichloromethane (371). In a few instances, further cleanup can also be achieved by submitting an organic extract to freezing at $-20°C$, a procedure that can precipitate dissolved matrix components (359, 366, 367).

Cleanup by solid-phase extraction has also been widely employed since it is a simple, fairly inexpensive, and easy-to-perform procedure for purification of the crude extract. The use of disposable solid-phase extraction columns is currently part of most, if not all, modern analytical methods for the determination of anthelminthics in biological matrices at residue levels. Both normal-phase columns based on silica (333–335, 340, 367, 372), alumina (346, 373–375), or aminopropyl (339, 365, 370) materials, and reversed-phase columns based on C_{18} (319, 323, 324, 328, 344, 346, 347, 349–351, 357–359, 364, 367) and cyclohexyl (329, 332, 360) sorbents have been described in analytical applications.

In some instances, combinations of normal- and reversed-phase columns can also be used for better purification of the crude extract. Combinations of C_{18} and alumina or C_{18} and silica solid-phase extraction columns have been successfully employed in the analysis of ivermectin residues in animal tissues (346) and bovine plasma (348), respectively. Elimination of coextracted materials and concentration of the analytes has also been accomplished using mixed-phase extraction columns. Such a copolymeric bonded silica column with both hydrophobic and cationic functions has been employed in the analysis of hygromycin B in plasma, serum and milk (326).

Matrix solid-phase dispersion has also been applied for the determination of ivermectin residues in bovine liver (373) and milk (372), moxidectin in bovine tissues (374), thiabendazole and mebendazole in meat (66), and five and seven benzimidazoles in bovine liver (375) and milk (322), respectively.

Online trace enrichment is another attractive route for increasing the resolving power of liquid chromatographic methods. An automated system by which nitroxynil in cattle muscle tissue could be loaded onto an anion-exchange precolumn and then eluted and chromatographed on a polymeric analytical column has been described (354). In practice, this is the online and higher performance analogue of conventional offline cleanup that typically employs a sequence of low-resolution chromatographic steps.

Ultrafiltration through a 30000 molecular mass cut-off cellulose membrane is another cleanup procedure that has been successfully applied in the analysis of luxabendazole residues in biological fluids (364). Although efficient, this technique was not used for treatment of urine samples since it would have implied working with low flow rates and a consequent increase in analysis time.

Immunoaffinity chromatography cleanup has also been applied as an ideal and reliable strategy for residue analysis. Immunoaffinity columns prepared by coupling the antibodies to a cyanogen bromide-activated support were used to analyze avermectin B1 residues in cattle tissues (359) and ivermectin in sheep serum (376). An immunoaffinity column prepared by an alternative activation/coupling procedure with carbonyl diimidazole was also employed to analyze ivermectin residues in swine liver (361) since the earlier-reported methods did not work well in the analysis of this matrix. This recent work demonstrated the high specificity of the antibody-mediated cleanup, but also showed that the immunoaffinity procedures could not always or completely eliminate matrix interference of samples. Therefore, application of additional cleanup steps before or after these procedures is often inevitable.

Although cleanup by immunoaffinity chromatography is an elegant approach that offers the advantage of specific recognition of a drug, it requires the production and purification of the specific antibodies, which can be an expensive process. Thus, affinity chromatography has further been suggested for the determination of hygromycin B in bovine plasma, serum, and milk (326). Unlike with immunoaffinity chromatography, any ligand that specifically recognizes and reversibly binds another molecule may be used for affinity chromatography. Lysozyme and α-lactalbumin were the proteins selected as the immobilized ligands for binding the aminoglycoside anthelminthic hygromycin B.

Following sample extraction and cleanup, anthelminthics can be separated by thin-layer, liquid, or gas chromatographic procedures. Direct mass spectrometric methods have also been described (Table 29.10).

A direct mass spectrometric method for simultaneous detection of five benzimidazoles including levamisole, thiabendazole, mebendazole, fenbendazole, and febantel in sheep milk was reported (377). The method, which involves injection of crude milk extracts and selection and collision of the most abundant ionic species obtained under electron impact ionization, was highly sensitive and rapid. Another direct mass spectrometric approach for rapid and quantitative determination of phenothiazine in milk was also described (323). This method involves an extraction step using a C_{18} microcolumn disc, followed by thermal desorption of the analyte from the disc directly into an ion trap mass spectrometer.

Thin-layer chromatographic methods are limited to the determination of hygromycin B and have been carried out on commercially available silica gel

TABLE 29.10 Physicochemical Methods for Anthelminthics in Biological Matrices

Compound(s)	Matrix	Sample preparation	Steps	Stationary phase	Mobile phase	Detection/ identification	Sensitivity/ recovery	Ref.
SPECTROMETRIC METHODS								
Phenothiazine	Milk	H₂O diln, cleanup on C₁₈ microcolumn extn disc	4	—	—	TD-IT-MS-MS	10 ppb/ 39 ± 4%	323
Five benzimida- zoles	Sheep milk	HCl addn, centrgn, ether/hexane extn, liq–liq partns	14	—	—	EI-CAD MIKE-MS	0.6–2.8 ppb/ 80–90%	377
THIN-LAYER CHROMATOGRAPHIC METHODS								
Hygromycin B	Plasma, serum	H₃PO₄ (plasma) or TCA (serum) diln, ion-exchange column cleanup	20	LHK-PD Silica gel	Acetone/EtOH/ NH₄OH	Fluorometric/ Fluorescamine	25–50 ppb/ >80%	327
	Plasma, serum, milk	H₃PO₄ diln, SPE cleanup, affinity column cleanup	15	LHK-PD Silica gel	Acetone/EtOH/ NH₄OH	Fluorometric/ Fluorescamine	~1 ppm/ >80%	326
GAS CHROMATOGRAPHIC METHODS								
Albendazole 2- aminosulfone	Bovine liver	Acid hydrolysis, EtOAc extn, liq–liq partns, SPE cleanup, derivatization with MTBSTFA (TMS derivative)	35	DB-5, 30 m, capillary	Helium	EI-MS and MID-MS	100 ppb/ 73–105%	318

(continued)

TABLE 29.10 Continued

Compound(s)	Matrix	Sample preparation	Steps	Stationary phase	Mobile phase	Detection/identification	Sensitivity/recovery	Ref.
Clorsulon	Bovine kidney	NH₃/hydroxylamine treatment, EtOAc extn, liq–liq partn, SPE cleanup, derivatization with methyl iodide, liq–liq partns	36	Supelcoport with 3% SP2100	Helium	EI-MS and MID-MS	200 ppb/ 97%	329
Coumaphos	Honey	H₂O diln, tandem SPE cleanup	8	BP-1, 12 m, capillary	Helium	SIM-MS	40 ppb/ 79–86%	324
Levamisole	Cattle and swine liver	NaOH soln addn, EtOAc extn, liq–liq partns	18	Methylsilicone, 15 m, capillary	Helium	EI-MS	10 ppb/ 61–100%	330
	Milk	NaOH soln addn, EtOAc extn, liq–liq partns	19	DB-1, 30 m, capillary	Helium	NPD	0.5 ppb/ 85–94%	331
	Milk	pH 4.6 adjustment, centrgn at 10°C, SPE cleanup, online LC purification on Spherisorb S5W normal phase silica column	7	DB-17, 30 m, capillary	Helium	FID & NPD	2.2–0.4 ppb/ 85–95%	328
Thiabendazole, 5-hydroxy-thiabendazole	Bovine tissues	Glusulase hydrolysis, EtOAc extn, liq–liq partns, on column methylation with trimethylanilinium	33	Gas-Chrom Q with 3% polysulfone	Helium	SIM-MS	100 ppb/ 81–112%	317

Liquid Chromatographic Methods

Albendazole 2-aminosulfone	Bovine liver	HCl hydrolysis, EtOAc extn, liq–liq partns, SPE cleanup	30	µBondapak C_{18} with Co-Pell ODS or LiChrosorb, 10 µm, guard column	0.02M KH_2PO_4, contg 10mM diethanolamine/MeOH/ACN (68:20:12)	Fluorometric, ex: 300 nm, em: 320 nm	200 ppb/ 73–105%	319
	Milk	H_3PO_4 hydrolysis, ACN extn, SPE cleanup, liq–liq partns	32	Econosphere ODS, 5 µm, with Brownlee RP-18, 10 µm, guard column	0.02M KH_2PO_4, contg 10mM diethanolamine/MeOH/ACN (60:30:10)	Fluorometric, ex: 300 nm, em: 320 nm	8 ppb/ 92–104%	320
Avermectin B_1	Bovine muscle and plasma	MeOH extn, SPE cleanup, cleanup by freezing, IAC cleanup	18	Spheri-5, RP-18	H_2O/MeOH (10:90)	UV 245 nm	6 ppb/ 80–86%	359
Clorsulon	Bovine kidney	NH_3/hydroxylamine treatment, EtOAc extn, liq–liq partn, SPE cleanup	20	Alltech C_{18}, with Spheri-5, RP-18 OD-GU, guard column	0.01M, pH 7, phosp. buffer/ACN (80:20), at 32°C	UV 265 nm	500 ppb/ 93–106%	332
	Milk	Hydroxylamine addn, MeOH extn, SPE cleanup	12	Econosphere C_{18}, 3 µm	Phosp. buffer, pH 7.0/ACN (75:25)	UV 265 nm	5 ppb/ 74–79%	360
Closantel	Animal tissues, plasma	ACN/HOAc extn, SPE cleanup	9	Nucleosil 100 C_{18}, 5 µm	H_2O/ACN (15:85), pH 2.5	Fluorometric, ex: 335 nm, em: 510 nm	10–50 ppb/ 71–88%	344

(continued)

TABLE 29.10 Continued

Compound(s)	Matrix	Sample preparation	Steps	Stationary phase	Mobile phase	Detection/ identification	Sensitivity/ recovery	Ref.
Eprinomectin	Bovine liver	Na$_2$SO$_4$ addn, DCM/acetone extn, SPE cleanup	13	Abzelute ODS-DB, 5 μm	H$_2$O/ACN (30:70), pH 5, at 40°C	PICI-MS-MS-ESP	2400 ppb/ NR	370
	Bovine tissues	Na$_2$SO$_4$ addn, DCM/acetone extn, SPE cleanup, on-line precolumn derivatization with trifluoroacetic anhydride	15	Zorbax RX-C8	H$_2$O/MeOH/ACN/ TEA/H$_3$PO$_4$ (15:55:30:0.1:0.1), at 35°C	Fluorometric, ex: 365 nm, em: 470 nm	2 ppb/ 87–100%	365
Fenbendazole	Bovine liver	Na$_2$SO$_4$/Na$_2$CO$_3$ addn, EtOAc extn, liq–liq partns, SPE cleanup	30	Alltech C$_{18}$, 5 μm, with Brownlee RP-18 Spheri-10 MPLC, guard column	0.01M, pH 7, amm. phosp. buffer/MeOH (30:70), (47:53) and (60:40)	UV 298 nm	800 ppb/ 83%	333, 334
	Milk	ACN extn, liq–liq partns	9	Nucleosil 120 C$_{18}$, 5 μm	0.01M H$_3$PO$_4$/ ACN (50:50) contg 10 mM octane-sulfonate, at 50°C	UV 300 nm	3 ppb/ 98–100%	345

Ivermectin	Animal tissues	Acetone/H$_2$O/isooctane extn, cleanup by freezing, precolumn derivatization with methylimidazole/acetic anhydride, SPE cleanup	29	Zorbax ODS, with Spheri-5 RP-18, 5 μm, guard column	H$_2$O/MeOH (3:97), at 30°C	Fluorometric, ex: 360 nm, em: 425 nm	1 ppb/ 74–77%	366
	Animal tissues	ACN extn, two SPE cleanups, precolumn derivatization with methylimidazole/acetic anhydride, SPE cleanup	20	Brownlee RP-18 OD-224, with Brownlee RP-18 guard column	H$_2$O/MeOH (3:97)	Fluorometric, ex: 365 nm, em: 425 nm	2 ppb/ 77–99%	346
	Animal tissues	ACN extn, SPE cleanup, cleanup by freezing, liq–liq partns, precolumn derivatization with methylimidazole/acetic anhydride, SPE cleanup	35	Supelcosil LC-18, 5 μm, with Supelguard LC-18, 5 μm, guard column	H$_2$O/MeOH (5:95)	Fluorometric, ex: 360 nm, em: 470 nm	2 ppb/ 68–88%	347
	Bovine liver	MSPD extn/ cleanup, SPE cleanup, precolumn derivatization with methylimidazole/acetic anhydride, SPE cleanup	23	Econosil C$_{18}$, 5 μm, with Newguard C$_{18}$, guard column	H$_2$O/MeOH (5:95), at 37°C	Fluorometric, ex: 364 nm, em: 418 nm	1 ppb/ 72–77%	373

(continued)

TABLE 29.10 Continued

Compound(s)	Matrix	Sample preparation	Steps	Stationary phase	Mobile phase	Detection/ identification	Sensitivity/ recovery	Ref.
	Bovine blood and plasma	EtOH and acetone extn, cleanup by freezing, liq–liq partns	19	μBondapak NH$_2$	Hexane/THF/ MeOH/DMSO (75:25:2)	UV 254 nm	5 ppb/ 77–104%	367
	Bovine serum	ACN extn, two SPE cleanups	7	Nova-Pak C$_{18}$, 4 μm	H$_2$O/ACN/MeOH (10:45:45)	UV 245 nm	2 ppb/ 95 ± 4%	348
	Bovine liver and muscle	ACN extn, SPE cleanup	11	Nova-Pak C$_{18}$, 5 μm	H$_2$O/ACN/MeOH (10:45:45)	UV 254 nm/PDA (220–300 nm), (>50 ppb)	5–10 ppb/ 65–89%	349
	Bovine tissues, blood and serum	ACN extn, SPE cleanup	7	Ultrasphere XL ODS, 3 μm	H$_2$O/ACN/MeOH (18:49:33), at 56°C	UV 245 nm	2 ppb/ 77%	350
	Meat, liver	ACN/H$_2$O extn, SPE cleanup, precolumn derivatization with methylimidazole/ trifluoroacetic anhydride	12	μBondapak C$_{18}$	H$_2$O/MeOH (5:95)	Fluorometric, ex: 364 nm, em: 470 nm	5 ppb/ 71–88%	351

Milk	27	NH₄OH/EtOH/EtOAc/isooctane extn, liq–liq partns, precolumn derivatization with methylimidazole/acetic anhydride, SPE cleanup	Econosil C₁₈, 5 µm, or Zorbax ODS, with Brownlee OD-GU guard column	H₂O/MeOH (95:5), at 30°C	Fluorometric, ex: 364 nm, em: 418 nm	1 ppb/ 59–99%	369
Milk	35	MSPD extn/ cleanup, SPE cleanup, precolumn derivatization with methylimidazole/acetic anhydride, SPE cleanup	Econosil C₁₈, 5 µm, with Newguard RP-18, guard column	H₂O/MeOH/THF (5:85:15)	Fluorometric, ex: 364 nm, em: 455 nm	1 ppb/ 81–91%	372
Sheep serum	7	MeOH/phosp. buffer diln, IAC cleanup	Spheri-5, RP-18, 5 µm	H₂O/MeOH (5:95)	UV 245 nm	2 ppb/ 90–99%	376
Swine liver	15	MeOH extn, IAC cleanup, liq–liq partn	Brownlee C₁₈, 5 µm	H₂O/ACN/MeOH (10:45:45)	UV 245 nm	5 ppb/ 85–102%	361
Luxabendazole Serum, urine	4–7	DMF extn, ultrafiltn or SPE cleanup	Nucleosil C₁₈, 5 µm, with Perisorb RP-18, 30–40 µm, pellicular guard column	0.05M, pH 7, phosp. buffer/ ACN (60:40)	UV 290 nm	15–25 ppb/ 60–116% or 84–108%	364
Mebendazole Eel muscle	14	Na₂SO₄/Na₂CO₃ addn, EtOAc extn, SPE cleanup	LiChrosorb RP-8, 5 µm, with pellicular RP, 40 µm, guard column	0.05M amm. phosp. buffer/ ACN (70:30), pH 6.7	UV 311 nm/PDA (200–360 nm)	10 ppb/ 62–83%	335

(continued)

TABLE 29.10 Continued

Compound(s)	Matrix	Sample preparation	Steps	Stationary phase	Mobile phase	Detection/ identification	Sensitivity/ recovery	Ref.
Moxidectin	Bovine tissues	ACN extn, liq–liq partns, precolumn derivatization with methylimidazole/ acetic anhydride, SPE cleanup	26	Zorbax ODS, 5 μm	H₂O/MeOH (2:98)	Fluorometric, ex: 364 nm, em: 470 nm/ LC-MS-TSP without derivatization and after LC conditions modification (>250 ppb)	10 ppb/ 89–99%	352
	Bovine tissues	MSPD extn/ cleanup, SPE cleanup, precolumn derivatization with methylimidazole/ trifluoroacetic anhydride	13	Supelcosil C₁₈, 3 μm	0.2% HOAc/ MeOH/ACN (8:30:62)	Fluorometric, ex: 383 nm, em: 447 nm	1 ppb/ 80–100%	374
	Plasma	ACN extn, SPE cleanup, precolumn derivatization with methylimidazole/ trifluoroacetic anhydride	9	Supelcosil C₁₈	0.2% HOAc/ MeOH/ACN (8:30:62)	Fluorometric, ex: 383 nm, em: 447 nm	0.1 ppb/ 77–86%	353

Nitroxynil	Bovine muscle	TEA/ACN extn, on line trace enrichment on Anagel-TSK DEAE-5PW, 10 μm, preconcn column and switching to analytical column	11	PLRP-S, 5 μm, analytical and guard column	0.01M, pH 7, phosp. buffer/ACN (80:20)	UV 273 nm	5 ppb/89–94%	354
	Milk	ACN/acetone extn, liq-liq partns	9	Lichrospher 100 RP-18, 5 μm	0.05M KH_2PO_4/ACN (80:20), pH 4, at 40°C	Electro-chemical	0.7 ppb/92–97%	368
Oxfendazole	Milk	Acetone extn, liq-liq partns	26	μBondapak C_{18}, with Co-Pell ODS guard column	H_2O/ACN (75.5:24.5)	UV 254 nm	5 ppb/100–105%	362
Praziquantel	Fish plasma and tissues	Acetone extn, liq-liq partns	10	Supelcosil LC-ABZ, 5 μm, analytical and guard column	H_2O/ACN (61:39)	UV 205 nm	5–20 ppb/81–100%	363
Thiabendazole	Meat	HCl hydrolysis, SPE cleanup	10	μBondapak C_{18}, 10 μm, with Bondapak C_{18}/Corasil, 37–50 μm, guard column	0.03M sodium acetate/MeOH (45:55), pH 7.6	UV 300 nm, and fluorometric, ex: 313 nm, em: 365 nm	5 ppb/62–75%	321

(continued)

TABLE 29.10 Continued

Compound(s)	Matrix	Sample preparation	Steps	Stationary phase	Mobile phase	Detection/ identification	Sensitivity/ recovery	Ref.
Thiabendazole, 5-hydroxy-thiabendazole	Milk	HCl hydrolysis, EtOAc extn, SPE cleanup	14	PartiSphere SCX, 5 μm	0.05M phosp. buffer/ACN (80:20), pH 3.8, at 25°C	Fluorometric, ex: 305 & 318 nm, em: 380 & 525 nm	50 ppb/ 90–108%	378
Thiabendazoe, levamisole	Meat	Na$_2$SO$_4$/KOH addn, EtOAc extn, liq–liq partns	11	μBondapak C$_{18}$, 10 μm, with Bondapak C$_{18}$/Corasil, 37–50 μm, guard column	0.03M sodium acetate/MeOH (35:65), pH 7.6	UV 240 and 300 nm/ PDA (200–400 nm)	5–25 ppb/ 63–75%	336
Thiabendazole, mebendazole	Meat	MSPD extn/ cleanup	6	Spherisorb C$_{18}$ ODS2, 5 μm	Solvent A: 0.01M, pH 5.2, acetate buffer Solvent B: ACN/ MeOH (70:30) Gradient from (56:44) to (36:64), at 35°C	UV 254 and 290 nm, and fluorometric, ex: 308 nm, em: 365 nm/ PDA (200–450 nm)	0.4–15 ppb/ 69–102%	66

Analyte	Matrix	Sample prep		Column	Mobile phase	Detection	LOD/Recovery	Ref.
Albendazole and two metabolites	Milk	NaOH addn, EtOAc extn, liq–liq partn	5	Nucleosil 120 C$_{18}$, 5 μm	0.01M H$_3$PO$_4$/ACN (80:20) contg 5 mM tetrabutyl-ammonium hydrogen sulfate, at 50°C	UV 292 nm	2–5 ppb/ 78–100%	337
Three albendazole metabolites	Cheese	ACN extn, liq–liq partns	8	Nucleosil 120 C$_{18}$, 5 μm	0.01M H$_3$PO$_4$/ACN (73:27) contg 20 mM octanesulfonate and 2.5 mM tetrabutyl-ammonium hydrogen sulfate, at 40°C	Fluorometric, ex: 290 nm, em: 320 nm	0.9–55 ppb/ 74–85%	355
	Milk	NaOH addn, EtOAc extn, liq–liq partn	6	Nucleosil 120 C$_{18}$, 5 μm	0.01M H$_3$PO$_4$/ACN (73:27) contg 20 mM octanesulfonate and 2.5 mM tetrabutyl-ammonium hydrogen sulfate, at 40°C	Fluorometric, ex: 290 nm, em: 320 nm	0.09–6 ppb/ 83–96%	338

(continued)

TABLE 29.10 Continued

Compound(s)	Matrix	Sample preparation	Steps	Stationary phase	Mobile phase	Detection/identification	Sensitivity/recovery	Ref.
Mebendazole and two metabolites	Eel muscle	NaOH addn, EtOAc extn, SPE cleanup	21	ChromSpher B C$_{18}$, 5 μm, with C$_{18}$, 20 μm, guard column	0.01M, pH 6.2, NaH$_2$PO$_4$ACN (70:30)	UV 289 nm	1–2 ppb/ 59–99%	339
Fenbendazole and two metabolites	Fish muscle	Na$_2$CO$_3$ soln addn, EtOAc extn, SPE cleanup	17	Two in series Lichrosorb RP 8, 5 μm, columns with pellicular C$_{18}$ 40 μm, guard column	0.05M, pH 5.0, amm. phosp buffer/ACN/ MeOH (55:28:17)	UV 297 nm	4–7 ppb/ 70–93%	340
Fenbendazole and three metabolites	Milk	ACN extn, liq–liq partns	11	Nucleosil 120 C$_{18}$, 5 μm	0.01M H$_3$PO$_4$/ ACN (70:30) contg 2.5 mM octanesulfonate and 5 mM tetrabutyl-ammonium hydrogen sulfate, at 50°C	UV 290 nm	2–5 ppb/ 82–91%	356
Fenbendazole and four metabolites	Liver, plasma	NH$_4$OH addn, SPE cleanup	6	Micro Pak MCH 10	H$_2$O/0.05N H$_3$PO$_4$/ACN (5:15:80) or 0.05N H$_3$PO$_4$/ ACN (22:78)	UV 290 nm	10 ppb/ 89–102%	371

Four benzimidazoles	Milk	Na$_2$SO$_4$ addn, EtOAc extn, liq–liq partns, SPE cleanup	30	LiChrosorb RP-18, 10 μm or Hypersil ODS, 5 μm, with pellicular C-8 guard pellicular C$_{18}$ guard column	0.01M, pH 7, amm. phosp. buffer/MeOH (30:70), (47:53), and (60:40)	UV 298 nm and 318 nm	0.5–30 ppb/ 56–94%	341
Five anthelminthics	Milk	ACN/acetone extn, liq–liq partn, SPE cleanup	8	Kaseisorb LC-300-5, 5 μm	0.05M KH$_2$PO$_4$/ ACN (45:55), pH 3, at 40°C	Electro-chemical	4–20 ppb/ 79–98%	357
Five benzimidazoles	Bovine liver	MSPD extn/ cleanup, SPE cleanup	10	Micro Pak, 10 μm	0.017M H$_3$PO$_4$/ ACN (60:40), at 45°C	UV 290 nm/ PDA (200–350 nm)	100 ppb/ 62–87%	375
Seven benzimidazoles	Milk	MSPD extn/ cleanup	9	Micro Pak, 10 μm	0.05N H$_3$PO$_4$ACN (60:40), at 45°C	UV 290 nm/ PDA (200–350 nm)	62.5 ppb/ 70–107%	322
Eight benzimidazoles	Animal tissues	Na$_2$SO$_4$/K$_2$CO$_4$ addn, EtOAc extn, liq–liq partns, SPE cleanup	20	Partisphere C$_{18}$, 5 μm	0.01M, pH 7, amm. phosp. buffer/MeOH (47:53) contg 10 mM TEA	UV 298 nm/ GC-EI-MS after derivatization with MTBSTFA (TMS derivatives)	50 ppb/ 81–99%	342

(continued)

TABLE 29.10 Continued

Compound(s)	Matrix	Sample preparation	Steps	Stationary phase	Mobile phase	Detection/identification	Sensitivity/recovery	Ref.
Eight benzimidazoles	Animal tissues	ACN extn, liq–liq partns, two SPE cleanups	24	Hewlett-Packard RP-18, 5 μm, with Kontron RP-18 Presat, 25–40 μm, guard column	0.01M pentane-sulfonate contg 0.5% TEA, pH 3.5/ACN (50:50)	UV 298 nm/ GC-NPD or GC-EI-MS or GC-Pulsed PICI-NICI-MS after derivatization with methyl iodine or pentafluoro-benzyl bromide	20–50 ppb/ 39–87%	358
Eight benzimidazoles	Bovine liver	Normal saline diln, MSPD extn/cleanup using diatomaceous earth, liq–liq partns	21	Micro Pak MCH 10	H_2O/0.05N H_3PO_4/ACN (6:6:88)	UV 290 nm	10–250 ppb/ 61–92%	325
Ten benzimidazoles	Milk	NaOH addn, EtOAc extn, liq–liq partn	5	Nucleosil 120 C_{18}, 5 μm	0.01M H_3PO_4/ACN (80:20) contg 5 mM tetrabutyl-ammonium hydrogen sulfate, at 50°C	UV 292 nm	2–40 ppb/ 59–100%	343

TD–IT, Thermal desorption–ion trap; CAD MIKE, collisionally activated decomposition mass-analyzed ion kinetic energy; MID, multiple ion detection; FID, flame ionization detector; NPD, nitrogen/phosphorus detector; SIM, selected ion monitoring; EI, electron impact; TMS, trimethylsilane; MTBSTFA, N-methyl-N-(tetr.-butyldimethylsilyl)trifluoroacetamide. Other abbreviations as in Tables 29.1 and 29.3.

plates (326, 327). Hygromycin B bands were derivatized at acidic pH with fluorescamine, and visualized under ultraviolet light. Unlike other aminoglycosides, hygromycin B exhibited a higher fluorescence in acidic solutions than in basic conditions. These methods generally lack the performance characteristics required to detect the low ppb levels likely to occur in animal tissues.

Liquid chromatographic methods have become the most widely used separation techniques for determining anthelminthic residues in edible animal products (Table 29.10). Separation is generally carried out on octadecyl, octyl, or polymeric reversed-phase columns, but normal-phase columns (367), such as μ-Bondapak NH_2, have also been employed. In reversed-phase separations, ion-suppressing or ionization-enhancing mobile phases are the most useful separation modes for analysis of multiple benzimidazole residues (338, 343). With mobile phases at neutral pH (341), where ionization of the analytes is suppressed, excessive retention and broadness of the late-eluting peaks often occur. By changing to acidic mobile phases, where ionization of benzimidazoles is enhanced, early-eluting peaks are readily separated, but the late-eluting peaks tail badly. Such behavior indicates some adsorptive interaction between protonated analytes and the negatively charged silanol groups on the silica-based stationary phase. Adding tetrabutylammonium cations to an acidic mobile phase greatly improves chromatography eliminating peak distortion and increasing peak heights (343).

Detection in liquid chromatography is mostly performed by fluorescence and/or ultraviolet absorption. In a few instances, electrochemical detection has also been employed (357, 368). For compounds that exhibit inherent intense fluorescence such as albendazole and metabolites (319, 320, 338, 355), closantel (344), and thiabendazole and metabolites (378), fluorometric detection is the preferred detection mode since it allows higher sensitivity. Compounds that do not fluoresce such as eprinomectin, moxidectin, and ivermectin, are usually converted to fluorescent derivatives prior to their injection into the liquid chromatographic analytical column. The derivatization procedure commonly applied for this group of compounds includes reaction with trifluoroacetic anhydride in presence of N-methylimidazole as a base catalyst in acetonitrile (346, 347, 351, 352, 366, 369, 372–374). The formation of the fluorophore is achieved in 30 s at 25°C and results in a very stable derivative of ivermectin and moxidectin (353) but a relatively unstable derivative of eprinomectin (365). However, the derivatized extracts are not pure enough, so that their injection dramatically shortens the life of the liquid chromatographic column unless a silica solid-phase extraction cleanup is finally applied.

Confirmatory analysis of suspected liquid chromatographic peaks can be accomplished by a photodiode array detector that continuously collects spectral data during the chromatographic separation and further compares the spectrum (200–450 nm) of the eluted suspected compound with that of a standard (66,

322, 335, 336, 349, 375). Although confirmation with a photodiode array detector is simple, specificity and sensitivity are not sufficient to determine or identify trace levels of residual anthelminthics in edible animal products.

Coupling of liquid chromatography with mass spectrometry can provide unequivocal on-line spectrometric identification of anthelminthic residues in animal-derived foods. Typical applications of such techniques include the confirmation of moxidectin residues in cattle fat by liquid chromatography–thermospray mass spectrometry (352), and the confirmation of eprinomectin residues in bovine liver tissue by liquid chromatography, electrospray ionization, and multiple reaction monitoring in the MS–MS mode with positive ion detection (370).

Gas chromatographic separation has not gained wide acceptance in spite of being quite sensitive and specific. This mode of separation is complicated by the necessity for derivatization of anthelminthics before analysis. Because the benzimidazoles are basic and exhibit low volatility, a derivatization procedure is inevitable. Only thiabendazole and triclabendazole are accessible by direct gas chromatography, although with a high detection limit. However, other anthelminthics such as organophosphates and levamisole are usually separated by direct gas chromatography with excellent detection limits (324, 328, 330, 331).

Among the derivatization reactions generally employed in the gas chromatographic determination of compounds with amino functions, acylation with trifluoroacetic anhydride, heptafluorobutyric anhydride, and N-methyltrifluoroacetamide; and alkylation with methyl iodide, pentafluorobenzyl bromide, and trimethylanilinium hydroxide are the most commonly used. On-column methylation using trimethylanilinium hydroxide in methanol has been employed in a combined gas–liquid chromatographic/mass spectrometric confirmatory assay for thiabendazole and 5-hydroxythiabendazole in animal tissues (317). For the gas chromatographic determination of albendazole-2-aminosulfone (318) or clorsulon (329) in bovine tissues, precolumn silylation with N-Methyl-N-(tetr.-butyldimethylsilyl)trifluoroacetamide or methylation with methyl iodide have been used, respectively. The confirmation of the derivatized analytes has been accomplished using a mass spectrometric detector operating in multiple ion detection or electron impact mode.

Methods for anthelminthic analysis that present attractive performance characteristics in terms of simplicity, selectivity, and sensitivity are those reported by Fletouris et al. (338, 343), and DeGroodt et al. (351).

A simple, rapid, and sensitive ion-pair liquid chromatographic method was described by Fletouris et al. (338) for the determination in milk of the sulfoxide, sulfone, and 2-aminosulfone metabolites that comprise the marker residue of albendazole. According to this method, a 1 ml aliquot of milk sample is alkalinized with sodium hydroxide solution, extracted with 7 ml ethyl acetate, and the extract is cleaned up by partition with 1 ml water. Following centrifugation, the top organic layer is collected, evaporated to dryness, and reconstituted in 0.5 ml mobile phase before liquid chromatography. Separation of the analytes is performed on a Hichrom column packed with Nucleosil 120, C_{18}, 5 μm material. The mobile phase consists of acetonitrile and 0.01M phosphoric acid, (27:73, v/v), and contained 20 mM octanesulfonate and 2.5 mM tetrabutylammonium ion pair reagents. Detection is carried out fluorometrically using excitation and emission wavelengths of 290 and 320 nm, respectively. Overall recoveries were 85.3 ± 9.0%, 96.4 ± 6.2%, and 83.4 ± 7.5% for the sulfoxide, sulfone, and 2-aminosulfone metabolites, respectively, while precision data, based on within- and between-days variation, suggested overall relative standard deviation values ranged from 2.9 to 6.0%. The good analytical characteristics of the method could allow limits of detection in the low ng/ml range to be realized (Table 29.10).

A multiresidue liquid chromatographic method was also reported by Fletouris et al. (343) for the quantitative screening of 10 benzimidazoles in milk including albendazole 2-aminosulfone, albendazole sulfoxide, oxibendazole, oxfendazole, albendazole sulfone, p-hydroxy-fenbendazole, albendazole, mebendazole, fenbendazole sulfone, and fenbendazole residues. According to this method, a 1 ml milk sample is alkalinized to pH 10 by addition of sodium hydroxide solution, and extracted with 6 ml ethyl acetate. The extract is cleaned up by partitioning with 1 ml water, evaporated to dryness, reconstituted with mobile phase, and analyzed isocratically on a Hichron column packed with Nucleosil 120, C_{18}, 5 μm material (Fig. 29.10.1). The mobile phase consists of acetonitrile and 0.01M phosphoric acid (20:80, v/v), containing 5 mM tetrabutylammonium hydrogen sulfate. Detection is carried out at 292 nm. Overall recoveries of most analytes ranged from 79 to 100%, while precision data, based on within- and between-days variation, suggested overall relative standard deviation values ranged from 2.0 to 5.8%.

DeGroodt et al. (351) described a liquid chromatographic method for the determination of ivermectin residues in meat and liver from cattle and swine. According to this method, a 4 g minced meat or liver sample is vortexed–mixed with 40 ml acetonitrile and 3.5 ml water. Following centrifugation, the precipitate is extracted again with 20 ml acetonitrile and 3.5 ml water. The combined extracts are evaporated to 6 ml and then diluted with 6 ml water. The diluted extract is loaded on a Bond Elut C_{18} cartridge and, following passing of the extract, the cartridge is dried by air aspiration. Ivermectin is eluted with 5 ml acetonitrile, which is then evaporated to dryness. Derivatization of ivermectin is performed in the dark by adding to the dried residue 150 μl trifluoroacetic anhydride/acetonitrile (1:2), and 100 μl N-methylimidazole/acetonitrile (1:1). Chromatographic analysis is accomplished on a C_{18} Bondapak reversed-phase column using a meth-

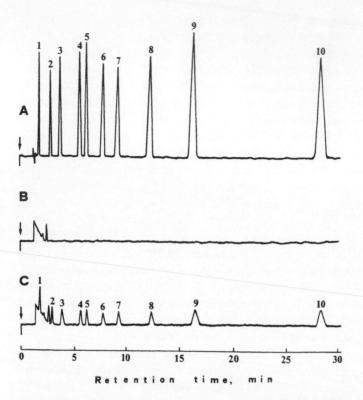

Fig. 29.10.1 Typical chromatograms of a mixed standard working solution (A), a control milk sample (B), and a control milk sample fortified with benzimidazoles at concentrations close to their detection limits (C). Peaks: 1, albendazole-2-aminosulfone; 2, albendazole sulfoxide; 3, oxibendazole; 4, oxfendazole; 5, albendazole sulfone; 6, p-hydroxyfenbendazole; 7, albendazole; 8, mebendazole; 9, fenbendazole sulfone; 10, fenbendazole. (From Ref. 343.).

anol–water (95:5) mobile phase (Fig. 29.10.2). Detection is carried out fluorometrically using excitation and emission wavelengths of 364 and 470 nm, respectively. Recovery ranged from 70 to 88%, and the quantification limit was as low as 5 ppb.

29.11 ANTICOCCIDIAL AND OTHER ANTIPROTOZOAL DRUGS

The first drugs used to treat coccidiosis were the sulfonamides. Subsequently, a wide range of compounds have replaced them. Many of these compounds, includ-

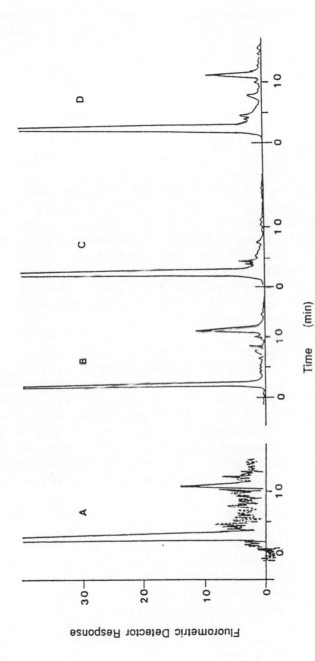

FIG. 29.10.2 Chromatograms of ivermectin. A, Absolute detection limit (250 pg); B, standard solution (3.6 ng); C, blank meat sample; D, spiked meat sample (22.5 ppb). (From Ref. 351.).

ing sulfonamides, nitrofurans, and tetracyclines, in addition to their role as coccidiostats are also used as antibacterials. Other drugs such as avoparcin, bacitracin,
carbadox, halquinol, nitrovin, roxarsone, and virginiamycin, are classified as
growth promoters. This section concentrates on those drugs whose primary function and use is as antiprotozoals. Included in this group of drugs are the benzamides, carbanilides, nitroimidazoles, polyether antibiotics, quinolone derivatives,
triazines, and some miscellaneous compounds. The majority of these drugs have
no common chemical structure and therefore no group tests can be used to screen
for residues in animal-derived foods.

Before an extraction procedure may commerce, the sample must be prepared so that it is in a condition for extraction of the analyte(s). This is particularly
relevant for complex matrices such as animal-derived foods, the nature of which
determines the kind of pretreatment step required. When analyzing semi-solid
food samples, such as muscle, liver, and skin, a pretreatment step may be required.
The analyte(s) must be exposed to extracting solvents to ensure maximum extraction. This may be accomplished by mechanical dispersion using a mincer/homog-
enizer. The most popular approach for tissue break-up is the homogenization of
samples in water or an aqueous buffer. Addition of anhydrous sodium sulfate to
the tissue samples, to combine with the water present, has been carried out for
facilitating the extraction of dimetridazole (379, 380).

For liquid samples, such as honey, a pretreatment dilution step with
acetonitrile/water, followed by filtration prior to liquid chromatographic analysis,
may be required (381). Addition of anhydrous sodium sulfate to egg homogenate,
prior to sample cleanup, is considered essential to remove part of the water and
facilitate the extraction of nicarbazin (382, 383) and halofuginone (384). Furthermore, it was found (382) that homogenizing eggs with acetic acid to adjust the
pH reduced the viscosity of the sample. This reduced viscosity, made the sample
more suitable for extraction, and improved the recovery. On the other hand,
homogenizing eggs with hydrochloric acid and saturated sodium chloride solution
has been considered essential (385) prior to liquid–liquid partitioning on diatomaceous earth column.

Extraction/deproteinization has been performed by either vortexing liquid
samples or homogenizing semisolid samples with acetonitrile (227, 382, 383,
386–392), methanol (14, 393–395), methanol/water mixtures (396–401), ethyl
acetate (384, 402–406), dichloromethane (379, 380, 407), and acetone (408, 409).
Nonpolar organic solvents, such as isooctane (410, 411) and toluene (407), have
also been reported to work extremely well for extracting salinomycin and dimetridazole from chicken tissues, respectively. Sample extraction with these nonpolar
solvents yields a cleaner extract and an easier workup than extraction with commonly used polar solvents. However, selecting an extraction solvent is critical
in establishing an analytical method because it is closely related to the cleanup
systems.

Using the previously mentioned extraction/deproteinization procedures, the obtained extracts often represent very dilute solutions of the analyte(s). These extracts may also contain coextractives that, if not efficiently separated prior to analysis of the final extract, will increase the background noise of the detector, making it impossible to determine the analyte(s) at the trace residue levels likely to occur in the analyzed samples. Hence, to reduce potential interferences and concentrate the analyte(s), the primary sample extracts are often subjected to some kind of additional sample cleanup such as liquid–liquid partitioning, solid-phase extraction, matrix solid-phase dispersion, online trace enrichment, and liquid chromatography. Extraction strategies needed for anticoccidial drugs generally depend upon the nature of the biomatrix. However, in many instances, more than one of these cleanup procedures may be applied in combination to allow greater purification of the analyte(s).

Liquid–liquid partitioning has been used for many years for the purification of anticoccidial drugs. The judicious use of multistep procedures involving extraction and back-extraction into organic and aqueous phases with appropriate use of pH and ionic strength can remove desired compounds from biological matrices as well as reducing the amount of interfering contaminants in the final extract. Quite different liquid–liquid partitioning approaches have been described, the selection being determined by the individual chemical properties of the drugs analyzed.

Polyether antibiotics are hydrophobic compounds that are characterized chemically by their low polarities and their instability under acidic conditions. These antibiotics can be quantitatively extracted from the primary organic extract into carbon tetrachloride (393–395). When partitioning from a sodium chloride solution into an organic solvent, high yields have been achieved using dichloromethane (396, 397), carbon tetrachloride (391, 399), and chloroform (14, 398) as extraction solvents. In a different approach, water extracts containing lasalocid residues have been purified by partitioning into the mobile phase, which was a complex mixture of tetrahydrofuran, methanol, n-hexane, and ammonia (387, 389, 390, 392). To remove lipids, sample extracts have often been partitioned with n-hexane.

Nitroimidazoles are polar compounds with characteristic amphoteric properties. They can easily be extracted from the primary organic sample extract into a strongly acidic aqueous solution and then back-extracted into dichloromethane under alkaline conditions (379, 402). In a different approach (385), on-column liquid–liquid partitioning is achieved using columns containing hydrophilic packing material (diatomaceous earth) to absorb and distribute egg homogenates over a large surface area, following which the analytes are eluted from the column with dichloromethane. Isooctane or n-hexane washing has often been used to remove lipids from sample extracts.

From the other anticoccidial drugs, benzamides can be readily extracted as ion-pairs into dichloromethane at strong alkaline conditions (pH 11) using tetrabutylammonium as pairing ion (257). Imidocarb residues have been partitioned into chloroform from alkaline water extracts containing sodium chloride (409), while ethopabate can be partitioned into ethyl acetate from water extracts containing sodium chloride without pH adjustment (388).

Removing proteins and other matrix constituents can also be accomplished with solid-phase extraction procedure. This procedure has become the method of choice in many laboratories for the isolation and/or cleanup of anticoccidial drugs from biological matrices. It is particularly advantageous because it requires low solvent usage, is generally less time-consuming and less labor-intensive, and has a variety of special properties that allow better extraction of these drugs.

Cleanup and concentration of both polar and nonpolar anticoccidial drugs from coextracted substances have mainly been accomplished with polar sorbents, such as silica (379, 391, 396, 398, 399, 402, 407, 410, 411), alumina (227, 257, 403, 404, 406, 412), or Florisil (388), since they provide high recovery of the analytes. However, in many cases, cation exchange sorbents (409), reversed-phase sorbents (405), or combinations of silica with reversed-phase sorbents (395, 400), alumina with Sephadex LH-20 (406), or alumina with Sephadex LH-20 and silica (397, 401) sorbents have been reported to be a powerful approach for the isolation and/or cleanup of these compounds. It is significant to note that cleanup systems using alumina are not suitable for isolation of lasalocid residues since they are irreversibly bound to the sorbent.

In contrast to the solid-phase extraction approach, only nonpolar C_{18} derivatized silica has been used as the sorbent in matrix solid-phase dispersion technique. This technique, which simplifies the overall methodology and removes most of the interfering compounds from animal-derived foods, has been successfully applied in the determination of nicarbazin residues in meat (66) and chicken tissues (412).

Online trace enrichment has also been described for the isolation/purification of nicarbazin residues from eggs (383), and salinomycin residues from chicken skin and fat (395). This technique involved trapping the analyte onto an LC preconcentration column, rinsing of coretained material to waste, and flushing of the concentrated analytes onto the analytical column. In a somewhat similar but seemingly different approach, liquid chromatographic cleanup was successfully employed in the determination of lasalocid in bovine liver (387). This involves loading of sample extract onto a normal-phase semipreparative column (Partisil 10 M9), elution with a proper mobile phase, collection of the narrow predetermined fraction of the chromatographic effluent containing this antibiotic, and reanalysis by pyrolysis gas chromatography.

Following their extraction and cleanup, anticoccidial drug residues in sample extracts can be detected after thin-layer, gas, or liquid chromatographic separation (Table 29.11).

TABLE 29.11 Physicochemical Methods for Anticoccidial and other Antiprotozoal Drugs in Edible Animal Products

Compound(s)	Matrix	Sample preparation	Steps	Stationary phase	Mobile phase	Detection/ identification	Sensitivity/ recovery		Ref.
THIN-LAYER CHROMATOGRAPHIC METHODS									
Monensin	Animal tissues	MeOH extn, liq–liq partns	14	Silica gel	CHCl$_3$/MeOH/ acetone/ glycerol	B. subtilis bioautography	5–10 ppm/ NR		14
	Chicken fat	ACN extn, liq–liq partns	10	Silica gel	CC14/benzene/ methyl cellosolve	FAB-MS	10 ppb/ NR		386
	Poultry tissues	MeOH extn, liq–liq partns	12	Silica gel LK5D	CHCl$_3$/MeOH/ acetone/ glycerol	B. subtilis bioautography	250 ppb/	93–97%	393
Salinomycin	Chicken liver	H$_2$O addn, isooctane extn, silica column cleanup	8	Silica gel GF	CHCl$_3$/MeOH/ NH$_4$OH	B. subtilis bioautography	25 ppb/	85–147%	410
	Rabbit tissues	Acetone extn, liq–liq partns	7	Silica gel G	Hexane/ether/ MeOH/ HOAc	B. stearo- thermophilus bioautography	10 ppb/	50–100%	408

(continued)

TABLE 29.11 Continued

Compound(s)	Matrix	Sample preparation	Steps	Stationary phase	Mobile phase	Detection/ identification	Sensitivity/ recovery	Ref.
Monensin, lasalocid, salinomycin	Animal tissues	MeOH extn, liq–liq partn	9	Silica gel	EtOAc/ACN	*B. subtilis* bioautography	0.45–1 ppm/ NR	394
Zoalene, nitromide, and metabolites	Chicken liver	CHCl₃/EtOAc extn, alumina column cleanup, liq–liq partn, ion-pair extn	13	Silica gel G	CHCl₃/EtOAc/ MeOH	Vis, after N-(1-naphthyl)-ethylenediamine derivatization	0.1–1 ppm/ 17–78%	257
GAS CHROMATOGRAPHIC METHODS								
Hydroxy dimetridazole	Swine muscle	K₂HPO₄/NaCl addn, EtOAc extn, liq–liq partns, SPE cleanup, esterification with HOAc/ H₂SO₄, liq–liq partns	34	Supelcoport with 3% OV-225	Argon/ methane	ECD	2 ppb/ 72–85%	402
Lasalosid	Bovine liver	ACN extn, liq–liq partns, LC purification on Partisil M9 column, derivatization with BSTFA (TMS derivative)	13	Gas-Chrom Q with 3% SE-30	Isobutane	PICI-MS	NR	387

LIQUID CHROMATOGRAPHIC METHODS

Drug	Matrix	Extraction/cleanup	No.	Column	Mobile phase	Detection	LOD/Recovery	Ref.
Dimetridazole	Bovine muscle	Na_2SO_4 addn, DCM extn, SPE cleanup, liq–liq partns	18	Novapak C_{18}, 4 μm	0.05M, pH 4.3, amm. acetate buffer/ACN (70:30)	UV 320 Nm/ PDA (240–360 nm)	5 ppb/ 78–87%	379
	Poultry tissues and eggs	DCM (muscle) or toluene (liver, egg) extn, SPE cleanup, liq–liq partn	16	Partisil 5 ODS 3, 5 μm	H_2O/ACN (50:50) contg 0.05M amm. acetate	PICI-MS-TSP	5 ppb/ 80%	407
Ethopabate	Chicken tissues	ACN extn, liq–liq partns, Florisil column cleanup	18	Zorbax ODS	0.01M KH_2PO_4/ ACN/TEA (59:40:1), pH 4.0, at 50°C	Fluorometric, ex: 306 nm, em: 350 nm	0.5 ppb/ 82–96%	388
Fumagillin	Honey	ACN/H_2O diln, filtn	2	Phenomenex IB-SIL 5 C_{18}, analytical and guard column	H_2O/ACN/ HOAc (50:50:0.15)	UV-Vis 350 nm	100 ppb	381
Halofuginone	Eggs	Na_2CO_3/Na_2SO_4 addn, EtOAc extn, Celite column cleanup	21	Waters C_{18}, 10 μm	H_2O/ACN/ 0.25M, pH 4.9, ammonium acetate buffer (60:25:15)	UV 243 nm	5 ppb/ 79–103%	384

(continued)

TABLE 29.11 Continued

Compound(s)	Matrix	Sample preparation	Steps	Stationary phase	Mobile phase	Detection/ identification	Sensitivity/ recovery	Ref.
Imidocarb	Bovine kidney	Acetone/Na$_2$CO$_3$ extn, liq–liq partns, SPE cleanup	17	Spherisorb S3W-C18, 3 μm	Solvent A: 0.01M sodium acetate–0.01M sodium trifluoroacetate/ ACN (85:15) Solvent B: 0.01M sodium acetate–0.01M sodium trifluoroacetate– 0.01M tetra- methylammonium chloride, pH 2/ ACN (90:10) Solvent A for 5 min and then solvent B for 15 min	UV 260 nm	1 ppb/ 72–83%	409

Lasalocid	Bovine liver	ACN extn, liq–liq partns	7	Two Partisil 10 PXS columns in series	Hexane/THF/MeOH (82:15:3) adjusted to alkaline pH with NH₄OH	Fluorometric, ex: 310 nm, em: 430 nm	25 ppb/ 54–88%	389
	Bovine liver	ACN extn, liq–liq partn	7	Two Partisil 10 PXS columns in series	Hexane/THF/MeOH (82:15:3) adjusted to alkaline pH with NH₄OH	Fluorometric, ex: 310 nm, em: 430 nm/ PICI-GC-MS after silylation	240 ppb/ 59–110%	390
	Bovine tissues and milk	MeOH/H₂O extn, liq–liq partns, SPE cleanup	13	Partisil 5 ODS-3 25	H₂O/MeOH/HOAc (6:94:0.1)	Vis 520 nm, postcolumn derivatization with vanillin	5–25 ppb/ 80–88%	396
	Chicken muscle and eggs	ACN extn, liq–liq partn, SPE cleanup	14	PLRP-S, 5 μm, analytical and guard column	0.01M, pH 10, disodium tetraborate/ACN (40:60)	Fluorometric, ex: 310 nm, em: 420–430 nm	2–10 ppb/ 60–88%	391
	Chicken skin	ACN extn, liq–liq partns	7	Partisil PXS 5/25	Hexane/THF/MeOH (82:15:3) adjusted to alk. pH with NH₄OH	Fluorometric, ex: 310 nm, em: 430 nm	150 ppb/ 67–113%	392

(continued)

TABLE 29.11 Continued

Compound(s)	Matrix	Sample preparation	Steps	Stationary phase	Mobile phase	Detection/ identification	Sensitivity/ recovery	Ref.
Monensin	Bovine liver	MeOH/H_2O extn, alumina column cleanup, liq–liq partns, Sephadex LH-20 column cleanup, acetylation with pyridine/acetic anhydride (1:1), liq–liq partns, precolumn derivatization with 9-anthryl-diazomethane, silica gel column cleanup	40	RP-C_8 or RP-C_{18}, 5 µm, with pellicular C_{18} guard column	Solvent A: ACN Solvent B: H_2O/ ACN (90:10) Isocratic (20:80), at 40°C	Fluorometric, ex: 365 nm, em: 418 nm	50 ppb/ 71–96%	397
	Chicken tissues	MeOH/H_2O extn, liq–liq partns, silica gel column cleanup, liq–liq partns, precolumn derivatization with 9-anthryl-diazomethane, SPE cleanup	27	µ-Porasil	DCM/MeOH (95:5)	Fluorometric, ex: 365 nm, em: 412 nm/ GC-MS after methylation	1 ppb/ 47–78%	398

Chicken tissues	MeOH/H_2O extn, liq–liq partns, SPE cleanup	13	Partisil 5 ODS-3 25	H_2O/MeOH/HOAc (6:94:0.1)	Vis 520 nm, postcolumn derivatization with vanillin	25 ppb/ 82–96%	399
Nicarbazin							
Chicken tissues	MSPD extn/ cleanup, SPE cleanup	14	Econosphere, 3 μm	H_2O/MeOH (25:75)	UV 340 nm	1–2 ppm/ 80–97%	412
Chicken tissues	EtOAc extn, liq–liq partns, cleanup on tandem alumina SPE columns	16	Phenomenex IB-SIL C_{18}, 3 μm	H_2O/MeOH (25:75)	UV 340 nm/ NICI-MS-TSP after LC conditions modification	4 ppm/ 75–98%	403
Chicken tissues	EtOAc extn, liq–liq partns, cleanup on tandem alumina SPE columns	23	C_{18}, 3 μm, column	H_2O/MeOH (25:75)	UV 340 nm/ NICI-MS-TSP after LC conditions modification	20 ppb/ 76–88%	404
Eggs	HOAc/Na_2SO_4 addn, ACN extn, SPE cleanup	14	Two ChromSpher C_{18}, 5 μm, columns in series, with pellicular RP, 30–40 μm, guard column	H_2O/0.02M, pH 4.8, acetate buffer/ACN (36:10:54)	UV-Vis 360 nm	2.5 ppb/ 88–116%	382

(continued)

TABLE 29.11 Continued

Compound(s)	Matrix	Sample preparation	Steps	Stationary phase	Mobile phase	Detection/ identification	Sensitivity/ recovery	Ref.
	Eggs	Na_2SO_4 addn, ACN extn, online trace enrichment on Chrompack reversed-phase preconcn column and switching to analytical column	9	ChromSpher C_{18}, 5 μm, with pellicular RP guard column	0.01M, pH 4.0, KH_2PO_4/ACN (50:50)	UV 343 nm	5 ppb/ 81–94%	383
	Meat	MSPD extn/ cleanup	6	Spherisorb C_{18} ODS2, 5 μm	Solvent A: 0.01 M, pH 5.2, acetate buffer Solvent B: ACN/ MeOH (70:30) Gradient from (56:44) to (36:64), at 35°C	UV 348 nm/ PDA (200– 450 nm)	1 ppb/ 52–55%	66
Salinomycin	Chicken skin and fat	MeOH extn, liq–liq partns, two SPE cleanups, pyridinium dichromate oxidation, liq–liq partns, silica gel column cleanup, on-line trace enrichment on MPLC C_{18}, 5 μm, preconcn column and switching to analytical column	30	Ultrasphere ODS, 5 μm	H_2O/THF/ACN/ H_3PO_4 (6:4:90:0.01)	UV 225 nm	100 ppb/ 95–102%	395

	Sample	Sample prep		Column	Mobile phase	Detection	Detection limit/recovery	Ref
	Chicken tissues	H$_2$O addn, isooctane extn, SPE cleanup, pyridinium dichromate oxidation, liq–liq partns, SPE cleanup	18	Ultrasphere ODS, 5 μm	H$_2$O/THF/ACN/H$_3$PO$_4$ (6:4:90:0.01)	UV 225 nm	5–20 ppb/ >90%	411
Semduramicin	Chicken liver	MeOH/NH$_4$OH extn, two SPE cleanups	18	Zorbax silica, with LC-Si, 40 μm, guard column	EtOAc/isooctane/HOAc/TEA/MeOH (65:35:0.4:0.2:0.1)	Vis 522 nm, postcolumn derivatization with vanillin	25 ppb/ 88–100%	400
Amprolium ethopabate	Chicken tissues	ACN extn, liq–liq partns, alumina column cleanup	16	L-column ODS	0.2M KH$_2$PO$_4$/ACN (85:15) contg 5mM hexanesulfonate (for amprolium), at 40°C. 0.01M, pH 5.0, phosp. buffer/ACN (79:21) (for ethopabate), at 40°C	UV 270 nm (ethopabate). Fluorometric, postcolumn derivatization with potassium ferricyanide, ex: 367 nm, em: 470 nm (amprolium)	2–4 ppb/ 86–100%	227

(continued)

TABLE 29.11 Physicochemical Methods for Anticoccidial and other Antiprotozoal Drugs in Edible Animal Products

Compound(s)	Matrix	Sample preparation	Steps	Stationary phase	Mobile phase	Detection/ identification	Sensitivity/ recovery	Ref.
Dimetridazole, hydroxy dimetridazole	Swine muscle	Na_2SO_4 addn, DCM extn, liq–liq partn, online deoxygenation and loading on Spheri-10 RP-18, 10 μm, column and switching to analytical column	15	Ultrasphere ODS, 5 μm	0.6M ammonium acetate, pH 5.0, buffer/ACN (85:15) contg 0.3% TEA	Electro-chemical	0.26 ppb/ 52–78%	380
Nitroimidazole metabolites	Swine and turkey muscle	K_2HPO_4/NaCl addn, EtOAc extn, liq–liq partn, SPE cleanup	15	Hibar RP-18, 5 μm	0.05M, pH 7–7.3, ammonium phosp. buffer/ ACN (83:17)	UV 325 nm	2 ppb/ 53–79%	405
Three nitroimidazoles and metabolites	Eggs	Saturated NaCl/HCl diln, SPE cleanup, liq–liq partn	12	LiChrosorb RP-18, 7 μm, with μBondapak C_{18}/ Corasil, 37–50 μm, guard column	0.25M K_3PO_4/ ACN/MeOH (90:4:6), pH 4.0	UV 313 nm/ PDA (225–400 nm)	5–10 ppb/ 80–98%	385

| Four polyether antibiotics | Bovine liver | 40 | MeOH/H_2O extn, alumina column cleanup, liq–liq partns, Sephadex LH-20 column cleanup, acetylation with pyridine/acetic anhydride (1:1), liq–liq partns, precolumn derivatization with 9-anthryldiazomethane, silica gel column cleanup | RP-C_8, 5 μm, with pellicular C_{18} guard column | Solvent A: ACN Solvent B: H_2O/ACN (90:10) Isocratic (20:80) for 9 min and gradient to (10:90), at 40°C | Fluorometric, ex: 365 nm, em: 418 nm | 15 ppb/ 48–99% | 401 |
| Five anticoccidials | Chicken liver | 24 | EtOAc extn, liq–liq partns, Sephadex LH-20 column cleanup, alumina column cleanup | Radial-Pak C_{18}, 5 μm | H_2O/ACN Isocratic (75:25) for 10 min and gradient to (45:55) | UV 260 nm | 50 ppb/ 57–97% | 406 |

TMS, trimethylsilane; BSTFA, N,O-Bis(trimethylsilyl)trifluoroacetamide. Other abbreviations as in Tables 29.1 and 29.3.

In thin-layer chromatography, which is mainly used for the determination of polyether antibiotics, anticoccidials are first separated on commercially available silica gel plates using various solvent mixtures as mobile phase, and subsequently detected by bioautography using *Bacillus subtilis* (14, 393, 394, 410) or *Bacillus stearothermophilus* (408) as test organisms. Visible photometric detection of benzamide anticoccidials after spraying with Bratton-Marshall reagent (257), and fast atom bombardment mass spectrometric detection of monensin (386), have also been reported. These methods, however, have limited application and are generally used for screening or qualitative analysis since they lack the performance characteristics required to detect the low ppb levels likely to occur in edible animal products.

Gas chromatographic separation has not gained wide acceptance in spite of being quite sensitive and specific. This mode of separation is complicated by the necessity for derivatization of anticoccidials before analysis. The hydroxy metabolite of dimetridazole is subjected to derivatization via esterification with acetic acid/sulfuric acid mixture (402), while lasalocid is derivatized via silylation with N,O-Bis(trimethylsilyl)trifluoroacetamide (BSTFA) (387). This derivatization step is required not only to form the volatile derivatives of these drugs but also to improve their chromatographic properties (thermal stability and decreased polarity).

Following separation on conventional gas chromatographic columns, electron-capture detector (402) has been used for the determination of the hydroxy metabolite of dimetridazole in swine muscle with good sensitivity and specificity. To confirm the presence of lasalocid residues in bovine liver, gas chromatography coupled with mass spectrometry via a chemical ionization interface (387) has been successfully applied.

At present, liquid chromatography has become the most widely used technique for determining anticoccidial drugs in edible animal products (Table 29.11). The separation of these drugs is generally done on nonpolar reversed-phase columns (octadecyl, octyl and phenyl), the preferred type being the octadecyl bonded silica. However, polar (389, 390, 392, 398, 400) columns have also been used for the determination of the polyether antibiotics in edible animal products.

As far as the type of the organic modifier is concerned, there has not been any particular reason for selecting methanol or acetonitrile in the preparation of the mobile phase. However, the concentration of the organic modifier used differs according to the polarity of the anticoccidial drugs analyzed, the applied derivatization technique, and the pH of the mobile phase. In general, when analyzing low-polarity compounds, such as polyether antibiotics, concentrations higher than 80% have been reported.

Although spectrophotometric, fluorometric, electrochemical, and mass spectrometric detectors have all been equally well used in liquid chromatographic analysis of anticoccidial drugs, the most popular is the ultraviolet photometric detector. The detection wavelength has been set at 243 nm for halofuginone, 260 nm for imidocarb and benzamides, 270 nm for ethopabate, 313–325 nm for nitroimidazoles, 350 nm for fumagillin, and 340–360 nm for nicarbazin. Polyether antibiotics do not have a specific ultraviolet chromophore and thus show an extremely weak absorption in the ultraviolet region. Therefore, postcolumn derivatization with vanillin (396, 399, 400) and detection at 520–522 nm, or precolumn derivatization with pyridinium dichromate (395, 411) and detection at 225 nm have been applied to the analysis of polyether antibiotic residues in tissues.

Fluorometric detection is generally preferred by many workers for the determination of polyether antibiotics in edible animal products because it confers the advantages of selectivity and sensitivity. The only intrinsically fluorescent polyether antibiotic is lasalocid, but this intrinsic fluorescence is highly pH-dependent. All of the liquid chromatographic-based assays that have been developed to determine the other polyether antibiotics in foods require derivatization to introduce a suitable fluorescent chromophore. The most common derivatizing reagent used is 9-anthryldiazomethane (397, 398, 401). Other anticoccidial drugs such as ethopabate (388) and amprolium (227) have also been monitored using fluorometric detection. The former exhibits inherent fluorescence, while the latter is subjected to postcolumn derivatization with potassium ferricyanide.

Electrochemical detection, in the reductive mode, has been successively applied by Carignan et al. (380) for the determination of underivatized dimetridazole residues in swine muscle. The major difficulty in this detection mode is the strong interference by oxygen, thus deoxygenation of the entire system is required.

To confirm anticoccidials in liquid chromatography-based methodologies, the photodiode array detector, which collects continuous spectral data during the analysis to check for interfering substances by comparing the spectrum of the sample with that of the standard, has been used (66, 379, 385). Although confirmation with a photodiode array detector is simple, specificity and sensitivity are not sufficient to determine or identify trace levels of residual anticoccidials in edible animal products.

Coupling of liquid chromatography with mass spectrometry provides unequivocal on-line spectrometric identification of an individual analyte at the very low residue concentrations that meet the regulatory enforcement requirements for confirmatory analysis of anticoccidial drugs in animal-derived foods. Online mass spectrometry has the advantage of being suited to analysis and identification of polar nonvolatile compounds without the necessity for derivatization procedures. Typical applications of mass spectrometry in confirming anticoccidial residues in edible animal products are through interfacing liquid chromatography with mass spectrometry via thermospray, using negative (403, 404) or positive-ion (407) detection. In liquid chromatography-based methodologies, the presence of incurred lasalocid and monensin residues in animal tissues can also be confirmed offline by analyzing the methylated (398) or silylated (390) residues by gas chromatography-mass spectrometry.

Cannavan and Kennedy (407), Tarbin and Shearer (391), Moran et al. (399), Boulaire et al. (66), and Gallicano et al. (406) described promising methods in terms of simplicity, selectivity, and sensitivity, for screening and even confirmation of anticoccidial residues in edible animal products.

Cannavan and Kennedy (407), described a confirmatory liquid chromatographic–mass spectrometric method for the determination of dimetridazole residues in poultry tissues and eggs. According to this method, 4 g homogenized sample is extracted twice with dichloromethane (muscle) or toluene (liver, eggs). After centrifugation, the extract is applied to a Bakerbond silica cartridge. Following cartridge washing with toluene (muscle extracts) or dichloromethane (liver and egg extracts) and hexane, dimetridazole is eluted with acetone and the eluate is evaporated to dryness. The residue is reconstituted in methanol/water (1:1), washed with hexane, and analyzed by liquid chromatography. Separation is performed on a 25 cm Partisil 5 ODS 3 (5 μm) analytical column, with a water/methanol (50:50) mobile phase, containing 50 mM ammonium acetate, at a flow-rate of 1 ml/min (Fig. 29.11.1). Under these conditions concentrations as low as

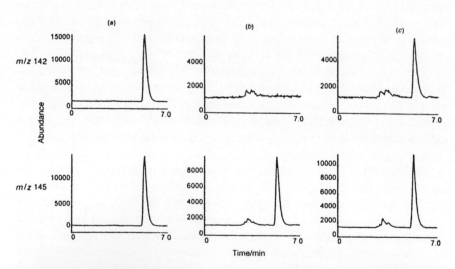

FIG. 29.11.1   SIM chromatograms of (a) a dimetridazole standard solution, (b) a blank egg extract, and (c) an incurred egg extract containing 16.1 ppb dimetridazole. Upper panel: (m/z 142) is the $[M + H]^+$ ion for dimetridazole; lower panel: (m/z 145) is the $[M + H]^+$ ion for D_3-dimetridazole. (From Ref. 407 — Reproduced by permission of The Royal Society of Chemistry.)

5 ppb could be determined in poultry tissues and eggs using thermospray mass spectrometric detection in the positive-ion chemical ionization mode.

Tarbin and Shearer (391), in another study, developed a liquid chromatographic method for the determination of lasalocid residues in chicken muscle and eggs. In the proposed method a 10 g tissue or egg sample is extracted twice with 50 ml acetonitrile. After centrifugation, saturated sodium chloride solution is added to the extract and lasalocid is partitioned into carbon tetrachloride. The extract is evaporated to dryness and the residue is reconstituted in hexane and applied to a Bond-Elut silica cartridge. Following cartridge washing with chloroform, lasalocid is eluted with chloroform/methanol (95:5) and the eluate is evaporated to dryness. The residue is reconstituted in mobile phase and analyzed by liquid chromatography onto a 25-cm PLRP-S (5 µm) analytical column protected by a guard column packed with the same packing material. Analysis is performed using a 0.01M, pH 10, disodium tetraborate/acetonitrile (40:60) mobile phase at a flow rate of 1 ml/min. Under these conditions, lasalocid concentrations as low as 2 ppb for muscle tissue and 10 ppb for eggs could be readily determined by fluorometric detection (310 nm for excitation and 420–430 nm for emission).

In another method developed by Moran et al. (399), quantitation of monensin residues in chicken tissues can be accomplished by liquid chromatography with postcolumn derivatization and photometric detection. A 20 g minced tissue is extracted with methanol/water (85:15) mixture. After centrifugation, 40 ml of 10% sodium chloride solution is added to the aqueous methanol extract and monensin is partitioned into three 25 ml portions of carbon tetrachloride. The extract is evaporated to dryness and the residue is reconstituted in chloroform and applied to a Sep-Pak silica cartridge. Following cartridge washing with chloroform and chloroform/hexane (9:1), monensin is eluted with chloroform/methanol (95:5) and the eluate is evaporated to dryness. The residue is reconstituted in mobile phase and analyzed by liquid chromatography on a 25 cm Partisil 5 ODS-3 analytical column. Using a water–methanol (94:6) mobile phase that contained 0.1% acetic acid, concentrations of monensin down to 25 ppb could be determined after postcolumn derivatization with vanillin and spectrophotometric detection (520 nm).

A specific cleanup procedure, based on matrix solid-phase dispersion, has been described by Boulaire et al. (66) for the liquid chromatographic determination of nicarbazin and 14 other drugs in meat. In this method, a 0.5 g ground tissue sample is blended in a mortar with C_{18} material and the resultant mixture is transferred to a 10 ml syringe barrel. Following syringe washing with hexane and dichloromethane, the analytes are eluted with 8 ml ethyl acetate and the eluate is evaporated to dryness. The residue is reconstituted in 0.25 ml of 0.01M, pH5.2, ammonium acetate buffer/acetonitrile/methanol (56:31:13) mixture, and analyzed by liquid chromatography. Separation is performed on a 25 cm Spherisorb C_{18} ODS II (5 μm) analytical column, with the mobile phase and the gradient elution program presented in Table 29.11, at a flow-rate of 0.5 ml/min and a column temperature of 35°C. Under these conditions concentrations down to 1 ppb could be readily determined in meat using an ultraviolet spectrometer monitored at 348 nm. Tentative confirmation of the presence of nicarbazin residues in the suspected samples can be achieved using a photodiode array detector.

A multiresidue liquid chromatographic method for simultaneously determining aklomide, dinsed, ethopabate, nitromide, and zoalene in chicken liver has been described by Gallicano et al. (406). According to this method, 10 g macerated liver is extracted with 100 ml ethyl acetate and the mixture is filtrated. The filtrate is concentrated to approximately 10 ml, washed with 7% sodium chloride solution, and dried over anhydrous sodium sulfate. The extract is evaporated to dryness, reconstituted in hexane/benzene (3:7), and applied to a Sephadex LH-20 column. Anticoccidials are eluted with methanol/benzene (1:9) and the eluate is evaporated to dryness. The residue is redissolved in hexane/dichloromethane (1:9) and applied to an alumina column. Following elution with methanol/dichloromethane (1:9), the eluate is evaporated to dryness and the residue is reconstituted in water/acetonitrile (7:3) and analyzed by liquid chromatography. Separation is performed on a Radial-Pak C_{18} (5 μm) analytical column under the chromatographic conditions presented in Table 29.11 (Fig. 29.11.2). Under these condi-

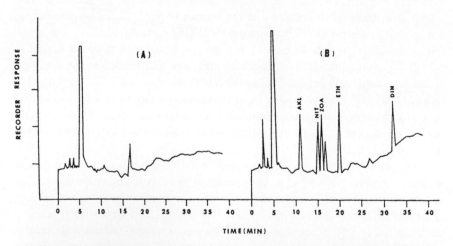

FIG. 29.11.2 Chromatograms of (A) blank liver sample and (B) blank liver fortified with 1000 ng each aklomide (AKL), nitromide (NIT), zoalene (ZOA), ethopabate (ETH), and dinsed (DIN). (Reprinted from Ref. 406. Copyright, (1988), by Assoc. Off. Anal. Chem.)

tions, concentrations as low as 50 ppb for all analytes could be determined in chicken liver using an ultraviolet spectrometer monitored at 260 nm.

29.12 ANTIMICROBIAL GROWTH PROMOTERS

Currently, the permitted antimicrobial growth promoters in the European Union are only four antibiotics (monensin, salinomycin, bambermycin, and avilamycin) and two synthetic antimicrobials (carbadox and olaquindox). In the United States, permitted antimicrobial growth promoters are several antibiotic and synthetic antimicrobial agents. The former group is composed of three aminoglycoside antibiotics (neomycin, streptomycin and bambermycin), three macrolide antibiotics (erythromycin, oleandomycin and tylosin) three polyether ionophore antibiotics (lasalocid, monensin, and salinomycin), two tetracycline antibiotics (chlortetracycline and oxytetracycline), three peptide antibiotics (avoparcin, bacitracin, and virginiamycin), and a series of miscellaneous antimicrobials including lincomycin, penicillin procaine, avilamycin, and tiamulin. Within the latter group, several compounds such as arsenical compounds, nitrofurans including furazolidone and nitrofurazone, sulfonamides including sulfamethazine, sulfathiazole, and sulfaquinoxaline, and quinoxaline-1,4-dioxides are included.

Since many of the above-mentioned compounds possess major anti-infectious activity in addition to their role as growth promoters, the methods of their determination in edible animal products have already been discussed in other sections of this chapter. Hence, this section concentrates on the remaining compounds within this group, namely the organic arsenicals, peptide antibiotics, quinoxaline-1,4-dioxides, and miscellaneous substances.

Quinoxaline-1,4-dioxides are synthetic antimicrobial agents; the best-known members are carbadox and olaquindox. Both compounds are rapidly metabolized to monoxy- and desoxy- compounds. The final product from carbadox and the one most often determined, mainly in liver (target tissue), is quinoxaline-2-carboxylic acid. Carbadox and olaquindox are light-sensitive compounds and sample manipulations should be performed only under the minimum of indirect incandescent illumination. Carbadox and desoxycarbadox are insoluble in water but are soluble in chloroform and methanol, while olaquindox is slightly soluble in water and some organic solvents. The solubility, however, of quinoxaline-2-carboxylic acid can be easily monitored by adjusting the pH because it is a strong carboxylic acid (pK$_a$ 2.88).

Carbadox, olaquindox, and their monoxy- and desoxy- metabolites are amenable to extraction from tissues and eggs with polar organic solvents. Sample extraction/deproteinization is usually accomplished with ethanol (413), acetonitrile (414, 415), and acetonitrile/methanol (416–418). To reduce interferences and concentrate the analyte(s), the primary sample extract is further subjected to various types of sample cleanup procedures such as conventional liquid–liquid partitioning, solid-phase extraction, and online trace enrichment (Table 29.12).

Liquid–liquid partitioning of sample extracts with isooctane (416) or hexane (413, 414) to remove lipids has been reported. Removing lipids and other matrix constituents can also be accomplished with solid-phase extraction columns. Cleanup and concentration of carbadox and olaquindox residues from coextracted substances have been accomplished with polar sorbents such as alumina (413–415), or alumina/Florisil (416–418), since they provide high recovery of the analytes. However, in many cases, cleanup on these polar materials seems to be not effective in removing interfering substances from the sample extract. Therefore, online trace enrichment has been reported to be a more powerful approach for the isolation and/or cleanup of these compounds. This involves purification by trapping the analytes onto a liquid chromatographic preconcentration column (Bondapak C_{18}/Corasil, Sep-Pak C_{18}, or Serdolit AD-4), rinsing coextracted materials to waste, and then flushing the concentrated analytes onto the analytical column (416–418).

Following extraction/cleanup, carbadox and olaquindox residues can be detected photometrically after liquid chromatographic separation. The separation of these drugs is generally done on nonpolar reversed-phase columns (octadecyl, octyl or polymeric), the preferred type being the octadecyl bonded silica. Following separation, carbadox and olaquindox residues have to be detected using a spectrophotometer monitored at wavelengths ranging from 335 to 374 nm. However, to increase selectivity in carbadox determination, postcolumn derivatization with sodium hydroxide solution and photometric detection at 420 nm (416) or 390 nm (417) has been reported.

A promising liquid chromatographic method in terms of simplicity, selectivity, and sensitivity has been described by Binnendijk et al. (417) for the determination of carbadox and some of its metabolites in swine tissues and eggs. According to this method, 10 g homogenized sample is extracted with 40 ml acetonitrile/ methanol (1 : 1). After centrifugation the supernatant is applied on an alumina/ Florisil column, and an aliquot of the eluate is concentrated under nitrogen to a volume of 0.9–1.1 ml to be further diluted to 4.0 ml with water. The resulting solution is partitioned with 2 ml isooctane and centrifuged. An aliquot (1 ml) of the separated aqueous layer is injected into the liquid chromatographic system and the analytes are trapped at the beginning of a 55–105 μm Sep-Pak C_{18} preconcentration column. Using an automated column-switching system, the trapped analytes are back-flashed into the analytical column (ChromSpher C_{18}, 5 μm) and analyzed using a 0.01M, pH 6, acetate buffer/acetonitrile (86 : 14) mobile phase. Analytes are detected at 390 nm after postcolumn derivatization with sodium hydroxide. Under these conditions concentrations down to 0.5–2 ppb could be readily determined in swine tissues and eggs.

TABLE 29.12 Physicochemical Methods for Antimicrobial Growth Promoters in Edible Animal Products

Compound(s)	Matrix	Sample preparation	Steps	Stationary phase	Mobile phase	Detection/ identification	Sensitivity/ recovery	Ref.
GAS CHROMATOGRAPHIC METHODS								
Avilamycin	Swine tissues	Alk hydrolysis, liq–liq partns, silica gel column cleanup, methylester derivative	22	Gas-Chrom Q with 3% silar 10C	Helium	ECD	100 ppb/ 70–95%	426
Quinoxaline-2-carboxylic acid (carbadox metabolite)	Swine liver	Alk hydrolysis, HCl addn (pH < 1), EtOAc extn, liq–liq partns, AG MP-50 column cleanup, liq–liq partns, methylester derivative, liq–liq partn	24	Gas-Chrom Q with 3% silar 10C	Helium	EI-MS	30 ppb/ 82 ± 6.7%	419
	Swine liver	Alk hydrolysis, HCl addn (pH < 1), EtOAc extn, liq–liq partns, AG MP-50 column cleanup, liq–liq partns, methylester derivative, TLC purification, EtOAc extn	29	DB-5, 19 m, capillary	Helium	IT-MS	3 ppb/ NR	420

(continued)

TABLE 29.12 Continued

Compound(s)	Matrix	Sample preparation	Steps	Stationary phase	Mobile phase	Detection/ identification	Sensitivity/ recovery	Ref.
	Swine tissues	Alk hydrolysis, liq–liq partns, HCl addn (pH < 1), EtOAc extn, 2nd alk hydrolysis, liq–liq partns, ethylester derivative, liq–liq partn	23	WCOT, 25 m, capillary coated with CP-Sil 5CB	Helium	SIM-MS	2 ppb/ NR	421
	Swine tissues	Alk3 hydrolysis, HCl addn (pH < 1), DCM extn, liq–liq partns, silica gel column cleanup, liq–liq partns, methylester derivative, liq–liq partn, silica gel column cleanup	29	Chromosorb W HP with 3.5% DEGS	Nitrogen	ECD	10 ppb/ 62–81%	422
	Swine tissues	Enzymatic digestion with subtilisin A, liq–liq partns, HCl addn (pH < 1), EtOAc extn, propylester derivative, LC purification on Hypersil-ODS, 3 μm, column, liq–liq partns	27	SE52, 25 m, capillary	Helium	SIM-MS	2 ppb/ NR	423

LIQUID CHROMATOGRAPHIC METHODS

Analyte	Matrix	Sample preparation		Column	Mobile phase	Detection	LOD/Recovery	Ref.
Carbadox, desoxycarbadox	Swine tissues	EtOH extn, metaphosphoric acid addn, liq–liq partns, alumina column cleanup	20	Brownlee RP-10A, C_6, 10 μm, with RP-GU MPLC, C_8, 10 μm guard column	0.01M amm. acetate/ACN/EtOH (70:25:5)	UV-Vis 350 nm	2 ppb/ 39–98%	413
Carbadox and metabolites	Swine tissues	ACN/MeOH extn, alumina/Florisil column cleanup, liq–liq partn, on-line trace enrichment on Bondapak C_{18}/Corasil, 37–50 μm, preconcn column and switching to analytical column	8	ChromSpher C_{18}, 5 μm, with Bondapak C_{18}/Corasil, 37–50 μm, guard column	0.01M, pH 6, acetate buffer/ACN (85:15)	Vis 420 nm, postcolumn derivatization with NaOH	1–5 ppb/ 81–87%	416
	Swine tissues, eggs	ACN/MeOH extn, alumina/Florisil column cleanup, liq–liq partn, on-line trace enrichment on Sep-Pak C_{18}, 55–105 μm, preconcn column and switching to analytical column	8	ChromSpher C_{18}, 5 μm	0.01M, pH 6, acetate buffer/ACN (86:14)	Vis 390 nm, postcolumn derivastization with NaOH	0.5–2 ppb/ 70–95%	417

(continued)

TABLE 29.12 Continued

Compound(s)	Matrix	Sample preparation	Steps	Stationary phase	Mobile phase	Detection/ identification	Sensitivity/ recovery	Ref.
Olaquindox	Swine muscle	ACN extn, alumina column cleanup	10	ChromSpher C$_{18}$, 5 μm, with Pellicular C$_{18}$, guard column	H$_2$O/ACN (90:10)	UV-Vis 374 nm	NR/ 54–79%	415
	Swine tissues	ACN extn, alumina column cleanup, liq–liq partn	11	Nucleosil C$_{18}$, 5 μm, with Nucleosil C$_{18}$, 10 μm, guard column	H$_2$O/ACN (95:5), at 30°C	UV-Vis 350 nm	20 ppb/ 54–86%	414
Olaquindox and metabolites	Eggs	ACN/MeOH extn, alumina/Florisil column cleanup, on-line trace enrichment on Serdolit AD-4 preconcn column and switching to analytical column	6	C-8 DB column	NR	UV-Vis 372 nm for olaquindox and UV 335 nm for the metabolites	1–3 ppb/ NR	418
Roxarsone	Swine tissues	EtOH/HOAc microwave extn	6	PRP-1, 10 μm, with 2 μm guard column	H$_2$O/isopropyl alcohol/TFA (94:6:0.1), at 30°C	Vis 410 nm, postcolumn derivatization with NaOH	250 ppb/ 75–82%	425

| Virginiamycin | Meat | MSPD extn/ cleanup | 6 | Spherisorb C$_{18}$ ODS2, 5 μm | Solvent A: 0.01M, pH 5.2, acetate buffer Solvent B: ACN/ MeOH (70:30) Gradient from (56:44) to (36:64), at 35°C | UV 254 nm/ PDA (200– 450 nm) | 2.5–7.5 ppb/ 78 ± 7.7% | 66 |
| | Swine tissues | 0.2M NH$_4$H$_2$PO$_4$ addn, MeOH extn, liq–liq partns | 7 | Supelcosil LC-18-DB, 5 μm, analytical and guard column | 0.01M NH$_4$H$_2$PO$_4$/ ACN Isocratic (80:20) for 2 min and gradient to (20:80) | UV 254 nm | 10 ppb/ 84–94% | 424 |

IT, ion trap.
Other abbreviations as in Tables 29.1 and 29.3.

Carbadox-related residues can also be monitored by conversion to quinoxaline-2-carboxylic acid. This conversion as well as its liberation are accomplished by alkaline hydrolysis of tissue, followed by isolation of the analyte from indigenous hydrolysis products through extraction and cleanup procedures (419–422). Enzymatic digestion of swine tissues with subtilisin A, which liberates quinoxaline-2-carboxylic acid from macromolecules, has also been reported (423).

After hydrolyzate acidification with hydrochloric acid at pH values lower than 1, quinoxaline-2-carboxylic acid is quantitatively extracted into ethyl acetate, chloroform, or dichloromethane, since at these strongly acidic conditions the ionization of their carboxylate moiety is suppressed (pK$_a$ 2.88), and then back-extracted into aqueous buffered solutions at pH 6.0 or higher. These liquid–liquid partitioning procedures isolate quinoxaline-2-carboxylic acid from a complex mixture of tissue hydrolysates, and provide an aqueous extract suitable for further purification by solid-phase extraction. This has been accomplished either with the strong cation-exchange resin AG MP-50 (419, 420) or with a polar silica column (422).

Following extraction/cleanup, quinoxaline-2-carboxylic acid can be detected by electron capture, or mass spectrometric techniques, after gas chromatographic separation on capillary or conventional columns. A prerequisite of quinoxaline-2-carboxylic acid analysis by gas chromatography is the derivatization of the molecule by means of esterification. Esterification has been accomplished with methanol (419, 420, 422), ethanol (421), or propanol (423) under sulfuric acid catalysis. Further purification of the alkyl ester derivative with solid-phase extraction on a silica gel column (422), thin-layer chromatography on silica gel plate (420), or liquid chromatography on Hypersil-ODS, 3 μm, column (423), has been reported.

Lynch et al. (420) have proposed a promising gas chromatographic–mass spectrometric method for the determination and even confirmation of quinoxaline-2-carboxylic acid in swine liver. In this method, 5 g liver is homogenized with 10 ml 3M sodium hydroxide and hydrolized by incubation at 95–100°C for 30 min. Following acidification of the hydrolysate with hydrochloric acid at pH < 1, quinoxaline-2-carboxylic acid is extracted three times with ethyl acetate and then back-extracted twice into 0.5M pH 6 citrate buffer. After hydrochloric acid addition, the aqueous extract is further purified using a cation exchange column (AGMP-50 resin). Following column washing with 1 N hydrochloric acid, elution of the analyte is effected with 10% methanol, and the eluate is acidified with hydrochloric acid to be further extracted twice with chloroform. The organic layer is evaporated to dryness and the residue is esterified using freshly prepared methanol-sulfuric acid. Following derivatization, quinoxaline-2-carboxylic acid methyl ester is partitioned into benzene to be further purified by thin-layer chromatography. After development the plate is scraped out at the position of the methyl ester, the sorbent is extracted with ethyl acetate, and the extract is analyzed on a DB-5 fused-silica capillary column with helium as the carrier gas. Using ion-trap mass-spectrometric detection, quinoxaline-2-carboxylic acid could be readily determined in swine liver at concentrations as low as 3 ppb.

Peptide antibiotics are large peptide molecules containing amino acids, which are covalently linked to other chemical entities, and consist of more than one component. They often contain D forms of amino acids, in contrast to naturally occurring proteins, which are built up from L-amino acids only. Avoparcin, bacitracin, efrotomycin, enramycin, thiopeptin, and virginiamycin are important members of this group. Very few reports have been published concerning the residue analysis of peptide antibiotics. In particular, no physicochemical method for residual bacitracin and avoparcin has been reported, while the existing methods concern the determination of virginiamycin in animal tissues.

Virginiamycin is a mixture of two components designated M_1 and S_1, which are both cyclic polypeptides. It is soluble in methanol, ethanol, acetic acid, ethyl acetate, acetone, chloroform, and benzene but is practically insoluble in water and dilute acid. It also dissolves in alkalis but is rapidly deactivated.

Moats and Leskinen (424) and Boulaire et al (66) have reported liquid chromatographic methods for determining residual virginiamycin in animal tissues. The former method was developed for detecting the M_1 factor in swine tissues. The sample (5 g) is blended with 15 ml 0.2M ammonium dihydrogen phosphate, mixed with an equal volume of methanol, and filtered. Following filtrate washing with petroleum ether, virginiamycin is partitioned into dichloromethane/petroleum ether (3:2). Water and acetonitrile are added, and the mixture is evaporated to 1–2 ml and taken up in water/acetonitrile (8:2) to be further analyzed by liquid chromatography. Separation is performed on a 15 cm Supelcosil LC-18-DB (5 μm) analytical column, protected with a guard column of the same sorbent, using the mobile phase and the gradient elution program presented in Table 29.12, at a flow rate of 1 ml/min. Under these conditions, concentrations down to 10 ppb could be readily determined in swine tissues using an ultraviolet spectrometer monitored at 254 nm.

A specific cleanup procedure, based on matrix solid-phase dispersion, has been described by Boulaire et al. (66) for the liquid chromatographic determination of virginiamycin and 14 other drugs in meat. In this method, a 0.5 g ground tissue sample is blended in a mortar with C_{18} material and the resultant mixture is transferred to a 10 ml syringe barrel. Following syringe washing with hexane and dichloromethane, the analytes are eluted with 8 ml ethyl acetate and the eluate is evaporated to dryness. The residue is reconstituted in 0.25 ml of 0.01M, pH5.2, ammonium acetate buffer–acetonitrile–methanol (56:31:13) mixture and analyzed by liquid chromatography. Separation is performed on a 25 cm Spherisorb C_{18} ODS II (5 μm) analytical column, with the mobile phase and the gradient elution program presented in Table 29.12, at a flow rate of 0.5 ml/min and a column temperature of 35°C. Under these conditions, concentrations ranging from

2.5 to 7.5 ppb could be readily determined in meat using an ultraviolet spectrometer monitored at 254 nm. Tentative confirmation of the presence of virginiamycin residues in the suspected samples can be achieved using a photodiode array detector.

Roxarsone and avilamycin are antimicrobial growth promoters for which methodology for tissue analysis is scarce. According to the liquid chromatographic method developed by Croteau et al. (425) for the determination of roxarsone, an organic arsenical, in swine tissues, a 1 g tissue sample is mixed with 25 ml ethanol and 0.5 ml acetic acid and extracted by microwave-assisted process. Following centrifugation the supernatant is evaporated to dryness and the residue is reconstituted in mobile phase to be further analyzed by liquid chromatography. Separation is performed on a 25 cm PRP-1 (10 μm) analytical column, protected with a guard column of the same sorbent, using a water/isopropyl alcohol/trifluoroacetic acid (94:6:0.1) mobile phase, at a flow-rate of 1 ml/min and a column temperature of 30°C (Fig. 29.12). Under these conditions concentrations down

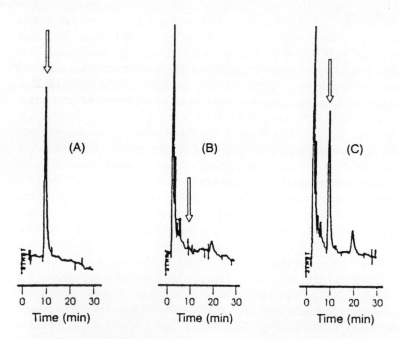

FIG. 29.12   Chromatograms of (A) roxarsone standard solution, (B) blank liver sample, and (C) spiked liver sample at a concentration of 4 ppm. (From Ref. 425.).

to 250 ppb could be readily determined in swine tissues after postcolumn derivatization with sodium hydroxide and detection at 410 nm.

Determination of avilamycin in swine tissues has been monitored using gas chromatography (426). In the proposed method avilamycin and its metabolites are converted by alkaline hydrolysis to dichloroisoeverninic acid. Following partition into chlorinated solvents and cleanup on a silica column, the derivative is methylated and determined at levels down to 100 ppb by gas chromatography using an electron-capture detector.

29.13 ANABOLIC HORMONAL-TYPE GROWTH PROMOTERS

In the field of residue analysis for illegal growth-promoting agents, the compounds used are frequently exogenous. In these cases, since there are no tolerance levels, only unambiguous identification is necessary. However, in such instances as forensic analyses for estradiol and testosterone, which are endogenous compounds also used for growth promotion, quantification is also necessary in addition to identification. These different objectives of an analysis impose different demands on the techniques and procedures used.

Liquid samples such as urine, plasma, bile, or milk are normally incubated in the presence of β-glucuronidase/sulfatase at 37°C for 2 h to deconjugate glucuronide and sulfate conjugates of the analytes (427–430). The most common preparation for this purpose is the juice of the snail *Helix pomatia*, which has sulfatase and glucuronidase activity. In some instances, dilution of urine with water (431), or dilution of plasma with phosphate buffer and centrifugation (432), may constitute the only pretreatment procedure applied.

Semisolid samples such as muscle and liver tissues can be homogenized by blending with water or an appropriate aqueous solution such as a buffer in a mechanical or an ultrasonic device to expose the residue to the extraction solvent. Fatty tissue samples are sometimes subjected to heating at 40 or 60°C until fat becomes liquid, prior to extraction of the analytes with hexane (433) or acetonitrile (434), respectively. An alternative pretreatment approach is the enzymatic digestion of the tissue by means of proteolytic enzymes such as subtilisin A (429, 435–437).

Anabolics in meat are present in the free unconjugated form, and therefore meat samples may not require the incubation step with β-glucuronidase/sulfatase necessary for urine samples (438). The necessity of an enzymatic hydrolysis to cleave steroid glucuronides or sulfates, which is required by several reference methods (439), has been questioned by several authors, especially for the analysis of anabolic androgens, estrogens, and progestogens in muscle and fatty tissues (440, 441). The proportion of cleavable conjugated testosterone in muscle tissue was reported to be in the range 0–17% (442), that of conjugated estrogens in the range 3–5% (443), and that of conjugated progesterone less than 5% (444). However, glucuronidase digestion has shown an eightfold increase in detection of incurred zeranol residues in bovine liver (427).

If hydrolysis of conjugates of the analytes is required, the homogenate as well as the digestive are then neutralized, spiked with β-glucuronidase/sulfatase solution, and subsequently kept overnight at 37°C to enable enzymatic cleavage of conjugates (429, 435, 445–447). When extraction of the analytes is to be carried out by supercritical fluid extraction, homogenization of the tissue samples into a smooth paste that is then submitted to freeze drying is the recommended procedure (213, 448). Because anabolic steroids are frequently injected into the animal in the form of esters, an incubation under alkaline conditions can also be applied (449).

Following sample pretreatment, extraction of the analytes from the sample matrix is usually accomplished with aqueous acetone (427), diethyl ether (435–437), acetonitrile (445), basified acetonitrile (430), or tert.-butyl methyl ether (449). Samples that have not been previously submitted to a particular treatment can also be directly partitioned with organic solvents to allow extraction of the anabolic residues from the matrix. Organic solvents most commonly used for this purpose include aqueous acetone (450), tetrahydrofuran (451), methanol (447, 452, 453), tert.-butyl methyl ether (438), acetonitrile (434), and chloroform–methanol (454).

The primary sample extract is subsequently subjected to cleanup using several different approaches including conventional liquid–liquid partitioning, solid-phase extraction, liquid chromatography, immunoaffinity chromatography, and supercritical fluid extraction cleanup. In some instances, more than one of these purification procedures can be applied in combination for better results.

Liquid–liquid partitioning cleanup is sometimes directed solely to the removal of fat from the sample extract. This has been accomplished through use of either hexane for the removal of fat from acetonitrile (451, 434) or aqueous methanol sample extracts (452), or isooctane from acetonitrile sample extracts (454). When hexane was used for the initial extraction of 30 anabolics from fatty tissue samples, partitioning against methanol-acetate buffer, pH 5.2 proved to be an efficient procedure for fat removal because the analytes were preferentially partitioned into the aqueous buffer layer (433); further extract purification could be readily accomplished by back extraction of the analytes into dichloromethane.

A three-phase liquid–liquid partitioning consisting of hexane, acetonitrile, and dichloromethane has also proven to be a preferred cleanup method for diethylstilbestrol and zeranol (455), trenbolone and epitrenbolone (445), trenbolone and nortestosterone (446), and melengestrol residues (456) in tissues. Following adjustment of the initial aqueous acetonitrile sample extract at pH 13, most of the polar and ionic acidic matrix components were directed into the aqueous layer during the partitioning process, while the low-polarity components were extracted into the upper hexane layer. Compounds such as the analytes that exhibit intermediate polarity were partitioned solely into the middle acetonitrile layer.

An alternative cleanup procedure is the partition of the raw extract, which often contains considerable amounts of lipid material, between an organic and an aqueous sodium hydroxide phase. With this partitioning scheme, the analytes are further fractionated into estrogens and nonestrogens. The presence of phenolic groups in the molecules of estrogens such as diethylstilbestrol and zeranol ensures their complete extraction from organic phases such as chloroform or tert.-butyl methyl ether into the aqueous sodium hydroxide phase (435, 438, 447). Further purification could be accomplished by neutralization of the sodium hydroxide solution and back-extraction of the contained diethylstilbestrol into diethyl ether (435), or adjustment of the pH of the sodium hydroxide solution to 10.6–10.8 and back-extraction of the contained zeranol into a chloroform phase (447).

Liquid–liquid partitioning cleanup on a hydrophilic matrix can also be employed for purification of the primary sample extract. This procedure was only applied in the determination of zearalenone and its metabolites in milk using a Chem Elut disposable column to partition an acidified aqueous milk extract into dichloromethane (430).

In earlier times, the method of choice for a more or less thorough purification of the crude extract was column chromatography. The sample extract was applied to the top of a glass column filled with an adsorptive material such as alumina and Celite (457). An organic solvent or a mixture of solvents was allowed to migrate through the adsorbent bed, during which an efficient separation of the analytes and the bulk of interferences was supposed to take place. Successful application of this technique has been described in the determination of seven steroid hormones in meat using a glass column filled with silica gel 60 (451).

Disposable solid-phase extraction columns allow a simple, fairly inexpensive, and easy-to-perform purification of the crude extract. The use of solid-phase extraction columns is part of most, if not all, modern analytical procedures for steroids at residue levels. Both normal-phase columns based on silica (431, 445, 453), alumina (427, 450), cyano (434), or amino (430) materials and reversed-phase columns based on C_{18} (431, 433, 437, 438, 445) or C_8 (452) sorbents have been described in analytical applications.

Cleanup on C_{18} solid-phase extraction cartridges or on Amberlite XAD-2 resin is particularly suitable for steroids with hydrophobic and neutral character. However, use of the C_{18} sorbent has led to low recovery for stanozolol (428). The presence of the pyrazole nucleus condensed to the androstane ring confers its ionizing properties on stanozolol. Stanozolol has two ionizable hydrogen atoms and therefore hydrogen binding may occur between labile hydrogens of stanozolol and the active sites of the column or glassware. Thus, efficient purification can be achieved on a solid-phase extraction cartridge that contains a mixed sorbent having both C_8 and benzene sulfonic acid functionality.

In some instances, combinations of C_{18} and silica columns are also used for better purification of the crude extracts (431, 445). A combination of C_8, silica, and amino solid-phase extraction columns has been successfully employed to fractionate anabolic and catabolic steroid hormone residues from meat in polar and nonpolar neutral and phenolic compounds, and to purify further each fraction effectively (452). Another combination of two solid-phase extraction columns, one using a graphitized carbon black sorbent and the other Amberlite resin in the hydroxyl form, allowed neutral anabolics to be isolated and separated from acidic anabolics and their metabolites (453). A combination of basic alumina column placed in tandem with an ion-exchange column has also been applied for the purification of the crude extracts in the determination of diethylstilbestrol and zeranol (427), and estradiol and zeranol in tissues (450).

Solid-phase extraction columns offer a rough cleanup of the crude extract, which might nevertheless not be sufficient for some detection systems such as mass spectrometry. Some authors have proposed a combination of solid-phase extraction and liquid chromatography columns for extract cleanup (440). Other methods appeal to liquid chromatography on C_{18} columns with automated fraction collection. Fractions containing the analyte of interest were evaporated to dryness, yielding a residue that in most cases was suitable for gas chromatographic detection after suitable derivatization (445, 437).

Column-switching techniques that offer an attractive route for increasing the resolving power of liquid chromatographic systems have also been described. In practice, this is the online and higher performance analogue of conventional offline cleanup, which typically employs a sequence of low-resolution chromatographic steps. Liquid chromatographic systems are readily assembled, although some care is necessary in the selection of compatible chromatographic modes to ensure refocusing of analyte peaks transferred between columns. In a pertinent application (446), a cattle liver extract was injected onto a gel permeation liquid chromatographic column, and the two fractions containing the steroids were diverted onto individual trace-enrichment silica columns, where the hormone residues were retained. The trapped trenbolone and nortestosterone residues were sequentially eluted onto a cyano column to be then driven through a second column-switching stage to a silica liquid chromatographic analytical column. Another example is offered by melengestrol acetate, which is a neutral, lipophilic steroid that is difficult to isolate by manual sample cleanup techniques such as solid-phase extraction (445). Since the selectivity and resolution afforded by solid-phase extraction were not sufficient to isolate this analyte from complex bovine tissue extracts, isolation of melengestrol acetate from the tissue matrix was performed by utilizing a phenyl liquid chromatographic column for the primary cleanup step instead of solid-phase extraction (456). Coupling a silica analytical column to the primary cleanup column through a silica trace-enrichment column allowed online screening, and sample purification suitable for subsequent GC-MS analysis.

For most of the analytes, cleanup by immunoaffinity chromatography is another elegant approach. Several laboratories have prepared their own immunoaffinity chromatography materials. For multiresidue methods, appropriate immunoaffinity chromatography materials can be combined. This approach is limited, however, to a small number of steroid hormones. Cleanup by immunoaffinity chromatography has been described in the analysis of diethylstilbestrol, dienestrol, and hexestrol in biological samples (432); nortestosterone, testosterone, and trenbolone in meat and urine samples (458); and nortestosterone in meat (436). In addition, online immunoaffinity chromatography cleanup has been reported in the analysis of nortestosterone and its epimetabolite in biological samples (429).

Supercritical fluid extraction, the relatively new analytical isolation technique, also offers some desirable advantages including processing at low temperature, recovery of a solvent-free extract, and rapid extraction. However, very limited studies have been published on the use of supercritical fluids for the isolation of anabolic agents from biological samples. A combination of supercritical fluid extraction and supercritical fluid chromatography has been employed for the detection of diethylstilbestrol, dienestrol, and hexestrol residues in pig kidney (213). During extraction with supercritical CO_2, the drugs were retained by the column while nonpolar endogenous material was not retained and thus passed to waste. Subsequent changes to the mobile phase composition eluted the drugs, which were then detected by tandem mass spectrometry.

The feasibility of supercritical fluid extraction to isolate seven growth-promoting anabolics directly from bovine tissues with CO_2 has also been investigated recently (448). It was shown that the recoveries of the polar drugs including dexamethasone, triamcinolone acetonide, and zeranol were poor, varying from 44% to 58%, while those of the nonpolar drugs including melengestrol acetate, medroxyprogesterone, and diethystilbestrol, were quite good, varying from 83 to 91%. Trenbolone could not be measured at all, due to interference from coeluting compounds. Fat and fat-related compounds coeluted and interfered with the interpretation of the liquid chromatographic peaks, especially in the case of the liver samples. Therefore, one should not expect supercritical fluid extraction to replace all other forms of sample preparation steps. Some sample cleanup may still have to be done after or before supercritical fluid extraction.

Following extraction and cleanup, anabolic compounds can be separated by thin-layer, liquid, or gas chromatographic methods. Thin-layer and gas chromatography are the principal separation techniques prior to the end-point measurement. Because most molecules are stable and volatile enough after appropriate derivatization, liquid chromatography has not been able to keep pace with gas chromatography techniques.

Thin-layer chromatographic methods are rapid, inexpensive, and suitable for screening residues prior to their analysis with other instrumental methods. Several multiresidue thin-layer analyses of estrogenic growth promoters have been reported (433, 457, 459–462). In an attempt to improve sensitivity of thin-layer chromatographic analysis and selectivity of visualizing agents for detection of estrogenic anabolic hormones, several dyes were screened for their chromogenic interactions with estrone, estradiol, diethylstilbestrol, zeranol, zearalanone, zearalenone, and zearalenol (427, 450). Diazonium dyes form diazo complexes with the phenolic and resorcyclic groups of these estrogens to give chromatograms of varying color intensity. Fast Corinth V and Fast Blue BB were identified as the salts giving the strongest color intensity.

In liquid chromatography, reversed-phase materials such as C_{18} and C_8 are the most commonly used sorbents (429, 430, 434, 438, 446, 447, 453, 454). Examples of baseline separations with reversed-phase columns of several groups of anabolics including stilbenes, resorcyclic acid lactones, and other, frequently used anabolics have been reported (463–466). In addition to reversed-phase separations normal-phase separations of anabolics using either Hypersil (467) and Brownlee (456) silica or diol-modified silica have been reported. Although not all analytes were completely separated, the latter column could be efficiently used to differentiate between estrogenic and androgenic compounds within a mixture of 15 anabolics and their metabolites (468).

Detection in liquid chromatography is often performed in the ultraviolet region. Although almost all anabolic compounds except testosterone and derivatives show absorption at 200 nm, this wavelength is less suitable for detection because of the increased sensitivity of other matrix components at this wavelength. Most of the anabolic compounds can be monitored with great sensitivity at 240 nm. If a sensitive ultraviolet detector is used, the androgens and gestagens can be detected at the 1 ppb level. Diethylstilbestrol has a submaximum at 240 nm, whereas the other stilbenes including dienestrol and hexestrol have submaxima at 230 and 225 nm, respectively. Completely different absorption spectra are observed for zeranol and trenbolone-like compounds. Zeranol shows three absorption maxima at 235, 275, and 315 nm with decreasing intensity, whereas trenbolone and derivatives show their maximum absorption at 350 nm and almost no absorption in the 200–300 nm region. Estrogenic compounds including 17β-estradiol and ethinylestradiol show their absorption maxima at 280 nm, but with a very low intensity.

The applications of liquid chromatography with online ultraviolet detection depend strongly on the matrix of analysis. For the detection of anabolic compounds at injection sites where relatively high concentrations of the parent compounds are usually present, liquid chromatography with diode array detection is very suitable with respect both to matrix interference and the sensitivity. However, in urine samples liquid chromatographic applications are limited due to the complex sample matrix. Poor sensitivity and interference from coextractives may appear at these low detection wavelengths unless sample extracts are extensively cleaned up and concentrated. This problem may be overcome by fluorescence detection, as in the case of 17α-methyltestosterone and metabolites in trout muscle (454), zearalenone and zearalenol in milk (430), and nine steroids in tissues (453). Voltammetric detection following LC of several growth-promoting hormones including zeranol and zearalenone has also been reported (469). Electrochemical detection is another selective technique that has been successfully applied in the analysis of zeranol, zearalenone, and their metabolites in tissues (447) and nine steroid hormones in tissues (453).

The number of detectors that are sensitive and selective enough to be applied online with LC is limited because the solvents used are not compatible, as in the case of immunochemical detection after reversed- or normal-phase LC. The technology of coupling is still under development and not yet available in a large number of laboratories not specialized in techniques such as LC-MS. Therefore, LC separations are frequently followed by offline detection. Confirmatory analysis of suspected liquid chromatographic peaks can be made possible by coupling liquid chromatography with mass spectrometry. Atmospheric-pressure chemical ionization LC-MS has been employed for the identification of six steroid hormones in bovine tissues (448).

Within residue analysis of steroids, immunochemical and mass spectrometric techniques are widely used, the latter most frequently in combination with GC. The principal advantage of gas chromatography is the ease with which detection can be carried out by electron impact mass spectrometry either by full scanning or by selected-ion monitoring. Because of the sensitivity and structure information that can be obtained with gas chromatography–mass spectrometry, this is also the method of choice for confirmation purposes. Most gas chromatographic methods seek a compromise between the length of sample preparation and the required specificity of analyte detection. Specificity in the analysis of the analytes that usually occur at sub-ppb levels can be achieved by either a lengthy sample preparation and cleanup to eliminate potential interference or by using a lower-quality cleanup but a more specific detector. As a direct consequence of the latter approach, increased mass spectrometry specificity is pursued by the use of chemical ionization mass spectrometry, both positive and negative, and by sophisticated mass spectrometers, which, unfortunately, are not available to most routine laboratories.

Because the choice of a particular derivative is a compromise between good mass spectrometric characteristics and good chromatographic characteristics such as volatility, stability, and absence of interference, heptafluorobutyryl derivatives have been preferred to trimethylsilyl ethers because of their higher mass gain, which made interference less likely to occur, and their favorable fragmentation pattern (428, 435, 436). Moreover, the former were more easily formed, although they lacked the stability of the trimethylsilyl derivatives (431).

Multiresidue methods that present attractive performance characteristics in the analysis of anabolic hormonal-type growth promoters in meat are those reported by Lagana and Marino (453), and Hartmann and Steinhart (452).

Lagana and Marino (453) described a liquid chromatographic method for the determination of trenbolone, testosterone, progesterone, estradiol, diethylstilbestrol, taleranol, zearalenol, zearalenone, and zeranol residues in chicken muscle and ox muscle and liver. According to this method, a 1 g sample is homogenized with 5 ml methanol and centrifuged. The extraction process is repeated with the remaining pellet, and the supernatants are pooled and diluted with water at a ratio of 85 : 15. The mixture is allowed to percolate through a Carbopack B column and the eluate is collected in test tube I. The column is then washed with methanol–water (85 : 15) and the eluate is collected in the same test tube I. Following column washing with methanol, all the analytes except diethylstilbestrol, which was already eluted in test tube I, are eluted with dichloromethane–methanol (70 : 30), and the eluate is collected in test tube II. Each of the solutions contained in the test tubes I and II is then allowed to percolate through individual Amberlite columns, and the eluate from the first column corresponding to test tube I is discarded. That from the second column is collected in a conical tube since it contains the nonretained neutral anabolics including testosterone, trenbolone, and progesterone. The first column is washed with methanol and 0.1M hydrochloric acid, and elution of the retained diethylstilbestrol is accomplished with 0.03M hydrochloric acid in acetonitrile–methanol (20 : 80). The second column is washed with methanol, the washing being added to the conical tube; and with 1M hydrochloric acid, the washing being discarded. Elution of the acidic anabolics taleranol, zearalenol, zeranol, zearalenone, and estradiol from the second column is carried out with 0.03M hydrochloric acid in acetonitrile–methanol (20 : 80). All three eluates containing the analytes of interest are evaporated to dryness, reconstituted in appropriate solvents, and analyzed by liquid chromatography. The mobile phases selected for the separation varied with the type of the analytes and the detection technique. Acetonitrile–0.01M potassium dihydrogen phosphate, pH 3 (48 : 52), was used for diethylstilbestrol determination by electrochemical detection. Acetonitrile–0.01M potassium dihydrogen phosphate, pH (46 : 54), was used for estradiol determination by fluorescence detection. Acetonitrile–methanol–tetrahydrofuran–0.01M potassium dihydrogen phosphate, pH 3 (21 : 7 : 12 : 60), was used for zeranol and zearalenone determination by electrochemical detection. Finally, for testosterone, trenbolone, and progesterone determination by ultraviolet detection, an acetonitrile–water gradient was used from 40% to 65% acetonitrile in 30 min. Other chromatographic conditions and the performance characteristics are shown in Table 29.13.

TABLE 29.13 Physicochemical Methods for Anabolic Hormonal-type Growth Promoters in Biological Matrices

Compound(s)	Matrix	Sample preparation	Steps	Stationary phase	Mobile phase	Detection/ Identification	Sensitivity/ Recovery	Ref.
THIN-LAYER CHROMATOGRAPHIC METHODS								
Diethyl-stilbestrol, zeranol	Bovine tissues and plasma	Enzymatic digestion with protease, β-glucuronidase hydrolysis, H_2O/acetone extn, cleanup on tandem basic alumina column and Bio-Rex anion-exchange membrane, liq–liq partns	21	HPTLC Kieselgel 60	DCM/MeOH/ PrOH	Vis/Fast Corinth V	25 ppb/ NR	427
Estradiol, zeranol	Animal tissues, bovine plasma	H_2O/acetone extn, cleanup on tandem basic alumina and Ag-MP-1 columns, liq–liq partns	19–24	HPTLC-GHL Silica gel	DCM/MeOH/ PrOH	Vis/Fast Corinth V	4–250 ppb/ 62–76%	450
Thirty steroid hormones	Bovine fatty tissues	Hexane extn, liq–liq partns, SPE cleanup	22	HPTLC Silica gel 60	$CHCl_3$/acetone and cyclohexane/ EtOAc/EtOH, in two opposite directions	UV-Vis 366 nm	1–10 ppb/ NR	433

(continued)

TABLE 29.13 Continued

Compound(s)	Matrix	Sample preparation	Steps	Stationary phase	Mobile phase	Detection/ Identification	Sensitivity/ Recovery	Ref.
Gas Chromatographic Methods								
Diethylstilbestrol	Meat	Enzymatic digestion with subtilisin A, β-glucuronidase/ arylsulfatase hydrolysis, ether extn, liq–liq partns, derivatization with heptafluorobutyric acid anhydride (HFB derivative)	19	25 m, capillary, coated with phenylmethyl-silicone	Helium	EI-MS	0.1 ppb/ 90 ± 2.2%	435
Nortestosterone, methyl-testosterone	Bovine muscle	Enzymatic digestion with subtilisin A, ether extn, SPE cleanup, IAC cleanup, liq–liq partns, derivatization with heptafluorobutyric acid anhydride (HFB derivatives), liq–liq partns,	25	DB-1, 30 m, capillary	Helium	NICI-MS	1 ppb/ 80 ± 6%	436

Analyte	Matrix	Method		Column	Carrier gas	Detection	LOD/Recovery	Ref
Zearalenone, α-zearalenol	Bovine and sheep urine	H_2O diln, two SPE cleanups, derivatization with Tri-Sil BT (TMS derivatives)	13	DB-5, 15 m, capillary	Helium	MS-MS	1 ppb/ 55–119%	431
Trenbolone, epitrenbolone	Bovine tissues	β-Glucuronidase hydrolysis, ACN extn, liq–liq partns, two SPE cleanups, LC purification on Perkin-Elmer, C_{18}, column, on-line derivatization with BSTFA (TMS derivatives)	27	30 m, capillary, coated with 100% methylsilicone	Helium	EI-MS	0.5 ppb/ NR	445
Diethylstilbestrol, dienestrol, hexestrol	Plasma, urine	Centrgn, phosp. buffer diln, IAC cleanup, derivatization with pentafluorobenzyl bromide (PFB derivatives)	10	CP Sil 5 CB, 25 m, capillary	Helium	NICI-MS	0.01 ppb/ 28–96%	432
19-Nor-testosterone, testosterone, trenbolone	Urine	IAC cleanup, derivatization with carboxymethoxylamine, pentafluorobenzyl bromide and BSTFA (PFBCMO-TMS derivatives)	11	CP Sil 5 CB, 25 m, capillary	Helium	NICI-MS	0.02–0.06 ppb/ 35–87%	458

(continued)

TABLE 29.13 Continued

Compound(s)	Matrix	Sample preparation	Steps	Stationary phase	Mobile phase	Detection/ Identification	Sensitivity/ Recovery	Ref.
Stanozolol and two hydroxy metabolites	Bovine urine	β-Glucuronidase/ sulfatase hydrolysis, SPE cleanup, deri- vatization with heptafluorobutyric acid anhydride (HFB derivatives)	10	OV-1, 30 m, capillary, and OPTIMA 5, 15 m, capillary	Helium	EI-MS	0.001 ppb/ 90 ± 6%	428
Seven steroid hormones	Meat	THF extn, liq–liq partns, silica column cleanup, derivatization with BSA (TMS derivatives)	19	10 m, capillary, coated with nonpolar silicone phase SE-54	Helium	EI-MS	1–5 ppb/ NR	451
Nine steroid hormones	Meat	Enzymatic digestion with subtilisin A, ether extn, SPE cleanup, LC purification on LiChrospher RP-18, 5 µm column, deri- vatization with heptafluorobutyric acid, anhydride (HFB derivatives), and MSTFA (TMS derivatives)	17	HP Ultra-2, 25 m, capillary	Helium	EI-MS	NR/ 85–99%	437

Thirteen steroid hormones	Bovine muscle	MeOH extn, liq–liq partns, SPE cleanup, derivatization with MSTFA (TMS derivatives)	40	BPX-5, 30 m, capillary, with deactivated fused-silica quard column	Helium	EI-MS	0.02–0.1 ppb/ 56–95% 452

LIQUID CHROMATOGRAPHIC METHODS

Diethylstilbestrol	Bovine muscle	Tetr.-butyl methyl ether extn, liq–liq partn, SPE cleanup	15	Nucleosil 5 C$_{18}$, 5 μm	0.05M, pH 3.5, phosp buffer/ MeOH (33:67)	Electro-chemical	0.2 ppb/ 66 ± 14% 438
Melengestrol	Bovine tissues	H$_2$O/ACN extn, liq–liq partn on-line cleanup on Spherisorb phenyl, 3 μm, column, trace enrichment on duPont silica, 5 μm, preconcn column and switching to analytical column	9	Brownlee, 5 μm, silica	DCM contg 5% MeOH and 0.1% H$_2$O/ hexane (14:86)	UV 287 nm/ GC-EI-MS after derivatization with HFAA	2–5 ppb/ 86 ± 9.8% 456

(continued)

TABLE 29.13 Continued

Compound(s)	Matrix	Sample preparation	Steps	Stationary phase	Mobile phase	Detection/ Identification	Sensitivity/ Recovery	Ref.
β-19-Nortestosterone, α-19-nortestosterone	Bovine tissues and urine	Tris buffer addn, enzymatic digestion with subtilopeptidase A (tissues), Amberlite XAD-2 addn, β-glucuronidase-arylsulfatase hydrolysis (urine, liver, kidney), on-line IAC cleanup, trace enrichment on Chrompack C₁₈, preconcn column and switching to analytical column	14–19	Chromspher C₁₈, 5 μm, with Chromsep guard column	H₂O/ACN (65:35)	UV 247 nm/ GC-MS after derivatization with BSTFA	0.05 ppb/ 44–82%	429
Trenbolone, 19-nortestosterone	Bovine liver	Acetate buffer, pH 4.1, extn, β-glucuronidase hydrolysis, liq–liq partns, cleanup on Bio-Beads S-X3 size exclusion chromatography column, online cleanup on PLgel,	23	Spherisorb S5CN, 5 μm, and Spherisorb S5W, 5 μm	2,2,4-trimethyl-pentane/propan-2-ol (85:15), at 30°C	UV 340 & 247 nm	0.1–0.3 ppb/ 38–61%	446

Analyte	Matrix	Sample preparation		Column	Mobile phase	Detection	LOD/Recovery	Ref.
		5 µm, gel-permeation column, trace enrichment on ChromSpher silica, 40 µm, preconcn columns and switching to analytical columns						
Melengestrol, megestrol, chlormadinone	Animal fat	ACN extn, liq–liq partns, SPE cleanup	32	C18, 5 µm, end-capped with 20% carbon load, analytical and guard column	H2O/ACN (30:70)	UV 291 nm	10 ppb/ 84–116%	434
17α-methyl-testosterone and two metabolites	Trout muscle	CHCl3/MeOH extn, liq–liq partns, cleanup on Lipidex 5000 column, SPE cleanup	23	Hypersil C8, 5 µm, and Nucleosil C18, 5 µm, columns in series, with ODS 2, 5 µm, guard column	H2O/MeOH (25:75)	Fluorometric, postcolumn enzymatic reaction with 3α-HSD, ex: 340 nm, em: 470 nm	1–5 ppb/ 91–94%	454
Zearalenone, α-zearalenol, β-zeralenol	Milk	β-glucuronidase/sulfatase hydrolysis, ACN extn, cleanup on a liquid-liquid extraction column, SPE cleanup	21	Ultra Teschsphere ODs, 5 µm, with Resolve C18, guard column	H2O/MeOH/ACN (35:61:4)	Fluorometric, ex: 236 nm, em: 470 nm	0.2–2 ppb/ 84–93%	430

(continued)

TABLE 29.13 Continued

Compound(s)	Matrix	Sample preparation	Steps	Stationary phase	Mobile phase	Detection/ Identification	Sensitivity/ Recovery	Ref.
Zeranol, zearalenone, and four metabolites	Animal tissues	MeOH extn, β-glucuronidase hydrolyis, liq–liq partns	27	Nova-Pak RP-C_{18}, 5 μm	0.09M, pH 6.9, sodium acetate buffer, contg 10 mM EDTA/ MeOH (50:50)	Electro-chemical/ GC–MS after derivatization with BSA	5 ppb/ 53–75%	447
Six steroid hormones	Bovine tissues	Lyophilization, SFE (CO_2) cleanup	5	Supelcosil, 5 μm	0.02M ammonium formate/ MeOH-ACN (1:1) Gradient from (95:5) to (5:95)	MS-APCI	100 ppb/ 44–91%	448

| Nine steroid hormones | Animal tissues | MeOH extn, Carbopack B, and Amberlite column cleanups | 24 | C_{18}, 5 μm, with Supelguard LC-18, 5 μm, guard column | Different according to the type of the molecules | UV (242 nm), electro-chemical, & fluorometric (ex: 280 nm, em: 308 nm) | 1 ppb/ 84–91% | 453 |

SUPERCRITICAL-FLUID CHROMATOGRAPHIC METHODS

| Diethylstilbestrol, dienestrol, hexestrol | Swine kidney | Lyophilization, SFE (CO_2) cleanup | 6 | Spherisorb 5 amino | CO_2/MeOH Isocratic (100:0) for 8 min and then gradient to (80:20) | MS-MS-TSP | 10000 ppb/ NR | 213 |

HFAA, heptafluorobutyric acid anyhydride; BSTFA, N,O-bis(trimethylsilyl)trifluoroacetamide; 3α-hydroxysteroid dehydrogenase; BSA, N,O-bis(trimethylsilyl)acetamide; MSTFA, N-methyl-N-(trimethylsilyl)trifluoroacetamide; TMS, trimethylsilane; SEA, supercritical-fluid extraction; PFBCMO, pentafluorobenzylcarboxymethoxime. Other abbreviations as in Tables 29.1 and 29.3.

Hartmann and Steinhart (452) developed a gas chromatographic–mass spectrometric method for the determination of steroid hormones including androstenedione, androsterone, testosterone, progesterone, estrone, estradiol, dehydroepiandrosterone, dihydrotestosterone, epitestosterone, hydroxytestosterone, epitestosterone, hydroxyprogesterone, pregnenolone, estriol, methyltestosterone, and medroxyprogesterone in bovine muscle tissue. According to this method, a 20 g sample is homogenized with 70 ml methanol and 20 ml water, and the homogenate is heated at 60°C for 15 min, allowed to cool, and centrifuged. The supernatant is then extracted twice with 20 ml hexane to remove fat, evaporated to constant volume, and the remaining aqueous layer is submitted to solid-phase extraction cleanup on a C_8 cartridge. Following cartridge washing with water and methanol–water (40:60), polar steroids (fraction I) are eluted with methanol–water (60:40), while nonpolar steroids (fraction II) are eluted with pure methanol. Cleanup of the polar steroids is effected by dissolving the dry residue of fraction I in ethyl acetate and filtering the solution through a silica solid-phase extraction cartridge. Separation of the nonpolar steroids into phenolics and neutral steroids is carried out by dissolving the dry residue of fraction II in chloroform and partitioning the solution against hexane and 0.25M sodium hydroxide. The sodium

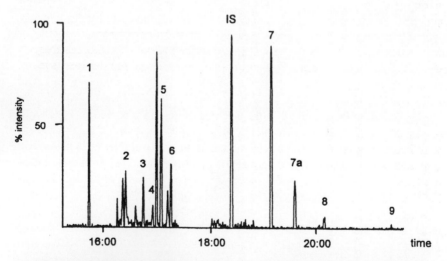

FIG. 29.13 GC–MS chromatogram of neutral steroids in meat. Androgens (fortified, 0.2–0.5 ppb): 1, a-androsterone; 2, dehydroepiandrosterone; 3, epitestosterone; 4, dihydrotestosterone; 5, androstenedione; 6, testosterone; IS, methyltestosterone. Progestogens (fortified): 7,7a, pregnenolone (2.1 ppb); 8, progesterone (0.4 ppb); 9, hydroxyprogesterone (0.3 ppb). (Reprinted from Ref. 452, with permission from Elsevier Science.)

hydroxide layer (fraction IIb) that contains the nonpolar phenolics is then neutralized with hydrochloric acid. The organic layer of the phenolate extraction (fraction IIa) is loaded on another silica solid-phase extraction cartridge, and following washing with hexane–ethyl acetate (90:10) the nonpolar neutral steroids are eluted with hexane–ethyl acetate (25:75). Cleanup of the nonpolar phenolics is accomplished by extracting the neutralized sodium hydroxide layer with diethyl ether, evaporating the ether phase, reconstituting it with ethyl acetate–methanol (80:20), and filtering the solution through an amino solid-phase extraction cartridge. All three eluates containing the polar, the nonpolar phenolics, and the nonpolar neutral steroids are evaporated to dryness, and derivatization of the analytes is performed by adding to the dry residues 40 μl of a mixture containing N-methyl-N-trimethylsilyltrifluoroacetamide, trimethyliodosilane, and 1,4-dithioerythritol, and heating at 40°C for 15 min. The derivatized solutions are then analyzed by gas chromatography–mass spectrometry under the conditions shown in Table 29.13 (Fig. 29.13).

29.14 β-ADRENERGIC AGONISTS

β-Agonists are relatively polar compounds that can be extracted from biological matrices using aqueous or organic solvents. These drugs fall into two major categories: substituted anilines, including clenbuterol; and substituted phenols, including salbutamol. This distinction is important because most methods for drugs in the former category depend upon pH adjustment to partition the analytes between organic and aqueous phases. This pH dependence is not valid, however, for drugs within the latter category, since phenolic compounds are charged under all pH conditions.

When analyzing liquid samples such as urine and plasma for residues of β-agonists, deconjugation of bound residues using β-glucuronidase/sulfatase enzyme hydrolysis prior to sample extraction is often recommended (470–476). Semisolid samples such as liver, muscle, hair and eye usually require more intensive sample pretreatment for tissue break-up. The most popular approach is sample homogenization in dilute hydrochloric acid (470, 471, 477–480), perchloric acid–EDTA (475), or aqueous buffer (481–483). In general, dilute acids allow high extraction yields for all categories of β-agonists, because the aromatic moiety of these analytes is uncharged under acidic conditions while their aliphatic amino group is positively ionized. Following centrifugation of the extract, the supernatant may be further treated with β-glucuronidase–sulfatase (470, 471) or subtilisin A (482) to allow hydrolysis of the conjugated residues.

The primary sample extract is subsequently subjected to cleanup using several different approaches including conventional liquid–liquid partitioning, diphasic dialysis, solid-phase extraction, immunoaffinity chromatography, and liquid chromatography cleanup. In some instances, more than one of these procedures is applied in combination in order to achieve better extract purification.

Liquid–liquid partitioning cleanup is generally carried out at alkaline conditions using ethyl acetate (481, 484), ethyl acetate/tert.-butanol mixture (482), diethyl ether (478), or tert.-butylmethyl ether/n-butanol (485) as extraction solvents. The organic extracts are then either concentrated to dryness (482), or repartitioned with dilute acid to facilitate back-extraction of the analytes into the acidic solution. A literature survey shows that liquid–liquid partitioning cleanup resulted in good recoveries of substituted anilines such as clenbuterol (478, 481, 484), but it was less effective for more polar compounds such as salbutamol (482).

Diphasic dialysis can also be used for purification of the primary sample extract. This procedure was only applied in the determination of clenbuterol residues in liver using tert.-butylmethyl ether as the extraction solvent (483).

Solid-phase extraction and immunoaffinity chromatography are alternative cleanup procedures that are, generally, better suited to the multiresidue analysis of β-agonists. Since these procedures are not time-consuming and labor-intensive, and require low solvent usage, they have become the methods of choice in many laboratories for isolation and/or cleanup of β-agonists from biological matrices. They are particularly advantageous because they allow better extraction of the more hydrophilic β-agonists including salbutamol.

β-Agonists are particularly suited to reversed-phase solid-phase extraction due, in part, to their relatively nonpolar aliphatic moiety, which can interact with the hydrophobic octadecyl- and octyl-based sorbents of the cartridge (472, 473, 475, 480, 486, 487). By adjusting the pH of the sample extracts at values greater than 10, optimum retention of the analytes can be achieved. Adsorption solid-phase extraction using a neutral alumina sorbent has also been described for improved cleanup of liver homogenates (482).

Ion-exchange solid-phase extraction is another cleanup procedure successfully used in the purification of liver and tissue homogenates (479). Significant improvements in terms of speed and simplicity were reported by workers who employed an Empore cation-exchange extraction membrane (488). Since multiresidue solid-phase extraction procedures covering β-agonists of different types present, in general, analytical problems, mixed-phase solid-phase extraction sorbents, which contained a mixture of reversed-phase and ion-exchange material, were also employed to improve the retention of the more polar compounds. Several different sorbents were designed, and procedures that utilized both interaction mechanisms were described (472, 474, 476, 482, 489).

Owing to its high specificity and sample cleanup efficiency, immunoaffinity chromatography has also received widespread acceptance for the determination of β-agonists in biological matrices (470, 471, 473, 475, 479, 487, 490). The potential of online immunoaffinity extraction for the multiresidue determination of β-agonists in bovine urine was recently demonstrated, using an automated column-switching system (490). In contrast, applications of extract cleanup by liquid chromatography are rather limited and concern solely the isolation of clenbuterol residues from urine samples (485).

Following extraction and cleanup, β-agonists can be detected in sample extracts by either direct nonchromatographic methods or by liquid and gas chromatographic methods (Table 29.14). Direct nonchromatographic methods are targeted to screening of β-agonist residues in urine extracts. Direct spectrometric detection of β-agonists in urine extracts has been achieved using either thermospray tandem mass spectrometry (476) or electrospray mass spectrometry (485).

In the liquid chromatographic methods, reversed-phase columns are commonly used for the separation of the β-agonists molecules due to their hydrophobic interaction with the C_{18} sorbent. Efficient reversed-phase ion-pair separation of β-agonists has also been reported using sodium dodecyl sulfate as the pairing ion (477).

Detection in liquid chromatography is often performed in the ultraviolet region at wavelengths of 245 (479) or 260 nm (486). However, poor sensitivity and interference from coextractives may appear at these low detection wavelengths unless sample extracts are extensively cleaned up and concentrated. This problem may be overcome by postcolumn derivatization of the aromatic amino group of the β-agonist molecules to the corresponding diazo dyes through a Bratton-Marshall reaction, and subsequent spectrophotometric detection at 494 nm (477).

Although spectrophotometric detection is generally acceptable, electrochemical detection seems to be more appropriate for the analysis of β-agonists, due to the presence on the aromatic part of their molecule of oxidizable hydroxyl and amino groups. This method of detection has been applied in the determination of clenbuterol residues in bovine retinal tissue with sufficient sensitivity for this tissue (478).

Confirmatory analysis of suspected liquid chromatographic peaks can be made possible by coupling liquid chromatography with mass spectrometry. Ion spray LC–MS–MS has been used to monitor five β-agonists in bovine urine (490), while atmospheric-pressure chemical ionization LC–MS–MS has been employed for the identification of ractopamine residues in bovine urine (472).

Gas chromatographic separation of β-agonist residues is generally complicated by the necessity of derivatization of their polar hydroxyl and amino functional groups. Silyl derivatives are preferentially prepared by treating sample extracts with N,O-bis(trimethylsilyl)trifluoroacetamide (470, 471, 473, 475, 483, 487), N-methyl-N-(trimethylsilyl)trifluoroacetamide (482) or N-methyl-N-(tert-butyldimethylsilyl)trifluoroacetamide (473, 487). Pentafluoropropionic anhydride (481), phosgene (484), trimethylboroxine (480), methyl- and butylboronic acid (489), or a combination of N,O bis(trimethylsilyl)trifluoroacetamide with

TABLE 29.14 Physicochemical Methods for β-Adrenergic Agonists in Biological Matrices

Compound(s)	Matrix	Sample preparation	Steps	Stationary phase	Mobile phase	Detection/identification	Sensitivity/recovery	Ref.
SPECTROMETRIC METHODS								
Clenbuterol	Bovine urine	Tert.-butylmethyl ether/BuOH extn, LC purification on Ultrabase C$_{18}$ column, liq–liq partns	12	—	—	MS-ESP	NR	485
Five β-agonists	Bovine urine	β-Glucuronidase/sulfatase hydrolysis, SPE cleanup	8	—	—	MS-MS-TSP	0.5–1 ppb/NR	476
GAS CHROMATOGRAPHIC METHODS								
Clenbuterol	Animal tissues	EtOAc extn, liq–liq partns, derivatization with phosgene, liq–liq partns	29	DB-5, 12 m, capillary	Helium	EI-MS	0.25 ppb/61–98%	484
	Bovine hair and urine	HCl extn (hair), SPE cleanup, derivatization with trimethyl-boroxine	9–14	CP-Sil-8 CB, 25 m, capillary	Helium	EI-MS	0.14–16 ppb/90–92%	480
	Bovine liver	Ba(OH)$_2$/BaCl$_2$ buffer addn, diphasic dialysis, derivatization with BSTFA (TMS derivative)	7	HP SP 5, 25 m, capillary	Helium	CI-MS	0.5 ppb/99.3%	483

	Bovine tissues and plasma	Sorensen buffer, pH 7 (tissue), or EtOAc (plasma) extn, liq–liq partns, derivatization with pentafluoro-propionic anhydride	6–12	OV-1701, 25 m, capillary	Helium	NICI-MS	0.01 ppb/ 95–106%	481
	Urine	IAC cleanup, SPE cleanup, derivatization with BSTFA (TMS derivatives) and MTBSTFA (tBDMS derivatives)	14	DB-5, 30 m, capillary	Helium	CI-MS and/or EI-MS	0.2 ppb/ NR	487
Clenbuterol, mabuterol, salbutamol	Bovine liver and urine	HCl extn (liver), β-glucuronidase/ sulfatase hydrolysis, SPE cleanup, IAC cleanup, derivatization with BSTFA (TMS derivatives)	13–16	CP-Sil-5 CB, 25 m, capillary	Helium	FT-IR	1–2.5 ppb/ NR	471

(continued)

TABLE 29.14 Continued

Compound(s)	Matrix	Sample preparation	Steps	Stationary phase	Mobile phase	Detection/ identification	Sensitivity/ recovery	Ref.
Four β-agonists	Bovine liver and urine	β-Glucuronidase/ sulfatase hydrolysis (urine), perchloric acid/EDTA extn (liver), SPE cleanup (liver), IAC cleanup, SPE cleanup, derivatization with BSTFA (TMS derivatives)	24–33	CP-Sil-5 CB, 25 m, capillary	Helium	EI–MS and/ or PICI–MS	1–3 ppb/ 59–110%	475
Five β-agonists	Bovine liver and urine	HCl extn (liver), β-glucuronidase/ sulfatase hydrolysis, SPE cleanup, IAC cleanup, derivatization with BSTFA (TMS derivatives)	13–16	Permabond SE-52, 25 m, capillary	Helium	EI–MS	1–2 ppb/ 40–100%	470
Six β-agonists	Bovine urine	β-Glucuronidase/ sulfatase hydrolysis, IAC cleanup, SPE cleanup, derivatization with BSTFA (TMS derivatives) and MTBSTFA (tBDMS derivatives)	14	DB-5, 30 m, capillary	Helium	CI–MS	0.2–0.4 ppb/ NR	473

Seven β-agonists	Bovine liver and urine	Tris buffer extn, subtilisin A addn (liver), liq–liq partns, two SPE cleanups, derivatization with MSTFA (TMS derivatives)	20	WCOT RSL 150BP, 30 m, capillary	Helium	PICI–MS–MS	0.5–5 ppb/ 3–85%	482
Eight β-agonists	Bovine urine	SPE cleanup, derivatization with methyl- and butylboronic acid	8	HP1, 15 m, capillary	Helium	EI–MS	0.3–3 ppb/ 23–91%	489
Nine β-agonists	Bovine urine	Filtn, cleanup on Empore cation-exchange extraction membrane	7	OV-1, 30 m, capillary	Helium	EI–MS and/ or PICI–MS	NR/10–80%	488
Thirteen β-agonists	Urine	β-Glucuronidase/ sulfatase hydrolysis, SPE cleanup, derivatization with BSTFA (TMS derivatives), or CMDMCS (cyclic DMS derivatives)	14	OV-1, 30 m, capillary	Helium	EI–MS and/ or PICI–MS	0.5–1 ppb/ 20–73%	474

(continued)

TABLE 29.14 Continued

LIQUID CHROMATOGRAPHIC METHODS

Compound(s)	Matrix	Sample preparation	Steps	Stationary phase	Mobile phase	Detection/ identification	Sensitivity/ recovery	Ref.
Clenbuterol	Bovine liver and muscle	HCl extn, SPE cleanup, IAC cleanup	18	Symmetry C$_{18}$	0.01M, pH 4.6, amm. acetate buffer/MeOH Gradient from (70:30) to (30:70)	UV 245 nm	0.3 ppb/ 53–74%	479
	Bovine retina	HCl extn, EDTA addn, liq–liq partns	14	LiChrospher 100 RP-18e, 5 μm, analytical and guard column	H$_2$O/MeOH (66:34) contg 1% formic acid, at 40°C	Electro-chemical	5 ppb/ 76 ± 7.5%	478
Ractopamine	Bovine urine	β-Glucuronidase hydrolysis, two SPE cleanups	17	Inertsil 5 ODS, 3 μm, analytical and guard column	0.01M amm. acetate/ MeOH Gradient from (95:05) to (20:80)	MS-MS-APCI	2 ppb/ NR	472
Clenbuterol, cimaterol	Animal tissues, urine, blood, plasma	HCl extn (tissue), SPE cleanup, liq–liq partn	7–12	Nova-pak C$_{18}$, 4 μm	0.02M HOAc contg 25 mM SDS, pH 3.5/ ACN (53:47)	Vis 494 nm, postcolumn derivatization (Bratton-Marshall)/ HPTLC & GC-SIM-MS	0.1–0.2 ppb/ 60–99%	477

Clenbuterol, salbutamol, cimaterol	Urine	5	SPE cleanup	LiChrospher RP-select B, 5 μm	0.02M KH_2PO_4, contg 30 μM EDTA, pH 3.9/MeOH (92.5:7.5), or 0.02M phosp. buffer/MeOH (75:25) for clenbuterol	UV 260 nm/ EIA	1 ppb/ 65–100%	486
Five β-agonists	Bovine urine	2	Diln with phosphate-buffered saline, purification by online sample cleanup on IAC column, and subsequent trace enrichment on Pellicular C_8, 30–40 μm, preconcn column and switching to analytical column	Spherisorb C_{18}, 3 μm, capillary or microbore column	Solvent A: H_2O/ACN/MeOH (95:2.5:2.5) contg 0.1% HOAc and 5mM amm. acetate Solvent B: H_2O/ACN/MeOH (5:47.5:47.5) contg 0.1% HOAc and 5mM amm. acetate Isocratic (28:72)	MS-MS-ISP	0.01–0.05 ppb/ 94–108%	490

Abbreviations: BSTFA, N,O-bis(trimethylsilyl)trifluoroacetamide; MTBSTFA, N-methyl-N-(tetr.-butyldimethylsilyl)trifluoroacetamide; DMS, 2-dimethylsilamorpholine; CMDMCS, chloromethyldimethylchlorosilane; TMS, trimethylsilane; EIA, enzyme immunoassay. Other abbreviations as in Tables 29.1 and 29.3.

chloromethyldimethylchlorosilane (474, 488) were also employed for derivatization of β-agonist residues isolated from biological samples.

Despite its inherent analytical difficulties, gas chromatography on capillary columns in combination with sensitive and specific mass spectrometry has been widely used for separation of these analytes. Typical examples of such applications are those interfacing gas chromatography with mass spectrometry via electron impact (470, 484, 480, 489), chemical ionization (481, 478, 483, 473), or both interfaces (474, 475, 487, 488). Apart from mass spectrometry, Fourier transform infrared spectrometry has also been suggested as an alternative very useful identification tool in the area of the β-agonist analysis. Capillary gas chromatography with Fourier transform infrared spectrometry was successfully employed to monitor clenbuterol, mabuterol, and salbutamol residues in bovine liver and urine (471).

Methods particularly useful for screening and even confirmation of β-agonists residues in biological matrices have been described by Lin et al. (478), Cai and Henion (490), and Montrade et al. (474).

Lin et al. (478) described a method for the determination of clenbuterol in bovine retinal tissue. According to this method, retinal tissue is homogenized and extracted with 5 ml 1M hydrochloric acid. After centrifugation, the supernatant is mixed with 5 ml 1M EDTA in 4M sodium hydroxide solution and the pH of the mixture is adjusted to 12.2. The mixture is extracted two times with 5 ml portions of diethyl ether, and the combined extracts are concentrated to dryness. The residue is reconstituted in 0.2 ml 1% formic acid to be further analyzed by liquid chromatography. Separation is performed on a 25 cm LiChrospher 100 RP-18e (5 μm) analytical column that is protected by a guard column with the same packing material. Using a mobile phase of water–methanol (66:34) containing 1% formic acid, concentrations down to 5 ppb could be determined by electrochemical detection.

A different approach was followed by Cai and Henion (490) in a capillary liquid chromatographic method for multiresidue determination of clenbuterol, methylclenbuterol, mabuterol, mapenterol, and tolubuterol in bovine urine. According to this method, a 10 ml sample is diluted with 4 volumes of phosphate-buffered saline, and purified online by loading the diluted urine onto an immunoaffinity extraction column. Following column washing with phosphate-buffered saline, the preconcentrated analytes are eluted with 2% acetic acid and trapped at the beginning of a 30–40 μm Pellicular C$_8$ column. Using an automated column switching system, the trapped analytes are back-flashed into the analytical column (320 μm × 150 mm, Spherisorb C$_{18}$, 3 μm, capillary, or 100 × 1.0 mm, Spherisorb C$_{18}$, 5 μm, microbore) and analyzed under the conditions shown in Table 29.14. Concentrations as low as 0.05 ppb for clenbuterol and methylclenbuterol, 0.02 ppb for mabuterol, and 0.01 ppb for mapenterol could be readily determined using ion-spray tandem mass spectrometric detection.

Montrade et al. (474) employed gas chromatography–mass spectrometry for the determination of 13 β-agonists in urine of meat-producing animals. In this method, the pH of a 10 ml sample of previously centrifuged urine is adjusted to 4.8, and the sample is incubated overnight at 40°C with β-glucuronidase/sulfatase. Following pH adjustment to 6.0, the treated sample is applied to a mixed-phase column (Clean Screen DAU). Column washing is carried out with diluted acetic acid and methanol, while the analytes are eluted with ethyl acetate containing 3% concentrated (32%) ammonia solution. After evaporation of the eluent, the analytes are derivatized to either their trimethylsilyl (TMS) or cyclic 2-(dimethyl)silamorpholine (DMS) derivatives by adding to the dry residue 50 μl of a N,O-bis(trimethylsilyl)trifluoroacetamide or chloromethyldimethylchlorosilane solution, respectively. The derivatized extract is then evaporated to dryness, redissolved with 25 μl of toluene, and analyzed on a OV-1 fused-silica capillary column (30 m × 0.25 mm i.d.), with helium as the carrier gas (Fig. 29.14). Using the TMS derivatives both for screening (electron impact mode) and confirmation (positive-ion chemical ionization mode) purposes, concentrations as low as 0.5–1 ppb of the 13 β-agonists could be readily determined in the urine.

29.15 DYE DRUGS

Dye drugs used in animal husbandry can be classified in terms of their chemical structure into triphenylmethanes, acridine, and phenothiazine congeners. Methyl derivatives of the triphenylmethane dyes comprise a series of basic drugs including gentian violet and malachite green. Acridine derivatives are yellow-color dyes that have been designated as flavines. These dyes possess either basic or neutral properties and include drugs such as acriflavine and proflavine. Commercially available acriflavine is a mixture of acriflavine and proflavine. Methylene blue constitutes the major drug within the phenothiazine group of dyes.

Dye drugs have recently been studied at some length. Analytical methods have been developed and are available for residue monitoring in a variety of matrices due to the knowledge or suspicion of unauthorized or extralabel use. Since metabolic data have shown that residues may be of either the "chromic" or "leuco" form, methodology destined for food control should be capable of detecting both forms.

Liquid samples such as milk do not normally require application of any pretreatment procedure. Semisolid samples such as muscle, liver, and fat tissues usually require more intensive sample pretreatment for tissue break-up. The most popular approach is grinding the sample in a food chopper or homogenization in a Waring blender to expose residues to the extraction solvent. Fatty tissue samples are usually warmed at 35°C until fat melts (491–493), or sometimes blended with immersion blender (494). A fat sample that has been blended with immersion blender melts to produce yellow oil, whereas oil does not separate

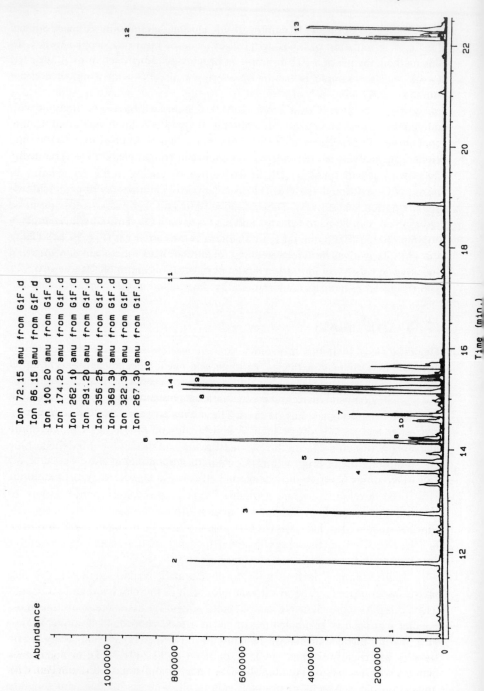

from fat ground in a food chopper (493). During sample pretreatment, special precautions are often required to avoid the presence of certain metal ions, such as those in rust, strong acids, and bases, since these agents can catalyze the oxidation of the leuco forms of the potentially present residues to the corresponding parent drugs.

A range of extraction techniques have been suggested, including several solvent homogenization and percolation systems. Their effectiveness appears to be limited by the strong binding of the dyes to the sample proteins, and the high lipid content (10–15%) of fish and fatty tissue samples that caused emulsion formation.

Thus, simple deproteinization of plasma with trichloroacetic acid, perchloric acid, phosphoric acid, or acetonitrile, followed by centrifugation and direct injection of the supernatants, yielded low recoveries of malachite green and leucomalachite green, probably due to insufficient debinding of the analytes (495). Acidification or alkalinization of plasma and subsequent extraction with ethyl acetate also resulted in poor recoveries. In contrast, protein denaturation with a mixture of either acetonitrile or methanol and citric acid could substantially improve the recovery of the analytes, possibly due to the pairing-ion function of the citrate ions.

Efficient ion-pair extraction has also been applied in the determination of methylene blue in catfish (496), the thionin metabolite of methylene blue in milk (497), gentian and leucogentian violet in catfish (498) and chicken (499) tissues, malachite and leucomalachite green in catfish (500–502), and gentian violet, malachite green, and their leuco metabolites in catfish (503, 504). Extraction is effected by homogenizing the sample with ammonium acetate buffer in the presence of the pairing ions hydroxylamine and *p*-toluene sulfonic acid and partitioning with acetonitrile.

In methods of tissue analysis in which ion-pair extraction procedures are not used, long extraction times have been shown to be necessary for extraction

---

FIG. 29.14 El-selected-ion current profiles of a TMS-derivatized urine extract obtained in the selected-ion monitoring mode: blank urine sample spiked with tolubuterol (1) TMS1 (m/z 86), mabuterol (2) TMS1 (86), methylmabuterol (3) TMS1 (100), metaproterenol (4) TMS3 (356), terbutaline (5) TMS3 (86, 356), clenbuterol (6) TMS1 (86, 262), cimaterol (8) TMS1 (72), methylcimaterol (10) TMS1 (86), salbutamol (7) TMS3 (86, 369), cimaterol (8) TMS2 (72, 291), metoprolol (14) TMS1 (72), methylclenbuterol (9) TMS1 (100, 262), methylcimaterol (10) TMS2 (86, 291), NA1141 (11) TMS2 (174), fenoterol (12) TMS4 (322), and ractopamine (13) TMS3 (267). Abundance in arbitrary units. (Reprinted from Ref. 474, with permission from Elsevier Science.)

of the analytes from the tissue matrix. Thus, overnight extraction has been recommended for efficient recovery of either malachite green from fish tissues when a mixture of acetonitrile, chloroform, and acetic acid is used as extractant (505), or gentian and leucogentian violet from chicken tissues using an acetonitrile–acetate buffer (499). In contrast, a 3 h extraction procedure was found to be sufficient for quantitative recovery of malachite and leucomalachite green from rainbow trout by a mixture of acetonitrile, dichloromethane, and perchloric acid (506).

Prolonged extraction was not required when acidified methanol was employed for the extraction of acriflavine and proflavine from catfish tissues (507), when acetonitrile was used for the extraction of methylene blue and four metabolites from milk (508), or when dichloromethane in presence of sodium sulfate was employed for the extraction of leucogentian violet from chicken fat (491–494).

Following extraction, the primary sample extract is subsequently subjected to some type of cleanup including conventional liquid–liquid partitioning and/ or solid-phase extraction. The liquid–liquid partitioning cleanup applied differs with the initial extraction system. Thus, for isolating fat from analytes, the primary dichloromethane sample extract was partitioned with 1N hydrochloric acid in the analysis of leucogentian violet in chicken fat (491–494). The acidic layer was then neutralized with trisodium citrate to facilitate back extraction of the analytes into dichloromethane.

In addition, for removing fat from an acetonitrile–chloroform–acetic acid extract of fish tissues, partitioning with hexane was carried out (505). Further cleanup could be effected by partitioning the extract against diethyl ether–hexane–sodium chloride solution, evaporating the organic layer that contained the malachite green analyte, reconstituting in methanol–phosphoric acid, freezing the solution at $-20°C$, and centrifuging.

When an ion-pair extraction was employed for analyzing methylene blue (496), gentian violet (498), and malachite and leucomalachite green (501, 502) in catfish, partitioning of the acetonitrile extracts with dichloromethane and water yielded good results. Cleanup of a primary acetonitrile extract from polar milk constituents was carried out by adding sodium chloride solution and partitioning with chloroform, thus transferring methylene blue and its metabolites, except thionin, into the chloroform layer (508). For thionin assay, the remaining aqueous layer was alkalinized at pH 10, and then thionin was extracted with chloroform.

Solid-phase extraction is also complementarily used in many analyses for improved extract cleanup. While cyano, diol, or cation exchange solid-phase extraction cartridges, alone, were found to be effective for the relatively simple concentration and cleanup of malachite and leucomalachite green during the analysis of water (509, 510) or plasma (495), most methods for analysis of fish tissue employed either solvent partitioning and washing (491–494, 511), or a combination of alumina and strong cation exchange solid-phase extraction (502) to separate interferences. There have been only two methods for fish analysis that employ a single reversed-phase solid-phase extraction (506, 507) or a cation exchange solid-phase extraction (495, 508). For GC–MS confirmation of leuco-malachite green in catfish tissue, a third cleanup on a cyano column has been further suggested (512).

Following extraction and cleanup, dye drugs can be separated by liquid or gas chromatographic methods. However, most methods reported in the scientific literature for dye drugs analyses in a variety of matrices employ liquid chromatography. Cyano- (491, 493, 496, 498–500, 502, 507, 508), C_{18-} (491, 494, 501, 506), and polymer-based (505) packing materials are mostly used in liquid chromatographic separations. Several column packing materials including Chromspher C_8 and C_{18}, Hypersil ODS, Microspher C_{18}, Lichrosorb RP-8 and Chromspher 5B, Polymer Lab. PLRP-S, and Hamilton PRP-1 have been tested for effective column efficiency and resolution of malachite green, leucomalachite green, and their demethylated metabolites (495). Nucleosil 5 C_{18}, Lichrosorb C_8, and Chromspher 5B showed the most effective column efficiency and resolution for these compounds.

Early liquid chromatographic methods have taken advantage of the strong and distinctive visible absorption of the parent compounds for detection and quantification of both them and their leuco metabolites. Initial methods for the determination of malachite and leucomalachite green in fish muscle tissue were based on indirect measurement of the analytes. Following extract cleanup by silica gel solid-phase extraction, the cleaned sample was splitted and half of the extract was oxidized with PbO_2 prior to its liquid chromatographic analysis (513, 514). In later studies, an on-line PbO_2 postcolumn oxidation reactor was introduced that opened the possibility for simultaneous monitoring of both analytes in a single liquid chromatographic analysis (515). The PbO_2 postcolumn reaction system oxidized the reduced leuco forms of gentian violet and malachite green to their respective parent chromophores, thus permitting detection at a selected visible wavelength that allowed increased specificity. As an alternative to the use of absorbance, electrochemical detection has also been described (491, 493, 499).

The performance of the postcolumn oxidation reactor with respect to its lifetime and the ability to convert the leuco form to malachite green was assessed (495). The relatively large size of the postcolumn oxidation reactor suggested by some authors (515) was probably the cause of band broadening such reactors are liable to produce. Reduction of the size of the reactor gave much sharper peaks, but the PbO_2 in the reactor depleted rapidly. Increasing the PbO_2 content from 10% to 25% markedly prolonged the lifetime of the reactor. The lifetime of the postcolumn oxidation reactor could be further prolonged by placing a guard oxidation reactor before the injector. In this way, oxidizable substances in the mobile phase that were originated from impurities of the solvents, such as ketones and aldehydes in acetonitrile, could be efficiently eliminated. As a result of this

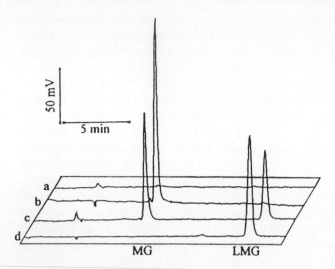

FIG. 29.15.1 Representative chromatograms of (a) blank rainbow trout sample, (b) 100 ppb malachite green standard, (c) rainbow trout sample fortified at 50 ppb with malachite green and leuco malachite green, and (d) 50 ppb leuco malachite green standard. (From Ref. 506.).

treatment, both malachite green and leucomalachite green were stable at room temperature in a so-treated mobile phase although not in an untreated mobile phase.

The use of coulometrically efficient electrochemical cell to oxidize leuco-malachite green to malachite green between the outlet of the liquid chromato-graphic column and the inlet of the visible detector was found to be an effective alternative way to overcome the problems associated with packing and maintaining a PbO_2 postcolumn reactor, while avoiding the band-broadening such reactors are liable to produce (Fig. 29.15.1). In addition, observations on the behavior of the carbon electrode in the amperometric detector, led to some investigations demonstrating that activated charcoal might be superior to PbO_2 for oxidation of leuco forms to the parent compounds.

Online electrochemical oxidation allows additional confidence in the identity of a peak eluting at the correct retention time. If the output of the electrochemical cell in monitored during the analysis, for example, of leucomalachite green, current flow reflecting the passage of an electroactive species will be observed shortly prior to detection of the compound at the visible detector. This would not occur if the peak was due to an already colored coextractive. Second, the size of the suspected leucomalachite green peak in the visible chromatogram should vary in a manner similar to that of a leuco standard when the electrode potential is manually altered. This would provide strong confirmation of the identity of the unknown, since would seem very unlikely that any coextracted compound would have the same retention time, hydrodynamic voltammogram, and colored oxidation product as leucomalachite green. In an alternative detection system (504), the coulometric electrochemical cell preceded a diode array detector that was followed in series by a fluorescence detector.

For complete analytical detection, mass spectral analysis is critical for unambiguous identification of suspect residues found in samples analyzed by determinative methods. Liquid chromatography combined with atmospheric pressure chemical ionization mass spectrometry and/or particle beam liquid chromatography–mass spectrometry are excellent confirmatory techniques (501, 516) but are not prevalent in laboratories due to their expense. Thermospray spectra of some dyes have recently been published that permit use of the existing liquid chromatographic methods for thermospray analysis. However, these spectra are limited to mostly MH and MNH_4 cations, thus limiting the usefulness of liquid chromatography–thermospray mass spectrometry.

Particle beam mass spectral analysis gives mass spectra similar to conventional electron ionization spectra, but can also be used for nonvolatile compounds. Eight triphenylmethane dyes including malachite green and its demethylated and leucomalachite green metabolites, gentian violet and its demethylated and leucogentian violet metabolites, and brilliant green were characterized by particle beam liquid chromatography–mass spectrometry (501). Aside from the reduction of the chromic form in the mass spectrometer source, the triphenylmethane dyes responded well using the particle beam interface. The electron ionization spectra of these spectra obtained by this technique exhibited similar fragmentation, with the formation of phenyl and substituted phenyl radicals, and loss of alkyl groups from the amines. It was observed that six cationic dyes were reduced in the mass spectrometer source to form the corresponding leuco compounds.

Although less expensive than liquid chromatography–mass spectrometry, confirmation by gas chromatography–mass spectrometry (492, 512) is applicable only to the volatile leuco forms and not to chromatic forms of the dyes. The reduced leuco forms of triphenylmethane dyes are volatile and thermally stable enough to be analyzed by gas chromatography–mass spectrometry (492, 512).

Gas and liquid chromatographic methods that are attractive in terms of performance and practicability for screening and confirmation of dye drug residues in foods of animal origin have been described by Rushing and Hansen (504), Munns et al. (493), and Wilson et al. (492).

Rushing and Hansen (504) described a sensitive analytical procedure for screening and confirmation of residues of malachite green, gentian violet, and their leuco analogs in catfish and trout tissues using liquid chromatographic separation and electrochemical, diode array, and fluorescence detection in series.

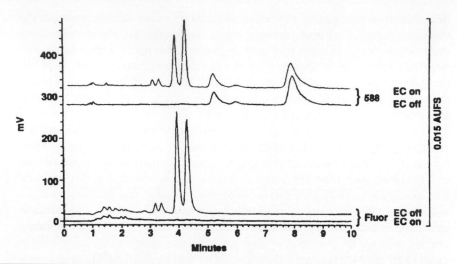

FIG. 29.15.2 Chromatograms of a 10 ppb fortified catfish tissue sample followed simultaneously in the 588 nm channel and the fluorescence channel. From left to right on the chromatogram: leuco malachite green, leuco gentian violet, malachite green, and gentian violet. (Reprinted from Ref. 504, with permission from Elsevier Science.)

According to this method, a 20 g fish sample is homogenized with 20 ml 0.1 M ammonium acetate buffer, pH 4.5, 5 ml 0.05 M p-toluenesulfonic acid, and 3 ml 0.25 g/ml hydroxylamine. Following homogenization, 90 ml acetonitrile was added and the sample was homogenized again. Basic alumina (20 g) was then added, and the homogenate was centrifuged. The supernatant was subsequently partitioned against a mixture consisting of 100 ml water, 50 ml dichloromethane, and 2 ml diethylene glycol. The separated bottom layer was evaporated, and the remaining residue was reconstituted in a mixture of 2 ml dichloromethane and 5 ml acetonitrile to be loaded on an alumina cartridge placed on top of a propylsylfonic acid cartridge using a suitable adapter. Following columns washing with 3 × 5 ml acetonitrile, the alumina cartridge was discarded. The propylsulfonic acid cartridge was further washed with 2 ml water and 1 ml acetonitrile–0.1M ammonium acetate buffer (1:1). Elution of the analytes was effected using 2 ml acetonitrile–0.1M ammonium acetate buffer (1:1). Liquid chromatographic separation of the analytes was carried out under the conditions shown in Table 29.15 (Fig. 29.15.2).

The detection system consisted of a coulometric electrochemical cell preceded by a diode array detector followed in series by a fluorescence detector.

When the coulometric detector was turned on, both leuco forms were completely oxidized to their nonfluorescing chromatic forms and thus vanished from the fluorescence channel. This disappearance was balanced by the arrearance of their chromatic forms in the diode array channel. The confirmation of malachite green, gentian violet, and their leuco analogs in catfish and trout tissue could be based, therefore, on the correct retention times, the observation of the natural fluorescence of the leuco forms when the coulometric detector was turned off, the absence of the leuco form peaks in the 588 nm channel when the coulometric detector was off, the disappearance of the fluorescence of the leuco forms when the coulometric detector was on, the appearance of peaks of parent drugs formed by oxidation of the leuco forms in the 588-nm diode array channel, and the correct ultraviolet-visible spectra maxima for all four peaks.

A determinative liquid chromatographic method followed by a gas chromatographic–mass spectrometric procedure for confirming the identity of leucogentian violet in chicken fat was developed by Munns et al. (493) and Wilson et al. (492) for regulatory applications. According to this method, 10 g ground fat is melted at 35°C and extracted with a total of 50 ml dichloromethane in the presence of anhydrous sodium sulfate. Following filtering, the extract is partitioned against 10 ml 1N hydrochloric acid, and the dichloromethane layer that contains the fat matrix is discarded. The aqueous acid layer is neutralized by the addition of 10 ml saturated trisodium citrate solution. Leucogentian violet is reextracted with two portions of 25 ml dichloromethane. Dichloromethane is then evaporated, and the residue is reconstituted in an acetonitrile–water solution that is filtered before liquid chromatography using a cyano column, an acetate buffer–acetonitrile mobile phase, and an electrochemical detector. The extract remaining after liquid chromatographic analysis was employed for gas chromatography–mass spectrometry. A 1 ml portion of this extract was vortex-mixed with 2 ml toluene and centrifuged. The upper organic layer was evaporated, and the dried residue reconstituted with acetonitrile to be injected for chromatography–mass spectrometry analysis. Chromatographic separation was performed on a DB-1 30 m capillary column coated with methyl silicone. The column temperature was held at 150°C for 1 min, ramped at 16°C/min to 300°C, and held for 20 min. Other gas and liquid chromatographic conditions along with performance characteristics are presented in Table 29.15.

29.16 SEDATIVES AND β-BLOCKERS

Sedatives and β-blockers commonly used in food-producing animals include basic compounds with apolar (promazines and the β-blocker carazolol) or polar properties (xylazine, azaperone, and haloperidol).

In analyzing liquid samples such as serum and urine, diethyl ether (517–519) or chloroform (520) have been mainly employed for extraction of the

TABLE 29.15 Physicochemical Methods for Dye Drugs in Biological Matrices

Compound(s)	Matrix	Sample preparation	Steps	Stationary phase	Mobile phase	Detection/ Identification	Sensitivity/ Recovery	Ref.
GAS CHROMATOGRAPHIC METHODS								
Leucogentian violet	Chicken fat	DCM diln, Na_2SO_4 addn, liq–liq partns	22	DB-1, 30 m, capillary, coated with methyl silicone	Helium	EI-MS	5 ppb/ NR	492
LIQUID CHROMATOGRAPHIC METHODS								
Leucogentian violet	Chicken fat	DCM diln, Na_2SO_4 addn, liq–liq partns	16	Altech Cyano, 5 μm (for EC detection), Zorbax ODS, 5 μm, with Supelco LC-18-DB guard column (for UV detection)	Sodium acetate, pH 4.5, buffer/ ACN (50:50), for EC detection, amm. acetate, pH 4, buffer/ MeOH (10:90), for UV detection	Electro-chemical or UV 265 nm	5 ppb/ 59–103%	491
	Chicken fat	DCM diln, Na_2SO_4 addn, liq–liq partns	21	Alltech Cyano, 5 μm	0.1M, pH 4.5, acetate buffer contg 25 mg EDTA/ACN (50:50)	Electro-chemical	5 ppb/ 78–84%	493

	Sample	Extraction/cleanup		Column	Mobile phase	Detection	LOD/Recovery	Ref.
	Chicken fat	DCM diln, Na_2SO_4 addn, liq–liq partns	16	Zorbax ODS, 5 μm, with Supelco LC-18-DB guard column	Amm. acetate, pH 4, buffer/MeOH (10:90)	UV 265 nm	2 ppb/ 70–83%	494
Malachite green	Fish tissues	ACN/$CHCl_3$/HOAc extn, liq–liq partns	15	PLRP-S, 5 μm, analytical and guard column	0.02M H_3PO_4/ACN/THF (49:40:11)	Vis 615 nm	1–10 ppb/ 101–116%	505
Thionin	Milk	Ion pair/ACN extn, HCl hydrolysis, liq–liq partn	9	Phenomenex CN	Acetate, pH 4.5, buffer/ACN (50:50)	Vis 603 nm	5 ppb/ 56 ± 10%	497
Methylene blue	Catfish muscle	Ion pair/ACN extn, basic alumina addn, liq–liq partns, tandem SPE cleanup	19	Ultremex 5CN, 5 μm	Sodium acetate, pH 4.5, buffer/ACN (65:35) contg 50 mM p-TSA	Vis 660–665 nm	10 ppb/ 75–90%	496
Methylene blue and four metabolites	Milk	ACN extn, liq–liq partns, SPE cleanup	20	Alltech Econosil/CN, 5 μm	Sodium acetate, pH 4.5, buffer/ACN (50:50)	Vis 627 nm	5–20 ppb/ 23–84%	508
Acriflavine, proflavine	Catfish muscle	MeOH/HOAc extn, SPE cleanup	14	Ultremex 5CN, 5 μm, with Zorbax CN, 5 μm, guard column	Sodium acetate, pH 4.0, buffer/ACN (75:25)	Vis 454 nm	5 ppb/ 86–95%	507

(continued)

TABLE 29.15 Continued

Compound(s)	Matrix	Sample preparation	Steps	Stationary phase	Mobile phase	Detection/ Identification	Sensitivity/ Recovery	Ref.
Gentian violet, leucogentian violet	Catfish muscle	Ion pair/ACN extn, basic alumina addn, liq–liq partns, tandem SPE cleanup	22	Supelco LC-CN, 5 μm, with pellicular CN guard column	0.125M, pH 4.5, amm. acetate buffer/ACN (40 : 60) contg 0.1% TEA	Vis 588 nm, postcolumn oxidation with PbO_2	1 ppb/ 78–95%	498
Malachite green, leucomalachite green	Catfish muscle and plasma	Ion pair/ACN extn, alumina addn (muscle), liq–liq partns, tandem SPE cleanup	7–22	Ultremex 5CN, 5 μm	0.1M, pH 4.5, sodium acetate buffer, contg 5mM p-TSA/ ACN (50 : 50)	Vis 618 nm, postcolumn oxidation with PbO_2	2–10 ppb/ 83–100%	500
	Catfish muscle	Ion pair/ACN extn, basic alumina addn, liq–liq partns, tandem SPE cleanup	20	Ultracarb C_{18}, 5 μm	0.1M, pH 4.5, amm. acetate buffer/ACN (20 : 80)	EI-MS	20 ppb/ NR	501
	Catfish muscle	Ion pair/ACN extn, basic alumina addn, liq–liq partns, tandem SPE cleanup	19	Ultremex 5CN, 5 μm	0.1M, pH 4.5, sodium acetate buffer, contg 5mM p-TSA/ ACN (50 : 50)	Vis 618 nm, postcolumn oxidation with PbO_2	5 ppb/ 70–88%	502

Eel plasma	MeOH/citric/ascorbic acid extn, SPE cleanup	13	Chromspher B, 5 μm, with pellicular, 40 μm, guard column	0.025M, pH 4.0, acetate buffer, contg 25mM pentane-sulfonate and 50mM sodium perchlorate/ACN (40:60)	Vis 610 nm, postcolumn oxidation with PbO_2	1–5 ppb/ 79–89%	495
Rainbow trout	ACN/DCM/perchloric acid extn, SPE cleanup	9	Econosphere C_{18}, 5 μm	0.05M H_3PO_4/ACN (6:94) contg 10mM pentane-sulfonic acid	Vis 610 nm, postcolumn oxidation with EC detector cell	3–6 ppb/ 73–98%	506
Malachite green, gentian violet, and their leuco metabolites; Catfish and trout muscle	Ion pair/ACN extn, basic alumina addn, liq–liq partns, tandem SPE cleanup	19	SynChropak, 5 μm, with pellicular C_{18} guard column	0.01M, pH 3.6 amm. acetate buffer/ACN (45:55) contg 0.1% TEA	Vis 588 nm, postcolumn oxidation with PbO_2	0.5–3 ppb/ 49–90%	503

(continued)

TABLE 29.15 Continued

Compound(s)	Matrix	Sample preparation	Steps	Stationary phase	Mobile phase	Detection/ Identification	Sensitivity/ Recovery	Ref.
	Catfish and trout muscle	Ion pair/ACN extn, basic alumina addn, liq–liq partns, tandem SPE cleanup	19	Synchropak, 5 μm, with pellicular C$_{18}$ guard column	0.01M, pH 3.6 amm. acetate buffer/ACN (45:55) contg 0.1% TEA	Vis 588 nm, postcolumn oxidation with coulometric EC cell/ PDA (250–800 nm), and fluorometric, ex: 265 nm, em: 360 nm	10 ppb/ 49–90%	504
Gentian violet and three metabolites	Chicken tissues	Acetate buffer, pH 4.5/ACN extn, liq–liq partn, alumina column cleanup, liq–liq partns, carboxylic acid column cleanup	30	Alltech Cyano, 5 μm	0.1M, pH 4.5, acetate buffer contg 25 mg EDTA/ACN (50:50)	Electro-chemical	1 ppb/ 66–93%	499

p-TSA, p-toluenesulfonic acid; EC, electrochemical.
Other abbreviations as in Tables 29.1 and 29.3.

polar xylazine under alkaline or salting-out (518) conditions. In analyzing urine and plasma at alkaline conditions, hexane has also been used for extraction of promazines and xylazine (521), whereas hexane–methyl butanol mixture has been used for extraction of carazolol (522).

Semisolid samples, such as kidney, liver, and muscle, often require more intensive sample pretreatment. A favorite approach for tissue break-up appears to be the homogenization in acetonitrile (519, 523, 524) or in an acetone–sulfuric acid mixture (521). Using chloroform for extraction of xylazine and its main metabolite from kidney tissue, high recovery values were attained (525). However, prior alkaline hydrolysis of the incurred samples at 95°C was considered essential when diethyl ether was used for extraction of the β-blocker carazolol and seven sedatives from kidney tissue (526).

Purification of the primary sample extracts can be achieved by application of conventional liquid–liquid partitioning and/or solid-phase extraction procedures. Liquid–liquid partitioning cleanup is generally carried out at alkaline conditions using diethyl ether (517, 519) or hexane (521) as extraction solvents. The drugs are then back-extracted into dilute acid to be subsequently re-extracted into chloroform either at a high pH value (519) or in the presence of the pairing ion octane-1-sulfonate (517). Liquid–liquid partitioning cleanup resulted in good recovery of polar compounds such as xylazine (517, 519) and carazolol (522). As an alternative to classic liquid–liquid partitioning, use of an acidic Celite column has been suggested for improved cleanup of kidney homogenates that contained xylazine and its major metabolite (525).

In contrast to liquid–liquid partitioning cleanup, which is particularly suitable for individual drugs or groups of drugs with similar chemical properties, solid-phase extraction is more appropriate for multiresidue analysis. On that account, solid-phase extraction in combination with liquid–liquid partitioning has become the method of choice in many laboratories for the purification of residues of sedatives and β-blockers that may occur in biological matrices. Purification is usually accomplished on reversed-phase solid-phase extraction columns. Optimum retention of seven sedatives and carazolol on a reversed-phase solid-phase extraction column was reported when 10% sodium chloride solution was added to the acetonitrile tissue extract prior to its solid-phase extraction cleanup (523, 524). A silica-based diol solid-phase extraction column was further suggested for efficient isolation of sedative and β-blocker residues from food extracts (526).

Separation and detection of sedatives and the β-blocker carazolol can be carried out by either gas chromatography and flame ionization or flame photometric detection, or liquid chromatography followed by spectrophotometric, fluorometric, or electrochemical detection. Unfortunately, a limited number of relevant gas chromatographic methods have been available in the literature (519, 521), although derivatization is not needed for such analytes. Gas chromatographic separation has been carried out using packed or capillary columns, whereas detection has been performed using flame ionization (519) or flame photometric detectors (521).

Liquid chromatographic separation of sedatives and β-blockers is usually performed using reversed-phase columns. The preferred type of reversed-phase material is C_{18}-bonded silica (Table 29.16), but phenyl-bonded silica has also been employed for separation of xylazine and its major metabolite (525). Ionpair liquid chromatography has also been suggested for separation of carazolol and xylazine residues, by addition to the mobile phase of dodecyl sulfate (522) or heptanesulfonate (520) pairing ions, respectively.

Ultraviolet spectrophotometric detection can be carried out at wavelengths in the range 220–254 nm (517, 518, 520, 524, 525, 526). Fluorometric detection, which is particularly suitable for azaperol and carazolol, confers the advantages of selectivity and sensitivity. This mode of detection has been employed for the determination of carazolol residues in serum and plasma, using excitation and emission wavelengths at 330 and 360 nm, respectively (522). Fluorometric detection has also been applied to monitor carazolol and azaperol residues in swine kidney with excitation and emission wavelengths of 246 and 351 nm, respectively (524).

Electrochemical detection has also been further recommended as an excellent alternative for the determination of seven sedatives and carazolol in swine liver and kidney (523). In this study, significant selectivity and sensitivity improvements compared to existing methods have been reported.

Tentative confirmation of suspected liquid chromatographic peaks has been achieved in the analysis of carazolol and seven sedatives in swine kidney, by using photodiode-array detection in the wavelength range of 220–320 nm. It was reported (526) that further identification could be made possible if the corresponding fractions of the eluate were submitted off-line to two-dimensional thin-layer chromatography.

Most promising for surveillance purposes appears to be the method of Rose and Shearer (523), which actually combines the extraction procedure reported by Keukens and Aerts (524) and the high performance liquid chromatographic procedure proposed by van Ginkel et al. (526). This multiresidue method permits determination of azaperone and its metabolite azaperol, xylazine, haloperidol, acepromazine, propionylpromazine, chlorpromazine, and carazolol in swine liver and kidney. According to this method, a 5 g tissue sample is homogenized and extracted with two volumes of acetonitrile. Following centrifugation, 7.5 ml supernatant is mixed with 40 ml 10% sodium chloride solution, and subjected to cleanup by a Bond-Elut C_{18} solid-phase extraction cartridge. Following cartridge washing with 0.85 ml 0.01 M sulfuric acid, the analytes are eluted with 3.5 ml acidified acetonitrile. The eluate is evaporated to dryness, dissolved in 0.3 ml 0.01 M sulfuric acid, and extracted with 1 ml hexane. The mixture is centrifuged, the lower aqueous phase is isolated, and 50 μl is injected into the liquid chromato-

TABLE 29.16 Chromatographic Methods for Sedatives and β-Blockers in Biological Matrices

Compound(s)	Matrix	Sample preparation	Steps	Stationary phase	Mobile phase	Detection/ identification	Sensitivity/ recovery	Ref.
GAS CHROMATOGRAPHIC METHODS								
Xylazine	Animal tissues and serum	ACN (tissues) or ether (serum) extn, liq–liq partns	15–26	Supelcoport with 3% SP-2250 DB or 5% SP-2401 DB or 20 m, capillary, coated with SP-1000	Helium	FID	4–5 ppb/ 93–100%	519
Four sedatives	Meat, urine, plasma	Acetone/H_2SO_4 (meat) or hexane (plasma, urine) extn, liq–liq partns	7–10	Chromosorb W HP with 3% OV-1	Nitrogen	FPD	NR/ 50–100%	521
LIQUID CHROMATOGRAPHIC METHODS								
Carazolol	Swine serum and plasma	Hexane/2-methyl-2-butanol extn, liq–liq partn	5	Hypersil ODS, 5 μm, with C_{18} guard column	0.1M, pH 4.5, amm. acetate buffer/PrOH/ ACN/SDS (61:25:14:0.05)	Fluorometric, ex: 330 nm, em: 360 nm	0.6 ppb/ 94 ± 1.5%	522
Xylazine	Blood	Ether extn	5	μBondapak C_{18}	0.001M HCl/ACN/ MeOH (30:65:5)	UV 254 nm	5 ppb/ 91–100%	518
Xylazine	Plasma	$CHCl_3$ extn	4	μBondapak C_{18}, 10 μm	H_2OMeOH/ heptanesulfonic acid (55:45:0.2) contg 2% HOAc, pH 3.5	UV 225 nm	20 ppb/ 76 ± 3.4%	520

(continued)

TABLE 29.16 Chromatographic Methods for Sedatives and β-Blockers in Biological Matrices

Compound(s)	Matrix	Sample preparation	Steps	Stationary phase	Mobile phase	Detection/ identification	Sensitivity/ recovery	Ref.
Xylazine, 2,6-dimethylaniline (xylazine metabolite)	Sheep and cattle plasma	Ether extn, liq-liq partn, ion-pair extn	8	Nucleosil 120, C$_{18}$, 5 μm	0.02N H$_3$PO$_4$/ACN (55:45), at 35°C	UV 220 nm	3 ppb/97–103%	517
	Bovine and swine kidney	CHCl$_3$ extn, celite column cleanup	22	μBondapak phenyl, 10 μm	H$_2$O/ACN/2M sodium acetate/1M HOAc (64:32::2:2)	UV 225 nm	25 ppb/75–97%	525
Carazolol, seven sedatives	Swine kidney	ACN extn, SPE cleanup, liq-liq partn	13	μBondapak C$_{18}$, with Bondapak C$_{18}$, 37–50 μm, guard column	Sodium acetate/ACN (45:55), pH 6.5	UV 240 nm, Fluorometric, ex: 246 nm, em: 351 nm	0.3–6 ppb/52–101%	524
Carazolol, seven sedatives	Swine kidney	NaOH soln addn, 95°C incubation, ether extn, SPE cleanup, liq-liq partn	16	SAS-Hypersil, 5 μm, with Chromquard guard column	H$_2$O/ACN/1M amm. acetate (54.5:44.5:1)	UV 235 nm/PDA (220–320 nm) & two-dimensional TLC	1–10 ppb/31–64%	526
Carazolol, seven sedatives	Swine liver and kidney	ACN extn, SPE cleanup, liq-liq partn	13	SAS-Hypersil C$_1$, 5 μm, analytical and guard column	0.02M amm. acetate/ACN (50:50)	Electro-chemical	2 ppb/62–90%	523

FPD, flame-photometric detector.
Other abbreviations as in Tables 29.1 and 29.3.

graphic system. Separation is performed on a 25-cm SAS Hypersil C_1 (5 μm) analytical column, protected by a SAS Hypersil C_1 quard column, with a mobile phase of 0.02M ammonium acetate–acetonitrile (50:50), at a flow rate of 2 ml/min (Fig. 29.16). Using electrochemical detection, concentrations as low as 2 ppb of each analyte could be readily analyzed.

29.17 CORTICOSTEROIDS

Corticosteroids potentially used in food-producing animals include a variety of compounds such as cortisone, cortisol, prednisone, prednisolone, methylprednisolone, betamethasone, dexamethasone, flumethasone, fluoroprednisolone, isoflupredone, and triamcinolone. Corticosteroid administration to feedlots as growth-promoting agents has been recently introduced illicitly in animal production because of their ability to promote water retention in the body. This use has been strongly enhanced for commercial reasons, in order to produce meat more appealing to consumers, due to the juicy and lean look. It is therefore crucial to rely on accurate, sensitive and specific analytical methods to measure residues in biological samples.

Very few methods have appeared in the literature with respect to the extraction, cleanup, and subsequent determination of corticosteroids in food samples (Table 29.17). Milk analysis usually requires a pretreatment step for fat elimination (527). Centrifugation for 20 min at about 7000 g at 4°C is the usually applied procedure for making the fat floating on the top of the sample. Tissue analysis also requires a pretreatment step for matrix break-up that can be accomplished by means of a mincing and/or a homogenizing apparatus.

When analyzing liver or urine for residues of corticosteroids, enzymatic hydrolysis of glucuronide and sulfate conjugates using β-glucuronidase/sulfatase prior to sample extraction is often recommended (527, 528). One of the major problems with the enzymatic hydrolysis is the slowness of the enzymatic reaction, which is a major concern in routine analysis. However, in certain situations, the hydrolysis process can be substantially speeded up by utilizing higher temperatures or prolonged incubation (527, 528). When extraction of the analytes is to be carried out by supercritical fluid extraction, homogenization of the tissue samples into a smooth paste that is then submitted to freeze drying is the recommended procedure (448).

Sample extraction and deproteinization is usually accomplished with non-polar organic solvents at a specified pH. Organic solvents such as chloroform for the determination of cortisol in milk (529); dichloromethane/hexane (4:1) for the determination of free cortisol and its 21-acetate in milk (530); ethyl acetate for the determination of prednisolone, fluoroprednisolone, triamcinolone, and betamethasone in animal tissues (531); methylprednisolone in milk (532); fluoroprednisolone in milk (533); and dexamethasone in milk (534); ethyl acetate in

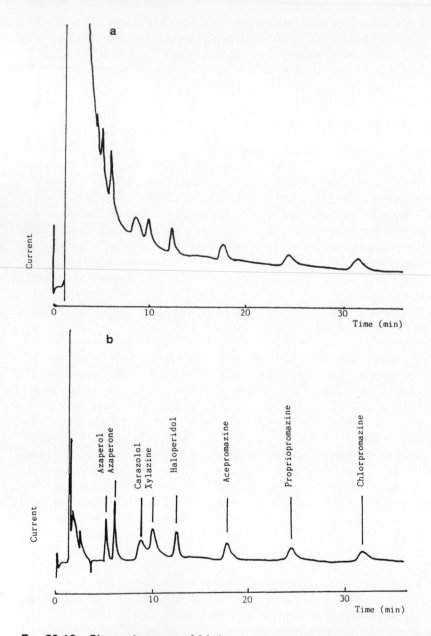

Fɪɢ. **29.16** Chromatograms of (a) tissue extract spiked with seven sedatives and carazolol at 2 ppb and (b) mixed standard equivalent to 2 ppb. (Reprinted from Ref. 523, with permission from Elsevier Science.)

TABLE 29.17 Physicochemical Methods for Corticosteroids, Thyreostatics, Diuretics and Non-Steroidal Anti-Inflammatory Drugs in Biological Matrices

Compound(s)	Matrix	Sample preparation	Steps	Stationary phase	Mobile phase	Detection/ Identification	Sensitivity/ Recovery	Ref.
THIN-LAYER CHROMATOGRAPHIC METHODS								
Six thyreostatics	Thyroid gland	MeOH extn, mercurated affinity column cleanup, derivatization with NBD-Cl, liq–liq partns	16	HPTLC Silica gel	DCM/MeOH & DCM/ propionic acid	Fluorometric/ alkaline cysteine, MS-MS-ESP	25–100 ppb/ NR	616
GAS CHROMATOGRAPHIC METHODS								
Indomethacin	Ovine plasma and urine	EtOAc extn, derivatization with MTBSTFA (tBDMS derivative)	9	HP Ultra-2, 25 m, capillary, coated with 5% phenyl-methyl silicone	Hydrogen	ECD/EI-MS	1 ppb/ 84–105%	589
Thiouracil, methylthiouracil, propylthiouracil	Bovine urine	MeOH extn, mercurated affinity column cleanup, methyl iodide methylation, liq–liq partn	12	Chrompack, 25 m, capillary coated with CP-Sil-8 CB or CP Sil-5 CB	Helium	NPD/SIM-MS	25 ppb/ NR	617
Five corticosteroids	Bovine muscle	MeOH extn, liq–liq partns, two SPE cleanups, derivatization with MSTFA (TMS derivatives)	24	BPX-5, 30 m, capillary, with deactivated fused-silica guard column	Helium	EI-MS	0.1 ppb/ 55–81%	452

(continued)

TABLE 29.17 Continued

Compound(s)	Matrix	Sample preparation	Steps	Stationary phase	Mobile phase	Detection/ Identification	Sensitivity/ Recovery	Ref.
Five corticosteroids	Bovine milk, liver, urine, feces	Centrgn (milk), β-glucuronidase hydrolysis, ACN (liver) ether (feces) extn, liq–liq partn (liver, feces), SPE cleanup, IAC cleanup, derivatization with pyridinium chlorochromate, liq–liq partn	26–33	HP5 MS, 30 m, capillary	Helium	NICI-MS	0.5 ppb/ 60–75%	527
Five thyreostatics	Bovine muscle	ACN extn, liq–liq partns, anion exchange column cleanup, on column methyl iodide methylation	18	HP Ultra 2, 25 m, capillary coated with 5% Ph-Me silicone	Helium	SIM-MS	15–25 ppb/ 51–90%	620
Six thyreostatics	Thyroid gland	NaOH extn, pentafluorobenzyl derivative, liq–liq partns, SPE cleanup, derivatization with MSTFA (TMS derivatives)	20	HP-1, 30 m, capillary	Helium	NICI-MS or PICI-MS	5 ppb/ 40–71%	621

Analyte	Sample	Sample preparation	Column no.	Column	Mobile phase/carrier	Detection	LOD/Recovery	Ref.
Seven anti-inflammatory drugs	Equine plasma and urine	DCM extn, derivatization with BSTFA (TMS derivatives)	4	Econocap SE-54, 30 m, capillary	Helium	EI-MS	20–50 ppb/ 97–107%	597
Seventeen anti-inflammatory drugs	Equine plasma and urine	Ether extn, liq–liq partn, methyl iodide methylation	7–10	HP, 25 m, capillary, coated with methyl silicone	Helium	EI-MS	5–25 ppb/ 23–100%	596
LIQUID CHROMATOGRAPHIC METHODS								
Dexamethasone	Bovine tissues	β-Glucuronidase hydrolysis, ACN extn, liq–liq partn, purification by on-line sample cleanup on Spherisorb phenyl-silica, 3 μm, subsequent trace enrichment on silica, 5 μm, prconcn column and switching to analytical column	10	Spherisorb cyanopropyl-silica, 3 μm	H_2O/HOAc/PrOH/hexane (0.1:0.1:12.8:87), at 30°C	UV 239 nm/ GC-EI-MS after derivatization with BSA	4–6 ppb/ 66–75%	528
	Bovine tissues	Lyophilization, SFE (CO_2) cleanup	5	Supelcosil, 5 μm	0.02M amm. formate/ MeOH/ ACN (50:50) Gradient from (95:5) to (5:95)	MS-APCI	100 ppb/ 57 ± 14%	448

(continued)

TABLE 29.17 Continued

Compound(s)	Matrix	Sample preparation	Steps	Stationary phase	Mobile phase	Detection/ Identification	Sensitivity/ Recovery	Ref.
	Bovine tissues	NaOH addn, EtOAc (tissues) or ether (fat) extn, liq–liq partns, SPE cleanup	22	Nova Pak C_{18}, 4 μm, with μBondapak guard column	H_2O/ACN/TEA (72:28:0.02)	UV 254 nm	10 ppb/ 72–116%	535
Flunixin	Equine urine	pH adjustment at 7.0, SPE cleanup	14	Hypersil SI, 5 μm, or Hypersil ODS, 5 μm	Isopropanol, contg 5% H_2O/ hexane Step gradient from (2:98) to (100:0), at 45°C or 1% HOAc/ ACN Isocratic (70:30) for 2 min and gradient to (0:100)	EI-MS-NICI-MS, PICI-MS, or MS-ESP	10 ppb/ 83–94%	582
	Milk	β-Glucuronidase hydrolysis, MSPD extn/ cleanup, liq–liq partns, SPE cleanup	16	Hypersil ODS, 5 μm, analytical and guard column	0.002M NaOH contg 5 mM tetrabutyl-ammonium hydrogen sulfate/MeOH (42:58), at 45°C	UV 285 nm/GC-EI-MS after methyl iodide methylation	1.7 ppb/ 70–74%	604

Drug	Matrix	Sample prep		Column	Mobile phase	Detection	LOD/Recovery	Ref
Furosemide	Milk	Centrgn, ACN extn	5	PRP-1, 5 μm, analytical and guard column	0.05M, pH 3, potassium phosp. buffer/ACN (70:30), at 35°C	Fluorometric, ex: 272 nm, em: 410 nm	5 ppb/ 95 ± 9%	556
Indomethacin	Chicken tissues	DCM extn	5	Spherisorb ODS-2, 5 μm	0.5% HOAc/ACN (50:50)	UV 254 nm	20 ppb/ 63–100%	601
Phenylbutazone	Milk	EtOH/NH$_4$OH extn, liq–liq partns	9	Ultracarb 5 ODS, with Supelcosil LC-18DB guard column	0.02M sodium phosp. buffer/MeOH (50:50), at 35°C	UV 264 nm	5.4 ppb/ 79–84%	602
Trichlormethiazide	Milk	Centrgn, lead acetate addn, ACN extn, liq–liq partns	9	PRP-1, 5 μm, analytical and guard column	0.05M, pH 3, potassium phosp. buffer/ACN (70:30), at 35°C	UV 225 nm	5 ppb/ 88–117%	559
Chlorothiazide, hydrochloro-thiazide	Milk	Centrgn, lead acetate addn, ACN extn, liq–liq partns	9	PRP-1, 5 μm, analytical and guard column	0.05M, pH 3, potassium phosp. buffer/THF/ACN (50:43:7), at 30°C	UV 225 mm	~22 ppb/ 87–99%	558

(continued)

TABLE 29.17 Continued

Compound(s)	Matrix	Sample preparation	Steps	Stationary phase	Mobile phase	Detection/ Identification	Sensitivity/ Recovery	Ref.
Phenylbutazone, oxyphenbutazone	Equine plasma	Phosp. buffer diln, SPE cleanup	8	Hypersil C_{18}, 5 μm	0.01M HOAc, contg 0.01% heptanesulfonic acid/ MeOH (40:60), at 40°C	UV 240 nm/PDA (230–350 nm), GC-MS after derivatization with MSTFA	1 ppm/ 43–63%	581
Five thyreostatics	Bovine plasma	EtOAc/EDTA extn	3	LiChrosorb RP-18, 10 μm, with LiChroprep RP-18 guard column	0.025M, pH 3, phosp. buffer/ MeOH Gradient from (90:10) to (30:70)	UV 276 nm & 258 nm	200 ppb/ 57–87%	625
Five thyreostatics	Urine, thyroid tissue	EDTA/2-mercaptoethanol addn, EtOAc/ Na_2SO_4 extn, SPE cleanup	13	Prodigy ODS3	Solvent A: 0.1% HFB Solvent B: H_2O/ MeOH (45:55) contg 0.1% HFB Gradient from (95:5) to (5:95)	PICI-MS-APCI	25 ppb/ 42–111%	626

| Seven anti-inflammatory drugs | Equine plasma and urine | DCM extn | 3 | Supelcosil LC-8, 3 μm | 0.05M H_3PO_4/ACN (55:45) | UV 235 nm and fluorometric ex: 235 nm, em: 405 nm/ PDA (209–402 nm) | 10–150 ppb/ 97–113% | 597 |
| Nine anti-inflammatory drugs | Plasma | HCl hydrolysis, SPE cleanup | 10 | Inertsil ODS II, 5 μm, analytical and guard column | 0.1M, pH 3, HOAc/ACN Gradient from (80:20) to (36:64), at 40°C | UV 240, 278 and 290 nm/PDA (240–400 mm) | 50 ppb/ 39–111% | 598 |

NBD-Cl, 7-chloro-4-nitrobenzo-2-oxa-1,3-diazole; MSTFA, N-methyl-N-(trimethylsilyl)trifluoroacetamide; BSA, N, O-bis(trimethylsilyl)acetamide; MTBSTFA, N-methyl-N-(tetr.-butyldimethylsilyl)trifluoroacetamide; BSTFA, N,O-bis(trimethylsilyl)trifluoroacetamide; HFB, heptafluorobutyric acid; SFE, supercritical-fluid extraction. Other abbreviations as in Tables 29.1 and 29.3.

presence of 0.1N sodium hydroxide for the determination of dexamethasone in bovine tissues (535); methanol for the determination of five corticosteroids in bovine muscle (452); acetonitrile for the determination of five synthetic cortico-steroids in bovine liver (527); and dexamethasone in bovine tissues (528); ethyl ether for the determination of nine synthetic corticosteroids in bovine feces (527); dichloromethane for the determination of fluoroprednisolone in animal fat (533); and acetone for the determination of fluoroprednisolone in animal liver, kidney, and muscle (533), have all been used with varying success for extraction of corticosteroid residues from biological samples. Extraction of corticosteroids from milk or urine samples can also be accomplished by simple dilution with water or acetate buffer (527).

To eliminate or reduce interference and concentrate the analyte(s), the pri-mary sample extract can further be subjected to various types of cleanup proce-dures including liquid–liquid partitioning, solid-phase extraction, immunoaffinity chromatography, and column-switching techniques (Table 29.17). In some in-stances, more than one of these procedures may be used in combination to enhance the cleanup efficiency.

Liquid–liquid partitioning cleanup may vary from a simple one-step solvent extraction to complicated back-extraction in other solvents. Generally, the type of extraction and amount of sample cleanup is determined by the efficiency and the selectivity of the chromatographic technique used for the analysis. The more specific and efficient the chromatographic system, the less sample extraction and cleanup are necessary to obtain the desired results. Sometimes the liquid–liquid partitioning steps are necessary to improve the sensitivity of the assay method by concentrating the analyte. The liquid–liquid partitioning methods eliminate most of the sample proteins and appropriate washes with sodium hydroxide also eliminate many of the interfering phenolic estrogens present in biological samples.

As an example, evaporated extracts with residues of methylprednisolone can be cleaned up by partitioning between hexane and acetonitrile, and then between hexane and water saturated with sodium sulfate, and finally into dichloro-methane (532). Evaporated extracts with residues of fluoroprednisolone can be cleaned up by partitioning between acetonitrile and hexane, then between hexane and water, and finally into dichloromethane (533). Ethyl acetate extracts with residues of prednisolone, fluoroprednisolone, triamcinolone, and betamethasone can be cleaned up by successive washing with aqueous acid and base to remove impurities (531). Ethyl acetate extracts containing residues of dexamethasone can be efficiently cleaned up by washing with aqueous sodium hydroxide (535).

In addition, residues of corticosteroids can be cleaned up through applica-tion of a three-phase liquid–liquid partition system consisting of acetonitrile, hexane, and dichloromethane. Since its inception, this procedure has been used successfully to perform a fast, crude fractionation of tissue components and drugs extracted from tissue homogenates into the aqueous acetonitrile supernatant. Nonpolar components partition into the hexane layer, polar and ionic components partition into the bottom aqueous layer, and corticosteroids along with other components of the tissue partition into the middle acetonitrile layer (527, 528).

Cleanup and concentration of corticosteroids from coextracted matrix constituents can also be accomplished using solid-phase extraction cartridges that contain nonpolar C_{18} (527, 535), or C_8 sorbents (452), as shown in Table 29.17. In addition, C_{18} cartridges have been used to extract endogenous and synthetic corticosteroids from swine plasma (536), and to isolate cortisol from plasma or serum samples (537). Other workers employed conventional columns containing deactivated Florisil to isolate cortisol in milk (529) or fluoroprednisolone in bovine tissues (533).

Immunoaffinity chromatography and column-switching techniques are alternative cleanup procedures in corticosteroid analysis. The former technique has been recently shown to improve tremendously the gas chromatographic–mass spectrometric profile of nine corticosteroid residues in different matrices including liver, milk, urine and feces; the combination of two antibodies facilitated the extraction and purification of almost all analytes (527). The combined use of immunoaffinity chromatography with gas chromatography–negative ion chemical ionization mass spectrometry has been described as a means of confirming flumethasone abuse in equines (538).

In addition, column-switching between three columns coupled together for sample cleanup, concentration of analyte, and analytical separation proved to be a rugged, automated means of isolating dexamethasone from bovine tissues (528). The analyte, along with co-eluting matrix components, was heart-cut from the first, phenyl-silica, column and collected on a second, silica, column. The second column was then backflushed with a stronger eluent onto the third, cyanopropyl-silica, column where the analyte was finally resolved from matrix components.

Supercritical fluid extraction, offers also some desirable advantages including processing at low temperature, recovery of a solvent-free extract, and rapid extraction. However, very limited studies have been published on the use of supercritical fluids for the isolation of corticosteroids from biological samples. A combination of supercritical fluid extraction and liquid chromatography has been employed for the detection of dexamethasone residues in bovine tissues (448).

Following extraction and cleanup, corticosteroid residues in sample extracts can be determined by thin-layer, liquid, or gas chromatographic methods. Spectrophotometric, fluorometric, electron capture, or mass spectrometric detection systems have all been successfully used in corticosteroids analysis.

Early applications of thin-layer chromatography in corticosteroid analysis were mainly based on use of phenylhydrazine in sulfuric acid as a spray reagent for derivatization of the analytes (529, 530). Later applications involved use of other spray reagents including phosphoric acid in methanol, tetrazolium blue,

p-toluenesulfonic acid, and 2,3,5-triphenyl-2H-tetrazolium chloride (539–542). Recently, a high-performance thin-layer chromatographic system was developed for screening injection sites for the presence of 29 corticosteroids (543). The development of the analytes on preloaded Kieselgel 60 plates with chloroform–methanol and their derivatization with a resorcylaldehyde spray yielded the best separation, color differentiation, and fluorescence at 366 nm for several analytes. The major drawback of these method is that they are not sensitive enough for regulatory purposes, and they are rather complicated by the need for derivatization.

Over the past 10 years, liquid chromatography coupled with ultraviolet detection appears to have become the method of choice for the determination of corticosteroids, offering the analyst both satisfactory selectivity and sensitivity. Both reversed-phase (544–547) and normal-phase (548) chromatography have been applied to the determination of dexamethasone in plasma, coupled with ultraviolet (UV) detection generally at 254 nm, and in bovine tissues (528, 535). A series of both reversed- and normal phase LC systems have also been used for the simultaneous determination of dexamethasone and other steroids. Two different liquid chromatographic separations have been described for the isolation and simultaneous separation of steroids in serum (549).

Normal-phase liquid chromatography was required for the separation of prednisone from cortisol when prednisone treatment was indicated. This strategy for the separation of steroids was applied to the determination of a number of steroids in the thymus, using a combination of anionic and C_{18} extraction cartridges for cleanup and concentration of samples (550). Goto et al. (551) also used a normal-phase chromatographic system to separate dexamethasone and cortisol in serum simultaneously. This method involves precolumn derivatization with 9-anthroylnitrile and final detection using a fluorescence spectrophotometer. A combination of solid-phase extraction cartridges was used to eliminate the unused reagent and for cleanup of the steroids in serum. In addition, normal-phase liquid chromatography has been reported for the simultaneous assay of cortisol, cortisone, dexamethasone, prednisolone, prednisone, and methyl prednisolone in plasma, with a lower limit of detection at 10 ppb (536). Confirmatory analysis of suspected liquid chromatographic peaks can be made possible by coupling liquid chromatography (LC) with mass spectrometry (MS) Atmospheric–pressure chemical ionization LC–MS has been employed for the identification of dexamethasone in bovine tissues (448). Confirmation of the suspected liquid chromatographic peaks in dexamethasone analysis has also been made by converting the analytes to the corresponding TMS–enol–TMS derivatives and analyzing them by gas chromatography–mass spectrometry (528).

Most early gas-chromatographic methods for corticosteroid analysis in foods involved use of an OV-17 275 cm column at high temperature and an electron capture detector for separation of the analytes in form of their TMS derivatives (531, 533). As an example, prednisolone, fluoroprednisolone, triamcinolone, and betamethasone residues required silylation with a mixture of N,O-bis(trimethylsilyl)acetamide, trimethylsilylimidazole, and trimethylchlorosilane at room temperature to give a single substance in all cases (531). The derivatization of all the oxygen functions with the silylation mixture obviated the protection of the C-3 and C-20 ketones. More recent methods are based on capillary columns and mass spectrometric detection. A TMS–enol–TMS derivative has been suggested for the analysis of dexamethasone (528), whereas derivatives oxidized with pyridinium chlorochromate for the analysis of several corticosteroids (527). In the latter case, the final derivative was a thermally stable trione that favored the generation of abundant ionic species and hence sensitivity in the selected ion recording mode.

A favorable screening, determinative, and confirmatory method for analyzing five corticosteroids including prednisolone, methylprednisolone, dexamethasone, flumethasone, and isoflupredone in liver, milk, urine, and feces has recently been described by Delahaut et al. (527). Milk extraction is performed by submitting a 10 ml milk sample to centrifugation at 4°C. The floating fat is eliminated, and the residual skimmed milk is diluted with an equivalent volume of water to be loaded on a C_{18} cartridge for cleanup. For liver extraction, a 5 g sample is homogenized in a mixture of 10 ml acetate buffer and *Helix pomatia* juice to be then incubated at 60°C for 2 h. After this hydrolysis step, the homogenate is extracted with 20 ml acetonitrile, centrifuged, and the supernatant is mixed with 8 ml hexane and 2 ml dichloromethane. Following shaking and centrifugation, the middle layer is collected, evaporated, and the residual is reconstituted in 1 ml ethanol, pending loading on the C_{18} cartridge for further cleanup. For urine extraction, a 5 ml sample is mixed with 2 ml of a pH 4.8 acetate buffer and *Helix pomatia* juice, and incubated overnight at 37°C. A 5 ml volume of phosphate-buffered saline is added to the incubate prior to its loading on the C_{18} cartridge. Feces extraction is performed by mixing vigorously a 5 g sample with 10 ml acetate buffer and 35 ml ethyl ether. After centrifugation, the ether layer is evaporated and the solid residue is dissolved in 3 ml ethanol to be further mixed with 12 ml water and 5 ml hexane. Hexane and solid material are removed by aspiration, and the aqueous layer is collected pending loading on the C_{18} cartridge for further cleanup.

Solid-phase extraction for milk, urine, and feces samples is carried out by washing the loaded C_{18} cartridge successively with 5 ml water, 5 ml acetone/water (20:80), 5 ml methanol/water (20:80), 5 ml dichloromethane/hexane (20:80), and 5 ml ethyl acetate/hexane (10:90). The corticosteroids are eluted with 3 ml ethyl acetate. The eluate is evaporated, and the residual is reconstituted in 0.5 ml ethanol and 5 ml phosphate-buffered saline, pending subsequent immunoaffinity column cleanup. The solid-phase extraction procedure differs for liver samples. In that case, washing of the cartridge is performed with 5 ml water, 5

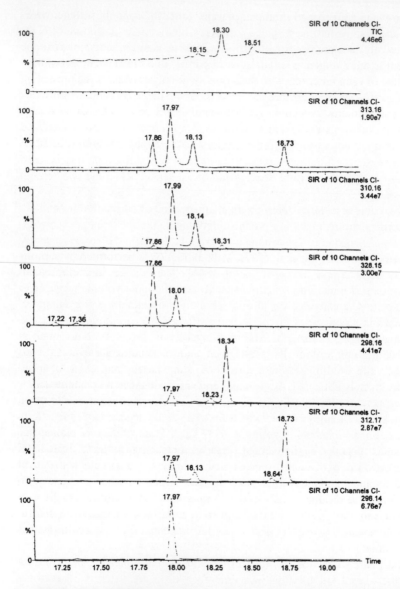

Fɪɢ. 29.17 TIC and SIR recordings collected from blank and spiked milk samples with 2 ppb of the various tested corticosteroids. From top to bottom: total ionic current; m/z 313, t_R: 17:97/18:13 min for dexamethasone $^2H_3$ (IS); m/z 310, t_R: 17:99/18:14 min for dexamethasone; m/z 328, t_R: 17:86/18:01 min for flumethasone; m/z 298, t_R: 18:34 min for prednisolone; m/z 312, t_R: 18:73 min for methylprednisolone; m/z 296, t_R: 17:97 min for isoflupredone. (Reprinted from Ref. 527, with permission from Elsevier Science.)

ml acetone-water (20:80), 5 ml methanol/water (20:80), and 5 ml hexane, while elution is carried out with 1 ml ethyl acetate.

Following solid-phase extraction, all extracts are adjusted in the pH range 7–7.5, and submitted to additional cleanup on an immunoaffinity column containing a mixture of dexamethasone- and prednisolone-specific gels. Column washing is performed with water, while elution of the analytes with 3 ml methanol/water (80:20). Aliquots of the eluates are submitted to oxidative reaction with pyridinium chlorochromate, and the oxidized corticosteroid derivatives are then analyzed by gas chromatography–mass spectrometry under the conditions shown in Table 29.17 (Fig. 29.17).

29.18 DIURETICS AND NONSTEROIDAL ANTI-INFLAMMATORY DRUGS

Diuretics are therapeutic agents used in certain pathological conditions to eliminate bodily fluids. Furosemide and the thiazide diuretics, chlorothiazide, hydrochlorothiazide, and trichlormethiazide are approved for use in dairy cattle for treatment of postparturient edema of the mammary gland and associated structures. The potential misuse of these diuretic drugs in cattle could lead to unacceptable residues in meat or milk destined for human consumption. Therefore, analytical methods sufficiently sensitive to monitor residue concentration levels in foods are valuable in preventing unapproved use of diuretics.

In determining diuretic residues in foods, it is often necessary to know their physicochemical characteristics. In general, the diuretics are soluble in methanol, ethanol, and water with the exception of hydrochlorothiazide that is insoluble in water (552, 553). Furosemide, which is a strongly acidic o-chlorosulfonamide compound, is the least stable among these diuretics. Its degradation proceeds with both a hydrolysis and a photochemical oxidation process. The major product generated is 4-chloro-5-sulfamoylanthranilic acid, which is further converted into 4-chloro-5-sulfoanthranilic acid. Acid hydrolysis of the furosemide also gives 4-chloro-5-sulfamoylanthranilic acid and furfuryl alcohol. Chlorothiazide, hydrochlorothiazide, and trichlormethiazide are all characterized by two ultraviolet absorbance maxima at 225 and 270 nm, whereas furosemide exhibits a natural fluorescence with excitation and emission wavelengths at 272 and 410 nm, respectively.

Extensive literature reviews (554, 555) have indicated that almost all reported analytical methods for the analysis of diuretics employ liquid chromatography. Most of these methods are limited, however, to assaying diuretics in urine and plasma. With the exception of a liquid chromatographic method for the determination of furosemide, another one for chlormethiazide, and a third method for chlorothiazide and hydrochlorothiazide residues in bovine milk, no chromatographic method has been reported in the literature for assaying diuretics in meat (Table 29.17).

In 1995, a liquid chromatographic method was reported for the determination of furosemide in bovine milk (556). This method involves a defatting step by milk centrifugation followed by deproteinization by acetonitrile. Following centrifugation, the supernatant is collected, acetonitrile is evaporated, and the remaining aqueous layer is directly analyzed by liquid chromatography. Separation is performed on a reversed-phase column using an isocratic phosphate–acetonitrile mobile phase, whereas detection by fluorescence at excitation and emission wavelengths of 272 and 410 nm, respectively. Performance characteristics were 95% for recovery, 9% for precision, and 3 ppb for the limit of detection.

The furosemide extraction procedure was later examined for potential application in the analysis of thiazide diuretics in milk. Since this procedure could not provide sufficiently clean extracts for thiazides, additional acidic and basic extraction procedures were evaluated (557). Thus, milk was deproteinized with trichloroacetic acid, phosphoric acid, or potassium dihydrogen phosphate and centrifuged. The supernatants were extracted with ethyl acetate, evaporated to dryness, reconstituted in mobile phase, and analyzed by liquid chromatography. The recoveries in most cases were low and widely variable. Basic extraction, on the other hand, with sodium bicarbonate/potassium carbonate mixture or potassium monohydrogen phosphate followed by extraction with ethyl acetate also gave poor recoveries in most cases. It appears that a significant degradation of chlorothiazide occurred under the basic conditions.

Solid-phase extraction was also evaluated for its potential to achieve the desired cleanup. Either C_{18} or C_8 cartridges were loaded with defatted and deproteinized milk extracts, washed with water or water–methanol, and elution of the analytes was performed with methanol (553). The recoveries in this case were also poor. These results of poor recovery for solid-phase extraction and both acidic and basic extractions are consistent with those reported in the literature (553, 557).

Much better results were obtained when lead acetate and sodium tungstate were employed in the cleanup procedure. The former is well known for its ability to precipitate pigments and a number of amino acids, whereas the latter is capable of binding with alkaloids and other products entering the milk, possibly through the diet.

On the basis of the above observations, a common extraction and cleanup procedure was developed and applied in two recently reported liquid chromatographic methods for the determination of either chlorothiazide and hydrochlorothiazide (558) or chlormethiazide (559) in bovine milk. Both of these methods involve a defatting step by milk centrifugation. The defatted milk (4.75 ml) is mixed with 2 ml 5% lead acetate solution and extracted with 9 ml acetonitrile. Following centrifugation, the supernatant is extracted with 25 ml water-saturated ethyl acetate and centrifuged. A portion of about 27–30 ml of the organic layer is removed, mixed with 4 ml 10% sodium tungstate solution, and centrifuged. A portion of about 25–27 ml of the organic layer is removed, evaporated to dryness, and reconstituted in 0.25–1.0 ml mobile phase to be analyzed by liquid chromatography (Fig. 29.18.1).

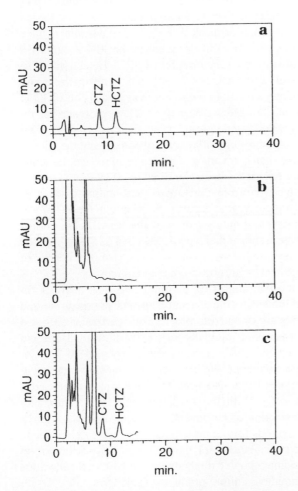

FIG. 29.18.1   Liquid chromatograms of (a) 50 ng each chlorothiazide (CTZ) and hydrochlorothiazide (HCTZ) standards, (b) control milk sample, and (c) 70 ng/ml fortified milk extract. (Reprinted with permission from Ref. 558. Copyright 1998 American Chemical Society.)

For chlorothiazide and hydrochlorothiazide analysis, separation is performed on a reversed-phase polymer PRP-I column using a mobile phase consisting of a 1:1 ratio of 14% acetonitrile/tetrahydrofuran in 0.05M potassium phosphate buffer of pH 3. Detection is carried out with a variable-wavelength detector set at 225 nm. Performance evaluation showed that recoveries were 97 and 89% for chlorothiazide and hydrochlorothiazide, respectively, with average precision of 6 and 5% for chlorothiazide and hydrochlorothiazide, respectively. The limit of detection and the limit of quantification were estimated to be 22 and 35 ppb, respectively, for both chlorothiazide and hydrochlorothiazide.

For trichlormethiazide analysis, separation is performed on a similar column using a mobile phase consisting of either 30% acetonitrile or 30% acetonitrile/tetrahydrofuran in 0.05M potassium phosphate buffer of pH 3. Detection is also carried out with a variable-wavelength detector set at 225 nm. Performance evaluation showed an average recovery of 101%, with an average precision of 13%.

The **nonsteroidal anti-inflammatory drugs** (NSAIDs) represent a heterogeneous group of compounds widely used in human and veterinary medicine for their ability either to suppress or reduce the inflammatory process and the clinical signs associated with it. These agents are often chemically unrelated, although most of them are organic acids. NSAIDs can be identified in salicylic acid derivatives, propionic acid derivatives, pyrazole derivatives, and aniline derivatives including nicotinic acid and anthranilic acid derivatives. Although the EU procedure for assigning maximum residue limits for most of the NSAIDs has not yet been completed, it can rightly be assumed that a permanent ban might be imposed on certain NSAIDs such as phenylbutazone, requiring more stringent control of a possible misuse of these substances in food-producing animals.

A literature survey shows that almost all reported analytical methods for the analysis of NSAIDs are limited to the detection of analytes in urine and plasma. Most of these methods are optimized to detect one particular drug and its metabolites in plasma and urine using liquid chromatography (560–581), liquid chromatography–mass spectrometry (582), gas chromatography (583–589), or gas chromatography–mass spectrometry (590–595). A few screening and/or confirmation multiresidue procedures have also been reported using either gas or liquid chromatography (596–600). With the exception of a liquid chromatographic method for the determination of indomethacin in chicken tissues (601), two liquid chromatographic methods for the determination of phenylbutazone in bovine milk (602, 603), and two methods for the determination of flunixin in bovine milk (604, 605), no chromatographic methods are available in the literature for assaying other NSAIDs in edible animal products (Table 29.17).

Determination of indomethacin residues in liver, muscle, and fat tissues of chicken can be carried out by homogenizing 5 g of the different tissues with 15 ml of a pH 3.5 phosphate buffer solution (601). Four ml aliquots of the homogenates are then extracted with 20 ml dichloromethane and centrifuged. The aqueous layer is discarded, while the organic layer is evaporated to dryness and reconstituted in 200 μl methanol to be analyzed by liquid chromatography. Separation is performed on a reversed-phase column using an isocratic 0.5% acetic acid/acetonitrile mobile phase, with determination by ultraviolet detection at 254 nm. Indomethacin detection limit was 20 ppb for the studied tissues.

There are two available methods for the determination of phenylbutazone in milk but they differ only slightly in the liquid–liquid partitioning cleanup. The original method (603) uses hexane while the modified version (602) suggests replacement of hexane with a tetrahydrofuran/hexane solution in order to inhibit gel formation during the partitioning process. Both methods are based on the fact than phenylbutazone is soluble in aqueous basic conditions and partitions quantitatively into the aqueous phase during extraction with organic immiscible solvents due to its weak, lipophilic acidic properties and its pK_a value, which, depending upon the solvent, lies between 4.5 and 5.8.

According to the modified procedure (602), milk is thoroughly mixed in its storage container immediately before transfer of the 1 ml aliquot in the extraction tube. This is necessary because approximately 50% of phenylbutazone in milk is associated with the cream. The sample is extracted with 2.4 ml diethyl ether and 2.4 ml petroleum ether in presence of 1 ml ethanol and 100 μl 25% ammonia solution. The organic layer that contains the milk lipids is discarded. Five ml hexane–tetrahydrofuran (4 : 1) is added to the aqueous layer, which is then acidified with hydrochloric acid and the layers are mixed. Under the acidic conditions, phenylbutazone partitions quantitatively into the organic layer, which is collected, evaporated, and dissolved in the mobile phase to be analyzed by liquid chromatography. Separation is performed on a reversed-phase column using an isocratic 0.02 M phosphate buffer/methanol mobile phase, and determination is by ultraviolet detection at 264 nm (Fig. 29.18.2). The limit of detection and limit of quantification were 3.0 and 5.4 ppb, respectively (Table 29.17).

Although two methods have been reported so far for the determination of flunixin in milk, the early published liquid chromatographic method (605) lacks some specific details and was not performed on incurred residues. The recent method (604) is a determinative liquid chromatographic method that allows confirmation by gas chromatography–mass spectrometry and selected ion monitoring. According to this method, a 5 ml milk sample is acidified to pH 3.0–3.5 with 1M hydrochloric acid. Following acidification, the sample is thoroughly mixed with 5.5 g silica gel until the silica is dry and mobile again and has no lumps. The mixture is packed into a chromatographic column, which is then defatted with water-saturated dichloromethane/hexane (30 : 70), and flunixin is eluted with ethyl acetate. The ethyl acetate extract is washed with water at pH 3.5, the water is discarded, and the ethyl acetate layer is then extracted with 0.1M sodium hydroxide. The aqueous layer is drained, passed through a primed C_{18} solid-phase extraction cartridge, and eluted with ethyl acetate. The ethyl acetate

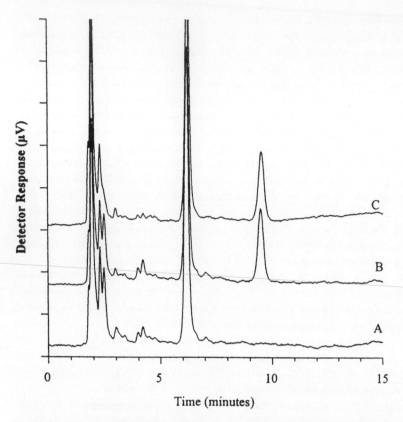

FIG. 29.18.2 Composite chromatograms of control milk (A), control milk fortified at 100 ng/ml with phenylbutazone (B), and incurred milk containing 70 ng
phenylbutazone/ml (C). (Reprinted from Ref. 602. Copyright, (1996), by AOAC
INTERNATIONAL.)

layer is evaporated, taken up in a solution of methanol/5 mM tetrabutylammonium
hydrogen sulfate plus 2 mM sodium hydroxide (50:50), sonicated, and filtered.
The analyte is determined by liquid chromatography using a C_{18} column, a mobile
phase of 58% methanol and 42% 5 mM tetrabutylammonium hydrogen sulfate
plus 2 mM sodium hydroxide, and a diode-array ultraviolet detector at 285 nm.
Performance characteristics of this method are presented in Table 29.17. The
presence of flunixin in suspect samples could be confirmed by gas chromatography–mass spectrometry with selected ion monitoring.

29.19 THYREOSTATIC DRUGS

Thyreostatics, also known as antihormones, belong to a category of drugs capable of inhibiting production of the thyroidal hormone thyroxine. In addition to their application in humans in treating hyperthyroidism, thyreostatics are also fraudulently utilized to fatten animals for slaughter because of their effect of enhancing water retention in tissues. Since this practice is not desirable from a fraud and health standpoint, a number of methods have been developed to control the illegal use of such compounds in food-producing animals. In regulatory control at the farm, plasma, urine, or feces may be sampled. At the retail level or in the case of import or export, sampling is restricted to tissue only. At the slaughterhouse, thyroid gland can be sampled since it contains the highest concentration of thyreostatic drugs.

The most important and powerful thyreostatic drugs used hitherto are the thiouracil analogues, such as thiouracil, methylthiouracil, propylthiouracil, and phenylthiouracil; and the mercaptoimidazole analogues such as tapazole or methimazole. New thyreostatics as mercaptobenzimidazole are said to have been misused recently in some EU countries.

Thyreostatic residues in biological samples are not easily amenable to quantitative analysis (Table 29.17). Successful separation of thyreostatics from coextracted matrix components is often hampered by their highly polar hydrophilic nature, which limits the applicability of techniques such as solvent partitioning and the more common solid-phase extraction cartridges. Thyreostatics are not easily soluble in the common organic solvents. The best organic solvents appear to be the organochlorine solvents.

Early methods applied for the detection of thiouracil were colorimetric; they were based on the reactivity of the thiol or thione functions (606–608). In 1967, Bruggemann and Schole (609) improved the analytical methodology by suggesting use of paper chromatography with n-butanol saturated with aqueous ammonia to spot the concentrated extracts and elute thiouracil, methylthiouracil, and propylyhiouracil. The spots were visualized with a specific colorimetric reaction using 2,6-dichloroquinone-chloroimide. Later, van Waes (610) further improved the analysis of thyreostatics by reporting a method in which methylthiouracil residues could be determined in meat by combining a methanol extraction with column chromatography on alumina using chloroform/methanol (1:1) as the eluent. Recoveries of added analyte at the 100 ppb level were sufficiently high if the analysis was carried out without delay.

Since interferences could not be adequately eliminated with the alumina column, Gissel and Schaal (611) proposed an alternative procedure for extract purification involving use of Kieselgel thin-layer chromatographic plates, elution with trichloroethane/ethanol (8:2), and detection at 254 nm. The detection limit for three thiouracil residues in thyroid glands was in the range 0.5–1.0 ppm.

A more comprehensive approach was reported in 1975 by Brabander and Verbeke (612). In this method, tissue samples were extracted with methanol and the acidified extract defatted with petroleum ether to be loaded onto a Dowex 50W-X8 anion-exchange resin. Following elution with aqueous methanol, the concentrated buffered extract was further defatted with diethyl ether. The sample was derivatized with 7-chloro-4-nitrobenzo-2-oxa-1,3-diazole (NBD-Cl) to be further spotted on a silica high-performance thin-layer chromatographic plate developed in two dimensions using chloroform/ethanol and chloroform/propionic acid consecutively as eluents. Detection of the propylthiouracil, phenylthiouracil, and tapazole residues was carried out on the basis of the fluorescence induction of the NBD derivatives of the drugs with an alkaline cysteine solution.

A substantial improvement of this method was reported in 1984 with the fixation in the anion-exchange column of mercury ions (613). Using the interaction between thiol groups present in the analytes, and immobilized organic mercury molecules, the thyreostatics were selectively retained and a high degree of sample cleanup could be obtained. Most of the analytes were extracted with high efficiency, except for tapazole and phenylthiouracil, which recovered at a level of less than 50%. Another major advantage with the mercurated affinity column was the possibility of omitting extraction of thyreostatics from urine samples. Owing to their high polarity, such an extraction is also possible with very polar solvents.

Later on, another pertinent method (614) allowed confirmation of the thin-layer chromatographic results by scraping of the suspect spots from the plate, silylating the analytes, and proceeding to gas chromatographic–mass spectrometric analysis in the positive chemical ionization mode with isobutane as the reagent gas. Since this new procedure increased the selectivity of the identification power of the method, a direct gas chromatographic–mass spectrometric method for the determination of thyreostatics in urine was also developed by the Brabander group (615).

The most recent modification of the NBD-Cl method involves a further improvement in its qualitative support (616). It involves the infusion of the extract employed for thin-layer chromatography via an electrospray interface into a mass spectrometer operating in the multiple-stage mass spectrometry mode, thus allowing confirmation of suspect results. The cleanup of the thyroid gland samples was also performed with a selective extraction procedure, based on the specific complex formation of the thiouracil, methylthiouracil, propylthiouracil and phenylthiouracil, tapazole, and mercaptobenzimidazole residues with mercury ions bound in a Dowex 1-X2 affinity column.

A mercurated affinity column was also employed by Schilt et al. (617) for sample cleanup in a method for the determination of residues of thiouracil, methylthiouracil, and propylthiouracil in cattle urine by gas chromatography and nitrogen phosphorous or mass spectrometry detection. The presence of nitrogen atoms in the thyreostatics provided the opportunity to use a nitrogen phosphorous detector for screening purposes. However, derivatization was necessary for gas chromatographic analysis, to decrease the polarity of the analytes. A variety of derivatization procedures, including alkylation with methyl iodide or pentafluorobenzyl bromide, has been described for these types of compounds (618, 619). Since most of the alkylation procedures are performed in nonaqueous media such as acetonitrile or dichloromethane, the analytes have to be extracted from the aqueous matrices, prior to derivatization. The high polarity of thyreostatics causes, however, low extraction yields with organic solvents. Hence, an extractive alkylation technique was applied in which the polar analytes were ionized by adding an alkaline solution. The ionized compounds were extracted with tetrabutylammonium hydrogen sulfate, a pairing-ion reagent, into dichloromethane and derivatized with methyl iodide, an alkylating reagent. During methylation, the thiouracil analogues formed two derivatives with an intensity ratio of about 1 : 10, probably due to methylation of different groups in the molecules. For tapazole, only a monomethyl derivative on the single sulfur atom was possible.

Modern gas chromatographic-mass spectrometric methods for the analysis of thyreostatics in biological materials have recently been described (620, 621). In one of these methods (620), resin-mediated alkylation was used as the basis of a simple, cost-effective procedure for the multiresidue determination at the ppb level of thiouracil and its analogues in beef muscle. Trapping and washing the analytes on an anion exchange resin prior to their release by derivatization with methyl iodide in acetonitrile solvent produced sufficiently clean extracts for their reproducible determination by gas chromatography–mass spectrometry. Another method is based on a liquid–liquid extraction of thyroid gland, derivatization with pentafluorobenzyl bromide, purification on a silica solid-phase extraction column, and final derivatization with N-methyl-N-(trimethylsilyl)trifluoroacetamide prior to gas chromatography–mass spectrometry (621). Using a quadrupole mass spectrometer with negative chemical ionization in the selected-ion monitoring acquisition mode, thiouracil, methylthiouracil, propylthiouracil, phenylthiouracil, benzylthiouracil, and tapazole residues could be detected at below the 1 ppb level.

Liquid chromatographic methods based on ultraviolet and/or electrochemical detection have also been developed (622–625). In the earliest of these methods (623), tissues were extracted with methanol/water (1:1), and the evaporated residue was taken up in dichloromethane. The extract was then injected on a Kieselgel Merckosorb SI-60 liquid chromatographic column, and eluted with dichloromethane/ethanol/water. Monitoring at 280 nm allowed 5 ppb thiouracils to be readily detected in the tissue samples. In the latest method (625), cattle plasma samples were extracted with ethyl acetate in presence of ethylenediaminetetraacetate (EDTA). The addition of EDTA could significantly improve the efficiency of the extraction process. Remarkable improvement of the ethyl acetate extraction efficiency was also recently reported in a method using liquid chromatography–atmospheric pressure ionization mass spectrometry for the determination of thyreostatics in urine and thyroid gland (626). It was found that the addition of anhydrous sodium sulfate to remove water led to a marked recovery improvement and the addition of EDTA, and 2-mercaptoethanol further improved the figures.

The most promising methods for screening and confirmation of thyreostatic residues in biological matrices are those reported by Gladys et al. (620) and Blanchflower et al. (626).

Gladys et al. (620) described a gas chromatographic–mass spectrometric method for screening and confirmation of residues of the thyreostatic substances

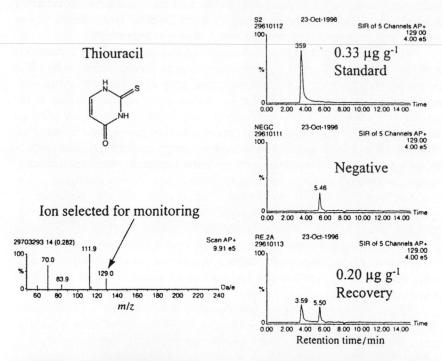

Fɪɢ. 29.19   LC–APCI–MS of thiouracil. Left: upper panel, structure of thiouracil; lower panel, full scan spectrum of thiouracil standard (2.5 μg) using a cone voltage of 35 V. Right: SIM spectra, cone voltage = 10 V, m/z 129, normalized to 4.00×10^5. Upper panel, standard, equivalent to 0.33 μg thiouracil/g thyroid; centre panel, known negative thyroid; lower panel, negative thyroid fortified with thiouracil at 0.20 μg/g. (From Ref. 626 — Reproduced by permission of The Royal Society of Chemistry.)

thiouracil, methylthiouracil, propylthiouracil, and phenylthiouracil in beef muscle. According to this method, a 5 g homogenized beef muscle sample is extracted with 10 ml acetonitrile and centrifuged. After a complementary second extraction with a further 5 ml of acetonitrile, the fat in the combined extracts is removed by partition with two portions of hexane followed by centrifugation and discarding of the hexane layer. The remaining layer is then evaporated to about 2 ml, made up to 10 ml with 0.1N sodium hydroxide, and loaded onto an anion-exchange resin AG MP-1. Methylation of the analytes is carried out in situ by adding a methyl iodide solution in acetonitrile to the resin bed and allowing to stand for 1 h at room temperature. The methylated products are eluted with two 0.5 ml portions of acetonitrile, and analyzed by gas chromatography–mass spectrometry with detection in the selected-ion monitoring mode.

A different approach was followed by Blanchflower et al. (626) in a liquid chromatographic–atmospheric pressure chemical ionization mass spectrometric method for screening and confirmation of thiouracil, methylthiouracil, propylthiouracil, phenylthiouracil, and tapazole residues in thyroid gland and urine. According to this method, a 3 g sample of thyroid gland or a 1 ml urine sample is extracted by homogenization with 10 ml or 5 ml, respectively, of ethyl acetate in presence of EDTA, 2-mercaptoethanol, and anhydrous sodium sulfate. Following centrifugation, the extracts are evaporated, reconstituted in 3 ml chloroform, and loaded on a silica Sep-Pak solid-phase extraction cartridge. Cartridge washing is performed with chloroform, and any thyreostatics present are eluted with methanol/chloroform (15:85). The eluates are evaporated to dryness, reconstituted in mobile phase, and analyzed by liquid chromatography–mass spectrometry in the selected-ion monitoring mode (Fig. 29.19).

REFERENCES

1. B. Shaikh and J. Jackson, J. Liq. Chromatogr., 12:1497 (1989).
2. P.J. Kijak, J. Jackson, and B. Shaikh, J. Chromatogr., 691:377 (1997).
3. P.G. Schermerhorn, P.S. Chu, and P.J. Kijak, J. Agric. Food Chem., 43:2122 (1995).
4. G. Morovjan, P. Csokan, and A. Romvary, in Residues of Veterinary Drugs in Food, Proc. Euroresidue III Conf., Veldhoven, May 6–8, 1996 (N. Haagsma and A. Ruiter, Eds.), Fac. Vet. Med., Univ. Utrecht, The Netherlands, p. 726 (1996).
5. D.J. Sweeney and M.R. Coleman, J. AOAC int., 81:1141 (1998).
6. V. Hormazabal and M. Yndestad, J. Liq. Chromatogr., 18:2695 (1995).
7. V. Hormazabal and M. Yndestad, J. Liq. Chromatogr., 20:2259 (1997).
8. F. Sar, P. Leroy, A. Nicolas, and P. Archimbault, Anal. Chim. Acta, 275:285 (1993).
9. K. Ng, P.D. Rice, and D.R. Bobbitt, Microchem. J., 44:25 (1991).
10. G.C. Gerhardt, C.D.C. Salisbury, and J.D. MacNeil, J. AOAC Int., 77:334 (1994).
11. G.C. Gerhardt, C.D.C. Salisbury, and J.D. MacNeil, J. AOAC Int., 77:765 (1994).
12. R.E. Hornish and J.R. Wiest, J. Chromatogr., 812:123 (1998).
13. A.A. Bergwerff, P. Scherpenisse, and N. Haagsma, Analyst, 123:2139 (1998).

14. C.D.C. Salisbury, C.E. Rigby, and W. Chan, J. Agric. Food Chem., 37:105 (1989).
15. B. Shaikh, E.H. Allen, and J.C. Gridley, J. Assoc. Off. Anal. Chem., 68:29 (1985).
16. B. Shaikh and J. Jackson, J. AOAC Int., 76:543 (1993).
17. V.P. Agarwal, J. Liq. Chromatogr., 12:613 (1989).
18. V.P. Agarwal, J. Liq. Chromatogr., 13:2475 (1990).
19. L.G. McLaughlin and J.D. Henion, J. Chromatogr., 591:195 (1992).
20. L.G. McLaughlin, J.D. Henion, and P.J. Kijak, Biol. Mass Spectrom., 23:417 (1994).
21. C. van de Water, D. Tebbal, and N. Haagsma, J. Chromatogr., 478:205 (1989).
22. V.M. Moretti, C. van de Water, and N. Haagsma, J. Chromatogr., 583:77 (1992).
23. W.J. Blanchflower, A. Cannavan, R.J. McCracken, S.A. Hewitt, and D.G. Kennedy, in Residues of Veterinary Drugs in Food, Proc. Euroresidue II Conf., Veldhoven, May 3–5, 1993 (N. Haagsma, A. Ruiter, and P.B. Czedik-Eysenberg, Eds.), Fac. Vet. Med., Univ. Utrecht, The Netherlands, p. 196 (1993).
24. K. Yoshida and F. Kondo, J. Liq. Chromatogr., 17:2625 (1994).
25. R.L. Epstein, C. Henry, K.P. Holland, and J. Dreas, J. AOAC Int., 77:570 (1994).
26. H.J. Keukens, W.M.J. Beek, and M.M.L. Aerts, J. Chromatogr., 352:445 (1986).
27. B. Johannes, K.-H. Korfer, J. Schad, and I. Ulbrich, Arch. Lebensmmitelhyg., 34: 1 (1983).
28. B. Yohannes, K.H. Korfer, J. Schad, and I. Ulbrich, Arch. Lebensmittelhyg., 34:1 (1983).
29. J.P. Abjean, J. AOAC Int., 80:737 (1997).
30. J.P. Abjean, J. AOAC Int., 77:1101 (1994).
31. J.R. Nelson, K.F.T. Copeland, R.J. Forster, D.J. Campbell, and W.D. Black, J. Chromatogr., 276:438 (1983).
32. L.A. van Ginkel, H.J. van Rossum, P.W. Zoontjes, H. van Blitterswijk, G. Ellen, E. van der Heeft, A.P.J.M. de Jong, and G. Zomer, Anal. Chim. Acta, 237:61 (1990).
33. M.H. Akhtar, C. Danis, A. Sauve, and C. Barry, J. Chromatogr., 696:123 (1995).
34. P.J. Kijak, J. AOAC Int., 77:34 (1994).
35. R.K. Munns, D.C. Holland, J.E. Roybal, J.M. Storey, A.R. Long, G.R. Stehly, and S.M. Plakas, J. AOAC Int., 77:596 (1994).
36. G.S.F. Bories, J.-C. Peleran, and J.-M. Wal, J. Assoc. Off. Anal. Chem., 66:1521 (1983).
37. M. Gips, M. Bridzy, S. Barel, and S. Soback, in Residues of Veterinary Drugs in Food, Proc. Euroresidue II Conf., Veldhoven, May 3–5, 1993 (N. Haagsma, A. Ruiter, and P.B. Czedik-Eysenberg, Eds.), Fac. Vet. Med., Univ. Utrecht, The Netherlands, p. 313 (1993).
38. J.M. Degroodt, B. Wyhowski de Bukanski, J. de Groof, H. Beernaert, and S. Srebrnik, J. Liq. Chromatogr., 15:2355 (1992).
39. B. Delepine and P. Sanders, J. Chromatogr., 582:113 (1992).
40. B. Roudaut, J. Liq. Chrom. & Rel. Technol., 19:1097 (1996).
41. J.-M. Wal, J.-C. Peleran, and G.F. Bories, J. Assoc. Off. Anal. Chem., 63:1044 (1980).
42. N. Haagsma, C. Schreuder, and E.R.A. Rensen, J. Chromatogr., 363:353 (1986).

43. J.E. Psomas and E.G. Iosifidou, J. Liq. Chromatogr., 16:2653 (1993).
44. E.G. Iosifidou and J.E. Psomas, J. Liq. Chromatogr., 18:1863 (1995).
45. T. Nagata and M. Saeki, J. Liq. Chromatogr., 15:2045 (1992).
46. M. Dagorn, J. Manceau, B. Delepine, and P. Sanders, Anal. Chim. Acta, 275:305 (1992).
47. L. Weber, in Residues of Veterinary Drugs in Food, Proc. Euroresidue Conf., Noordwijkerhout, May 21–23, 1990 (N. Haagsma, A. Ruiter, and P.B. Czedik-Eysenberg, Eds.), Fac. Vet. Med., Univ. Utrecht, The Netherlands, p. 394 (1990).
48. J.M. Wal, J.C. Peleran, and G. Bories, J. Chromatogr., 168:179 (1979).
49. R. Malisch, Z. Lebensm. Unters. Forsch., 182:385 (1986).
50. Th. Gude, A. Preiss, and K. Rubach, J. Chromatogr., 673:197 (1995).
51. A.P. Pfenning, M.R. Madson, J.E. Roybal, S.B. Turnipseed, S.A. Gonzales, J.A. Hurlbut, and G.D. Salmon, J. AOAC Int., 81:714 (1998).
52. C. Hummert, B. Luckas, and H. Siebenlist, J. Chromatogr., 668:53 (1995).
53. M. Ramos, Th. Reuvers, A. Aranda, and J. Gomez, J. Liq. Chromatogr., 17:385 (1994).
54. G. Samouris, B. Nathanael, H. Tsoukali-Papadopoulou, and N. Papadimitriou, Vet. Human Toxicol., 35:406 (1993).
55. M. Chevalier, M.F. Pochard, and B. Bel, Food Addit. Contam., 12:101 (1995).
56. M. Petz, Z. Lebensm. Unters. Forsch., 176:289 (1983).
57. M. Petz, Arch. Lebensmittelhyg., 35:51 (1984).
58. M.M.L. Aerts, H.J. Keukens, and G.A. Werdmuller, J. Assoc. Off. Anal. Chem., 72:570 (1989).
59. H.J. Keukens, M.M.L. Aerts, W.A. Traag, J.F.M. Nouws, W.G. de Ruig, W.M.J. Beek, and J.M.P. den Hartog, J. AOAC Int., 75:245 (1992).
60. C. van de Water and N. Haagsma, J. Chromatogr., 411:415 (1987).
61. A.M. Di Pietra, V. Piazza, V. Andrisano, and V. Cavrini, J. Liq. Chromatogr., 18:3529 (1995).
62. V. Hormazabal, I. Steffenak, and M. Yndestad, J. Chromatogr., 616:161 (1993).
63. U.R. Tjaden, D.S. Stegehuis, B.J.E.M. Reeuwijk, H. Lingeman, and J. van der Greef, Analyst, 113:171 (1988).
64. S. Fabiansson, T. Nilsson, and J. Backstrom, J. Sci. Fd Agric., 27:1156 (1976).
65. A. Simonella, L. Torreti, and C. Filipponi, J. High Res. Chromatogr., 555:555 (1989).
66. S. Le Boulaire, J.-C. Bauduret, and F. Andre, J. Agric Food Chem., 45:2134 (1997).
67. A.R. Long, L.C. Hsieh, A.C. Bello, M.S. Malbrough, C.R. Short, and S.A. Barker, J. Agric. Food Chem., 38:427 (1990).
68. J. Bayo, M.A. Moreno, J. Prieta, S. Diaz, G. Suarez, and L. Dominguez, J. AOAC Int., 77:854 (1994).
69. J.A. Tarbin, W.H.H. Farrington, and G. Shearer, Anal. Chim. Acta, 318:95 (1995).
70. K.O. Dasenbrock and W.R. LaCourse, Anal. Chem., 70:2415 (1998).
71. L.K. Sorensen, B.M. Rasmussen, J.O. Boison, and L. Keng, J. Chromatogr., 694:383 (1997).
72. R.F. Straub and R.D. Voyksner, J. Chromatogr., 647:167 (1993).
73. K.L. Tyczkowska, R.D. Voyksner, K.L. Anderson, and A.L. Aronson, J. Chromatogr., 614:123 (1993).

74. J. Keever, R.D. Voyksner, and K.L. Tyczkowska, J. Chromatogr., 794:57 (1998).
75. K.L. Tyczkowska, R.D. Voyksner, R.F. Straub, and A.L. Aronson, J. AOAC Int., 77:1122 (1994).
76. R.F. Straub, M. Linder, and R.D. Voyksner, Anal. Chem., 66:3651 (1994).
77. K.L. Tyczkowska, R.D. Voyksner, and A.L. Aronson, J. Vet. Pharmacol. Ther., 14:51 (1991).
78. K. Tyczkowska, R.D. Voyksner, and A.L. Aronson, J. Chromatogr., 490:101 (1989).
79. R.D. Voyksner, K.L. Tyczkowska, and A.L. Aronson, J. Chromatogr., 567:389 (1991).
80. H. Terada and Y. Sakabe, J. Chromatogr., 348:379 (1985).
81. A.I. MacIntosh, J. Assoc. Off. Anal. Chem., 73:880 (1990).
82. P.J. McNeilly, V.B. Reeves, and E.J.I. Deveau, J. AOAC Int., 79:844 (1996).
83. W. Luo, E.B. Hansen, C.Y.W. Ang, J. Deck, J.P. Freeman, and H.C. Thompson, J. Agric. Food Chem., 45:1264 (1997).
84. W.A. Moats, J. Agric. Food Chem., 31:880 (1983).
85. W.A. Moats, J. Chromatogr., 317:311 (1984).
86. W.A. Moats, J. Chromatogr., 507:177 (1990).
87. W.A. Moats, in Residues of Veterinary Drugs in Food, Proc. Euroresidue Conf., Noordwijkerhout, May 21–23, 1990 (N. Haagsma, A. Ruiter, and P.B. Czedik-Eysenberg, Eds.), Fac. Vet. Med., Univ. Utrecht, The Netherlands, p. 280 (1990).
88. W.A. Moats and R. Malisch, J. AOAC Int., 75:257 (1992).
89. W.A. Moats, J. Chromatogr., 593:15 (1992).
90. H.-E. Gee, K.-B. Ho, and J. Toothill, J. AOAC Int., 79:640 (1996).
91. C.-C. Hong, C.-L. Lin, C.-E. Tsai, and F. Kondo, Am. J. Vet. Res., 56:297 (1995).
92. S. Lihl and M. Petz, Z. Lebensm. Unters Forsch, 199:229 (1994).
93. K. Takeba, K. Fujinuma, T. Miyazaki, and H. Nakazawa, J. Chromatogr., 812:205 (1998).
94. P.G. Schermerhorn, P.-S. Chu, and M.A. Ngoh, J. AOAC Int., 81:973 (1998).
95. U. Meetschen and M. Petz, Z. Lebensm. Unters. Forsch., 193:337 (1991).
96. K. Berger and M. Petz, in Residues of Veterinary Drugs in Food, Proc. Euroresidue Conf., Noordwijkerhout, May 21–23, 1990 (N. Haagsma, A. Ruiter, and P.B. Czedik-Eysenberg, Eds.), Fac. Vet. Med., Univ. Utrecht, The Netherlands, p. 119 (1990).
97. U. Meetschen and M. Petz, J. Assoc. Off. Anal. Chem., 73:373 (1990).
98. B. Perez, C. Prats, E. Castells, and M. Arboix, J. Chromatogr., 698:155 (1997).
99. S. Lihl, A. Rehorek, and M. Petz, J. Chromatogr., 729:229 (1996).
100. C.Y.W. Ang and W. Luo, J. AOAC Int., 80:25 (1997).
101. T. Nagata and M. Saeki, J. Assoc. Off. Anal. Chem., 69:448 (1986).
102. H. Yoshimura, O. Itoh, and S. Yonezawa, Jpn. J. Vet. Sci., 43:833 (1981).
103. V. Hormazabal and M. Yndestad, J. Liq. Chromatogr., 18:2467 (1995).
104. R. Bossuyt, R. van Renterghem, and G. Waes, J. Chromatogr., 124:37 (1976).
105. D.J. Fletouris, J.E. Psomas, and A.J. Mantis, J. Agric. Food Chem., 40:617 (1992).
106. W.A. Moats, J. AOAC Int., 76:535 (1993).
107. W.A. Moats, J. AOAC Int., 77:41 (1994).
108. W.A. Moats and R. Harik-Khan, J. AOAC Int., 78:49 (1995).

109. R. Harik-Khan and W.A. Moats, J. AOAC Int., 78:978 (1995).

110. W.A. Moats and R.D. Romanowski, J. Chromatogr., 812:237 (1998).

111. W.A. Moats and R.D. Romanowski, J. Agric. Food Chem., 46:1410 (1998).

112. J.O.K. Boison, C.D.C. Salisbury, W. Chan, and J.D. MacNeil, J. Assoc. Off. Anal. Chem., 74:497 (1991).

113. H. Terada, M. Asanoma, and Y. Sakabe, J. Chromatogr., 318:299 (1985).

114. W. Chan and C.D.C. Salisbury, in Residues of Veterinary Drugs in Food, Proc. Euroresidue II Conf., Veldhoven, May 3–5, 1993 (N. Haagsma, A. Ruiter, and P.B. Czedik-Eysenberg, Eds.), Fac. Vet. Med., Univ. Utrecht, The Netherlands, p. 236 (1993).

115. J.O.K. Boison, L.J.-Y Keng, and J.D. MacNeil, J. AOAC Int., 77:565 (1994).

116. P. Kubalec, E. Brandsteterova, and A. Bednarikova, Z. Lebensm. Unters Forsch., 205:85 (1997).

117. C.Y.W. Ang, W. Luo, E.B. Hansen, J.P. Freeman, and H.C. Thompson, J. AOAC Int., 79:389 (1996).

118. W. Luo, C.Y.W. Ang, and H.C. Thompson, J. Chromatogr., 694:401 (1997).

119. V. Hormazabal and M. Yndestad, J. Liq. Chromatogr. Rel. Technol., 21:3099 (1998).

120. D.J. Everest, S.J. Everest, and R. Jackman, Anal. Chim. Acta, 275:249 (1993).

121. J.O. Boison and L.J.-Y. Keng, J. AOAC Int., 81:1113 (1998).

122. J.O. Boison and L.J.-Y. Keng, J. AOAC Int., 81:1267 (1998).

123. E. Verdon and P. Couedor, J. Chromatogr., 705:71 (1998).

124. M.G. Beconi-Barker, R.D. Roof, L. Millerioux, F.M. Kausche, T.J. Vidmar, E.B. Smith, J.K. Callahan, V.I. Hubbard, G.A. Smith, and T.J. Gilbertson, J. Chromatogr., 729:229 (1996).

125. D. Hurtaud-Pessel and B. Delepine, in Residues of Veterinary Drugs in Food, Proc. Euroresidue III Conf., Veldhoven, 1996 (N. Haagsma and A. Ruiter, Eds.), Fac. Vet. Med., Univ. Utrecht, The Netherlands, p. 526 (1996).

126. B. Gala, A. Gomez-Hens, and D. Perez-Bendito, Talanta, 44:1883 (1997).

127. D.J. Fletouris, J.E. Psomas, and A.J. Mantis, Chromatographia, 32:436 (1991).

128. J.O. Miners, J. Liq. Chromatogr., 8:2827 (1985).

129. W.A. Moats, J. Chromatogr., 366:69 (1986).

130. W.A. Moats and L. Leskinen, J. Chromatogr., 386:79 (1987).

131. A.M. Lipezynski, Analyst, 112:411 (1987).

132. J. Martin, R. Mendez, and A. Negro, J. Liq. Chromatogr., 11:1707 (1988).

133. M.A. Ngoh, J. AOAC Int., 79:652 (1996).

134. E. Usleber, M. Straka, and E. Martlbauer, Archiv Lebensmittelhyg., 48:73 (1997).

135. H.J. Keukens, M.J.H. Tomassen, and A. Boekestein, in Residues of Veterinary Drugs in Food, Proc. Euroresidue III Conf., Veldhoven, May 6-8, 1996 (N. Haagsma and A. Ruiter, Eds.), Fac. Vet. Med., Univ. Utrecht, The Netherlands, p. 616 (1996).

136. W.A. Moats, E.W. Harris, and N.C. Steele, J. Assoc. Off. Anal. Chem., 68:413 (1986).

137. W. Chan, G.C. Gerhardt, and C.D.C. Salisbury, J. AOAC Int., 77:331 (1994).

138. T. Nagata and M. Saeki, J. Assoc. Off. Anal. Chem., 69:644 (1986).

139. M. Janecek, M.A. Quilliam, M.R. Bailey, and D.H. North, J. Chromatogr., 619:63 (1993).

140. D.N. Heller, J. AOAC Int., 80:975 (1997).

141. D.N. Heller, J. AOAC Int., 79:1054 (1996).

142. R.E. Hornish, A.R. Cazers, S.T. Chester, and R.D. Roof, J. Chromatogr., 674:219 (1995).

143. M. Petz, R. Solly, M. Lymburn, and M.H. Clear, J. Assoc. Off. Anal. Chem., 70: 691 (1987).

144. K. Takatsuki, S. Suzuki, N. Sato, I. Ushizawa, and T. Shoji, J. Assoc. Off. Anal. Chem., 70:708 (1987).

145. M. De Liguoro, P. Anfossi, R. Angeletti, and C. Montesissa, Analyst, 123:1279 (1998).

146. W.A. Moats, J. Agric. Food Chem., 39:1812 (1991).

147. M. Horie, K. Saito, R. Ishii, T. Yoshida, Y. Haramaki, and H. Nakazawa, J. Chromatogr., 812:295 (1998).

148. A.R. Barbiers and A.W. Neff, J. Assoc. Off. Anal. Chem., 59:849 (1976).

149. P. Sanders, P. Guillot, G. Moulin, B. Delepine, and D. Mourot, in Residues of Veterinary Drugs in Food, Proc. Euroresidue Conf., Noordwijkerhout, May 21–23, 1990 (N. Haagsma, A. Ruiter, and P.B. Czedik-Eysenberg, Eds.), Fac. Vet. Med., Univ. Utrecht, The Netherlands, p. 315 (1990).

150. B. Delepine, D. Hurtaud-Pessel, and P. Sanders, J. AOAC Int., 79:397 (1996).

151. B. Delepine, D. Hurtaud-Pessel, and P. Sanders, in Residues of Veterinary Drugs in Food, Proc. Euroresidue III Conf., Veldhoven, May 6–8, 1996 (N. Haagsma, and A. Ruiter, Eds.), Fac. Vet. Med., Univ. Utrecht, The Netherlands, p. 372 (1996).

152. L.J.-Y Keng and J.O.K. Boison, J. Liq. Chromatogr., 15:2025 (1992).

153. J. Okada and S. Kondo, J. Assoc. Off. Anal. Chem., 70:818 (1987).

154. W. Luo, E.B. Hansen, C.Y.W. Ang, and H.C. Thompson, J. AOAC Int., 79:839 (1996).

155. M.M.L. Aerts, W.M.J. Beek, and U.A. Th. Brinkman, J. Chromatogr., 500:453 (1990).

156. T.G. Diaz, L.L. Martinez, M.M. Galera, and F. Salinas, J. Liq. Chromatogr., 17: 457 (1994).

157. K. Yoshida and F. Kondo, J. AOAC Int., 78:1126 (1995).

158. J.P. Heotis, J.L. Mertz, R.J. Herrett, J.R. Diaz, D.C. VanHart, and I. Olivard, J. Assoc. Off. Anal. Chem., 63:720 (1980).

159. T. Juszkiewicz, A. Posyniak, S. Semeniuk, and J. Niedzielska, in Residues of Veterinary Drugs in Food, Proc. Euroresidue II Conf., Veldhoven, May 3–5, 1993 (N. Haagsma, A. Ruiter, and P.B. Czedik-Eysenberg, Eds.), Fac. Vet. Med., Univ. Utrecht, The Netherlands, p. 401 (1993).

160. G.R. Stehly, S.M. Plakas, and K.R. El Said, J. AOAC Int., 77:901 (1994).

161. H.S. Rupp, R.K. Munns, and A.R. Long, J. AOAC Int., 76:1235 (1993).

162. L. Kumar, J.R. Toothill, and K-B Ho, J. AOAC Int., 77:591 (1994).

163. H.S. Rupp, R.K. Munns, A.R. Long, and S.M. Plakas, J. AOAC Int., 77:344 (1994).

164. J.J. Laurensen and J.F.M. Nouws, J. Chromatogr., 472:321 (1989).

165. M. Petz, Dtsch. Lebensm.-Rundsch., 78:396 (1982).

166. R. Draisci, L. Giannetti, L. Lucentini, L. Palleschi, G. Brambilla, L. Serpe, and P. Gallo, J. Chromatogr., 777:201 (1997).

167. N.M. Angelini, O.D. Rampini, and H. Mugica, J. AOAC Int., 80:481 (1997).
168. W.M.J. Beek and M.M.L. Aerts, Z. Lebensm. Unters. Forsch., 180:211 (1985).
169. L.H.M. Vroomen, M.C.J. Berghmans, and T.D.B. Van Der Struijs, J. Chromatogr., 362:141 (1986).
170. W. Winterlin, G. Hall, and C. Mourer, J. Assoc. Off. Anal. Chem., 64:1055 (1981).
171. N.A. Botsoglou, J. Agric. Food Chem., 36:1224 (1988).
172. G. Carignan, A.I. MacIntosh, and S. Sved, J. Agric. Food Chem., 38:716 (1990).
173. T. Galeano Diaz, A. Guiberteau Cabanillas, M.I. Acedo Valenzuela, C.A. Correa, and F. Salinas, J. Chromatogr., 764:243 (1997).
174. R.J. McCracken and D.G. Kennedy, J. Chromatogr., 691:87 (1997).
175. O.B. Samuelsen, J. Chromatogr., 528:495 (1990).
176. W.J. Blanchflower, R.J. McCracken, and D.G. Kennedy, in Residues of Veterinary Drugs in Food, Proc. Euroresidue II Conf., Veldhoven, May 3–5, 1993 (N. Haagsma, A. Ruiter, and P.B. Czedik-Eysenberg, Eds.), Fac. Vet. Med., Univ. Utrecht, The Netherlands, p. 201 (1993).
177. M. Horie, K. Saito, Y. Hoshino, N. Nose, H. Nakazawa, and Y. Yamane, J. Chromatogr., 538:484 (1991).
178. M. Kuhne, A. Kobe, R. Fries, and A. Ebrecht, Arch. Lebensmittelhyg., 43:59 (1992).
179. O.W. Parks, J. Assoc. Off. Anal. Chem., 72:567 (1989).
180. A.R. Long, L.C. Hsieh, M.S. Malbrough, C.R. Short, and S.A. Barker, J. Assoc. Off. Anal. Chem., 74:292 (1991).
181. A.R. Long, L.C. Hsieh, M.S. Malbrough, C.R. Short, and S.A. Barker, J. Agric. Food Chem., 38.430 (1990).
182. N. Haagsma, M. van Roy, and B.G.M. Gortemaker, in Residues of Veterinary Drugs in Food, Proc. Euroresidue II Conf., Veldhoven, May 3–5, 1993 (N. Haagsma, A. Ruiter, and P.B. Czedik-Eysenberg, Eds.), Fac. Vet. Med., Univ. Utrecht, The Netherlands, p. 337 (1993).
183. L. Larocque, M. Schnurr, S. Sved, and A. Weninger, J. Assoc. Off. Anal. Chem., 74:608 (1991).
184. S. Sved, L. Larocque, A. Weninger, M. Schnurr, and D. Vas, in Residues of Veterinary Drugs in Food, Proc. Euroresidue Conf., Noordwijkerhout, May 21–23, 1990 (N, Haagsma, A. Ruiter, and P.B. Czedik-Eysenberg, Eds.), Fac. Vet. Med., Univ. Utrecht, The Netherlands, p. 356 (1990).
185. G. Carignan, L. Larocque, and S. Sved, J. Assoc. Off. Anal. Chem., 74:906 (1991).
186. J.M. Degroodt, B. Wyhowski de Bukanski, and S. Srebrnik, J. Liq. Chromatogr., 17:1785 (1994).
187. Y. Ikai, H. Oka, N. Kawamura, M. Yamada, K.-I. Harada, M. Suzuki, and H. Nakazawa, J. Chromatogr., 477:397 (1989).
188. J.E. Roybal, A.P. Pfenning, S.B. Turnipseed, C.C. Walker, and J.A. Hurlbut, J. AOAC Int., 80:982 (1997).
189. AOAC, Official Methods of Analysis (K. Helrich, Ed.), 15th Edition, Association of Official Analytical Chemists, Arlington, Virginia, Section 970.84 (1990).
190. R.S. Browning and E.L. Pratt, J. Assoc. Off. Anal. Chem., 53:464 (1970).
191. K. Takatsuki, J. AOAC Int., 75:982 (1992).
192. B. Roudaut, and J. Boisseau, in Residues of Veterinary Drugs in Food, Proc. Euroresidue Conf., Noordwijkerhout, May 21-23, 1990 (N, Haagsma, A. Ruiter, and P.B.

Czedik-Eysenberg, Eds.), Fac. Vet. Med., Univ. Utrecht, The Netherlands, p. 311 (1990).

193. G.Y. Eng, R.J. Maxwell, E. Cohen, E.G. Piotrowski, and W. Fiddler, J. Chromatogr., 799:349 (1998).

194. N. Nose, Y. Hoshino, Y. Kikuchi, M. Horie, K. Saitoh, T. Kawachi, and H. Nakazawa, J. Assoc. Off. Anal. Chem., 70:714 (1987).

195. A.P. Pfenning, R.K. Munns, S.B. Turnipseed, J.E. Roybal, D.C. Holland, A.R. Long, and S.M. Plakas, J. AOAC Int., 79:1227 (1996).

196. R.K. Munns, S.B. Turnipseed, A.P. Pfenning, J.E. Roybal, D.C. Holland, A.R. Long, and S.M. Plakas, J. AOAC Int., 78:343 (1995).

197. M. Horie, K. Saito, Y. Hoshino, N. Nose, E. Mochizuki, and H. Nakazawa, J. Chromatogr., 402:301 (1987).

198. M. Horie and H. nakazawa, J. Liq. Chromatogr., 15:2057 (1992).

199. H. Pouliquen, D. Gouelo, M. Larhantec, N. Pilet, and L. Pinault, J. Chromatogr., 702:157 (1997).

200. S. Horii and H. Nakazawa, J. Liq. Chromatogr., 388:459 (1987).

201. V. Hormazabal and M. Yndestad, J. Liq. Chromatogr., 17:3775 (1994).

202. J.R. Meinertz, V.K. Dawson, W.H. Gingerich, B. Cheng, and M.M. Tubergen, J. AOAC Int., 77:871 (1994).

203. N. Haagsma, L.M.J. Mains, W. van Leeuwen, and H.W. van Gend, in Residues of Veterinary Drugs in Food, Proc. Euroresidue Conf., Noordwijkerhout, May 21–23, 1990 (N, Haagsma, A. Ruiter, and P.B. Czedik-Eysenberg, Eds.), Fac. Vet. Med., Univ. Utrecht, The Netherlands, p. 206 (1990).

204. H.H. Thanh, A.T. Andersen, T. Agasoster, and K.E. Rasmussen, J. Chromatogr., 532:363 (1990).

205. V. Hormazabal and M. Yndestad, J. Liq. Chromatogr., 17:2911 (1994).

206. H.H. Jarboe and K.M. Kleinow, J. AOAC Int., 75:428 (1992).

207. M. Sanchez Pena, F. Salinas, M.C. Mahedero, and J.J. Aaron, J. Pharm. Biomed. Anal., 10:805 (1992).

208. J. Unruh, E. Piotrowski, D.P. Schwartz, and R.A. Barford, J. Chromatogr., 519: 179 (1990).

209. M.M.L. Aets, W.M.J. Beek, and U.A.Th. Brinkman, J. Chromatogr., 435:97 (1988).

210. J. Sherma, W. Bretschneier, M. Dittamo, N. DiBiase, D. Huh, and D.P. Schwartz, J. Chromatogr., 463:229 (1989).

211. P. Vinas, C.L. Erroz, A.H. Canals, and M.H. Cordoba, Chromatographia, 40:382 (1995).

212. F. Salinas, A. Espinosa Mansilla, and J.J. Berzas Nevado, Microchem. J. 43:244 (1991).

213. E.D. Ramsey, J.R. Perkins, D.E. Games, and J.R. Startin, J. Chromatogr., 464:353 (1989).

214. M.J.B. Mengelers, J.F. Staal, M.M.L. Aerts, H.A. Kuiper, and A.S.J.P.A.M. van Meirt, in Residues of Veterinary Drugs in Food, Proc. Euroresidue Conf., Noordwijkerhout, May 21–23, 1990 (N, Haagsma, A. Ruiter, and P.B. Czedik-Eysenberg, Eds.), Fac. Vet. Med., Univ. Utrecht, The Netherlands, p. 276 (1990).

215. M.J.B. Mengelers, A.M.M. Polman, M.M.L. Aerts, H.A. Kuiper, and A.S.J.P.A.M. van Miert, J. Liq. Chromatogr., 16:257 (1993).

216. E. Brandsteterova, P. Kubalec, and L. Machackova, Z. Lebensm. Unters Forsch., 204:341 (1997).

217. N. Takeda and Y. Akiyama, J. Chromatogr., 607:31 (1992).

218. G. Suhren and W. Heeschen, Anal. Chim. Acta, 275:329 (1993).

219. P. Vinas, C.L. Erroz, N. Campillo, and M.H. Cordoba, J. Chromatogr., 726:125 (1996).

220. M.D. Smedley, J. AOAC Int., 77:1112 (1994).

221. J. Abian, M.I. Churchwell, and W.A. Korfmacher, J. Chromatogr., 629:267 (1993).

222. E. Zomer, S. Saul, and S.e. Charm, J. AOAC Int., 75:987 (1992).

223. G. Carignan and K. Carrier, J. Assoc. Off. Anal. Chem., 74:479 (1991).

224. K. Takatsuki and T. Kikuchi, J. Assoc. Off. Anal. Chem., 73:886 (1990).

225. M. Nishikawa, Y. Takahashi, and Y. Ishihara, J. Liq. Chromatogr., 16:4031 (1993).

226. M. Petz, J. Chromatogr., 423:217 (1987).

227. Y. Takahashi, T. Sekiya, M. Nishikawa, and Y.S. Endoh, J. Liq. Chromatogr., 17: 4489 (1994).

228. C.-E., Tsai and F. Kondo, J. Liq. Chromatogr., 18:965 (1995).

229. Y.S. Endoh, Y. Takahashi, and M. Nishikawa, J. Liq. Chromatogr., 15:2091 (1992).

230. C.-E., Tsai and f. Kondo, J. AOAC Int., 78:674 (1995).

231. T.A. Gehring, L.G. Rushing, and H.C. Thompson, J. AOAC Int., 80:751 (1997).

232. R. Malisch, Z. Lebensm. Unters. Forsch., 182:385 (1986).

233. J.O.K. Boison and L.J.-Y Keng, J. AOAC Int., 77:558 (1994).

234. J.d. Weber and M.D. Smedley, J. Assoc. Off. Anal. Chem., 72:445 (1989).

235. J.D. Weber and M.d. Smedley, J. AOAC Int., 76:725 (1993).

236. M.A. Alawi and H.A. Russel, Fresenius Z. Anal. Chem., 307:382 (1981).

237. J.O. Boison and L.J.-Y. Keng, J. AOAC Int., 78:651 (1995).

238. E.J. Simeonidou, N.A. Botsoglou, I.E. Psomas, and D.J. Fletouris, J. Liq. Chromatogr., 19:2349 (1996).

239. N. Takada and Y. Akiyama, J. Chromatogr., 558:175 (1991).

240. M.D. Smedley and J.D. Weber, J. Assoc. Off. Anal. Chem., 73:875 (1990).

241. M.H. Thomas, R.L. Epstein, R.B. Ashworth, and H. Marks, J. Assoc. Off. Anal. Chem., 66:884 (1983).

242. M. Dagorn and J.M. Delmas, Anal. Chim. Acta, 285:353 (1994).

243. G.K. Kristiansen, R. Brock, and G. Bojesen, Anal. Chem., 66:3253 (1994).

244. Y. Ikai, H. Oka, N. Kawamura, J. Hayakawa, M. Yamada, K.-I. Harada, M. Suzuki, and H. Nakazawa, J. Chromatogr., 541:393 (1991).

245. E. Neidert, Z. Baraniak, and A. Sauve, J. Assoc. Off. Anal. Chem., 69:641 (1986).

246. N. Haagsma, B. Dieleman, and B. G. M. Gortemaker, Vet. Q., 6:8 (1984).

247. M. Horie, K. Saito, N. Nose, and H. Nakazawa, J. AOAC Int., 75:786 (1992).

248. S. Pleasance, P. Blay, and M.A. Quilliam, J. Chromatogr., 558:155 (1991).

249. C.P. Barry and G.M. MacEachern, J. Assoc. Off. Anal. Chem., 66:4 (1983).

250. N.P. Milner, M.R. Johnson, and K.J. Perry, J. AOAC Int., 77:875 (1994).

251. G. Weiss, P.D. Duke, and L. Gonzales, J. Agric. Food Chem., 35:905 (1987).

252. S.C. Mutha, T.L. Brown, B. Chamberlain, and C.E. Lee, J. Agric. Food Chem., 25:556 (1977).

253. AOAC, Official Methods of Analysis (K. Helrich, Ed.), 15th Edition, Association of Official Analytical Chemists, Arlington, Virginia, Section 982.40 (1990).

254. J.E. Matusik, C.G. Guyer, J.N. Geleta, and C.J. Barnes, J. Assoc. Off. Anal. Chem., 70:546 (1987).
255. O.W. Parks, J. Assoc. Off. Anal. Chem., 65:632 (1982).
256. A.E. Mooser and H. Koch, J. AOAC Int., 76:976 (1993).
257. O.W. Parks, J. Assoc. Off. Anal. Chem., 68:20 (1985).
258. J. Unruh, E. Piotrowski, D.P. Schwartz, and R.A. Barford, J. Chromatogr., 519: 179 (1990).
259. J. Unruh, D.P. Schwartz, and R.A. Barford, J. AOAC Int., 76:335 (1993).
260. M. Horie, K. Saito, Y. Hoshino, N. Nose, N. Hamada, and H. Nakazawa, J. Chromatogr., 502:371 (1987).
261. A. Cannavan, S.A. Hewitt, W.J. Blanchflower, and D.G. Kennedy, Analyst, 121: 1457 (1996).
262. D.P. Schwartz and A.R. Lightfield, J. AOAC Int., 78:967 (1995).
263. N. Haagsma and C. van de Water, J. Chromatogr., 333:256 (1985).
264. G.J. Reimer and A. Suarez, J. Chromatogr., 555:315 (1991).
265. A.R. Long, L.C. Hsieh, M.S. Malbrough, C.R. Short, and S.A. Barker, J. Assoc. Off. Anal. Chem., 73:868 (1990).
266. C.C. Walker and S.A. Barker, J. AOAC Int., 77:1460 (1994).
267. G.J. Reimers and A. Suarez, J. AOAC Int., 75:979 (1992).
268. L.V. Walker, J.R. Walsh, and J.J. Webber, J. Chromatogr., 595:179 (1992).
269. A.R. Long, L.C. Hsieh, M.S. Malbrough, C.R. Short, and S.A. Barker, J. Agric. Food Chem., 38:423 (1990).
270. A.R. Long, C.R. Short, and S.A. Barker, J. Chromatogr., 502:87 (1990).
271. J.E. Matusik, R.S. Sternal, C.J. Barnes, and J.A. Sphon, J. Assoc. Off. Anal. Chem., 73:529 (1990).
272. K. Smilde, A. Knevelman, and P.M.J. Coenegracht, J. Chromatogr., 369:1 (1986).
273. N.A. Botsoglou, D.J. Fletouris, E.J. Simeonidou, and I.E. Psomas, Chromatographia, 46:477 (1997).
274. R.F. Cross, J. Chromatogr., 478:422 (1989).
275. V. Hormazabal and A. Rogstad, J. Chromatogr., 583:201 (1992).
276. L.V. Bui, J. AOAC Int., 76:966 (1993).
277. A. Cannavan, S.A. Hewitt, S.D. Floyd, and D.G. Kennedy, Analyst, 122:1379 (1997).
278. M.C. Carson, J. AOAC Int., 76:329 (1993).
279. M.C. Carson, and W. Breslyn, J. AOAC Int, 79:29 (1996).
280. M.C. Carson, M.A. Ngoh, and S.W. Hadley, J. Chromatogr., 712:113 (1998).
281. C.-L. Chen and X. Gu, J. AOAC Int, 78:1369 (1995).
282. A.L. Savage, S.H. Sarijo, and J. Baird, Anal. Chim. Acta, 375:1 (1998).
283. H. Oka, Y. Ikai, N. Kawamura, K. Uno, M. Yamada, K.-I. Harada, and M. Suzuki, J. Chromatogr., 400:253 (1987).
284. M.H. Thomas, J. Assoc. Off. Anal. Chem., 72:564 (1989).
285. B. Roudaut, and M. Garnier, in Residues of Veterinary Drugs in Food, Proc. Euroresidue II Conf., Veldhoven, May 3–5, 1993 (N. Haagsma, A. Ruiter and P.B. Czedik-Eysenberg, Eds.), Fac. Vet. Med., Univ. Utrecht, The Netherlands, p. 596 (1993).
286. G.J. Reimer and L.M. Young, J. Assoc. Off. Anal. Chem., 73:813 (1990).

287. Y. Ikai, H. Oka, N. Kawamura, M. Yamada, K.-I. Harada, and M. Suzuki, J. Chromatogr., 411:313 (1987).

288. J.D. MacNeil, V.K. Martz, G.O. Korsrud, C.D.C. Salisbury, H. Oka, R.L. Epstein, and C.J. Barnes, J. AOAC Int, 79:405 (1996).

289. J.R. Walsh, L.V. Walker, and J.J. Webber, J. Chromatogr., 596:211 (1992).

290. E. Brandsteterova, P. Kubalec, L. Bovanova, P. Simko, A. Bednarikova, and L. Machackova, Z. Lebensm. Unters Forsch., 205:311 (1997).

291. H. Oka, H. Matsumoto, K. Uno, K.-I. Harada, S. Kadowaki, and M. Suzuki, J. Chromatogr., 325:265 (1985).

292. H. Oka, Y. Ikai, Y. Ito, J. Hayakawa, K. Harada, M. Suzuki, H. Odani, and K. Maeda, J. Chromatogr., 693:337 (1997).

293. H. Oka, Y. Ikai, J. Hayakawa, K. Masuda, K.-I. Harada, and M. Suzuki, J. AOAC Int., 77:891 (1994).

294. S.M. Croubels, H. Vermeersch, P. De Backer, M.D.F. Santos, J.P. Remon, and C.H. Van Peteghem, J. Chromatogr., 708:145 (1998).

295. S.M. Croubels, K.E.I. Vanoosthuyze, and C.H. Van Peteghem, J. Chromatogr., 690:173 (1997).

296. J.M. Degroodt, B. Wyhowski de Bukanski, and S. Srebrnik, J. Liq. Chromatogr., 16:3515 (1993).

297. D.J. Fletouris, J.E. Psomas, and N.A. Botsoglou, J. Agric. Food Chem., 38:1913 (1990).

298. W.A. Moats, J. Chromatogr., 358:253 (1986).

299. C.R. White, W.A. Moats, and K.L. Kotula, J. AOAC Int., 76:549 (1993).

300. S. Horii, J. Liq. Chromatogr., 17:213 (1994).

301. R.G. Aoyama, K.M. McErlane, H. Erber, D.D. Kitts, and H.M. Burt, J. Chromatogr., 588:181 (1991).

302. H. Poiger and Ch. Schlatter, Analyst, 101:808 (1976).

303. G. Carignan, K. Carrier, and S. Sved, J. AOAC Int., 76:325 (1993).

304. H. Bjorklund, J. Chromatogr., 432:381 (1988).

305. A.D. Cooper, G.W.F. Stubbings, M. Kelly, J.A. Tarbin, W.H.H. Farrington, and G. Shearer, J. Chromatogr., 812:321 (1998).

306. W.J. Blanchflower, R.J. McCracken, and D.A. Rice, Analyst, 114:421 (1989).

307. W.J. Blanchflower, R.J. McCracken, A.S. Haggan, and D.G. Kennedy, J. Chromatogr., 692:351 (1997).

308. N.A. Botsoglou, B.N. Vassilopoulos, and D.C. Kufidis, Chimica Chronika, New Series, 13:37 (1984).

309. S. Kawata, K. Sato, Y. Nishikawa, and K. Iwama, J. AOAC Int, 79:1463 (1996).

310. N. Haagsma and M.J.B. Mengelers, Z. Lebensm. Unters. Forsch., 188:227 (1989).

311. A.R. Long, L.C. Hsieh, M.S. Malbrough, C.R. Short, and S.A. Barker, J. Assoc. Off. Anal. Chem., 73:379 (1990).

312. W.A. Moats, and L. Leskinen, J. Assoc. Off. Anal. Chem., 71:776 (1988).

313. V.B. Reeves, J. AOAC Int., 78:55 (1995).

314. Y. Ikai, in Chemical Analysis for Antibiotics Used in Agriculture (H. Oka, H. Nakazawa, K.-I. Harada, and J.D. MacNeil, Eds.), AOAC International, Arlington, VA, USA, p. 407 (1995).

315. J.R. Markus and J. Sherma, J. AOAC Int., 76:451 (1993).
316. J.R. Markus and J. Sherma, J. AOAC Int., 76:459 (1993).
317. W.J.A. VandenHeuvel, J.S. Wood, M. DiGiovanni, and R.W. Walker, J. Agric. Food Chem., 25:386 (1977).
318. J. Markus and J. Sherma, J. AOAC Int., 75:1135 (1992).
319. J. Markus and J. Sherma, J. AOAC Int., 75:1129 (1992).
320. P.S. Chu, R.Y. Wang, T.A. Brandt, and C.A. Weerasinghe, J. Chromatogr., 620: 129 (1993).
321. B.W. de Bukanski, J.M. Degroodt, and H. Beernaert, Z. Lebensm. Unters Forsch., 193:130 (1991).
322. A.R. Long, L.C. Hsieh, M.S. Malbrough, C.R. Short, and S.A. Barker, J. Assoc. Off. Anal. Chem., 72:739 (1989).
323. S.A. Barshick and M.V. Buchanan, J. AOAC Int., 77:1428 (1994).
324. M.A.F. Muino and J.S. Lozano, Analyst, 118:1519 (1993).
325. S.A. Barker, T. McDowell, B. Charkhian, L.C. Hsieh, and C.R. Short, J. Assoc. Off. Anal. Chem., 73:22 (1990).
326. N.F. Campbell, L.E. Hubbard, R.S. Mazenko, and M.B. Medina, J. Chromatogr., 692:367 (1997).
327. M.B. Medina and J.J. Unruh, J. Chromatogr., 663:127 (1995).
328. C.G. Chappell, C.S. Creaser, and M.J. Shepherd, J. Chromatogr., 626:223 (1992).
329. J. Markus and J. Sherma, J. AOAC Int., 75:942 (1992).
330. S.J. Stout, A.R. daCunha, R.E. Tondreau, and J.E. Boyd, J. Assoc. Off. Anal. Chem., 71:1150 (1988).
331. F.J. Schenck, L.V. Podhorniak, and R. Wagner, Food Addit. Contam., 15:411 (1998).
332. J. Markus and J. Sherma, J. AOAC Int., 75:937 (1992).
333. L.W. LeVan and C.J. Barnes, J. Assoc. Off. Anal. Chem., 74:487 (1991).
334. K. Helrich (Ed.), AOAC, Official Methods of Analysis 15th ed., Association of Official Analytical Chemists, Arlington, VA, Sec. 991.17 (1991).
335. J.G. Steenbaar, C.A.J. Hajee, and N. Haagsma, J. Chromatogr., 615:186 (1993).
336. B.W. de Bukanski, J.M. Degroodt, and H. Beernaert, Z. Lebensm. Unters Forsch., 193:545 (1991).
337. D.J. Fletouris, N.A. Botsoglou, I.E. Psomas, and A.I. Mantis, J. Chromatogr., 687: 427 (1996).
338. D.J. Fletouris, N.A. Botsoglou, I.E. Psomas, and A.I. Mantis, Anal. Chim. Acta, 345:111 (1997).
339. C.A.J. Hajee and N. Haagsma, J. AOAC Int., 79:645 (1996).
340. E.G. Iosifidou, and N. Haagsma, J. Liq. Chrom. & Rel. Technol., 19:1819 (1996).
341. S.S.C. Tai, N. Cargile, and C.J. Barnes, J. Assoc. Off. Anal. Chem., 73:368 (1990).
342. R.T. Wilson, J.M. Groneck, A.C. Henry, and L.D. Rowe, J. Assoc. Off. Anal. Chem., 74:56 (1991).
343. D.J. Fletouris, N.A. Botsoglou, I.E. Psomas, and A.I. Mantis, J. AOAC Int., 79: 1281 (1996).
344. G. Stoev, J. Chromatogr., 710:234 (1998).
345. D.J. Fletouris, N.A. Botsoglou, I.E. Psomas, and A.I. Mantis, Analyst, 119:2801 (1994).

346. C.D.C. Salisbury, J. AOAC Int., 76:1149 (1993).

347. G. Dusi, M. Curatolo, A. Fierro, and E. Faggionato, J. Liq. Chrom. & Rel. Technol., 19:1607 (1996).

348. D.D. Oehler and J.A. Miller, J. Assoc. Off. Anal. Chem., 72:59 (1989).

349. Th. Reuvers, R. Diaz, M. Martin de Pozuelo, and M. Ramos, Anal. Chim. Acta, 275:353 (1993).

350. C.M. Dickinson, J. Chromatogr., 528:250 (1990).

351. J.M. Degroodt, B.W. De Bukanski, and S. Srebrnik, J. Liq. Chromatogr., 17:1419 (1994).

352. A. Khunachak, A.R. Dacunha, and S.J. Stout, J. AOAC Int., 76:1230 (1993).

353. M. Alvinerie, J.F. Sutra, M. Badri, and P. Galtier, J. Chromatogr., 674:119 (1995).

354. J.A. Tarbin and G. Shearer, J. Chromatogr., 613:347 (1993).

355. D.J. Fletouris, N.A. Botsoglou, I.E. Psomas, and A.I. Mantis, J. Dairy Sci., 80: 2695 (1997).

356. D.J. Fletouris, N.A. Botsoglou, I.E. Psomas, and A.I. Mantis, J. Agric. Food Chem., 44:3882 (1996).

357. K. Takeda, T. Itoh, M. Matsumoto, H. Nakazawa, and S. Tanabe, J. AOAC Int., 79:848 (1996).

358. A.M. Marti, A.E. Mooser, and H. Koch, J. Chromatogr., 498:145 (1990).

359. J. Li and C. Qian, J. AOAC Int., 79:1062 (1996).

360. F.J. Schenck, R. Wagner, and W. Bargo, J. Liq. Chromatogr., 16:513 (1993).

361. J.S. Li, X.W. Li, and H.B. Hu, J. Chromatogr., 696:166 (1997).

362. I.W. Tsina and S.B. Matin, J. Pharm. Sci., 70:858 (1981).

363. V. Hormazabal, and M. Yndestad, J. Liq. Chromatogr., 18:589 (1995).

364. M.L. Alvarez-Bujidos, A. Ortiz, R. Balana, J.C. Cubria, D. Ordonez, and A. Negro, J. Chromatogr., 578:321 (1992).

365. L.D. Payne, V.R. Mayo, L.A. Morneweck, M.B. Hicks, and T.A. Wehner, J. Agric. Food Chem., 45:3501 (1997).

366. K.P. Reising, J. AOAC Int., 75:751 (1992).

367. H.J. Schnitzerling and J. Nolan, J. Assoc. Off. Anal. Chem., 68:36 (1985).

368. K. Takeda, M. Matsumoto, and H. Nakazawa, J. Chromatogr., 596:67 (1992).

369. P.J. Kijak, J. AOAC Int., 75:747 (1992).

370. J.M. Ballard, L.D. Payne, R.S. Egan, T.A. Wehner, G.S. Rahn, and S. Tom, J. Agric. Food Chem., 45:3507 (1997).

371. S.A. Barker, L.C. Hsieh, and C.R. Short, Anal. Biochem., 155:112 (1986).

372. F.J. Schenck, J. Liq. Chromatogr., 18:349 (1995).

373. F.J. Schenck, S.A. Barker, and A.R. Long, J. AOAC Int., 75:655 (1992).

374. M. Alvinerie, J.F. Sutra, D. Capela, P. Galtier, A. Fernandez-Suarez, E. Horne, and M. O'Keeffe, Analyst, 121:1469 (1996).

375. A.R. Long, M.S. Malbrough, L.C. Hsieh, C.R. Short, and S.A. Barker, J. Assoc. Off. Anal. Chem., 73:860 (1990).

376. J. Li and S. Zhang, J. AOAC Int., 79:1300 (1996).

377. R.M. Facino, M. Carini, and P. Traldi, Biolog. Mass Spectrom., 21:195 (1992).

378. R.V. Arenas and N.A. Johnson, J. AOAC Int., 78:642 (1995).

379. M. Ramos, A. Aranda, Th. Reuvers, and R. Jimenez, Anal. Chim. Acta, 275:317 (1993).

380. G. Carignan, W. Skakum, and S. Sved, J. Assoc. Off. Anal. Chem., 71:1141 (1988).
381. H.I. Assil and P. Sporns, J. Agric. Food Chem., 39:2206 (1991).
382. M.H. Vertommen, A. Van Der Laan, and H.M. Veenendaal-Hesselman, J. Chromatogr., 481:452 (1989).
383. J.A. Tarbin and G. Shearer, J. Chromatogr., 613:354 (1993).
384. D.C. Holland, R.K. Munns, J.E. Roybal, J.A. Hurlbut, and A.R. Long, J. AOAC Int., 78:37 (1995).
385. R.M.L. Aerts, I.M. Egberink, C.A. Kan, H.J. Keukens, and W.M.J. Beek, J. Assoc. Off. Anal. Chem., 74:46 (1991).
386. G.B. Blomkvist, K.M. Jansson, E.R. Ryhage, and B.-G. Osterdahl, J. Agric. Food Chem., 34:274 (1986).
387. G. Weiss, M. Kaykaty, and B. Miwa, J. Agric. Food Chem., 31:78 (1983).
388. T. Nagata, M. Saeki, H. Nakazawa, M. Fujita, and E. Takabatake, J. Assoc. Off. Anal. Chem., 68:27 (1985).
389. G. Weiss, N.R. Felicito, M. Kaykaty, G. Chen, A. Caruso, E. Hargroves, C. Crowley, and A. MacDonald, J. Agric. Food Chem., 31:75 (1983).
390. D.R. Newkirk, and C.J. Barnes, J. Assoc. Off. Anal. Chem., 72:581 (1989).
391. J.A. Tarbin and G. Shearer, J. Chromatogr., 579:177 (1992).
392. L.R. Frank and C.J. Barnes, J. Assoc. Off. Anal. Chem., 72:584 (1989).
393. P.A. Vanderkop and J.D. MacNeil, J. Assoc. Off. Anal. Chem., 72:735 (1989).
394. P.A. VanderKop and J.D. MacNeil, J. Chromatogr., 508:386 (1990).
395. G.P. Dimenna, J.A. Creegan, L.B. Turnbull, and G.J. Wright, J. Agric. Food Chem., 34:805 (1986).
396. J.W. Moran, J.M. Turner, and M.R. Coleman, J. AOAC Int., 78:668 (1995).
397. E.E. Mertinez and W. Shimoda, J. Assoc. Off. Anal. Chem., 68:1149 (1985).
398. K. Takatsuki, S. Suzuki, and I. Ushizawa, J. Assoc. Off. Anal. Chem., 69:443 (1986).
399. J.W. Moran, J.M. Rodewald, A.L. Donoho, and M.R. Coleman, J. AOAC Int., 77:885 (1994).
400. J.F. Ericson, A. Calcagni, and M.J. Lynch, J. AOAC Int., 77:577 (1994).
401. E.E. Mertinez and W. Shimoda, J. Assoc. Off. Anal. Chem., 69:637 (1986).
402. D.R. Newkirk, H.F. Righter, F.J. Schenck, J.L. Okrasinski, and C.J. Barnes, J. Assoc. Off. Anal. Chem., 73:702 (1990).
403. M.G. Leadbetter and J.E. Matusik, J. AOAC Int., 76:420 (1993).
404. J.L. Lewis, T.D. Macy, and D.A. Garteiz, J. Assoc. Off. Anal. Chem., 72:577 (1989).
405. E.T. Mallinson, A.C. Henry, and L. Rowe, J. AOAC Int., 75:790 (1992).
406. K.D. Gallicano, H. Park, J. Yee, L.M. Young, and P.W. Saschenbrecker, J. Assoc. Off. Anal. Chem., 71:48 (1988).
407. A. Cannavan and G. Kennedy, Analyst, 122:963 (1997).
408. K. Heil, F. Peter, and V. Cicleszky, J. Agric. Food Chem., 32:997 (1984).
409. J.A. Tarbin and G. Shearer, J. Chromatogr., 577:376 (1992).
410. G.P. Dimenna, B.E. Walker, L.B. Turnbull, and G.J. Wright, J. Agric. Food Chem., 34:472 (1986).
411. G.P. Dimenna, F.S. Lyon, F.M. Thompson, J.A. Creegan, and G.J. Wright, J. Agric. Food Chem., 37:668 (1989).

412. F.J. Schenck, S.A. Barker, and A.R. Long, J. AOAC Int., 75:659 (1992).

413. A.I. MacIntosh and G.A. Neville, J. Assoc. Off. Anal. Chem., 67:958 (1984).

414. T. Nagata and M. Saeki, J. Assoc. Off. Anal. Chem., 70:706 (1987).

415. K. Sinigoj Gacnik, V. Cerkvenik, and M. Komar, in Residues of Veterinary Drugs in Food, Proc. Euroresidue II Conf., Veldhoven, May 3–5, 1993 (N. Haagsma, A. Ruiter and P.B. Czedik-Eysenberg, Eds.), Fac. Vet. Med., Univ. Utrecht, The Netherlands, p. 637 (1993).

416. M.M.L. Aerts, W.M.J. Beek, H.J. Keukens, and U.A.Th. Brinkman, J. Chromatogr., 456:105 (1988).

417. G.M. Binnendijk, M.M.L. Aerts, H.J. Keukens, and U.A.Th. Brinkman, J. Chromatogr., 541:401 (1991).

418. H.J. Keukens, C.A. Kan, and M.J.H. Tomassen, in Residues of Veterinary Drugs in Food, Proc. Euroresidue III Conf., Veldhoven, 1996 (N. Haagsma, and A. Ruiter, Eds.), Fac. Vet. Med., Univ. Utrecht, The Netherlands, p. 611 (1996).

419. M.J. Lynch and S.R. Bartolucci, J. Assoc. Off. Anal. Chem., 65:66 (1982).

420. M.J. Lynch, F.R. Mosher, R.P. Schneider, H.G. Fouda, and J.E. Risk, J. Assoc. Off. Anal. Chem., 74:611 (1991).

421. G.J. de Graaf, Th.J. Spierenburg, and A.J. Baars, in Residues of Veterinary Drugs in Food, Proc. Euroresidue Conf., Noordwijkerhout, May 21–23, 1990 (N. Haagsma, A. Ruiter, and P.B. Czedik-Eysenberg, Eds.), Fac. Vet. Med., Univ. Utrecht, The Netherlands, p. 203 (1990).

422. M.G. Lauridsen, C. Lund, and M. Jacobsen, J. Assoc. Off. Anal. Chem., 71:921 (1988).

423. L.A. van Ginkel, P.L.W.J. Schwillens, M. Jaquemijns, and G. Zomer, in Residues of Veterinary Drugs in Food, Proc. Euroresidue Conf., Noordwijkerhout, May 21–23, 1990 (N. Haagsma, A. Ruiter, and P.B. Czedik-Eysenberg, Eds.), Fac. Vet. Med., Univ. Utrecht, The Netherlands, p. 189 (1990).

424. W.A. Moats and L. Leskinen, J. Agric. Food Chem., 36:1297 (1988).

425. L.G. Croteau, M.H. Akhtar, J.M.R. Belanger, and J.R.J. Pare, J. Liq. Chromatogr., 17:2971 (1994).

426. G. Formica and C. Giannone, J. Assoc. Off. Anal. Chem., 69:763 (1986).

427. M.B. Medina and N. Nagdy, J. Chromatogr., 614:315 (1993).

428. V. Ferchaud, B. Le Bizec, M.-P. Montrade, D. Maume, F. Monteau, and F. Andre, J. Chromatogr., 695:269 (1997).

429. W. Haasnoot, R. Schilt, A.R.M. Hamers, F.A. Huf, A. Farjam, R.W. Frei, and U.A.Th. Brinkman, J. Chromatogr., 489:157 (1989).

430. P.M. Scott, and G.A. Lawrence, J. Assoc. Off. Anal. Chem., 71:1176 (1988).

431. J. Plasencia, C.J. Mirocha, R.J. Pawlosky, and J.F. Smith, J. Assoc. Off. Anal. Chem., 73:973 (1990).

432. R. Bagnati, M.G. Castelli, L. Airoldi, M.P. Oriundi, A. Ubaldi, and R. Fanelli, J. Chromatogr., 527:267 (1990).

433. L. Van Look, Ph. Deschuytere, and C. Van Peteghem, J. Chromatogr., 489:213 (1989).

434. M.T. Andresen and A.C.E. Fesser, J. AOAC Int., 79:1037 (1996).

435. C.H. Van Peteghem, M.F. Lefevere, G.M. Van Haver, and A.P. De Leenheer, J. Agric. Food Chem., 35:228 (1987).

436. L.A. Van Ginkel, R.W. Stephany, H.J. Van Rossum, H.M. Steinbuch, G. Zomer, E. Van De Heeft, and A.P.J.M. De Jong, J. Chromatogr., 489:111 (1989).

437. E. Daeseleire, A. De Guesquiere, and C. Van Peteghem, J. Chromatogr., 562:673 (1991).

438. Th. Reuvers, E. Perogordo, and R. Jimenez, J. Chromatogr., 564:477 (1991).

439. B. Bergner-Lang and M. Kachele, Dtsch. Lebensm. Rundsch. 77:305 (1981).

440. E.A.I. Daeseleire, A. de Guesquiere, and C. van Peteghem, J. Chromatogr. Sci., 30:409 (1992).

441. F. Busico, G. Moretti, G.P. Cartoni, and F. Rosati, J. High Resol. Chromatogr., 15: 94 (1992).

442. B. Hoffman and E. Rattenberger, J. Anim. Sci., 46:635 (1977).

443. T.G. Dunn, C.C. Kaltenbach, D.R. Koritnik, D.L. Turner, and G.D. Niswender, J. Anim. Sci., 46:659 (1977).

444. V.L. Estergreen, M.T. Lin, E.L. Martin, G.E. Moss, A.L. Branen, L.O. Luedecke, and W. Shimoda, J. Anim. Sci., 46:642 (1977).

445. S.H. Hsu, R.H. Eckerlin, and J.D. Henion, J. Chromatogr., 424:219 (1988).

446. G.W. Stubbings and M.J. Shepherd, J. Liq. Chromatogr., 16:241 (1993).

447. J.E. Roybal, R.K. Munns, W.J. Morris, J.A. Hurlbut, and W. Shimoda, J. Assoc. Off. Anal. Chem., 71:263 (1988).

448. R.P. Huopalahti and J.D. Henion, J. Liq. Chrom. & Rel. Technol., 19:69 (1996).

449. L.A. van Ginkel, E.H.J.M. Jansen, R.W. Stephany, P.W. Zoontjes, P.L.W.J. Schwillens, H.J. van Rossum, and T. Visser, J. Chromatogr., 624:389 (1992).

450. M.B. Medina and D.P. Schwartz, J. Chromatogr., 581:119 (1992).

451. H.-J. Stan and B. Abraham, J. Chromatogr., 195:231 (1980).

452. S. Hartmann and H. Steinhart, J. Chromatogr., 704:105 (1997).

453. A. Lagana and A. Marino, J. Chromatogr., 588:89 (1991).

454. J.P. Cravedi and G. Delous, J. Chromatogr., 564:461 (1991).

455. T.R. Covey, G.A. Maylin, and J.D. Henion, Biomed. Mass Spectrom., 12:274 (1985).

456. T.M.P. Chichila, P.O. Edlund, J.D. Henion, R. Wilson, and R.L. Epstein, J. Chromatogr., 488:389 (1989).

457. R. Verbeke, J. Chromatogr., 177:69 (1979).

458. R. Bagnati and R. Fanelli, J. Chromatogr., 547:325 (1991).

459. H.O. Gunther, Fresenius Z. Anal. Chem., 290:389 (1978).

460. B. Wortberg, R. Woller, and T. Chulamorakot, J. Chromatogr., 156:205 (1978).

461. W.G. de Ruig, H. Hooijerink, and J.M. Weseman, Fresenius Z. Anal. Chem., 320: 749 (1985).

462. M.B. Medina and D.P. Schwartz, J. Agric. Food Chem., 34:907 (1986).

463. E.H.J.M. Jansen, R. Both-Miedema, H. van Blitterswijk, and R.W. Stephany, J. Chromatogr., 299:450 (1984).

464. J.O. de Beer, J. Chromatogr., 489:139 (1989).

465. H.H.D. Meyer, F.X. Hartman, and M. Rapp, J. Chromatogr., 489:173 (1989).

466. E.H.J.M. Jansen, L.A. van Ginkel, R.H. van der Berg, and R.W. Stephany, J. Chromatogr., 580:111 (1992).

467. E.H.J.M. Jansen, R.H. van der Berg, G. Zomer, R. Both-Miedema, C. Enkelaar-Willemsen, and R.W. Stephany, Anal. Chim. Acta, 170:21 (1985).

468. E.H.J.M. Jansen, H. van Blitterswijk, P.W. Zoontjes, R. Both-Miedema, and R.W. Stephany, J. Chromatogr., 347:375 (1985).

469. C.G.B. Frischkorn, M.R. Smyth, H.E. Frischkorn, and J. Golimowski, Fresenius Z. Anal. Chem., 300:407 (1980).

470. L.A. van Ginkel, R.W. Stephany, and H.J. van Rossum, J. AOAC Int., 75:554 (1992).

471. T. Visser, M.J. Vredenbregt, A.P.J.M. de Jong, L.A. van Ginkel, H.J. van Rossum, and R.W. Stephany, Anal. Chim. Acta, 275:205 (1993).

472. C.T. Elliott, C.S. Thompson, C.J.M. Arts, S.R.H. Crooks, M.J. van Baak, E.R. Verheij, and G.A. Baxter, Analyst, 123:1103 (1998).

473. J.A. van Rhijn, H.H. Heskamp, M.L. Essers, H.J. van de Wetering, H.C.H. Kleijnen, and A.H. Roos, J. Chromatogr., 665:395 (1995).

474. M.-P. Montrade, B. Le Bizec, F. Monteau, B. Siliart, and F. Andre, Anal. Chim. Acta, 275:253 (1993).

475. R. Schilt, W. Haasnoot, M.A. Jonker, H. Hooijerink, and R.J.A. Paulussen, in Residues of Veterinary Drugs in Food, Proc. Euroresidue Conf., Noordwijkerhout, May 21–23, 1990 (N. Haagsma, A. Ruiter, and P.B. Czedik-Eysenberg, Eds.), Fac. Vet. Med., Univ. Utrecht, The Netherlands, p. 320 (1990).

476. J.A. van Rhijn, M. O'Keeffe, H.H. Heskamp, and S. Collins, J. Chromatogr., 712: 67 (1995).

477. D. Courtheyn, C. Desaeven, and R. Verhe, J. Chromatogr., 564:537 (1991).

478. I.A. Lin, J.A. Tomlinson, and R.D. Satzger, J. Chromatogr., 762:275 (1997).

479. J.F. Lawrence and C. Menard, J. Chromatogr., 696:291 (1997).

480. Y. Gaillard, A. Balland, F. Doucet, and G. Pepin, J. Chromatogr., 703:85 (1997).

481. J. Girault and J.B. Fourtillan, J. Chromatogr., 518:41 (1990).

482. L. Leyssens, C. Driessen, A. Jacobs, J. Czech, and J. Raus, J. Chromatogr., 564: 515 (1991).

483. P. Gonzalez, C.A. Fente, C. Franco, B. Vazquez, E. Quinto, and A. Cepeda, J. Chromatogr., 693:321 (1997).

484. R.T. Wilson, J.M. Groneck, K.P. Holland, and A.C. Henry, J. AOAC Int., 77:917 (1994).

485. L. Debrauwer, and G. Bories, Anal. Chim. Acta, 275:231 (1993).

486. H.H.D. Meyer, L. Rinke, and I. Dursch, J. Chromatogr., 564:551 (1991).

487. J.A. van Rhijn, W.A. Traag, and H.H. Heskamp, J. Chromatogr., 619:243 (1993).

488. K. Vanoosthuyze, and C. van Peteghem, in Residues of Veterinary Drugs in Food, Proc. Euroresidue III Conf., Veldhoven, May 6–8, 1996 (N. Haagsma and A. Ruiter, Eds.), Fac. Vet. Med., Univ. Utrecht, The Netherlands, p. 958 (1996).

489. F. Ramos, C. Santos, A. Silva, and M.I.N. da Silveira, J. Chromatogr., 716:366 (1998).

490. J. Cai and J. Henion, J. Chromatogr., 691:357 (1997).

491. P.G. Schermerhorn, and R.K. Munns, J. AOAC Int., 77:1454 (1994).

492. R.T. Wilson, J. Wong, J. Johnston, R. Epstein, and D.N. Heller, J. AOAC Int., 77: 1137 (1994).

493. R.K. Munns, J.E. Roybal, J.A. Hurlbut, and W. Shimoda, J. Assoc. Off. Anal. Chem., 73:705 (1990).

494. D.N. Heller, J. AOAC Int., 75:650 (1992).
495. C.A.J. Hajee and N. Haagsma, J. Chromatogr., 669:219 (1995).
496. S.B. Turnipseed, J.E. Roybal, S.M. Plakas, A.P. Pfenning, J.A. Hurlbut, and A.R. Long, J. AOAC Int., 80:31 (1997).
497. J.E. Roybal, R.K. Munns, D.C. Holland, J.A. Hurlbut, and A.R. Long, in Residues of Veterinary Drugs in Food, Proc. Euroresidue II Conf., Veldhoven, May 3–5, 1993 (N. Haagsma, A. Ruiter, and P.B. Czedik-Eysenberg, Eds.), Fac. Vet. Med., Univ. Utrecht, The Netherlands, p. 601 (1993).
498. L.G. Rushing, S.F. Webb, and H.C. Thompson, J. Chromatogr., 674:125 (1995).
499. J.E. Roybal, R.K. Munns, J.A. Hurlbut, and W. Shimoda, J. Assoc. Off. Anal. Chem., 73:940 (1990).
500. S.M. Plakas, K.R. El Said, G.R. Stehly, and J.E. Roybal, J. AOAC Int., 78:1388 (1995).
501. S.B. Turnipseed, J.E. Roybal, H.S. Rupp, J.A. Hurlbut, and A.R. Long, J. Chromatogr., 670:55 (1995).
502. J.E. Roybal, A.P. Pfenning, R.K. Munns, D.C. Holland, J.A. Hurlbut, and A.R. Long, J. AOAC Int., 78:453 (1995).
503. L.G. Rushing and H.C. Thompson, J. Chromatogr., 688:325 (1997).
504. L.G. Rushing and E.B. Hansen, J. Chromatogr., 700:223 (1997).
505. V. Hormazabal, I. Steffenak, and M. Yndestad, J. Liq. Chromatogr., 15:2035 (1992).
506. A. Swarbrick, E.J. Murby, and P. Hume, J. Liq. Chromatogr. Rel. Technol., 20:2269 (1997).
507. S.M. Plakas, K.R. El Said, E.L.E. Jester, F.A. Bencsath, and W.L. Hayton, J. AOAC Int., 80:486 (1997).
508. R.K. Munns, D.C. Holland, J.E. Roybal, J.G. Meyer, J.A. Hurlbut, and A.R. Long, J. AOAC Int., 75:796 (1992).
509. J.L. Allen, J.R. Meinertz, and J.E. Gofus, J. Assoc. Off. Anal. Chem., 75:646 (1992).
510. K. Sagar, M.R. Smyth, J.G. Wilson, K. McLaughlin, J. Chromatogr., 659:329 (1994).
511. J.L. Allen, J.E. Gofus, and J.R. Meinertz, J. AOAC Int, 77:553 (1994).
512. S.B. Turnipseed, J.E. Roybal, J. Hurlbutt, and A.R. Long, J. AOAC Int., 78:971 (1995).
513. K. Bauer, H. Dangschat, H.-O. Knoppler, and J. Neudegger, Arch. Lebensm. Hyg., 39:97 (1988).
514. E. Klein, M. Edelhauser, and R. Lippold, Dtsch. Lebensm. Rundsch., 87:350 (1991).
515. J.L. Allen and J.R. Meinertz, J. Chromatogr., 536:217 (1991).
516. D.R. Doerge, M.I. Churchwell, L.G. Rushing, and S. Bajic, Rapid Commun. Mass Spectrom., 10:1479 (1996).
517. J.E. Psomas and D.J. Fletouris, J. Liq. Chromatogr., 15:1543 (1992).
518. A. Akbari, B.J. Gordon, P.B. Bush, and J.N. Moore, J. Chromatogr., 426:207 (1988).
519. A. Rogstad and M. Yndestad, J. Chromatogr., 216:350 (1981).
520. M. Alvinerie and P.L. Toutain, J. Chromatogr., 222:308 (1981).
521. L. Laitem, I. Bello, and P. Gaspar, J. Chromatogr., 156:327 (1978).
522. F. Kadir and J. Zuidema, J. Chromatogr., 527:461 (1990).
523. M.D. Rose and G. Shearer, J. Chromatogr., 624:471 (1992).

524. H.J. Keukens and M.M.L. Aerts, J. Chromatogr., 464:149 (1989).

525. D.C. Holland, R.K. Munns, J.E. Roybal, J.A. Hurlbut, and A.R. Long, J. AOAC Int., 76:720 (1993).

526. L.A. Van Ginkel, P.L.W.J. Schwillens, and M. Olling, Anal. Chim. Acta, 225:137 (1989).

527. Ph. Delahaut, P. Jacquemin, Y. Colemonts, M. Dubois, J. De Graeve, and H. Deluyker, J. Chromatogr., 696:203 (1997).

528. L.G. McLaughlin and J.D. Henion, J. Chromatogr., 529:1 (1990).

529. M.W. Trucksess, J. Donoso, and Craig, J. Assoc. Off. Anal. Chem., 52:932 (1969).

530. R.P. Mooney and N.R. Pasarela, J. Agric. Food Chem., 14:12 (1966).

531. P.M. Simpson, J. Chromatogr., 77:161 (1973).

532. L.F. Krzeminski, B.L. Cox, P.N. Perrel, and R.A. Schiltz, J. Agric. Food Chem., 20:970 (1972).

533. L.F. Krzeminski, B.L. Cox, D.D. Hagg, J. Agric. Food Chem., 22:882 (1974).

534. A.M. de Paolis, G. Schnabel, S.E. Katz, and J.D. Rosen, J. Assoc. Off. Anal. Chem., 60:210 (1977).

535. P. Shearan, M. O 'Keeffe, and M.R. Smyth, Analyst, 116:1365 (1991).

536. V.K. Prasad, B. Ho, and C. Haneke, J. Chromatogr., 378:305 (1986).

537. B.T. Hofreiter, A.G. Mizera, J.P. Allen, A.M. Masi, and W.C. Hicok, Clin. Chem., 29:1808 (1983).

538. S.M.R. Stanley, B.S. Wilhelmi, J.P. Rodgers, and H. Bertschinger, J. Chromatogr., 614:77 (1993).

539. G. Szepesi and M. Gazdag, in Handbook of Thin-Layer Chromatography (J. Sherma and B. Fried, Eds.), Marcel Dekker, New York, p. 907 (1991).

540. G. Windhorst, J. Keller, and J.P. de Kleijn, J. Planar Chromatogr., 3:300 (1990).

541. M. Okamoto and M. Ohta, J. Chromatogr., 369:403 (1986).

542. R. Neher, in Thin-Layer Chromatography. A Laboratory Handbook (E. Stahl, Ed.), Springer, Berlin, p. 311 (1969).

543. K.E. Vanoosthuyze, L.S.G. van Poucke, A.C.A. Deloof, and C.H. van Peteghem, Anal. Chim. Acta, 275:177 (1993).

544. B.E. Cham, B. Sadowski, J.M. O'Hagan, C.N. de Wytt, F. Bochner, and M.J. Eadie, Ther. Drug Monit., 2:373 (1980).

545. D. Lamiable, R. Vistelle, H. Millart, V. Sulmont, R. Fay, J. Caron, and H. Choisy, J. Chromatogr., 378:486 (1986).

546. P.M. Plezia and P.L. Berens, Clin. Chem., 31:1870 (1985).

547. H. Derendorf, P. Rohdewald, G. Hochhaus, and H. Mollmann, J. Pharm. Biomed. Anal., 4:197 (1986).

548. M. Alvinerie and P.L. Toutain, J. Pharm. Sci., 71:816 (1982).

549. J.M. Pomoell, H. Kopu, and H. Adlercreutz, Anal. Chem. Symp. Ser., 23:499 (1985).

550. J. Reisch and J. Norrenbrock, J. Pharm. Sci., 55:81 (1987).

551. J. Goto, F. Shamsa, and T. Nambora, Jpn. Clin. Chem., 12:327 (1983).

552. F. de Croo, W. van de Bossche, and P. de Moerloose, J. Chromatogr., 325:395 (1985).

553. P. Campins-Falco, R. Herraez-Hernandez, and A. Sevillano-Cabeza, J. Liq. Chromatogr., 14:3575 (1991).

554. R. Herraez-Hernandez, P. Campins-Falco, and A. Sevillano-Cabeza, Chromatographia, 33:177 (1992).
555. B. Shaikh, in Veterinary Drug Residues (W.A. Moats and M.B. Medina, Eds.), American Chemical Society, Washington, DC, p. 161 (1996).
556. B. Shaikh, J. Agric. Food Chem., 43:2117 (1995).
557. S.F. Cooper, R. Masse, and R. Dugal, J. Chromatogr., 489:65 (1989).
558. B. Shaikh and N. Rummel, J. Agric. Food Chem., 46:1039 (1998).
559. B. Shaikh and N. Rummel, J. Chromatogr., 709:137 (1998).
560. A.J. Higgins, P. Lees, S.C. Sharma, and J.B. Taylor, Equine Vet. J., 19:303 (1987).
561. J. Sato, E. Owada, K. Ito, Y. Niida, A. Wakamatsu, and M. Umetsu, J. Chromatogr., 493:239 (1989).
562. F.T. Delbeke, M. Debackere, and L. Vynckier, J. Vet. Pharmacol. Ther., 14:145 (1991).
563. I.M. Johansson, P. Kallings, and M. Hammsrlund-Udenaes, J. Vet. Pharmacol. Ther., 14:235 (1991).
564. M.C. Rouan, J. Campestrini, J.B. Lecaillon, and J. Godbillon, J. Chromatogr., 577:387 (1992).
565. T.B. Vree, M. van den Biggelar-Martea, and C.P.W.G.M. Verwey-van Wissen, J. Chromatogr., 578:239 (1992).
566. M.C. Caturla and E. Cusido, J. Chromatogr., 581:101 (1992).
567. M. Castillo and P.C. Smith, J. Chromatogr., 614:109 (1993).
568. T.B. Vree, M. van den Biggelar-Martea, and C.P.W.G.M. Verwey-van Wissen, J. Chromatogr., 616:271 (1993).
569. R. Brent Miller, J. Chromatogr., 616:283 (1993).
570. F.T. Delbeke, L. Vynckier, and M. Debackere, J. Vet. Pharmacol. Ther., 16:283 (1993).
571. M.S. Bernstein, M.A. Evans, J. Chromatogr., 229:179 (1982).
572. A.A. Al-Angary, Y.M. El-Sayed, M.A. Al-Meshal, and K.M. Lufti, J. Clin. Pharm. Ther., 15:257 (1990).
573. J.B. Taylor, P. Lees, and E.L. Gerring, Equine Vet. J., 13:201 (1981).
574. P. Lees, J.B. Taylor, A.J. Higgins, and S.C. Sharma, J. Vet. Pharmacol. Ther., 9:204, (1986).
575. A. Avgerinos and S. Malamataris, J. Chromatogr., 495:309 (1989).
576. Y.L. Brown, R.J. Mandrotas, J.B. Douglas, and P. Gal, J. Chromatogr., 459:275 (1988).
577. D. de Zeeuw, J.L. Leinfelder, and D.C. Bruter, J. Chromatogr., 380:157 (1986).
578. P. Hubert, M. Renson, and J. Crommen, J. Pharm. Biomed. Anal., 7:1819 (1992).
579. A.G. Johnson and J.E. Ray, Ther. Drug Monit., 14:61 (1992).
580. A.K. Singh, Y. Yang, U. Mishra, and K. Granley, J. Chromatogr., 568:351 (1991).
581. M.R. Taylor and S.A. Westwood, J. Chromatogr., 697:389 (1995).
582. S.M.R. Stanley, N.A. Owens, and J.P. Rodgers, J. Chromatogr., 667:95 (1995).
583. A. Arbin, J. Chromatogr., 144:85 (1977).
584. M.A. Evans, J. Pharm. Sci., 69:19 (1980).
585. C. Giachetti, S. Canali, and G. Zanolo, J. Chromatogr., 279:587 (1983).
586. P. Guissou, G. Cuisinaud, and J. Sassard, J. Chromatogr., 277:368 (1983).

587. K.M. Jensen, J. Chromatogr., 153:195 (1978).
588. R. Nishioka, T. Harimoto, I. Umeda, S. Yamamoto, and N. Oi, J. Chromatogr., 526:210 (1990).
589. R. Krishna, K.W. Riggs, M.P.R. Walker, E. Kwan, and D.W. Rurak, J. Chromatogr., 674:65 (1995).
590. Ph. Jaussaud, D. Courtot, J.L. Guyot, and J. Paris, J. Chromatogr., 423:123 (1987).
591. M. Johansson and E.L. Anler, J. Chromatogr., 427:55 (1988).
592. J. Segura, M. Mestres, J. Aubets, R. de la Torre, B. Ugena, and J. Cami, Biomed. Environ. Mass Spectron., 16:361 (1988).
593. A. Sioufi, F. Pommier, and J. Godbillon, J. Chromatogr., 571:87 (1991).
594. Ph. Jaussaud, D. Guieu, D. Courtot, B. Babier, and Y. Bonnaire, J. Chromatogr., 573:136 (1992).
595. E. Benoit, P. Jaussaud, S. Besse, B. Videmann, D. Courtot, P. Delatour, and Y. Bonnaire, J. Chromatogr., 583:167 (1992).
596. G. Gonzalez, R. Ventura, A.K. Smith, R. de la Torre, and J. Segura, J. Chromatogr., 719:251 (1996).
597. A.K. Singh, Y. Jang, U. Mishra, and K. Granley, J. Chromatogr., 568:351 (1991).
598. P. Gowik, B. Julicher, and S. Uhlig, J. Chromatogr., 716:221 (1998).
599. E.G. de Jong, J. Kiffers, and R.A.A. Maes, J. Pharm. Biomed. Anal., 7:1617 (1989).
600. S.G. Owen, M.S. Roberts, and W.T. Friesen, J. Chromatogr., 416:293 (1987).
601. C. Cristofol, B. Perez, M. Pons, J.E. Valladares, G. Marti, and M. Arboix, J. Chromatogr., 709:310 (1998).
602. E.J. Ian De Veau, J. AOAC Int., 79:1050 (1996).
603. K. Martin, M.I. Stridsberg, and B.M. Wiese, J. Chromatogr., 276:224 (1983).
604. H.S. Rupp, D.C. Holland, R.K. Munns, S.B. Turnipseed, and A.R. Long, J. AOAC Int., 78:959 (1995).
605. C.A. Neff-Davis and K. Bosch, J. Vet. Pharmacol. Ther., 8:331 (1985).
606. L.C. Chesley, J. Biol. Chem., 152:571 (1944).
607. H. van Genderen, K.L. Lier, and J. Debeus, Biochim. Biophys. Acta, 2:482 (1948).
608. R.A. Allister, and K.W. Howells, J. Pharm. Pharmacol., 4:259 (1952).
609. J. Bruggermann, and J. Schole, Landwirdsch. Forsch. Sonderh., 21:134 (1967).
610. H. van Waes, Rev. Agr., 26:435 (1973).
611. C. Gissel and M. Schaal, Arch. Lebensmittelhyg., 25:8 (1974).
612. H.F. de Brabander and R. Verbeke, J. Chromatogr., 108:141 (1975).
613. H.F. de Brabander and R. Verbeke, Trends Anal. Chem., 3:162 (1984).
614. H.F. de Brabander, P. Batjoens, and J. van Hoof, J. Planar Chromatogr., 5:124 (1992).
615. P. Batjoens, H.F. de Brabander, and K. de Wasch, J. Chromatogr., 750:127 (1996).
616. K. De Wasch, H.F. De Brabander, L.A. van Ginkel, A. Spaan, S.S. Sterk, and H.D. Meiring, J. Chromatogr., 819:99 (1998).
617. R. Schilt, J.M. Weseman, H. Hooijerink, H.J. Korbee, W.A. Traag, M.J. van Steenbergen, and W. Haasnoot, J. Chromatogr., 489:127 (1989).
618. J. Buhlert, Dtsch. Lebensm. Rundsch., 82:146 (1986).
619. S. Floberg, K. Lambeck, and B. Lindstrom, J. Chromatogr., 182:63 (1980).
620. G.Y.F. Yu, E.J. Murby, and R.J. Wells, J. Chromatogr., 703:159 (1997).

621. B. Le Bizec, F. Monteau, D. Maume, M.P. Montrade, C. Gade, and F. Andre, Anal. Chim Acta, 340:201 (1997).
622. H. Hooijerink and W.G. de Ruig, J. Chromatogr., 394:403 (1987).
623. W. Wildanger, Chromatographia, 8:42 (1975).
624. M.F. Pochard, M. Karageorgis, M. Chevalier, J. Chromatogr., 298:183 (1984).
625. G. Moretti, P. Betto, P. Cammarata, F. Fracassi, M. Giambenedetti, and A. Borghese, J. Chromatogr., 616:291 (1993).
626. W.J. Blanchflower, P.J. Hughes, A. Cannavan, M.A. McCoy, and D.G. Kennedy, Analyst, 122:967 (1997).

30

Future Trends

The number of drugs legally administered in food-producing animals is large and becomes huge when one includes the plethora of other drugs used illegally. Many of the main metabolites of the drugs are not known and, if known, the analytical methods used usually measure only the parent compound. This is particularly important whenever the drugs are rapidly metabolized or a metabolite has a high toxicity. There is also a need for more research on the effects of temperature as experienced in cooking and pasteurizing, and of prolonged storage, on residues in foods. Therefore, control of drug residues, achieved through measurements, is now essential to meet the required levels of food quality to ensure consumer safety and to fulfill food protection goals. Nano- pico- and even femtogram levels of residues and contaminants have become important, and need to be measured accurately.

The ever-increasing demand for improved quality control and more thorough food monitoring requires sophisticated technologies for the determination of analytes of various structures and very low concentrations in extremely complex biological matrices. Furthermore, food protection advocates, such as the general public and governments, attempt to protect human health by forcing analysts to use complex chromatographic methodology and instrumentation that, perhaps, would not have been considered previously. As a consequence, analysts have learned to use technologies that operate very close to the theoretical limits of performance. All of these complex analytical measurements require trained personnel with skills and experience well beyond those acquired in college. The weakness of some chemical determinations is their length, often involving difficult and intricate manipulations necessitating experienced personnel to ensure high rates of reproducibility.

Analysis of drug residues in foods is a challenging task and numerous methods have been developed for the direct screening of meat, milk, eggs, and honey. The analyst has a wide range of extraction, enrichment, and instrumental techniques to choose from. There is no best method, and the analyst's choice will depend on the nature of the sample matrix, whether it is solid or liquid, fatty or nonfatty, and the expected range and levels of the analytes. The instruments available for the confirmation and quantification of the individual residues will also influence the choice of enrichment and quantification method.

The cost, tedium, and instrumentation requirements of the conventional methods for determining drug residues have created pressures to lower analytical costs and increase sample throughput. The result is a trend toward simpler, miniaturized, and automated extraction and cleanup procedures.

Research into the optimization and use of selective extraction procedures such as supercritical fluid extraction may help both to lower the cost of sample extraction and yield a cleaner extract that requires less enrichment. In addition, the various configurations of the newly developed solid-phase extraction discs offer advantages over conventional solid-phase extraction packed columns, attributable primarily to their combination of reduced bed mass, large flow area, and rigid structure. The low bed mass in a format that eliminates channeling requires significantly less sample, solvent, and processing time than packed solid-phase extraction columns. It also results in high analyte recoveries with less interference from low-affinity material.

The use of small columns such as microbore liquid chromatographic columns, requiring smaller sample size, and computer-controlled solvent delivery and collection systems should lead to the development of fully integrated and automated cleanup systems. Small sample sizes facilitate miniaturization of sample preparation procedures, which in turn brings several benefits including reduced solvent and reagent consumption, reduced processing time, less demand for bench space, and ease of automation.

The innovative use of bioassays based on biological molecules such as antibodies is changing the way analysts approach many traditional problems. The current tendency within residue analysis is toward the development of either fast screening procedures that are optimized for maximum sample throughput and a minimum chance of obtaining false-negative results, or confirmatory methods.

Microbiological assays can be used to identify and rank samples that contain biologically relevant levels of drug residues. Immunochemical assays can also help screen out negative samples and prioritize samples for mass spectrometry. Both microbiological and immunochemical assays can play important roles in the analytical laboratory of the future and have the potential to reduce overall costs and expedite studies that may not otherwise be possible.

However, there will remain a need to support these assays by reasonably specific isolation and quantification methods that can provide rapid identification and/or a degree of confirmation of the analytes. Liquid and gas chromatographic methods that are amenable to automation and are thus compatible with the rapid screening tests in terms of sample throughput and turnaround time have been developed, but there is no consensus as to the best method to use for individual residues. Most of these methods appear to be simple and precise, but only a few have been subjected to international collaborative study trials for ruggedness and practicability. One of the pitfalls in method development, regardless of whether it involves liquid chromatography, gas chromatography, or other techniques, is the use of recovery studies based on fortification. The practice of casually stirring the fortifying chemical into the biological sample is illusory and particularly questionable. Recovery of the residue from treated, weathered, and aged samples should be tried with exhaustive extraction. There is still some way to go, therefore, before physicochemical reference methods will be available for most drugs.

During recent years, however, the distinction between these two types of methods has become less clear because of the improved methods of sample cleanup that allow selective isolation of groups of compounds. Mixed-mechanism solid-phase extraction procedures and multi-immunoaffinity techniques are clear examples of liquid chromatographic developments that have contributed greatly to the current state of the art within residue analysis.

A reference method should be able to yield direct structure information on the compound detected. The remarkable progress made in hyphenation techniques during recent years has turned chromatography into one of the most important and powerful tools used in analytical chemistry. Nearly every day, analysts are confronted with the demand for increasingly faster, more and more reliable analyses at lower and lower concentration levels. Very often, the only efficient way to tackle these kinds of problems is by combining chromatographic separation possibilities with the power of one or more sophisticated detection systems such as mass spectrometry, and Fourier transform infrared and diode array detection. Only these powerful hyphenated systems offer the required possibilities for enhanced selectivity and sensitivity. So far mass spectrometry is the only technique suitable in cases of international dispute. Liquid chromatography–mass spectrometry has found only a limited number of applications within residue analysis. In the near future this situation is likely to change. The use of immunoaffinity chromatography, column-switching procedures, and the further advancement of liquid chromatography-mass spectrometry will be areas of future development.

The need to use drugs in animal husbandry will continue well into the future and, therefore, monitoring of edible animal products for violative residues will remain an area of increasing concern and importance due to the potential impact on human health. The next decade may open up new avenues for the analysis of drug residues in foods, with the routine use of new technologies in immunochemistry, chromatography, electrophoresis and mass spectrometry being currently explored in many laboratories. These, together with further development in the automation of sample preparation, measurement, and data handling, will provide analysts with a unique opportunity for further innovation and improvements to meet the ever-expanding requirements in the field of the analysis of antibacterial residues in edible animal products.

In the area of separations, the need for ever-faster turnaround time is a continuing driving force, and the use of short, fast columns will become more the rule rather than the exception. Commercially available fast gas chromatographic systems have proven to be very powerful analytical tools, but have not yet gone far enough down the road to miniaturization. Furthermore, currently used gas chromatographic phases have to be upgraded to meet today's quality demands, particularly the reproducibility of retentive properties and the thermal stability. The new generation of stationary phases should include phases in which different types of functional groups, such as phenyl and cyanopropyl, are simultaneously present.

Emerging separation technologies such as capillary electrophoresis may lead to the improved and cost-effective resolution of complex mixtures of drug residues. This is a valuable tool that is finding its place as a workhorse technique in the analytical laboratory. Capillary electrophoresis is expected to provide a wide variety of new methods that may well prove superior to currently available technology.

Capillary electrochromatography is also an emerging technique, combining the selectivity of high-performance liquid chromatography with the efficiency of capillary electrophoresis. The transfer of some of those promising techniques from the research to the routine laboratory will enhance the range of tools available to the analyst and should also help to improve the accuracy and precision of drug residues data.

The trend towards more online applications will surely continue for the next few years. If the proper online instrumentation is not available, existing laboratory instrumentation will be converted to do the job. Open-architecture instrumentation will become necessary, enabling systems to be connected remotely to a central chromatographic information-management system that will handle all the real-time data acquisition, control, and troubleshooting.

The demand for multidimensional techniques providing maximum information content will continue to increase. The fact that more bench-top liquid chromatography-, gas chromatography- and capillary electrophoresis–mass spectrometry instruments are being introduced shows great promise for the future. These instruments are not only becoming less expensive, but are also performing in a more sensitive and faster manner. Mass spectrometry has become a standard tool in every modern laboratory, but there will be a growing need for even more sophisticated couplings. In addition, less common detection techniques will become more widely available to many more scientists and laboratories. Tools such as liquid chromatography–nuclear magnetic resonance spectroscopy, liquid chromatography–nuclear magnetic resonance spectroscopy–mass spectroscopy, liquid chromatography–Raman spectroscopy, and others will become routine, with detection limits only dreamed of in the past.

Index

Printed and bound by CPI Group (UK) Ltd, Croydon, CR0 4YY

23/10/2024

01778268-0001